WS 115 SHA   £59.50

Clinical Paediatric Dietetics

Clinical Paediatric Dietetics

EDITED BY

Vanessa Shaw

and

Margaret Lawson

Third edition

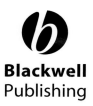

Blackwell
Publishing

Blackwell Publishing editorial offices:
Blackwell Publishing Ltd, 9600 Garsington Road, Oxford OX4 2DQ, UK
    Tel: +44 (0)1865 776868
Blackwell Publishing Professional, 2121 State Avenue, Ames, Iowa 50014-8300, USA
    Tel: +1 515 292 0140
Blackwell Publishing Asia Pty Ltd, 550 Swanston Street, Carlton, Victoria 3053, Australia
    Tel: +61 (0)3 8359 1011

First edition published 1994
Second edition published 2001
Third edition published 2007

1   2007

ISBN: 978-14051-3493-4

Library of Congress Cataloging-in-Publication Data
Clinical paediatric dietetics / edited by Vanessa Shaw and Margaret Lawson. — 3rd ed.
        p. cm.
    Includes bibliographical references and index.
    ISBN-13: 978-1-4051-3493-4 (hardback : alk. paper)
    ISBN-10: 1-4051-3493-3 (hardback : alk. paper)
    1. Diet therapy for children.   I. Shaw, Vanessa.   II. Lawson, Margaret, MSc.
RJ53.D53C58 2007
615.8′54083—dc22

                                                                                2006034442

A catalogue record for this title is available from the British Library

Set in 9.5/11.5pt Palatino
by Graphicraft Limited, Hong Kong
Printed and bound in Singapore
by COS Printers Pte Ltd

For further information on Blackwell Publishing, visit our website:
www.blackwellpublishing.com

Contents

Contributors

Liz Allott
Senior Lecturer in Dietetic Practice,
Faculty of Health and Social Work, University
of Plymouth, Peninsula Allied Health Centre,
College of St Mark and St John, Derriford Road,
Plymouth PL6 9BH

Sarah Almond
Senior Paediatric Dietitian,
Chailey Heritage Clinical Services, Beggars
Wood Road, North Chailey, East Sussex
BN8 4JN

Eleanor Baldwin
Refsum's Research Dietitian,
Nutrition & Dietetic Department, Chelsea &
Westminster Hospital, 369 Fulham Road,
London SW10 9NH

Zoe Connor
Community Paediatric Dietitian, Bromley NHS
PCT, St Paul's Cray Clinic, Mickleham Road,
Orpington, Kent BR5 2RJ

Katie Elwig
Chief Paediatric Dietitian,
St Mary's Hospital, Praed Street, London W2 1NY

Marjorie Dixon
Specialist Dietitian,
Great Ormond Street Hospital for Children NHS
Trust, London WC1N 3JH

Stephanie France
Former Chief Paediatric Dietitian, Kings College
Hospital, Denmark Hill, London SE5 9RS

Kate Grimshaw
Research Dietitian, University Child Health,
Southampton General Hospital, Tremona Road,
Southampton SO16 6YD

Joanne Grogan
Senior Dietitian, Royal Liverpool Children's NHS
Trust, Eaton Road, Liverpool L2 2AP

Claire Gurry
Senior Paediatric Dietitian, Central Manchester
and Manchester Children's University Hospitals
NHS Trust, Charlestown Road, Blackley,
Manchester M9 7AA

Kate Hall
Freelance Dietitian, kate-hall@tiscali.co.uk

Lesley Haynes
Specialist Dietitian, Great Ormond Street Hospital
for Children NHS Trust, London WC1N 3JH

David Hopkins
Specialist Dietitian, Bristol Royal Hospital for
Children, Paul O'Gorman Building, Bristol BS2 8BJ

Tracey Johnson
Specialist Dietitian, The Birmingham Children's
Hospital NHS Trust, Steelhouse Lane, Birmingham
B4 6NH

Alison Johnston
Lead Clinical Specialist Dietitian (Diabetes),
Royal Hospital for Sick Children, Yorkhill,
Glasgow G3 8SJ

Caroline King
Clinical Lead and Specialist Neonatal Dietitian,
Hammersmith Hospital, Du Cane Road, London
W12 0HS

Julie Lanigan
Clinical Trials Co-ordinator/Specialist Research
Dietitian, Institute of Child Health, 30 Guilford
Street, London WC1N 1EH

Margaret Lawson
Former Nestlé Senior Research Fellow,
Institute of Child Health, 30 Guilford Street,
London WC1N 1EH

Helen McCarthy
Lecturer in Dietetics, School of Biomedical
Sciences, University of Ulster, Cromore Road,
Coleraine BT52 1SA

Anita MacDonald
Consultant Dietitian in Inherited Metabolic
Disorders, The Birmingham Children's Hospital
NHS Trust, Steelhouse Lane, Birmingham
B4 6NH

Sarah Macdonald
Specialist Dietitian, Great Ormond Street Hospital
for Children NHS Trust, London WC1N 3JH

Gwynneth McGrath
Senior Dietitian, The Birmingham Children's
Hospital NHS Trust, Steelhouse Lane, Birmingham
B4 6NH

Rosan Meyer
Paediatric Research Dietitian, Room 252 Norfolk
Place, Imperial College St Mary's Campus,
London W2 1BG

Judy More
Freelance Paediatric Dietitian, London,
www.child-nutrition.co.uk

Liz Neal
Research Dietitan, Institute of Child Health,
30 Guilford Street, London WC1N 1EH

Dasha Nicholls
Consultant Child and Adolescent Psychiatrist,

Head of Feeding and Eating Disorders Service,
Great Ormond Street Hospital for Children NHS
Trust, London WC1N 3JH.

Carolyn Patchell
Head of Dietetic Services, The Birmingham
Children's Hospital NHS Trust, Steelhouse Lane,
Birmingham B4 6NH

Julie Royle
Chief Dietitian, Central Manchester and
Manchester Children's University Hospitals
NHS Trust, Pendlebury, Manchester
M27 4HA

Patricia Rutherford
Former Chief Dietitian, Royal Liverpool
Children's NHS Trust, Eaton Road, Liverpool,
L12 2AP. Now Clinical Information Manager,
Vitaflo International Ltd, 11–16 Century
Building, Liverpool L3 4BL

Marian Sewell
Senior Dietitian, Great Ormond Street Hospital for
Children NHS Trust, London WC1N 3JH

Vanessa Shaw
Head of Dietetics, Great Ormond Street
Hospital for Children NHS Trust, London
WC1N 3JH

Zofia Smith
Community Paediatric Dietitian, Parkside
Community Health Centre, 311 Dewsbury Road,
Beeston, Leeds LS11 5LQ

Laura Stewart
Community Paediatric Dietitian,
Royal Hospital for Sick Children, Sciennes Road,
Edinburgh EH9 1LF

Carina Venter
Senior Allergy Dietitian
(Research and Clinical), The David Hide Asthma
and Allergy Research Centre, St Mary's Hospital,
Newport, Isle of Wight

Evelyn Ward
Senior Paediatric Dietitian, St James
University Hospital NHS Trust, Beckett Street,
Leeds LS9 7TF

Ruth Watling
Head of Dietetics, Royal Liverpool Children's NHS
Trust, Eaton Road, Liverpool L2 2AP

Fiona White
Chief Metabolic Dietitian, Central Manchester
and Manchester Children's University
Hospitals NHS Trust, Pendlebury,
Manchester M27 4HA

Vivien Wigg
Senior Dietitian, Great Ormond Street Hospital for
Children NHS Trust, London WC1N 3JH

Sue Wolfe
Chief Paediatric Dietitian, St James University
Hospital NHS Trust, Beckett Street, Leeds LS9 7TF

Foreword

It gives me great pleasure to write the foreword for the third edition of *Clinical Paediatric Dietetics*. This edition clearly shows the diversity of areas paediatric dietitians work within, from clinical dietetics to community nutrition. The new structure recognises the important extent of the role dietitians play in the health care of sick infants and children.

Recognition should be given to The Paediatric Group of the British Dietetic Association for their evidence based and practical approach. Vanessa and Margaret should once again be sincerely congratulated for managing contributions from almost 40 dietitians with valued input from a significant number of others – a task that would overwhelm many.

The value of this book is recognised not only by dietitians but also by many other health professionals as an excellent source of reliable information to ensure optimal nutritional care is given to sick infants and children.

Dame Barbara Clayton DBE
Honorary Research Professor in Metabolism,
University of Southampton
Honorary President, The British Dietetic Association

Preface

The aim of this manual is to provide a very practical approach to the nutritional management of a wide range of paediatric nutritional disorders that may benefit from nutritional support or be ameliorated or resolved by dietary manipulation. The text will be of particular relevance to professional dietitians, dietetic students and their tutors, paediatricians, paediatric nurses and members of the community health team involved with children requiring therapeutic diets. The importance of nutritional support and dietary management in many paediatric conditions is increasingly recognised and is reflected in new text for this edition.

The authors are largely drawn from practising paediatric dietitians around the United Kingdom, with additional contributions from academic research dietitians and a psychiatrist. The text has been reorganised for this edition and includes a thorough review of the scientific and medical literature to support practice wherever available. The major part of the text concentrates on nutritional requirements of sick infants and children in the clinical setting. Normal dietary constituents are used alongside special dietetic products to provide a prescription that will control progression and symptoms of disease whilst maintaining the growth potential of the child. There is a new section on community nutrition including healthy eating throughout childhood. We acknowledge that the distinction between clinical dietetics and nutrition in the community is rather arbitrary since many clinical conditions are dealt with in the community, and the principles of healthy eating underpin many clinical interventions.

New topics have been added: nutrition support in critical care, autistic spectrum disorders, prevention of food allergy. There has been an expansion of the range of disorders and treatments described in many chapters, e.g. gastroenterology, liver disease, gut transplantation, cardiac conditions, fatty acid oxidation defects; and new recommendations and guidelines for parenteral nutrition, feeding preterm infants and assessing children with neurodisabilities.

Arranged under headings of disorders of organ systems rather than type of diet, and with much information presented in tabular form and with worked examples, the manual is easy to use. Appendices list the many and varied special products described in the text, together with details of their manufacturers. The appendices are not exhaustive, but include the products most commonly used in the UK. The most recent information and data has been used in the preparation of this edition, but no guarantee can be given of the validity or availability at the time of going to press.

Vanessa Shaw
Margaret Lawson

Acknowledgements

We would like to thank a number of the contributors to the first edition, who were unable to contribute to the second edition, but whose work formed the basis for the following chapters:

Chapter 2, Provision of Nutrition in a Hospital Setting: Christine Clothier
Chapter 3, Enteral Feeding: Debra Woodward
Chapter 4, Parenteral Nutrition: Alison Macleod
Chapter 6, The Gastrointestinal Tract: Sheena Laing
Chapter 8, The Liver and Pancreas: Jane Ely
Chapter 14, Ketogenic Diet for Epilepsy: Jane Eaton
Chapter 18, Lipid Disorders: Anne Maclean
Chapter 22, Eating Disorders: Bernadette Wren and Bryan Lask
Chapter 25, Burns: Judith Martin

We would like to thank a number of the contributors to the second edition, who were unable to contribute to this third edition, but whose work has formed the basis for the following chapters:

Chapter 4, Parenteral Nutrition: Janice Glynn
Chapter 12, The Kidney: Janet Coleman
Chapter 13, The Cardiothoracic System: Marion Noble
Chapter 14, Food hypersensitivity: Christine Carter
Chapter 15, HIV and AIDS: Jayne Butler
Chapter 15, Immunodeficiency Syndromes: Dona Hileti-Telfer
Chapter 21, Refsum's Disease: June Brown
Chapter 25, Burns: Dearbhla Hunt
Chapter 30, Feeding Children with Neurodisabilities: Karen Jeffereys
Chapter 31, Obesity: Mary Deane

Part 1

Principles of Paediatric Dietetics

1 Nutritional Assessment, Dietary Requirements, Feed Supplementation

Vanessa Shaw & Margaret Lawson

Introduction

This text provides a practical approach to the dietary management of a range of paediatric disorders. The therapies outlined in Parts 2 and 3 describe dietetic manipulations and the nutritional requirements of the infant and child in a clinical setting, illustrating how normal dietary constituents are used alongside special dietetic products to allow for the continued growth of the child while controlling the progression and symptoms of disease. Nutrition for the healthy child and nutritional care most often provided in the community setting is addressed in Part 4.

Dietary principles

The following principles are relevant to the treatment of all infants and children and provide the basis for many of the therapies described later in the text.

Assessment of nutritional status

Assessment and monitoring of nutritional status should be included in any dietary regimen, audit procedure or research project where a modified diet has a role. There are a number of methods of assessing specific aspects of nutritional status, but no one measurement will give an overall picture of status for all nutrients. There are several assessment techniques, some of which should be used routinely in all centres while others are still in a developmental stage or are suitable only for research. Figure 1.1 outlines the techniques that can be used for nutritional assessment.

Dietary intake

For children over the age of 2 years food intake is assessed in the same way as for adults: using a recall diet history, a quantitative food diary over a number of days, a weighed food intake over a number of days or a food frequency questionnaire [1]. For most clinical purposes an oral history from the usual carers (or from the child if appropriate) will provide sufficient information on which to base recommendations. As well as assessing the range and quantity of foods eaten it is also useful to assess whether the texture and presentation of food is appropriate for the age and developmental level of the child. For instance, does the child use an infant feeding bottle or a cup; is the child able to self-feed or need a lot of help; is the food of normal consistency, as eaten by the family, or is it a smooth purée, chopped or mashed?

The assessment of milk intake for breast fed infants is difficult and only very general estimations can be made. Infants can be test-weighed before and after a breast feed and the amount of milk consumed can be calculated. This requires the use of very accurate scales (±1–2 g) and should be

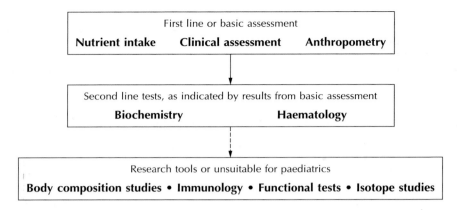

Figure 1.1   Nutritional assessment methods.

carried out for all feeds over a 24-hour period as the volume consumed varies throughout the day. Test-weighing should be avoided if at all possible as it is disturbing for the infant, engenders anxiety in the mother and is likely to compromise breast feeding. Studies have shown that the volume of breast milk consumed is approximately 770 mL at 5 weeks and 870 mL at 11 weeks [2]. In general, an intake of 850 mL is assumed for infants who are fully breast fed and over the age of 6 weeks, with additional intake from food at the appropriate weaning age. Estimation of food intake is particularly difficult in infants, as it is not possible to assess accurately the amount of food wasted through, for example, spitting or drooling.

Conversion of food intake into nutrient values for young children may involve the use of manufacturers' data if the child is taking proprietary infant foods and/or infant formula. The composition of breast milk varies and food table values may be inaccurate by up to 20% because of individual variation.

Assessment of the adequacy of an individual calculated nutrient intake for sick and for healthy infants and children is discussed in the section on Dietary Reference Values (see p. 10).

Anthropometry

Measurement of weight and height or length is critical as the basis for calculating dietary requirements as well as monitoring the effects of dietary intervention. Other anthropometric measurements are summarised in Table 1.1.

Head circumference

Head circumference is a useful measurement in children under the age of 2 years, particularly where it is difficult to obtain an accurate length measurement. After this age head growth slows and is a less useful indicator of somatic growth. A number of genetic and acquired conditions will affect head growth (e.g. neurodevelopmental delay) and measurement of head circumference will not be a useful indicator of nutritional status in these conditions. Head circumference is measured using a narrow, flexible, non-stretch tape. Details of a suitable disposable paper tape are available from the Child Growth Foundation (see p. 20). Measurement should be made just above the eyes to include the maximum circumference of the head, with the child supported in an upright position and looking straight ahead.

Weight

Measurement of weight is an easy and routine procedure using an electronic digital scale or a beam balance. Ideally, infants should be weighed nude and children wearing just a dry nappy or pants, but if this is not possible it is important to record whether the infant is weighed wearing a nappy, and the amount and type of clothing worn by older children. For weighing infants up to 10 kg, scales should be accurate to 10 g; for children up to 20 kg, accuracy should be ±20 g and over 20 kg it should be about 50–200 g. A higher degree of accuracy is required for the assessment of sick children than for routine measurements in the community. Frequent weight monitoring is important for the sick infant

Table 1.1   Anthropometric measurements.

Measurement	Derived indices	Comments
Head circumference	Head circumference for age	Easy to measure; useful up to the age of 2 years; useful as proxy for length increase; does not normally change rapidly Affected by medical condition; may not indicate nutritional status
Weight	Weight for age Weight for age z score	Easy to measure; useful on a day to day basis Does not differentiate between lean tissue, oedema and body fat
Length/height	Length/height for age Length/height for age z score Height age	Not easy to measure accurately – needs more than one person to measure; does not change rapidly Best overall indicator of nutritional wellbeing
	Weight for stature Body mass index (W/H²) Body mass index z score	Useful for children with low height age BMI indicates relative weight for height, but does not differentiate between lean and fat tissue
Mid arm circumference	Mid arm circumference for age Mid arm circumference z score	Easy to measure; useful up to the age of 5 years Less likely to be affected by water retention or fat deposition than body weight
Skinfold thickness (SFT)	Triceps SFT for age	Difficult to measure accurately; unpleasant procedure for children Usually triceps only are used in children Distinguishes between lean and fat tissue
Waist circumference	Waist circumference for age	Easy to measure, although requires removal of clothes Distinguishes between high weight due to muscle bulk and that due to fat
Hip circumference	Waist : hip ratio	Easy to measure No standards for children

or child and hospitalised infants should be weighed daily if there are problems with fluid balance, otherwise on alternate days; children over the age of 2 years in hospital should be weighed at least weekly. Recommendations for the routine measurement of healthy infants where there are no concerns about growth are given in Table 1.2 [3]. If there are concerns about weight gain that is too slow or too rapid, measurement of weight should be carried out more frequently.

Height

Height or length measurement requires a stadiometer or length-board. Details of suitable equipment, which may be fixed or portable, are available from the Child Growth Foundation. Measurement of length using a tape measure is too inaccurate to be of use for longitudinal monitoring of growth, although an approximate length may be useful as a single measure (e.g. for calculating body mass index). Under the age of about 2 years supine length is measured; standing height is usually measured

Table 1.2   Recommendations for routine measurements for healthy infants and children.

Weight	Length/Height	Head Circumference
Birth 2 months	Birth 6–8 weeks if birthweight <2.5 kg or if other cause for concern	Birth or neonatal period 6–8 weeks
3 months 4 months 8 months		
Additional weights at parent's request, not more frequently than 2 weekly under the age of 6 months, monthly 6–12 months 12–15 months School entry	No other routine measurement of length/height School entry	No other routine measurement of head circumference

Source: After Health for all Children [3].

over this age or whenever the child can stand straight and unsupported. When the method of measurement changes there is likely to be a difference in length, and measurements should be made by both methods on one occasion when switching from supine length to standing height. Measurement of length is difficult and requires careful positioning of the infant, ensuring that the back, legs and head are straight, the heels are against the footboard, the shoulders are touching the baseboard and the crown of the head is touching the headboard. Two people are required to measure length – one to hold the child in position and one to record the measurement. Positioning of the child is also important when measuring standing height and care should be taken to ensure that the back and legs are straight, the heels, buttocks, shoulder blades and back of head are touching the measurement board and that the child is looking straight ahead.

Sick infants should be measured every month and older children whenever they attend a clinic. Healthy infants have a length measurement at birth (although this is notoriously inaccurate) and no further height checks are recommended until the pre-school check [3]. Whenever there are concerns about growth or weight gain a height measurement should be made more often, although there is little point in measuring height more frequently than every 3 months.

Body mass index
A body mass index (BMI) measurement can be calculated from the weight and height measurements: BMI = weight (kg)/height (m)^2. This provides an indication of fatness or thinness. In adults, body fatness is largely unrelated to age and high BMI measurements are related to health risks. In children, the amount and distribution of body fat is dependent on age, and does not appear to be related to health. At the extremes of centiles, BMI does not differentiate well between heaviness resulting from lean tissue (e.g. high muscle mass) and weight resulting from excess fat deposition, and further interpretation is necessary.

Proxy measurements for length/height
In some cases it is difficult to obtain length or height measurements (e.g. in very sick or preterm infants and in older children with scoliosis). A number of proxy measurements can be used which are useful to monitor whether longitudinal growth is progressing in an individual, but there are no recognised centile charts as yet and indices such as BMI cannot be calculated. In adults, arm span is approximately equivalent to height, but body proportions depend upon age and this measurement is not generally useful. Measurements of lower leg length or knee–heel length have been used and are a useful proxy for growth. For infants and small children, a kneemometer has been developed which displays knee–heel length digitally [4]. For older children knee–heel length is measured with the child in a supine position (if possible) with the knee bent at a 90° angle using a caliper with a blade at either end. One blade is fitted under the heel of the foot and the other onto the knee, immediately behind the patella, using the outside surface of the leg. Total leg length is rarely measured outside specialist growth clinics and is calculated as the difference between measured sitting height and standing height. A number of other measures have been used in children with cerebral palsy as a proxy for height, but numbers are too small for reference standards to be established [5]. Formulas for calculating height from proxy measurements are further discussed in Chapter 29.

Supplementary measurements
The measurement of weight and length or height forms the basis of anthropometric assessment. However, these measurements on their own do not indicate whether weight increments are due to lean and fat tissue, or whether weight gained is merely fat. Supplementary measurements that can be used include mid upper arm circumference (MUAC). This is a useful measurement in children under the age of 5 years, as MUAC increases fairly rapidly up until this age. Age related standards exist for children over the age of 1 year [6]. Increases in MUAC are more likely to comprise muscle and less likely to be affected by oedema than body weight. In order to fully differentiate between lean and fat, measurement of triceps skinfold thickness (TSF or SFT) is necessary. This can be an unpleasant procedure for young children, who are afraid of the skinfold caliper and may not remain still for long enough for accurate measurements to be taken. The equipment and technique are identical to those used in adults and the measurement is subject to the same observer

Table 1.3 Arm fat and arm muscle area.

$$\text{Arm muscle area (mm}^2) = \frac{[MAC - (\pi \times TSF)]^2}{4 \times \pi}$$

$$\text{Arm fat area (mm}^2) = \frac{TSF \times MAC}{2} - \frac{\pi \times (TSF)^2}{4}$$

MAC = mid arm circumference in mm^2
TSF = triceps skinfold thickness in mm

Worked example for a boy aged 6 years:
MAC = 180 mm   (50th centile* for age)
TSF = 16 mm   (95th centile* for age)

Arm muscle area = 1340 mm^2 (<5th centile* for age)
Arm fat area = 1238 mm^2 (90–95th centile* for age)
Although all measurements are within the normal range for age, this boy is severely depleted in muscle and may be depleted in all lean tissue

* Reference standards taken from Gibson [6].

error. Skinfold thickness is not used as a routine anthropometric measure but provides valuable data in research studies. Reference data for children over the age of 1 year are available [6] and the World Health Organization (WHO) will publish reference norms for children aged 1–5 in the near future. Arm muscle and arm fat area can be calculated and compared to reference data [6]. A calculation of arm fat and muscle area is shown in Table 1.3.

Measurement of the waist circumference can help distinguish between a high weight for age that is caused by high body lean tissue or high body fat. In general, children with a high weight for height or high BMI who have a high muscle bulk (usually resulting from sports training) will have a low waist circumference centile, while overweight and obese children will have a high waist centile. The waist : hip ratio in children has not proved to be a useful predictor of obesity in pre-pubertal children [7], and reference data do not exist at present for European children.

Growth charts

Measurements should be regularly plotted on the relevant centile chart using a dot rather than a cross or a circle. All children in the UK are issued with a growth centile chart as part of the personal child health record that is held by parents and completed by health care professionals whenever the child is weighed or measured. UK centile charts are avail-

able for weight, length/height, head circumference and BMI and the standard ones in use are based on the UK 1990 data [8]. These data were based on a cohort of infants who were largely formula fed during the first 6 months of life. The growth of breast fed infants differs from that of artificially fed infants, and breast fed infants tend to be longer and leaner at age 3 months [9]. Centile charts for fully breast fed infants are available from the Child Growth Foundation, and can be used for both breast and formula fed infants; however, they are based on a very small cohort of 120 infants who had solids introduced at a mean age of 15 weeks and only 40% were still receiving breast milk at 1 year of age. The WHO has produced growth charts based on a sample size of 8440 children for longitudinal and cross-sectional study from ethnically diverse populations across the globe [10]. These children were raised in optimal conditions including exclusive or predominant breast feeding for at least 4 months, introduction of complementary foods by 6 months of age and continued partial breast feeding to at least 12 months of age. These charts may be more suitable than the standard UK 1990 charts for infants and children who are recent immigrants to the UK.

Age related centile charts for BMI have been developed [11] and indicate how heavy the child is relevant to their height and age. Waist circumference centile charts are also available for British children over the age of 3 years [12]. Some medical conditions have a significant effect on growth, and where sufficient data exist, for instance in Down's syndrome, Turner's syndrome and sickle cell disease, separate growth charts have been developed for these conditions [13], and are available from the Child Growth Foundation.

Evaluation of anthropometric measurements

There are a number of problems associated with accurate plotting on charts that can lead to inaccuracies in monitoring. Charts may give time increments in months or may require the decimal age to be calculated using the decimal age calendar on the centile charts, and it is important to check which type of chart is being used. In a clinic or a centre where a number of people are involved in plotting measurements, agreement should be reached over whether values that fall between centiles should be rounded up or rounded down. Variations in procedures can result in relatively large errors, particularly in infants, and deviations from centiles can be missed. When assessing height it is important to take parental height into consideration, and the genetic height potential for the child can be approximately estimated using the mid-parental height +7 cm for boys, and the mid-parental height –7 cm for girls. This calculation is not appropriate if either parent is not of normal stature. The UK 1990 growth charts give example calculations for adult height potential. (For definitions of obesity and failure to thrive see Chapters 29 and 31.)

It is difficult to assess progress or decide upon targets where a measurement falls outside the centile lines: either <0.4th centile or >99.6th centile. Amended weight charts showing up to ±5 standard deviations for monitoring children with slow weight gain are available [14]; details from the Child Growth Foundation. 'Thrive lines' have also been developed to aid interpretation of infants with either slow or rapid weight gain. The 5% thrive lines define the slowest rate of normal weight velocity in healthy infants. If an infant is growing at a rate parallel to or slower than a 5% thrive line, weight gain is abnormally slow. The 95% thrive lines define the most rapid rate of normal weight gain in healthy infants and weight gain that parallels or is faster than the 95% thrive line is abnormally rapid [14]. Thrive lines are in the form of an acetate sheet which overlays either the standard A4 weight centile charts or charts in the personal child health record. Acetates are available from the Child Growth Foundation.

There are a number of methods of overcoming problems in plotting onto charts, which involve converting the weight and height into a finite proportion of a reference or standard measurement. Calculation of the standard deviation score (SDS) or z score for length/height, weight and BMI gives a numerical score indicating how far away from the 50th centile for age the child's measurements falls. A child on the 0.4th centile will have a SDS of –2.65 SD. A child on the 99.6th centile will have a SDS of +2.65 SD, while a measurement that falls exactly on the 50th centile will have a z score of 0. Because of the distribution of the data, calculation of z scores by hand is extremely laborious. A computer software program is available from the Child Growth Foundation that will calculate z scores from height, weight and age data. The z score is also used when

Table 1.4   Height for age, height age and weight for height.

Worked example – six-year-old girl with cerebral palsy referred with severe feeding problems

Visit 1   Decimal age = 6.2 years
Height = 93 cm (<0.4th centile)
Weight = 10 kg (<0.4th centile)
50th centile for height for a girl aged
6.2 years = 117 cm
Height for age $= \dfrac{93}{117} = 79.5\%$ height for age

Height age is the age at which 93 cm (measured height) falls on 50th centile = 2.7 years
50th centile for weight for 2.7 years = 14 kg
Weight for height $= \dfrac{10}{14} = 71\%$ weight for height

Visit 2   (after intervention) Decimal age = 6.8 years
Height = 95.5 cm (<0.4th centile)
Weight = 12 kg (<0.4th centile)
50th centile for height for age 3.1 years = 121 cm
Height for age $= \dfrac{95.5}{121} = 79\%$ height for age

Height age = 3.1 years
50th centile for weight for age 3.1 years = 14.5 kg
Weight for height $= \dfrac{12}{14.5} = 82.7\%$ weight for height

Conclusions: the child has shown catch-up weight gain – weight for height has increased from 71% to 83%. She has continued to grow in height, but has not had any catch-up – her height continues to be about 79% of that expected for her chronological age

comparing groups of children of different genders or ages, when a comparison of the measurements themselves would not be useful.

The calculation of height for age, height age and weight for height are useful when assessing nutritional status initially or when monitoring progress in children who are short for their chronological age. Table 1.4 shows examples of calculations for these measurements. Calculation of height age is necessary when determining nutrient requirements for children who are much smaller (or larger) than their chronological age (see p. 12).

A number of methods of classification of malnutrition have been used in developing countries. The Waterlow classification [15] may be of use when assessing children in the UK with severe failure to thrive. An adaptation of the classification is shown in Table 1.5. The WHO defines malnutrition as moderate if the weight for age z score is less than

Table 1.5   Classification of malnutrition.

Acute malnutrition (wasting)	Chronic malnutrition (stunting ± wasting)
Weight for height	Height for age
80–90% standard – grade 1	90–95% standard – grade 1
70–80% standard – grade 2	85–90% standard – grade 2
<70% standard – grade 3	<80% standard – grade 3

Source: After Waterlow [15].

−0.2 and severe if the weight for age z score is less than −0.3 [16].

Clinical assessment

Clinical assessment of the child involves a medical history and a physical examination. The medical history will identify medical, social or environmental factors that may be risk factors for the development of nutritional problems. Such factors include parental knowledge and money available for food purchase, underlying disease, changes in weight, food allergies and medications. Clinical signs of poor nutrition, revealed in the physical examination, only appear at a late stage in the development of a deficiency disease and absence of clinical signs should not be taken as indicating that a deficiency is not present. Typical physical signs associated with poor nutrition that have been described in children in western countries are summarised in Table 1.6. Physical signs represent very general changes and may not be caused by nutrient deficiencies alone. Other indications such as poor weight gain and/or low dietary intake are needed in order to reinforce suspicions, and a blood test should be carried out to confirm the diagnosis.

Food and nutrient intake, anthropometric measurements and clinical examination and history form the basis of routine nutritional assessment. None of these are diagnostic tests and can only predict which nutrients may be deficient and which children need further investigation. If a nutrient deficiency (or excess) is suspected as a result of the first line assessment tools, then confirmation using other objective measures should be sought.

Biochemistry and haematology

Methods of confirming suspicion of a nutritional

Table 1.6   Physical signs of nutritional problems.

Assessment	Clinical sign	Possible nutrient(s)
Hair	Thin, sparse	Protein and energy, zinc, copper
	Colour change – 'flag sign'	
	Easily plucked	
Skin	Dry, flaky	Essential fatty acids B vitamins
	Rough, 'sandpaper' texture	Vitamin A
	Petechiae, bruising	Vitamin C
Eyes	Pale conjunctiva	Iron
	Xerosis	Vitamin A
	Keratomalacia	
Lips	Angular stomatitis Cheilosis	B vitamins
Tongue	Colour changes	B vitamins
Teeth	Mottling of enamel	Fluorosis (excess fluoride)
Gums	Spongy, bleed easily	Vitamin C
Face	Thyroid enlargement	Iodine
Nails	Spoon shape, koilonychia	Iron, zinc, copper
Subcutaneous tissue	Oedema Over-hydration	Protein, sodium
	Depleted subcutaneous fat	Energy
Muscles	Wasting	Protein, energy, zinc
Bones	Craniotabes Parietal and frontal bossing Epiphyseal enlargement Beading of ribs	Vitamin D

problem include analysis of levels of nutrients or nutrient-dependent metabolites in body fluids or tissues, or measuring functional impairment of a nutrient-dependent metabolic process.

The most commonly used tissue for investigation is the blood. Whole blood, plasma, serum or blood cells can be used, depending on the test. Tests may be static (e.g. levels of zinc in plasma) or may be functional (e.g. the measurement of the activity of glutathione peroxidase, a selenium-dependent enzyme, as a measure of selenium status). Although an objective measurement is obtained from a blood test, there are a number of factors that can affect the validity of such biochemical or haematological investigations. Age specific normal ranges need to be established for the individual centre unless the laboratory participates in a regional or national quality control scheme. Recent food intake and time of sampling can affect levels and it may be necessary to take a fasting blood sample for some nutrients. Physiological processes such as infection, disease or drugs may alter normal levels. Contamination from exogenous materials such as equipment or endogenous sources such as sweat or interstitial fluid is important for nutrients such as trace elements, and care must be taken to choose the correct sampling procedure. A fuller review of the subject is given by Clayton & Round [17]. A summary of some biochemical and haematological measurements is given in Table 1.7.

Urine is often used for adult investigations, but many tests require the collection of a 24-hour urine sample and this is difficult in babies and children. The usefulness of a single urine sample for nutritional tests is limited and needs to be compared with a standard metabolite, usually creatinine. However, creatinine excretion itself is age dependent and this needs to be taken into consideration. Hair and nails have been used to assess trace element and heavy metal status in populations, but a number of environmental and physiological factors affect levels and these tissues are not routinely used in the UK. Tissues that store certain nutrients, such as the liver and bone, would be useful materials to investigate, but sampling is too invasive for routine clinical use.

Other tests

A number of other tests that are indicative of nutritional status may provide useful information but are not available routinely. Measurement of body composition using isotope dilution or imaging techniques is particularly useful for the clinical dietitian as most methods of assessment do not indicate whether growth consists of normal ratios of fat and protein or whether excess amounts of adipose tissues are being accumulated. Body composition measurements are described by Ruxton et al. [18]. The use of bioimpedance (BIA) in assessing body composition in adults has increased since

the development of relatively inexpensive and user friendly equipment ('Body Fat Analysers'). However, this method assumes a constant state of hydration, which has shown not to be true for obese individuals. In addition the method has not been validated for use in children and young people under the age of 18 years [19].

Tests that are not routinely carried out but that may be useful research tools are summarised in Table 1.8.

Expected growth in childhood

The 50th centile birthweight for infants in the UK is 3.5 kg. There is some weight loss during the first 5–7 days of life while feeding on full volumes of milk is established; birthweight is normally regained by the 10th to 14th day. Thereafter, average weight gain is as follows:

- 200 g per week for the first 3 months
- 150 g per week for the second 3 months
- 100 g per week for the third 3 months
- 50–75 g per week for the fourth 3 months

Increase in length during the first year of life: 25 cm.

During the second year, the toddler following the 50th centile for growth velocity gains approximately 2.5 kg in weight and a further 12 cm in length. Average growth continues at a rate of approximately 2 kg per year and 10 cm per year, steadily declining to 6 cm per year until the growth spurt at puberty.

Dietary Reference Values

The 1991 Department of Health Report on Dietary Reference Values [20] provides information and figures for requirements for a comprehensive range of nutrients and energy. The requirements are termed dietary reference values (DRV) and are for normal, healthy populations of infants fed artificial formulas and for older infants, children and adults consuming food. DRVs are not set for breast fed babies as it is considered that human milk provides the necessary amounts of nutrients. In some cases, the DRVs for infants aged up to 3 months who are formula fed are in excess of those that would be expected to derive from breast milk; this is because

Table 1.7 Biochemical and haematological tests.

Nutrient	Test	Normal values in children	Comments
Biochemical tests			
Protein	Total plasma protein	55–80 g/L	Low levels reflect long term not acute depletion
	Albumin	30–45 g/L	
	Caeruloplasmin	0.18–0.46 g/L	Low levels indicate acute protein depletion, but are acute phase proteins which increase during infection
	Retinol binding protein	2.6–7.6 g/L	
Thiamin	Erythrocyte transketolase	1–1.15	High activity coefficient (>1.15) indicates thiamin activity coefficient deficiency
Vitamin B_{12}	Plasma B_{12} value	263–1336 pmol/L	Low levels indicate deficiency
Riboflavin	Erythrocyte glutathione reductase activity coefficient	1.0–1.3	High activity coefficient (>1.3) indicates deficiency
Vitamin C	Plasma ascorbate level	8.8–124 µmol/L	Low levels indicate deficiency
Vitamin A	Plasma retinol level	0.54–1.56 µmol/L	Low level indicates deficiency
Vitamin D	Plasma 25-hydroxy cholecalciferol level	30–110 nmol/L	Low level indicates deficiency
Vitamin E	Plasma tocopherol level	α tocopherol 10.9–28.1 µmol/L	Low levels indicate deficiency
Copper	Plasma level	70–140 µmol/L	Low levels indicate deficiency
Selenium	Plasma level	0.76–1.07 µmol/L	Low levels indicate deficiency
	Glutathione peroxidase activity	>1.77 µmol/L	Low levels indicate deficiency
Zinc	Plasma level	10–18 µmol/L	Low levels indicate deficiency
Haematology tests			
Folic acid	Plasma folate	7–48 nmol/L	Low levels indicate deficiency
	Red cell folate	429–1749 nmol/L	Low levels indicate deficiency
Haemoglobin	Whole blood	104–140 g/L	Levels <110 g/L indicate iron deficiency
Red cell distribution width	Whole blood	<16%	High values indicate iron deficiency
Mean corpuscular volume	Whole blood	70–86 fL	Small volume (microcytosis) indicates iron deficiency. Large volume (macrocytosis) indicates folate or B_{12} deficiency
Mean cell haemoglobin	Whole blood	22.7–29.6 pg	Low values indicate iron deficiency
Percentage hypochromic cells	Whole blood	<2.5%	High values (>2.5%) indicate iron deficiency
Zinc protoporphyrin	Red cell	32–102 µmol/mol haem	High levels indicate iron deficiency
Ferritin	Plasma level	5–70 µg/L	Low levels indicate depletion of iron stores. Ferritin is an acute phase protein and increases during infection

Table 1.8   Other tests.

Measurement	Method
Body composition	Total body potassium using ^{40}K Total body water using water labelled with stable isotopes (^2H_2O, $H_2^{18}O$, $^2H_2^{18}O$) Ultrasound Bioelectrical impedance Computerised tomography Dual X-ray absorptiometry
Functional tests	Muscle strength using dynamometer to assess protein energy malnutrition Taste acuity to assess zinc status Dark adaptation test to assess vitamin A adequacy These tests require the co-operation of the subject and none have been used extensively in children
Immunological tests	Leucocyte function, delayed cutaneous hypersensitivity reaction These tests are affected by infection and are age dependent There is no reference data for children and immunological tests are not normally used as a measure of nutritional status in paediatrics

of the different bioavailability of some nutrients from breast and artificial formulas.

It is important to remember that these are recommendations for groups, not for individuals; however, they can be used as a basis for estimating suitable intakes for the individual, using the Reference Nutrient Intake (RNI). This level of intake should satisfy the requirements of 97.5% of healthy individuals in a population group. A summary of these DRVs for energy, protein, sodium, potassium, vitamin C, calcium and iron is given in Table 1.9. The DRVs for other nutrients may be found in the full report. The WHO has recently published new recommendations for energy intakes that are lower than those formerly used [21]. A number of other bodies, including the European Union, have also published estimated requirements which include children, and these have been summarised [22].

When estimating requirements for the individual sick child it is important to calculate energy and nutrient intakes based on actual body weight, and not expected body weight. The latter will lead to a proposed intake that is inappropriately high for the child who has an abnormally low body weight. In some instances it may be more appropriate to consider the child's height age rather than chronological age when comparing intakes with the DRVs as this is a more realistic measure of the child's body size and hence nutrient requirement. An estimation of requirements for sick children is given in Table 1.10.

Fluid requirements in the newborn

Breast feeding is the most appropriate method of feeding the normal infant and may be suitable for sick infants with a variety of clinical conditions. Demand breast feeding will automatically ensure that the healthy infant gets the right volume of milk and hence nutrients. If the infant is too ill or too immature to suckle (the suck–swallow–breathe sequence that allows the newborn infant to feed orally is usually well developed by 35–37 weeks' gestation), the mother may express her breast milk; expressed breast milk (EBM) may be modified to suit the sick infant's requirements. If EBM is unavailable or inappropriate to feed in certain circumstances, infant formula milks must be used (Table 1.11). After the age of 6 months, a follow-on milk may be used (Table 1.12). These milks are higher in protein, iron and some other minerals and vitamins than formulas designed to be given from birth and may be useful for infants with a poor intake of solids or who are fluid restricted. Organic infant formulas and follow-on milks are also available.

Low birthweight and preterm infants

Chapter 6 gives a full account of the special requirements of these babies.

Infants over 2.5 kg birthweight

Fluid offered per 24 hours: 150–200 mL/kg. On the first day, if bottle fed, approximately one-seventh of the total volume should be offered, divided into eight feeds and fed every 2–3 hours. The volume offered should be gradually increased over the following days to give full requirements by the

Table 1.9 Selected dietary reference values.

| | Weight* | Fluid | | Energy (EAR) | | | RNI | | | | | | | | |
Age	kg	ml/kg	kJ/d	kJ/kg/d	kcal/d	kcal/kg/d	Protein g/d	g/kg/d	Sodium mmol/d	mmol/kg/d	Potassium mmol/d	mmol/kg/d	Vitamin C mg/d	Calcium mmol/d	Iron µmol/d
Males															
0–3 months	5.9	150	2280	480–420	545	115–100	12.5	2.1	9	1.5	20	3.4	25	13.1	30
4–6	7.7	150	2890	400	690	95	12.7	1.6	12	1.6	22	2.8	25	13.1	80
7–9	8.9	120	3440	400	825	95	13.7	1.5	14	1.6	18	2.0	25	13.1	140
10–12	9.8	120	3850	400	920	95	14.9	1.5	15	1.5	18	1.8	25	13.1	140
1–3 years	12.6	90	5150	400	1230	95	14.5	1.1	22	1.7	20	1.6	30	8.8	120
4–6	17.8	80	7160	380	1715	90	19.7	1.1	30	1.7	28	1.6	30	11.3	110
7–10	28.3	60	8240	–	1970	–	28.3	–	50	–	50	–	30	13.8	160
11–14	43.1	50	9270	–	2220	–	42.1	–	70	–	80	–	35	25.0	200
15–18	64.5	40	11510	–	2755	–	55.2	–	70	–	90	–	40	25.0	200
Females															
0–3 months	5.9	150	2160	480–420	515	115–100	12.5	2.1	9	1.5	20	3.4	25	13.1	30
4–6	7.7	150	2690	400	645	95	12.7	1.6	12	1.6	22	2.8	25	13.1	80
7–9	8.9	120	3200	400	765	95	13.7	1.5	14	1.6	18	2.0	25	13.1	140
10–12	9.8	120	3610	400	865	95	14.9	1.5	15	1.5	18	1.8	25	13.1	140
1–3 years	12.6	90	4860	400	1165	95	14.5	1.1	22	1.7	20	1.6	30	8.8	120
4–6	17.8	80	6460	380	1545	90	19.7	1.1	30	1.7	28	1.6	30	11.3	110
7–10	28.3	60	7280	–	1740	–	28.3	–	50	–	50	–	30	13.8	160
11–14	43.8	50	7920	–	1845	–	42.1	–	70	–	80	–	35	20.0	260
15–18	55.5	40	8830	–	2110	–	45.4	–	70	–	90	–	40	20.0	260

EAR, Estimated average requirement; RNI, Reference nutrient intake.
* Standard weights for age ranges [20]

Table 1.10   General guide to oral requirements in sick children.

	Infants 0–1 year (based on actual weight, not expected weight)	Children
Energy	High: 130–150 kcals/kg/day (545–630 kJ/kg/day) Very high: 150–220 kcals/kg/day (630–920 kJ/kg/day)	High: 120% EAR for age Very high: 150% EAR for age
Protein	High: 3–4.5 g/kg/day Very high: 6 g/kg/day 0–6 months, increasing to maximum of 10 g/kg/day up to 1 year	High: 2 g/kg/day, actual body weight It should be recognised that children may easily eat more than this
Sodium	High: 3.0 mmol/kg/day Very high: 4.5 mmol/kg/day A concentration >7.7 mmol Na/100 mL of infant formula will have an emetic effect	For severely underweight children, initially an energy and protein intake based on weight, not age, is used
Potassium	High: 3.0 mmol/kg/day Very high: 4.5 mmol/kg/day	

Table 1.11   Infant milk formulas.

Whey based	Casein based	Manufacturer
Aptamil First*	Aptamil Extra*	Milupa Ltd
Cow & Gate Premium*	Cow & Gate Plus*†	Cow & Gate Nutricia Ltd
Farley's First Milk	Farley's Second Milk	HJ Heinz Co Ltd
SMA Gold	SMA White	SMA Nutrition

All formulas contain nucleotides and beta-carotene.
* Contains prebiotics.
† Does not contain long chain polyunsaturated fatty acids.

Table 1.12   Follow-on milks suitable from 6 months.

	Manufacturer
Farley's Follow-on Milk	HJ Heinz Co Ltd
Forward	Milupa Ltd
Progress	SMA Nutrition
Step-up, Next Steps*	Cow & Gate Nutricia Ltd

* From 9 months.

seventh day of life, or sooner if the infant is feeding well. Breast fed infants will regulate their own intake of milk. Bottle fed babies should also ideally be fed on demand.

Fluid requirements in the first few weeks

The normal infant will tolerate 4-hourly feeds, six times daily once a body weight of more than 3.5 kg is reached. By the age of 3–6 weeks (body weight approximately 4 kg), the infant may sleep longer through the night and drop a feed. A fluid intake of 150 mL/kg should be maintained to provide adequate fluids, energy and nutrients. Infants should not normally be given more than 1200 mL of feed per 24 hours as this may induce vomiting and, in the long term, will lead to an inappropriately high energy intake. Sick infants may need smaller, more frequent feeds than the normal baby and,

according to the clinical condition, may have increased or decreased fluid requirements. Breast fed infants will continue to regulate their own intake of milk and feeding pattern.

Fluid requirements in older infants and children

Once solids are introduced around 6 months of age (p. 525) the infant's appetite for milk will lessen. For the older infant aged 7–12 months fluid requirements decrease to 120 mL/kg, assuming that some water is also obtained from solids. At 1 year, the child's thirst will largely determine how much fluid is taken.

Very few authorities publish fluid requirements for healthy populations. European recommendations for fluid intakes are summarised [22]. Table 1.13 gives recommendations in the USA [23].

If all a child's nutrition comes from feed and there is no significant contribution to fluid intake from foods, then fluid requirements may be estimated using the following guideline:

Table 1.13   Recommended intakes of water by age group.

	Total water intake per day, including water contained in food	Water obtained from drinks per day
Infants 0–6 months	700 mL, assumed to be from human milk	
7–12 months	800 mL from milk and complementary foods and beverages	600 mL
Children 1–3 years	1300 mL	900 mL
4–8 years	1700 mL	1200 mL
Boys 9–13 years	2400 mL	1800 mL
Girls 9–13 years	2100 mL	1600 mL

Source: Adadpted from USA dietary recommendations [23].

Body weight	Estimated fluid requirement
11–20 kg	100 mL/kg for the first 10 kg + 50 mL/kg for the next 10 kg
20 kg and above	100 mL/kg for the first 10 kg + 50 mL/kg for the next 10 kg + 25 mL/kg thereafter

Worked example for a child weighing 22 kg:

100 mL/kg for the first 10 kg	= 1000 mL
+ 50 mL/kg for the next 10 kg	= 500 mL
+ 25 mL/kg for the final 2 kg	= 50 mL
Total	= 1550 mL
	= 70 mL/kg

It is important to remember that not all of this fluid needs to be given as feed if nutritional requirements are met from a smaller volume; the remaining fluid requirement may simply be given as water. Estimates of fluid requirements using this guideline and standard body weights for age groups are given in Table 1.9.

Supplementing feeds for infants with faltering growth or who are fluid restricted

Supplements may be used to fortify standard infant formulas and special therapeutic formulas to achieve the necessary increase in energy and protein required by some infants. Expressed breast milk can also be fortified using a standard infant formula powder in term babies (Table 1.14) or a breast milk fortifier in preterm infants (see p. 80). Care needs to be taken not to present an osmotic load of more than 500 mOsm/kg H_2O to the normal functioning gut, otherwise an osmotic diarrhoea will result. If the infant has malabsorption, an upper limit of 400 mOsm/kg H_2O may be necessary. Infants who are fluid restricted will need to meet their nutritional requirements in a lower volume of feed than usual and the following feed manipulations can also be used for these babies.

Concentrating infant formulas

Normally, infant formula powders, whether whey and casein based formulas or specialised dietetic products, should be diluted according to the manufacturers' instructions as this provides the correct balance of energy, protein and nutrients when fed

Table 1.14   Examples of energy and nutrient dense formulas for infants per 100 mL.

	Energy		Protein (g)	CHO (g)	Fat (g)	Na (mmol)	K (mmol)	Osmolality (mOsm/kg H_2O)	P : E ratio
	kcal	kJ							
12.7% SMA Gold	67	280	1.5	7.2	3.6	0.7	1.8	294	9.0
15% SMA Gold	79	330	1.8	8.5	4.3	0.8	2.1	347	9.0
EBM + 3% SMA Gold	84	353	1.7	8.9	4.9	0.7	1.8	–	8.1
SMA High Energy	91	382	2.0	9.8	4.9	1.0	2.3	415	8.8
Infatrini	100	420	2.6	10.3	5.4	1.1	2.4	310	10.4
15% C&G Premium + Maxijul to 12% CHO + Calogen to 5% fat	100	420	1.6	12.0	5.0	0.9	2.1	–	6.4

P : E, protein:energy; EBM, expressed breast milk.

at the appropriate volume. However, there are occasions when, to achieve a feed that is denser in energy, protein and other nutrients, it is necessary to concentrate the formula. Most normal baby milks in the UK are made up at a dilution of approximately 13%. By making the baby milk up at a dilution of 15% (15 g powder per 100 mL water), more nutrition can be given in a given volume of feed, e.g. energy content may be increased from 67 kcal (280 kJ) per 100 mL to 77 kcal (325 kJ) per 100 mL and protein content from 1.5 g per 100 mL to 1.7 g per 100 mL. Similarly, special therapeutic feeds that are usually made up at a dilution of, say, 15% may be concentrated to a 17% dilution. This concentrating of feeds should only be performed as a therapeutic procedure and is not usual practice. Table 1.14 shows an example of a 15% feed.

The protein : energy ratio of the feed should ideally be kept within the range 7.5–12% for infants (i.e. 7.5–12% energy from protein) and 5–15% in older children. In order for accelerated or 'catch-up' growth to occur, it is necessary to provide about 9% energy from protein [24]. In some clinical situations it is not possible to preserve this protein : energy ratio as carbohydrate and fat sources alone may be added to a feed to control deranged blood biochemistry, for example. In these situations it is important to ensure that the infant is receiving at least the RNI for protein.

If infants are to be discharged home on a concentrated feed the recipe may be translated into scoop measures for ease of use. This will mean that more scoops of milk powder will be added to a given volume of water than recommended by the manufacturer. As this is contrary to normal practice the reasons for this deviation should be carefully explained to the parents and communicated to primary health care staff.

Nutrient-dense ready-to-feed formulas

There are two nutrient-dense ready-to-feed formulas available for hospital use and in the community, Infatrini and SMA High Energy (Table 1.14). They are nutritionally complete formulas containing more energy, protein and nutrients per 100 mL than standard infant formulas. They are suitable for use from birth and are designed for infants who have increased nutritional requirements or who are fluid restricted. They obviate the need for carers to make up normal infant formulas at concentrations other than the usual one scoop of powder to 30 mL water.

Energy and protein modules

There may be therapeutic circumstances when energy and/or protein supplements need to be added to normal infant formulas or special formulas without necessarily the need to increase the concentration of the base feed. Sometimes a ready-to-feed formula does not meet the needs of the individual child. Energy and protein modules and their use are described.

Carbohydrate
Carbohydrate provides 4 kcal/g (16 kJ/g). It is preferable to add carbohydrate to a feed in the form of glucose polymers, rather than using mono- or disaccharides, because they exert a lesser osmotic effect on the gut. Hence, a larger amount can be used per given volume of feed (Table 1.15). Glucose polymers should be added in 1% increments each 24 hours (i.e. 1 g per 100 mL feed per 24 hours). This will allow the point at which the infant becomes intolerant (i.e. has loose stools) to the concentration of the extra carbohydrate to be identified. Tolerance depends on the age of the infant and the maturity and absorptive capacity of the gut. As a guideline, the following percentage concentrations of carbohydrate (g total carbohydrate per 100 mL feed) should be tolerated if glucose polymer is used:

- 10–12% carbohydrate concentration in infants under 6 months (i.e. 7 g from formula, 3–5 g added)
- 12–15% in infants aged 6 months to 1 year
- 15–20% in toddlers aged 1–2 years
- 20–30% in older children

If glucose or fructose needs to be added to a feed where there is an intolerance of glucose polymer, an upper limit of tolerance may be reached at a total carbohydrate concentration of 7–8% in infants and young children.

Fat
Fat provides 9 kcal/g (37 kJ/g). Long chain fat emulsions are favoured over medium chain fat emulsions because they have a lower osmotic effect on the gut and provide a source of essential fatty

Table 1.15   Energy supplements.

Per 100 g	Ingredients	Energy* kcal	Energy* kJ	Na (mmol)	K (mmol)	PO$_4$ (mmol)
Glucose polymers						
Caloreen (Nestle Clinical)	Hydrolysed corn starch	390	1630	<1.8	0.3	–
Super Soluble Maxijul (SHS)	Hydrolysed corn starch	380	1615	<0.86	<0.12	<0.16
Polycal (Nutricia Clinical)	Hydrolysed corn starch	380	1615	2.2	1.3	2.3–4.2
Polycose (Abbott Laboratories)	Hydrolysed corn starch	376	1598	4.8	0.26	0.39
Vitajoule (Vitaflo Ltd)	Hydrolysed corn starch	380	1610	<1.9	<0.2	–
Fat emulsions						
Calogen (SHS)	Canola oil, sunflower oil	450	1850	0.9	0.5	
Liquigen (SHS)	Coconut oil	450	1850	1.2	–	
Combined fat and carbohydrate supplements						
Super Soluble Duocal (SHS)	Glucose syrup, canola oil, coconut oil, safflower oil	492	2061	<0.9	<0.1	
MCT Duocal (SHS)	Cornstarch, coconut oil, walnut oil, canola oil, palm oil	497	2082	<1.3	<0.5	

* As quoted by manufacturers

acids. Medium chain fats are incorporated where there is malabsorption of long chain fat (Table 1.15).

Fat emulsions should be added to feeds in 1% increments each 24 hours, so providing an increase of 0.5 g fat per 100 mL per 24 hours. Infants will tolerate a total fat concentration of 5–6% (i.e. 5–6 g fat per 100 mL feed) if the gut is functioning normally. Children over 1 year of age will tolerate more fat, although concentrations above 7% may induce a feeling of nausea and cause vomiting. Medium chain fat will not be tolerated at such high concentrations, and may be the cause of abdominal cramps and osmotic diarrhoea if not introduced slowly to the feed.

There are combined carbohydrate and fat supplements using both long and medium chain fats (Table 1.15). Again, these must be introduced to feeds in 1% increments to determine the child's tolerance of the product. A schedule for the addition of energy supplements to infant formulas is given in Table 1.16.

Protein
Protein may be added to feeds in the form of whole protein, peptides or amino acids (Table 1.17). Protein

supplementation is rarely required without an accompanying increase in energy consumption.

Protein supplements are added to feeds to provide a specific amount of protein per kilogram

Table 1.16   Schedule for the addition of energy supplements to infant formulas.

Day	Energy source added	Additional CHO/fat per 100 mL feed	Energy added per 100 mL kcal	Energy added per 100 mL kJ
1	1% Glucose Polymer	1 g CHO	4	17
2	2% Glucose Polymer	2 g CHO	8	33
3	3% Glucose Polymer	3 g CHO	12	50
4	3% Glucose Polymer + 1% Fat Emulsion	3 g CHO 0.5 g Fat	17	69
5	3% Glucose Polymer + 2% Fat Emulsion	3 g CHO 1 g Fat	21	88
6	4% Glucose Polymer + 2% Fat Emulsion	4 g CHO 1 g Fat	25	105
7	5% Glucose Polymer + 2% Fat Emulsion	5 g CHO 1 g Fat	29	121
8	5% Glucose Polymer + 3% Fat Emulsion	5 g CHO 1.5 g Fat	34	140

Table 1.17   Protein supplements.

Per 100 g	Energy		Protein (g)	CHO (g)	Fat (g)	Na (mmol)	K (mmol)
	kcal	kJ					
Vitapro whole protein (Vitaflo Ltd)	360	1506	75	9.0	6.0	<13	18.0
ProMod whole protein (Abbott)	426	1794	76	10.2	9.12	16.5	17.5
Protifar whole protein (Nutricia Clinical)	373	1580	88.5	1.5	1.6	1.3	1.2
Peptide Module 767 peptides from hydrolysed meat and soya (SHS)	346	1469	86.4	–	–	–	–
Complete Amino Acid Mix Code 124 L-amino acids (SHS)	328	1394	82	–	–	–	–

actual body weight of the child. It is rarely necessary to give intakes of greater than 6 g protein/kg; if intakes do approach this value, blood urea levels should be monitored twice weekly to avoid the danger of uraemia developing. Supplements should be added in small increments as they can very quickly and inappropriately increase the child's intake of protein. The osmotic effect of whole protein products will be less than that of peptides, and peptides less than the effect of amino acids.

Vitamin and mineral requirements

Vitamin and mineral requirements for populations of normal children are provided by the DRVs and some are shown in Table 1.9. In disease states, requirements for certain vitamins and minerals will be different and are fully described in the dietary management of each clinical condition. The prescribable vitamin and mineral supplements that are most often used in paediatric practice are given in Tables 1.18–1.20.

Table 1.18   Vitamin supplements.

	Healthy Start[‡] Children's Vitamin Drops (SSL)	Abidec (Chefaro)	Dalivit (LPC)	Ketovite (Paines & Byrne)
	5 drops for all infants from 6 months of age[†]	0.3 mL <1 year 0.6 mL >1 year*	0.6 mL	5 mL liquid[†] 3 tablets
Thiamin (B$_1$) (mg)	–	0.4	1	3.0
Riboflavin (B$_2$) (mg)	–	0.8	0.4	3.0
Pyridoxine (B$_6$) (mg)	–	0.8	0.5	1.0
Nicotinamide (mg)	–	5	5	9.9
Pantothenate (mg)	–	–	–	3.5
Ascorbic acid (C) (mg)	20	40	50	50
Alpha-tocopherol (E) (mg)	–	–	–	15.0
Inositol (mg)	–	–	–	150
Biotin (mg)	–	–	–	0.5
Folic acid (mg)	–	–	–	0.8
Acetomenaphthone (K) (mg)	–	–	–	1.5
Vitamin A (µg)	233	400	1500	750
Vitamin D (µg)	7.5	10	10	10
Choline chloride (mg)	–	–	–	150
Cyanocobalamin (B$_{12}$) (µg)	–	–	–	12.5

* Values relate to 0.6 mL dose.
† Unless taking >500 mL infant formula or follow-on milk.
‡ Eligibility under the Healthy Start Scheme, p. 531.

Table 1.19   Mineral supplements.

	1.5 g/kg/day up to full dose of 8 g/day* Metabolic Mineral Mixture (SHS)
Sodium (mmol)	14
Potassium (mmol)	17
Chloride (mmol)	4
Calcium (mmol)	16
Phosphorus (mmol)	15
Magnesium (mmol)	3.2
Iron (mg)	5
Zinc (mg)	4
Iodine	trace
Manganese (mg)	0.4
Copper (mg)	1
Molybdenum	trace
Cobalt	–
Aluminium	trace

* Values relate to 8 g dose.

Prescribing products for paediatric use

The majority of specialised formulas, supplements and special dietary foods can be prescribed for specific conditions. The Advisory Committee on Borderline Substances recommends suitable products and defines the conditions for which they can be used. Prescriptions from the general practitioner (FP10; GP10 in Scotland) should be marked 'ACBS' to indicate that the prescription complies with recommendations. A list of prescribable items for paediatric use appears in the *BNF (British National Formulary) for Children* under the Borderline Substances Appendix and is also available on line at www.bnf.org. Children under the age of 16 years in the UK are exempt from prescription charges.

Table 1.20   Vitamin and mineral supplements.

Daily dose	Paediatric Seravit (powder) Unflavoured 17 g powder	Forceval Junior Capsules 2 capsules
Sodium (mmol)	0.15	–
Potassium (mmol)	trace	–
Chloride (mmol)	1.12	–
Calcium (mmol)	11.7	–
Phosphorus (mmol)	9.4	–
Magnesium (mmol)	2.5	0.08
Iron (mg)	4	10.0
Zinc (mg)	2.7	10.0
Iodine (mg)	0.06	0.15
Manganese (mg)	0.78	2.5
Copper (mg)	0.78	2.0
Molybdenum (mg)	0.06	0.1
Selenium (mg)	0.02	0.05
Chromium (mg)	0.02	0.1
Vitamin A (µg)	714	750
Vitamin E (mg)	3.6	10.0
Vitamin C (mg)	68	50
Thiamin (mg)	0.54	3.0
Riboflavin (mg)	0.75	2.0
Pyridoxine (mg)	0.58	2.0
Nicotinamide (mg)	5.95	15.0
Pantothenic acid (mg)	2.89	4.0
Inositol (mg)	119	–
Choline (mg)	59.5	–
Vitamin D_3 (µg)	9.44	10.0
Vitamin B_{12} (µg)	1.46	4.0
Folic acid (mg)	0.05	0.2
Biotin (mg)	0.04	0.1
Vitamin K (mg)	0.03	0.05
Carbohydrate	glucose polymer 75 g/100 g	
Osmolality	216 mOsm/kg H_2O at 10% dilution	

References

1 Lanigan JA, Wells J, Lawson MS *et al.* Number of days needed to assess energy and nutrient intake in infants and young children. *Eur J Clin Nutr*, 2004, **58** 745–50.

2 Lucas A, Ewing G, Roberts SB, Coward WA How much energy does the breast-fed infant consume and expend? *Br Med J*, 1987, **295** 75–7.

3 Hall D, Elliman D Growth monitoring and nutrition. In: *Health For All Children*, 4th edn. Oxford: Oxford University Press, 2003, pp. 170–95.

4 Michaelson KF Short-term measurements of linear growth in early life: infant kneemometry. *Acta Paediatr*, 1997, **86** 551–3.

5 Stevenson RD Use of segmental measures to estimate stature in children with cerebral palsy. *Arch Pediatr Adolesc Med*, 1995, **149** 658–62.

6 Gibson RS *Principles of Nutritional Assessment*, 2nd edn. New York: Oxford University Press, 2005.

7 Sangi H, Mueller WH Which measure of body fat distribution is best for epidemiological research among adolescents. *Am J Epidemiol*, 1991, **133** 870–3.

8   Freeman JV, Cole TJ, Chinn S *et al.* Cross sectional stature and weight reference curves for the UK. 1990. *Arch Dis Child*, 1995, **73** 17–24.

9   Cole TJ, Paul AA, Whitehead RG Weight reference charts for British long-term breast-fed infants. *Acta Paediatr*, 2002, **91** 1296–300.

10 www.WHOint/growthstandards Accessed August 2006.

11 Cole TJ, Freeman JV, Preece MA Body mass index curves for the UK, 1990. *Arch Dis Child*, 1995, **73** 25–9.

12 McCarthy HD, Jarrett KV, Crawley HF The development of waist circumference percentiles in British children aged 5.0–16.9 years. *Eur J Clin Nutr*, 2001, **55** 902–7.

13 Styles ME, Cole TJ, Dennis J *et al.* New cross sectional stature, weight and head circumference references for Down's syndrome in the UK and republic of Ireland. *Arch Dis Child*, 2002, **87** 104–8.

14 Cole TJ Conditional reference charts to assess weight gain in British infants. *Arch Dis Child*, 1995, **73** 8–16.

15 Waterlow JC Some aspects of protein calorie malnutrition. *Br Med J*, 1972, **3** 556–69.

16 WHO Multicenter Growth Reference study group: WHO child growth standards based on length/height, weight and age. *Acta Paediatr*, 2006, suppl. **450** 76–85.

17 Clayton BE, Round JM (eds) *Chemical Pathology and the Sick Child*. Oxford: Blackwell Science, 1994.

18 Ruxton CH, Reilly JJ, Kirk TR Body composition of healthy 7- and 8-year-old children and a comparison with the 'reference child'. *Int J Obes*, 1999, **23** 1276–81.

19 Haroun D, Wells JCT, Williams JE Composition of the fat-free mass in obese and non-obese children: matched case–control study. *Int J Obes*, 2005, **29** 29–36.

20 Department of Health. Report on Health and Social Subjects No 41. *Dietary Reference Values for Food Energy and Nutrients for the United Kingdom*. London: The Stationery Office, 1991.

21 Human Energy Requirements. Report of a joint FAO/WHO/UNU expert committee. World Health Organization, Rome, 2005.

22 Lawson MS Children: Nutritional requirements. In: Caballero B, Allen L, Prentice A (eds) *Encyclopedia of Human Nutrition*, 2nd edn. London: Elsevier, 2005, pp. 357–69.

23 Dietary Reference Values for water, potassium, sodium, chloride and sulfate. Washington DC: Institute of Medicine of the National Academies, 2004.

24 Jackson AA, Wooton SA The energy requirements of growth and catch-up growth. In: Scrimshaw NS, Scűrch B (eds) *Activity, Energy Expenditure and Energy Requirements of Infants and Children*. Lausanne, Switzerland: IDECG, 1990, pp. 185–214.

Further reading

Gibson RS *Principles of Nutritional Assessment*, 2nd edn. Oxford: Oxford University Press, 2005.

Talbot J (ed) *Infant Feeding in the First Year*. London: Profile Productions Ltd, 1989.

Thompson JM *Nutritional Requirements of Infants and Young Children*. Oxford: Blackwell Science, 1998.

Wardley BL, Puntis JWL, Taitz LS *Handbook of Child Nutrition*, 2nd edn. Oxford: Oxford University Press, 1997.

Hall DMB, Elliman D *Health for All Children*, 4th edn. Oxford: Oxford University Press, 2003.

Morgan JB, Dickerson JWT (eds) *Nutrition in Early Life*. Chichester: Wiley, 2003.

Useful address

Child Growth Foundation
2 Mayfield Avenue, Chiswick, London W4 1PW. Tel. 020 8994 7625/8995 0257, e-mail: cgflondon@aol.com
www.childgrowthfoundation.org

2 Provision of Nutrition in a Hospital Setting

Ruth Watling

Introduction

Children in hospital are likely to be particularly vulnerable and susceptible to the effects of under-nutrition. There are few current data on actual incidence of acute and chronic malnutrition but older studies indicated that this was significant and possibly more common in children with already established disease [1–4].

The organised and effective delivery of nutrition and fluid to children in hospital has two main aims. First, to ensure that children eat sufficient food to meet their nutritional requirements and, secondly, to encourage good healthy eating habits [5]. The first of these aims cannot be overstated and the achievement of this aim is the subject of a number of key UK government resolutions and policies [6–8].

To meet the nutritional needs of the range of hospitalised paediatric patients, a variety of services are required including:

- Facilitation of breast feeding
- Ready-to-feed (RTF) infant milks
- Enteral feeds
- Provision of parenteral nutrition
- Ordinary food including provision for therapeutic diets

Provision of nutrition in a hospital setting requires effort and the close collaboration of nurses, doctors, dietitians, catering staff, the child or young adult and their carers.

Infant and enteral feeds

Infant milks

Many hospitalised infants, who are not breast fed, will simply require an adequate volume of infant milk. To minimise infection risk and ensure uniform composition this is best provided in an RTF form. The need to recommend the use of RTF milk, unless clinically contraindicated, has been further strengthened by concerns regarding the risk of *Enterobacter sakazakii* infections [9]. A selection of whey and casein based milks should be available to meet the personal preference of the family. If RTF milks are not available, the guidance for preparation of adapted or specialised formulas apply.

Adapted infant milks and specialised formulas

To prepare adapted infant milks (e.g. thickened or energy supplemented milk, or specialised infant formulas), a designated feed-making area is required.

Children receiving such feeds are likely to be those at greatest nutritional risk, therefore feeds must be made accurately to ensure the prescribed nutritional content is achieved.

Hygiene standards in feed preparation are of paramount importance as they are generally prepared for infants or for older children who are immunologically compromised as a result of illness.

Enteral feeds

The range and presentation of paediatric enteral feeds continues to expand, increasing the possibility that feeds in a sterile ready-to-hang presentation could be available at ward level. In situations where enteral feeds require adaptation (e.g. energy supplementation or decanting into enteral feeding bottles), again, these processes should be carried out in a designated feed-making area.

Designated feed-making area

In large hospitals preparing in excess of 15–20 feeds daily, a feed-making unit will be required, normally consisting of three separate areas for storage, preparation and cleaning. For units requiring less than 15 feeds daily, a designated feed-making room or a specific area of the ward kitchen should be available.

Any feed-making operation must comply with the requirements of the Food Safety Act 1990 [10]. The American Dietetic Association has produced comprehensive guidelines on preparation of formula and these are an essential reference standard for a safe, effective and efficient designated feed-making area [11]. The manager of such an operation has a legal obligation to ensure that it operates to acceptable standards of hygiene. To establish and monitor such standards, a hazard analysis and critical control point (HACCP) system is recommended [12]. Such a system will ensure that all aspects of feed production are subjected to rigorous assessment for potential hazards and risks, and that adequate control points are incorporated into the process.

Structural design of feed-making areas

A designated feed-making area should be an independent unit or room whose access is restricted to authorised personnel. Designed to prevent the entrance and harbouring of vermin and pests and constructed to be easily cleaned, it must be operated to the highest standards of hygiene.

It is desirable to separate the unit into three main areas:

- *Storage area:* situated adjacent to the feed preparation area, where bulk goods are delivered, unpacked and stored. It should be large enough to accommodate adequate storage racks which are constructed and sited to permit segregation of commodities, stock rotation and effective cleaning. Items must be stored on racks or shelves, not directly on the floor. The temperature should be maintained between 10°C and 15°C and should be monitored daily. Entry to this area is restricted to unit and delivery staff.
- *Feed preparation area:* where very clean conditions prevail and access is strictly limited to feed preparation staff; entry should be via an anteroom containing a wash-hand basin and storage facilities for outer protective clothing. Bulk storage of items (e.g. large cardboard cartons) is not recommended. There should be sufficient space to allow clean equipment and small quantities of ingredients to be stored, preferably on wheel-mounted stainless steel solid shelving, leaving worktops clear. During the preparation of feeds, all other activities in the area should cease and the doors should be closed and secured against all staff who are not involved in the preparation process. If it is necessary for staff to leave the preparation area they must, on re-entry, wash their hands again, according to the correct handwashing procedure.
- *Utility area for equipment washing and administrative work:* a unit reusing feeding bottles will require a designated space, adjoining the feed preparation area, with a separate access for the delivery of dirty bottles. The utility area can also be used to house computer equipment for feed labelling. Storage of cleaning materials should be separated from ingredients and equipment and requires a designated clean, dry room or cupboard.

A cloakroom with a separate changing room for feed unit staff should be conveniently sited but segregated from the feed-making area. The cloakroom should have a toilet and wash-hand basin with foot or elbow operated taps.

Recommendations for construction of special feeds units are as follows:

Plant
- *Walls, floors and ceilings:* hardwearing, impervious, free from cracks and open joints. Smooth surfaces to permit ease of cleaning and coved junctions between floors, walls and ceilings to prevent collection of dust and dirt. Light-coloured sheen finish to reflect light and increase illumination.
- *Doors in the production area:* self-closing with glass observation panel.
- *Windows:* sealed to prevent opening.
- *Lighting level:* to allow staff to work cleanly and safely without eye strain, and to expose dirt and dust. Light fixtures flush with wall or ceiling.
- *Ventilation in the production area:* mechanical means; air supply filtered with temperature (and preferably humidity) control to give optimum working environment and control bacterial and dust contamination. Steam-producing equipment such as sterilisers, dishwashers and pasteurisers should be fitted with a canopy and exhaust fan system to draw off steam and fumes.
- *Wash-hand basins:* one hand basin provided in each utility and preparation area. Hot and cold water with foot or elbow operated taps. Adjacent soap dispenser and either single use disposable towels or a hot air hand dryer.
- *Water supply:* of potable quality from a rising main. Softened water supply to equipment is preferable to prevent calcium deposition, but water softened by ion exchange should not be used in feeds because of its increased sodium content.

The Department of Health has not advised against the use of tap water in feed preparation, unlike the USA [11]. Where tap water is used it should be provided from a fixed device such as a gas or electric water boiler to dispense water above 80°C. The alternative is to use sterile water and this decision will require a cost–benefit and risk analysis in conjunction with microbiological advice.

Large equipment
- Large equipment such as shelving, tables and refrigerators should be castor mounted with wheel brakes to allow easy access for cleaning.

Smooth impervious surfaces free from sharp internal corners, which may act as dirt traps, which can be easily cleaned and disinfected (e.g. stainless steel) are recommended.
- One or more refrigerators which operate at a temperature between 1–4°C are a necessity; the temperature should be monitored and recorded twice daily.
- A blast chiller to allow rapid cooling of all feeds to 4°C within 1 hour of preparation [11].
- A deep freeze which operates at −18°C will be necessary if expressed breast milk is to be stored for more than a few hours. Both the refrigerator and freezer should be self-defrosting and have shelves that are easy to clean. An alarm which is activated if the door is left open accidentally or the internal temperature rises is also useful.
- Pasteurisation equipment that is suitable for the range of procedures carried out (see p. 24) and that includes a method of monitoring and recording pasteurisation cycles is desirable.
- Thermal sterilisation or disinfection equipment is desirable in a small unit and essential in a large centralised unit. This can be a dishwasher adapted for bottle and equipment washing, with a rinse cycle that holds a temperature of 85°C for 2 minutes. This ensures a surface temperature of 80°C for 1 minute, which is an effective disinfectant. A drying cycle is useful [13].
- A feed delivery trolley.

Small equipment
- Mixing and measuring equipment including jugs, measures, cutlery and whisks should be made from plastic or stainless steel. They must be easily washed and cleaned.
- Weighing equipment should be easy to clean, easy to use and of the appropriate accuracy for the task. It may be battery or electrically operated.
- Feed bottles are available in glass, polycarbonate or plastic polythene in 50–240 mL sizes. Glass is a hazardous material prone to cracking and chipping; polycarbonate shrinks if autoclaved at temperatures greater than 119°C and bottles become scratched or crazed after some time in use. Reusable bottles require washing, sanitising by heat or chemical means; sealing discs or caps need to undergo a similar treatment and are likely to become lost or misshapen

with continuous use. Disposable sterile poly-thene bottles reduce the workload in the unit. The decision to use disposable or reusable bottles is a matter for each individual unit based on cost–benefit analysis and risk analysis of possible contamination from inadequately cleaned bottles. Single-use enteral feeding containers will also be required for larger prepared volumes or for decanted sterile RTF formulas. The use of tamper-proof seals on all bottles produced in a special feeds unit is recommended.

Staffing

Feed provision is usually required 365 days a year and staffing levels should take this fact and the workload into consideration. Part-time employment of some staff may be particularly appropriate. In large units, the dietitian may be managerially responsible for staff and feed preparation. In small areas attached to a ward, the supervision and management may be the responsibility of the nursing staff with the dietitian acting in an advisory capacity. As identified in the Food Safety Act [10], all food handlers should hold a Basic Food Hygiene Certificate. No other specific qualifications are required for feed preparation staff, provided that adequate instruction and supervision are provided, although given the nature of the work they must have good literacy and numeracy skills.

Training should cover personal hygiene, prevention of bacterial and foreign matter contamination, preparation procedures, and basic knowledge of the feed composition and clinical indication.

Suitable protective uniforms and a satisfactory laundry service are required. A disposable plastic apron should be worn during feed preparation and a disposable head covering should completely cover the hair. Shoes should be flat-heeled and cover the foot; jewellery (with the exception of a wedding ring and stud type earrings) is not allowed. Appointment of staff should be subject to a satisfactory medical examination; bacteriological screening of faecal specimens should take place prior to appointment, and after a gastrointestinal illness.

Feed preparation

There are three key components of safe feed preparation: appropriate ingredients, safe and accurate preparation, and limitation of microbial growth.

All ingredients received into a feed-making area should be of the required standards and specification. Goods received should be checked and stock rotated according to date. Tins and packets of powdered formula should be dated when opened and any remaining powder discarded after a specified time according to local policy. Opened tins or packets (e.g. from the patient's home) should not be accepted into the feed-making area. If pasteurised cow's milk is used (e.g. to reconstitute powdered supplements), it should be stocked according to its dated shelf-life and if opened any unused should be discarded at the end of the working day. Expressed breast milk will require an agreed procedure for its safe storage and use [11,14].

Details of each feed to be prepared should be in a clearly written or printed form including the patient's name, date of birth and hospital number, the weight or volume of each feed ingredient, the total fluid volume, the number and volume of each feed required. All ingredients should be weighed or measured accurately. Prepared feeds should be decanted into the appropriate number and size of bottles and each bottle labelled. The label must include details of the patient's name, ward, feed type, preparation date and preferably advice to refrigerate and discard after 24 hours.

Finally, limitation of microbial growth is critical to safe feed provision. The type of feeds prepared will readily support the growth of harmful microorganisms, particularly if stored at temperatures above 5°C. Pasteurisation can limit potential microbiological contamination and will destroy *Staphylococcus aureus*, *Enterobacter* sp. and *Salmonella* sp., but may be less effective against all potential pathogens (e.g. *Bacillus* sp.) (Anderton A, personal communication, 1998). There are no regulations to govern the pasteurisation of infant formula powders in special feeds units, but culture results may be referenced to the standard proposed in the Dairy Products (Hygiene) Regulations [15].

There are two methods of pasteurisation commonly used:

1 Holder method for expressed breast milk where the temperature is raised to 62.5°C for 30 minutes followed by rapid cooling to less than 10°C.
2 Flash method for prepared feeds where the temperature is raised to 67.5°C for 4 minutes followed by rapid cooling to less than 10°C.

Blast chilling is an effective method of achieving one of the most important steps in limiting microbial growth in prepared feeds (i.e. cooling rapidly to below 5°C). Both pasteurisers and blast chillers should be fitted with data loggers to show the temperature and process time. Following preparation, and/or pasteurisation, blast chilling feeds should be placed in a holding refrigerator at less that 5°C until delivery to wards.

Delivery

Feed delivery to wards should be compatible with food safety requirements of being refrigerated at less than 5°C without avoidable delay. If the preparation unit is some distance from wards this may require a refrigerated trolley. Feeds should be checked and placed in a designated refrigerator at ward level; this refrigerator should be reserved for milk feeds and should not contain items of food. The temperature of ward refrigerators should be 1–4°C and should be checked twice daily.

Cleaning procedures

Sterilisation (the destruction of all microorganisms and their spores) is not attainable in a special feeds unit. Sanitisation or disinfection of small equipment can be achieved by autoclaving, by a dishwasher or by chemical means.

Autoclaving, although effective, has a number of disadvantages: equipment first has to be washed, dried, packed and sealed; this is costly and time consuming. In addition water condensation forms and remains in feeding bottles, where it can induce bacterial activity.

Thermal disinfection in a dishwasher requires less time and the inclusion of a drying cycle will ensure that all equipment is dry and ready for storage. To achieve thermal disinfection, the water in the dishwasher should reach a minimum temperature of 85°C for 2 minutes.

Chemical disinfection (e.g. hypochlorite) reduces levels of harmful bacteria to acceptable levels and is also satisfactory for small (non-metallic) equipment, provided recommendations are followed; heat sanitisation is the preferred method. Chemical disinfection will only be effective if:

- The equipment is adequately cleaned; residual organic matter inactivates the chlorine content of the disinfectant.

- The disinfectant is freshly and correctly prepared with all air bubbles removed to ensure the solution comes into contact with all surfaces of the equipment.
- The equipment remains in the disinfectant for the recommended length of time. After disinfection, the equipment should be rinsed free of contaminated hypochlorite with clean water.

Regardless of the method used, feed equipment should be covered with sterile paper and used within 24 hours of disinfection. Equipment that is stored for longer than this should be re-disinfected before use.

Walls of a special feeds unit should be washed every 6 months, floors cleaned daily and all cleaning procedures documented.

Microbiological surveillance

The aim of a designated feed-making area is to minimise the risk of microbial contamination in prepared infant formulas, enteral feeds or oral supplements. Adherence to the principles outlined here and other published guidelines [11] will support this aim. To ensure satisfactory standards of working practice are maintained, a microbiological surveillance policy can be a useful component of quality control. The following samples should be sent for microbiological analysis once each month: each type of feed; water from boiler, tap and pasteuriser; a swab from work surfaces, sinks, shelving, mixing equipment and feeding bottles. An air sample should be taken if *Staphylococcus aureus* is identified.

Procedures and documentation

To comply with legislative requirements, clear written procedures are required for every aspect of feed preparation. This includes guidelines for personal hygiene and prevention of cross-infection, procedures for ordering supplies, feed preparation, instructions for pasteurisation and blast chilling, cleaning and disinfection, procedures for microbiological surveillance and accident procedures. Information about equipment maintenance and emergency telephone numbers in case of breakdown should also be displayed.

Currently, there are no accepted published standards for the preparation of enteral feeds for the paediatric age range. Operational practices should be based on standards identified for food products [10,12].

Normal diet in a hospital setting

Good practice principles have been published [8] and in summary are as follow:

- Nutritionally, the focus should be on energy and menus should meet the Estimated Average Requirement (EAR) [16] by increasing the energy density of foods and frequency of meals and the availability of favourite foods around the clock.
- Meet the Reference Nutrient Intake (RNI) [16] for protein. This is almost always achieved if EAR for energy is met.

- A wide variety of portion sizes will be required to meet the requirements of the paediatric population (Table 2.1).
- The service should be delivered in a manner and in an environment that encourages the child to eat. Crockery and utensils appropriate to age should be used.
- Children in hospital should be provided with breakfast, two main meals and 2–3 snacks daily and the following should be available to all: 200 mL fruit juice for vitamin C, 350–500 mL full fat milk for calcium (semi-skimmed available as required for children over 2 years), fresh fruit.
- Accurate records of a child's food and drink intake should be kept.
- Choices should be available to vegetarians, vegans and those whose eating habits are based on religious and cultural beliefs.

Table 2.1 Food portion sizes for different age groups.

	1 year	2–3 years	3–5 years	10 years
Meal pattern	3 small meals and 3 snacks plus milk	3 meals and 2–3 snacks or milky drinks	3 meals and 1–2 snacks or milky drinks	3 meals and 1–2 snacks or milky drinks
Meat, fish, egg	1/2–1 tablespoon (15–25 g) minced/ finely chopped, with gravy/sauce; 1/2–1 hard cooked egg	1 1/2 tablespoons (20–30 g) chopped; 1 fish finger; 1 sausage; 1 egg	2–3 tablespoons (40–80 g); 1–2 fish fingers/sausages; 1 egg	90–120 g; 3–4 fish fingers/sausages; 2 eggs
Cheese	20 g grated	25–30 g cubed or grated	30–40 g	50–60 g
Potato	1 tablespoon (30 g) mashed	1–2 tablespoons (30–60 g); 6 smallish chips	2–3 tablespoons (60–80 g); 8–10 chips	4–6 tablespoons (100–180 g); 100–150 g chips
Vegetables	1 tablespoon (30 g) soft or mashed	1–2 tablespoons (30–60 g) or small chopped salad	2–3 tablespoons (60–80 g)	3–4 tablespoons (100–120 g)
Fruit	1/2–1 piece (40–80 g)	1 piece (80–100 g)	1 piece (100 g)	1 piece (100 g)
Dessert (e.g. custard/yoghurt)	2 tablespoons (60 g)	2–3 tablespoons (60–80 g)	4 tablespoons (120 g); 1 carton yoghurt (150 g)	6 tablespoons (180 g)
Bread	1/2–1 slice (20–30 g)	1 large slice (40 g)	1–2 large slices (40–80 g)	2–4 large slices (80–160 g)
Breakfast cereal	1 tablespoon (15 g); 1/2 Weetabix	1–1 1/2 tablespoons (15–20 g); 1 Weetabix	2–3 tablespoons (20–30 g); 1 Weetabix	3–4 tablespoons (30–40 g); 2 Weetabix
Drinks	3/4 teacup (100 mL)	1 teacup (150 mL)	1 teacup (150 mL)	1 mug (200 mL)
Milk	500 mL whole milk/day	350 mL whole or semi-skimmed/day	350 mL whole or or semi-skimmed/day	350 mL whole, semi-skimmed or skimmed/day

For children in all age groups: 6–8 drinks per day including milk drinks.

Modified diet in a hospital setting

The major role of the dietitian is to liaise with the medical and nursing staff and to advise on the appropriate therapeutic regimen. The advice and education given to children requiring modified diets and to their carers is the responsibility of the dietitian. In addition to this, the dietitian assists in the provision of modified diets within the hospital. Usually, this is in an advisory capacity to diet cooks employed by the caterer, but rarely dietitians may also be managerially responsible for the diet kitchen. In the majority of cases, design and maintenance of the diet preparation area, staff management, supply of provisions and responsibility for hygiene will rest with the catering manager. If these are the responsibility of the dietitian, the same principles apply as previously described for feed-making areas [10].

Staff involved in the preparation of modified diets must be aware of the need for accuracy, appropriate portion size for age, consistency of nutrient content and variety. For those on a modified diet, the food provided in hospital is taken as an example and must therefore be correct. It is advisable that staff employed to prepare modified diets should have as a minimum qualification City and Guilds 706/2 and have attended a diet cookery course. In-service training of diet cooks should be undertaken by the dietitian particularly to ensure that staff are kept up-to-date with changes to dietary treatment.

The dietitian should specify to the caterer standards of quality and suitability of provisions for use in the diet preparation area. Stocks of specific dietary products such as gluten-free and low-protein products should be available and those working in the area should be familiar with the use of these products.

Appropriate equipment for preparation of small quantities of food must be available for the diet cooks. Specifically, a sturdy industrial liquidiser, small pots and pans and accurate scales are all essential items. Freezer space is also required, as it is useful to keep frozen portions of special items (e.g. vegetable casserole for low-protein diets; low-protein bread; milk, egg, wheat and soya-free baked goods).

The dietitian should always provide the diet cooks with clear written and verbal instructions for each individual diet being prepared. The written information should include the patient's name, age and ward, the diet required and specific instructions regarding the composition of the diet and the portion size required.

A suitable plating system for diets must be used. The diet meals should be clearly labelled with the patient's name, ward and type of diet. Where a bulk catering system is operated food may be delivered to the ward in individual foil containers which must be clearly labelled with the type of diet the food item is suitable for.

Within the diet preparation area there should be a diet manual. This should include instructions regarding commonly requested modified diets and appropriate recipes. It is also useful to include details of any patients on particularly unusual diets if they are likely to be admitted. This manual should be regularly updated.

To ensure consistency and accuracy, the provision of modified diets should be monitored regularly. The following should all be considered: the quality, freshness and suitability of the provisions; the storage methods; the preparation of raw ingredients; and the presentation to the patient. Regular monitoring should ensure a high-quality product.

Immunosuppression and 'clean' meal provision

Children with a number of conditions (including acute megaloblastic leukaemia, stage IV neuroblastoma, relapsed acute lymphoblastic leukaemia and immunodeficiency syndromes) requiring a bone marrow transplant or autograft, receive drug therapy that causes severe immunosuppression and neutropenia. They require protective isolation in the immediate post-transplant period. Food is a potential source of infection and generally procedures will be in place to limit the potential of food-borne infection [17]. In immunosuppressed patients even normally non-pathogenic organisms may cause problems. Particular attention should be paid to personal hygiene in the food handler, and to food purchase, storage and preparation.

There is limited evidence on the use and effectiveness of 'clean' diets. Practice is variable and in general there has been a move away from stringent sterile diets [18]. Three levels of 'clean' diet are generally recognised: sterile diet, clean diet and common sense food hygiene guidelines.

Sterile meals

In some units, food production may be a sterile or near-sterile method incorporating the use of gamma-irradiated and canned foods prepared in a filtered laminar airflow system. Such a system requires specialised facilities and equipment and is labour-intensive and costly. Irradiation adversely affects food flavour and texture and consequently patient acceptability of food [19].

'Clean' diet

A practical and acceptable alternative to sterile meals is the use of a reduced bacterial diet or 'very clean food regimen'. Such regimens avoid the use of raw foods, reheated dishes and foods known to contain high levels of pathogenic and non-pathogenic bacteria, such as soft cheese, chicken and pâté. Details of foods allowed and forbidden are given in Table 2.2. Practice between centres can vary; for example, some allow all meat and poultry providing it is well cooked and served immediately.

Other centres follow common sense food hygiene guidelines and avoid high risk foods only (Table 2.3).

Purchasing

1   Many chilled and frozen foods contain unacceptably high levels of microorganisms for the immunosuppressed patient. Before allowing them to be included, a sample of the product should be tested. Canned and sterilised products are generally suitable.
2   The 'Best Before' date should be checked on manufactured foods.
3   Individual portions of foods (e.g. jams, butter/margarine, breakfast cereals, juices, sugar) should be purchased where these are available.
4   Foods should be purchased as fresh as possible and cooked shortly after purchase.

Storage

1   Temperatures of refrigerators and freezers must be checked regularly.
2   Food for 'clean' meals should be stored in a separate refrigerator; where this is not practical the top shelf should be used.
3   Food that is to be eaten cold must be transferred to the refrigerator as quickly as possible; all foods stored in the refrigerator should be covered or wrapped. Leftover food should be disposed of quickly; leftovers and reheated foods should not be used.

Preparation

1   Hands must be washed thoroughly with soap and water and dried with a hand dryer or a clean paper towel before handling food.
2   In the hospital setting, the food handler should wear a fresh plastic apron over the usual kitchen dress.
3   Clean utensils, containers and chopping boards must have been through a disinfecting dishwasher before use.
4   In a hospital kitchen, work surfaces should be wiped with a suitable disinfectant solution before 'clean' meals are prepared. This precaution should be unnecessary at home.
5   Wooden utensils (e.g. chopping boards) must not be used.
6   A fresh packet or tin should be used for each meal to avoid re-opening containers. Large packets (e.g. a loaf of bread, a pint of milk) can be divided into convenient size portions and individually wrapped at the beginning of each day.
7   Before opening packages such as tins, the top should be wiped with a clean cloth or paper towel.
8   Tin openers should be washed daily, preferably in a disinfecting dishwasher.
9   Cooking methods employed should ensure a minimum core temperature of 70°C, and this temperature should be maintained until the food is eaten.
10   There should be minimum delay between food being cooked and consumed.

The 'clean' diet should be fully explained to the patient and carers prior to transplant as it should be

Table 2.2   Foods for a 'clean' diet.

Food	Allowed	Not allowed
Water	Sterile water Boiled tap water	Mineral water Unboiled water
Drinks	Fruit juice and soft drinks – individual cartons or cans Ice cubes and ice lollies – made with sterile water High energy packaged drinks (e.g. Polycal Liquid) Tea, coffee, cocoa etc. – individual sachets	Squashes unless prepacked and pasteurised
Milk and dairy products	Milk – UHT, pasteurised, condensed or sterilised in individual portions Cheeses – individually vacuum wrapped portions; cheese spread portions; processed cheese Yoghurt – pasteurised Butter/margarine – individual portions Cream – UHT or sterilised Ice cream – individually wrapped portions	Unpasteurised milk Soft cheeses Unwrapped hard cheese Blue cheeses Unpasteurised or 'live' yoghurt Fresh cream
Cereals	Breakfast cereals – individual packets Bread from newly opened loaf Biscuits and cakes – individual portions Rice – well cooked Pasta – tinned or dried	Cereals with added milk powder; sugar coated cereals Unwrapped bread Cream cakes Slow-cooked rice (e.g. rice pudding) Fresh pasta
Meat and poultry	Pork, lamb, beef, veal – fresh or frozen, well cooked Tinned meats; chicken, sausages, ham, corned beef Meat paste in individual jars	Chicken, turkey – fresh or frozen Sausages Pies (unless home made) Take away meals (e.g. hamburgers) Salami Liver pâté, liver sausage
Fish	Freshly-cooked fresh or frozen fish Tinned fish Fish fingers, fish paste	Shellfish
Eggs	Hard boiled egg Fried egg	Raw egg, soft-cooked egg
Vegetables	Fresh leafy vegetables – well washed and cooked Root vegetables, washed, peeled and cooked Jacket potato; oven chips Beans and lentils – well cooked or tinned Tomato and cucumber – raw, peeled Tinned and frozen vegetables	Salad vegetables which cannot be peeled (e.g. lettuce, radish) Raw root vegetables
Fruit	Fresh fruit that can be peeled Tinned fruit	Unpeeled fruit Dried fruit
Snacks and soups	Crisps, sweets etc. – individual packets Tinned soups, packet soups – made with boiled water	Unwrapped sweets
Miscellaneous	Cooking oils Puddings, pies, custards – freshly made Jelly – made with sterile/boiled water Salt, salad cream, sauces – individual portions Pepper – gamma-irradiated	Instant puddings made with cold water Herbs and spices

Table 2.3   High risk foods.

Mineral water
Raw eggs and cooked egg dishes
Soft and blue-veined cheeses
Pâté
Live and bio yoghurts
Take-away foods
Reheated chilled meals
Ready-to-eat poultry
Shellfish
Soft whip ice cream
Nuts and dried fruit

commenced as soon as the patient is able to take anything orally. Prior discussion also allows time to obtain supplies of favourite or unusual foods and to liaise with the catering department regarding provision of supplies.

At discharge, neutrophil counts may still be below normal so care to avoid food-borne infection is required. Food hygiene advice and avoidance of high risk foods (Table 2.3) are required. Comprehensive food safety advice is available from the Food Standards Agency [20].

References

1   Moy RJD, Smallman S, Booth IW Malnutrition in a UK children's hospital. *J Hum Nutr Diet*, 1990, **3** 93–100.
2   Merritt RJ, Suskind RM Nutritional survey of the hospitalised paediatric patient. *Am J Clin Nutr*, 1979, **32** 1320–25.
3   Hendrickse WK, Reilly JJ, Weaver LT Malnutrition in a children's hospital. *Clin Nutr*, 1997, **16** 13–18.
4   Cameron JW, Rosenthal A, Olson AD Malnutrition in hospitalized children with congenital heart disease. *Arch Pediatr Adolesc Med*, 1995, **149** 1098–1102.
5   Department of Health. *Getting the Right Start. The National Service Framework for Children. Standards for Hospital Services*, 2003.
6   Council of Europe. *Food and Nutrition Care in Hospitals. How to Prevent Undernutrition*. www.coe.int Accessed 8 March 2006.
7   Food, Fluid and Nutritional Care in Hospitals. NHS Quality Improvement Scotland, 2003.
8   NHS Estates. Better Hospital Food Programme: Services for Children and Young Adults, 2003.
9   Food and Drug Administration. Health professionals' letter on *Enterobacter sakazakii* infections associated with use of powdered infant formulas. www.cfsan.fda.gov Accessed 8 March 2006.
10   The Food Safety Act. London: The Stationery Office, 1990.
11   Robbins ST, Becker LT *Infant Feedings: Guidelines for Preparation of Formula and Breastmilk in Healthcare Facilities*. American Dietetic Association, 2005. www.eatright.org Accessed 8 March 2006.
12   *Assured Safety Catering: A Management System for Hazard Analysis*. London: The Stationery Office, 1993.
13   Health Technical Memorandum 2030: *Washer-disinfectors*, NHS Estates. London: The Stationery Office, 1997.
14   Department of Health and Social Security Report on Health and Social Subjects No 22. *The Collection and Storage of Human Milk*. London: The Stationery Office, 1981.
15   Greenwood M, Rampling A *A guide to the Dairy Products (Hygiene) Regulations 1995 for Public Health microbiologists*. Public Health Laboratory Service Microbiology Digest, 1995, 12.
16   Department of Health Report on Health and Social Subjects No. 41. *Dietary Reference Values for Food. Energy and Nutrition for the United Kingdom*. London: The Stationery Office, 1991.
17   Dezenhall A *et al*. Food and nutrition services in bone marrow transplant centres. *J Am Diet Assoc*, 1987, **87** 1351–3.
18   Pattinson AJ Review of current practice in 'clean' diets in the UK. *J Hum Nutr Diet*, 1993, **6** 3–11.
19   Aker SN, Cheney CU The use of sterile and low microbial diets in ultra isolation environments. *J Parent Ent Nutr*, 1983, **7** 390.
20   www.food.gov.uk/safereating Accessed 8 March 2006.

Part 2

Nutrition Support and Intensive Care

3 Enteral Nutrition

Tracey Johnson

Enteral nutrition is the method of supplying nutrients to the gastrointestinal tract. Although enteral nutrition is the term often used to describe nasogastric, gastrostomy and jejunostomy feeding, it also includes food and drink taken orally.

Enteral feeding is the preferred method of providing nutritional support to children who have a functioning gastrointestinal tract, with parenteral nutrition (PN) reserved for children with severely compromised gut function. It is safer and easier to administer than PN both in hospital and at home and can be adapted to meet the individual requirements of infants and children of all ages.

Some children receive their full nutritional requirements via a nasogastric, gastrostomy or jejunostomy tube, whereas others require nutritional support to supplement poor oral intake or to meet increased nutritional requirements. Enteral feeding may be short term but for many children it can be a long term or even life-long method of feeding. As a result, regimens need to be adaptable to ensure each child receives the vital nutrients they require for normal growth and development.

Tube feeding of children requires the expert input of a paediatric dietitian who, along with a specialist multidisciplinary team, has the knowledge to use feeds and feeding equipment appropriate to the individual requirements and clinical condition of the patient. Indications for enteral feeding are given in Table 3.1.

Table 3.1 Indications for enteral feeding.

Indication	Example
Inability to suck or swallow	Neurological handicap and degenerative disorders Severe developmental delay Trauma Critically ill child requiring ventilation
Anorexia associated with chronic illness	Cystic fibrosis Malignancy Inflammatory bowel disease Liver disease Chronic renal failure Congenital heart disease Inherited metabolic disease
Increased requirements	Cystic fibrosis Congenital heart disease Malabsorption syndromes (e.g. short gut syndrome, liver disease)
Congenital anomalies	Tracheo-oesophageal fistula Oesophageal atresia Orofacial malformations
Primary disease management	Crohn's disease Severe gastro-oesophageal reflux Short bowel syndrome Glycogen storage disease Very long chain fatty acid disorders

Choice of feeds

The choice of feed is dependent on a number of factors:

- Age
- Gut function
- Dietary restrictions and specific nutrient requirements
- Route of administration
- Prescribability and cost

Infants under 12 months

Many infants requiring tube feeding may be given the same feed they would otherwise be taking orally. Children who are breast fed may be able to continue breast milk and there are physiological and psychological advantages to this. Mother's expressed breast milk (EBM) may be given to her own baby or pasteurised donor breast milk may be available. The principal benefits of using breast milk are the presence of immunoglobulins, antimicrobial factors and lipase activity. In addition, there is a psychological benefit to the mother if she is able to contribute to the care of her sick child by providing breast milk. These benefits may be outweighed by the possible poorer energy density of EBM, particularly if the fore milk is used which is lower in fat than the hind milk. If the infant fails to gain weight on breast milk alone, it can be supplemented with a commercial human milk fortifier (see p. 80 for the premature infant) or with standard infant formula powder (see p. 15 for the term infant).

Pasteurisation of a mother's EBM remains a controversial issue. Pasteurisation will destroy a percentage of the antimicrobial, hormonal and enzymic factors within the milk [1] but may protect against bacterial contamination. The vitamin content of breast milk can also be affected by pasteurisation [2]. Currently, there are no national guidelines and individual hospitals and units have developed their own local protocols. The cleanliness of the collection technique can be assessed by microbial analysis and a decision then made as to whether the milk can be used raw or whether it needs to be pasteurised.

Standard infant formulas are suitable for enteral feeding from birth to 12 months of age for those children with normal gut function and normal nutritional requirements. They provide an energy density of 65–70 kcal (270–290 kJ)/100 mL and meet the European Community Regulations for Infant Formulae [3]. Follow-on formulas may also be used after 6 months of age if their higher protein and iron content is thought to be more beneficial to the child. Many infants requiring enteral feeding will have increased nutritional requirements. Nutrient dense infant formulas such as Infatrini and SMA High Energy are commercially available and have been shown to promote better growth than standard formulas with added energy supplements (glucose polymer powders and fat emulsions) [4]. Concentrating standard infant formulas achieves a feed that is more nutrient dense and retains an appropriate protein : energy ratio similar to the commercial nutrient dense formulas (see p. 15).

Standard infant formulas are based on cow's milk protein, lactose and long chain fat. Infants with impaired gut function who do not tolerate whole protein feeds frequently benefit from the use of hydrolysed protein or amino acid based feeds. Such feeds are hypoallergenic and are free of cow's milk protein and lactose. Many of these formulas also have a proportion of the fat content as medium chain triglycerides (MCT) which can be beneficial where there is fat malabsorption, e.g. liver disease, short gut syndrome (see Table 7.7).

If the specific requirements of an infant cannot be met by a commercial infant formula, it is possible to formulate a feed from separate ingredients. These modular feeds allow a choice of protein, fat and carbohydrate and give the flexibility to meet the needs of individual patients. However, they are expensive and time consuming to prepare and there is a greater risk of bacterial contamination and mistakes during their preparation. It will take several days to establish a child on a full strength modular feed (see Table 7.25). Consequently, modular feeds should only be used if a ready-made feed is unsuitable and, in the hospital setting, should ideally be prepared in a dedicated special feed preparation area.

Children 1–12 years (8–45 kg body weight)

Specialist paediatric feeds are available for children 1–12 years of age or who weigh 8–45 kg.

Department of Health guidelines [5] indicate children have differing nutritional requirements according to their age and consequently specifically designed feeds for these age groups are recommended to ensure provision of appropriate levels of protein, micronutrients and electrolytes to optimise growth. Although nutritional profiles of paediatric feeds are designed to meet the specific requirements of children, it is still important to assess requirements and intakes for the individual.

Feeds are available for children within three age bands:

- 1–6 years
- 1–10 years
- 7–12 years

Feeds for younger children were originally based on guidelines published in 1988 [6]. All feeds are categorised as Dietary Foods for Special Medical Purposes and must comply with the 1999 EC Directive [7]. Standard paediatric feeds are based on cow's milk protein but are lactose free and provide three levels of energy density: 100 kcal (420 kJ)/ 100 mL, 120 kcal (510 kJ)/100 mL and 150 kcal (630 kJ)/100 mL. A lower energy feed, 75 kcal (315 kJ)/100 mL, is also available. Most product ranges are formulated either with or without added fibre.

Constipation is common in exclusively tube fed children, particularly those with neurological impairment [8]. A normal diet contains fibre and with an improved knowledge of the role of dietary fibre it is now common practice for children to receive a fibre-containing feed as the standard. Studies have shown the use of fibre-enriched feeds reduces the incidence of constipation and laxative use [9,10].

Children with neurological impairment form the largest single diagnostic group who have long term enteral feeding at home [11]. This group of children frequently have a low energy expenditure and if a standard feed is provided in adequate volumes to meet recommendations for protein and micronutrients, they may show excessive weight gain. Lower energy feeds with appropriate protein and micronutrient profiles are available to meet the specific requirements of this group of children (see p. 581).

The range of paediatric enteral feeds is outlined in Table 3.2.

For children with abnormal gut function, as with infants, hydrolysed protein feeds are also available (see Table 7.12). It is also sometimes necessary, as with infants, to use a modular feed (see Table 7.26).

Table 3.2 Paediatric enteral feeds.

	Age (Weight)	Energy kcal (kJ)/100 mL	Protein g/100 mL	Fibre g/100 mL
Nutrini (Nutricia)	1–6 years (8–20 kg)	100 (420)	2.7	–
Paediasure (Abbott)	1–10 years (8–30 kg)	101 (422)	2.9	–
Clinutren Junior Powder (Nestle)	1–6 years (8–20 kg)	100 (420)	2.97	–
		150 (630)	4.46	–
Frebini Original (Fresenius)	1–10 years (8–30 kg)	100 (420)	2.5	–
Nutrini Multifibre (Nutricia)	1–6 years (8–20 kg)	100 (420)	2.7	0.75
Paediasure Fibre (Abbott)	1–10 years (8–30 kg)	101 (422)	2.9	0.5
Frebini Original Fibre (Fresenius)	1–10 years (8–30 kg)	100 (420)	2.5	0.75
Isosource Junior (Novartis)	1–6 years (8–20 kg)	120 (510)	2.7	–
Nutrini Energy (Nutricia)	1–6 years (8–20 kg)	150 (630)	4.1	–
Paediasure Plus (Abbott)	1–10 years (8–30 kg)	151 (632)	4.2	–
Frebini Energy (Fresenius)	1–10 years (8–30 kg)	150 (630)	3.75	–
Nutrini Energy Multifibre (Nutricia)	1–6 years (8–20 kg)	150 (630)	4.1	0.75
Paediasure Plus Fibre (Abbott)	1–10 years (8–30 kg)	151 (632)	4.2	0.75
Frebini Energy Fibre (Fresenius)	1–10 years (8–30 kg)	150 (630)	3.75	1.1
Nutrini Low Energy Multifibre (Nutricia)	1–6 years (8–20 kg)	75 (315)	2.05	0.75
Tentrini (Nutricia)	7–12 years (21–45 kg)	100 (420)	3.3	–
Tentrini Multifibre (Nutricia)	7–12 years (21–45 kg)	100 (420)	3.3	1.1
Tentrini Energy (Nutricia)	7–12 years (21–45 kg)	150 (630)	4.9	–
Tentrini Energy Multifibre (Nutricia)	7–12 years (21–45 kg)	150 (630)	4.9	1.1

Children over 12 years (>45 kg body weight)

The requirements of children over 12 years of age may still be met by a paediatric feed designed for 7–12-year-olds; individual assessment is necessary. Standard adult feeds may also be used and are available with energy densities of 1 kcal (4 kJ)/mL and 1.5 kcal (6 kJ)/mL, with and without fibre. Some adult feeds have a protein content of 6 g/100 mL or more, so care should be taken when using such feeds for children, even if they are over 12 years of age, as they may provide excessively high amounts of protein. Intakes of copper, chromium, molybdenum and vitamins E, C, B_6 and B_{12} will also be high. Adult peptide based and elemental feeds can be used for children with impaired gut function and it is also necessary in special circumstances to employ the flexibility of a modular feed.

The choice of feeds suitable for children is given in Table 3.3.

Feed thickeners

Feed thickeners can be a useful dietary intervention for children with gastro-oesophageal reflux. In

Table 3.3 Choice of feeds for enteral feeding.

	Normal gut function	Impaired gut function
Infants	*Normal energy requirements* Breast milk or standard infant formula *High energy requirements* Breast milk + BMF/standard infant formula Concentrated infant formula Nutrient dense infant formula (e.g. Infatrini, SMA High Energy)	Hydrolysed protein formula, e.g. Pepti-Junior (Cow & Gate), Nutramigen 1, 2 (Mead Johnson) Amino acid infant formula, e.g. Neocate (SHS) Modular feed
1–6 years (8–20 kg)	*Normal energy requirements* Standard paediatric enteral feed e.g. Nutrini (Nutricia), Paediasure (Abbott) +/– fibre *High energy requirements* High energy paediatric enteral feed e.g. Nutrini Energy (Nutricia), Paediasure Plus (Abbott) +/– fibre *Low energy requirements* Low energy paediatric feed e.g. Nutrini Low Energy Multifibre (Nutricia)	Hydrolysed protein formula, e.g. Pepdite 1⁺ (SHS), Peptamen Junior (Nestlé) Amino acid formula, e.g. Neocate Advance (SHS) Modular feed
6–12 years (20–45 kg)	*Normal energy requirements* Standard paediatric enteral feed e.g. Tentrini (Nutricia), Paediasure (Abbott) +/– fibre *High energy requirements* High energy paediatric enteral feed e.g. Tentrini Energy (Nutricia) , Paediasure Plus (Abbott)	Hydrolysed protein formula, e.g. Pepdite 1⁺ (SHS), Peptamen (Nestlé) Amino acid formula, e.g. E028/E028 Extra (SHS) Modular feed
12 years + (>45 kg)	*Normal energy requirements** Standard adult enteral feed +/– fibre e.g. Nutrison Standard (Nutricia), Osmolite (Abbott) *High energy requirements** High energy adult enteral feed +/– fibre Nutrison Energy (Nutricia), Ensure Plus (Abbott)	Hydrolysed protein feed, e.g. Peptamen (Nestlé), Nutrison Pepti (Nutricia) Amino acid feed, e.g. E028/E028 Extra (SHS) Modular feed

BMF, breast milk fortifier.
* Paediatric feed designed for 6–12-year-olds may be suitable.

addition to anti-reflux medication, feed thickeners can help to reduce vomiting and minimise the risk of aspiration. Feed thickeners can also be added to enteral feeds that would otherwise separate out when left to stand (e.g. modular feeds).

There is a wide range of commercial products that are suitable for thickening enteral feeds (see Table 7.27). Thickened feeds may be difficult to give as a bolus via a fine bore nasogastric tube, so syringe feeding or pump feeding may be necessary. It is also important to consider the energy contribution of some of the thickening agents. The thickeners based on modified starch given at a concentration of 3 g/100 mL may result in an increased energy content of more than 10%.

Routes of administration

Nasogastric feeding

Nasogastric is the most common route for enteral feeding and, unless prolonged enteral nutrition is anticipated, it would usually be the route of choice. Passing a nasogastric tube can be distressing for both parents and children and careful preparation is beneficial [12]. Frank discussions and a clear explanation of the procedure can help older children, and play therapy with the use of dolls, mannequins [13] and picture books has been shown to alleviate anxieties in the younger age group. Older children, particularly teenagers, are naturally sensitive about their body image and they may be reluctant to start nasogastric feeding. Some children successfully pass their own nasogastric tube at night and remove their tube in the daytime, which can be a successful way of administering supplementary feeds without the embarrassment of a permanent nasogastric tube *in situ*.

Nasogastric feeding is a lifeline for many children, but it is not without its complications. Some of the more serious complications are related to dislodgement, poor placement and migration of tubes. Following a number of deaths, the National Patient Safety Agency published a report suggesting conventional methods to check tube placement were inaccurate. The common method to aspirate the tube and test with blue litmus paper is not sensitive enough to distinguish between gastric and bronchial secretions; auscultation of air or observation of gastric contents is also considered ineffective. Radiology and testing of gastric aspirate with pH paper are the only acceptable methods of confiming nasogastric tube position [14].

Long term nasogastric feeding in some children can cause inflammation and irritation to the skin where the nasogastric tube is secured to the face. Use of DuoDerm or Granuflex (ConvaTec, Ickenham, Middx) placed onto the skin can improve this. Another common problem, particularly with fine bore tubes, is tube blockage. Regular flushing of tubes can help to prevent this problem and the use of carbonated liquids can clear and prevent the build-up of feed within the lumen of the tube.

Gastrostomy feeding

Gastrostomy is a widely used route of feeding when longer term enteral nutrition is indicated [15]. Gastrostomy feeding is generally well accepted in children as it is more comfortable, obviates the need for frequent tube changes and is cosmetically more acceptable. Indications are not solely for long term feeding; in certain situations gastrostomy feeding is the route of choice. This includes children with congenital abnormalities such as tracheo-oesophageal fistula and oesophageal atresia and children with oesophageal injuries (e.g. following the ingestion of caustic chemicals). It has been suggested that a contraindication for gastrostomy is severe gastro-oesophageal reflux. This can be exacerbated with the introduction of a gastrostomy tube [16] and gastrostomy placement in such children is generally performed in combination with a fundoplication (p. 129).

The most popular technique for placing a gastrostomy tube is the percutaneous endoscopic gastrostomy (PEG) method [17]. This does not require open surgery and is therefore completed with a shorter anaesthetic time, making it a quicker technique with fewer complications than a surgically placed gastrostomy tube. After about 3 months, once the tract is formed, a child can be fitted with a gastrostomy button that sits almost flush against the skin. This is far more discreet than the tubing associated with a conventional gastrostomy catheter and is a popular choice, particularly with teenagers.

Gastrostomy tubes and buttons require less frequent changes than nasogastric tubes. A device secured by a deflatable balloon is easier to change than one secured by an internal bumper bar or disc. If a tube is inadvertently removed it should be replaced within 6–8 hours or the tract will start to close.

The main complication of gastrostomy feeding is leakage from around the gastrostomy site. This can cause severe inflammation and skin irritation and patients and parents should be taught about skin care.

Feeding into the jejunum

Indications for feeding into the jejunum include:

- Congenital gastrointestinal anomalies
- Gastric dysmotility
- Severe vomiting resulting in failure to thrive
- Children at risk of aspiration

When children are fed directly into the jejunum, feed enters the intestine distal to the site of release of pancreatic enzymes and bile. Whole protein feeds may be well tolerated but if malabsorption occurs the use of a hydrolysed protein feed is recommended. Feeds delivered into the jejunum should always be given by continuous infusion. The stomach acts as a reservoir for food in the normally fed child, regulating the amount of food that is delivered into the small intestine. Feed given as a bolus into the small intestine can cause abdominal pain, diarrhoea and dumping syndrome, resulting from rapid delivery of a hyperosmolar feed into the jejunum.

Placement of a nasojejunal tube is difficult and maintaining the position of the tube causes numerous problems. The position of the tube can be checked using pH paper. The tube can spontaneously resite into the stomach or can be inadvertently pulled back, and weighted tubes do not seem to be of much value in preventing this occurrence [18]. For longer term feeding, a surgical jejunostomy tube or a gastrojejunal tube is usually a more successful route for nutritional support.

Complications can include bacterial overgrowth, malabsorption, bowel perforation and tube blockage. Like nasogastric and gastrostomy tubes, jejunostomy tubes need regular flushing to maintain patency and it is recommended that sterile water is always used.

The routes of enteral feeding are shown in Fig. 3.1. The advantages and disadvantages of the routes of feed administration are given in Table 3.4.

Orogastric feeding

This route is principally used for feeding neonates where nasal access is not feasible or where

Table 3.4 Advantages and disadvantages of various routes of feed administration.

Nasogastric feeds	Gastrostomy feeds	Jejunostomy feeds
Advantages		
No surgical procedure required	Percutaneous endoscopic gastrostomy tubes can be inserted with a short anaesthetic	No possibility of aspiration
Placement can be easily taught		No nightly insertion of tube
Non-invasive	No nightly insertion of tube	
Disadvantages		
Nausea	Nausea	Nausea
Dislodgement of the tubes with coughing	Vomiting associated with coughing and reflux	Tube blockage
Vomiting associated with coughing and reflux	Local infection	Feeling of satiety
Feeling of satiety	Leakage around the tube causing granuloma formation	Placed under general anaesthesia
Difficulty in inserting nasogastric tube	Possibility of aspiration	Increase risk of nutrient malabsorption
Irritation to the nose and throat	Tube blockage	Leakage around the tube causing granuloma formation
Possibility of aspiration	Local infection	
Visible	Tube dislodgement	

By kind permission of A. MacDonald.

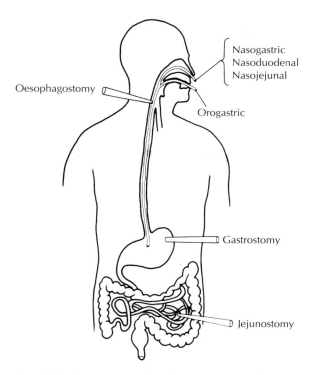

Figure 3.1 Routes of enteral feeding.

breathing would be compromised. The tube is passed via the mouth into the stomach. If all feeds are given via the orogastric tube it can be taped in place, but if the infant is taking some breast or bottle feeds the tube can be passed as required and removed between feeds.

Gastrostomy coupled with oesophagostomy

Following surgery in infants born with tracheo-oesophageal fistulas or oesophageal atresia, it is not always possible to join the upper and lower ends of the oesophagus in continuity. When the baby has grown, surgical reconnection will be considered at a later date. Until this time the child receives nutrition via a gastrostomy tube but is encouraged to feed orally to learn normal feeding skills. The food that is taken orally is collected at an oesophagostomy site and is commonly referred to as a 'sham feed' (see p. 127).

Continuous versus bolus feeding

Enteral feeds can be given continuously via an enteral feeding pump, or as boluses, or a combination of both. A regimen should be chosen to meet the individual requirements of the child and in most cases can be tailored to the most practical method of feeding to cause minimum disruption to the child's lifestyle and that of their family. Certain situations will dictate a preferred feeding regimen, but a flexible approach to feeding should be taken wherever possible. This enables the child to maintain their usual day-to-day activities and for the family to experience minimal disruption to their lifestyle and routines. Flexibility is especially important in children with a need for long term tube feeding who, as time passes, will need a feed that is appropriate to their age and changing nutritional requirements and a regimen that is adaptable as they grow and develop.

Continuous feeding

Generally, children will tolerate a slow, continuous infusion of feed better than bolus feeds and this method is sometimes chosen when enteral feeding is first started. Potentially, there are fewer problems with intolerance when small feed volumes are infused continuously and there is a smaller time commitment for ward staff and for parents and carers at home. Mobility is affected but is minimised by the use of portable feeding pumps, particularly for children who are on continuous feeding for longer than 12 hours. These portable pumps can be carried by older children as backpacks and for infants can be carried by their parents, carers or attached to a pram or pushchair. Children under 6 years are often too small to carry a heavy backpack, yet cannot be kept still for long periods of continuous feeding. In these children the extra hours of feeding can sometimes be achieved during daytime sleeps and when they are occupied with quieter tasks or watching television and DVDs.

There are situations where continuous feeding is essential. Feeds given through a nasojejunal tube or feeding jejunostomy should always be delivered by continuous infusion. Severe gastro-oesophageal reflux can be managed with a slow continuous infusion of feed as an adjunct to anti-reflux medication and positioning. Infants and children with malabsorption will also benefit from a continuous infusion of feed. This will slow transit time and may improve symptoms of diarrhoea, steatorrhoea and abdominal cramps and help to promote weight gain. In children with protracted diarrhoea and short bowel syndrome, continuous enteral feeding with a specialised formula often forms the basis of medical management; continuous tube feeding is also a well-established treatment option for children with Crohn's disease to induce remission of disease. Infants and children with glycogen storage disease type I require a frequent supply of dietary glucose to maintain their blood glucose levels within normal limits. A continuous overnight nasogastric infusion of glucose polymer solution or standard feed will maintain blood sugars when the child is asleep.

Intermittent bolus feeding

Bolus tube feeding is successfully used in many children requiring enteral feeding both in hospital and at home. Boluses given 3–4-hourly throughout the day via the nasogastric or gastrostomy tube mimics a physiologically normal feeding pattern and can be adapted to fit in with family mealtimes. It is more time consuming than continuous feeding but is the preferred method for many families with children requiring long term feeding as it gives them greater freedom and mobility.

There are situations in which bolus feeding is recommended. Neonates requiring small volumes may need to be given their feed by hourly bolus as the length of tubing between the reservoir and child creates a 'dead space' holding feed. This can be particularly relevant in infants fed EBM as some fat can be lost by adherence to the sides of the burette and tubing [19]. Children who have had a surgical anti-reflux procedure are unable to vomit. Large volumes of feed from a continuous infusion can accumulate in the stomach and remain undetected in children who have gastric stasis or poor gastrointestinal motility. This can lead to gastric rupture. Bolus feeding with a gravity feeding pack will prevent over-filling of the stomach as tubes are routinely aspirated before each feed and further feed will be prevented from entering the stomach from the feeding chamber if the stomach is already full.

Children who frequently try to remove their nasogastric tube risk aspiration if the end of the tube is dislodged into the airways. They will benefit from bolus feeding as they can be constantly supervised during the feed. Children with an oesophagostomy who are sham fed should preferably receive bolus feeds to coincide with their oral feeds. Finally, the continuous delivery of enteral feeds may interfere with the absorption of medication. Bolus feeding will provide periods of rest when medication can be given on an empty stomach to allow optimal absorption.

A schedule of feeding regimens is given in Table 3.5.

Enteral feeding equipment

Nasogastric feeding tubes

There is a wide range of paediatric feeding tubes available. The tubes are of varying lengths and gauges to meet the requirements of children of all ages. All tubes should conform to British Standards BS 6314 with a male Luer connection to avoid connection with intravenous lines and should be radio-opaque to help confirm position. For children, an ideal tube should be of a small gauge with a large internal diameter to make the tube more comfortable and cosmetically acceptable. All tubes will have a syringe adaptor to use for flushing, aspiration or administration of drugs. Some tubes may also have separate side ports.

Polyvinylchloride (PVC) tubes are used for short term enteral feeding. They are for single use only and require changing every week as the tubes stiffen over time and may cause tissue damage. These tubes are less likely to be displaced than a polyurethane tube so can also be used for children who are prone to vomiting.

Fine bore polyurethane or silicone tubes are designed for longer term nasogastric feeding and are very much softer and more comfortable than PVC tubes. Each tube comes with a guidewire or stylet to give the tube rigidity when passed. As a general guide tubes can usually remain *in situ* for 4–6 weeks but manufacturers' instructions regarding usage should always be followed. Unlike PVC tubes which are for single use and must not be repassed, these tubes can be removed during the

Table 3.5 Choosing a suitable feeding regimen.

Regimen	Example
Bolus top-up feeding	*Congenital heart disease* Bottle feeds are not completed due to breathlessness: the remaining feed is topped up via the nasogastric tube
Exclusive bolus feeding	*Long term feeding for children with a neurological handicap* Daytime bolus feeding can allow flexibility and mobility and provide a regimen that can fit in with family mealtimes *Post-fundoplication* Bolus feeding is usually the method of choice for children following a surgical anti-reflux procedure *Sham feeding* Children who are sham fed should receive a bolus feed to coincide with oral feeds
Combination of bolus and continuous feeding	*Chronic illness* Children with anorexia associated with chronic illness may receive a large proportion of their nutrition via a nasogastric or gastrostomy tube. Daytime boluses allow for a normal meal pattern and overnight feeding with a feeding pump reduces the time commitment at night for parents and ward staff
Overnight feeding only	*Supplementary nutrition* Children who require enteral feeding to supplement their poor oral intake or to meet their increased nutritional requirements are usually fed overnight only. This allows the children to maintain a normal daytime eating pattern while still providing the nutritional support they require
Continuous feeding only	*Primary disease management* Gastro-oesophageal reflux Malabsorption syndromes (e.g. short gut) Crohn's disease Glycogen storage disease

daytime and repassed at night if storage and cleaning instructions are carefully adhered to.

When passing polyurethane tubes there is a high risk of tracheal intubation in children who have an impaired swallow or who are ventilated. In these children PVC tubes may be preferable despite the need for longer term feeding.

Gastrostomy devices

Gastrostomy devices evolved considerably in the 1990s with an increasing amount of equipment entering the specialised paediatric market. Gastrostomy tubes, whether inserted by an open procedure or a percutaneous endoscopic method, are manufactured from pliable, biocompatible silicone. PEG tubes are held in place by a cross bar or bumper preventing inadvertent removal and require repeat endoscopy for change of tube or replacement with a gastrostomy button once the tract has formed. Surgically placed gastrostomy tubes are secured by an inflated balloon which allows easy replacement of the tube. They also have a skin level retention disc preventing migration of the tube. Foley catheters are not ideal but may be used as gastrostomy tubes. They require strapping securely in place, as they have no retention disc and may easily migrate into the duodenum. Children requiring long term gastrostomy feeding will usually elect to have a gastrostomy button once a tract has been established. These devices are secured within the stomach by an inflated balloon facilitating removal and replacement.

Enteral feeding pumps

Choice of feeding pumps will depend on the requirements of individual hospitals and individual children but there are a number of features that are either essential or desirable:

- Occlusion and low battery alarms
- Easy to operate
- Durable
- Tamper-proof
- Easy to clean
- Low noise
- Small and lightweight if designed to be portable
- Long battery life if designed to be portable
- Accurate flow rate setting (5–10%)
- Small flow rate increments (1 mL/hour preferable)
- Option of bolus feeding
- Good servicing back-up

Reservoirs

Many standard paediatric feeds are now available in pre-filled containers which can be connected directly to the giving set. This reduces the need for decanting and the risk of bacterial contamination.

If it is necessary to decant a feed into a reservoir there are many different flexible and rigid containers on the market for this purpose. Generally, children require smaller reservoirs than adults, especially when using a portable system. Infants requiring small volumes of feed may have their feed decanted into a burette, which has a small capacity and is principally for hospital use.

Studies have shown that feed contamination is common [20,21] so feed should always be decanted in a clean environment. Whatever choice is made, the reservoir and giving set should be changed every 24 hours and discarded. Any practice of sterilisation and re-use potentially leads to infection and is not recommended.

The length of time a feed can safely be left 'hanging' varies. Sterile ready-to-use feeds may be hung and delivered over a period of up to 24 hours. Local policy will vary but hanging time for reconstituted feeds is much shorter and generally no longer than 4 hours in the hospital setting.

Home enteral feeding

When a decision is made to commence enteral feeding at home it is important that the parents undergo a training programme that will teach them to look after all aspects of feeding and equipment safely. Correct procedures and adherence to safety are paramount and all parents and carers will require help and supervision to become familiar with the techniques involved prior to hospital discharge [22]. Pictorial teaching aids may be used to help families for whom English is not their first language and those unable to read and follow written guidelines [23]. It is essential to identify and liaise with community teams who will be sharing care when a child is discharged; they will have a key role in supporting the child and family. While it is essential that the child receives adequate nutrition, the enteral feeding regimen should be planned to fit in as much as possible with the family's lifestyle.

Home enteral feeding companies can supply both feeds and feeding equipment directly to the home. With more companies providing a home delivery service, the market has become competitive and hospital and community trusts are benefiting from improved deals. The companies may insist on the use of their own brand of pumps and feeds so it is important to ensure the child gets a suitable infusion pump and the feed that has been prescribed.

The National Institute for Health and Clinical Excellence (NICE) gives recommendations for infection control during enteral feeding in the community [24]. These include guidelines for education of patients, their carers and health care personnel; preparation, storage and administration of feeds; and care of feeding devices. They recommend that prepackaged ready-to-use feeds should be used in preference to feeds requiring decanting, reconstitution or dilution, and that reconstituted feeds when used should be administered over a maximum 4-hour period. They acknowledge that the recommendations need to be adapted and incorporated into local practice guidelines.

The social and emotional aspects of tube feeding are often overlooked. Studies have shown that families experience frequent problems with enteral feeding at home related to sleep disturbance, tube dislodgement, tube blockage and difficulties with home delivery of feed and equipment [25,26]. Dietitians and community nurses need to explore solutions to the common problems associated with overnight feeding. Regular review is necessary in long term patients to continue to identify and minimise problems.

Table 3.6   Feed intolerance.

Symptom	Cause	Solution
Diarrhoea	Unsuitable choice of feed in children with impaired gut function	Change to hydrolysed formula or modular feed
	Fast infusion rate	Slow infusion rate and increase as tolerated to provide required nutritional intake
	Intolerance of bolus feeds	Frequent, smaller feeds or change feeding regimen to continuous infusion
	High feed osmolality	Build up strength of feeds and deliver by continuous infusion
	Contamination of feed	Use sterile commercially produced feeds wherever possible and prepare other feeds in clean environments
	Drugs (e.g. antibiotics, laxatives)	Consider drugs as a cause of diarrhoea before feed is stopped or reduced
Nausea and vomiting	Fast infusion rate	Slowly increase rate of feed infusion or give over a longer period of time
	Slow gastric emptying	Correct positioning and prokinetic drugs
	Psychological factors	Address behavioural feeding issues
	Constipation	Maintain regular bowel motions with adequate fluid intakes, fibre containing feeds and laxatives
	Medicines given at the same time as feeds	Allow time between giving medicines and giving feeds or stop continuous feed for a short time when medicines are given
Regurgitation and aspiration	Gastro-oesophageal reflux	Correct positioning, anti-reflux drugs, feed thickener, fundoplication
	Dislodged tubes	Secure tube adequately and test position of tube regularly
	Fast infusion rate	Slow infusion rate
	Intolerance of bolus feeds	Smaller, more frequent feeds or continuous infusion

Enteral feeds are prescribed by the general practitioner although the costs for disposable equipment may be funded by a number of different agencies. These include hospital, community and dietetic budgets.

Feed administration and tolerance

The way in which a feed is administered ultimately depends on the clinical condition of the individual child so there are no set rules for starting enteral feeds. Neonates may need to be started on just 1 mL/hour infusion rates whereas older children may tolerate rates of 100 mL/hour. In most cases feeds can be started at full strength with the volume being gradually increased in stages either at an increased infusion rate or as a larger bolus.

Gastrointestinal symptoms are the most common complications of enteral feeding but with the wide choice of feeds, administration techniques and enteral feeding devices it should be possible to minimise gastrointestinal symptoms.

Some causes of feed intolerance and their resolution are given in Table 3.6.

Monitoring children on enteral feeds

Children who are commenced on enteral feeds require monitoring and review. There are presently no standards for the monitoring of children on long term enteral feeding at home in the UK.

At the initiation of enteral feeding, goals must be set with respect to the aim of the nutritional intervention (e.g. an improvement in nutritional status, control of symptoms, palliative care), and the expected growth of the child, taking into account their underlying clinical disorder. Regular follow-up is required to monitor both short term and longer term progress. Anthropometry, blood monitoring and control of any symptoms should be included in the monitoring procedure. As children gain weight and get older, their requirements change and follow-up is essential to ensure they continue to receive adequate nutrition. Although enteral feeds are formulated to be nutritionally complete it is wise to check nutritional status with blood tests, particularly if tube feeding is the sole source of nutrition [27]. Routine checks of albumin, electrolytes and haemoglobin are useful as well as assessment of micronutrient status. Blood tests can also be helpful in assessing response to nutritional therapy; for example, monitoring of inflammatory markers as well as assessment of symptoms can measure the success of feeding in children with active Crohn's disease. Both hospital and community staff have a part to play in monitoring the child's progress and helping the family cope with tube feeding at home. The needs of a young infant are quite different from those of a toddler or teenager and the individual needs of each child should be considered at different stages of their development.

Regular follow-up is also important for the family as well as the child. Home enteral feeding has a big impact on family life, resulting in both psychological and practical problems which should be addressed regularly. Good communication between the family, hospital and community teams is essential and the family must be given a contact for professional help in the case of any emergency.

Another important aspect of follow-up is the encouragement to maintain oral feeding skills. Children who miss out on early experiences of taste and texture are much more likely to develop feeding problems [28]. Offering a small amount of food gives children the chance to use the lips and tongue and develop their oral motor skills while experiencing a range of tastes. This is particularly important around the time of weaning when children are often more willing to accept different foods. Studies have also shown that in long term tube fed children even tactile stimulation of the face and mouth alone can help re-establish oral feeding [29].

References

1 Balmer SE *et al. Guidelines for the collection, storage and handling of mother's breast milk to be fed to her own baby on a neonatal unit.* London: British Association of Perinatal Medicine, 1997.

2 Van Zoeren-Grobben D, Shrijver J, Van den Berg *et al.* Human milk vitamin content after pasteurisation, storage, or tube feeding. *Arch Dis Child,* 1987, **62** 161–5.

3 *Infant Formula and Follow-on Regulations.* Statutory Instrument No. 77. London: The Stationery Office, 1995.

4 Clarke SE, MacDonald A, Booth IW Impaired growth and nitrogen deficiency in infants receiving an energy supplemented standard infant formula. Proceedings of the Royal College of Paediatrics and Child Health Annual Spring Meeting 1998. Abstract G132, 2–75.

5 Department of Health Report on Health and Social Subjects No. 41. *Dietary Reference Values for Food Energy and Nutrients for the United Kingdom.* London: The Stationery Office, 1991.

6 Russell C *et al. Paediatric Enteral Feeding Solutions and Systems.* Report by the joint working party of the Paediatric Group and Parenteral and Enteral Nutrition Group of the British Dietetic Association. Birmingham: BDA, 1988.

7 Commission Directive 199/21/EC on Dietary Foods for Special Medical Purposes. Official Journal of the European Communities 17.4.1999.

8 Sullivan PB Gastrointestinal problems in the neurologically impaired child. *Baillieres Clin Gastroenterol,* 1997, **11** 529–46.

9 Trier E, Wells JCK, Thomas AG Effect of a multifibre supplemented paediatric feed on gastrointestinal function. *J Pediatr Gastroenterol Nutr,* 1999, **28** 595.

10 Daly A, Johnson T, MacDonald A Is fibre supplementation in paediatric sip feeds beneficial? *J Hum Nutr Diet,* 2004, **17** 365–70.

11 Provisional Executive Summary of British Artificial Nutrition Survey (BANS) Data, 2004. British Association for Parenteral and Enteral Nutrition. Published online www.bapen.org.uk

12 Holden CE, MacDonald A, Ward M *et al.* Psychological preparation for nasogastric feeding in children. *Br J Nurs,* 1997, **6** 376–85.

13 Sexton E, Holden CE The hungry mannequin. *Nurs Times,* 2000, **96** (17 Suppl) 8–9.

14 National Patient Safety Agency. Reducing the harm caused by misplaced nasogastric feeding tubes. Patient Safety Alert, 21 February 2005.

15 Payne-James J Enteral nutrition: tubes and techniques of delivery. In: Payne-James J, Grimble G, Silk D (eds) *Artificial Nutritional Support in Clinical Practice,* 2nd edn. Cambridge: Cambridge University Press, 2001, pp. 281–302.

16 Khattak IU, Kimber C, Kiely EM *et al.* Percutaneous endoscopic gastrostomy in paediatric practice: complications and outcome. *J Pediatr Surg,* 1998, **33** 67–72.

17 Caulfield MP Percutaneous endoscopic gastrostomy placement in children. *Gastrointest Endosc Clin N Am,* 1994, **4** 179–93.

18 Rees RGP, Payne-James JJ, King C *et al.* Spontaneous transpyloric passage and performance of fine bore

polyurethane feeding tubes. A controlled clinical trial. *J Parent Ent Nutr*, 1998, **12** 469–72.

19 Brook OG, Barley J Loss of energy during continuous infusions of breast milk. *Arch Dis Child*, 1978, **53** 344–5.

20 Patchell CJ Bacterial contamination of enteral feeds. *Arch Dis Child*, 1994, **170** 327–30.

21 McKinlay J, Wildgoose A, Wood W *et al*. The effect of system design on bacterial contamination of enteral tube feeds. *J Hosp Infect*, 2001, **47** 138–42.

22 Holden C, Johnson T, Caney D Nutritional Support for Children. In: Holden C, MacDonald A (eds). *The Community in Nutrition and Child Health*. London: Bailliere Tindall, 2000, pp. 177–222.

23 Sexton E, Paul L, Holden C A pictorial assisted teaching tool for families. *Pediatr Nurs*, 1996, **8** 24–6.

24 National Institute for Clinical Excellence. *Prevention of healthcare-associated infections in primary and community care*. Clinical Guideline 2 June 2003.

25 Evans S, MacDonald A, Holden C Home enteral feeding audit. *J Hum Nutr Diet*, 2004, **17** 537–42.

26 Evans S, MacDonald A, Holden C Home enteral feeding audit 1 year post-initiation. *J Hum Nutr Diet*, 2006, **19** 27–9.

27 Johnson T, Janes SJ, MacDonald A *et al*. An observational study to evaluate micronutrient status during enteral feeding. *Arch Dis Child*, 2002, **86** 411–15.

28 Mason S, Harris G, Blisset J Tube Feeding in Infancy: Implications for the Development of Normal Eating and Drinking Skills. *Dysphagia*, 2005, **20** 46–61.

29 Senez C, Guys JM, Mancini J *et al*. Weaning children from tube to oral feeding. *Childs Nerv Syst*, 1996, **12** 590–4.

Support group

Patients on Intravenous and Nasogastric Nutrition Therapy (PINNT) is a support group for patients receiving parenteral or enteral nutrition, with a sub-group HALF PINNT for children. The group promotes public awareness and encourages contact between patients receiving similar treatment. As well as providing general support, the group provides assistance with claiming benefits and can provide members with portable equipment for holidays.

Useful address

PINNT
PO Box 3126, Christchurch, Dorset, BH23 2XS.
www.pinnt.com

4 Parenteral Nutrition

Joanne Grogan

Introduction

Intravenous feeding was one of the major medical developments of the 20th century. Parenteral nutrition (PN) first became available for general use in the 1960s. Problems with infusion of high concentration carbohydrate solutions into peripheral veins meant that severe phlebitis limited the length of time PN could be used, because of lack of access. However, in 1968 Wilmore *et al.* [1] described the provision of intravenous nutrients to an infant via a central venous catheter. Since that time lipid solutions have been developed, improving energy density in iso-osmolar solutions. The 1970s saw the development of crystalline amino acid solutions, reducing the risk of anaphylaxis.

Parenteral nutrition is now an established therapy, to which many patients of all ages owe their lives. It has transformed the outcome for many conditions including feeding the preterm infant and for post-surgical neonates with short gut syndrome [2].

The composition of PN continues to be developed and refined. As with many life-saving procedures, PN is not without its risks and is associated with fatal complications (Table 4.1). PN should therefore not be used casually but in a disciplined and organised manner in carefully selected patients [3,4]. PN should be prescribed only where there are experienced clinicians, dietitians, pharmacists and nurses available to contribute to the provision and monitoring of PN therapy. Improvement in outcome of PN has been demonstrated where multidisciplinary nutrition teams are involved [5,6].

Nutrition support teams

Parenteral feeding requires considerable clinical, pharmaceutical and nursing skills, and the use of special laboratory facilities for the biochemical monitoring of small blood samples. Children who require PN should be cared for by staff who are experienced in the prescription, production and care of PN and its equipment.

A multidisciplinary nutrition team often facilitates this and many centres now follow this principle [4]. The team usually plans regimens and provides training in the care, prescription and monitoring of patients on PN.

The nutrition support team is usually monitored by a nutrition steering committee, which produces protocols and procedures and organises audit and reviews of the PN service. Core members of the multidisciplinary nutrition team vary from centre to centre. Good interdisciplinary communication is paramount if patient care is to be of the highest standard. Core members are usually as follow:

- *Consultant* – oversees patient care
- *Surgeon* – inserts feeding lines and advises regarding surgical management as required

- *Medical registrar* – advises on prescription of PN and many other aspects of care
- *PN pharmacist* – production of solutions, stability, checking of solutions
- *Intravenous therapy/PN nurse* – trains carers and staff, co-ordinates patient care
- *Biochemist* – advises on monitoring and interpretation of blood biochemistry
- *Dietitian* – in recent guidelines a specialist dietitian is cited as a key member of the nutrition support team [7]

The role of the dietitian is to ensure the child's nutritional requirements are met in order to maintain adequate growth and development. The dietitian sets targets for enteral and parenteral feeding and devises a feeding plan. The dietitian monitors that correct volumes of prescribed feeds/PN are received and uses centile charts to plot the child's height, weight and head circumference (up to 2 years of age). It is imperative that inadequate growth is recognised and discussed with the team at the earliest opportunity. The dietitian advises regarding suitable adjustments to feeding regimens to enhance intake and absorption and, if necessary, advises on changes to feeds in cases of malabsorption or feed intolerance. As part of the multidisciplinary team, the dietitian reviews the nutritional biochemistry and contributes to the discussion and decision making with regard to nutrient intakes and adjustments to the PN.

Nutrition teams usually review the child's progress at least weekly, with reviews by some individual members daily. In centres where nutrition teams have been established, reported benefits include a reduction in mechanical line problems, reduced sepsis, fewer metabolic complications, shorter courses of PN (as a result of faster transition to appropriate enteral formulas) and savings on the cost of providing PN [5,6].

Indications for parenteral nutrition in children

Intestinal failure

- Functional immaturity
- Surgical gastrointestinal abnormalities (e.g. gastroschisis, intestinal atresia)
- Short bowel syndrome

- Necrotising enterocolitis
- Protracted diarrhoea
- Malabsorption syndromes
- Inflammatory bowel disease
- Chronic pseudo-obstruction

Other common indications

- Crohn's disease
- Chemotherapy-related intestinal failure
- Pancreatitis

Patients requiring additional nutrition support

- Trauma, burns
- Renal failure
- Liver disease
- Malignant disease

This is not an exhaustive list. In children, PN is a hazardous and expensive form of nutritional support and is indicated only where enteral nutrition cannot prevent or reverse growth failure. PN is associated with many complications (Table 4.1) and for this reason it is widely accepted that enteral feeding should always be used when possible. If the gut works, it should be used, even if only minimal feeds are possible [8]. Absence of luminal nutrients has been associated with atrophic changes in the gut mucosa and it is well recognised that enteral feeding is the single most effective way of preventing many gut-related complications.

Nutritionally insignificant volumes of enteral nutrition have been found to have a trophic effect on the gut, encouraging intestinal adaptation, and have been linked to enhanced gut motility, decreased incidence of PN-induced cholestasis and bacterial translocation [9–11]. Unless contraindicated, breast milk (if available) is the feed of choice for infants. Short, frequent breast feeds or small boluses of as little as 1–2 mL/hour is beneficial. Choice of feed is dictated by the clinical condition of the child. Breast milk or standard infant formulas are indicated unless there is evidence of malabsorption and/or feed intolerance. Indicators of malabsorption include watery frequent stools which on analysis are positive for fat and reducing substances. It may be advantageous to deliver the feed

Table 4.1   Some complications of parenteral nutrition.

Gut related	Solution related	Line related
Villous atrophy	Over/under delivery of nutrients	Sepsis
Decreased digestive enzyme activity	Hyperglycaemia	Catheter occlusion
Cholestasis	Hyperlipidaemia	Accidental line removal
Bacterial overgrowth/bacterial translocation	Micronutrient toxicity	Site infection
Fluid/electrolyte imbalance	Toxic effects of non-nutrient components of solutions	
Metabolic bone disease	Growth failure	
	Refeeding syndrome	
	Cholestasis	
	Metabolic bone disease	

continuously via a feeding pump to aid absorption (most enteral feeding pumps will not deliver at a rate lower than 5 mL/hour). If malabsorption is present, hydrolysed protein feeds which are lactose free and have a proportion of medium chain fat are indicated (e.g. Pregestimil or Pepti-Junior).

The timing and duration of PN is dependent upon the child's nutritional reserves, expected duration of starvation and severity of illness. PN is normally built up over 2–4 days and therefore it is it is neither reasonable nor clinically indicated to prescribe PN for less than 5 days [12].

Considerations in paediatric parenteral nutrition

Growth

Malnutrition in children results in impaired growth and development. This is particularly true in infants because of already limited energy reserves. A preterm infant weighing 1 kg has only 1% body fat and may survive for only 4 days if starved [13].

Nutritional requirements vary considerably with age and size, with growth being fastest in infancy and puberty. The majority of brain growth occurs in the last trimester of pregnancy and the first 2 years of life. Special care should be taken to avoid malnutrition and biochemical abnormalities at this time (e.g. hypernatraemia or hyperaminoacidaemia) [14,15] as poor nutrition at critical periods not only results in slowing and stunting of growth, but may permanently affect neurological development.

Infants are at considerable risk and the commencement of PN in a small infant who cannot tolerate enteral feeds is a matter of urgency.

Adolescents are at significant risk of not achieving their growth potential if nutrient requirements are not met during this critical period.

Liver disease

The prevalence of PN-associated liver disease is much greater in children than in adults. It has been reported that up to 65% of infants on PN develop abnormal liver function tests within 2–3 weeks of starting PN [16]. PN-associated cholestasis is related to prematurity, immature enterohepatic circulation, underlying disease, number of infections, number of surgeries and number of blood transfusions [17,18].

PN solutions themselves may have a part to play in the development of liver disease. Lipid emulsions have been implicated [19] and over-feeding of glucose has been associated with hepatic steatosis [20] (p. 52).

The aetiology of PN-associated liver disease is multifactorial and can progress to cirrhosis and end-stage liver failure in some cases [20]. The early introduction of enteral feeding is the most important measure that can be taken to help reduce the risk of cholestasis. [3]. Enteral feeding is commonly withheld in preterm neonates in order to help prevent necrotising enterocolitis developing; however, a review failed to determine whether or not minimal enteral feeding was beneficial in this group [21].

Essential nutrients

Amino acid requirements differ in children compared with adults. In infancy, because of immature metabolic pathways, some non-essential amino acids become conditionally essential. Histidine is an essential amino acid in infancy in addition to the eight required by older children and adults and arginine, cysteine, glycine, proline, taurine and tyrosine may also be conditionally essential [7]. Because of low stores, essential fatty acid deficiency can occur within 72 hours of birth [22].

Fluid

Infants have immature organ systems and require high volumes of fluid in order to excrete electrolytes sufficiently. Young children are physiologically unable to concentrate urine as effectively as adults. Maximum urine concentrations are 550 mOsm/L in preterm infants and 700 mOsm/L in term infants compared with 1200 mOsm/L in adults [23]. Dehydration and metabolic acidosis can occur; care should always be taken that adequate fluid requirements are met (Table 4.2).

Oral hypersensitivity

This occurs when the oral route is not used for feeding for lengthy periods of time. Lack of stimulation together with unpleasant procedures and/or experiences around the mouth area such as intubations, suction, vomiting, choking may lead to long term feeding problems. Wherever possible use of dummies, sips, tastes should be employed to maintain oral function, especially in infancy.

Table 4.2 Summary of parenteral fluid and electrolyte requirements for children.

Age/weight	Fluid (mL/kg/day)	Na (mmol/kg/day)	K (mmol/kg/day)
<1500 g	140–180	2.0–3.0	1.0–2.0
>1500 g	140–160	3.0–5.0	1.0–3.0
Preterm–2 m	140–160	2.0–5.0	1.5–5.0
2 m–1 year	120–180	2.0–3.0	1.0–3.0
1–2 years	80–150	1.0–3.0	1.0–3.0
3–5 years	80–100	1.0–3.0	1.0–3.0
6–12 years	60–80	1.0–3.0	1.0–3.0
13–18 years	50–70	1.0–3.0	1.0–3.0

Source: After Koletzko *et al.* [7]

In cases of refusal to feed or distress during feeding time, involvement of a specialist speech therapist to advise regarding oral desensitisation is recommended.

Nutrient requirements and solutions

Nutrient intakes vary at different centres and tend to be based on clinical experience [4,12,24,25]. European guidelines have recently been published [7] based on current available evidence. The main recommendations for macronutrient intake are summarised in Table 4.3.

Daily fluid requirements and factors affecting fluid needs are described in detail elsewhere [7]. Table 4.2 summarises the recommendations. Age, size, fluid balance, the environment and clinical conditions are all factors affecting fluid

Table 4.3 Summary of recommended daily intakes of macronutrients from parenteral nutrition.

Energy		Amino acids		Lipid		CHO	
Age	kcal/kg	Age	g/kg	Age	g/kg	Weight (kg)	g/kg
Prem	110–120	Prem	1.5–4	Prem	3–4	Up to 3	Up to18
0–1 years	90–100	Term	1.5–3	Infants	3–4	3–10	16–18
1–7 years	75–90	2 m–3 years	1.0–2.5			10–15	12–14
7–12 years	60–75					15–20	10–12
						20–30	<12
12–18 years	30–60	3–18 years	1.0–2.0	Older children	2–3	>30	<10

Source: After Koletzko *et al.* [7]
CHO, carbohydrate; Prem, preterm.

requirements. Cardiac impairment, renal disease and respiratory insufficiency are examples of conditions that may limit available fluid volumes, whereas high fluid losses due to diarrhoea, high output fistula/stoma and fever may all increase fluid needs. Additional fluid may be needed if radiant heaters or phototherapy is used.

When ordering PN, the available fluid allowance should be considered initially. It should be noted that some of this fluid allowance may be taken up by medications. The available fluid volume for PN may influence the choice of nutrient solutions and the route of delivery. If concentrated PN solutions are needed to provide adequate nutrition (due to fluid restrictions), then the peripheral route may be contraindicated, as there is a risk that concentrated solutions will cause thrombophlebitis. Children who are severely fluid restricted will only receive adequate nutrition if the concentrated PN is delivered via a central venous catheter (p. 54).

Fluid and electrolytes

Electrolyte requirements vary with age, clinical condition and blood biochemistry. Electrolyte solutions are usually added to the PN in response to each individual child's blood biochemistry.

Due to very tight homoeostatic mechanisms, sodium depletion is not always reflected in blood biochemistry. Monitoring of urinary sodium excretion to assess total body sodium is useful especially in cases of high sodium losses such as high output fistula or cystic fibrosis. A low urinary sodium excretion will indicate the need for increased enteral/parenteral sodium provision.

Macronutrients

Energy

Many well infants and children will achieve their expected growth rate if the energy intakes shown in Table 4.3 are provided. In illness these requirements will vary. An appropriate gain in weight for the age, sex and size of the individual child, taking the clinical condition into consideration, is likely to indicate that the prescription is adequate. All children on PN should be weighed and measured regularly and these measurements recorded and

plotted on growth charts to ensure appropriate growth is maintained. Research suggests that actual energy requirements for many children are less than originally thought [26]. It is recommended that energy intakes should be adapted for disease states that have been found to increase resting energy expenditure (REE) (e.g. head injury, burn injury, pulmonary and cardiac disease) [7]. Uncomplicated surgery has been found not to significantly increase energy requirements [27,28]. In critically ill children, energy requirements vary from day to day [29]. The very sick child may not have significantly increased REE as the catabolic process inhibits growth [30]. Extremely low birthweight neonates requiring ventilation have been found to have significantly increased rates of energy expenditure [31]. Recommendations specifically relating to neonates can be found elsewhere [7,32].

Whatever estimate of energy requirement is used for an individual child, it is essential to monitor closely to ensure appropriate growth is achieved without adverse biochemical consequences.

Nitrogen

Crystaline L-amino acid solutions are used as the nitrogen source for PN. The amino acid composition of the products for adult and older children is based on high biological value protein. The products designed for use in infants, at the time of writing, are Vaminolact, which is based on breast milk amino acid profile, and Primene, which is based on the profile of cord blood. The ideal amino acid profile for PN solutions for infants and children is still unclear. A solution that contains insufficient quantities of essential amino acids will inhibit protein synthesis and may limit growth [33].

A solution that contains excessive amounts of an amino acid may result in hyperaminoacidaemia and metabolic complications, which can cause coma and brain injury. Plasma aminograms should be checked if insufficient or excess amino acids are administered. Estimates of protein requirements are often based on 10–20% of the total energy intake. Recent guidelines are based on amounts required to maintain nitrogen balance and growth [7]. Utilisation of nitrogen requires sufficient energy intake and 30–40 kcal (125–165 kJ)/g protein or 250 kcal (1.05 MJ)/g nitrogen is recommended [34].

Glutamine

A systematic review found there was no evidence for the routine supplementation of glutamine in preterm infants and there is no evidence for its routine use in paediatric PN [35].

Carnitine

Carnitine is a nitrogen-based compound and plays a part in the beta-oxidation of long chain fatty acids, which it transports across the mitochondrial membrane in the form of carnitine esters.

Carnitine is present in breast milk and formula feeds but current PN formulations do not contain it. Carnitine can usually be synthesised in the liver from lysine and methionine and the ability to synthesise it is age dependent [36]. Non-supplemented parenterally fed infants have very low tissue carnitine levels [37]. Relative carnitine deficiency may impair fatty acid oxidation. However, a recent review has failed to find evidence to support the routine supplementation of parenterally fed neonates with carnitine [38] and further studies in this group are required.

It is recommended that carnitine supplementation should be considered on an individual basis in infants on exclusive PN for more than 4 weeks [7].

Fat/lipid

Intravenous lipids provide essential fatty acids (EFA) and improve net nitrogen balance when compared with glucose alone as a source of non-protein energy [20].

Lipid preparations provide a concentrated source of energy in an isotonic solution: 2 kcal (8 kJ)/mL in a 20% lipid solution compared with 0.8 kcal (3 kJ)/mL in a 20% carbohydrate solution. If the fluid intake is not restricted, the use of a lipid emulsion via a peripheral vein will help to provide sufficient energy for growth, avoiding the complications associated with central venous access, and it may prolong the life of peripheral lines in infants [39].

Intravenous lipid particles in solution resemble endogenously produced chylomicrons in terms of size and are hydrolysed by lipoprotein lipase.

When the fluid volume is limited, maximum energy intake can only be achieved via a central venous catheter by using dextrose and fat mixtures.

Lipid emulsions normally contribute 25–40% of non-protein energy.

In the UK, a range of intravenous lipid emulsions are available that have undergone trials in paediatric patients. They contain soybean oil (e.g. Intralipid), coconut oil plus soy bean oil (Lipofundin MCT/LCT) and olive oil plus soy bean oil (ClinOleic). All solutions contain glycerol and phospholipids and are available as 10%, 20% and 30% emulsions.

Higher concentrations are advantageous where there is fluid restriction and they also deliver less phospholipid per gram of triglyceride, leading to more normal plasma phospholipid and cholesterol levels [40]. It is recommended that 20% or higher concentrations of lipid solutions are used because of the higher phospholipids : triglyceride ratio found in 10% emulsions [7].

Lipid emulsions currently used are either based on long chain triglycerides (LCT) or long chain and medium chain triglycerides (MCT) mixed together. MCT has the advantage of carnitine-independent uptake by the mitochondria, therefore they were thought to have a more rapid clearance from the plasma after infusion [41,42]. Both are considered safe to use in paediatric patients.

There are concerns over the effect of the highly polyunsaturated, unphysiological fatty acid supply from soybean oil. Soya oil/olive oil-based solutions may produce more physiological levels of linoleic and oleic acid and better antioxidant status [43]. However, there is currently not enough evidence to recommend one particular solution above another.

Structured lipids are new lipid emulsions manufactured from synthetically produced triglycerides. At the time of writing no trials have been completed in the paediatric population.

Serum lipid levels are monitored to ensure adequate clearance and hence utilisation. Clearance of lipids from the plasma is limited by the rate of activity of lipoprotein lipase. The amount of fat infused should be adapted to the lipid oxidation capacity, approximately 3–4 g/kg/day [3,7]. Hyperlipidaemia will result if the enzyme is saturated by excessive doses of fat or by rapid infusion [44]. Gradually increasing the volume of the lipid emulsion by 1 g/kg/day over 3–4 days and maintaining a steady rate of infusion helps prevent possible hypertriglyceridaemia. Tolerance of lipid emulsions has been found to be improved if given continuously in preterm infants [45], although it is usual practice to give 4 hours off the infusion per 24 hours to allow all administered fat to clear the circulation before the next infusion begins. Serum lipids should be monitored as the volume of fat increases and should always be taken 4 hours after the infusion is completed. Peak levels of triglyceride and free fatty acids normally occur towards the end of the infusion, returning to fasting levels 2–4 hours later. Once they are stable, weekly monitoring is likely to be sufficient.

In malnourished children, it is good practice to assess baseline serum lipids prior to starting PN as children who have failed to thrive or lost weight frequently have raised triglyceride levels that return to normal when sufficient energy is provided. Restricting lipid, and therefore energy, would not be beneficial in this case. A reduced lipid dose may be indicated for children with a marked risk of hyperlipadaemia (e.g. low birthweight infants, sepsis, catabolism) [7]. Essential fatty acid deficiency can be prevented with as little as 0.5–1.0 g/kg lipid/day [46], although suboptimal energy intake will be the limiting factor.

In some cases, medication may be given in fat emulsions (e.g. the sedative propofol or the antifungal amphotericin). Consideration should be made of the fat content of this.

Carbohydrate

The major source of non-protein calories in PN is D-glucose (dextrose). Carbohydrate normally provides 60–70% of the total non-protein energy intake. Glucose is an essential fuel for infants and is the most important substrate for brain cell metabolism; a continuous supply is essential for normal neurological function. Excessive intravenous glucose administration can lead to hyperglycaemia, hepatic steatosis, excessive carbon dioxide production, essential fatty acid deficiency (in the absence of lipid) and impaired protein metabolism [20]. Insulin resistance may occur in some situations (e.g. steroid use, very low birthweight, sepsis, trauma and stress). Glucose infusion rates may need to be reduced in order to prevent hyperglycaemia. In critically ill adults it is accepted practice to use insulin infusions to manage hyperglycaemia; in children this has not been sufficiently researched and should only be considered when reduction of glucose infusion has failed [7].

Glucose should be administered gradually, increasing over 3–4 days to maximum infusion rates. Rates of glucose oxidation vary significantly with age and clinical status. It is recommended in term neonates and children up to 2 years that glucose intake should not exceed 18 g/kg/day [7,47]. Infusion rates exceeding glucose oxidative capacity result in conversion of carbohydrate to fatty acids and can consume up to 15% of the available energy from carbohydrate [48].

Cyclical PN refers to the intermittent administration of intravenous fluids with a regular break in each 24-hour period. There may be advantages in terms of changes in insulin–glucagon balance and decreased lipogenesis, time off to allow for physical activity and reduction in the risk of development of liver disease [49]. If the infusion rate is increased it should be less than 1.2 g carbohydrate/kg/hour in order not to exceed the maximum glucose oxidation rate [7]. A stepwise increase and decrease of infusion at commencement and cessation of PN may also be considered to prevent hypo- or hyperglycaemia [7].

Micronutrients and minerals

A summary of reasonable intakes of micronutrients for paediatric PN can be found in Tables 4.4 and 4.5. These are a guide and should be used in conjunction with the document from which they are taken [7]. Requirements for intravenous vitamins in infants and children remain unclear. The last major publication on parenteral vitamin requirements in children was in 1988 [50]. A Cochrane review [51] in premature (<32 weeks' gestation) infants found an association between supply of vitamin A and a reduction in death or oxygen requirement at 1 month of age and of oxygen requirement at 38 weeks post menstrual age. Current knowledge is based on the historical use of available vitamin and mineral solutions and the apparent lack of deficiencies or complications associated with this. Optimal requirements in children have not been determined and there has been little published research on this topic in the last 20 years.

Following the guidelines currently in use appears to maintain blood levels within acceptable ranges for infants and children and is based on expert opinion [3,7,50]. The amount of intravenous vitamins given is usually recommended to be

Table 4.4 Ranges of reasonable intakes of vitamins.

Vitamin	Infants (per kg/day)	Children (dose/day)
A (µg)	150–300	150
D (µg)	0.8 (32 IU)	10 (400 IU)
E (mg)	2.8–3.5	7.0
K (µg)	10	200
C (mg)	15–25	80
Thiamine (mg)	0.35–0.5	1.2
Riboflavin (mg)	0.15–0.2	1.4
Pyridoxine(mg)	0.15–0.2	1.0
Niacin (mg)	4.0–6.8	17
B_{12} (µg)	0.3	1.0
Pantothenic acid (mg)	1.0–2.0	5.0
Biotin(µg)	5.0–8.0	20
Folic acid (µg)	56	140

Source: After Koletzko et al. [7]

NB No upper limits are given; care must be taken to avoid over delivery of individual nutrients. Where nutrient mixtures are used manufacturers' guidelines should be followed.

higher than that given enterally. This is to allow for losses of the vitamins by adsorption onto the PN bag and giving set or biodegradation re-

sulting from light exposure, thus reducing the available intake. Vitamin A is most affected by these problems [52]. Addition of the vitamins to the lipid bag and protecting lipids from direct sunlight is the best method of preserving the vitamin concentration. Artificial light has little effect on the stability of the vitamins [7]. There are few commercially available vitamin solutions for preterm infants and neonates. Daily administration is recommended with the exception of vitamin K which may be given weekly [7]. Thiamine requirements may be higher than previously recommended [53] and guidelines have therefore been increased [7].

Current commercially available paediatric mineral solutions do not contain iron. Intravenous iron supplementation is controversial because of the risk of adverse side effects [54]. Parenterally administered iron bypasses the normal homoeostatic mechanism of the intestine and excess iron may lead to iron overload syndrome. Iron enhances the risk of Gram-negative septicaemia [55] and also has powerful oxidative properties; it may therefore increase demand for antioxidants. Monitoring

Table 4.5 Recommended intakes of trace elements.

Trace element	Dose	Comment
Chromium	0.2 µg/kg/day (max 5µg/kg/day)	Present as a contaminant, therefore not usually added to PN
Copper	20 µg/kg/day	Requirements may increase with high gastrointestinal losses or thermal injuries. Toxicity risk in cholestasis
Iodine	1 µg/day	
Manganese	1 µg/kg/day (max 50 µg/day)	In toxicity CNS deposition of manganese can occur without symptoms. Monitor regularly
Molybdenum	LBW: 1 µg/kg/day Infant and child: 0.25 µg/kg/day (max 5 µg/day)	
Selenium	Preterm/LBW: 2–3 ng/kg/day Infant and child: 1–3 ng/kg/day	Optimal dose remains unclear
Zinc	Preterm: 450–500 µg/kg/day Infant <3 m: 250 µg/kg/day Infant >3 m: 100 µg/kg/day Child: 5 µg/kg/day (max 5 mg/day)	Preterm infants, and children with thermal injuries may have increased requirements
Iron	Preterm: Up to 200 µg/kg/day Infant and child: 50–100 µg/kg/day	Not necessary in short term PN (<3 weeks' duration) Monitor carefully to avoid toxicity (see text)

Source: After Koletzko et al. [7]

NB No upper limits are given; care must be taken to avoid over delivery of individual nutrients. Where nutrient mixtures are used manufacturers' guidelines should be followed.

CNS, central nervous system; LBW, low birthweight; PN, parenteral nutrition.

Table 4.6   Suggested intakes of parenteral calcium, phosphorus and magnesium.

Age	Ca mg (mmol)/kg	P mg (mmol)/kg	Mg mg (mmol)/kg
0–6 months	32 (0.8)	14 (0.5)	5.0 (0.2)
7–12 months	20 (0.5)	15 (0.5)	4.2 (0.2)
1–13 years	11 (0.2)	6 (0.2)	2.4 (0.1)
14–18 years	7 (0.2)	6 (0.2)	2.4 (0.1)

Source: After Koletzko *et al.* [7]
NB Where upper limits are not given care must be taken to avoid over delivery of individual nutrients. Where nutrient mixtures are used manufacturers' guidelines should be followed.

of serum ferritin and reduction or removal of iron supplementation, if levels become too high, is recommended [7]. Iron preparations may be added to the intravenous solution with care because of poor solubility and risk of anaphylaxis; additional iron is usually given by week three of receiving PN [7]. Top-up blood transfusions may be given when required, if oral or intravenous supplementation fails.

Calcium, phosphorus and magnesium are usually added as individual solutions and the suggested intakes are listed in Table 4.6.

Cholestatic patients with obstructive jaundice can accumulate copper and manganese (normally excreted in bile). Renal patients may not be able to excrete selenium, molybdenum, zinc and chromium [50,56]. High fluid losses result in greater losses of magnesium and zinc. Individual preparations of some trace elements are available where there is a particular need to exclude or increase doses of single trace elements. Iron deficiency may lead to increased blood manganese levels [57]. In the absence of iron, manganese binds to transferrin [58] and iron deficiency up-regulates both iron and manganese absorption from the intestine [57].

Administration of parenteral nutrition

A more detailed account of the techniques of PN administration is available in other publications [4,7]. PN may be infused via a peripheral vein, or via a central venous catheter. Each route has advantages and disadvantages [59].

Peripheral lines

A needle or short catheter is placed into a subcutaneous vein to gain peripheral access. Peripheral lines are rarely associated with septicaemia and are useful in short term PN (7–10 days' duration) where the fluid allowance is not restricted and concentration of PN solutions is <600 mOsm/L, and where venous access is good. They are often used in neonates. One major disadvantage is the risk of thrombophlebitis caused by the hypertonic solutions used. A maximum concentration of glucose used with these lines is 12%. Infiltration is also a common problem: the peripheral line may penetrate the surrounding tissues resulting in leaking of the infusion. This leakage is known as extravasation and if undetected can cause tissue necrosis and severe scarring. Drip sites must be inspected frequently to avoid this. Drips that fail must be resited quickly to avoid the risks of rebound hypoglycaemia and suboptimal nutritional intake.

Central venous catheters

A central venous catheter (CVC) (e.g. Broviac or Hickman catheter) is a catheter that is tunnelled beneath the skin and inserted into the superior or inferior vena cava or outside the right atrium via a subclavian vein.

Central venous catheters can be inserted either surgically or percutaneously. They are made of silicone which helps decrease sepsis rates and inhibits fibrin production and is therefore less likely to block. They have a Dacron cuff planted subcutaneously which serves to fix the line in place and also inhibits the migration of microorganisms from the skin.

A CVC can remain *in situ* for months. The major disadvantages of CVCs are the risks associated with insertion and catheter care. Complications include sepsis, occlusion, infection of the line site and accidental removal. Loss of venous access can be a life-limiting factor in PN-dependant children (e.g. those with intestinal failure). It is therefore imperative that these lines are cared for. The more frequently a line is accessed the greater the risk of infection. Only PN or fluid (not drugs) should be given via a single lumen catheter [4,59].

For blood samples, blood products or medication separate venous access should be organised. Multiple lumen catheters are usually inserted when frequent intravenous drug therapy is required as well as PN and where the child is critically unwell (e.g. bone marrow transplants or intensive care). The rate of infection of these catheters is higher compared with single lumen catheters [60] and this is probably a reflection of more frequent catheter manipulation.

Portacath

Portacath is a totally implantable device, which requires needle sticking for vascular access. It has limited value for PN but is useful for vascular access for frequent medications (e.g. prophylactic antibiotics in cystic fibrosis).

Delivery methods

Parenteral nutrition can be delivered by a variety of systems. Infants and children usually have a system in which amino acids and dextrose are mixed and delivered over 24 hours. The fat emulsion is delivered from a separate container but mixed with the amino acid and dextrose solution as close as possible to the peripheral or central line. All the components are compounded in a specialist pharmacy unit under aseptic conditions in an isolator. Computer based programs are available for use by specialist pharmacists to ensure that the nutrient content of the bag is appropriate for the child's age, condition and biochemistry. They also help to ensure that nutrient stability is assessed and drug–nutrient interactions avoided [61].

'All-in-one' mixes (containing amino acids, dextrose and lipids) are available. They are used more commonly in adults but products are now available that can be used in children who are relatively stable, e.g. OliClinomel. These products do not contain vitamins and if used long term will require the addition of vitamins. The stability of 'all-in-one' PN relies upon the stability of the nutrient solutions and the formulations cannot be varied greatly. They are not suitable for unstable patients or patients with unusually low or high requirements. As the mixing of the lipid and aqueous solutions shortens the 'shelf life' of PN, some solutions come in separate chambers which can be rolled together and mixed just before use, e.g. NuTRIflex. The composition of these bags must be scrutinised prior to consideration for use in paediatric patients.

PN is supplied from the manufacturing pharmacy in a pre-mixed collapsible bag with an opaque cover to protect nutrients in the solution from photodegradation. When low rates of infusion are prescribed and the solution remains in the burette for long periods, light protective sets may also be used although these have limited effectiveness and are most useful if solutions are exposed to direct sunlight [7]. Some of the solutions available for paediatric PN can be found in Tables 4.7–4.10. Manufacturers' guidelines advise on dosage and administration.

Equipment

A steady flow rate should be maintained when infusing PN. Hyperglycaemia and hyperlipidaemia will result if infusions are delivered too quickly. If the line blocks or the infusion stops suddenly, hypoglycaemia may occur [4]. Volumetric pumps are sufficiently accurate for use in children; these deliver measured volumes via a cassette with a syringe mechanism ensuring accuracy. Syringe

Table 4.7   Amino acid solutions.

Name	Manufacturer	Nitrogen (g/L)	Cysteine (g/L)	Tyrosine (g/L)	Taurine (g/L)	Comment
Primene (10%)	Baxter	15	1.89	0.45	0.6	
Vamin 9 Glucose	Fresenius Kabi	9.5	1.4	0.5	0	Glucose 100 g/L
Vaminolact	Fresenius Kabi	9.3	1.0	0.5	0.3	

Table 4.8   Lipid emulsions (20%).*

Name	Manufacturer	Composition	TG (g/L)	Soya oil (g/L)	Olive oil (g/L)	% MCT
Intralipid (20%)	Fresenius Kabi	Soya	200	200	0	0
ClinOleic (20%)	Baxter	80% Olive 20% Soya	200	40	160	0
Lipofundin MCT/LCT (20%)	B Braun	50% Soya 50% Coconut	200	100	0	50

LCT, long chain triglycerides; MCT, medium chain triglycerides; TG, triglycerides.
*10% Solutions are available but are not recommended due to the high phospholipid:TG ratio [7].

Table 4.9   Trace element solutions.

Trace element	Additrace (Fresenius Kabi) (μmol/10 mL)	Peditrace (Fresenius Kabi) (μg/1 mL)
Iron	20	0
Zinc	100	250
Copper	20	20
Manganese	5	1
Chromium	0.2	0
Selenium	0.4	2
Iodine	1	1
Fluoride	50	57
Molybdenum	0.2	0

Table 4.10   Vitamin solutions.

Vitamin	Solvito (Fresenius Kabi) per vial	Vitlipid Infant (Fresenius Kabi) per vial
A	0	2300 IU
D	0	400 IU
E	0	7.0 IU
K	0	200 μg
B_1	2.5 mg	0
B_2	3.6 mg	0
B_6	4.0 mg	0
B_{12}	5.0 μg	0
C	100 mg	0
Niacin	40 mg	0
Pantothenic acid	15 mg	0
Biotin	60 μg	0
Folic acid	0.4 mg	0

pumps are used instead of volumetric pumps when small volumes are required. These have a linear drive mechanism and can be set to deliver as little as 0.5 mL/hour. Filters are needed to remove any bacterial or fungal contamination and prevent air embolism and entry of particulate matter. It is considered good practice to filter all amino acid and dextrose solutions using a filter with a pore size of 0.22 μm, and 1.2 μm for 'all-in-one' bags and lipids.

Weaning off parenteral nutrition

Ideally, some degree of enteral nutrition will be maintained during the period on PN via the most appropriate route and type of feed. The concentration and rate of delivery of enteral feed will be gradually increased in line with tolerance and growth parameters. If fluid restriction is not a major issue, once enteral feeds or diet provide at least 25% of the total requirements a corresponding

reduction can be made to the PN solution. Once 50% of requirements are met enterally the PN can be decreased to 50%, with a further decrease to 25% once the enteral route meets 75% of requirements. When more than 75% of requirements are achieved by enteral nutrition the PN could be stopped in most cases [62]. These reductions are dependent upon satisfactory growth and development of the child. If the PN is provided as separate lipid and aqueous (carbohydrate and nitrogen) solutions it is important to decrease each solution proportionally in order to maintain an adequate energy : nitrogen ratio.

If fluid restriction is a complicating factor the PN will usually need to be decreased by each millilitre that the enteral nutrition is increased (although a greater fluid volume is usually tolerated via the enteral route than the parenteral route). Care and attention to actual intake must be employed in these cases to ensure maximum nutrition is achieved, as enteral feeds are often less concentrated than PN. This is especially important in infancy or for malnourished children.

References

1 Wilmore DM, Dudrick SJ Growth and development of an infant receiving all nutrients via vein. *J Am Med Assoc*, 1968, **203** 860–4.

2 Evans TJ, Cockburn F Parenteral feeding. In: McLaren DS, Burman D (eds) *Textbook of Paediatric Nutrition*, 2nd edn. Edinburgh: Churchill Livingstone, 1990, pp. 337–54.

3 Puntis JWL Update on intravenous feeding in children. Guidelines to regimes and techniques for TPN. *Br J Int Care*, 1993, **3** 299–305.

4 Milla PJ, Bethune K, Hill S *et al. Current perspectives on paediatric parenteral nutrition.* A report by the working party for the British Association for Parenteral and Enteral Nutrition, Maidenhead, Berks, 2000.

5 Jonkers CF, Prins F, Van Kempen A *et al.* Towards implementation of optimum nutrition and better clinical nutrition support. *Clin Nutr* 2001, **20** 361–6.

6 Puntis JWL Establishing a nutrition support team. *Baillieres Clin Paediatr*, 1997, **5** 189–99.

7 Koletzko B, Goulet O, Hunt J *et al.* Guidelines on paediatric parenteral nutrition of the European Society of Paediatric Gastroenterology, Hepatology and Nutrition (ESPGHAN) and the European Society for Clinical Nutrition and Metabolism (ESPEN), supported by the European Society of Paediatric Research (ESPR). *J Paediatr Gastroenterol Nutr*, 2005, **41** S1–4.

8 Williamson RC Intestinal adaptation (first of two parts) structural, functional and cytokinetic changes. *N Engl J Med*, 1978, **298** 1393–402.

9 McClure RJ, Newell SJ Randomised controlled trial of trophic feeding and gut motility. *Arch Dis Child, Fetal Neonatal Ed*, 1999, **80** F54–8.

10 Pierro A Cholestatic jaundice in newborn infants receiving parenteral nutrition. *Semin Neonatol*, 1996, **1** 231–9.

11 Andorskey DJ, Lund DP, Lillehei W *et al.* Nutritional and other post operative management of neonates with short bowel syndrome correlates with clinical outcomes. *J Pediatr*, 2001, **139** 27–33.

12 Ball PA, Booth IW, Holden CE *et al. Paediatric Parenteral Nutrition.* Milton Keynes: Pharmacia Ltd, 1998.

13 Heird WC, Driscoll JM, Schullinger JN *et al.* Intravenous alimentation in paediatric patients. *J Pediatr*, 1972, **80** 351–72.

14 Payne J, Grimble G, Silk D Metabolic complications of parenteral nutrition. In: Nordenstrom J (ed) *Artificial Nutrition Support in Clinical Practice*. London: Edward Arnold, 1995, pp. 343–58.

15 Wigglesworth JS Malnutrition and brain development. *Dev Med Child Neurol*, 1969, **11** 791–803.

16 Grant JP, Cox CE, Kleinman LM *et al.* Serum hepatic enzyme and bilirubin elevations during parenteral nutrition. *Surg Gynecol Obstet*, 1997, **145** 573–80.

17 Drongowski RA, Corain AG An analysis of factors contributing to the development of parenteral nutrition induced cholestasis. *J Parenter Enteral Nutr*, 1989, **13** 586–89.

18 Beath SV, Davies P, Papadopolou A *et al.* Parenteral nutrition related cholestasis in post surgical neonates: multivariate analysis of risk factors. *J Pediatr Surg*, 1996, **31** 604–6.

19 Colomb V Role of lipid emulsions in cholestasis associated with long term parenteral nutrition in children. *J Parenter Enteral Nutr*, 2000, **24** 345–50.

20 Bresson JL, Narcy P, Putet G *et al.* Energy substrate utilisation in infants receiving total parenteral nutrition with different glucose fat ratios. *Pediatr Res*, 1989, **25** 645.

21 Tyson JE, Kennedy KA Trophic feedings for parenterally fed infants. *Cochrane Database Syst Rev*, 1997, **4** Art No. CD000504.

22 Friedman Z, Danon A, Stahlman MT *et al.* Rapid onset of essential fatty acid deficiency in the newborn. *Pediatrics*, 1976, **58** 640–9.

23 Chevalier R Developmental renal physiology of the low birth weight pre-term newborn. *J Urol*, 1996, **156** 714–19.

24 Candy DCA Parenteral nutrition in paediatric practice a review. *J Hum Nutr*, 1980, **34** 287–96.

25 Nutritional Support Committee *Parenteral Nutrition Manual*, 4th edn. Children's Hospital of Pittsburgh. One Children's Place, 3705 Fifth Avenue, Pittsburgh PA, 1996.

26 Gorran MI, Broemeling L, Herndon DN *et al.* Estimating energy requirements in burned children a new approach derived from measurements of resting energy expenditure. *Am J Clin Nutr*, 1991, **54** 35–40.

27 Pierro A, Jones MO, Hammond P *et al.* A new equation to predict resting energy expenditure of surgical infants. *J Pediatr Surg*, 1994, **29** 1103–8.

28 Lloyd DA Energy requirements of surgical newborn infants requiring parenteral nutrition. *Nutrition*, 1998, **14** 101–4.

29 White MS, Shepherd RW, McEniery JA Energy expenditure measurements in ventilated critically ill children within and between day variability. *J Parenter Enteral Nutr*, 1999, **23** 300–4.

30　Chwals WJ Overfeeding the criticaly ill child: fact or fantasy? *New Horiz*, 1994, **2** 147–55.

31　Carr B, Denne S, Leitch C Total energy expenditure in extremely premature and term infants in early post natal life. *Pediatr Res*, 2000, **47** 284A.

32　King C The Hammersmith Hospital NHS Trust Nutrition and Dietetic Department Neonatal Unit Parenteral Nutrition Policy. December, 1998.

33　Hanning RM, Zlotkin SH Nitrogen needs of the parenterally fed neonate. In: Yu V, McMahon B (eds) *Intravenous Feeding of the Neonate*. Kent, England: Hodder and Stoughton, 1992, p. 32.

34　Lucas A, Baker BA, Morley RM Hyperphenylalaninaemia and outcome in intravenously fed pre-term neonates. *Arch Dis Child*, 1989, **64** 939.

35　Tubman T, Thompson S, McGuire W Glutamine supplementation to prevent morbidity and mortality in preterm infants. *Cochrane Database Syst Rev*, 2005, Art. No. CD001457.

36　Borum PR Carnitine in neonatal nutrition. *J Child Neurol*, 1995, **10** (suppl 2) S25–31.

37　Dahllstrom KA, Ament ME, Moukarzel A *et al.* Low blood and plasma carnitine levels in children receiving long term parenteral nutrition. *J Pediatr Gastroenterol Nutr*, 1990, **11** 375.

38　Cairns PA, Stalker DJ Carnitine supplementation of parenterally fed neonates. *Cochrane Database Syst Rev*, 2000, Art. No. CD000950.

39　Phelps SJ, Cochrane EC, Kamper CA Peripheral venous line infiltration in infants receiving 10% dextrose, 10% dextrose/amino acids, 10% dextrose/amino acids/fat emulsion. *Pediatr Res*, 1987, **21** (Abstract 67A).

40　Haemont D, Decklebaum RJ, Richelle M *et al.* Plasma lipid and plasma lipoprotein concentrations in low birth weight infants given parenteral nutrition with twenty or ten percent lipid emulsion. *J Pediatr*, 1989, **115** 787–93.

41　Donnell SC, Nunn A, Lloyd DA *et al.* Intravenous medium chain triglycerides in surgical neonates: effects on energy metabolism and fat utilization. British Association for Parenteral and Enteral Nutrition, 1995.

42　Deckelbaum RJ, Hamilton JA, Moser A *et al.* Medium chain versus long chain triacylglycerol emulsion hydrolysis by lipoprotein lipase and hepatic lipase: implications for the mechanism of lipase action. *Biochemistry*, 1990, **29** 1136–42.

43　Gobel Y, Koletzko B, Bohles HJ *et al.* Parenteral fat emulsions based on olive and soya bean oils: a randomised clinical trial in pre-term infants. *J Pediatr Gastroenterol Nutr*, 2003, **37** 167–70.

44　Brans YW, Andrews DS, Carillo DW *et al.* Tolerance of fat emulsions in very low birthweight neonates. *Am J Dis Child*, 1988, **142** 145–52.

45　Andrew G, Chan G, Schiff D Lipid metabolism in the neonate. The effects of intralipid infusion plasma triglyceride and free fatty acid concentrations in the neonate. *J Pediatr*, 1976, **88** 273–8.

46　Cooke R, Yeh YY, Gibson D *et al.* Soybean oil emulsion administration during parenteral nutrition in the pre-term infant: effect on essential fatty acid, lipid and glucose metabolism. *J Pediatr*, 1987, **111** 767–75.

47　Jones MO, Pierro A, Hammond P *et al.* Glucose utilization in the surgical newborn infant receiving total parenteral nutrition. *J Pediatr Surg*, 1993, **28** 1121–5.

48　Sauer P, Van Aerde J Smith J *et al.* Substrate utilization of newborn infants fed intravenously with or without fat emulsion. *Pediatr Res*, 1984, **18** 804 (Abstract 46).

49　Hwang TL, Lue MC, Chen LL Early use of cyclic total parenteral nutrition prevents further deterioration of liver functions for the TPN patients with impaired liver function. *Hepatogastroenterol*, 2000, **47** 1347–50.

50　Greene HL *et al.* Guidelines for the use of vitamins, trace elements, calcium, magnesium and phosphorus in infants and children receiving total parenteral nutrition: Report of the subcommittee on paediatric parenteral nutrient requirements from the committee on clinical practice issues of the American Society for Clinical Nutrition. *Am J Clin Nutr*, 1988, **48** 1324–42.

51　Darlow BA, Graham PJ Vitamin A supplementation for preventing morbidity and mortality in very low birthweight infants. *Cochrane Database Syst Rev*, 2002, **4** Art. No. CD000501.

52　Allwood MC Compatability and stability of TPN mixtures in big bags. *J Clin Hosp Pharm*, 1984, **9** 181–98.

53　Friel JK, Bessie JC, Belkhule SL *et al.* Thiamine, riboflavin, pyridoxine and vitamin C status in premature infants receiving parenteral and enteral nutrition. *J Pediatric Gastroenterol Nutr*, 2001, **33** 64–9.

54　Kumpf KJ Parenteral iron supplementation. *Nutr Clin Pract*, August 1996, **11** 139–46.

55　Barry DM, Reeve AW Increased risk of gram negative neonatal sepsis with intramuscular iron administration. *Pediatrics*, 1997, **60** 908–12.

56　Fell JM, Reynolds AP, Meadows N *et al.* Manganese toxicity in children receiving long term parenteral nutrition. *Lancet*, 1996, **347** 1218–21.

57　Finley JW Manganese absorption and retention by young women is associated with serum ferritin concentration. *Am J Clin Nutr*, 1997, **70** 33–7.

58　Davidsson L, Lonnerdal B, Sandstrom B *et al.* Identification of transferrin as the major plasma carrier for manganese introduced orally or intravenously or after *in vitro* addition in the rat. *J Nutr*, 1989, **119** 1461–4.

59 Hansell D Intravenous nutrition: the central or peripheral route? *Int Ther Clin Mon*, 1989, **10** 184–90.

60 Clark-Christoff N, Watters WA, Sparkes W *et al.* Use of triple lumen catheters for administration of total parenteral nutrition. *J Parenter Enteral Nutr*, 1992, **16** 403–7.

61 Cole D, Thickson N, Oruck J Computer assisted compounding of neonatal/pediatric parenteral nutrition solutions. *Can J Hosp Pharm*, 1991, **44** 229–33.

62 Braunschweig CL, Wesley JR, Mercer N Rationale and guidelines for parenteral and enteral transition feeding of the 3–30 kg child. *J Am Diet Assoc*, 1988, **88** 479–82.

5 Nutrition in Critically Ill Children

Rosan Meyer & Katie Elwig

Introduction

Nutritional support in critically ill children (CIC) is unique when compared with feeding the child on a general paediatric ward. In addition to minimising the starvation effects associated with suboptimal alimentation, preventing overfeeding and nutritional deficiencies, its goal is to sustain organ function and prevent dysfunction of the cardiovascular, respiratory and immune systems until the acute-phase inflammatory response resolves [1]. Both under- and overnutrition have the potential to compromise this goal and significantly complicate and increase the stay in an intensive care unit [2,3]. Overfeeding can lead to increased carbon dioxide production, resulting in difficulties with weaning from mechanical ventilator support, as well as diarrhoea associated with electrolyte imbalances and other well-documented metabolic and physiological complications [4]. Underfeeding, however, is a more common occurrence in CIC, with 16–20% developing significant, acute protein energy malnutrition (PEM) within 48 hours of admission to a paediatric intensive care unit (PICU) [2]. This leads to impaired muscle strength [5], reduced wound healing as a result of altered immunity and increased rates of sepsis [6]. Ensuring optimal nutrition in these patients is therefore crucial [7].

Assessment of nutritional status

Anthropometrics, biochemical markers, clinical and dietary review form part of the nutritional assessment in CIC [8]. However, this process is notoriously difficult because of a multitude of factors including oedema, ascites and severity of disease, which often renders patients too unstable to be weighed. In addition, the emotional impact of having a child on the PICU frequently makes the diet history unreliable. It is quite common practice in PICUs in the UK to estimate the weight (in kilograms) of a critically ill child in the absence of an accurate weight, using the Advanced Paediatric Life Support formula: (age + 4) × 2 [9]. This method has been shown to correlate reasonably well with actual weight, but has significant outliers, especially in underfed and overweight children as well as teenagers [10]. An accurate (admission) weight is therefore always superior to an estimated weight as it is not only used in the assessment of nutritional status and calculating energy requirements, but also used for estimating fluid requirements and medication dosages. Transfer and hospital notes, as well as the individual's personal child health record (the 'red/blue book'), may have a recent accurate weight (often height and head circumference as well) which can be used. It is important that available accurate weight, height and head circumference is plotted on an appropriate growth chart [11].

The use of both triceps skin fold thickness (TSF) as well as mid-arm circumference (MAC) have been documented in this population. Their use is limited by oedema and by the relative short average length of stay (4–5 days) on a PICU. They are most helpful when followed over time and measured by the same trained person [8,11]. Hulst [8] studied the feasibility of routinely performing nutritional assessments using non-invasive methods in CIC. It was found that anthropometrics were reliably obtained within 24 hours of admission in 56–91% of patients. Unfortunately, the more seriously ill patients were those where measurements were less feasible but who might have benefited the most. Both TSF and MAC are therefore more useful in patients who are on PICU for longer periods of time and with no oedema.

Most laboratory markers of nutritional status are affected by the acute inflammatory response, renal impairment and fluid shifts. The prevalence of hypomagnesaemia, hypertriglyceridaemia, uraemia and hypoalbuminaemia were 20%, 25%, 30% and 52%, respectively, in a study on CIC performed by Hulst *et al.* [12]. Except for uraemia, no significant associations between the biochemical parameters and anthropometric measurements were found. Serum urea levels can indicate the degree of catabolic stress and levels of protein breakdown associated with illness, surgery and trauma, but are often not reliable because of impaired renal function, dehydration, polyuria and severe sweating on admission. Children with sepsis or cardiac anomalies in this study showed the highest prevalence of uraemia, which can be explained by the degree of catabolism and impairment of renal function. Although pre-albumin, retinol binding protein, transferrin and nitrogen balance studies have also been used in research on nutritional status in CIC, their accuracy and the value of routine use have been questioned by several authors [12]. It is therefore important to select biomarkers for the assessment of nutritional status in the critically ill patient with care and interpret them accordingly.

Diet history taking often gets neglected on PICU [11]. Although manipulation of oral intake is not possible and also not practical on the intensive care unit, many acute and chronic nutrition-related problems can be identified on admission and can assist the dietitian in the planning of dietary input during their admission period. Long term problems (e.g. obesity, constipation) can be addressed once the patient is extubated and transferred to a ward or local hospital.

Energy expenditure and substrate utilisation

Traditionally, nutritional support has been withheld in children on PICU until metabolic and cardiopulmonary stability has been established. However, many units have changed their protocols and guidelines to include nutritional support at an earlier stage. Knowledge of metabolic changes and fuel utilisation during physiological stress can assist dietitians in commencing nutritional support at the appropriate time, using a suitable feed and starting at the correct rate.

Critical illness is characterised by a cascade of endocrine and metabolic reactions, affecting all major organs (Fig. 5.1; Table 5.1) [13]. The reaction of the body to physiological stress is not a static process and changes over time. The acute phase response can be divided into the ebb phase which is characterised by the body's attempt to maintain normal perfusion and mobilisation of stress hormones, and the flow phase which is the dynamic state of acute injury and affects substrate metabolism (protein catabolism is at its highest). The final phase, the anabolic phase, is characterised by the slow re-accumulation of protein and body fat after the metabolic response to injury subsides [14–18].

Several studies have focused on the relation between a critically ill child's metabolic state, their nutritional intake, substrate utilisation and nitrogen balance. In a similar way to critically ill adults, the stress response and the severity of disease is characterised by protein catabolism. In contrast to adults, in children fat is the preferred fuel source for oxidation and carbohydrates are poorly utilised during critical illness. Maximal glucose oxidation occurs at a glucose intake of 5 mg/kg/minute. If intake exceeds 8 mg/kg/minute, lipogenesis takes place leading to an increase in triglyceride levels, fat deposition in the liver and an increase in fat instead of lean body mass [16]. It is therefore important to

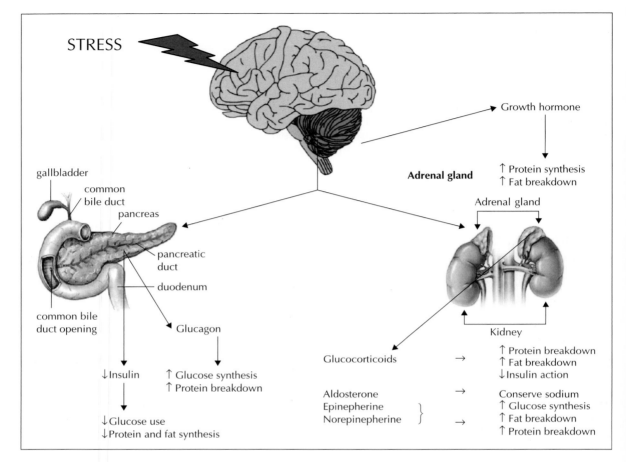

Figure 5.1   The metabolic response to stress [13]. Adjusted from Krause *et al.* [13].

Table 5.1   The effect of critical illness on the major organs.

Gastrointestinal system	Cardiovascular system	Respiratory system	Renal system
Gastroparesis (motility affected due to medication, e.g. morphine, inotropic agents and antibiotics, as well as the disease process itself) [18] Impaired digestive enzyme secretion [18] Cholestasis Impaired lipid metabolism due to affected liver function [16] Increased intestinal permeability Poor gut perfusion [18]	Tachycardia [16] High cardiac output Fluid shift from the intracellular to the extracellular compartments [14]	Respiratory deterioration leading to artificial ventilation [17]	Mild renal impairment to acute renal failure requiring haemofiltration [16]

Table 5.2 Factors that influence energy expenditure.

Factor	Influence on energy expenditure
Sedation	↓ Energy expenditure (reduced brain activity)
Muscle relaxants	↓ Energy expenditure but not significantly
Ventilation (with humidified air)	↓ Energy expenditure (reduces the workload of breathing as well as heat loss)
Thermoneutral environment (environment adjusted according to patient's temperature)	↓ Insensible losses, therefore lowers energy expenditure
Pyrexia	↑ Energy expenditure (8–12% increase in energy expenditure per 1°C above normal)
Severity of disease	Inconclusive evidence
Diagnosis and severity of disease (using PRISM scoring)	No difference in energy expenditure in different diagnoses

PRISM, paediatric risk of mortality score.

ensure that carbohydrate intake in CIC is monitored, especially if parenteral nutrition (PN) is used.

Some older studies have suggested a hypermetabolic state during the acute phase of illness [15]; new evidence points towards hypometabolism, which can be explained by both the treatment as well as the unique nature of fuel utilisation in CIC [15–19]. Several factors (sedation, muscle relaxants, ventilation, environment, severity of disease, temperature) have been shown to impact on energy expenditure. Table 5.2 summarises the influences on requirements.

In addition to the factors listed in Table 5.2, many authors have speculated that during the acute phase, growth does not take place and this energy is diverted into the recovery processes [19–21]. Although the verdict on energy expenditure is still pending, it is clear that substrate metabolism needs to be taken into account when calculating the energy requirements and choosing feeds for these patients.

Nutritional requirements

Energy requirements

Several predictive equations have been used in the paediatric critical setting to calculate energy requirements. They include Harris–Benedict, the World Health Organization, Talbot, Schofield and PICU regression equations [20–24] (Table 5.3). A number of studies confirmed the inaccuracy of these equations for the ventilated CIC with most of them grossly overestimating energy requirements, except for the regression equation developed by

White & Shepherd [22] which significantly underestimates requirements [19,23]. They also require the addition of stress and activity factors, which have been based mainly on adult data and are dependent on the subjective opinion of a dietitian or clinician [24]. Most authors have found that the actual energy expenditure is closer to the basal metabolic rate (BMR) with an increase of 8–10% in requirements for every 1°C above the norm in body temperature [19,20,25].

The Schofield equation is used most commonly in the UK, with some evidence of reasonable correlation with ventilated CIC. In the absence of routine indirect calorimetry, which is the gold standard for measuring energy expenditure, the BMR calculated by Schofield (using the formula that requires an accurate weight) plus 10% for every 1°C above 37.3°C (Table 5.3) is a useful alternative while a child is being ventilated on the intensive care unit, and new research in this area is awaited [26].

Example: 1-year-old boy weighing 10 kg with a temperature of 38.5°C

$$= (59.512 \times 10) - 30.4$$
$$= 564.72 + 10\%$$
$$= 621 \text{ kcal}$$

Protein requirements

Although there are no specific guidelines on protein requirements in ventilated CIC, research has shown that patients with an adequate energy and protein intake have a positive nitrogen balance, unlike patients who are underfed. Nitrogen (N) balance correlates with energy expenditure; feeding

Table 5.3   Predictive equations for calculating basal metabolic rate (BMR) in critically ill children.

Name of equation	Equation (kcal/24 hours)
Schofield (if accurate weight is available)	*Males* <3 years: $(59.512 \times W) - 30.4$ 3–10 years: $(22.7 \times W) + 504.3$ 10–18 years: $(17.5 \times W) + 651$ *Females* <3 years: $(58.317 \times W) - 31.1$ 3–10 years: $(22.706 \times W) + 485.9$ 10–18 years: $(17.686 \times W) + 692.6$
Schofield (if accurate weight and height are available)	*Males* <3 years: $(0.167 \times W) + (1517.4 \times H) - 616.6$ 3–10 years: $(19.59 \times W) + (130.3 \times H) + 414.9$ 10–18 years: $(16.25 \times W) + (137.2 \times H) + 515.5$ *Females* <3 years: $(16.252 \times W) + (1023.3 \times H) - 413.5$ 3–10 years: $(16.969 \times W) + (161.8 \times H) + 371.2$ 10–18 years: $(8.365 \times W) + (465 \times H) + 200.0$
World Health Organization	*Males* 0–3 years: $(60.9 \times W) - 54$ 3–10 years: $(22.7 \times W) - 495$ 10–18 years: $(17.5 \times W) + 651$ *Females* 0–3 years: $(61 \times W) - 51$ 3–10 years: $(22.5 \times W) + 485.9$ 10–18 years: $(17.686 \times W) + 658.2$
White *et al.**	EE (kJ/day) $= (17 \times A) + (48 \times W) + (292 \times T) - 9677$

A, age (years); EE, energy expenditure; H, height (m); T, temperature (°C); W, weight (kg).
* Equation published in kilojoules only.

to total measured energy expenditure correlates with a positive N balance [27]. Agus & Jaksic [28] suggest that the critically ill infant and child should receive 2–3 g/kg and 1.5 g/kg protein, respectively, and in the severely stressed states may require even more. In the absence of specific guidelines, CIC should receive a minimum of the Recommended Nutrient Intake (RNI) for protein and a sufficient amount of energy to prevent gluconeogenesis and to ensure that the body utilises these effectively. Disease-specific protein recommendations (e.g. renal failure, cystic fibrosis) also provide useful guidelines for children on the PICU.

Vitamins and minerals

Vitamins and trace mineral metabolism in the critically ill and postoperative paediatric patient is not a well-researched area. As a result, no specific recommendations exist for the ventilated patient on the PICU. The pharmacological use of vitamins and trace minerals in paediatric illness is controversial because of reports of toxicity [28]. When energy and fluid requirements are met by commercial enteral tube feeds, CIC should receive sufficient vitamins and minerals to meet the RNI for both. However, many patients require additional supplementation, depending on diagnosis and treatment modality (e.g. prematurity, haemofiltration). This should be carried out under supervision and monitored with blood biochemistry.

Early implementation of enteral nutrition

The concept of early feeding has mainly been developed in adult surgical patients. In paediatric patients most authors agree to the definition of 'early enteral nutrition' as the initiation of enteral feed within 24–48 hours of PICU admission. Others describe patients receiving immediate feeding, but unfortunately this term does not come with a clear definition [29,30].

Four main hypotheses could justify the use of early feeding in CIC:

- Fasting has a deleterious effect on these patients
- Energy supply has an important role in the promotion of energy metabolism
- The delivery of nutrients is important for gut maintenance
- Specific nutrients provide support for organ and system functions [29]

Several studies have been published showing a delay in commencement of nutritional support ranging from 2 to 3 days from admission on a PICU [31]. The prevalence of significant PEM within 48 hours of admission therefore comes as no surprise. Early enteral nutrition (within 12 hours of admission) has been successfully used by numerous PICUs, in a variety of diagnoses and in the absence of any bowel sounds and has resulted in an improved nitrogen balance [30,32].

The combination of decreased blood flow and

interactions with drugs can also lead to a reduction of nutrient absorption and gastric motility, failure of gastric acid secretion and increase in intestinal permeability and bacterial translocation [18]. Early enteral nutritional support may reverse these effects by reducing catabolism, promoting wound healing and most likely decreasing the frequency of clinical sepsis.

Routes and methods of enteral feeding on PICU

Despite the ongoing debate on enteral versus parenteral nutrition in the critically ill population, research is now focusing on how nutrients can be delivered most effectively and safely, using the most appropriate route. In general it is deemed safe to initiate nutritional support when the patient is haemodynamically stable and this will include stabilisation of critical organ function, optimising haemodynamics and perfusion, and ensuring life-sustaining gas exchange [33].

Standard protocols for initiating and progressing nutritional support have been shown to be useful in both improving the time taken to initiate nutritional support as well as the progression to full feeds [34–36]. Enteral feeding protocols guide medical and nursing staff through the choice of tube feeds, the feeding rates dependent on the child's age and weight, as well as guidelines for the continuous monitoring process (Fig. 5.2) [37].

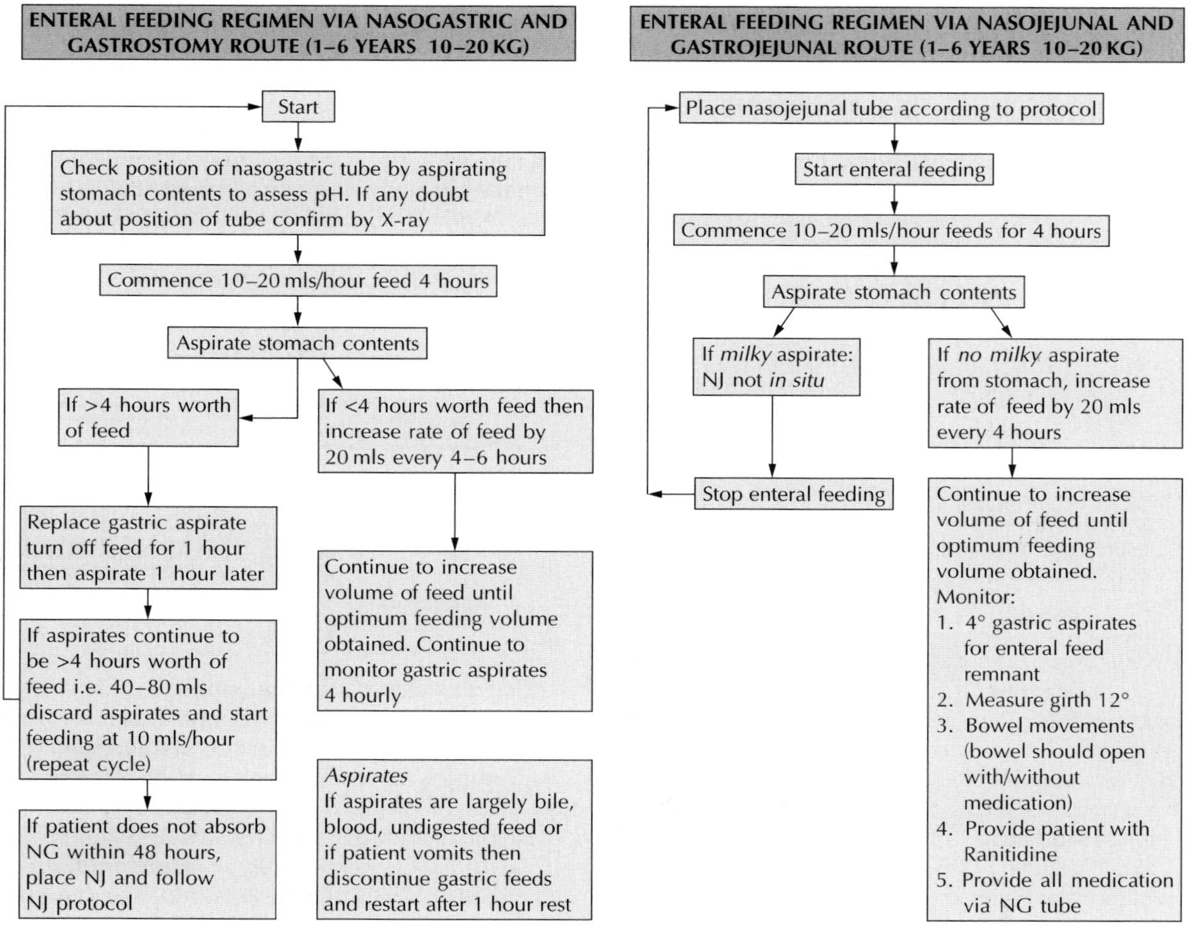

ENTERAL FEEDING REGIMEN VIA NASOGASTRIC AND GASTROSTOMY ROUTE (1–6 YEARS 10–20 KG)

Start

Check position of nasogastric tube by aspirating stomach contents to assess pH. If any doubt about position of tube confirm by X-ray

Commence 10–20 mls/hour feed 4 hours

Aspirate stomach contents

If >4 hours worth of feed

If <4 hours worth feed then increase rate of feed by 20 mls every 4–6 hours

Replace gastric aspirate turn off feed for 1 hour then aspirate 1 hour later

If aspirates continue to be >4 hours worth of feed i.e. 40–80 mls discard aspirates and start feeding at 10 mls/hour (repeat cycle)

If patient does not absorb NG within 48 hours, place NJ and follow NJ protocol

Continue to increase volume of feed until optimum feeding volume obtained. Continue to monitor gastric aspirates 4 hourly

Aspirates
If aspirates are largely bile, blood, undigested feed or if patient vomits then discontinue gastric feeds and restart after 1 hour rest

ENTERAL FEEDING REGIMEN VIA NASOJEJUNAL AND GASTROJEJUNAL ROUTE (1–6 YEARS 10–20 KG)

Place nasojejunal tube according to protocol

Start enteral feeding

Commence 10–20 mls/hour feeds for 4 hours

Aspirate stomach contents

If *milky* aspirate: NJ not *in situ*

If *no milky* aspirate from stomach, increase rate of feed by 20 mls every 4 hours

Stop enteral feeding

Continue to increase volume of feed until optimum feeding volume obtained.
Monitor:
1. 4° gastric aspirates for enteral feed remnant
2. Measure girth 12°
3. Bowel movements (bowel should open with/without medication)
4. Provide patient with Ranitidine
5. Provide all medication via NG tube

Figure 5.2   Example of a feeding protocol. From Department of Nutrition and Dietetics, St Mary's Hospital [37]. NJ, nasojejunal; NG, nasogastric.

Nasogastric versus nasojejunal feeding

Nasogastric (NG) feeding is the most widely used and is usually safe and well tolerated in CIC [1,34,38]. However, gastric delivery of enteral feed is frequently poorly tolerated because of disordered gastric motility which may lead to aspiration. The use of gastric residual volume as marker of tolerance of NG feeding has a poor evidence base and has often been blamed for inadequate delivery of feed [39]. Therefore, interest has focused on postpyloric feeding. Nasojejunal (NJ) feeding has been shown by several centres to be safe and effective in this subset of patients, enabling adequate delivery of energy in a shorter period of time. There is a reduction in the incidence of hyperglycaemia and hypertriglyceridaemia, and maintenance of normal hepatic function, both associated with PN [40,41]. In addition, a recent study in children has shown that postpyloric feeding can safely be continued even during ventilatory weaning and tracheal extubation. This enables the child to be fed up to the time of extubation without losing any feeding time while waiting for gastric emptying [42]. Many units avoid postpyloric feeding, as NJ tubes are notoriously difficult to

place and get dislodged very easily [43]. Several blind (non-radiological guided) bedside techniques have been developed in recent years using weighted or unweighted polyurethane NG tubes with hydrophilic guide wires. These methods have relied on a combination of estimating the postpyloric length, auscultation, aspiration and pH monitoring and blue dye testing. The blue dye test entails the administration of blue dye via the placed NJ tube and aspiration via the inserted NG tube. If no blue dye is present in the gastric aspirate, then the NJ tube placement was successful. This test has been shown to be extremely accurate in confirming the correct placement of NJ tubes and therefore preventing unnecessary exposure to abdominal X-rays for placement confirmation (Fig. 5.3) [44,45].

Continuous feeds versus bolus feeding

Both continuous as well as bolus feeding have been used in the paediatric critical care setting. The pros and cons of both the above are well studied in the neonatal setting, but remain a subject of unit preference in infants and children [46]. Although bolus

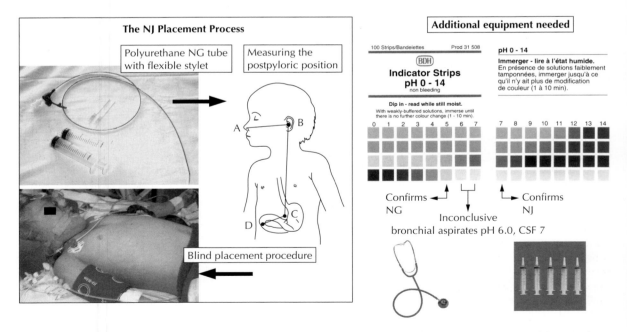

Figure 5.3 The blind nasojejunal (NJ) procedure. Approximation of length of the NJ tube: nose (A) to ear (B) to umbilicus (C) for gastric placement and to iliac crest (D) for jejunal length. NG, nasogastric. From Meyer *et al.* [45].

feeding is more physiological, difficulties with monitoring the tolerance as well as the additional nursing input has led to many units preferring continuous feeding. On the other hand, continuous feeding (less time consuming and easier to monitor) may delay gastric emptying in the adult intensive care setting [47] and reduce gallbladder contraction [48]. In the absence of substantial clinical evidence, consensus exists that the adequate delivery of nutritional support should be the main goal in feeding the CIC and should not be hampered by the feeding route [35,49].

Immunonutrition

The use of immune enhancing enteral feeding formulas is a well known phenomenon in adult intensive care. In addition to the normal macro- and micronutrients, these feeds may contain: a mixture of omega-3 and omega-6-fatty acids, with pro- and anti-inflammatory properties; additional arginine and/or glutamine, which become essential amino acids during increased physiological stress; increased levels of the antioxidants selenium and beta-carotene [50].

Although these enteral feeding formulas have all the ingredients to improve outcome, results in the adult population have been conflicting. A meta-analysis of 15 studies of immune enhancing diets in critically ill patients after trauma, sepsis or major surgery showed that enteral immunonutrition decreased the incidence of infection, number of ventilator days and length of hospital stay, but had no effect on stay in the intensive care unit [50]. More recent, multicentred randomised studies have shown conflicting results with higher mortality rates in the immunonutrition group among patients with severe sepsis or septic shock [51].

The only documentation of an immune enhancing enteral feeding formula being used in the paediatric critical care setting is by Briassoulis et al. [52], who used an adult feed, because of the unavailability of immune enhancing paediatric formulas. Preliminary results showed that the immune enhancing formula achieved a positive nitrogen balance by day 5, which the normal formula did not achieve, but was associated with an exacerbated metabolic response in a stressed state compared with the control group [52,53].

This area of paediatric critical care nutrition is still very new and the limited evidence does not yet support routine use of immune enhancing feeds or supplementation because of possible deleterious effects. Until such data are available specifically for the CIC, these ad hoc additions to feeds or future immune enhancing feeds should be used with caution [53].

Probiotics

A probiotic is a live microbial feed supplement that beneficially affects the host by improving its intestinal microbial balance [54]. Altering enteric flora is a concept gaining popularity throughout the world and the use of probiotic bacteria on the PICU is developing too. Intestinal permeability is increased during critical illness particularly after burns, major trauma and sepsis. In addition, bacterial translocation has been demonstrated in patients with bowel obstruction. The administration of some probiotic strains has been associated with a reduction in bacterial translocation and intestinal inflammation [55].

In the critically ill, the main concern remains the possibility of septicaemia related to the provision of live bacteria to patients who are relatively immunocompromised. Several studies using probiotics in the adult ICU setting show not only their beneficial effects, but also their safe use [55,56]. Routine use of probiotics on PICU is not common, but its safe use has been shown in a recent study [57], which excluded patients with human immunodeficiency virus, bone marrow transplants and other patients with neutropenia. No adverse effects (including septicaemia) were related to its routine use over 2 years during the study [57]. Additional complicating factors with the routine use of probiotics on a PICU are antibiotic use and the sensitivity of many of the commercially available strains to these. In the absence of disease-specific probiotic research in CIC, the most practical way of choosing a suitable probiotic is by matching the antibiotic to a resistant probiotic with a pathogenic inhibition capacity (Table 5.4) [58].

Probiotics may benefit children on the PICU. Although their safe use has been shown in patients who are not immunocompromised, more research is needed before they are routinely used in CIC.

Table 5.4   Probiotics and antibiotic resistance, sensitivity and pathogen inhibition.

	Bifido infantis (e.g. Biocare)	Lactobacillus acidophillus (e.g. Biocare)	Lactobacillus casei (e.g. Yakult, Actimel)	Lactobacillus plantarum (e.g. ProViva)	Lactobacillus rhamnosus (e.g. Lactobacillus GG)
Antibiotic sensitivity					
Amoxicillin	S	S	S	S	S
Ampicillin	S	S	S	S	S
Ceftazidime	S	I	R	R	R
Chloramphenicol	I	I	R	R	I
Ciprofloxacin	R	R	R	R	R
Clindamycin	I	I	I	S	S
Cloxacillin	S	S	I	R	S
Dicloxacillin	S	S	S	R	S
Erythromycin	I	S	I	I	S
Gentamicin	R	R	R	R	R
Imipenem	R	R	R	R	R
Kanamycin	R	R	R	R	R
Neomycin	R	R	R	R	R
Nitrofurantoin	R	R	R	R	R
Penicillin G	S	S	S	R	S
Polymixin B	R	R	R	R	R
Rifampicin	S	S	S	S	S
Streptomycin	R	R	R	R	R
Sulfamethoxazole	R	R	R	R	R
Tetracycline	R	R	S	R	I
Trimethoprim	R	R	R	R	R
Vancomycin	S	S	R	R	R
Pathogen inhibition					
Clostridium difficile	NA	NA	NA	NA	NA
Escherichia coli	+++	+++	++++	++	+++
Listeria monocytogenes	+	+	++	++	++
Salmonella	+	+	++	++	++
Staphylococcus aureus	+	+	++		++

I, inconclusive; NA, not available; R, resistant; S, sensitive.
Source: Gibson et al. [58].

References

1   Irving S, Derengowski Simone S, Hicks FW Nutrition for the critically ill child: enteral and parenteral support. *AACN Clin Issues*, 2000, **11** 541–58.
2   Pollack MM, Wiley J, Holbrook PR Early nutritional depletion in critically ill children. *Crit Care Med*, 1981, **9** 580–3.
3   Letton RW, Chwals WJ, Jamie A *et al*. Early postoperative alterations in infant energy use increase the risk of overfeeding. *J Pediatr Surg*, 1995, **30** 988–92; discussion 992–3.
4   Klein CJ, Stanek GS, Wiles CE Overfeeding macronutrients to critically ill adults: metabolic complications. *J Am Diet Assoc*, 1998, **98** 795–806.

5   Corke C Enteral nutrition in the critically ill. (Online) Available: www.nda.ox.ac.uk/wfsa/dl/html/papers/pap009.htm.   1996.   Accessed September 2005.
6   Chandra RK Nutrition and Immunology: from the clinic to cellular biology and back again. *Proc Nutr Soc*, 1999, **58** 681–3.
7   Pena D, Pujol M, Pallares R *et al*. Estimation of cost attributable to nosocomial infection: prolongation of hospitalization and calculation of alternative costs. *Med Clin (Barc)*, 1996, **106** 441–4.
8   Hulst JM Nutritional assessment of critically ill children: the search for practical tools. PhD Thesis, 2004, Erasmus University of Rotterdam, Holland.
9   Mackway-Jones K, Molyneux E, Phillips B *et al*.

Advanced Paediatric Life Support, 4th edn. Oxford: Blackwell Science, 2003, p. 9.

10 Argall JAW, Wright N, Mackway-Jones K *et al*. A comparison of two commonly used methods of weight estimation. *Arch Dis Child*, 2003, **88** 789–90.

11 Bettler J, Roberts KE Nutrition assessment of the critically ill child. *AACN Clin Issues*, 2000, **11** 498–506.

12 Hulst JM, Van Goudoever JB, Zimmermann LJI *et al*. The role of initial monitoring of routine biochemical nutritional markers in critically ill children. *J Nutr Biochem*, 2006, **17** 57–62.

13 Krause MV, Mahan LK, Arlin M Physiological stress: trauma, sepsis, burns and surgery. In: *Krause's Food, Nutrition and Diet Therapy*, 10th edn. Philadelphia: WB Saunders Company, 2002, p. 492.

14 Chiolero R, Revelly J Energy metabolism in sepsis and injury. *Nutrition*, 1997, **13** 45S–51S.

15 Coss-Bu JA, Klish WJ, Walding D *et al*. Energy metabolism, nitrogen balance, and substrate utilization in critically ill children. *Am J Clin Nutr*, 2001, **74** 664–9.

16 Turi R, Petros A, Eaton S *et al*. Energy metabolism of infants and children with systemic inflammatory response syndrome and sepsis. *Ann Surg*, 2001, **233** 581–7.

17 Haber BA, Deutschman CS Nutrition and metabolism in the critically ill child. In: Rogers MC, Nichols DG (eds) *Textbook of Pediatric Intensive Care*, 3rd edn. Boston: Lippincot Williams, 1996, pp. 1141–60.

18 Dobb GJ The role of the gut in critical illness. *Curr Anasth Crit Care*, 1996, **7** 62–8.

19 Taylor RM, Cheeseman P, Preedy V *et al*. Can energy expenditure be predicted in critically ill children. *Pediatr Crit Care Med*, 2003, **4** 176–9.

20 Vazquez Martinez JL, Martinez-Romillo PD, Sebastian JD *et al*. Predicted versus measured energy expenditure by continuous, online indirect calorimetry in ventilated critically ill children during the early post injury period. *Pediatr Crit Care Med*, 2004, **5** 19–27.

21 Briassoulis G, Ventkataranman S, Thompson AE Energy expenditure in critically ill children. *Crit Care Med*, 2000, **28** 1160–72.

22 White MS, Shepherd RW Energy expenditure in 100 ventilated, critically ill children: improving the accuracy of predictive equations. *Crit Care Med*, 2000, **28** 2307–12.

23 Hardy CM, Dwayer J, Snelling LK *et al*. Pitfalls in predicting resting energy requirements in critically ill children: a comparison of predictive methods to indirect calorimetry. *Nutr Clin Pract*, 2002, **17** 182–9.

24 Muller P, Bosy-Westphal A, Klaus S *et al*. World Health Organization equations have shortcomings for predicting resting energy expenditure in persons from a modern, affluent population: generation of a new reference standard from a retrospective analysis of a German database of resting energy expenditure. *Am J Clin Nutr*, 2004, **80** 1370–90.

25 Argent A From energy to nutrition intervention. *Pediatr Crit Care Med*, 2003, **4** 262–3.

26 Meyer R, Elwig K, Lang A Too much is not necessary better: an overview on calorie requirements in the critically ill child. *Care Crit Ill*, 2002, **10** 22–30.

27 Joosten KF, Verhoeven JJ, Hazelzet JA Energy expenditure and substrate utilization in mechanically ventilated children. *Nutrition*, 1999, **15** 444–8.

28 Agus MSD, Jaksic T Nutritional support of the critically ill child. *Curr Opin Pediatr*, 2002, **14** 470–81.

29 Chiolero RL, Tappy I, Berger MM Timing of nutritional support. *Nestle Clin Nutr: Early Intervention*, 2002, **7** 151–68.

30 Briassoulis G, Tsorva A, Zavras N *et al*. Influence of an aggressive early enteral nutrition protocol on nitrogen balance in critically ill children. *J Nutr Biochem*, 2002, **13** 560–5.

31 Chellis MJ, Sanders SV, Dean JM *et al*. Bedside transpyloric tube placement in the pediatric intensive care unit. *J Parenter Enteral Nutr*, 1996, **20** 88–90.

32 Hulst J, Joosten K, Zimmerman L *et al*. Malnutrition in critically ill children: from admission to 6 months after discharge. *Clin Nutr*, 2004, **23** 223–32.

33 Lin L, Cohen N Early nutritional support for the ICU patient: does it matter? *Contemp Crit Care*, 2005, **2** 1–10.

34 Briassoulis G, Zavras N, Hatzis T Effectiveness and safety of a protocol for promotion of early intragastric feeding in critically ill children. *Pediatr Crit Care Med*, 2001, **2** 113–21.

35 Meyer R The impact of ongoing audit on nutritional support in paediatric intensive care. Masters Thesis, 2004. University of Stellenbosch, South Africa.

36 Petrillo-Albarano T, Pettignano R, Asfaw M, Easley K Use of a feeding protocol to improve nutritional support through early, aggressive, enteral nutrition in the pediatric intensive care unit. *Pediatr Crit Care Med*, 2006, **7** 340–4.

37 Paediatric Dietitians Nasogastric and Nasojejunal Feeding Tubes. Paediatric Enteral Feeding Protocol, St. Mary's Hospital. London, 2002.

38 American Society for Parenteral and Enteral Nutrition (ASPEN) Board of Directors and the Clinical Guidelines Task Force Guidelines for the use of parenteral and enteral nutrition in adult and pediatric patients. *J Parenter Enteral Nutr*, 2002, **26** (S).

39 McClave CC, Snider HL, Lowen CC *et al*. Use of residual volume as a marker for enteral feeding intolerance: prospective blinded comparison with physical examination and radiographic findings. *J Parenter Enteral Nutr*, 1992, **16** 99–105.

40 Heyland DK, Drover JW, Dhaliwal R, Greenwood J Optimising the benefits and minimising the risk of

enteral nutrition in the critically ill: role of small bowel feeding. *J Parenter Enteral Nutr*, 2002, **26** S51–5.

41   Panadero E, Lopez-Herce J, Caro L *et al.* Transpyloric enteral feeding in critically ill children. *J Pediatr Gastroenterol Nutr*, 1998, **26** 43–8.

42   Jacobs B, Brilli R, Lyons K *et al.* Transpyloric feeding during ventilatory weaning and tracheal extubation is safe and effective in children. *Crit Care Med*, 1999, **27** 159–62.

43   De Lucas C, Moreno M, Lopez-Herce J *et al.* Transpyloric enteral nutrition reduces the complication rate and cost in the critically ill child. *J Pediatr Gastroenterol Nutr*, 2000, **30** 75–80.

44   Neuman DA, DeLegge MH Gastric versus small-bowel tube feeding in the intensive care unit: A prospective comparison of efficacy. *Crit Care Med*, 2002, **30** 1436–8.

45   Meyer R, Harrison S, Mehta C How to guide bedside placement of nasojejunal tubes in children. *Care Crit Ill*, 2001, **17** 23–4.

46   Premji S, Chessell L Continuous nasogastric milk feeding versus intermittent bolus milk feeding for premature infants less than 1500 grams. *Cochrane Database Syst Rev*, 2001, CD001819.

47   Soulsby C, Evans D, Powell-Tuck J Measurement of gastric volume in critically ill patients. *Care Crit Ill*, 2004, **20** 85–9.

48   Jawaheer G, Shaw N, Pierro A Continuous enteral feeding impairs gallbladder emptying in infants. *J Pediatr*, 2001, **138** 6–8.

49   Grant J, Denne S Effect of intermittent versus continuous enteral feeding on energy expenditure in premature infants. *J Pediatr*, 1994, **6** 118.

50   Kazamias P, Kotzampassi K, Koufogiannis D *et al.* Influence of enteral nutrition-induced splanchnic hyperemia on the septic origin of splanchnic ischaemia. *World J Surg*, 1998, **22** 6–11.

51   Bertolini G, Iapichino G, Radrizzani D *et al.* Early enteral immunonutrition in patients with severe sepsis: results of an interim analysis of a randomized multicentre clinical trial. *Intensive Care Med*, 2003, **2** 824.

52   Briassoulis G, Filippou O, Hatzi E *et al.* Comparative effects of early randomized immune or non-immune-enhancing enteral nutrition on cytokine production in children with septic shock. *Intensive Care Med*, 2005, **3** 851–8.

53   Briassoulis G, Filippou O, Hatzi E *et al.* Early enteral administration of immunonutrition in critically ill children: results of a blinded randomized controlled clinical trial. *Nutrition*, 2005, **21** 799–807.

54   Bengmark S Use of some pre-, pro and synbiotics in critically ill patients. *Best Pract Res Clin Gastroenterol*, 2003, **17** 833–48.

55   Klarin B, Johannsson M, Molin G *et al.* Adhesion of the probiotic bacterium *Lactobacillus plantarum* 299v onto the gut mucosa in crtically ill patients: a randomized open trial. *Crit Care*, 2005, **9** R285–93.

56   McNaught CE, Woodcock NP, Anderson ADG *et al.* A prospective randomized trial of probiotics in critically ill patients. *Clin Nutr*, 2005, **24** 211–19.

57   Srinivasan R, Meyer R, Ramnarayan P *et al.* Clinical safety of *Lactobacillus casei shirota* as a probiotic in critically ill children. *J Pediatr Gastroenterol Nutr*, 2005, **42** 171–3.

58   Gibson GR, Rouzaud G, Brostoff J *et al.* Final technical report for the FSA project ref G01022: *An evaluation of probiotic effects in the human gut: microbial aspects*. Food Standards Agency, London, 1998.

Part 3

Clinical Dietetics

continued

6 Preterm Infants

Caroline King

Definitions

A preterm infant is one born before 36 or 37 weeks' completed gestation, depending on source of definition. An infant born <2500 g is termed low birthweight (LBW) regardless of gestation, <1500 g very low birthweight (VLBW) and those <1000 g extremely low birthweight (ELBW). Categorisation of infants born smaller than expected is more contentious; however, they are often divided into small for gestational age (SGA) and intrauterine growth restricted (IUGR). Classification of SGA infants is usually as <10th or <3rd percentile for weight at birth (depending on source of definition) and probably constitute a heterogeneous group (i.e. those destined to be born small because of genetic influences and those who are IUGR). The former group tends to be proportionally small. Those who are IUGR will have similarly low birthweight, but may show head and/or length sparing depending on the timing of intrauterine nutrient restriction. These infants are at high risk of both perinatal and later problems [1].

The prevalence of IUGR is reported to be up to 7% of all deliveries [2]; however, this is made up by a disproportionately large number of preterm infants [3].

This chapter deals predominantly with the nutritional needs of preterm infants. Early nutritional management may be vital to later outcome, but can be hampered by an immature or dysfunctional gastrointestinal tract and poor tolerance of parenteral nutrition. Small term infants in general are mature with respect to oral motor function and can usually grow well if allowed breast or standard formula *ad lib*. Only where there are existent co-morbidities may small term infants need specialised nutritional input.

Nutritional requirements

Preterm infants have limited stores of many nutrients as accretion occurs predominantly in the last trimester [4]. They are poorly equipped to withstand inadequate nutrition; theoretically, endogenous reserves in a 1000 g infant are only sufficient for 4 days if unfed [5]. In addition, oral reflexes are immature, thus it is generally accepted that most infants <1000 g and many <1500 g will need some parenteral nutrition while enteral feeds are gradually increased to ensure an adequate nutritional intake.

The following is a brief discussion of the requirements for the major nutrients via the enteral route, unless otherwise specified. The most recent comprehensive review and recommendations, at the time of writing, are those of Tsang *et al.* [6] published in 2005. The interested reader is strongly advised to refer to this book for further information.

Table 6.1 Recommended enteral nutrient intakes for growing infants 1000–1500 g birthweight.

Nutrient	Recommended amount per kg
Protein (g)	26–30 weeks PCA 3.8–4.2*
	30–36 weeks PCA 3.4–3.6*
	36–40 weeks PCA 2.8–3.2*
Fat (g)	5.3–7.2
DHA (mg)	≥18 (0.2–0.5% total fat)
AA (mg)	≥24 (0.3–0.7% total fat)
AA : DHA	1.2–2 : 1
LA (mg/100 kcal)	352–1425
ALA (mg/100 kcal)	77–228
LA : ALA	6–16
Carbohydrate (g)	3.4–4.2
Minerals	
Sodium (mg)	69–115 (161[†])
Potassium (mg)	78–117
Chloride (mg)	107–249
Calcium (mg)	100–220
Phosphorus (mg)	60–140
Magnesium (mg)	7.9–15
Iron (mg)	2–4
Zinc (μg)	1000–3000
Copper (μg)	120–150
Iodine (μg)	10–60
Manganese (μg)	0.7–7.5
Selenium (μg)	1.3–4.5
Vitamins	
Vitamin A (μg)	210–450
Vitamin D (μg)	3.75–10 (min. 5, max. 25/day)
Vitamin E (mg)	6–12 (max 25 mg/day)
Vitamin K (μg)	8–10
Thiamin B_1 (μg)	180–240
Riboflavin B_2 (μg)	250–360
Niacin (mg)	3.6–4.8
Panthothenic acid (mg)	1.2–1.7
Pyridoxine B_6 (μg)	150–210
Folic acid (μg)	25–50
Vitamin B_{12} (μg)	0.3
Biotin (μg)	3.6–6
Vitamin C (mg)	18–24
Choline (mg)	14.4–28
Taurine (mg)	4.5–9
Inositol (mg)	32–81
Carnitine (mg)	~2.9
Nucleotides	see text
Beta-carotene	not specified

Source: Tsang *et al.* [6].
AA, arachidonic acid; ALA, α linolenic acid;
DHA, docosahexaenoic acid; LA, linoleic acid;
PCA, post-conceptional age.
* More may be needed for catch-up growth.
[†] May be needed if late hyponatraemia.

A summary of their recommendations is presented in Table 6.1. In this publication, precise requirements for infants born between 1.5 and 2.5 kg are not given. This has led to varying interpretations of the weight cut-offs for feeding preterm formula or fortifying breast milk. Higher nutrient density feeds are not routinely recommended for term SGA infants so gestational age as well as birthweight should be taken into account when deciding on local feeding policy. In practice, most infants born below 2 kg will benefit from the higher nutrient intakes recommended for infants born below 1.5 kg.

A further source of information is a review of recommendations for preterm infant formulas by Klein [7] which is available on the Internet.

Fluid

During the initial phase of adaptation to extrauterine life, fluid management is complicated as there is a delicate balance between matching high transcutaneous losses and avoiding fluid overload resulting from renal immaturity (although the latter should be minimised by appropriate nursing techniques). An extracellular fluid contraction is desirable over the first few days but this should not be excessive (i.e. more than around 7% birthweight). Early fluid management can lead to restricted volumes for feeding, particularly in the very sick preterm infant, but nutritional intakes should always be optimised within the fluid allowed and restrictions lifted as soon as clinical condition allows. In many neonatal units, current nutritional management leads to a large nutrient deficit when compared with recommended intakes [8], although it is not yet clearly established how this affects outcome.

Energy

The components contributing to energy requirements are summarised in Table 6.2 and demonstrate the wide range of intakes that may be necessary for maintenance and growth. In general, the upper extremes should be avoided. As measurement of individual energy expenditure remains a research tool, energy intake should be adjusted according to indirect measures (i.e. growth and serum biochemistry). Recommended

Table 6.2 Energy requirements.

	kcal/kg/day (multiply by 4.18 for kJ)		
	Acute phase	Intermediate phase	Convalescence
Resting energy expenditure (REE)*	45	50–60	50–70
Cold stress	0–10	0–10	5–10
Activity/handling[†]	0–10	5–15	5–15
Stool losses[‡]	0–10	10–15	10–15
Specific dynamic action[§]	0	0–5	10
Growth	0	20–30	20–30
Total[¶]	50–80	85–135	105–150

* The lower level applies to babies with normal REE, upper limit to those with diseases associated with increased REE (e.g. cardiac abnormalities/chronic lung disease).
[†] Zero if paralysed/heavily sedated.
[‡] Zero if on total parenteral nutrition.
[§] 10% of calories infused if on total parenteral nutrition.
[¶] Upper limit probably not physiological and should not be necessary.

energy intakes vary according to the baby's birthweight and postnatal age [6]. Table 6.3 shows requirements for babies <1.5 kg birthweight. Intakes above the individual baby's requirements will lead to higher weight gain, but this will usually be a result of fat deposition in excess of uterine accretion rate [9] and will lead to a higher metabolic rate [10]. There are no advantages in giving an energy intake higher than requirements for lean body mass or skeletal growth, particularly when protein intake is already >4 g/kg/day. Energy requirements may be decreased in very sick babies whose growth is slowed because of the stress response as the energy cost of growth is normally a substantial part of total

requirements [10,11]. Higher energy requirements may be necessary in some circumstances such as increased respiratory rate (as seen in chronic lung disease) [11], low body temperature [12] and excessive methylxanthine levels [13]. Some IUGR babies may have increased needs but this will vary between individuals and can only be established by monitoring progress and adjusting prescribed nutrient intakes accordingly. As discussed later, the concerns over the long term effects of excessive early growth need to be taken into consideration.

Protein

Recommended protein intakes vary in the same way as energy [6] (Tables 6.1 and 6.3). Between 27 and 35 weeks' gestation daily accretion of protein is around 2 g/kg. This can be achieved postnatally as long as the above protein intakes are accompanied by sufficient energy. Protein gain increases in a linear fashion up to an intake of around 4 g/kg/day after which it will reach a limit. The capacity for protein gain above the intrauterine rate may be useful when catch-up growth is occurring. In other circumstances, feeding over 4–5 g/kg/day should be approached with caution in case of additional metabolic stress on the vulnerable immature infant [14,15].

Hepatic immaturity leads to the need for exogenous supplies of cysteine, glycine and taurine normally considered non-essential in older babies.

Currently, there is much discussion concerning the potential benefits of providing more than the recommended equivalent of 2 g protein/kg within the first 24 hours following delivery. Studies evaluating this strategy have not yet found any benefits [16].

Table 6.3 Guidelines for energy and protein intakes for infants born <1500 g.

	Parenteral			Enteral		
	Day 1	Transition	Growing	Day 1	Transition	Growing
Energy (kcal/kg)*	40–50	60–85	90–115	50–60	75–100	110–150
Protein (g/kg)	2.0	3.5	3.2–4.0	2.0	3.5	3.4–4.4

Source: Tsang *et al.* [6].
NB the smaller the infant the higher the amount recommended.
* Multiply by 4.18 for kJ.

Fat

Fat absorption can vary between individuals but the more immature the infant the higher the risk for malabsorption because of low bile salt pools [17] and reduced pancreatic lipase levels [18]. Despite this, the fat component of both enteral and parenteral nutrition is crucial to attain the high energy requirements of preterm infants. Non-heat-treated breast milk has the advantage of an endogenous lipase (bile salt stimulated lipase) which ensures optimum fat absorption [19].

For many years, studies have investigated the theory that enteral medium chain triglycerides (MCT) would lead to improved fat absorption. However, a recent systematic review found no consistent advantage [20]. Despite this, some preterm formulas in North America have a high proportion of MCT but this is not the case in the UK.

It has been recommended that the long chain polyunsaturated (LCP) derivatives of linoleic and α linolenic acids, namely arachidonic (AA) and docosahexaenoic (DHA) acids are provided in the diet of preterm infants [6]. However, controversy remains concerning their role with a systematic review concluding that there were few significant benefits except some improved visual indices at 4 months, but not later in infancy [21].

Preterm infants, particularly those born VLBW and ELBW, will develop essential fatty acid deficiency very rapidly without an exogenous supply. This can be obtained from as little as 0.5 g/kg/day of one of the current parenteral lipid emulsions [22].

Carbohydrate

Many preterm formulas contain a mixture of lactose and glucose polymer to overcome the low lactase levels observed in preterm infants. Some work has been carried out looking at the addition of lactase to feeds but a systematic review concluded that there is no evidence of benefit and that more studies are needed [23]. Other data indicate that feeding a lactose containing milk will aid precocious development of lactase activity and hence feed tolerance [24]. In this study, human milk was more effective than formula milk. Poor tolerance of intravenous glucose infusion is common in sick preterm infants.

Folic acid

Requirements for folic acid have long been established [25] and preterm formulas are all fortified appropriately [6]. Many units still use a folic acid supplement and, although not seen as toxic, the appearance of unmetabolised folic acid in the serum may be undesirable, particularly in infants given a large weekly dose [26].

Fat-soluble vitamins

A note of caution is warranted when interpreting studies on enteral fat-soluble vitamin supplementation. Because of relatively poor enteral fat digestion and absorption (as discussed above), very high doses are often needed to normalise status [27]. Digestive capacity appears to develop rapidly in term infants [28] and dietary fat supplementation can enhance gastric lipase in preterm infants [29].

Vitamin A

Many preterm infants are born with poor vitamin A stores [30] and there is some evidence that high dose enteral supplementation (1500 µg/5000 IU/day) is needed to normalise serum levels [31]. There are data showing a small but significant reduction in rates of chronic lung disease (CLD) with early large doses of vitamin A [32]. However, there has been a low uptake of this strategy as it involves intramuscular injections and these could be considered unethical in small infants if the benefit derived is seen as relatively small [33,34]. In addition, CLD rates appear to be falling independent of changes in vitamin A intakes, probably because of a widespread use of prenatal steroids, postnatal surfactant administration and less aggressive ventilation techniques.

Vitamin D

Very high enteral intakes were thought necessary to avoid development of bone disease of prematurity, but experimental trials of high vs. lower doses did not improve outcome [35]. A recent study demonstrated that even a population from northerly latitudes, likely to have a lower range of vitamin D status at birth, did well on 10 µg/day [36]. A daily enteral intake of 5 µg (200 IU) to a maximum of 25 µg (1000 IU) total per day is recommended by Tsang *et al.* [6]. The upper limit is not encouraged, but is included as the upper tolerable amount recommended for term infants. The levels of vitamin D in Table 6.1 refer to those in the summary tables of Tsang *et al.* [6].

Vitamin E

There has been debate concerning the need for routine supplementation of preterm infants as some maintain an adequate status on unfortified breast milk. Interest in prevention of diseases thought to be associated with insufficient antioxidant defences led to trials of pharmacological doses. Nevertheless, a recent systematic review concluded that this strategy was not to be recommended [37].

Between 6 and 12 mg (6–12 IU) vitamin E/kg is recommended, with a minimum of 1 mg/g of linoleic acid and 0.7 mg/100 kcal (418 kJ) [6].

Calcium, phosphorus and magnesium

The fetus acquires 80% of the normal term body levels of calcium during the last trimester [38] and preterm infants have very high requirements for calcium and other minerals needed for bone formation. It has been suggested it is desirable to supply these minerals at the same levels as those that cross the placenta, although intrauterine retention rates may be achieved with lower intakes [39]. Contrary to earlier assumptions, inadequate mineral supply may be more important with respect to bone health in preterm infants than vitamin D [40]. Low plasma phosphate levels in particular seem to indicate higher risk of bone disease in this group and the aim should be to keep levels >1.8 mmol/L where possible [41]. Excessive calcium supplementation should be avoided because of the risk of interaction with fatty acids leading to calcium soap formation in the gut, particularly in formula fed babies. Calcium soaps are a risk for both intestinal bolus obstruction and reduced fat absorption [42,43].

Although a specific calcium : phosphorus ratio is not recommended [6], the authors discuss factors influencing the optimal ratio. In human milk it is 1.6 molar (2 by weight) and most preterm formulas are close to this. However, when supplements are added, their solubility will affect the relative amounts given. It is worth remembering that while there are several restraints on calcium absorption, phosphorus economy is controlled largely at the renal level and, because of the high soft tissue requirements for phosphorus, it may be needed in large amounts [44]. An important adjunct to appropriate nutrition for bone health may prove to be controlled physical activity [45] but this needs further careful evaluation.

Iron

Iron stores are low in preterm infants and without supplementation they will become depleted by 8 weeks [46]. Current recommendations are that supplements should start from 2 weeks as either a supplemented formula or medicinal iron at a level of 2–4 mg/kg/day [6]. Although the early anaemia of prematurity is not affected by iron supplementation, there is some evidence that infants supplemented by 2 weeks have better iron status at discharge [47]. For infants receiving human recombinant erythropoietin (EPO) a level of 6 mg/kg is recommended because of higher red blood cell production [6]. Despite high ferritin levels after blood transfusions this stored iron may not be readily available for haemopoiesis, therefore (although not stipulated by Tsang *et al.*) it is recommended by others that enteral iron supplementation continues regardless of transfusion status [48]. In well, moderately preterm infants a standard formula with an iron content of 0.5 mg/100 mL seems to meet iron needs post-discharge [49]. However, more may be needed for those who were smallest at birth and those who were sickest, because of lower iron stores and higher iron losses through multiple blood tests. As a result of the interactions of iron, copper and zinc during absorption, excessive amounts of each individual nutrient should be avoided.

Zinc

Zinc is an important component of many enzyme

systems and is essential for subcellular metabolism. Skeletal muscle stores are low in preterm compared with term infants and skeletal muscle accounts for 40% of body zinc stores [50]. Guidelines for intakes should ensure deficiency is avoided [6]. Renal losses may be high because of repeated acute phase protein responses [51] and diuretic therapy [52].

Selenium

Selenium is a component of the antioxidant enzyme glutathione peroxidase and is important in thyroid metabolism [53]. Selenium status is low at birth in preterm infants [54] and in theory puts them at risk of diseases thought to be related to oxidative damage. However, a large trial found no differences in markers of oxidative stress between supplemented and unsupplemented groups [55]. A systematic review concluded that supplementation was associated with a small reduction in sepsis rates, but no other benefit [56]. Nevertheless, it is important to ensure that guidelines are followed to prevent deficiency [6].

Iodine

The only major role of iodine is in thyroid metabolism, but as hypothyroidism is associated with poor neurodevelopmental outcome it is essential to ensure a good status. There is risk of deficiency with unsupplemented preterm formulas [57], although the relative role of iodine supply compared with other factors related to preterm birth are not yet clear [58].

Conditionally essential nutrients

Beta-carotene

No recommendations for the addition of beta-carotene to preterm formula exist although its presence in human milk, its role as an antioxidant and its provitamin-A activity have prompted some infant formula manufacturers to add it. Beta-carotene comprises only approximately 25% of the total carotenoid activity of human milk and its

levels vary greatly depending on time and number of lactations [59]. In adult studies, supplementation has led to adverse effects [60]. Intake should not be increased above that available from current formulas until evidence on outcome is available.

Nucleotides

Nucleotides are a constant component of mammalian milks and may be conditionally essential for the gut and immune system during times of stress [61]. Studies have been published describing reduction of diarrhoea in term infants [62] and improved growth in SGA infants [63]. Although no recommendations were made by Tsang et al. [6], there are figures in a summary table. This reflects the fact that the European Union has recognised nucleotides as semi-essential components of initial formula. However, in the preterm population supplemented formula requires further evaluation [64].

Glutamine

Glutamine is an important fuel for the small intestine and immune system and possibly becomes rate limiting during increased demand [65]. A large series of controlled trials have now been conducted to allow a conclusive systematic review which recommends that supplemental glutamine is of no benefit to preterm infants [66].

Parenteral nutrition

With increased survival, preterm infants have become major recipients of parenteral nutrition (PN). Initiation of some PN within the first 48 hours and subsequent increase to full requirements has been shown to be well tolerated in stable infants [67].

Because of high energy requirements, up to 12 mg/kg/minute glucose and 0.15 g/kg/hour lipid infusions are optimal and are well tolerated in stable infants [68,69] although the latter study evaluated only appropriately grown infants who were born over 27 weeks' gestation.

Above a 12 mg/kg/minute glucose infusion

rate there is likely to be a plateauing of glucose oxidation [68,70], indicating that no additional adenosine triphosphate (ATP) is being produced to support synthesis and growth. The unoxidised glucose would be used for lipogenesis which is an inefficient use of energy. However, raised blood glucose and triglyceride levels are common in sick preterm infants. Insulin is often given, but should not be used to aid tolerance of >12 mg/kg/minute glucose.

Reduction of lipid infusion in response to lipaemia should be as brief as possible to minimise suboptimal energy, fat-soluble vitamin and essential fatty acid intake. A systematic review of early vs. late intravenous lipid found no difference in clinical outcome [71].

There is a high risk of bone disease of prematurity when solutions containing inadequate levels of calcium and phosphate are given. For this reason, interest is growing in organic mineral salts such as glycerophosphate which allow larger amounts of mineral to be delivered because of their high solubility. Greene et al. [72,73] give a good review of parenteral mineral and vitamin requirements.

Parenteral solutions should be protected from high light exposure and this should help to minimise photodegradation of susceptible nutrients and production of toxic hydroperoxides. Despite the theories that many of the diseases found in preterm infants may be linked to oxidative stress, there is much contradictory evidence and more work is needed [74], but it still seems advisable to reduce a large oxidative load. Mixing the intravenous vitamin preparations with the lipid helps reduce degradation [75] and increase delivery of some of the vitamins and may protect against lipid oxidation [34].

Of the microminerals, zinc has not always been given with short term PN for preterm infants. However, there is now greater awareness of the high risk of zinc deficiency so it should always be included. In addition, zinc can be lost in large quantities via the renal route when given parenterally [6,76].

Enteral nutrition

The advantages of early and minimal enteral feeding have been shown in many studies although a recent systematic review concluded that further work was needed to completely exclude the possibility of increased risk of necrotising enterocolitis (NEC) [77] (see p. 83).

Human milk

Human milk has been evaluated for the feeding of preterm infants in many studies, but in a systematic review most were excluded because of methodological flaws in both design and execution, leaving just one to review [78]. When NEC was examined separately it was found that human milk did significantly reduce risk [79]. A significant problem is the difficulty in randomising infants to human milk, and this is not possible with mother's own milk. The milk of choice undoubtedly remains mother's own freshly expressed breast milk (EBM) [80]. Advantages include improved feed tolerance [81], reduced risk of NEC [82–84] and reduced risk of sepsis [81,85]. The latter two studies showed a dose-dependent reduction of risk. There may be long term neurodevelopmental advantages in feeding human milk [86,87]. Banked donor breast milk retains some immunological advantages and protects against NEC [79], although heat labile vitamins, bile salt stimulated lipase and live cells are reduced or destroyed in donor milk because it is pasteurised and it is recommend for initiation of feeds only in the absence of mother's own milk.

Human milk may be nutritionally adequate in many respects for infants >1500 g when fed in sufficient volumes (i.e. up to 220 mL/kg in well infants), although an iron supplement will be needed. However, in infants <1500 g several nutrients may be limiting, particularly protein, and some minerals and vitamins. Serum phosphate levels should be kept >1.5 mmol/L (preferably >1.8 mmol/L), but below serum calcium levels. When phosphate is <1.5 mmol/L, a supplement is required: 0.5 mmol twice a day has been given with a successful outcome [88]. Individual requirements can vary considerably so the dose should be titrated according to serum biochemistry.

Zinc bioavailability is greater from human milk than cow's milk based formula [89], but additional supplements are advised to ensure that high demands are met [6].

Breast milk during the first 2–3 weeks of lactation may have higher protein levels [90], although this is not a consistent finding and wide variations have been reported [91]. An indirect measure of protein intake is serum urea level. This was found to drop below 1.6 mmol/L in most cases when human milk protein intake fell <3 g/kg/day [92]. Protein fortification can be considered once serum urea reaches 2 mmol/L after a consistent fall. A commercially produced human milk fortifier has many advantages over supplementing with liquid formula, as this will allow use of full volumes of mother's milk. Although not all fortifiers have undergone sufficiently large trials, one North American product supported growth and was well tolerated [93]. A systematic review of available studies concluded that fortifiers promote short term growth, and that despite a lack of longer term outcome data it was unlikely that further trials would be carried out with an unfortified breast milk group [94]. Choosing a fortifier that brings human milk nutritional composition to within the Tsang guidelines will negate the need for separate additions of most minerals, vitamins and protein. However, a separate iron supplement will still be necessary. Fortification should occur as close to feeding time as possible to minimise interference with immunological factors [95]. Table 6.4 gives the composition of breast milk fortifiers available in the UK.

Routine supplementation of human milk with energy alone is not advised as there is a risk of reducing the protein : energy ratio to an unacceptably low level, particularly after the first 2 weeks of lactation. Occasionally, expressing technique may need improving to ensure all the hind milk is removed at each expression, thus avoiding a low fat and therefore low energy milk. When a mother is expressing milk of a lower fat content than average, a result can be that her infant has poor weight gain despite a serum urea level in the normal range. As yet there is not a bedside method for evaluating breast milk composition, although one group has shown improved weight gain when the latter half of each milk expression is fed preferentially [96]. There are no firm guidelines on how long fortification should continue and criteria include until the infant is feeding fully from the breast and thriving, or around a weight of 2.0–2.5 kg.

Preterm formulas

For those infants <2000 g birthweight who do not have access to human milk the feed of choice is a preterm formula. In addition, those infants whose mothers' milk supply is inadequate should be supplemented with preterm formula. However, it is not advisable to mix and store human milk and formula for prolonged periods. There has been some work suggesting that hydrolysed protein formulas lead to shorter gastrointestinal transit times compared with whole protein [97] and might be preferable. This has resulted in reduced time taken to reach full feeds in one trial [98], although breast milk led to the largest cumulative feeding volume when compared with either milk formulas [99].

Preterm formulas are highly specialised feeds designed to meet the increased nutritional needs of preterm infants without exceeding volume tolerance. Although they all generally follow Tsang et al.'s [6] guidelines they do still differ significantly in some aspects. Table 6.5 gives the composition of preterm formulas currently available in the UK.

Of note are the differing levels of iron, fat-soluble vitamins and some of the 'conditionally' essential nutrients (e.g. arachidonic acid, docosohexaenoic acid, nucleotides, inositol and beta-carotene). Some formulas will need supplementing with iron in order to comply fully with the most recent guidelines, and although all contain sufficient folic acid many units appear to continue giving supplements. There is a wide variation between neonatal units as to the age and weight at which preterm formula is stopped. A suggested range is between 2.0 and 2.5 kg body weight, or discharge from hospital, whichever is sooner. Using the upper weight limit may shorten time to achieve catch-up growth and allow infants to achieve the nutrient intake they need without having to take very large feed volumes [100]. It is important to remember that at any age or weight each individual baby may need assessment to decide on the optimum formula.

Aggressive nutrition

There has been much speculation that early nutritional support followed by an 'aggressive' approach will give clinical benefits [101]. However,

Table 6.4   Composition of human milk and breast milk fortifiers available in the UK.

Composition of recommended dose	Nutriprem breast milk fortifier (Cow & Gate)	SMA breast milk fortifier (SMA)*	Mature human milk[†]
Recommended dose (g/100 mL breast milk)	4.2	4	–
Protein (g)	0.8[‡]	1.0	1.3
Casein : whey	50 : 50	0 : 100	60 : 40
Energy (kcal) (kJ)[§]	15 (63)	14.6 (61)	69 (288)
Minerals (mg)			
Calcium	64	90	34
Phosphorus	44	46	15
Magnesium	6	3	3
Sodium	10	18	15
Potassium	8	28	58
Chloride	7	17	42
Trace elements (µg)			
Zinc	400	260	300
Copper	30	NP	40
Manganese	8	4.6	Tr
Iodine	11	NP	7
Vitamins (µg)			
Vitamin A	130	270	58
Vitamin C (mg)	12	40	4
Vitamin D	5	7.6	Tr
Vitamin E (mg)	2.6	3	0.34
Vitamin K	6.3	11	–
Biotin	2.5	1.5	0.7
Folic acid	50	30	5
Niacin (mg)	2.3	3.6	0.2
Vitamin B_{12}	0.2	0.3	Tr
Pyridioxine B_6	110	260	10
Riboflavin B_2	170	260	30
Thiamin	130	220	20
Pantothenic Acid B_5	750	900	250
Beta-carotene	NP	15	(24)
Presentation	2.1 g sachet powder	2 g sachet powder	

Figures for breast milk fortifiers only correct at time of publication; check manufacturers' data.
NP, not present.
* Available on request to company.
[†] Food Standards Agency. *McCance and Widdowson's The Composition of Foods*, 6th summary edn. Cambridge: Royal Society of Chemistry, 2002. The composition of breast milk is variable and these figures should be used with caution when considering the individual infant.
[‡] Hydrolysed protein.
[§] Energy source carbohydrate.

several studies investigating this approach have not shown any clinical advantages, just faster growth [16,102,103].

When looking at the data for long term outcome there is evidence that early very poor growth is detrimental to later development, but that breast milk can ameliorate these effects [86,87,104], hence reinforcing the recommendation that wherever possible breast milk should be used. In addition, recent data indicate that early rapid growth may

Table 6.5   Composition of preterm formulas in the UK.

Nutrients per 100 mL	Pre-Aptamil (Milupa)	Nutriprem 1 (Cow & Gate)	SMA Gold Prem (SMA)	Pre Nan (Nestlé)	Osterprem (Farley's)
Energy (kcal) (kJ)	80 (334)	80 (334)	82 (343)	80 (334)	80 (334)
Protein (g)	2.5	2.5	2.2	2.3	2.0
Fat (g)	4.4	4.4	4.4	4.2	4.6
MCT (g)	0.8	0.8	12.5%	26%	NP
LCP	AA/DHA/GLA	AA/DHA/GLA	AA/DHA	AA/DHA/GLA	DHA/GLA
Linoleic acid (g)	0.58	0.58	0.7	0.63	0.54
Linolenic acid (g)	0.08	0.08	0.064	0.07	0.06
Carbohydrate (g)	7.6	7.6	8.4	8.6	7.6
Fibre (g) (prebiotics)	0.8	0.8	NP	NP	NP
Minerals					
Sodium (mg)	50	50	42	33	42
Potassium (mg)	72	72	85	95	72
Chloride (mg)	66	66	60	51	60
Calcium (mg)	120	120	101	99	110
Phosphorus (mg)	66	66	61	54	63
Ca : P ratio (by weight)	2 : 1	2 : 1	1.7 : 1	1.8 : 1	1.7 : 1
Magnesium (mg)	8	8	8.2	8.0	5
Iron (mg)	1.4	1.4	0.8	1.2	0.04
Zinc (mg)	0.9	0.9	0.8	1.0	0.9
Copper (µg)	80	80	90	80	96
Iodine (µg)	25	25	10	20	20
Manganese (µg)	4.4	4.4	10	6.0	3
Selenium (µg)	1.9	1.9	1.7	1.7	1.4*
Vitamins					
Vitamin A (µg)	180	180	185	84	100
Vitamin D (µg)	3	3	3.4	2	2.4
Vitamin E (mg)	3.0	3.0	2.5	1.3	10
Vitamin K (µg)	6	6	8.0	6.4	7.0
Thiamin B_1 (mg)	0.14	0.14	0.135	0.056	0.1
Riboflavin B_2 (mg)	0.2	0.2	0.2	0.12	0.18
Niacin (mg NE)	3.2	3.2	2.87	0.8	1.0
Panthothenic acid (mg)	1.0	1.0	1	0.36	0.5
Pyridoxine B_6 (mg)	0.12	0.12	0.1	0.06	0.1
Folic acid (µg)	28	28	34	56	50
Vitamin B_{12} (µg)	0.18	0.18	0.3	0.24	0.2
Biotin (µg)	3.0	3.0	2.4	1.8	2.0
Vitamin C (mg)	13	13	16	13	28
Other					
Choline (mg)	13	13	15	12	5.6
Taurine (mg)	5.5	5.5	6	6.4	5.1
Inositol (mg)	40	40	30	5.2	3.2
Carnitine (mg)	1.8	1.8	2.6	1.7	1.0
Nucleotides (mg)	3.2	3.2	NP	NP	4.1
Beta-carotene (µg)	NP	NP	4	NP	24
Osmolality (mOsmol/kg/H_2O)	305	305	291	325	300

Figures for preterm formulas only correct at time of publication; check manufacturers' data.

AA, arachidonic acid; DHA, docosahexaenoic acid; GLA, gamma-linolenic acid; LCP, long chain polyunsaturated fatty acids; MCT, medium chain triglycerides; NP, not present.

* Naturally present.

lead to increased risk factors for cardiovascular disease later in life [105,106]. More evidence is needed before a truly aggressive nutritional approach is employed routinely.

Method of enteral feeding

Because of an immature suck–swallow–breathe pattern, preterm infants require tube feeding until around 35–37 weeks' gestation, some longer. There are advantages and disadvantages to both bolus and continuous gastric tube feeding with a recent systematic review unable to give a firm recommendation of one method over the other [107]. Boluses have been associated with less feed intolerance [83], but they may lead to a deterioration in respiratory function (resulting from gastric distension) in very compromised infants when compared with continuous feeds [108]. Continuous feeding of human milk can lead to excessive fat loss [109] and risk of sedimentation of added minerals. An alternative method has been shown to work well; this involves 2-hour slow infusion every 3 hours and has led to improved feed tolerance [110]. Transpyloric feeding is not recommended for routine use because of adverse outcomes in preterm infants [111]. There is evidence that rapid advancement of enteral feeds is associated with increased risk of NEC [112,113]. A limit of 20 mL/kg/day increase in feed volume has been recommended in those felt to be at high risk of NEC.

For some infants, particularly those who have been very unwell, the transition to nipple feeding, either breast or bottle, is very difficult. Liaison with an experienced speech and language therapist is invaluable in these circumstances. Some mother–infant pairs benefit from specialist advice on establishing breast feeding and, with support, infants born as young as 24 weeks can leave neonatal units fully breast feeding.

Feeding issues in special conditions

Necrotising enterocolitis

Necrotising enterocolitis is a serious inflammatory disease of the bowel occurring predominantly in preterm infants. Although it is relatively rare, there can be large variations between neonatal units in its prevalence, suggesting that modifiable factors are involved [113]. There has been much investigation into its aetiology because of its high mortality and morbidity rates. It appears to be triggered by a combination of one or all of the following factors: prematurity, hypoxia, gut ischaemia, gut bacterial overgrowth, disturbance of gut bacterial balance, sepsis, feeding of formula milk and over rapid advancement of enteral feeds. Although one single set of guidelines has not been identified, it does appear that institution of a standardised feeding protocol leads to large reductions in the incidence of NEC [114].

Chronic lung disease

Chronic lung disease, previously known as bronchopulmonary dysplasia, is a disease first described following the survival of mechanically ventilated infants. It appears that this condition is on the decrease as a result of several factors, including more widespread use of prenatal steroids to help accelerate maturation of the infant's lungs, postnatal surfactant administered directly into the infant's lungs to improve compliance and, more recently, more rapid transfer from mechanical intratracheal ventilation to nasal continuous positive airway pressure (CPAP). It is now only the most immature and compromised at birth who sustain this disease. Lung damage probably results from the barotrauma of ventilation, and possibly oxygen toxicity, although strategies to enhance antioxidant defences have not been effective in reducing CLD [55]. The result is a requirement for prolonged ventilatory support and possible discharge home on nasal prong oxygen. Elevated energy expenditure has been closely associated with respiratory status in one study [11], but not in another [115]. There is evidence for some increase in energy requirements with CLD [116]. The doubly labelled water technique has shown far more variable expenditures in those with CLD [117]. Thus, routine energy supplementation is not recommended in CLD but individual assessment is advised. Interestingly, intervention studies where infants were randomised to have increased nutritional intake have not prevented the disease [102] or improved respiratory outcome or growth [118,119].

As a result of long term adverse effects, use of steroids to aid weaning from ventilatory support has now virtually stopped, thus eliminating the major negative impact they have on growth in preterm babies.

Babies with CLD can show growth failure resistant to nutritional intervention and other factors should be considered (e.g. sodium depletion) [120], particularly if on diuretics, and the effect of inadequate oxygen therapy [121].

Post-discharge nutrition

All mothers should be encouraged to breast feed their infants on demand wherever possible after discharge from hospital, with close attention to growth monitoring. Infants who are breast feeding on discharge will need iron and a multivitamin supplement (containing vitamin D). For those mothers who cannot breast feed, a post-discharge formula is recommended. Nutrient enriched post-discharge formula (NEPDF) was developed following observations that preterm infants take up to 300 mL/kg of term formula post-discharge [100]. There are two brands available on prescription in the UK:

- Nutriprem 2 75 kcal (310 kJ)/100 mL; 2.0 g protein/100 mL
- PremCare 72 kcal (301 kJ)/100 mL; 1.85 g protein/100 mL

Although limited, there are data showing improved growth and bone mineralisation (the latter mainly in boys) in infants taking NEPDF, but no developmental advantages [122]. However, there are practical advantages in using a NEPDF such as providing additional vitamins and minerals, particularly iron, negating the need for separate supplements. Babies discharged on these formulas should on the whole take lower volumes that they would if on a term formula, and this can help parents cope with caring for their baby at home.

These formulas are prescribable to 6 months of age although major advantages of feeding them for this length of time are yet to be shown [122]. Achievement of catch-up growth may be used as a guide as to when to stop using them. Use of NEPDF for a period should speed up achievement of more normal bone mineralisation. Although NEPDF are currently prescribable for low birth weight as well as preterm infants there is no evidence that they are of any benefit to small term infants [123].

After NEPDF is stopped, a term formula can be used up to 12–18 months of age. Iron status should be adequately maintained without supplements on this formula [49], although some infants with limited dietary intakes may still need them. When formula or breast milk is changed to unmodified cow's milk at 12–18 months, the infant should be started on Healthy Start Children's Vitamin Drops as per Department of Health guidelines [124] (see Table 1.18).

Weaning onto solids

Introduction of solids is not recommended before 6 months for the general population, but the government guidelines are not intended for special groups such as preterm babies [125]. In this group there is very little published work to guide advice although anecdotal reports indicate that introduction at 5 months post-delivery is successful. Advice is not to start earlier than this unless there are exceptional circumstances. A suggested upper limit to start weaning is 7 months post-delivery. Although many infants will be at a relatively young post-conceptional age, there is evidence that preterm delivery leads to accelerated maturation of many organ systems, thus protecting the preterm infant against adverse effects associated with 'early' weaning. For example, the introduction of milk feeds leads to a precocious development of digestion and motility in the gastrointestinal tract [24,126]. There is no evidence for increased risk of allergy [127]. On the other hand, preterm infants seem to have a higher prevalence of behavioural feeding problems [128] particularly associated with chronic health problems [129]. This may be because of solids (particularly lumps) being delayed beyond a critical period for their acceptance. Direct evidence for this is lacking but case studies [130] and other observational data indicate a link [131]. Once weaning has started it should proceed according to current guidelines [124], with added advice provided in a booklet produced specifically to advise on weaning preterm infants produced by BLISS, a London based charity for the premature babies [132].

References

1   Pallotto EK, Kilbride HW Perinatal outcome and later implications of intrauterine growth restriction. *Clin Obstet Gynecol*, 2006, **49** 257–69.

2   Galbraith RS, Karchmar EJ, Piercy WN *et al.* The clinical prediction of intrauterine growth retardation. *Am J Obstet Gynecol*, 1979, **133** 281–6.

3   Sparks JW Human intrauterine growth and nutrient accretion. *Semin Perinatol*, 1984, **8** 74–93.

4   Friss-Hanson B Body composition during growth: *in vivo* measurements and biochemical data correlated to differential anatomical growth. *Pediatrics*, 1971, **47** 264–74.

5   Heird WC, Driscoll JM, Jr, Schullinger JN *et al.* Intravenous alimentation in pediatric patients. *J Pediatr*, 1972, **80** 351–72.

6   Tsang RC, Uauy R, Koletzko B *et al. Nutrition of the Preterm Infant: Scientific Basis and Practical Guidelines*, 2nd edn. Cincinnati, Ohio: Digital Educational Publishing, 2005.

7   Klein CJ Nutrient requirements for preterm infant formulas. *J Nutr*, 2002, **132** (Suppl 1) 1395S–577S.

8   Embleton NE, Pang N, Cooke RJ Postnatal malnutrition and growth retardation: an inevitable consequence of current recommendations in preterm infants? *Pediatrics*, 2001, **107** 270–3.

9   Kashyap S, Schulze KF, Forsyth M *et al.* Growth, nutrient retention, and metabolic response in low birth weight infants fed varying intakes of protein and energy. *J Pediatr*, 1988, **113** 713–21.

10 Brooke OG Energy balance and metabolic rate in preterm infants fed with standard and high-energy formulas. *Br J Nutr*, 1980, **44** 13–23.

11 de Meer K, Westerterp KR, Houwen RH *et al.* Total energy expenditure in infants with bronchopulmonary dysplasia is associated with respiratory status. *Eur J Pediatr*, 1997, **156** 299–304.

12 Sauer PJ, Dane HJ, Visser HK Longitudinal studies on metabolic rate, heat loss, and energy cost of growth in low birth weight infants. *Pediatr Res*, 1984, **18** 254–9.

13 Bauer J, Maier K, Linderkamp O *et al.* Effect of caffeine on oxygen consumption and metabolic rate in very low birth weight infants with idiopathic apnea. *Pediatrics*, 2001, **107** 660–3.

14 Raiha NCR, Heinonen K, Rassin DK *et al.* Milk protein quantity and quality in low birth weight infants: I metabolic responses and effects on growth. *Pediatrics*, 1976, **57** 659–74.

15 Svenningsen NW, Lindroth M, Lindquist B Growth in relation to protein intake of low birth weight infants. *Early Hum Dev*, 1982, **6** 47–58.

16 Ibrahim HM, Jeroudi MA, Baier RJ *et al.* Aggressive early total parenteral nutrition in low-birth-weight infants. *J Perinatol*, 2004, **24** 482–6.

17 Signer E, Murphy GM, Edkins S, Anderson CM Role of bile salts in fat malabsorption of premature infants. *Arch Dis Child*, 1974, **49** 174–80.

18 Hamosh M Lipid metabolism in premature infants. *Biol Neonate*, 1987, **52** (Suppl 1) 50–64.

19 Morgan C, Stammers J, Colley J *et al.* Fatty acid balance studies in preterm infants fed formula milk containing long-chain polyunsaturated fatty acids (LCP) II. *Acta Paediatr*, 1998, **87** 318–24.

20 Klenoff-Brumberg HL, Genen LH High versus low medium chain triglyceride content of formula for promoting short term growth of preterm infants. *Cochrane Database Syst Rev* 2003: CD002777.

21 Simmer K, Patole S Longchain polyunsaturated fatty acid supplementation in preterm infants. *Cochrane Database Syst Rev* 2004: CD000375.

22 Cooke RJ, Yeh YY, Gibson D *et al.* Soybean oil emulsion administration during parenteral nutrition in the preterm infant: effect on essential fatty acid, lipid, and glucose metabolism. *J Pediatr*, 1987, **111** 767–73.

23 Tan-Dy CR, Ohlsson A Lactase treated feeds to promote growth and feeding tolerance in preterm infants. *Cochrane Database Syst Rev* 2005, **2** CD004591.

24 Shulman RJ, Schanler RJ, Lau C *et al.* Early feeding, feeding tolerance, and lactase activity in preterm infants. *J Pediatr*, 1998, **133** 645–9.

25 Ek J, Behncke L, Halvorsen KS *et al.* Plasma and red cell folate values and folate requirements in formula fed premature infants. *Eur J Pediatr*, 1984, **142** 78–82.

26 Kelly P, McPartland J, Goggins M *et al.* Unmetabolised folic acid in serum: acute studies in subjects consuming fortified food and supplements. *Am J Clin Nutr*, 1997, **65** 1790–5.

27 Delvin EE, Salle BL, Claris O *et al.* Oral vitamin A, E and D supplementation of pre-term newborns either breast-fed or formula-fed: a 3-month longitudinal study. *J Pediatr Gastroenterol Nutr*, 2005, **40** 43–7.

28 Manson W, Dale E, Harding M *et al.* Functional capacity of the newborn to digest dietary fats. *J Pediatr Gastroenterol Nutr*, 1996, **22** 427A.

29 Pereira G, Barsky D, Hamosh M *et al.* Dietary fat supplements enhances gastric lipase activity in premature neonates. *Pediatr Res*, 1995, **37** 316A.

30 Mupanemunda RH, Lee DS, Fraher LJ *et al.* Postnatal changes in serum retinol status in very low birth weight infants. *Early Hum Dev*, 1994, **38** 45–54.

31 Landman J, Sive A, De V *et al.* Comparison of enteral and intramuscular vitamin A supplementation in preterm infants. *Earl Hum Dev*, 1992, **30** 163–70.

32 Tyson JE, Wright LL, Oh WOM *et al.* Vitamin A supplementation for extremely-low-birth-weight infants. *N Engl J Med*, 1999, **340** 1962–8.

33 Darlow BA, Graham PJ Vitamin A supplementation for preventing morbidity and mortality in very low birthweight infants. *Cochrane Database Syst Rev* 2002, **4** CD000501.

34 Mactier H, Weaver LT Vitamin A and preterm infants: what we know, what we don't know, and what we need to know. *Arch Dis Child Fetal Neonatal Ed*, 2005, **90** F103–8.

35 Evans JR, Allen AC, Stinson DA *et al.* Effect of high-dose vitamin D supplementation on radiographically detectable bone disease of very low birth weight infants. *J Pediatr*, 1989, **115** 779–86.

36 Backstrom MC, Maki R, Kuusela AL *et al.* Randomised controlled trial of vitamin D supplementation on bone density and biochemical indices in preterm infants. *Arch Dis Child*, 1999, **80** F161–6.

37 Brion L, Bell E, Raghuveer T Vitamin E supplementation for prevention of morbidity and mortality in preterm infants. *Cochrane Database Syst Rev* 2003, **4** CD003665.

38 Ziegler EE, O'Donnell AM, Nelson SE *et al.* Body composition of the reference fetus growth. *Growth*, 1976, **40** 329–41.

39 Pittard WB, Geddes KM, Sutherland SE *et al.* Longitudinal changes in the bone mineral content of term and premature infants. *Am J Dis Child*, 1990, **144** 36–40.

40 Koo WW, Sherman R, Succop P *et al.* Serum vitamin D metabolites in very low birth weight infants with and without rickets and fractures. *J Pediatr*, 1989, **114** 1017–22.

41 Aiken CG, Sherwood RA, Lenney W Role of plasma phosphate measurements in detecting rickets of prematurity and in monitoring treatment. *Ann Clin Biochem*, 1993, **30** 469–75.

42 Flikweert ER, La Hei ER, De Rijke YB *et al.* Return of the milk curd syndrome. *Pediatr Surg Int*, 2003, **19** 628–31.

43 Chappell JE, Clandinin MT, Kearney VC *et al.* Fatty acid balance studies in premature infants fed human milk or formula: effect of calcium supplementation. *J Pediatr*, 1986, **108** 439–47.

44 Mize CE, Uauy R, Waidelich D *et al.* Effect of phosphorus supply on mineral balance at high calcium intakes in very low birth weight infants. *Am J Clin Nutr*, 1995, **62** 385–91.

45 Litmanovitz I, Dolfin T, Friedland O *et al.* Early physical activity intervention prevents decrease of bone strength in very low birth weight infants. *Pediatrics*, 2003, **112** 15–19.

46 Olivares M, Llaguno S, Marin V *et al.* Iron status in low-birth-weight infants, small and appropriate for gestational age: a follow-up study. *Acta Paediatr*, 1992, **81** 824–8.

47 Yuen D, Kim J, Brazeau Gravelle P Early iron (Fe) supplementation of low birth weight (LBW) infants improves erythropoiesis. *Pediatr Res*, 1996, **39** 322A.

48 Ehrenkranz RA Iron requirements of preterm infants. *Nutrition*, 1994, **10** 77–8.

49 Griffin IJ, Cooke RJ, Reid MM *et al.* Iron nutritional status in preterm infants fed formulas fortified with iron. *Arch Dis Child*, 1999, **81** F45–9.

50 Aggett PJ Trace elements of the micropremie. *Clin Perinatol*, 2000, **27** 119–29.

51 Askari A, Long CL, Blakemore WS Urinary zinc, copper, nitrogen, and potassium losses in response to trauma. *J Parenter Enteral Nutr*, 1979, **3** 151–6.

52 Wester PO Tissue zinc at autopsy: relation to medication with diuretics. *Acta Med Scand*, 1980, **208** 269–71.

53 Daniels LA Selenium metabolism and bioavailability. *Biol Trace Elem Res*, 1996, **54** 185–99.

54 Lockitch G, Jacobson B, Quigley G *et al.* Selenium deficiency in low birth weight neonates: an unrecognized problem. *J Pediatr*, 1989, **114** 865–70.

55 Winterbourn CC, Chan T, Buss IH *et al.* Protein carbonyls and lipid peroxidation products as oxidation markers in preterm infant plasma: associations with chronic lung disease and retinopathy and effects of selenium supplementation. *Pediatr Res*, 2000, **48** 84–90.

56 Darlow BA, Austin NC Selenium supplementation to prevent short-term morbidity in preterm neonates. *Cochrane Database Syst Rev* 2003, **4** CD003312.

57 Ares S, Quero J, Duran S *et al.* Iodine content of infant formulas and iodine intake of premature babies: high risk of iodine deficiency. *Arch Dis Child Fetal Neonatal Ed*, 1994, **71** F184–91.

58 Ares S, Escobar-Morreale HF, Quero J *et al.* Neonatal hypothyroxinemia: effects of iodine intake and premature birth. *J Clin Endocrinol Metab*, 1997, **82** 1704–12.

59 Patton S, Canfield LM, Huston GE *et al.* Carotenoids of human colostrum. *Lipids*, 1990, **25** 159–65.

60 Rowe PM Beta-carotene takes a collective beating. *Lancet*, 1996, **347** 249.

61 Schlimme E, Martin D, Meisel H Nucleosides and nucleotides: natural bioactive substances in milk and colostrum. *Br J Nutr*, 2000, **84** (Suppl 1) S59–S68.

62 Brunser O, Espinoza J, Araya M *et al.* Effect of dietary nucleotide supplementation on diarrhoeal disease in infants. *Acta Paediatr*, 1994, **83** 188–91.

63 Cosgrove M, Davies DP, Jenkins HR Nucleotide supplementation and the growth of term small for gestational age infants. *Arch Dis Child Fetal Neonatal Ed*, 1996, **74** F122–5.

64 Carver JD, Stromquist CI Dietary nucleotides and preterm infant nutrition. *J Perinatol*, 2006, **26** 443–4.

65 Powell-Tuck J Glutamine, parenteral feeding, and intestinal nutrition. *Lancet*, 1993, **342** 451–2.

66 Tubman TR, Thompson SW, McGuire W Glutamine supplementation to prevent morbidity and mortality in preterm infants. *Cochrane Database Syst Rev* 2005, **1** CD001457.

67 Murdock N, Crighton A, Nelson LM *et al.* Low birthweight infants and total parenteral nutrition immediately after birth. II. Randomised study of biochemical tolerance of intravenous glucose, amino acids, and lipid. *Arch Dis Child Fetal Neonatal Ed*, 1995, **73** F8–12.

68 Bresson JL, Narcy P, Putet G *et al.* Energy substrate utilization in infants receiving total parenteral nutrition with different glucose to fat ratios. *Pediatr Res*, 1989, **25** 645–8.

69 Brans YW, Andrew DS, Carrillo DW *et al.* Tolerance of fat emulsions in very-low-birth-weight neonates. *Am J Dis Child*, 1988, **142** 145–52.

70 Jones MO, Pierro A, Hammond P *et al.* Glucose utilisation in the surgical newborn infant receiving total parenteral nutrition. *J Pediatr Surg*, 1993, **28** 1121–5.

71 Simmer K, Rao SC Early introduction of lipids to parenterally-fed preterm infants. *Cochrane Database Syst Rev* 2005, **2** CD005256.

72 Greene HL, Smith R, Pollack P *et al.* Intravenous vitamins for very-low-birth-weight infants. *J Am Coll Nutr*, 1991, **10** 281–8.

73 Greene HL, Hambidge KM, Schanler R *et al.* Guidelines for the use of vitamins, trace elements, calcium, magnesium, and phosphorus in infants and children receiving total parenteral nutrition: report of the Subcommittee on Pediatric Parenteral Nutrient Requirements from the Committee on Clinical Practice Issues of the American Society for Clinical Nutrition [published errata appear in *Am J Clin Nutr*, 1989, **49** 1332 and 1989, **50** 560]. *Am J Clin Nutr*, 1988, **48** 1324–42.

74 Pitkanen OM Parenteral lipids and the preterm infant: between Scylla and Charybdis. *Acta Paediatr*, 2004, **93** 1028–30.

75 Neuzil J, Darlow BA, Inder TE *et al.* Oxidation of parenteral lipid emulsion by ambient and phototherapy lights: potent toxicity of routine parenteral feeding. *J Pediatr*, 1995, **126** 785–96.

76 Zlotkin SH, Buchanan BE Meeting zinc and copper intake requirements in the parenterally fed preterm and full-term infant. *J Pediatr*, 1983, **103** 441–6.

77 Tyson JE, Kennedy KA Trophic feedings for parenterally fed infants. *Cochrane Database Syst Rev* 2005, **3** CD000504.

78 McGuire W, Anthony MY Formula milk versus preterm human milk for feeding preterm or low birth weight infants. *Cochrane Database Syst Rev* 2001, **3** CD002972.

79 McGuire W, Anthony MY Donor human milk versus formula for preventing necrotising enterocolitis in preterm infants: systematic review. *Arch Dis Child Fetal Neonatal Ed*, 2003, **88** F11–14.

80 Jones E, King C *Feeding and Nutrition in the Preterm Infant*. China: Elsevier Churchill Livingstone, 2005.

81 Uraizee F, Gross SJ Improved feeding tolerance and reduced incidence of sepsis in sick very low birth weight (VLBW) infants fed maternal milk. *Pediatr Res*, 1989, **25** 298A.

82 Schanler RJ, Shulman RJ, Lau C Feeding strategies for premature infants: beneficial outcomes of feeding fortified human milk versus preterm formula. *Pediatrics*, 1999, **103** 1150–7.

83 Schanler RJ, Shulman RJ, Lau C *et al.* Feeding strategies for premature infants: randomized trial of gastrointestinal priming and tube-feeding method. *Pediatrics*, 1999, **103** 434–9.

84 Lucas A, Cole TJ Breast milk and neonatal necrotising enterocolitis. *Lancet*, 1990, **336** 1519–23.

85 Hylander MA, Strobino DM, Dhanireddy R Human milk feedings and infection among very low birth weight infants. *Pediatrics*, 1998, **102** E38.

86 Lucas A, Morley R, Cole T Randomised trial of early diet in preterm babies and later intelligence quotient. *Br Med J*, 1998, **317** 1481–7.

87 Lucas A, Morley R, Cole TJ *et al.* A randomised multicentred study of human milk vs formula and later development in preterm infants. *Arch Dis Child*, 1994, **70** F141–6.

88 Holland P, Wilkinson A, Diez J *et al.* Prenatal deficiency of phosphate, phosphate supplementation and rickets in very low birth weight infants. *Lancet*, 1990, **335** 697–701.

89 Sandstrom B, Cederblad A, Lonnerdal B Zinc absorption from human milk, cow's milk, and infant formulas. *Am J Dis Child*, 1983, **137** 726–9.

90 Lucas A, Hudson GJ Preterm milk as a source of protein for low birth weight infants. *Arch Dis Child*, 1984, **59** 831–6.

91 Velona T, Abbiati L, Beretta B *et al.* Protein profiles in breast milk from mothers delivering term and preterm babies. *Pediatr Res*, 1999, **45** 658–63.

92 Polberger SKT, Axelsson IE, Raitia NCR Urinary and serum urea as indicators of protein metabolism in very low birth weight infants fed varying human milk protein intakes. *Acta Paediatr Scand*, 1990, **79** 737–42.

93 Lucas A, Fewtrell MS, Morley R Randomised outcome trial of human milk fortification and developmental outcome in preterm infants. *Am J Clin Nutr*, 1996, **64** 142–51.

94   Kuschel CA, Harding JE Multicomponent fortified human milk for promoting growth in preterm infants. *Cochrane Database Syst Rev* 2004, **1** CD000343.

95   Quan R, Yang C, Rubinstein S *et al.* The effect of nutritional additives on anti-infective factors in human milk. *Clin Pediatr (Phila)*, 1994, **33** 325–8.

96   Vasan U, Meier P, Meier W *et al.* Individualizing the lipid content of own mothers milk: effect of weight gain for extremely low birth weight (ELBW) infants. *Pediatr Res*, 2004, **43** 270A.

97   Mihatsch WA, Hogel J, Pohlandt F Hydrolysed protein accelerates the gastrointestinal transport of formula in preterm infants. *Acta Paediatr*, 2001, **90** 196–8.

98   Mihatsch WA, Franz AR, Hogel J *et al.* Hydrolyzed protein accelerates feeding advancement in very low birth weight infants. *Pediatrics*, 2002, **110** 1199–203.

99   Mihatsch WA, von Schoenaich P, Fahnenstich H *et al.* Randomized, multicenter trial of two different formulas for very early enteral feeding advancement in extremely-low-birth-weight infants. *J Pediatr Gastroenterol Nutr*, 2001, **33** 155–9.

100 Lucas A, King F, Bishop NB Post discharge formula consumption in infants born preterm. *Arch Dis Child*, 1992, **67** 691–2.

101 Ziegler EE, Thureen PJ, Carlson SJ Aggressive nutrition of the very low birthweight infant. *Clin Perinatol*, 2002, **29** 225–44.

102 Wilson DC, Cairns P, Halliday HL *et al.* Randomised controlled trial of an aggressive nutritional regimen in sick very low birthweight infants. *Arch Dis Child Fetal Neonatal Ed*, 1997, **77** F4–11.

103 Dinerstein A, Nieto RM, Solana CL *et al.* Early and aggressive nutritional strategy (parenteral and enteral) decreases postnatal growth failure in very low birth weight infants. *J Perinatol*, 2006, **26** 436–42.

104 Lucas A, Morley R, Cole TJ *et al.* Early diet in preterm babies and developmental status at 18 months. *Lancet*, 1990, **335** 1477–81.

105 Singhal A, Cole TJ, Fewtrell M *et al.* Is slower early growth beneficial for long-term cardiovascular health? *Circulation*, 2004, **109** 1108–13.

106 Cianfarani S, Germani D, Branca F Low birthweight and adult insulin resistance: the 'catch-up growth' hypothesis. *Arch Dis Child*, 1999, **81** F71–3.

107 Premji S, Chessell L Continuous nasogastric milk feeding versus intermittent bolus milk feeding for premature infants less than 1500 grams. *Cochrane Database Syst Rev* 2003, **1** CD001819.

108 Macagno F, Demarini S Techniques of enteral feeding in the newborn. *Acta Paediatr Suppl*, 1994, **402** 11–13.

109 Narayanan I, Singh B, Harvey D Fat loss during feeding of human milk. *Arch Dis Child*, 1984, **59** 475–7.

110 de Ville K, Knapp E, Al Tawil Y *et al.* Slow infusion feedings enhance duodenal motor responses and gastric emptying in preterm infants. *Am J Clin Nutr*, 1998, **68** 103–8.

111 McGuire W, McEwan P Transpyloric versus gastric tube feeding for preterm infants. *Cochrane Database Syst Rev* 2002, **3** CD003487.

112 McKeown RE, Marsh D, Amarnath U Role of delayed feeding and of feeding increments in necrotising enterocolitis. *J Pediatr*, 1992, **121** 764–70.

113 Uauy RD, Fanaroff AA, Korones SB Necrotising entercolitis in very low birth weight infants. Biodemographic and clinical correlates. *J Pediatr*, 1991, **119** 630–8.

114 Patole SK, de Klerk N Impact of standardised feeding regimens on incidence of neonatal necrotising enterocolitis: a systematic review and meta-analysis of observational studies. *Arch Dis Child Fetal Neonatal Ed*, 2005, **90** F147–51.

115 Kao LC, Durand DJ, Nickerson BG Improving pulmonary function does not decrease oxygen consumption in infants with bronchopulmonary dysplasia. *J Pediatr*, 1988, **112** 616–21.

116 Denne SC Energy expenditure in infants with pulmonary insufficiency: is there evidence for increased energy needs? *J Nutr*, 2001, **131** 935S–7S.

117 Leitch CA, Ahlrichs JA, Karn CA *et al.* Total energy expenditure is not increased in premature infants with broncopulmonary dysplasia. *Pediatr Res*, 1995, **37** 313A.

118 Moyer-Mileur L, Chan GM, Ammon BB *et al.* Growth and tolerance of calorically dense, high fat feeding in infants with bronchopulmonary dysplasia (BPD). *Pediatr Res*, 1994, **35** 317A.

119 Fewtrell MS, Adams C, Wilson DC *et al.* Randomized trial of high nutrient density formula versus standard formula in chronic lung disease. *Acta Paediatr*, 1997, **86** 577–82.

120 Chance CW, Raddle IC, Willis DM *et al.* Postnatal growth of infants <1.3 kg birth weight: effects of metabolic acidosis, of caloric intake and of calcium, sodium and phosphorus supplementation. *J Pediatr*, 1977, **91** 787–93.

121 Groothuis JR, Rosenberg AA Home oxygen promotes weight gain in infants with bronchopulmonary dysplasia. *Am J Dis Child*, 1987, **141** 992–5.

122 Henderson G, Fahey T, McGuire W Calorie and protein-enriched formula versus standard term formula for improving growth and development in preterm or low birth weight infants following

hospital discharge. *Cochrane Database Syst Rev* 2005, **2** CD004696.

123   Morley R, Fewtrell MS, Abbott RA *et al.* Neuro-development in children born small for gestational age: a randomized trial of nutrient-enriched versus standard formula and comparison with a reference breastfed group. *Pediatrics*, 2004, **113** 515–21.

124   Department of Health. Report on Health and Social Subjects No. 45. *Weaning and the weaning diet*. London: The Stationery Office, 1994.

125   Scientific Advisory Committee on Nutrition (SACN). Minutes 2nd Meeting 27th Sept 2001. agenda item 5, paragraph 18.

126   Berseth CL Effect of early feeding on maturation of the preterm infant's small intestine. *J Pediatr*, 1992, **120** 947–53.

127   Siltanen M, Kajosaari M, Pohjavuori M *et al.* Prematurity at birth reduces the long-term risk of atopy. *J Allergy Clin Immunol*, 2001, **107** 229–34.

128   Douglas JE, Bryon M Interview data on severe behavioural eating difficulties in young children. *Arch Dis Child*, 1996, **75** 304–8.

129   Martin M, Shaw NJ Feeding problems in infants and young children with chronic lung disease. *J Human Nutr*, 1997, **10** 271–5.

130   Illingworth R, Lister J The critical or sensitive period with special reference to certain feeding problems in infants and children. *J Pediatr*, 1964, **65** 839–49.

131   Northstone K, Emmett P, Nethersole F The effect of age of introduction to lumpy solids on foods eaten and reported feeding difficulties at 6 and 15 months. *J Hum Nutr Diet*, 2001, **14** 43–54.

132   King C, Marriott L, Foote KD *Weaning your Premature Baby*, 3rd edn. London: BLISS, 2006.

Further reading

Jones E, King C *Feeding and Nutrition in the Preterm Infant*. China: Elsevier Churchill Livingstone, 2005.

Useful addresses

BLISS (Baby Life Support Systems) – the premature baby charity
www.bliss.org.uk

British Association of Perinatal Medicine
www.bapm.org

7 Gastroenterology

Sarah Macdonald

Introduction

Gastroenterology is one of the most interesting and challenging areas in paediatric dietetics. The medical conditions encountered are diverse and require an understanding of normal gastrointestinal (GI) function before correct dietetic advice can be given. Problems as varied as diarrhoea, constipation and GI dysmotility can affect normal intake and absorption of nutrients. Manipulation of feeds and diet is often the primary treatment for the underlying condition and carers need careful explanation of the principles of the feed and diet prescribed.

Nutritional requirements

These vary according to the underlying disorder. For GI disorders that do not result in malabsorption, normal requirements for most nutrients will suffice, with additional energy and protein required for catch-up growth.

When malabsorption is present, requirements for all nutrients are raised to cover stool losses, particularly fluid, energy, protein and electrolytes. Most infants will have high to very high requirements. Careful monitoring of nutritional status, by anthropometric and biochemical means, is needed.

Table 7.1 can be used as a guide for requirements for infants with malabsorption who are fed

Table 7.1 Suggested requirements for infants with malabsorption.

Energy	High	130–150 kcal/kg/day (540–630 kJ/kg/day)
	Very high	150–220 kcal/kg/day (630–900 kJ/kg/day)
Protein	High	3–4 g/kg/day
	Very high	Maximum 6 g/kg/day
Sodium	High	3.0 mmol/kg/day
Potassium	Very high	4.5 mmol/kg/day
Fluid	High	180–220 mL/kg/day

enterally and are based on actual rather than expected weight.

Fluid and dietary therapy of acute diarrhoea

Acute diarrhoea remains one of the leading causes of childhood morbidity and mortality in developing nations, with an estimated 5–18 million deaths attributed to this cause each year. In industrial nations the mortality rate is much lower. Infants and children are particularly vulnerable to the effects of acute diarrhoea because of their greater relative fluid requirements and their susceptibility to faecal–oral agents.

The causative mechanisms in the GI tract are:

- Increased secretion
- Decreased absorption

Often these co-exist to produce an increased fluid load that exceeds the colonic absorptive capacity, resulting in diarrhoea. Both viral and bacterial pathogens can affect the gut in this way.

Transport of glucose and amino acids is an active process and requires the presence of a sodium gradient across the brush border membrane maintained by the Na^+–K^+ ATPase pump. The movement of water in the gut is a passive event driven by the movement of solute. The regulation of electrolye transport is controlled by several mediators and inhibition of these pathways results in poor absorption and active chloride secretion into the gut.

In infective diarrhoea, decreased absorption is not necessarily caused by reduced villous size. With increased cell loss, immature epithelial cells replace fully differentiated, mature absorptive cells. These cells have defective electrolyte and nutrient transport and functional impairment may be severe. This situation is worsened by cycles of fasting and starvation commonly seen in infants and children with acute diarrhoea in developing countries.

Oral rehydration solutions

Oral rehydration therapy is used to correct dehydration and maintain hydration. The sodium–glucose coupled transport mechanism stimulates water and electrolyte transport. This process is preserved in acute diarrhoeal disorders.

Specific recommendations for the composition of oral rehydration solutions (ORS) for children were published by the European Society of Paediatric Gastroenterology and Nutrition (ESPGAN) in 1992 [1]:

- Carbohydrate should be present as either glucose or glucose polymer at concentrations between 74 and 111 mmol/L
- ORS should contain 60 mmol/L sodium (compared with 90 mmol/L recommended by the World Health Organization [WHO] in developing countries) to minimise the risk of hypernatraemia

Table 7.2 Oral rehydration solutions (ORS) available in the UK.

	mmol/L			
	Na^+	K^+	Cl^-	CHO
Dioralyte (powder) (Aventis Pharma)	60	20	60	90 (glucose)
Electrolade (Baxter)	50	20	40	111 (glucose)
Rapolyte (Provalis)	60	20	50	110 (glucose)
Dioralyte Relief* (Aventis Pharma)	60	20	50	30 g (rice starch)
WHO Formulation Oral Rehydration Salts	75	20	65	75 (glucose)

* Effervescent and flavoured preparations are not suitable for young infants.

- Potassium should be added to replace stool losses
- Osmolality should be low (200–250 mOsm/kg H_2O) to ensure optimal water absorption

Systematic reviews have confirmed that this is still the best composition of ORS to use in children admitted to hospital with diarrhoea [2]. There is no evidence of benefit in reduction of stool loss by the use of ORS containing rice powder in non-cholera diarrhoea [3]. ORS available in the UK are summarised in Table 7.2.

Feeding during acute diarrhoea

For many years it was common practice to stop feeds during diarrhoeal episodes. It was thought that decreased lactase activity, chiefly associated with rotavirus gastroenteritis, would cause lactose malabsorption if milk feeds were introduced too early and that food proteins could be transported across an impaired mucosal barrier and cause sensitisation [4]. Consequently, bottle fed infants with gastroenteritis were fed ORS alone for 24 hours followed by the introduction of dilute feeds. This advice resulted in a reduced nutritional intake at a time when requirements were increased because of infection [5].

A meta-analysis of randomised clinical trials published in 1994 showed that the routine dilution of milk feeds and use of lactose free formula was not justified in the treatment of infants and children with acute diarrhoea [6]. A multicentre European study has shown that the complete resumption of a child's normal feeding after 4 hours of rehydration with ORS led to a significantly greater weight gain during hospitalisation and did not result in worsening or prolonged symptoms [7]. This is especially important in developing countries where children may already be malnourished.

In 1997, ESPGAN published recommendations that management of gastroenteritis should consist of oral rehydration with a low osmolar ORS for 4 hours (100 mL/kg over 4–6 hours in moderately dehydrated patients), followed by resumption of normal feeding [8]. Supplementing the usual feeds with ORS (10 mL/kg/liquid stool) can prevent further dehydration. Breast feeding should be continued at all times with supplementation of ORS.

Use of lactose free formula

There is no evidence to support the use of lactose reduced or cow's milk protein free formula in infants and children with acute diarrhoea, even if the infective agent is rotavirus. A very small minority of patients who show signs of feed intolerance (defined as worsening of diarrhoea with acidic stools containing >0.5% reducing substances) may need the temporary use of a lactose free formula (Table 7.3).

A multicentre study performed in 29 European countries showed that only a minority of physicians were following the ESPGAN guidelines. Children were still being fed ORS alone for inappropriately long periods of time and over 50% of physicians were prescribing lactose free formulas routinely following a diarrhoeal illness [9]. Guidelines for the optimal management of gastroenteritis need to be promoted to primary care physicians, health care workers and parents.

Table 7.3 Lactose free, cow's milk protein based formula available on prescription in the UK.

Galactomin Formula 17 (Scientific Hospital Supplies)
Enfamil Lactofree (Mead Johnson)
SMA LF (SMA Nutrition)

Congenital chloride losing diarrhoea

This is a selective defect in intestinal chloride transport in the ileum and colon which is inherited as an autosomal recessive trait. Life-long secretory diarrhoea occurs with high chloride concentrations. It has been reported in most populations including Britain; however, it is most commonly seen in Finland and the Arabian Gulf.

In the past it generally resulted in severe lethal dehydration. Watery diarrhoea is present from birth but often goes unnoticed as the fluid in the nappy is thought to be urine. Dehydration occurs rapidly followed by disturbances in electrolyte concentration causing hyponatraemia and hypochloraemia with mild metabolic acidosis.

Treatment

As the intestinal defect cannot be corrected, treatment requires replacement of the diarrhoeal losses of chloride, sodium and water. Initially, this may need to be given intravenously but this should gradually be changed to the oral route. Dietary manipulation is not required in this disorder other than to ensure a normal intake for age in conjunction with the prescribed electrolyte and fluid therapy.

Food allergy in gastroenterology

It is thought that the relatively high incidence of adverse reactions to food proteins seen in infancy is the result of immaturity of local and systemic immune systems, often in association with increased gut permeability to large molecules. One common cause of this is the post-enteritis syndrome where a loss of barrier function and the breakdown of normal immune tolerance follows an enteric infection. Deficiency of immunoglobulin A (IgA), which is involved in the immune defence of mucosal surfaces, is a common associated finding in allergic infants.

Food allergy may broadly be classified as either antibody mediated (e.g. IgE mediated: immediate GI hypersensitivity and oral allergy syndrome) or cell mediated (e.g. T-cell mediated: dietary protein enteropathy, protein induced enterocolitis and

Table 7.4 Gastrointestinal disorders that can be caused by allergy to dietary proteins.

Oral allergy syndrome
Eosinophilic oesophagitis
Eosinophilic gastroenteropathy (food protein induced enterocolitis)
Eosinophilic colitis
Enteropathy
Proctocolitis

proctocolitis) [10]. In some patients both mechanisms can co-exist (eosinophilic gastroenteropathy). Cells and mediators of the immune system such as eosinophils and lymphocytes can be found in biopsies of inflamed sites.

Allergic reactions can affect GI secretion, absorption (with or without mucosal damage) and motility. Interactions between the allergic cells and the mucosal nervous system is important in mediating alterations in secretion and motility. Both interleukin-5 (IL-5), a Th2 produced cytokine, and the chemokine eotaxin have a role in allergic responses that can present as delayed gastric emptying, gastro-oesophageal reflux and constipation [11].

Gastrointestinal conditions caused by allergic reactions to dietary proteins are summarised in Table 7.4. Often in the clinical setting dietary manipulations are used to treat symptoms before any formal investigations are carried out. An algorithm of suggested management is given in Fig. 7.1.

Although the most common foods to cause GI food allergic problems are cow's milk, egg, wheat and soya, any food ingested could be a culprit [12,13]. The current tests available (skin prick tests, patch tests and specific IgE) are of limited use in identifying food allergens causing GI disease. The prescribed exclusion diet is generally based on an underlying family history of atopy (hay fever/allergic rhinitis, asthma, eczema), allergies and organ-specific autoimmunity combined with the age of presentation of symptoms with food intake at that time. Sometimes a number of dietary manipulations need to be tried before the correct dietary restriction for the individual is achieved. In the presence of multiple food allergies, a few foods diet approach or exclusive use of a hypoallergenic feed may be needed with subsequent single food introductions to identify the causative food allergens.

Exclusion diets are difficult to manage at home and are expensive. Selection of suitable patients is important. Use of anti-allergic or anti-inflammatory drugs as a therapeutic alternative to dietary restriction might be considered in situations where the family will not cope with a strict exclusion diet.

When multiple foods are excluded from the diet at one time it is important to challenge sequentially with the excluded foods to identify those the child is reacting to in order to avoid over-restricting the diet.

Exclusion of cow's milk protein

Cow's milk is the most common food to cause a reaction in infants and the incidence of cow's milk protein intolerance (CMPI) or allergy reported in developed countries is between 2% and 3%; 0.5% of breast fed infants are reported to be food allergic or intolerant, reacting to exogenous food proteins secreted into the mother's milk. When an alternative infant formula is tried it is necessary to persist with this formula for a reasonable length of time, observing symptoms carefully, before abandoning it in favour of a different feed. Delayed reactions to dietary proteins can occur several days after their ingestion.

Prognosis is good with remission in approximately 50% of infants by 1 year of age, 75% at 2 years and 90% at 3 years of age. Less than 1% of infants maintain a life-long food allergy [14].

Alternative infant formulas

It is vital that an infant is given a nutritionally complete milk substitute to replace a formula based on cow's milk protein. In breast fed infants the mother's diet needs to be modified by the removal of cow's milk and any other foods allergenic to the infant, ensuring that the maternal diet continues to include adequate amounts of calcium, fluid, energy and protein. It has been found that breast fed infants can be sensitised to multiple allergens, including egg, soy, wheat and fish [15].

Mammalian milks

Mammalian milk is not suitable to be used as an infant feed without modification because of its high

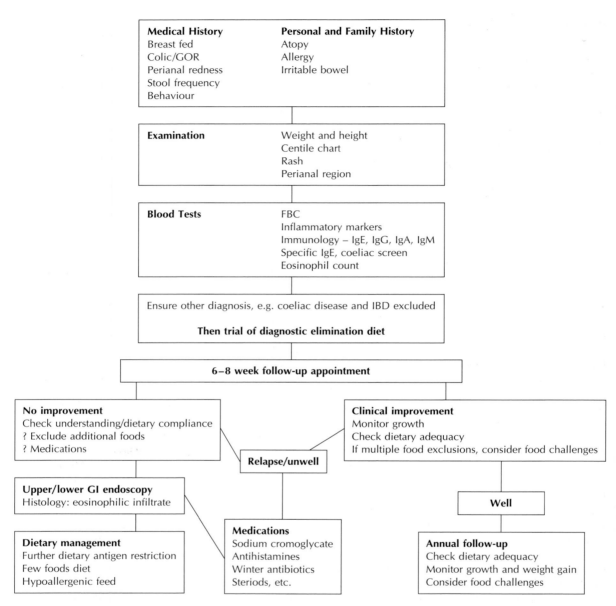

Figure 7.1   Suggested management of food allergy in gastroenterology. FBC, full blood count; GI, gastrointestinal; GOR, gastro-oesophageal reflux; IBD, inflammatory bowel disease; Ig, immunoglobulin.

renal solute load and inadequate vitamin and mineral content. The proteins in goat's and sheep's milks share antigenic cross-reactivity with cow's milk proteins. Infant formulas based on these milks are not recommended for use in GI food intolerances [16]. Infant milks based on goat's milk are not available in the UK.

Soy protein based formulas

A soy protein based formula was used for the first time in 1929 to feed infants with cow's milk protein allergy. Today these feeds are based on a soy protein isolate supplemented with L-methionine to give a suitable amino acid profile for use in infancy.

Table 7.5 Composition of soy infant formula available in the UK, per 100 mL.

Name and manufacturer	Dilution (%)	Energy (kcal)	(kJ)	CHO (g)	Protein (g)	Fat (g)	Osmolality (mOsm/kg H$_2$O)
InfaSoy (Cow & Gate)	12.7	66	277	6.7	1.8	3.6	200
SMA Wysoy (SMA Nutrition)	13.2	67	280	6.9	1.8	3.6	189
Farley's Soya Formula (Farley's)	13.7	70	294	7.0	2.0	3.8	210
ProSobee (Mead Johnson)	13.0	68	285	6.7	1.8	3.7	180
Isomil (Abbott)	13.1	68	285	6.9 (35% sucrose)	1.8	3.7	250

They are lactose free, with the carbohydrate generally being present as glucose polymer (Table 7.5). The fat is a mixture of vegetable oils that provide long chain fatty acids, including essential fatty acids. Feeding modern soy formulas to infants is associated with normal growth, protein status and bone mineralisation [17].

Use of soy protein in infancy

The Committee on Toxicity of Chemicals in Food, Consumer Products and the Environment (COT) published a final report on phytoestrogens and health in May 2003 [18]. Phytoestrogens are natural chemicals produced by some edible plants that can mimic or block the action of human oestrogens, although they are much less potent. COT felt that there was evidence of potential risk to the long-term reproductive health of infants from the biological activity of these molecules. Infants during the first 6 months of life are particularly sensitive developmentally and consume large quantities of isoflavones from soya feeds (up to 4 mg/kg/day) compared with an adult using soy products who might ingest 3 mg/day isoflavones.

They concluded that soy based infant formulas should only be fed to infants when indicated clinically. This was echoed by another independent advisory body, the Scientific Advisory Committee on Nutrition (SACN) who also felt that 'the use of soy-based infant formulas is of concern and that there was little evidence to support health benefits over products based on cow's milk protein isolate'.

The Paediatric Group of the British Dietetic Association published a position statement on the use of soya protein in infancy using a pragmatic approach to the advice given by these expert bodies [19]. They recommend that the use of soy formulas in children with atopy or allergy should be discouraged in the first 6 months of life. However, there is still a clinical need to use soy formulas in the following groups of infants as any potential risk is outweighed by the risk of withholding the formula: infants with cow's milk allergy who refuse extensively hydrolysed or elemental formulas, vegan mothers who are unable to breast feed and infants with galactosaemia.

There appears to be less risk to the infant after 6 months of age as the dose of isoflavones per kilogram body weight will be reduced as dependence on formula as a source of nutrition decreases. The infant's potentially vulnerable organ systems are likely to have matured by that age. More research in this area is needed.

Use of soy formulas in gastrointestinal disorders

Soy protein has a very large molecular weight and after digestion can generate a large number of potential allergens. Severe GI reactions to soy protein formula have been described for more than 30 years and include enteropathy, enterocolitis and proctitis. It is suggested that an intestinal mucosa damaged by cow's milk protein allows increased uptake and increased immunologic reaction to soy protein. A reported 60% of infants with cow's milk protein induced enterocolitis are equally sensitive to soy. For these reasons soy protein based formulas are not recommended in the management of cow's milk protein enteropathy or enterocolitis [17].

Older infants with documented IgE-mediated allergy to cow's milk protein can do well on soy protein based formula [20,21]. In other GI manifestations of possible cow's milk allergy, such as constipation or vomiting, where the mucosa is not damaged, soy feeds can be used. Soy formula has the benefit of being at least half the cost of hydrolysed protein formula and is much more palatable. Soy infant formulas available in the UK are summarised in Table 7.5.

Milk free diet

It is important that carers of infants requiring a cow's milk protein free feed are given appropriate advice to enable them to exclude cow's milk from solids. The following ingredients indicate the presence of cow's milk in a manufactured food: casein, hydrolysed caseinates, whey, hydrolysed whey, lactose, milk solids, non-fat milk solids, butter fat. Parents should be taught to recognise these in lists of ingredients and exclude foods containing them from the diet. A recent change in the law (Directive 2003/89/EC, November 2005) regarding labelling of ingredients now means that products containing milk must be clearly identifiable. Milk free dietary information is summarised in Table 7.6.

Feeds based on protein hydrolysates

Infants with cow's milk allergy and proven or

suspected soy intolerance need an alternative type of formula. The allergenicity or antigenicity of a particular protein is a function of the amino acid sequences present and the configuration of the molecule. An epitope is the area of a peptide chain capable of stimulating antibody production. During the manufacture of a hydrolysate the protein is denatured by heat treatment and hydrolysed by proteolytic enzymes leaving small peptides and free amino acids. The enzymes are then inactivated by heat and, along with residual large peptides, are removed by filtration [22].

The proteins used to make a hydrolysate vary and production methods also differ between manufacturers. The profile of peptide chain lengths between different feeds will not be identical, even when the initial protein is the same.

Potential problems with hydrolysate formulas
Despite the rigorous conditions employed in the manufacture of these feeds there are still potential sequential epitopes present that can be recognised by sensitive infants. Extensively hydrolysed protein based feeds vary considerably in their molecular weight profile and hence in their residual allergenic activity. Feeds with peptides of >1500 Da have been demonstrated to have residual allergenic activity [23,24]. The degree of hydrolysis does not predict the immunogenic or the allergenic effects in

Table 7.6   Milk free diet.

Foods permitted	Foods to be excluded	Check ingredients
Milk substitute Vegetable oils Custard made with milk substitute, sorbet	All mammalian milks, cheese, yoghurt, fromage frais, ice cream, butter	Margarines
Meat, fish, eggs, pulses		Sausages, pies, foods in batter or breadcrumbs Baked beans
All grains, dry pasta, flour Bread, most breakfast cereals	Pasta with cheese or milk sauce, milk bread, nan bread Cream cakes, chocolate biscuits	Tinned pasta Bought cakes or biscuits
Fruit and vegetables		Instant mashed potato
Plain crisps, nuts		Flavoured crisps
Sugar, jam, jelly Marmite	Milk chocolate, toffee	Plain chocolate Ketchup, salad dressings, soups
Milk shake syrups and powder Pop, juice, squash	Malted milk drinks	

Table 7.7   Extensively hydrolysed infant feeds available in UK.

Name and manufacturer	Dilution (%)	Energy (kcal)	(kJ)	CHO (g)*	Protein (g)	Fat (g)†	Na⁺ (mmol)	K⁺ (mmol)	Osmolality (mOsm/kg H_2O)
Casein									
Nutramigen 1 (Mead Johnson)	13.5	68	280	7.5	1.9	3.4	1.4	2.1	290
Nutramigen 2‡ (Mead Johnson)	14.6	72	300	7.8	2.3	3.5	1.6	2.3	342
Pregestimil (Mead Johnson)	13.5	68	280	6.9	1.9	3.8 (55%)	1.3	1.9	330
Whey									
Pepti-Junior (Cow & Gate)	12.8	67	280	6.9 trace lactose	1.8	3.6 (50%)	0.9	1.7	200
Pepti (Cow & Gate)	12.6	66	275	6.8 38% lactose	1.6	3.6	0.8	1.8	240
Pork collagen and soya									
Prejomin (Milupa)	15	75	313	8.6	2.0	3.6	1.4	2.0	193
Pepdite (SHS)	15	71	297	7.8	2.1	3.5 (3%)	1.5	1.5	237
MCT Pepdite (SHS)	15	68	286	8.8	2.0	2.7 (75%)	1.5	1.5	290

SHS, Scientific Hospital Supplies.
* Carbohydrate is present as glucose polymers derived from different sources unless otherwise stated.
† Figures in parenthesis indicate the percentage of fat present as medium chain triglycerides (MCT).
‡ Suitable from 6 months of age.

the recipient infant. It has been recommended that dietary products for treatment of cow's milk protein allergy in infants should be tolerated by at least 90% of infants with documented cow's milk allergy [16]. In instances where an infant is not malnourished and fails to tolerate one hydrolysate formula, a second hydrolysate from a different protein source can be tried.

Table 7.7 shows the composition of extensively hydrolysed infant formulas available in the UK. Feed choice may be influenced by:

- Palatability, which is affected by the presence of bitter peptides. This is particularly important in infants older than 3 months of age
- Co-existing fat malabsorption, where a feed with some of the fat as medium chain triglycerides (MCT) may be indicated
- Cost, some hydrolysates being twice as expensive as others
- Religion and culture, where parents do not wish their children to be given products derived from pork

Feed introduction

Hydrolysate feeds should be introduced slowly to infants with severe GI symptoms as they have a higher osmolality than normal infant formula. Feeds containing a high percentage of MCT should also be introduced gradually to ensure tolerance. The speed of introduction depends on clinical symptoms; a minimum of 12 hours on a half strength feed before the introduction of full strength formula is suggested. If the diarrhoea is very severe then it may be necessary to introduce

Table 7.8 Suggested plan for introducing hydrolysate feeds to older infants fed orally.

Day number	Percentage own feed	Percentage new hydrolysate feed
1	75	25
2	50	50
3	25	75
4	0	100

quarter strength feeds, grading up to full strength feeds over 4 days. If severe diarrhoea is present in an older infant it is preferable to stop all solids while a new feed is being introduced, to assess tolerance.

In an outpatient setting, where symptoms may be less severe, full strength formula can usually be introduced from the outset. In infants older than 6 months there may be an advantage in initially mixing the hydrolysate with their usual formula to slowly introduce the new taste and encourage acceptance. A suggested regimen is shown in Table 7.8. Milk shake flavourings at 2–4% concentration can also be used in this age group if sucrose is not contraindicated.

If an infant refuses to drink the hydrolysate feed a nasogastric tube needs to be passed to ensure adequate feed volumes are taken. Where failure to thrive co-exists, feeds can be fortified in the usual manner by the addition of fat, carbohydrate or an increase in formula concentration. All changes should be made slowly to ensure they are tolerated.

Pepti-Junior and Pepti both have sodium contents similar to standard infant formula which may not be sufficient for an infant with increased stool losses. Low urinary sodium (<20 mmol/L) alongside a normal plasma sodium concentration indicates sodium depletion and supplementation with sodium chloride will be required.

Amino acid based infant formula

Only pure amino acid mixtures are considered to be non-allergenic as there are no peptide chains present to act as epitopes. In infants who fail to tolerate a hydrolysate this is the next logical step, so long as there is not a co-existing fat or carbohydrate intolerance. In these situations a modular feeding approach should be used (see p. 109). At present there is only one such feed for infants in the UK, Neocate (Table 7.9). Studies have shown this to be effective in a number of clinical settings where protein hydrolysates have not been tolerated [13,24]. The sodium content of Neocate is relatively low for infants with chronic diarrhoea and may need further supplementation.

Introduction of solids

Weaning should take place at the recommended age of around 6 months and not before 17 weeks. It is important to ensure that food offered is free of cow's milk protein. Other dietary proteins that are most commonly implicated and may therefore need to be excluded include egg, soy and wheat. In very sensitive infants it may be wise to introduce new foods singly.

Exclusion of soy protein
In conditions where soy intolerance is present in addition to CMPI, foods containing soy and milk protein should be excluded from the diet (Tables 7.6 and 7.10). Vegetable or soy oils and soya lecithin are normally tolerated by individuals sensitive to soy protein and should not need to be excluded from the diet except in severely affected individuals.

Milk, egg, wheat and soy exclusion diets
In conditions where a simple exclusion diet has not worked or where there is a diet history suggestive

Table 7.9 Infant formula based on amino acids available in the UK, per 100 mL.

Name and manufacturer	Dilution (%)	Energy (kcal)	Energy (kJ)	CHO (g)	Protein equivalent (g)	Fat (g)	Na+ (mmol)	K+ (mmol)	Osmolality (mOsm/kg H₂O)
Neocate (Scientific Hospital Supplies)	15	71	298	8.1	2.0	3.5 (5% MCT)	0.8	1.6	360

MCT, medium chain triglycerides.

Table 7.10 Foods containing soya protein.

All soy based products including tofu and soy sauce
Texturised vegetable proteins
Breads, biscuits and cakes which contain soy flour
Baby foods containing soy protein
Soy margarines

of multiple food intolerances this dietary regimen may be tried. Families need a lot of help and information about commercial foods to enable them to adhere to this regimen. Suitable wheat free products that are available via the Advisory Committee on Borderline Substances (ACBS) cannot be prescribed for wheat allergy and a separate letter to the GP requesting help is often required. In addition to looking for milk, egg and soy based ingredients on food labels any unidentified starches, rusk and batter also needs to be excluded (Table 7.11).

Suitable feeds for older children

A suitable infant formula should be continued for as long as is nutritionally indicated in children on an exclusion diet and is preferable under the age of 2 years. In situations where a large percentage of the child's nutrition comes from a formula it will either need fortification to meet nutritional requirements or a feed designed for older children should be used. The feeds in Table 7.12 have been designed to meet the requirements of older children requiring hypo-allergenic feeds. Adult feeds based on soy or hydrolysed protein should be used with care in older children and may require modification or vitamin and mineral supplementation.

In children over the age of 2 years consuming a well-balanced diet and tolerating soy protein, supermarket 'adult' liquid soy milks can be given as an alternative to cow's milk. Those with added calcium help to ensure an adequate intake of this

Table 7.11 Milk, egg, wheat and soya free diet.

Foods permitted	Foods to be excluded	Check ingredients
Milk substitute Vegetable oils	All mammalian milks and products, soya milks and soy products, shredded suet Eggs	Margarines
All meat, poultry, fish, shellfish (fresh or frozen), pulses	Meat or fish dishes with pastry, breadcrumbs or batter Tofu, tempeh, soy beans, Quorn	Sausages, beef and vegetarian burgers, hot dogs, ready meals
Rice, rice noodles or pasta, maize corn pasta, cornflour, tapioca, sago, arrowroot, buckwheat, barley, oats, gram flour, potato flour, ground almonds, carob	Wheat, rye and soya flour, spelt flour, wheat bran or germ, semolina, couscous, tabouleh, pancakes, batter, pizza, stuffing mixes, ordinary pasta, e.g. spaghetti	Gluten free bread, cakes, biscuits, pasta; oatcakes
Breakfast cereals made from rice, corn and oats, poppadoms, rice and corn cakes	Wheat based breakfast cereals Bread, crispbreads, crackers, chapatti, croissants, biscuits, cake, cheesecake, instant desserts	
Jelly, custard or blancmange powders, rice, tapioca or sago pudding (made with milk substitute)		Pies, pastries, mousse, trifle, sorbet
Fruit and vegetables	Potato croquettes	Vegetables in dressing, e.g. coleslaw; potato waffles, instant mashed potato
Plain crisps		Flavoured potato crisps
Marmite, Bovril	Mayonnaise, salad cream, soy sauce	Stock cubes, gravy mixes, soups, sauces
Sugar, jam, honey, syrup, plain fruit lollies, milk shake syrup and powder, cocoa powder	Chocolate spread, lemon curd, milk chocolate, instant milk drinks	Plain chocolate, jelly sweets, marshmallows, baking powder, chocolate, malted drinks

Table 7.12   Hydrolysate and amino acid based feeds for older children per 100 mL.

Name	Dilution (%)	Energy (kcal)	(kJ)	CHO* (g)	Protein equivalent (g)	Fat[†] (g)	Na+ (mmol)	K+ (mmol)	Osmolality (mOsm/kg H_2O)
Hydrolysate feeds									
Pepdite 1+ (SHS)	23	100	423	13	3.1	3.9 (35)	2.1	3	465
MCT Pepdite 1+ (SHS)	20	91	380	11.8	2.8	3.6 (75)	1.8	2.6	460
Peptamen Junior (Nestlé)	22	100	418	13.8	3	3.8	2.9	3.5	310
Amino acid feeds									
Neocate Advance[§] (unflavoured) (SHS)	25	100	420	14.6	2.5	3.5 (35)	2.6	3.0	610
Neocate Active[§**] (unflavoured) (SHS)	21	100	420	11.3	2.8	4.8 (4)	1.3	1.5	520
Elemental 028[‡§] (unflavoured) (SHS)	20	78	328	14.4	2.0	1.3 (5)	2.6	2.4	496
Elemental 028[‡§] Extra (unflavoured) (SHS)	20	89	374	11.8	2.5	3.5 (35)	2.7	2.4	502
Emsogen [‡§¶] (unflavoured) (SHS)	20	88	370	12	2.5	3.3 (83)	2.6	2.4	539

SHS, Scientific Hospital Supplies. * All present as glucose polymer derived from different sources. [†] Figures in parenthesis show percentage fat present as MCT. [‡] Use with caution for children between 1–5 years. [§] Flavoured versions of these feeds are also available. [¶] Patients who are receiving a significant proportion of their nutritional requirements from Emsogen may need to supplement their intake of α linolenic acid to meet UK DRVs 1991 [25] and ESPGAN guidelines 1991 (p. 148). ** Neocate Active is designed as a dietary supplement rather than a complete feed.

nutrient. For children intolerant of soy and cow's milk, alternative 'milks' made from oat, rice, nut and pea are available in health food shops and supermarkets; they can be a useful social replacement for cow's milk. Some are fortified with calcium. Calcium supplements (Table 18.14) may be needed to achieve the reference nutrient intake (RNI) [25]. Most of these drinks contain very little protein so high protein foods must be eaten twice a day.

Calcium intakes below recommended intakes have been identified in a number of children limiting cow's milk in their diet, which may affect bone density [26]. One study showed that children aged between 31 and 37 months on milk free diets had significantly lower intakes of energy, fat, protein, calcium, riboflavin and niacin than age-matched controls. Careful monitoring of dietary adequacy with calcium and vitamin supplementation if needed is required [27].

Coeliac disease

This is an autoimmune disease primarily affecting the proximal small intestine characterised by an abnormal small intestinal mucosa and associated with a permanent intolerance to gluten. Coeliac disease (CD) is associated with other autoimmune disorders and a low IgA. There are at least two prerequisites for developing CD: a genetic predisposition and ingestion of gluten. More than one member of a family may be affected. The incidence was previously estimated to be 1 in 300 in England although a recent study suggested this could be as high as 1 in 100 [28,29]. There is considerable variation in the age of onset and in the mode of presentation, with patients now being diagnosed well into adulthood.

CD is an immunological disorder with local and systemic production of autoantibodies against structural proteins of the small intestine mucosa and other organs, in association with a specific pattern of cell-mediated damage in the small intestine. Anti-tissue transglutaminase (tTG) and anti-endomysial antibodies (the same antibody measured by different methods) are specific markers of CD, although they may not be raised in IgA deficient individuals [30]. These can also be raised in healthy first degree relatives with a normal small intestinal biopsy, perhaps implying that these individuals have a latent form of the disease.

The 'gold standard' for diagnosis remains a small intestinal biopsy demonstrating mucosal damage followed by a clinical response to gluten withdrawal [30,31]. It is important that patients with suspected CD continue on a normal diet until the diagnostic biopsy has been performed and a clear diagnosis made.

Treatment

CD is treated by excluding all dietary sources of gluten, a protein found in wheat, rye and barley. The gluten can be divided into four subclasses: gliadin, glutenins, albumins and globulins. In wheat the injurious constituent is the prolamin fraction of α-gliadin. The equivalent in rye is secalin and in barley hordein. Enzymatic degradation studies have suggested that the damaging fraction is an acidic polypeptide with a molecular weight of <1500 Da.

Gluten free diet

All possible sources of wheat, rye and barley need to be excluded from the diet which needs to be followed for life (Table 7.13). This excludes a number of staple foods such as bread, pasta, biscuits and cakes and parents need support and help in finding suitable substitutes that their child will eat. Wheat flour is commonly used in processed foods as a binding agent, filler or carrier for flavourings and spices. Recent testing using a more sensitive analysis method has shown that some breakfast cereals containing malt flavourings derived from barley exceed the accepted threshold allowed by the international Codex Standard and are no longer considered suitable for inclusion in the gluten free diet. Parents and children with CD need to be taught to

Table 7.13 Gluten free diet.

Foods permitted	Foods to avoid	Check ingredients
Milk, butter, cream, cheese		Cheese spreads, yoghurts, custard
Meat, fish, eggs, pulses	Products with pastry, thickened gravies and sauces, breadcrumbs, batter	Sausages, tinned meats
Rice, corn (maize), buckwheat, millet, tapioca, soya, gram flour, arrowroot	Wheat, rye, barley, bread, crumpets, cakes, biscuits, crackers, crispbread, chapattis, nan bread, pasta, noodles, semolina, couscous	Oats*
Special gluten free flours, breads, biscuits and pasta	Wheat based cereals, e.g. Weetabix, Shredded Wheat	Corn and rice based cereals
Vegetables, potato, fruit and nuts	Potato croquettes	Flavoured potato crisps, dry roasted nuts
Sugar, jam, honey, some chocolates	Liquorice	Filled chocolates, boiled sweets
Tea, coffee, drinking chocolate, fizzy drinks, juice, squash	Malted milk drinks, e.g. Horlicks and Ovaltine Barley water, beer	

* Exclusion may be necessary.

identify sources of the offending cereals in lists of food ingredients. A recent change to the food labelling legislation (Directive 2003/89/EC, November 2005) means that all foods containing gluten or wheat must be clearly labelled; exemptions to ingredient listing of compound ingredients have largely been abolished.

Children tend to be the highest consumers of savoury snack foods and processed foods which need to be excluded on this diet. The Food and Drink Directory produced annually by Coeliac UK and updated monthly on their website using data from supermarkets and manufacturers is an important resource for all individuals with CD. Increased variety of foods allowed will improve patient compliance. Young children should be taught to check with parents before eating foods outside the home or offered by siblings or friends. Where possible meals should be prepared that are suitable for the whole family so that the child does not feel different. Children's parties are a source of concern to parents and the coeliac child should be sent with suitable foods of their own to eat.

Commercially produced gluten free foods

A large number of proprietary gluten free foods are available, some based on wheat starch. In ordinary manufactured foods containing wheat starch the latter is not pure enough to be included in a gluten free diet. However, specially manufactured foods that comply with the International Gluten Free Standard up to 200 ppm (WHO Codex Alimentarius 1981) are suitable for inclusion in the diets of most people with CD. A number of staple food items have been passed as prescribable for patients with CD by ACBS, while the more luxurious items such as fruit cakes can be purchased via pharmacies or health food shops. Some supermarkets produce their own ranges of gluten free foods.

A prescribing guide for the gluten free diet has been produced by BSPGHAN (British Society of Paediatric Gastroenterology, Hepatology and Nutrition) to define the minimum monthly gluten free food prescription requirements for children and adults with CD [32]. Good dietary compliance is aided by the ease with which patients can obtain suitable amounts of gluten free foods on prescription. A large number of companies produce such foods and a complete list can be found in the *British National Formulary* (BNF) or in Coeliac UK's Food and Drink Directory. Products vary and patients should be encouraged to try different food items. Some of the larger companies will send newly diagnosed patients trial packs of their own products on application.

Oats

The inclusion of oats in the gluten free diet remains controversial. It is unclear whether the prolamin in oats, called avenin, contains the amino acid sequences that trigger the histological changes in the small intestinal mucosa. The quantity of avenin in oats is much less than the prolamins in other cereals, thus a larger quantity of the product may be required to produce an effect. Problems with earlier studies included small patient numbers, insensitive functional tests and small intestinal biopsies which were often difficult to interpret [33]. Coeliac UK's Medical Advisory Council published interim guidelines stating that moderate amounts of oats may be consumed by most adult coeliacs without risk, although the situation is less clear with children. Highly sensitised coeliacs should at present not be allowed oats and patients should be carefully followed up [34].

Two papers purport to show the safety of oats when ingested by adults and children with CD. The adult data showed no harm at 5 years, yet a significant number (33%) of the original subjects did not include oats in their diet during the follow-up period [35]. The randomised double blind paediatric study had a high number of withdrawals in both the group that ate oats (26%) and those whose diet remained free of oats (11%). At the end of the study the children consuming oats were taking smaller amounts than prescribed which, in some, may have resulted in too little avenin to cause an effect [36].

A further complicating factor is that oats can be contaminated with wheat at various stages of production: in fields, transportation, storage, milling and processing. Care should therefore be taken to avoid contaminated sources. The author's current practice is to initially advise avoidance of oats at the start of the gluten free diet but to review this at a later date once the patient is responding to the diet. Oat products are now included in an appendix to Coeliac UK's annual food list.

Bone health

One of the main complications of CD in adults is reduced bone mineral density leading to osteoporosis. It is unclear if this is caused by calcium malabsorption for prolonged periods prior to diagnosis. Studies in children found that while the bone mineral content of coeliacs was significantly lower than control subjects at diagnosis, after 1 year on a gluten free diet it had returned to normal. The calcium intake of the children was not assessed during this time [37]. Although there are no formal recommendations it would appear sensible to ensure that children's intake is at least equal to the RNI for calcium for their age [25]. Some gluten free products are fortified with calcium.

Coeliac UK

This is an independent registered charity with free membership which all parents of children with CD should be encouraged to join. The society acts as an invaluable resource on all aspects of management of the gluten free diet including topics as diverse as eating out to travelling abroad. It also produces many helpful publications: www. coeliac.co.uk.

Gluten challenge

ESPGHAN guidelines for the diagnosis of CD are currently being reviewed to include up-to-date serology testing. The 1990 guidelines state that gluten challenge is only necessary when there is some doubt at the time of initial diagnosis, for instance if the initial biopsy was atypical or if a gluten free diet was started before the biopsy with a clinical response [31]. For challenge purposes gluten can be introduced into the diet in two forms: either as gluten powder that can be mixed in foods such as yoghurt, or as gluten containing foods. Both need to be given daily in sufficient amounts to ensure an adequate challenge. Two slices of bread a day for older children has been suggested by one author [31]. The author's practice has been to give the children a normal diet for the duration of the challenge. Parents are often anxious that the inclusion of normal foods in the diet will make returning to gluten free diet difficult if the diagnosis of CD is confirmed. Reassurance is required and an explanation of the procedure to the child is very important in ensuring its success.

Associated food intolerances

Although a secondary disaccharidase deficiency can be demonstrated at the time of diagnosis it is rarely necessary to exclude lactose from the diet of a newly diagnosed individual with CD. However, some infants seem to be intolerant of cow's milk protein and benefit from a temporary dietary exclusion in addition to avoidance of gluten. They should be rechallenged with cow's milk 2–3 months after the commencement of the gluten free diet.

If patients remain symptomatic on a strict gluten free diet it may be necessary to exclude products containing traces of gluten such as gluten free wheat starch and all foods containing malt extract and flavouring. Patients responding to such dietary manipulations are described as super-sensitive.

Carbohydrate intolerances

Sugar malabsorption increases the osmotic load of GI fluid, draws water into the small intestine and stimulates peristalsis, resulting in diarrhoea. The severity depends on the quantity of ingested carbohydrate, the metabolic activity of colonic bacteria (which is reduced after antibiotic therapy) and the absorptive capacity of the colon for water and short chain fatty acids.

The infant is at a disadvantage compared with the adult as the small intestine is shorter and the reserve capacity of the colon to absorb luminal fluids is reduced. Because of a faster gut transit time there is less time for alternative paths of carbohydrate digestion to be effective. The undigested sugar is either excreted unchanged or is fermented by bacteria in the colon to short chain fatty acids and lactic acid.

Disaccharidase deficiencies

In the brush border of the small intestine there are four disaccharidase enzymes, with the highest level

Table 7.14 Brush border enzyme activity in the small intestine.

Enzyme	Substrate	Product
Sucrase-isomaltase (accounts for 80% maltase activity)	Sucrose α1–6 glucosidic bonds in starch molecule (approx. 25%) Isomaltose Maltose Maltotriose	Glucose Fructose
Maltase-glucoamylase (accounts for 20% maltase activity)	Maltose Maltotriose Starch	Glucose
Lactase	Lactose	Glucose Galactose
Trehelase	Trehalose	Glucose

Table 7.15 Low sucrose, low starch solids (<1 g/100 g).

Protein	Meat, poultry, egg*, fish
Fats	Margarine, butter, lard, vegetable oils
Vegetables	Most vegetables *except* potato, parsnip, carrot, peas, onion, sweet potato, sweetcorn, beetroot [39]
Fruits	Initially use fruits with <1 g sucrose per 100 g fruit (Table 7.16) Most fruits contain negligible amounts of starch
Milk	Breast milk, infant formula (free of glucose polymer and sucrose) Cow's milk, unsweetened natural yoghurt, cream
Others	Marmite, Bovril, vinegar, salt, pepper, herbs, spices, 1–2 teaspoons of tomato purée can be used in cooking, gelatine, essences and food colourings, sugar free jelly, sugar free drinks, fructose, glucose

* Soft eggs should not be given to babies under 1 year of age.

of activity occurring in the jejunum (Table 7.14). Deficiencies of these enzymes can be primary in nature resulting from a congenital enzyme defect or can be secondary to some other GI insult.

Congenital sucrase-isomaltase deficiency

Congenital sucrase-isomaltase deficiency (CSID) is an autosomal recessively inherited disease which is a rare, but frequently misdiagnosed, cause of chronic diarrhoea in infants and children. There is wide phenotypic variation. All CSID patients have an absence of intestinal sucrase activity; however, isomaltase activity varies from very little to almost normal. Although considered rare, the prevalence of CSID may have been underestimated and it is likely that the disease remains undiagnosed in numerous patients with a history of chronic diarrhoea, some of whom are diagnosed with CSID as adults.

While being breast fed or given a normal infant formula the infant remains asymptomatic and thrives. The introduction into the diet of starch or sucrose in weaning foods, or the change in formula to one containing sucrose or starch (found in pre-thickened formulas), initiates symptoms. The clinical presentation of CSID is very variable. Chronic watery diarrhoea and failure to thrive are common findings in infants and toddlers. A delay in the diagnosis may be related to the empirical institution of a low sucrose diet by parents, which controls

symptoms. Some children attain relatively normal growth with chronic symptoms of intermittent diarrhoea, bloating and abdominal cramps before diagnosis. In older children such symptoms may result in the diagnosis of irritable bowel syndrome.

One retrospective study suggests that a change in infant feeding practices in the last 20 years has resulted in the delayed introduction and decreased ingestion of sucrose and isomaltose in infancy. This has modified the course and the symptoms of the disease resulting in milder forms of chronic diarrhoea which may not start until a few weeks after the introduction of solids compared with a more acute onset of symptoms previously observed [38].

Treatment

In the first year of life this usually requires the elimination of sucrose from the diet. Starch is excluded initially and then introduced to tolerance (Table 7.15). The lactose in normal infant formula, breast milk and cow's milk is tolerated.

Care needs to be taken to ensure an adequate vitamin intake and it may be beneficial to continue an infant formula after 1 year of age. All medications should be sucrose free; a suitable complete carbohydrate free vitamin supplement is Ketovite liquid and tablets.

With increasing age the tolerance of starch and the lower sucrose containing foods should improve until, by the age of 2–3 years, the restriction of

Table 7.16 Sucrose content of some common fruits (per 100 g edible portion) [39].

<1 g sucrose	<3 g sucrose	<5 g sucrose
Bilberries, blackcurrants, cherries, damsons, gooseberries, grapes, lemons, loganberries, lychees, melon (except Gallia), pears, raisins, raspberries, redcurrants, rhubarb,strawberries, sultanas	Gallia melon, grapefruit, kiwi fruit, passion fruit, plums	Apples, apricots, oranges, clementines, satsumas

starch should no longer be needed. Tolerance can be titrated against dietary intake; if the capacity to absorb carbohydrate is exceeded this will cause osmotic diarrhoea or a recurrence of abdominal symptoms. Reducing the carbohydrate to the previously tolerated level will result in normal stool production. The sucrose content of fruits is shown in Table 7.16. Fruits containing higher amounts of sucrose can be added to the diet according to tolerance. If children have problems tolerating starch in reasonable quantities, soy flour can be used in recipes to replace wheat flour as it only contains 15 g starch per 100 g compared with 75 g per 100 g in wheat flour. Parents need reassurance that occasional dietary indiscretions will not cause long term problems.

Newly diagnosed older children should initially be advised to avoid dietary sources of sucrose only. If this does not lead to a prompt improvement in symptoms then the starch content of the diet can be reduced, particularly those foods with a high amylopectin content such as wheat and potatoes. Advice needs to be given to increase energy from protein and fat to replace the loss in dietary energy from reducing carbohydrate foods. Glucose tablets and Lucozade may be included in the diet. There is an international support group that tracks children with CSID and also provides further information on this disorder: www.csidinfo.com.

Enzyme substitution therapy
Sacrosidase, a liquid preparation containing high concentrations of yeast derived invertase (sucrase), has been used with good results and is available on prescription (Sucraid, Orphan Medical Inc). It is stable if refrigerated and tasteless when mixed with water. This formulation has also been shown to be resistant to acidic pH. Degradation by intragastric pepsin is buffered by taking the enzyme with protein foods. Unlike human intestinal sucrase-isomaltase, it has no activity on oligosaccharides containing $\alpha1-6$ glucosidic bonds.

A controlled, double blind trial of sacrosidase in 14 patients with CSID showed symptoms of diarrhoea, abdominal cramps and bloating were prevented or ameliorated in patients consuming a sucrose containing diet. The dosage recommended is 1 mL with each meal in patients weighing <15 kg, and 2 mL for those weighing >15 kg. This allows the consumption of a more normal diet by children with CSID and decreases the high incidence of chronic gastrointestinal complaints seen in this condition [40,41].

Lactase deficiency

Congenital lactase deficiency is very rare, the largest group of patients being found in Finland. Severe diarrhoea starts during the first days of life, resulting in dehydration and malnutrition, and resolves when either breast milk or normal formula are ceased and a lactose free formula is given (Table 7.3).

Primary adult type hypolactasia is found in a large proportion of the world's populations. Lactase levels are normal during infancy but decline to about 5–10% of the level at birth during childhood and adolescence. These population groups are common in East and South-East Asia, tropical Africa and native Americans and Australians. The age of onset of symptoms varies but is generally about 3 years or later, and only if a diet containing lactose is offered. In the majority of Europeans lactase levels remain high and this pattern of a declining tolerance of lactose with age is not seen.

In other ethnic groups with this problem a moderate reduction of dietary lactose will be sufficient, using either lactose reduced milks available from the supermarket or soy milks. It is important to ensure that children meet their requirements for calcium.

Secondary disaccharidase deficiency

Carbohydrate malabsorption can occur secondary to any insult causing damage to the GI mucosa.

Table 7.17   Composition of Galactomin 19 per 100 mL.

	Dilution (%)	Energy (kcal)	(kJ)	Protein (g)	CHO (g)	Fat (g)	Na$^+$ (mmol)	K$^+$ (mmol)	Osmolality (mOsm/kg H$_2$O)
Galactomin 19 Formula (Scientific Hospital Supplies)	12.9	69	288	1.9	6.4	4.0	0.9	1.5	407

This can present at any age, with onset of symptoms occurring shortly after the primary injury, for instance in cow's milk protein enteropathy, rotavirus infection, Crohn's disease, short gut syndrome and immunodeficiency syndromes.

Lactase deficiency is the most common secondary enzyme deficiency to be seen, probably because it has a lower activity than the other intestinal enzymes and is located on the distal end of the villous tip making it more susceptible to damage. However, a secondary sucrase-isomaltase deficiency can also occur.

Treatment

Treatment is to eliminate the offending carbohydrates and treat the primary disorder causing the mucosal damage. Clinical course depends on the underlying disease but studies in infants with rotavirus infections have shown an incidence of 30–50% lactose intolerance which recovers 2–4 weeks after the infection.

Children requiring a lactose free formula and diet can use either lactose free, cow's milk protein based formula (Table 7.3) or soy formula (Table 7.5). A milk free diet (Table 7.6) is necessary although mature cheese can be included. Medications need to be checked as these can contain lactose as a filler.

Monosaccharide malabsorption: glucose–galactose malabsorption

This is an extremely rare congenital disorder resulting from a selective defect in the intestinal glucose and galactose/sodium co-transport system in the brush border membrane. Glucose, galactose, lactose, sucrose, glucose polymers and starch are all contraindicated in this disorder. It presents in the neonatal period with the onset of severe, watery, acidic diarrhoea leading to dehydration

and metabolic acidosis. It is a heterogeneous condition in its expression and older children seem to have considerable variation in their tolerance of the offending carbohydrates.

Treatment

Initial intravenous rehydration is required. The use of ORS, all of which are glucose or starch based, is contraindicated. A fructose based complete infant formula, Galactomin 19, should be introduced slowly, initially as quarter and half strength formula with intravenous carbohydrate and electrolyte support, to avoid metabolic acidosis (Table 7.17).

Once the infant is established on feeds and gaining weight, it is important to discuss with the child's doctor a suitable protocol for oral rehydration should the child become unwell. Plain water or a 2–4% fructose solution can be given, but this does not have the same effect on water absorption as ORS. In severe infectious diarrhoea the infant may need intravenous fluids.

Fructose is available on prescription for this condition and can be used to sweeten foods for older children and as an additional energy source. It is important to ensure that all medicines are carbohydrate free.

Introduction of solids

Initially weaning solids should contain minimal amounts of starch, sucrose, lactose or glucose (Table 7.18). Manufactured baby foods are not suitable and it is necessary for weaning solids to be prepared at home. All foods should be cooked without salt and initially blended to a very smooth texture. To save time parents can prepare foods in advance and freeze in clean ice cube trays. Recipes are available from the author for egg custard sweetened with fructose and for fructose meringues.

With increasing age children gradually begin to absorb more of the offending carbohydrates due to

Table 7.18 Foods allowed in children with glucose–galactose malabsorption (<1 g glucose and galactose per 100 g).*

Protein	Meat, poultry, egg,[†] fish
Fats	Margarine, butter, lard, vegetable oils
Vegetables	Ackee (canned), asparagus, bamboo shoots, beansprouts (canned only), broccoli, celery, cucumber, endive, fennel, globe artichoke, lettuce, marrow, mushrooms, spinach, spring greens, steamed tofu, watercress, preserved vine leaves
Fruits	Avocado pear, rhubarb, lemon juice
Milk substitute	Galactomin 19 Formula
Others	Marmite, Bovril, vinegar, salt, pepper, herbs, spices, 1–2 teaspoons of tomato purée can be used in cooking, gelatine, essences and food colourings, sugar free jelly, sugar free drinks, fructose

* The lists of foods have been compiled calculating the amount of glucose and galactose as: g starch + g glucose + g lactose + 0.5 g sucrose [39].
[†] Soft eggs should not be given to babies under 1 year of age.

colonic salvage. The foods in Table 7.19 are grouped to allow a gradual increase in the amount of glucose and galactose in the diet. These lists can be used as a guide by parents. Small amounts of new foods can be introduced cautiously and increased as tolerated. Too much of these foods will exceed the individual's tolerance and cause diarrhoea. In this situation the child should return to the diet previously well tolerated and try introductions again a few months later.

Infants and children are very dependent on Galactomin 19 to meet their requirements for energy and parents should be encouraged to continue this formula for as long as possible. It can also be useful for older children entering adolescence who find it difficult to meet their increased energy requirements from eating a low starch diet. If sufficient formula is taken a vitamin supplement should not be needed.

Fat malabsorption

Intestinal lymphangiectasia

This is characterised by dilated enteric lymphatic vessels which rupture and leak lymphatic fluid into the gut, leading to protein loss. The presentation is variable but diarrhoea and hypoproteinaemic oedema are commonly seen. Failure to thrive can

Table 7.19 Glucose and galactose content of foods (per 100 g edible portion [39]).

1–2 g glucose + galactose	2–3 g glucose + galactose	3–5 g glucose + galactose
Protein		
Quorn, all 'hard' cheeses, cream cheese, brie, camembert		
Vegetables		
Aubergine, beans – french and runner, brussel sprouts, cabbage, cauliflower, celeriac, courgettes, gherkins (pickled), leeks, okra, onions (boiled), green peppers, radish, spring onions, swede, tomatoes (including tinned), turnip	Carrots	Sugar snap peas, butternut squash, mange tout
Fruits		
Gooseberries, redcurrants	Apples – cooking (sweeten with fructose or artificial sweetener), blackberries, loganberries, melon (all types), pears, raspberries, strawberries	Apricots, blackcurrants, cherries, clementines, peaches, pineapple, grapefruit, nectarines, oranges, satsumas, tangerines
Other		
Ordinary mayonnaise (retail) – not reduced calorie	Double cream	Whipping cream

also be a significant problem. Children usually present in the first 2 years of life although cases diagnosed as late as 15 years of age are documented [42]. The diagnosis is definitively established by a small intestinal biopsy demonstrating the characteristic lymphatic abnormality although, as the lesion is a patchy one, negative biopsy does not exclude the diagnosis [43]. Development of a video capsule that passes through the small intestine will aid diagnosis in this disorder.

Treatment

Treatment is by diet unless the lesion is localised enough to allow surgical excision of the involved part of the intestine. A reduced long chain triglyceride (LCT) diet is needed to control symptoms. This reduces the volume of intestinal lymphatic fluid and the pressure within the lacteals. It is recommended that the amount of LCT should be restricted to 5–10 g/day [43]. A very high protein intake may also be needed to maintain plasma levels of albumin. Intakes of protein as high as 6 g/kg/day with sufficient energy to ensure its proper utilisation have been suggested, although these guidelines are not evidence based. If the intestinal leakage can be stopped by reducing the lymphatic flow then such a high intake of protein should not be required. Enteric protein loss can be monitored by measuring faecal α_1-antitrypsin levels. MCT can be used as an energy source and to increase the palatability of the diet as these are absorbed directly into the portal system and not via the lymphatics.

Suitable feeds in infancy and early childhood are Monogen, MCT Step 1 or Caprilon, the first two being preferable because of their higher protein and energy content and lower LCT content (Table 7.20). If additional protein needs to be given to

maintain plasma albumin levels, this can be added to a complete feed (e.g. or Vitapro). The fat and electrolyte content of these products should be calculated in addition to the quantities supplied by the feed.

Minimal fat diet

Minimal fat weaning solids should initially be introduced and gradually expanded aiming to keep the total LCT intake below 10 g/day, certainly in the first 2 years of life. Details of minimal fat diets are given elsewhere (see pp. 251, 427). Attention needs to be given to protein intake and extra very low fat, high protein foods may be included.

As the problem is life-long it is necessary to continue dietary restrictions, certainly until the end of the pubertal growth spurt, although maintaining such a low intake of fat becomes increasingly difficult as the child becomes older. There is no information about the degree of fat restriction required in older children and some relaxation of the diet should be possible so long as symptoms are controlled and growth is adequate. Nutritional supplements such as Build Up made with skimmed milk, Fortijuce, Enlive Plus and Provide Xtra may be useful to ensure adequate protein intake in older children (see Table 11.3).

As the dietary restrictions are long term it is particularly important to ensure that the recommended amounts of essential fatty acids (EFAs) are included in the diet once the volume of complete infant formula is reduced. Walnut oil provides the most concentrated source of EFAs and can be given as a measured amount as a dietary supplement daily. Recommended amounts would be at least 0.1 mL per 56 kcal (234 kJ) provided from foods and drinks not supplemented with EFAs (see p. 427); however, there are no data as to how well this is

Table 7.20 Composition of minimal fat, cow's milk protein based infant formulas per 100 mL.

	Dilution (%)	Energy (kcal)	(kJ)	Protein (g)	CHO (g)	Fat (g)	Na+ (mmol)	K+ (mmol)	Osmolality (mOsm/kg H$_2$O)
Monogen (Scientific Hospital Supplies)	17.5	74	310	2.0	12.0	2.0 (90% MCT)	1.5	1.6	280
MCT Step 1 (Vitaflo)	17.5	7.4	310	2.1	12.0	2.1 (90% MCT)	1.4	1.6	238
Caprilon (Scientific Hospital Supplies)	12.7	66	275	1.5	7.0 (12% lactose)	3.6 (75% MCT)	0.8	1.7	233

MCT, medium chain triglycerides.

absorbed in this disorder. It may be prudent to give double the normal amount of walnut oil as a divided dose mixed with food or as a medicine. This needs to be included in the daily fat allowance.

Fat-soluble vitamin supplements (A, D, E) to meet at least the RNI for age should be given separately. If the above nutritional supplements are used they are fortified with these vitamins so separate vitamin supplements may not be required. Blood levels should be monitored at outpatient clinics.

Neonatal enteropathies and protracted diarrhoea

The causes of protracted diarrhoea in the first few months of life are mostly post-infectious enteropathies and food allergic enteropathies. Rare, and usually early onset, causes include microvillous inclusion disease, tufting enteropathy and auto-immune enteropathy [44]. Congenital glucose–galactose malabsorption, congenital chloride losing diarrhoea and congenital sodium losing diarrhoea will also manifest from birth, although villus morphology is normal in these babies.

Microvillous inclusion disease is a severe and intractable enteropathy that requires parenteral nutrition (PN) for fluid and nutritional maintenance. The genetic basis is unknown and for some reason it does not manifest *in utero* with hydramnios (as a result of intrauterine diarrhoea), but becomes apparent usually in the first few postnatal days. A late onset presentation is also recognised. Microvillous atrophy is almost invariably fatal without the intervention of PN or intestinal transplantation. Early onset syndromes are characterised by secretory diarrhoea (typically 200–250 mL/kg/day) and intolerance of any oral nutrition. Many babies in this group have early onset cholestatic liver disease.

Tufting and auto-immune enteropathies have a better outcome. Infants require PN support, but there appears to be a range of severity in these disorders with some children becoming less dependent on, and even stopping PN as they progress through childhood. The enteral management of tufting enteropathy is limited to the exclusion of major food allergens if there is concurrent inflammation in the gut biopsies. Auto-immune enteropathies are usually treated with immunosuppression, hypoallergenic feeds and dietary exclusion, but where there is evidence of an underlying primary immunodeficiency haematopoietic stem cell transplantation might be considered.

Modular feeds for use in intractable diarrhoea or short gut syndrome

Intractable diarrhoea can be defined as chronic diarrhoea in the absence of bacterial pathogens of >2 weeks' duration, together with failure to gain weight. Some infants with severe enteropathy or short gut syndrome fail to respond to feed manipulation using protein hydrolysates or amino acid based formulas as previously described and a modular feed becomes the feed of choice [45]. This allows individual manipulation of ingredients resulting in a tailor-made feed for a child. Careful assessment and monitoring is important to prevent nutritional deficiencies and to evaluate the response to feed manipulation. This approach can also assist in the diagnosis of the underlying problem.

Theories as to why modular feeds work include:

- The omission of an ingredient that is poorly tolerated
- The very slow mode of introduction which allows time for gut adaptation to take place
- The delay in adding fat to the feed (traditionally the last ingredient to be added) which may alter the inflammatory response in the gut

None of these theories have been proven but clinical experience has demonstrated the approach can be effective.

Feed ingredients

Some of the possible choices of feed ingredients and their advantages and disadvantages are listed in Tables 7.21–7.24. Before starting there needs to be a discussion with the medical staff regarding the appropriate feed composition for the individual baby and to establish good medical support for the dietitian managing the baby's nutrition. The aim is to produce a feed that is well tolerated and meets the infant's nutritional requirements. The following parameters need to be considered:

- Total energy content and appropriate energy ratio from fat and carbohydrate
- Protein, both type used and quantity

Table 7.21   Protein sources for use in modular feeds.

Product	Protein type	Suggested dilution (g/100 mL)*	Protein equivalent (g/100 mL)	ACBS prescribable	Comments
Hydrolysed Whey Protein/ Maltodextrin Mixture (SHS)	Hydrolysed whey	4	2	N	At this dilution: 1.5 g glucose polymer 0.8 mmol Na + 0.6 mmol K
Pepdite Module (Code 767) (SHS)	Hydrolysed pork and soya	2.5	2.2	N	At this dilution: 1 mmol Na + 0.4 mmol K
Complete Amino Acid Mix (SHS)	L-amino acids	2.5	2.0	N	Amino acids increase feed osmolality No electrolytes

ACBS, Advisory Committee on Borderline Substances.
* This is a suggested dilution only. Quantities can be varied according to the desired protein intake, age of child and feed tolerance.

Table 7.22   Carbohydrate sources for use in modular feeds.

Product	Suggested concentration (g/100 mL)	ACBS prescribable	Comments
Glucose polymer,* e.g. Maxijul (SHS), Polycal (Nutricia)	10–12	Y	Carbohydrate of choice as has the lowest osmolality
Glucose	7–8	Y	Use when glucose polymer intolerance is present. A combination of the two monosaccharides can be used to utilise two transport mechanisms
Fructose	7–8	Y	Monosaccharides will increase final feed osmolality

ACBS, Advisory Committee on Borderline Substances.
* Intolerance to glucose polymers has been documented in the literature [46]. This may be caused by a deficiency of pancreatic amylase or of the disaccharidase glucoamylase. Monosaccharides become the carbohydrates of choice in this situation. It may be possible to use sucrose as an alternative carbohydrate.

Table 7.23   Fat sources for use in modular feeds.

Product	Suggested concentration (g/100 mL*)	Comments
Calogen (canola, sunflower oil emulsion) (SHS)	6–10	Contains linoleic acid (C18 : 2) + α-linolenic acid (C18 : 3)
Liquigen (MCT emulsion) (SHS)	4–8	MCT increases feed osmolality. Does not contain EFAs
Vegetable oils, e.g. olive, sunflower†	3–5	Not water miscible. An emulsion can be prepared by mixing 50 mL oil with 50 mL water and liquidising with 1–2 g gum acacia

EFA, essential fatty acids; MCT, medium chain triglycerides.
* The amount of fat used will depend on tolerance.
† These ingredients are not Advisory Committee on Borderline Substances (ACBS) listed.

Table 7.24 Vitamins and mineral supplements for use in modular feeds.

Metabolic Mineral Mixture (SHS) + Ketovites 5 mL liquid + 3 tablets (Paines and Byrne)	Provide electrolytes. Does not contain selenium or chromium. Vitamins should be given separately Recommended dose of MMM is 1 g/100 mL up to a maximum 8 g dose. Doses >1.5 g/kg body weight/day may result in excessive electrolyte intake
Paediatric Seravit (SHS)	Contains glucose polymer which may be contraindicated. Does not contain electrolytes

- Essential fatty acid intake
- Full vitamin and mineral supplementation, including trace elements
- Suitable electrolyte concentrations
- Feed osmolality

Practical details

- Accurate feed calculation and measurement of ingredients is required to make the necessary small daily feed alterations. Scoop measurements are not accurate enough and ingredients should be weighed on electronic scales.

- Infants with protracted diarrhoea or short gut syndrome will tolerate frequent small bolus feeds given 1–2 hourly, or continuous feeds via a nasogastric tube, better than larger bolus feeds.
- Attention needs to be given to the combination of ingredients as these will affect the feed osmolality. The smaller the molecular size the greater the osmotic effect. Most hospital chemical pathology laboratories will analyse feed osmolality on request.
- Infants requiring a modular feeding approach will have high requirements for all nutrients.
- Paediatric Seravit and Metabolic Mineral Mixture used in conjunction with a fat emulsion, such as Calogen or Liquigen, causes the fat to separate out. For feeds given as a continuous infusion it is recommended that these products are administered separately.

Introduction of modular feeds

Depending on the clinical situation feeds are often introduced very slowly and the concentration of the individual components are gradually increased (Table 7.25). Occasionally, if an infant is already taking a full strength complete feed such as Neocate and the necessary dietary change is to use a modular feed with, say, the same profile as

Table 7.25 Example of slow introduction of a modular feed based on complete amino acid mix.

Time	Complete amino acid mix	NaCl/KCl	Maxijul	Liquigen*	Volume
Day 1–3	½ strength increasing to full strength	Full strength	4%	Nil	As prescribed*
Day 4–9	Full strength	Full strength	Increase in 1% increments daily to total of 10%	Nil	No change
Day 10–15	Full strength	Full strength	10%	Add in 1% increments to 6%	No change
Day 16†	Full strength	Full strength	10%	6%	Increase volume

A vitamin and mineral supplement such as Paediatric Seravit is required to make a complete feed. This should be administered separately if the feed contains a fat emulsion and is being fed continuously.

* Liquigen does not contain EFAs. This feed needs walnut oil given separately.

† If the child is having total parenteral nutrition (TPN) 10–20 mL/kg/day of feed should be given until a full energy feed is established, after which the feed volume can be increased in 2–5 mL/kg daily increments and the parenteral nutrition reduced in tandem.

Neocate with the exception of MCT as the source of fat rather than the usual LCT, then the modular feed may be started at full strength rather than going through this slow increase in concentration.

- Before starting a modular feed it is necessary to assess the infant's symptoms and current nutritional support. If PN is not available feeds should be introduced more rapidly to prevent long periods of inadequate nutrition.
- In the absence of intravenous glucose, the carbohydrate content of the feed should never be less than 4 g/100 mL because of the risk of hypoglycaemia. A higher percentage of energy from fat than from carbohydrate may result in excessive ketone production.
- An example of the slow introduction of an amino acid based modular feed (Tables 7.25 and 7.26) can be applied to other protein sources. Suggested incremental changes can take place every 24 hours. If well tolerated this process can be accelerated.
- The infant's response to each change of feed should be assessed daily before making any further alterations. Where possible making more than one alteration at a time should be avoided.

Preparing and teaching for home

After a period of time on a modular feed it may be worth trying a nutritionally complete feed again to see if this is now tolerated. The formula nearest in composition to the modular feed should be chosen and challenged slowly. If this is not possible, the aim should be to simplify feed ingredients as much as possible for home.

- Ingredients need to be converted into scoop measurements, using the minimum number of different scoops possible to avoid confusion, or scales can be used that measure in 1 g increments.
- A 24-hour recipe should be given to reduce inaccuracies in feed reconstitution, paying due care to issues of hygiene and refrigeration of feed until it is used. It is important to demonstrate the method for making the feed to the infant's carers on at least one occasion before discharge.
- Consideration should be given to providing a laminated recipe and wipe off pen for home use.
- Not all the suggested ingredients for modular feeds are ACBS listed. A separate letter to the child's general practitioner will be needed to arrange a supply of the product. A supply of these items may need to be given from the hospital.

Introduction of solids

Solids should preferably be introduced after the infant or child is established on a nutritionally complete feed. The restrictions imposed will depend on the underlying diagnosis. Often it is necessary to introduce food items singly to determine tolerance of different foods.

Inflammatory bowel disease

Crohn's disease

Crohn's disease (CrD) is caused by a chronic transmural inflammatory process that may affect any

Table 7.26   Example of a full strength modular feed using Complete Amino Acid Mix (per 100 mL).

	Energy		Protein (g)	CHO (g)	Fat (g)	Na$^+$ (mmol)	K$^+$ (mmol)
	(kcal)	(kJ)					
2.5 g Complete Amino Acid Mix	8	34	2	–	–	–	–
10 g Maxijul	38	160	–	9.5	–	–	–
6 mL Liquigen	27	113	–	–	3	0.1	–
1.4 mL NaCl (1 mmol/mL)	–	–	–	–	–	1.4	–
0.8 mL KCl (2 mmol/mL)	–	–	–	–	–	–	1.6
Final feed/100 mL	73	307	2	9.5	3.0	1.5	1.6

A vitamin and mineral supplement such as Paediatric Seravit is required to make a complete feed. This should be administered separately if the feed contains a fat emulsion and is being fed continually.

part of the GI tract from the mouth to the anus. It is an extremely heterogeneous disorder with great anatomical and histological diversity. The small intestine is involved in 90% of cases. The aggressive inflammatory process can cause fibrosis of the small bowel, stricture formation and ulceration leading to fistula formation. The aetiology of CrD is not yet fully understood but is now thought to be the result of an inappropriate immune response to the antigens of the normal bacterial flora in a genetically susceptible individual [47].

The presentation of CrD in children depends largely on the location and extent of the inflammation. In most cases it is insidious in onset with non-specific GI symptoms and growth failure often leading to an initially incorrect diagnosis [48]. It can also be associated with other inflammatory conditions affecting the joints, skin and eyes.

Over time, the disease causes nausea, anorexia and malabsorption. The mean energy intake of patients with active CrD has been found to be up to 420 kcal/day (1.75 MJ/day) lower than in age-matched controls [49]. The energy and protein deficit is reflected as weight loss (occurring in over 80% children) and a decreased height velocity [50]. Growth failure occurs in 15–40% children with CrD. In addition to a reduced oral intake, the pro-inflammatory cytokines that are increased in CrD have been shown to adversely affect growth [51]. Specific nutrient deficiencies such as calcium, magnesium, zinc, iron, folate, B_{12} and fat-soluble vitamins are common findings. During periods of active inflammation there is often enteric leakage of protein resulting in hypoalbuminaemia. Accompanying this is retarded bone mineralisation and development and delayed puberty [52,53].

Treatment

CrD is a chronic and as yet incurable disease and its management requires a combination of nutritional support, judicious use of drugs and appropriate surgery.

Enteral feeds as primary therapy
Nutrition as a treatment for CrD was identified in the 1970s. Since then many trials have been completed with the aim of establishing its efficacy as a primary therapy. These have compared enteral feeds with corticosteroids, a pharmacological treatment known to be effective in the treatment of CrD. They have also compared the effectiveness of different types of feed (elemental, hydrolysate and polymeric).

A systematic review published in 2001 aimed to evaluate the available evidence. The authors concluded that steroids were more effective than enteral nutrition in inducing remission in active CrD, although the latter was effective in inducing disease remission in a significant number of patients. There was no evidence to support an advantage of elemental formulas, the traditional feeds used in CrD, over polymeric (whole protein) feeds [54].

Confounding factors were that in adult studies, nasogastric tubes are not used in patients unable to complete the enteral feeds orally, which affected the results on an intention to treat basis. A CrD activity index has been used to assess clinical response to treatment. These indices are based on a combination of clinical and biochemical data and it is known that steroids favour the clinical index as they cause a feeling of wellbeing in patients [47]. A less rigorous meta-analysis of paediatric trials suggested that nutritional treatment and steroids were equally effective in children [55].

Although it is agreed that enteral feeds work for a significant number of patients, their mode of action is still not understood. Hypotheses include:

- Improvement in mucosal permeability leading to decreased antigen uptake and less stimulation of the gut-associated immune system
- Improved cell-mediated immunity
- Nutritional repletion in a malnourished patient
- Reduction in the intestinal synthesis of inflammatory mediators secondary to the low LCT content of some feeds used
- Altered bowel flora

Modulen IBD is a feed that has been designed specifically for patients with CrD. This has reported immunomodulatory effects brought about by the presence of transforming growth factor β (TGF-β), an anti-inflammatory cytokine present in casein. There are no published trials to date comparing this feed with other polymeric feeds.

The current evidence for enteral feeds as a treatment in active CrD is far from clear [50]. Most paediatric centres use enteral feeds as a primary therapy despite the increased cost compared with steroids and the potential difficulty following the treatment prescribed. As children with CrD are often chronically malnourished, enteral feeds are important for nutritional repletion. Feeds are also preferable as a first line of treatment because of the deleterious effect of steroids on growth. There is currently only low quality evidence to confirm the benefits of feeds on growth in children [51].

Protocol for enteral feeding in Crohn's disease

Although there is convincing evidence that polymeric feeds are as effective a treatment as hydrolysate or elemental feeds, the author's current protocol uses two different feed types, the choice of which is decided by a history of atopy in either the patient or first degree relatives. For those patients with no history suggestive of possible food allergy, a polymeric, whole protein, casein based feed is used while in the atopic individuals a feed based on amino acids is used. Polymeric feeds have the advantage of being more palatable and are cheaper than the elemental alternatives.

Stopping food during the treatment period has been previously recommended without any supportive evidence. A recent randomised paediatric study compared children having 100% nutrition from enteral feeds (total enteral nutrition, TEN) with a second group who received 50% of their requirements from feeds and were allowed to eat normally (partial enteral nutrition, PEN). On analysis, nutritional parameters improved equally in both groups; however, blood indices of inflammation failed to improve in the PEN group, showing that significant amounts of food affects the anti-inflammatory response to enteral feeds [56]. The effect of allowing small amounts of food while having 100% nutritional requirements from feeds has never been examined.

For all feeds the following protocol can be applied:

- Feeds should be gradually introduced over 3–5 days depending on symptoms.
- The enteral feed should provide complete nutrition for a 4–8 week period. If the feed is well tolerated but the child has difficulty managing the volume, the concentration of powdered feeds may be increased to decrease the volume of enteral feed required.
- Clear fluids, boiled sweets and chewing gum are allowed orally by some centres to improve compliance.

- All solid food should be stopped for the duration of the treatment.

As patients with CrD are generally adolescents they find this particularly difficult and require a high degree of support and motivation to complete the treatment. Despite this, feeds are well tolerated by most patients and the full 6 weeks generally adhered to, with 72% of patients in one study reporting it as a preferred treatment or as acceptable as steroid therapy [57].

If the patient is sure that they will be able to manage orally, feeds can be introduced at home. If a nasogastric feeding regimen is required this is best started as an inpatient. Once the feed choice and prescribed volumes have been decided the aim is to give as much control to the patient as possible. Feeds should be tried orally with different flavourings and the volume required daily explained carefully. Patients are given the option of drinking the feed or using a nasogastric tube. If the former is decided on it is important that they understand that the prescribed volume needs to be completed every day as compliance can become an issue. If a tube is chosen patients are taught to pass this each night and remove it in the morning to cause minimum inconvenience to their daily routine. Some patients choose to drink the full volume even of hydrolysate feeds; others opt for a combination approach (a percentage orally and the remainder via the tube); some opt for solely nocturnal nasogastric feeds.

Nutritional requirements and monitoring

Most studies have failed to show increased basal energy requirements in patients with CrD unless the patient has a fever [52,58]. A recent study confirmed that measured resting energy expenditure (REE) in children with CrD fed with PN correlated well with the predicted REE using FAO/WHO/UNU equations and was not increased [59]. However, a prospective study showed that the median energy intake of enterally fed children with CrD was 117.5% of estimated average requirement (EAR) for energy for age [60].

The initial aim should be to provide 100–120% EAR for age for energy and the RNI for protein from the full feed, checking that all vitamins and minerals are present in amounts at least equivalent to the RNI [25]. It should be explained that childen are allowed to take a larger feed volume if they are still hungry. They should be weighed weekly and monitored by telephone contact. A follow-up appointment should be arranged 2–3 weeks after discharge to ensure that the patient is responding to treatment and that weight gain is being achieved.

Introduction of foods and discontinuation of feeds
There is no agreement about the best methods of food introduction to patients completing a period of enteral feeds. In the UK, two main centres have published data with conflicting results. The East Anglian study found that a large number of patients were food intolerant, the most common foods cited as causing problems being corn, wheat, yeast, egg, potato, rye, tea and coffee [61]. This trial has been criticised as patients only completed 2 weeks of an elemental diet before foods were introduced which would not have been long enough to allow for full disease remission. This approach has been modified and a reduced allergen, low fat, low fibre diet devised to be introduced at the end of the 2–3 week period of enteral feeds with subsequent food reintroductions [62].

The group at Northwick Park Hospital introduced foods singly over 5-day periods after 4–8 weeks on complete enteral feeds. Food sensitivities could only be identified in 7% of the patients by double blind challenge. Most importantly, there was no significant difference in the duration of remission between patients who did or did not identify food sensitivities [63].

Beattie and Walker-Smith [64] concluded that neither study confirmed that intolerance to foodstuffs is seen in CrD and that no particular foods are known to exacerbate symptoms in a large group of patients.

Until there is further evidence it would appear prudent to reduce feed volume over a period of 2–4 weeks and gradually introduce a normal diet, ensuring that continued weight gain is maintained. Single food introductions do not seem worthwhile in the majority of patients and merely prolong the resumption of a normal diet. Patients found to be atopic and requiring a hydrolysate or amino acid based feed should be advised to exclude suspected food allergens, ensuring an adequate energy and calcium intake. Patients with a tight stricture in the ileum may require a low fibre diet to control symptoms until the stricture is surgically removed.

Long term outcome in Crohn's disease

Some patients require continued nutritional support either by nasogastric tube, gastrostomy or orally if appetite remains poor. It has also been reported that continued use of supplementary feeds in addition to a normal diet is associated with prolonged periods of disease remission and improved linear growth [57,65]. Studies have not been randomised and patient numbers are small. This is not current practice in UK centres at the time of writing.

A pilot study looking at quality of life (QOL) in a small group of children with apparently stable disease showed the impact of CrD. Difficulties in taking holidays, staying at friends' houses and inability to engage in school sports (because of lack of energy or presence of a stoma) were reported as well as frequently missing school. Future studies of treatment in children should attempt to assess the impact on the child's health-related QOL [66].

Ulcerative colitis

Like CrD, ulcerative colitis (UC) is a chronic, relapsing, inflammatory disease of the intestine which is confined to the colonic and rectal mucosa. It also has an unknown aetiology with evidence for an inherited predisposition to the disease alongside other, possibly environmental, factors. Tissue injury is most likely a result of non-specific activation of the immune system with some evidence that this has an auto-immune aetiology.

Drug therapy is used to induce and maintain disease remission. There is no evidence to support the use of enteral nutrition as a primary therapy in UC. The nutritional problems found in CrD are not as severe in UC because of the lack of involvement of the small intestine [53].

Nutritional support is needed if there is growth failure or weight loss and this can be given as a high energy diet and oral sip feeds.

Disorders of altered gut motility

Gastro-oesophageal reflux

Gastro-oesophageal reflux (GOR) refers to the inappropriate opening of the lower oesophageal sphincter (LOS) releasing gastric contents into the oesophagus. It is not a diagnosis and can be caused by differing pathologies. Approximately 50% of infants regurgitate at least once a day and, in the majority of children, this can be considered as an uncomplicated self-limiting condition which spontaneously resolves by 12–15 months of age. This is because of the lengthening of the oesophagus and the development of the gastro-oesophageal sphincter.

More severe forms of this problem are found when an infant with regurgitation does not respond to simple treatment and develops gastro-oesophageal reflux disease. Acid induced lesions of the oesophagus and oesophagitis develop and are associated with other symptoms such as failure to thrive, haematemesis, respiratory symptoms, apnoea, irritability, feeding disorders and iron deficiency anaemia. GOR is a common finding in infants with neurological problems.

Treatment

Parental reassurance is very important and may preclude the need for any other measures. However, recurrent symptoms of inconsolable crying or irritability, feeding or sleeping difficulties, persistent regurgitation or vomiting may lead to unnecessary parental distress, recurrent medical consultations and may need further treatment.

Positioning
Postural treatment of infants has been demonstrated to help and a prone elevated position at 30° is the most successful in reducing GOR [67]. It is no longer possible to recommend this as several studies have shown an increased risk of sudden infant death syndrome (SIDS) in the prone sleeping position. It also requires the purchase of a special cot in which the baby has to be tied up to be kept in place, which is not always possible [68]. A systematic review concluded that raising the head of the cot was not beneficial to infants lying in the supine position [69]. A more practical approach is to avoid positions that exacerbate the situation. Young infants tend to slump when placed in a seat, which increases pressure on the stomach and makes the reflux worse. It is better to place them in a seat that reclines or to lie them down.

Feeding
The infant must not be overfed and should be offered an age-appropriate volume of milk. Small

volume, frequent feeds may also be beneficial by reducing gastric distension (e.g. 150 mL formula/kg/day as 6–7 feeds). In practice frequent feeds may be difficult for parents to manage and reduced feed volumes may cause distress in a hungry baby.

The use of feed thickeners has been proven to reduce vomiting in infants, although pH monitoring shows that the gastro-oesophageal reflux index is not reduced [69,70]. Thickeners are well tolerated with very few side effects reported and should be used as a first line treatment in infants with regurgitation [68,69]. Caution has been urged by ESPGHAN that the indiscriminate use of thickening agents and pre-thickened formula should be avoided in healthy thriving infants who spit up feeds as the effects on nutrient bioavailability, metabolic and endocrine responses and frequency of allergic reactions to thickening agents are unknown [71].

Enfamil AR and SMA Staydown are nutritionally complete pre-thickened infant formulas based on cow's milk protein and are available on prescription (ACBS). Enfamil AR contains a high amylopectin, pre-gelatinised rice starch. It should be made with boiled water that has been cooled to room temperature to avoid lumps forming and the bottle then requires rolling between the hands to ensure proper mixing. SMA Staydown contains pre-cooked cornstarch and should be mixed with cold, previously boiled water. Both feeds thicken on contact with the acid pH of the stomach. The EC Scientific Committee for Food has accepted the addition of starch to a maximum of 2 g/100 mL in infant formula. Recommendations suggest that labelling should make it clear that 'AR' stands for 'Anti-Regurgitation' and not for 'Anti-Reflux' [72].

A variety of manufactured feed thickeners are on the market in the UK, based either on carob seed or modified maize starch (Table 7.27). Of the former, Instant Carobel has an advantage over Nestargel in that it thickens the feed without the need to be cooked. The complex carbohydrates in both products are non-absorbable and can lead, in a minority of infants, to the passage of frequent loose stools. Both products have the added flexibility of being mixed as a gel and fed from a spoon before breast feeds.

Where failure to thrive is a problem a starch based thickener can be used to provide extra energy. The lowest amount of thickener recommended should be added initially and the amount

Table 7.27 Feed thickeners for use in infancy available in the UK.

Product (Manufacturer)	Thickening agent	Suggested dilution (g/100 mL)	Added energy per 100 mL		ACBS prescribable
			(kcal)	(kJ)	
Instant Carobel (Nutricia Clinical)	Carob seed	1–3	3–8	13–33	Y
Nestargel* (Nestlé)	Carob seed	0.5–1	Negligible		Y
Thick and Easy (Fresenius Kabi) Thixo-D (Sutherland) Vitaquick (Vitaflo)	Pre-cooked maize starch	1–3	4–12	17–50	Y[†]

ACBS, Advisory Committee on Borderline Substances.
* Product requires cooking before use.
[†] Only prescribable for <1 year in cases of failure to thrive.

gradually increased to the maximum level if there is no resolution of symptoms. Feeding through a teat with a slightly larger hole, or a variable flow teat, is recommended. Ordinary cornflour can also be used as a thickening agent for infant feeds but has the inconvenience of requiring cooking. This should be done in approximately half of the volume of water required for the final feed recipe and cooled before the formula powder is added. Such feeds generally require sieving before use.

Comfort First Infant Milk and Follow-on Milk are thickened infant and follow-on formulas made from partially hydrolysed whey protein that contain prebiotic oligosaccharides. They are designed for bottle fed babies with minor feeding problems.

Food allergy

In more complicated GOR that fails to respond to simple treatment, a therapeutic change of formula should be considered as it has been demonstrated that GOR can be secondary to food allergy. Two studies have demonstrated that 30–40% of infants with GOR resistant to treatment have cow's milk allergy, with symptoms significantly improving on a cow's milk protein free diet [73,74]. In food sensitive patients cow's milk has been shown to cause gastric dysrhythmia and delayed gastric emptying which may exacerbate GOR and induce reflux vomiting [75]. The use of protein hydrolysate feeds in these infants for a trial period should be considered as a treatment option (Table 7.7).

Medical treatment

Medications that can be used to treat GOR range

from antacids to H_2 antagonists, such as ranitidine which reduces gastric acid secretion; proton pump inhibitors such as omeprazole; and prokinetic agents, such as domperidone, which elevates the LOS pressure and increases gastric emptying. A combination of these is often given to control symptoms.

In extreme cases that do not respond to the above treatments, surgery may be needed to correct the problem. A fundoplication which wraps the fundus of the stomach around the LOS creates an artificial valve and prevents GOR (see p. 129). A gastrostomy is usually inserted for venting gas from the stomach and, occasionally, for feeding purposes. There is considerable morbidity associated with this operation.

Feeding problems in GOR

Feeding difficulties are common in this disorder and are characterised by oral motor dysfunction, episodes of dysphagia and negative feeding experiences by both mother and baby. Infants with GOR are significantly more demanding and difficult to feed and have been found to ingest significantly less energy than matched infants without GOR [76]. These problems often persist after medical or surgical treatment with the continuing aversive behaviour being caused by associating pain with previous feeding experiences.

Where there are severe feeding problems it may be necessary to instigate feeding via a nasogastric tube or gastrostomy to ensure an adequate nutritional intake. Wherever possible an oral intake, however small, should be maintained to minimise later feeding problems. The child's feed should be administered as oral or bolus day feeds with continuous feeds overnight at a slow rate to avoid feed aspiration. The feed volume may need to be reduced below that recommended for age to ensure tolerance, with feeds fortified in the usual way to ensure adequate nutrition for catch-up growth. If using a fine bore nasogastric tube to administer bolus feeds, thickening agents should be kept to the minimum concentration recommended to prevent the tube blocking and an inappropriate length of time being taken to administer the feed. There is no evidence that reduced fat feeds promote gastric emptying and reduce GOR in these infants [72].

The requirement for tube feeding can continue for prolonged periods of time, as long as 36 months in one study [77]. Parents of infants with feeding problems secondary to GOR need a great deal of support. Optimal management should employ a multidisciplinary feeding disorder team including a psychologist with experience of children with these problems, a paediatrician, a dietitian and a speech and language therapist.

Constipation

Constipation is a symptom rather than a disease and can be caused by anatomical, physiological or histopathological abnormalities. Idiopathic constipation is not related to any of these and is thought to be most often caused by the intentional or subconscious withholding of stool after a precipitating acute event. Constipation has been found to account for 3% of visits to general paediatric outpatient clinics and 10–25% of visits to a paediatric gastroenterologist, so is a sizeable problem.

Average stool frequency has been estimated to be four stools per day in the first week of life, two per day at 1 year of age, decreasing to the adult pattern of between three per day and three per week by the age of 4 years. Within these patterns there is a great variation. The Paris Consensus on Childhood Constipation Terminology (PACCT) Group [78] defined chronic constipation as the occurrence of two or more of the following characteristics during the last 8 weeks:

- Less than three bowel movements per week
- More than one episode of faecal incontinence per week

- Large stools in the rectum or palpable on abdominal examination
- Passing of stools so large they obstruct the toilet
- Retentive posturing and withholding behaviour
- Painful defaecation

In idiopathic constipation prolonged stretching of the anal walls associated with chronic faecal retention leads to an atonic and desensitised rectum. This perpetuates the problem as large volumes of faeces must be present to initiate the call to pass a stool. Faecal incontinence (previously described as encopresis or soiling) is mostly as a result of chronic faecal retention and rarely occurs before the age of 3 years.

Treatment

Acute simple constipation is usually treated with a high fibre diet, sufficient fluid intake, filling out a stool frequency diary and toilet training. Treatment of chronic constipation is based on four phases:

- Education of the family to explain the pathogenesis of constipation
- Disimpaction using oral or rectal medication
- Prevention of re-accumulation of faeces using dietary interventions, behavioural modifications and laxatives (a mixture of osmotic laxatives such as lactulose, stimulants such as senna and mineral oils can be used)
- Follow-up [79]

Dietary fibre can be classified into water soluble and insoluble forms. The former includes pectins, fructo-oligosaccharides (FOS), gums and mucilages that are fermented by colonic bacteria to produce short chain fatty acids. This has been shown to increase stool water content and volume. Insoluble fibre mainly acts as a bulking agent in the stool by trapping water in the intestinal tract and acting like a sponge. Both soften and enlarge the stool and reduce GI transit times.

Surveys have shown that constipated children often eat considerably less fibre than their non-constipated counterparts. Even when advised to increase their fibre intake by a physician the fibre intake was only half of the amount of the control population. It appears that families can only make the necessary changes with specific dietary counselling [80]. Children with chronic constipation have also been shown to have lower energy intakes and a higher incidence of anorexia. It is difficult to know if this existed previously and predisposed to the condition or whether it is caused by early satiety secondary to constipation [81].

There are currently no guidelines in the UK for appropriate fibre intakes in children. In the USA recommendations are for children older than 2 years to consume daily a minimum number of grams of dietary fibre equal to their age in years plus 5 g/day (e.g. a 4-year-old should have a minimum of 4 + 5 = 9 g fibre/day) [82]. In infancy and childhood it is important to ensure that adequate fluids are taken. As a guide children should have 6–8 drinks a day preferably as water or juice and including any milk. For children who continue to drink insufficient amounts foods with a high fluid intake should be encouraged such as ice lollies, jelly and sauces. Fruit, vegetables and salad have a high fluid content as well as being desirable because of their fibre content.

In babies, the addition of carbohydrate to feeds can induce an osmotic softening of the stool but is not to be encouraged as a general public health message. Once solids are introduced these should include fruit and vegetables, with wholegrain cereals being introduced after the age of 6 months. Bran should not be used in infancy and with caution in older children.

In the 1999 American evidence based guidelines, no randomised controlled trial was found that showed an effect on stools in constipated children of any of the above dietary measures [79]. The fact that constipation is uncommon in societies that consume a high fibre diet has been used to justify this treatment. More recently, a double blind randomised control trial (DBRCT) studying the effects of infant cereal supplemented with FOS in normal infants showed that this resulted in more frequent and softer stools [83]. Another DBRCT using glucomannan as a water-soluble fibre supplement in the diet of children aged 4 or older with chronic constipation showed a beneficial outcome [84]. There are currently no confirmed positive effects of the use of probiotics in constipation.

Food allergy

In a select group of children with constipation who fail to respond to conventional treatment, cow's milk protein free diets have been shown to be beneficial [85]. Motility studies in these patients have indicated that the delay in faecal passage is a consequence of stool retention in the rectum and not of a generalised motility disorder [86]. It has therefore been proposed that all children with chronic constipation that fails to respond to normal treatment as outlined above should be considered for a trial of a cow's milk free diet (Table 7.6), especially if they are atopic [87]. A recent study showed that, of 52 patients with chronic constipation, 58% had an eosinophilic proctitis caused by an underlying food allergy. This was confirmed by double blind food challenges. The majority were intolerant of cow's milk protein; however, six patients had multiple food intolerances identified by the use of a few foods diet [88].

Gut motility disorders

Integration of the digestive, absorptive and motor functions of the gut is required for the assimilation of nutrients. In the mature gut, motor functions are organised into particular patterns of contractile activity that have several control mechanisms.

After swallowing, a bolus of fluid or food is propelled down the oesophagus by peristalsis; this action differs from the motility of the rest of the intestine in that it can be induced voluntarily. The LOS relaxes to allow food or fluid to pass into the stomach which acts as a reservoir and also initiates digestion. It has a contractile action that grinds food to 1–2 mm particle size. Gastric emptying can be modulated by feed components via hormonal secretion. LCTs have been found to inhibit gastric emptying. Different dietary proteins also have an effect with whey hydrolysates emptying more rapidly than whole protein feeds [89].

In the small intestine, motor activity is effected by smooth muscle contraction which is controlled by myogenic, neural and chemical factors. In the fasting state the gut has a contractile activity (the migrating motor complex) that keeps the luminal bacteria in the colon. Abnormalities of this phasic activity can result in bacterial overgrowth of the small intestine and malabsorption. Post-prandial activity is initiated by hormones and food eaten to produce peristalsis in the gut, relaxation of the muscle coats below and contraction above the bolus of food through the intestine. Disturbances in this co-ordinated system can occur at all levels.

Toddler diarrhoea

Toddler diarrhoea, also known as chronic non-specific diarrhoea, is the most frequent cause of chronic diarrhoea in children between the ages of 1 and 5 years of age. Symptoms include frequent watery stools containing undigested foodstuffs in a child who is otherwise well and thriving. Despite the children generally presenting in a good nutritional state, parental anxiety is high. The diarrhoea ceases spontaneously, generally between 2 and 4 years of age.

Proposed mechanisms
A primary problem has still not been identified. Children with this disorder are known to have a rapid gut transit time and intestinal motility is generally thought to be abnormal, although it is unsure whether this is caused by a reduced colonic transit time or a disturbance of small intestinal motility.

Carbohydrate malabsorption, particularly of fructose, has been extensively investigated in this disorder. Fructose is known to be slowly absorbed in the small intestine and is often present in large amounts in fruit juice. In recent years, the diets of children in this age group have undergone changes with an increase in the amount of fruit squash and fruit juices and a decrease in water taken as drinks [90]. As apple juice particularly has been implicated as causing toddler diarrhoea, studies have been completed using hydrogen breath tests to measure carbohydrate malabsorption. What now seems to be evident is that non-absorbable monosaccharides and oligosaccharides such as galacturonic acid are produced by enzymatic treatment of the fruit pulp in clear fruit juices, including apple, grape and bilberry juices. It is thought that these may cause problems in sensitive individuals, rather than fructose [91].

Treatment
All sources agree that parental reassurance is of primary importance. The role of diet in this disorder is controversial [43,92]. Advice is needed to correct any dietary idiosyncracies. Excessive fluid intake, particularly of fruit juices and squash, should be discouraged. Fibre intake has frequently been reduced by parents in an attempt to normalise stools, therefore increasing this to normal levels should be recommended. Fat intake may also have been reduced, either because of the excessive consumption of high carbohydrate fruit drinks or for health reasons, and should be increased to 35–40% of total dietary energy. Often parents have tried excluding foods from the child's diet, mistakenly believing the problems to be brought about by food intolerance. Once the diagnosis is established these foods should be reintroduced.

Chronic idiopathic pseudo-obstruction disorder

This term embraces a heterogeneous group of disorders that cause severe intestinal dysmotility with recurrent symptoms of intestinal obstruction in the absence of mechanical occlusion. Gut transit time is generally in excess of 96 hours. The cause is usually an enteric myopathy or neuropathy that can also affect the urinary tract [93]. It is an extremely rare disorder with a high morbidity and mortality.

Nutritional support is vital for these children. In one series of 44 patients, 72% required parenteral nutrition for a relatively long period of time, seven children dying of PN related complications with a further 10 remaining dependent on long term home PN [94].

Full enteral nutrition is possible to achieve in some patients but needs to be started slowly, with a gradual decrease in PN volume as the enteral nutrition is increased. Particular attention needs to be paid to fluid and electrolyte requirements. Many of the children have an ileostomy to decompress the gut. The loss of sodium rich effluent through the stoma generally results in high sodium requirements (up to 10 mmol/kg/day). Enteral feed can be pooled in the intestine for a prolonged period of time before passing through the stoma, resulting in a lack of appreciation of the relatively high fluid requirements of these children. In certain children (especially those with a migrating motor complex), jejunal feeding may be successful if a trial of gastric feeds have failed [95].

Treatment
The following suggestions for the nutritional management of these patients have proved beneficial:

- Liquids are easier for the dysmotile gut to process than highly textured foods. Aim to give full requirements from the feed or PN, or a combination of the two, to minimise intake of solids.
- Enteral feeds are more likely to be tolerated as a continuous infusion than as bolus feeds.

- Whey hydrolysates have been found to empty more rapidly from the stomach and form the mainstay of treatment [89].
- Care should be taken to ensure that enteral feeds are made as cleanly as possible to prevent the introduction of organisms into the gut, which could contribute to bacterial overgrowth. In older children the use of sterile feeds is preferable.
- Fluid and sodium requirements should be accurately assessed and supplements given as needed.
- Where solids are taken these should be low in fibre so as not to cause obstruction. Semi-solid or bite-dissolvable consistencies such as purées, mashed potato and puffed rice cereal will be more easily digested.

In these children weight measurements are not always accurate because of distended loops of gut pooling large quantities of fluid. They should be used in conjunction with other anthropometric measurements such as mid-arm circumference or skinfold thicknesses to assess nutritional state.

References

1 Recommendations for Composition of Oral Rehydration Solutions for the Children of Europe. Report of an ESPGAN Working Group. *J Pediatr Gastroenterol Nutr*, 1992, **14** 113–15.

2 Hahn S *et al.* Reduced osmolarity oral rehydration solution for treating dehydration caused by acute diarrhea in children. *Cochrane Database Syst Rev*, 2002, **1** CD002847.

3 Fontaine O *et al.* Rice-based oral rehydration solution for treating diarrhoea. *Cochrane Database Syst Rev*, 2000, **2** CD001264.

4 Sandhu B *et al.* Rationale for Early Feeding in Childhood Gastroenteritis. *J Pediatr Gastroenterol Nutr*, 2001, **33** S13–16.

5 Kaila M, *et al.* Treatment of acute diarrhoea in practice. *Acta Paediatr*, 1997, **86** 1340–4.

6 Brown KH *et al.* Use of non-human milks in the dietary management of young children with acute diarrhoea: a meta-analysis of clinical trials. *Pediatrics*, 1994, **93** 17–27.

7 Sandhu BK *et al.* Early feeding in childhood gastroenteritis. A multicente study on behalf of the European Society of Paediatric Gastroenterology and Nutrition working group on acute diarrhoea. *J Pediatr Gastroenterol Nutr*, 1997, **24** 522–7.

8 Walker-Smith JA *et al.* Recommendations for feeding in childhood gastroenteritis. European Society of Paediatric Gastroenterology and Nutrition. *J Paediatr Gastroenterol Nutr*, 1997, **24** 619–20.

9 Szajewska H *et al.* Management of acute gastroenteritis in Europe and the impact of the new recommendations: a multicenter study. *J Pediatr Gastroenterol Nutr*, 2000, **30** 522–7.

10 Johansson SGO *et al.* A revised nomenclature for allergy. *Allergy*, 2001, **56** 813–24.

11 Murch S. Allergy and Intestinal Dysmotility-Causal or Coincidental Links? *J Pediatr Gastroenterol Nutr*, 2005, **41** S14–16.

12 Nowak-Wegrzyn A *et al.* Food protein-induced enterocolitis syndrome caused by solid food proteins. *Pediatrics*, 2003, **111** 829–35.

13 Latcham F *et al.* A consistent pattern of minor immunodeficiency and subtle enteropathy in children with multiple food allergy. *J Pediatr*, 2003, **143** 39–47.

14 Wyllie R Cow's milk protein allergy and hypoallergenic formulas. *Clin Pediatr*, 1996, **35** 497–500.

15 de Boissieu D *et al.* Multiple food allergy: a possible diagnosis in breastfed infants. *Acta Paediatr*, 1997, **86** 1042–6.

16 Host A *et al.* Dietary products used in infants for treatment and prevention of food allergy. Joint statement of the ESPACI Committee on allergenic formulas and the ESPGAN Committee on nutrition. *Arch Dis Child*, 1999, **81** 80–4.

17 American Academy of Pediatrics Committee on Nutrition Soy protein-based formulas: recommendations for use in infant feeding. *Paediatrics*, 1998, **101** 148–53.

18 COT (2003): Phytoestrogens and health. FSA www.foodstandards.gov.uk/multimedia/pdfs/phytoreport0503

19 Paediatric Group Position Statement on the use of soya protein for infants, British Dietetic Association, Birmingham, 2003.

20 Zeiger RS *et al.* Soy allergy in infants and children with IgE-associated cow's milk allergy. *J Pediatr*, 1999, **134** 614–22.

21 Businco L *et al.* Allergenicity and nutritional adequacy of soy protein formulas. *J Pediatr*, 1992, **121** S21–8.

22 Lee YH Food processing approaches to altering allergenic potential of milk based formula. *J Pediatr*, 1992, **121** S47–50.

23 Wahn U *et al.* Comparison of the residual allergenic activity of six different hydrolyzed protein formulas. *J Pediatr*, 1992, **121** S80–4.

24 Vanderhoof JA *et al.* Intolerance to protein hydrolysate infant formulas: an under-recognised cause of gastrointestinal symptoms in infants. *J Pediatr*, 1997, **131** 741–4.

25 The Department of Health Report on Health and Social Subjects No. 41, Dietary Reference Values for Food Energy and Nutrients for the United Kingdom. London: The Stationery Office, 1991.

26 Madsen CD, Henderson RC Calcium intake in children with positive IgG RAST to cow's milk. *J Paediatr Child Health*, 1997, **33** 209–12.

27 Henriksen C *et al.* Nutrient intake among two-year-old children on cows' milk-restricted diets. *Acta Paediatr*, 2000, **89** 272–8.

28 Ciclitira P Guidelines for the management of Patients with Coeliac Disease, 2002. Available from: http://www.bsg.org.uk/clinical_prac/guidelines/coeliac.htm

29 Bingley PJ *et al.* Undiagnosed coeliac disease at age seven: population based prospective birth cohort study. *Br Med J*, 2004, **328** 322–3.

30 Hill ID *et al.* Guidelines for the diagnosis and treatment of celiac disease in children: recommendations of the North American Society for Paediatric Gastroenterology, Hepatology and Nutrition. *J Pediatr Gastroenterol Nutr*, 2005, **40** 1–19.

31 Revised criteria for diagnosis of coeliac disease. Report of working group of ESPGAN. *Arch Dis Child*, 1990, **65** 909–11.

32 Gluten-free foods: a prescribing guide, 2004. Available from: Good Relations Healthcare, Suite 2, Cobb House, Oyster Lane, Byfleet, Surrey, KT14 7DU.

33 Schmitz J Lack of oats toxicity in coeliac disease. *Br Med J*, 1997, **314** 159–60.

34 The Coeliac Society Guidelines on coeliac disease and oats. High Wycombe: Coeliac Society, 1998.

35 Janatuinen EK *et al.* No harm from five year ingestion of oats in coeliac disease. *Gut*, 2002, **50** 332–5.

36 Hogberg L *et al.* Oats to children with newly diagnosed coeliac disease: a randomized double blind study. *Gut*, 2004 **53** 649–54.

37 Berera G *et al.* Longitudinal changes in bone metabolism and bone mineral content in children with celiac disease during consumption of a gluten-free diet. *Am J Clin Nutr*, 2004, **79** 148–54.

38 Baudon JJ *et al.* Sucrase-isomaltase deficiency: changing pattern over two decades. *J Pediatr Gastroenterol Nutr*, 1996, **22** 284–8.

39 McCance & Widdowson's *The Composition of Foods*, 6th summary edn. Food Standards Agency 2002.

40 Treem WR Congenital sucrase-isomaltase deficiency. *J Pediatr Gastroenterol Nutr*, 1995, **21** 1–14.

41 Treem WR *et al.* Sacrosidase therapy for congenital sucrase-isomaltase deficiency. *J Pediatr Gastroenterol Nutr*, 1999, **28** 137–42.

42 Vardy PA *et al.* Intestinal lymphangiectasia: a reappraisal. *Pediatr*, 1975, **55** 842–51.

43 Walker Smith J, Murch S *Diseases of the Small Intestine in Childhood*, 4th edn. New York: Isis Medical Media Ltd, 1999.

44 Sherman PM *et al.* Neonatal enteropathies: defining the causes of protracted diarrhea of infancy. *J Pediatr Gastroenterol Nutr*, 2004, **38** 16–26.

45 Walker-Smith JA Nutritional management of enteropathy. *Nutr*, 1998, **14** 775–9.

46 Fisher SE *et al.* Chronic protracted diarrhea: intolerance to dietary glucose polymers. *Pediatrics*, 1981, **67** 271–2.

47 Beattie M *et al.* Childhood Crohn's disease and the efficacy of enteral diets. *Nutr*, 1998, **14** 345–50.

48 Walker-Smith JA Management of growth failure in Crohn's disease. *Arch Dis Child*, 1996, **75** 351–4.

49 Thomas AG *et al.* Dietary intake and nutritional treatment in childhood Crohn's disease. *J Pediatr Gastroenterol Nutr*, 1993, **17** 75–81.

50 Griffiths AG Inflammatory bowel disease. *Nutr*, 1998, **14** 788–91.

51 Newby EA *et al.* Interventions for growth failure in childhood Crohn's disease. *Cochrane Database Syst Rev*, 2005, **3** CD003873.

52 Hyams JS Crohn's disease in children. *Pediatr Clin North Am*, 1996, **43** 255–77.

53 Boot AM *et al.* Bone mineral density and nutritional status in children with chronic inflammatory bowel disease. *Gut*, 1998, **42** 188–94.

54 Zachos M *et al.* Enteral nutritional therapy for induction of remission in Crohn's disease. *Cochrane Database Syst Rev*, 2001, **3** CD000542.

55 Heuschkel R *et al.* Enteral nutrition and corticosteroids in the treatment of acute Crohn's disease in children. *J Pediatr Gastroenterol Nutr*, 2000, **31** 8–15.

56 Johnson T *et al.* Treatment of active Crohn's disease in children using partial enteral nutrition with liquid formula: a randomised controlled trial. *Gut*, 2006, **55** 356–61.

57 Wilschanski M *et al.* Supplementary enteral nutrition maintains remission in paediatric Crohn's disease. *Gut*, 1996, **38** 543–8.

58 Azcue M *et al.* Energy expenditure and body composition in children with Crohn's disease: effect of enteral nutrition and treatment with prednisolone. *Gut*, 1997, **41** 203–8.

59 Cormier K *et al.* Resting energy expenditure in the parenterally fed pediatric population with Crohn's disease. *J Parenteral Enteral Nutr*, 2005, **29** 102–7.

60 Gavin J *et al.* Energy intakes of children with Crohn's disease treated with enteral nutrition as primary therapy. *J Hum Nutr Diet*, 2005, **18** 337–42.

61 Riordan AM *et al.* Treatment of active Crohn's disease by exclusion diet: East Anglian multicentre controlled trial. *Lancet*, 1993, **342** 1131–4.

62 Woolner JT *et al.* The development and evaluation of a diet for maintaining remission in Crohn's disease. *J Hum Nutr Diet*, 1998, **11** 1–11.

63 Pearson M *et al.* Food intolerance and Crohn's disease. *Gut*, 1993, **34** 783–7.

64 Beattie RM, Walker-Smith JA Treatment of active Crohn's disease by exclusion diet. *J Pediatr Gastroenterol Nutr*, 1994, **19** 135–6.

65 Verma S *et al.* Oral nutritional supplementation is effective in the maintainance of remission in Crohn's disease. *Dig Liver Dis* 2000, **32** 769–74.

66 Akoberg AK *et al.* Quality of Life in Children with Crohn's Disease: A Pilot Study. *J Pediatr Gastroenterol Nutr*, 1999, **28** S37–9.

67 Orenstein SR *et al.* Positioning for prevention of infant gastroesophageal reflux. *J Paediatr*, 1983, **103** 534–7.

68 Vandenplas Y *et al.* Current concepts and issues in the management of regurgitation of infants: a reappraisal. *Acta Paediatr*, 1996, **85** 531–4.

69 Craig WR *et al.* Metoclopramide, thickened feedings and positioning for gastro-oesophageal reflux in children under two years. *Cochrane Database Syst Rev*, 2004, **3** CD003502.

70 Orenstein SR *et al.* Thickening of infant feedings for therapy of gastroesophageal reflux. *J Pediatr*, 1987, **110** 181–6.

71 Aggett PJ *et al.* Antireflux or antiregurgitation milk products for infants and young children: a commentary by the ESPGHAN Committee on Nutrition. *J Pediatr Gastroenterol Nutr*, 2002, **34** 496–8.

72 Vandenplas Y *et al.* Dietary treatment for regurgitation – recommendations from a working party. *Acta Paediatr*, 1998, **87** 462–8.

73 Cavataio F *et al.* Clinical and pH-metric characteristics of gastro-oesophageal reflux secondary to cow's milk protein allergy. *Arch Dis Child*, 1996, **75** 51–6.

74 Cavataio F *et al.* Gastroesophageal reflux and cow's milk allergy in infants: a prospective study. *J Allergy Clin Immunol*, 1996, **97** 822–7.

75 Ravelli AM *et al.* Vomiting and gastric motility in infants with cow's milk allergy. *J Pediatr Gastroenterol Nutr*, 2001, **32** 59–64.

76 Mathisen B *et al.* Feeding problems in infants with gastro-oesophageal reflux disease: a controlled study. *J Paediatr Child Health*, 1999, **35** 163–9.

77 Dellert SF *et al.* Feeding resistance and gastroesophageal reflux in infancy. *J Pediatr Gastroenterol Nutr*, 1993, **17** 66–71.

78 Benninga M *et al.* The Paris Consensus on Childhood Constipation Terminology (PACCT) Group. *J Pediatr Gastroenterol Nutr*, 2005, **40** 273–5.

79 Baker SS *et al.* Constipation in infants and children: evaluation and treatment. *J Pediatr Gastroenterol Nutr*, 1999, **29** 612–26.

80 McClung HJ *et al.* Constipation and dietary fiber intake in children. *Pediatrics*, 1995, **96** 999–1000.

81 Roma E *et al.* Diet and chronic constipation in children: the role of fiber. *J Pediatr Gastroenterol Nutr*, 1999, **28** 169–74.

82 Williams CL *et al.* A new recommendation for dietary fiber in childhood. *Pediatrics*, 1995, **96** 985–8.

83 Moore N *et al.* Effects of fructo-oligosaccharide-supplemented infant cereal: a double-blind, randomized trial. *Br J Nutr*, 2003, **90** 581–7.

84 Leoning-Baucke V *et al.* Fiber (glucomannan) is beneficial in the treatment of childhood constipation. *Pediatrics*, 2004, **113** 259–64.

85 Iacona G *et al.* Intolerance of cow's milk and chronic constipation in children. *N Engl J Med*, 1998, **339** 1100–4.

86 Shah N *et al.* Cow's milk and chronic constipation in children (letter). *N Engl J Med*, 1999, **340** 891–2.

87 Loening-Baucke V Constipation in children. *N Engl J Med*, 1998, **339** 1155–6.

88 Carroccio A *et al.* Chronic constipation and food intolerance: a model of proctitis causing constipation. *Scand J Gastroenterol*, 2005, **40** 33–42.

89 Tolia V *et al.* Gastric emptying using three different formulas in infants with gastroesophageal reflux. *J Pediatr Gastroenterol Nutr*, 1992, **15** 297–301.

90 Petter LPM *et al.* Is water out of vogue? A survey of the drinking habits of 2–7 year olds. *Arch Dis Child*, 1995, **72** 137–40.

91 Hoekstra JH Toddler diarrhoea: more a nutritional disorder than a disease. *Arch Dis Child*, 1998, **79** 2–5.

92 Kneepekens CMF, Hoestra JH Chronic non-specific diarrhoea of childhood, pathophysiology and management. *Paediatr Clin North Am*, 1996, **43** 375–90.

93 Rudolph CD *et al.* Diagnosis and treatment of chronic intestinal pseudo-obstruction in children: Report of Consensus Workshop. *J Pediatr Gastroenterol Nutr*, 1997, **24** 102–12.

94 Heneyke S *et al.* Chronic intestinal pseudo-obstruction: treatment and long term follow up of 44 patients. *Arch Dis Child*, 1999, **81** 21–7.

95 Di Lorenzo C *et al.* Intestinal motility and jejunal feeding in children with chronic intestinal pseudo-obstruction. *Gastroenterology*, 1995, **108** 1379–85.

Further reading

Guandalini S. *Textbook of Pediatric Gastroenterology and Nutrition*. London: Taylor & Francis, 2004.

Walker WA *et al. Pediatric Gastrointestinal Disease. Pathophysiology, Diagnosis and Management*, 3rd edn, Vols 1 & 2. Philadelphia: BC Decker Inc, 2000.

Walker Smith J, Murch S *Diseases of the Small Intestine in Childhood*, 4th edn. Oxford: Isis Medical Media Ltd, 1999.

Resource

Dietitians working in paediatric gastroenterology in the UK are encouraged to join the Associate Members group of the British Society of Paediatric Gastroenterology, Hepatology and Nutrition (BSPGHAN) www.bspghan.org.uk.

Useful addresses

Coeliac UK
Suites A–D, Octagon Court, High Wycombe, Bucks, HP11 2HS
Tel 01494 437278
www.coeliac.co.uk

CICRA (Crohn's in Childhood Research Association)
Parkgate House, 356 West Barnes Lane, Motspur Park, Surrey, KT3 6NB
Tel 020 8949 6209
www.cicra.org

Gut Motility Disorders Network
Westcott Farm, Oakford, Tiverton, EX16 9EZ
Tel: 01398 351173

Half PINNT (For children on intravenous and nasogastric feeding)
PO Box 3126, Christchurch, Dorset, BH23 2XS
www.pinnt.co.uk

NACC (National Association for Colitis and Crohn's Disease)
4 Beaumont House, Sutton Road, St Albans, Herts, ALI 5HH
Tel 0845 130 2233
www.nacc.org.uk

8 Surgery in the Gastrointestinal Tract

Vanessa Shaw

Introduction

There are a number of congenital malformations requiring surgery in the neonatal period. These malformations affect the oesophagus, stomach, duodenum and the small and large intestines. The type of feed and the method by which it is given will be governed by the area of gut affected and the surgery performed to correct the defect.

Oesophageal atresia and tracheo-oesophageal fistula

Oesophageal atresia (OA) occurs in about 1 in 3000 births [1]. The oesophagus ends blindly in a pouch so that there is no continuous route from the mouth to the stomach. This means that at birth the infant cannot swallow saliva and is seen to froth at the mouth. Aspiration of this saliva causes choking and cyanotic attacks. The obstruction usually occurs 8–10 cm from the gum margin. Eighty-six per cent of neonates with OA also have a distal tracheo-oesophageal fistula (TOF) [1] where the proximal end of the distal oesophagus is confluent with the trachea (Fig. 8.1). In this case any reflux of stomach contents will enter the trachea and, hence, the lungs. Isolated 'pure' OA without a fistula with the trachea occurs in 7% of babies and the rarer fistula between oesophagus and trachea without OA ('H' fistula) occurs in 4% [2].

OA is associated with other anomalies. Myers *et al.* [3] reviewed 618 patients over a 44-year period and found the most common associated anomalies in babies with OA to be: cardiac (20.7%), urinary (21.6%), gastrointestinal (22.7%), orthopaedic (15.7%); lesser associations were with the central nervous system, eye and chromosomal anomalies. Similar incidences were found in reports from other authors [4,5]. These other anomalies occur in more than 50% of babies with OA and are described as the VACTERL sequence (vertebral, anorectal, cardiac, tracheo-oesophageal, renal and limb defects) and the CHARGE association (coloboma, heart defects, choanal atresia, retarded development, genital hypoplasia and ear abnormalities) [6]. The survival of babies with a birth weight >1500 g and with no major heart problems is nearing 97%; mortality is most commonly associated with major congenital cardiac malformations and very low birth weight (<1500 g) where survival is only 22% [2].

Obviously, the infant cannot be fed via the enteral route until the lesion is corrected surgically and will therefore require parenteral nutrition initially. A Replogle tube will be passed through the nose into the oesophagus to drain any saliva. The tube also increases the size of the pouch at the blind end of the upper oesophagus. Treatment of OA, whether associated with TOF or not, is undertaken as soon as possible after birth. It involves the repair of the oesophagus by anastomosing the upper and

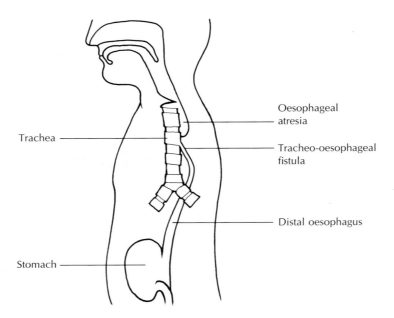

Trachea

Stomach

Oesophageal
atresia

Tracheo-oesophageal
fistula

Distal oesophagus

Figure 8.1   Oesophageal atresia and tracheo-oesophageal fistula.

lower ends, after closing any TOF if present, so that both the oesophagus and trachea are separate and continuous. This is possible in about 90% of affected babies.

Feeding the baby with oesophageal atresia and tracheo-oesophageal fistula

A primary anastomosis is performed when the distance between the proximal and distal ends of the oesophagus is short enough for the two to be joined in one procedure. Most surgeons pass a transanastomotic tube (TAT) to decompress the stomach the first few days post-surgery and to allow nasogastric feeding to commence. Some babies routinely have a chest drain inserted for up to 1 week. Infants can be feeding orally within 48–72 hours of corrective surgery, ideally being breast fed, or receiving expressed breast milk or infant formula. Puntis *et al.* [7] found that 50% of infants undergoing a primary anastomosis were breast fed for a median period of 3 months. If a chest drain has been inserted postoperatively, nasogastric feeding via the TAT may be prolonged for 7 days or so until contrast studies show that the oesophagus is intact prior to the commencement of oral feeding.

A study by Patel *et al.* [8] reviewed a 12-year period of a more simplified management of OA with TOF where chest drains, TAT and contrast studies were not routinely used. Seventeen babies were managed without a TAT and 23 with a TAT. The time to establishment of full oral feeding was 2–8 (average 3.9) days in the babies without a TAT, and 2–12 (average 5.9) days in those with a TAT. They concluded that a sizeable minority of babies do not require a TAT and that early introduction of oral feeds in this group is not associated with an increased risk of complications, such as developing strictures.

In some babies the distance between the upper and lower ends of the oesophagus exceeds 3 cm (or more than two vertebral bodies) and this is termed 'long gap OA'. It is technically impossible to join the upper and lower ends of the oesophagus so a staged procedure is required. The oesophagus is temporarily abandoned and a cervical oesophagostomy may be formed to allow the infant to swallow saliva. The oesophagus is left for 3–6 months before attempting to join the upper and lower ends. Although cervical oesophagostomy prevents growth in the upper pouch of the oesophagus, the lower pouch hypertrophies and shortens the distance between the two ends. Alternatively, the upper oesophagus is left intact with a double lumen Replogle tube *in situ* for 6–8 weeks, through which continuous low pressure suction can be applied to remove accumulating saliva; the upper pouch probably lengthens in this case and hypertrophies. A gastrostomy is formed to allow enteral feeding to proceed. If a TOF is present it must be disconnected and the defect in the trachea closed. Feeding babies undergoing a staged repair presents more of a challenge.

The gastrostomy feed will be either expressed breast milk (EBM) or infant formula and should be given at the same volume and frequency as the infant would receive orally. In order for the baby to experience normal oral behaviour, sham feeding should begin as soon as possible. To allow for normal development and co-ordination, the sham feed should be of the same volume as the gastrostomy feed, and the feed should be of the same duration and frequency so that the baby learns to associate sucking with hunger and satiety. It is also important that a similar taste is offered in the sham feed as that being put into the gastrostomy so that there is no refusal of feeds on the grounds of taste once the infant has an intact gut. The sham feed seeps out of the oesophagostomy, along with saliva and is usually dealt with by wrapping a towel or other absorbent material around the baby's neck (Fig. 8.2). Puntis *et al.* [7] report that 38% of babies with oesophagostomies were breast fed for a median duration of 2.5 months. It is now more regular practice for mothers who wish to give their babies breast milk to express their milk so that this can be given via the gastrostomy; the baby would be given infant formula by mouth for the sham feed. There are, however, problems with sham feeding:

- It is difficult to co-ordinate holding the baby, feeding from a bottle and mopping up feed from the oesophagostomy while giving a gastrostomy feed. This event may defeat nursing staff let alone the mother coping single-handedly at home.
- One-third of babies with OA suffer from cardiovascular complications and may need ventilating, making sham feeding impossible.
- The baby may tire quickly and not be able to suck for long enough to take the same volume orally as is going through the gastrostomy.
- Many babies have small stomachs and initially require small volumes of gastrostomy feed very

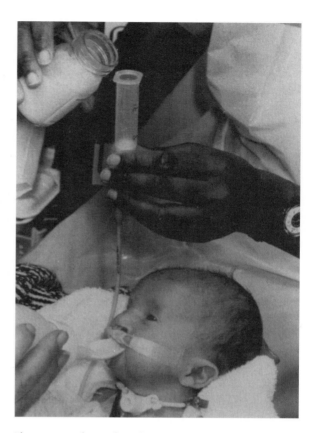

Figure 8.2   Infant with tracheo-oesophageal fistula and cervical oesophagostomy receiving oral sham feeds while being fed via a gastronomy tube. The infant also has a tracheostomy and cleft palate and takes oral feeds from a Rosti bottle.

frequently (e.g. 2 hourly), making it difficult to co-ordinate sham with gastrostomy feeding. However, this problem rapidly corrects itself as the feed volume is increased.

There may be no route for sham feeding if an oesophagostomy has not been formed as part of the initial corrective surgical procedure. Infants deprived of oral feedings for the first weeks to months of life can experience great difficulty in establishing sucking. This should not be a major problem if oral feeding is established within 2–3 months of life, but if oral feeding is delayed any longer than this, it is associated with gagging and vomiting; the baby may avert its head at the very sight of the bottle or push out the teat with the tongue. Desensitisation to this oral aversion is a long, slow process. It is important to remember that feeding is not just a process of providing nutrition; babies are very alert at feeding time and develop cognitive and motor abilities while feeding.

Babies with OA with or without TOF can grow well on breast milk and normal infant formulas if adequate volume of feed is taken. If there is a problem with weight gain, feeds can be concentrated and supplemented or commercial nutrient-dense feeds may be indicated (see Table 1.14).

Feeding the older baby and toddler

In order to promote normal development, these babies should be weaned at the appropriate age of around 6 months. It has been observed that weaning in babies who have undergone a primary anastomosis is certainly delayed to 6 months of age and the introduction of lumpy solids to 12 months of age [7]. Weaning solids should be sham fed if the oesophagus has not yet been joined up. There has been controversy in the past over what should go down the gastrostomy tube at this stage. A nutritionally adequate feed must be given in preference to weaning solids. In order to get strained weaning foods of the right consistency to go down the tube they have to be watered down, so diluting their energy and nutrient content. If this practice is continued in the long term, failure to thrive results. In the study published by Spitz et al. [5] in 1987, of 148 children with oesophageal atresia, 27% of the patients were below the third centile for height and weight at 6 months and 5 years. A contribution to this could well have been the practice of inappropriate solids being administered down gastrostomy tubes, as was common practice then. A more recent review in 2006 of 15 children with OA and TOF who had primary repair at birth found that all were between the 50th and 75th percentile of expected growth at 12 years of age [9].

If gagging is experienced when weaning solids are introduced, oral intake may be reduced to just tastes of food rather than giving large boluses in order to dispel the association between solid food and gagging. Foods need to be moist and fibrous foods should be avoided. Fluid should be given at mealtimes to help the food go down. Both mother and child need to build up confidence about eating.

In babies with long gap OA the attempt to join the oesophagus to the rest of the gastrointestinal tract may occur as early as 12 weeks of life and the native oesophagus should be used wherever possible. The proximal and distal oesophageal remnants undergo lengthening procedures such as circular myotomy and serial dilatation. If radiological study shows that it is still not possible to join the two ends of oesophagus then the baby is considered for an oesophageal substitution procedure, which may occur as early as 9 months of age but may be delayed to as late as 3–4 years. Until joined up, sham feeding of age-appropriate foods should continue with nutritionally adequate feeds through the gastrostomy. Fortified baby milks, such as concentrated infant formula, high energy formulas (SMA High Energy, Infatrini), may safely be used up to the age of 1 year or so, but will need to be replaced by a more nutritionally dense feed such as Paediasure or Nutrini to maintain good growth in the older child (see Table 3.2).

Oesophageal substitution procedures

There are various methods of correcting a long gap OA: colon interposition, gastric tube oesophagoplasty, gastric transposition and, less commonly, jejunal interposition and gastric elongation [10].

Colon interposition involves removing a piece of the colon and transposing it into the chest between the oesophagus above and the stomach below. This is the most common procedure and has the advantages of the length of the graft required not posing a problem and the diameter of the lumen of the transposed colon is appropriate for joining to the oesophagus. The disadvantages of this procedure are the blood supply to the colon is not good; the transposed colon does not have very good peristaltic function to propel food down to the stomach; there is a high incidence of leakage around the anastomoses in 30% of patients; 20% of patients will develop strictures; with time, the transposed colon may lose its muscular activity.

Gastric tube oesophagoplasty is where a longitudinal segment, formed from the greater curve of the stomach, is moved up into the chest and joined to the lower pouch of the oesophagus. The size of the graft is appropriate and the blood supply is good, but there is a high incidence of leakage (70%), there is a high stricture rate (50%) and gastro-oesophageal reflux (GOR) is common.

In a gastric transposition procedure the whole stomach is mobilised and moved into the chest. The proximal end of the oesophagus is joined to the top of the stomach in the neck. The blood supply is excellent and the rate of both leakage and strictures is much lower than in the procedures described above, each occurring in only 6% of patients. A review of gastric transposition by Spitz *et al.* [11] in 32 babies with OA showed graft survival of 100% and the outcome was excellent in 81% of the surviving patients. The procedure does have its disadvantages: poor gastric emptying; the fact that the bulk of the stomach is in the chest reduces respiratory capacity; GOR can be a problem; dumping can occur (see p. 131). Despite these problems, a more recent review of 41 babies, 26 of whom had OA undergoing gastric transposition at age 3.3 ± 0.6 years, concluded that this procedure was an appropriate alternative to colon interposition for oesophageal replacement in infants and children [12].

Feeding post-oesophageal substitution

The oesophagostomy, if present, is closed at the time of the oesophageal substitution. A feeding jejunostomy may be formed as a route for nutrition while the child is sedated post-surgery for gastric transposition as the pre-existing gastrostomy can no longer be used. Gastrostomy feeding can continue if colon interposition or gastric tube oesophagoplasty has been performed. Oral nutrition is introduced as soon as possible, but supplementary overnight gastrostomy/jejunostomy feeds may be indicated until an adequate intake is taken by mouth. Oesophageal replacement procedures have their problems when feeding recommences as indicated above. The advantage of the gastric transposition is that there is only one join in the gastrointestinal tract, but the stomach is now sited in a much smaller place in the thorax than it usually occupies in the abdomen. The volume of feed or meals that can be taken comfortably may be greatly reduced, imposing a feeding regimen of little and often. The problem with colon interposition is that two areas of the gut have undergone surgery and joining. The transplanted

colon makes a rather 'baggy' oesophagus because of the nature of its musculature, and the repaired oesophagus may not have normal peristaltic function. The colon may suffer temporary dysfunction because of surgical trauma and malabsorption may ensue, necessitating a change to a hydrolysed feed (Table 7.7). Gastric tube oesophagoplasty procedure has a high incidence of GOR. The end result of these surgical interventions may be oesophageal continuity, but not necessarily normal oesophageal function.

Problems with oesophageal function following repair

GOR is common following repair, with an incidence of at least 25% [13]. It may respond to medical management (e.g. thickening fluids; see Table 7.27), positioning the baby appropriately after feeding or the administration of drugs such as metoclopromide and domperidone. These are dopamine antagonists that stimulate gastric emptying and small intestinal transit, and enhance the strength of oesophageal sphincter contraction. H_2 receptor antagonists, cimetidine or ranitidine, may be administered to reduce the acidity of the stomach so that the reflux does less damage to the oesophageal mucosa. If GOR is severe and unresolved by these methods, surgical correction may be required by performing a fundoplication.

There are various anti-reflux operations (Nissen, Thal, Boix–Ochoa, Belsey) and the choice depends on what the surgeon believes to be the best procedure for the individual child. The Nissen fundoplication is the most common and involves mobilising the fundus of the stomach and wrapping it around the lower oesophagus, thus fashioning a valve at the junction of the oesophagus and stomach. Between 18% and 45% of children undergoing repair for OA have significant GOR, leading to life-threatening aspiration of feed, and require such anti-reflux surgery [5,14]. Following unsuccessful medical management of GOR, 45% of the 31 babies described by Curci and Dibbins [14] required Nissen fundoplication. Together with children with neurological dysfunction, infants and children who have a repaired oesophageal atresia and TOF comprise the majority of patients needing such a procedure.

The anti-reflux surgery is not without its post-operative complications. While preventing reflux into the oesophagus, the fundoplication may also stop the child from burping and gas bloat can be very uncomfortable in the stomach. Parents need to be taught to 'wind' their child through the gastrostomy tube. Although the child can no longer vomit, they often experience severe retching, which is very distressing for both child and parent, but this usually disappears after a few weeks or months. Fundoplication can also cause dumping (see p. 131). Occasionally, the valve created by the procedure weakens with time (usually a number of years, but sometimes after a few months) and GOR returns. If this cannot be managed medically then the Nissen's has to be 're-done'.

The change from receiving full nutrition from a gastrostomy/jejunostomy feed to maintaining an adequate intake orally is slow and there is often a long period where the child needs supplementary tube feeds while learning to eat normally. Prior to being joined up, the child has not experienced the sensation of a bolus of food passing the entire length of the oesophagus. Although the child should have been exposed to sham feeding, this method of feeding does not always lead to successful swallowing. Therefore, many children panic when offered any food other than in liquid form and the establishment of normal feeding has to proceed through stages of gradually altering the consistency of foods from purées to finely minced and mashed foods and then to the normal diet.

After repair, whether the child has undergone a primary repair in the first few days of life or whether a staged procedure has been performed, a circular scar will form where the upper and lower segments of the oesophagus are sutured together. With perfect healing the scar will have the same diameter as the oesophagus and will grow with the child. However, if the gap between the upper and lower pouches is >3 cm the two ends of the oesophagus have to be stretched to meet and this puts the repair under tension. This reduces the blood supply to the forming scar tissue, causing the tissue to shrink and form a stricture. Stricture occurs in about one-third of babies and children and the normal passage of food is impeded. Bread, meat and poultry, apple and raw vegetables are the foods most often cited as getting stuck.

If there is reflux of stomach contents up into the oesophagus the acid will inflame the healing scar, which may also lead to stricture formation. Sometimes the anastomosis joining the ends of the oesophagus leaks and this also causes a stricture to form. Children with these problems show difficulty in feeding and a reluctance to swallow; they will choke and splutter. Strictures require repeated dilatations to soften the scar tissue and allow the easier passage of solid food. The oesophagus may also go into spasm at the site of the join and particulate foods like mince and peas get stuck.

The frightening experience of repeated choking leads to fraught mealtimes which both parents and children come to dread. One-third of parents of babies with primary repair in Puntis et al.'s [7] study reported problems with choking or coughing, 17% with vomiting and 20% with feed refusal at feeding times at least twice a day in the first year of life. A similar frequency was seen in children after closure of oesophagostomy. The introduction of solids in the delayed repair children was significantly later than in both controls and children with primary repair, solid foods being introduced at 12 months and lumpy foods as late as 18 months. It is often easier to abandon the feeding of solids and go back to a completely liquid diet. If this is not supervised, the diet can quickly become very poor nutritionally.

Children often become bored with food; if meals are liquidised to stop them getting stuck in the throat there is the danger that every meal will end up looking the same brown unappetising mush. This can be improved by liquidising the foods separately so that tastes and colours can be distinguished. Mealtimes can become very antisocial; choking and vomiting are common at meals and children may need hefty pats on the back or turning upside down to dislodge food that has stuck. Eating can be a very slow process for the child as foods have to be thoroughly chewed before swallowing can be attempted. Parents understandably feel inhibited about eating out of the home, which curtails the social experience of the child. It is often difficult for parents and carers to understand the problems with swallowing following repair of OA and force feeding the child may be a temptation.

Adequate nutrition can usually be achieved with small frequent meals that are energy dense, and the provision of fluids at mealtimes to help wash down the food. Such are the problems associated with eating that families need help, advice and encouragement from all professionals with appropriate experience, including dietitians, speech therapists and clinical psychologists as well as the medical and nursing professions. The Tracheo-Oesophageal Fistula Support Group (TOFS) is a self-help organisation where carers of these children can share their experiences and offer advice.

Dysphagia may remain a problem for many years after repair, but improves with time. Half of the children in Puntis et al.'s [7] study experienced feeding difficulties at the age of 7 years. Anderson et al. [15] looked at the long-term follow-up of children undergoing either colon interposition or gastric tube interposition to see if one method of oesophageal replacement had an advantage over the other. Most of the children fell at or below the 10th percentile for height and weight, half needed to eat slowly and to avoid certain meats, and dysphagia was rare. There was no apparent difference between the two groups. Davenport et al. [16] studied the long-term effects of gastric transposition in 17 children who had undergone the procedure more than 5 years previously. They concluded that gastric transposition is compatible with life and allowed satisfactory growth and nutrition for the majority of subjects. They suggest that all children should have oral iron supplementation after the procedure to correct or prevent any defect in iron absorption because low ferritin levels were found in all children tested; one-third were anaemic. Iron absorption is facilitated by the presence of acid in the stomach, and the high incidence of hypochlorhydria seen in some adults after gastric transposition suggests this as a mechanism for defective iron absorption.

Outcome

Chetcuti et al. [17] interviewed 125 adults born with OA with or without TOF before 1969 to see how their congenital disease had affected their quality of life. Dysphagia and symptoms of GOR was present in over half of the adults, but most enjoyed a normal diet provided they drank fluids with their meals. Their social achievements and failures matched that of the rest of the population. This favourable long term outcome has been confirmed by Little et al. [18] in a group of 69 infants with a mean follow-up of 125 months (10.4 years). Dysphagia, frequent respiratory infections, GOR disease and growth delays were common in the first 5 years, but these all improved as the children matured.

Dumping following oesophageal replacement and Nissen fundoplication

Dumping syndrome is often seen in infants and young children following gastric transposition and is most probably brought about by rapid gastric emptying [19]. Ravelli et al. [20] studied gastric emptying in 12 children who had undergone gastric transposition using electrical impedance tomography. Gastric emptying was normal in one patient, delayed in seven and accelerated in four. Like the repaired oesophagus, the transposed stomach does not behave normally. The stomach retains its function as a reservoir but its emptying is extremely irregular. Spitz [19] found that the dumping experienced in the early postoperative period was short lived, although it lasted for as long as 6 months in some children and recurred periodically in one child.

Dumping can occur in children following Nissen fundoplication for severe GOR. Gastric emptying can be accelerated, with the result that hyperosmolar foodstuffs leave the stomach very rapidly and hence draw large quantities of fluid into the small bowel. This produces the 'early' symptoms of distension, discomfort, nausea, retching, tachycardia, pallor, sweating and dizziness. This may be associated with hyperglycaemia. 'Late' symptoms may occur from 1–4 hours later as a result of hypoglycaemia and may be indistinguishable from early symptoms [21].

There are no large studies on children with dumping syndrome and most of the published papers are case histories; all workers regard it as difficult to treat. Various dietary manoeuvres have been tried to overcome the symptoms of dumping and no one treatment is recommended. The aim is to avoid swings in blood sugar levels. Some children respond to a combination of treatments. In summary these are:

- Giving small frequent meals [19,21]
- Taking fluids separately from solid foods [19,22]

- Avoiding a high glucose intake [19,22]
- Adding uncooked cornstarch to feeds at a concentration of 3.5–7% [22] or 50 g/L feed [23]
- Adding pectin to the diet: 5–10 g (<12 years) or 10–15 g (>12 years) divided into six doses [22]
- Administering continuous feeds with added fat (both long chain and medium chain fats are used) or small frequent meals enriched with fat [23–25]

Borovoy *et al.* [26] described eight children with dumping syndrome fed by gastrostomy and found that uncooked cornstarch controlled glucose shifts, resolved most of the symptoms, allowed bolus feedings and enhanced weight gain. A guideline for the administration of uncooked cornstarch could be taken from the treatment of glycogen storage disease (see p. 395).

Duodenal atresia

Duodenal atresia is a cause of congenital intestinal obstruction and occurs in about 1 in 10 000 births. In most cases the atresia occurs below the ampulla of Vater. A plain X-ray demonstrates the typical 'double-bubble' of the dilated stomach and duodenum proximal and distal to the atresia. Duodenal atresia presents as significant vomiting after the first oral feed is given; the vomitus is usually bile-tinged as secreted bile cannot pass down the intestine. The obstruction is corrected by cutting the blind end of the duodenum and connecting it to the lower intestine. There are other anomalies associated with this atresia: Down's syndrome, OA, imperforate anus and cardiac malformations occur in over 50% of babies with duodenal atresia. Mortality is related to the severity of the associated anomalies. Mooney *et al.* [27] report an improvement in survival from 72% in 1973 to 100% in 1983.

Parenteral nutrition (PN) is used routinely to feed these babies in the first days of life. Once the amount of bile aspirate decreases (indicating that the lower gut is patent) and bowel sounds return, enteral feeding can be commenced. A TAT may be passed in the early days post-surgery to help in the delivery of feeds, although jejunal feeding tubes are associated with perforation and are easily dislodged. Mooney *et al.* [27] found that TATs prolonged the time until oral feeding was tolerated by 10 days: babies without the tube tolerated oral

feeds at 5.3 days; babies with the tube at 15.7 days. In a more recent study of 17 babies undergoing upper gastrointestinal surgery (10 with duodenal atresia, six with malrotation and one with jejunal atresia), enteral feeding was started via transgastric transanastomotic feeding jejunostomy tubes by day 2 post-surgery in 14 cases; the authors concluded that transgastric transanastomotic feeding jejunostomy was well tolerated and preferable to PN [28].

Breast feeding should be possible within a week of surgery; if bottle fed, EBM or normal infant formula should be given and, if administered correctly, should provide adequate nutrition. If weight gain is poor the usual methods of feed fortification can be used. These same feeds should be used if enteral feeding needs to be continued.

Feeding problems post-surgery

The feeding problems following repair of duodenal atresia are usually associated with the motility of the duodenum. *In utero*, the duodenum proximal to the atresia is stretched because ingested material cannot get past the atretic area of gut. The musculature does not function properly once the obstruction is removed, resulting in a baggy proximal duodenum. The infant may feed normally, but milk will accumulate in the lax duodenum rather than continuing its passage down the gut. This can result in huge vomits, up to 200 mL at a time. Feeds need to be small and frequent to overcome this problem.

If GOR is present, feeds can be thickened and the baby should be positioned correctly after feeding. As the gut grows and matures with the infant, problems should resolve so that the older child will feed normally.

Hirschsprung's disease

Hirschsprung's disease, also known as congenital megacolon or aganglionic megacolon, is an anomaly where there is a total absence of ganglion cells in the affected part of the large intestine resulting in a loss of peristalsis. It has an incidence of 1 in 5000 infants, with a higher incidence in boys than girls (4 : 1). In 75% of cases the rectosigmoid colon is involved and in 8% there is total colonic involvement [29]. Presentation occurs before 3 months of age in the majority and 80% of cases present by 1 year of age. The aganglionic parts of the colon cannot pass faeces so some affected neonates present with complete intestinal obstruction, bilious vomiting and profound abdominal distension, with a delayed passage of meconium. Other infants present with constipation, abdominal distension, vomiting, diarrhoea and poor growth after the neonatal period. Surgery aims to clear the obstruction by fashioning a colostomy as the initial procedure. When appropriate, the stoma is closed, the non-functioning segment of colon is removed, and a pull-through procedure is performed which connects the functioning bowel to the anus. In some cases the pull-through can be performed as a primary procedure.

Some children, aged 3–14 years, present later with intractable constipation alternating with diarrhoea which may be treated symptomatically with a high fibre diet. Constipation may persist in 10–20% of children despite successful surgery.

In long segment Hirschsprung's disease there is small intestinal involvement; resection of aganglionic bowel will be necessary, leaving the infant with a shortened length of bowel. The dietary management is as described for short bowel syndrome below.

Exomphalos and gastroschisis

These conditions are not abnormalities of the gastrointestinal tract, but are abdominal wall defects involving the exposure of the infant's intestine to the outside world. The incidence of exomphalos is 2–3 per 10 000 births. There is a risk of associated malformations and chromosomal abnormalities in babies with exomphalos. The incidence of gastroschisis is 4.4 in 10 000 births in Britain (2004), showing an increasing incidence compared with 1994 when the incidence was 2.5 in 10 000 births [30]. This increasing incidence has been seen in other countries and has been associated with lower maternal age and seems to be associated with tobacco smoking and recreational drugs around the time of conception.

An exomphalos can be small or large and occurs when the lateral folds of the abdominal wall fail to meet *in utero*, resulting in incomplete closure of the abdominal wall and herniation of the midgut. Not only bowel, but also solid viscera such as the liver, spleen, ovaries or testes are exposed, contained in a translucent membrane made of amnion and peritoneum. Emergency surgery is necessary as fluids and body heat are crucially lost through the exposed intestines. If the exomphalos is small, the bowel can be placed back inside the abdomen in one procedure, the abdominal wall is closed and a navel is fashioned. If the exomphalos is large, the surgeon may need to use a patch if there is not enough skin to close the abdomen. If the exomphalos is too large for this procedure, a staged repair is performed. The exposed intestines and other organs are covered with a prosthetic mesh sac to protect them. The sac is suspended above the child and is tightened regularly as the intestine gradually moves back into the abdominal cavity by gravity. The abdomen is then closed and a navel fashioned.

In gastroschisis, a rupture of the umbilical cord *in utero* in early pregnancy allows the intestine to escape outside the abdominal wall; in this case, unlike in exomphalos, the intestine has no covering membrane. Again, the bowel is put back inside the abdomen in one procedure if possible, or may need the staged procedure, tightening the prosthetic sac gradually as described above [31]. Both Silastic and Prolene prostheses and primary fascial closure are considered acceptable procedures; the primary closure has the advantage of avoiding additional operations [32]. In Sharp *et al*.'s [33] group of 70 cases of gastroschisis over a 10-year period, primary closure was achieved in 86% of babies and mean age at repair was 5.04 hours (range 2–14.5 hours). Outcome is not significantly differerent by type of surgery [34].

Feeding the infant with abdominal wall defects

The pressure of the prosthetic sac or the closed abdominal wall forces the intestine back into the abdomen, but this continual pressure will upset its normal function and the gut may suffer a prolonged paralytic ileus. Most of these infants will need PN for several weeks or months before bowel function returns and the use of PN is of major importance in the survival of these infants [35]. Adam *et al*. [36] found that delayed closure of the abdomen in exomphalos leads to more readily established enteral feeding. However, Sauter *et al.* [32] found no difference in the time taken to establish enteral feeding in babies with gastroschisis and exomphalos whether they underwent primary repair or a delayed procedure. Kitchanan *et al.* [34] found that neonates with gastroschisis had significant delays in reaching full enteral feeds compared with those with exomphalos (24 vs. 8 days) and required prolonged support with PN (23 vs. 6 days). The age at which the infant with gastroschisis is first given enteral feeds affects the length of stay in hospital and the duration of PN; each day delay in starting enteral feeds was associated with an increase hospital stay of 1.05 days and increased PN duration of 1.06 days [33]. Median day of first enteral feeds was day 8 post-surgery (range 3–40 days) [33].

Enteral feeding is considered when bowel sounds return. Expressed breast milk or infant formula is usually tolerated if given as small frequent bolus feeds. Large boluses are not tolerated as the intestinal tract is under constant pressure and cannot accomodate a large amount of fluid at once. If the baby can be handled normally and does not need to be nursed flat, breast feeding is possible. In one study 70% of babies were breast fed on discharge, 28% were bottle fed and 2% were on solids (median hospital stay 24 days, range 6–419 days) [33]. If there is malabsorption, then a hydrolysed feed is indicated. Babies with gastroschisis may have persistent intestinal dysmotility.

Exomphalos and gastroschisis were fatal abnormalities prior to the 1970s. The advent of PN and temporary prosthetic sacs, which allow delayed abdominal closure, has allowed the good survival rates seen today [31].

Outcome

A study of 40 patients published in the early 1990s shows 90% of babies with gastroschisis surviving [37]. A 10-year review of neonatal outcome of gastroschisis (21 babies) and exomphalos (five babies) published in 2000 gives survival rates of 91% and 100%, respectively [34]. Davies and Stringer [38] followed up 23 survivors of gastroschisis who were born between 1972 and 1984. They found that despite experiencing intrauterine growth retardation children with uncomplicated gastroschisis eventually achieve relatively normal growth. Other authors have shown that catch-up growth occurs throughout childhood, mostly within the first 5 years. Most babies surviving infancy after repair of gastroschisis can expect to become healthy adults [38].

Intestinal atresia occurs in 10–20% of babies with gastroschisis and they may also have intestinal necrosis, leading to short bowel syndrome. The management of this is described below.

Short Bowel Syndrome

Tracey Johnson

Short bowel syndrome (SBS) is a collection of disorders where a loss of intestinal length has occurred that compromises the ability to digest and absorb nutrients. Short bowel syndrome in children may occur at any age, but the majority of cases result following extensive bowel resection in the early neonatal period. Resection may be required in infants born with congenital abnormalities (e.g. gastroschisis, bowel atresias and malrotation), or in infants who develop necrotising enterocolitis (NEC). In older children, SBS may result from extensive resection following volvulus, trauma, intestinal malignancy or Crohn's disease. Even in the absence of resection, children may have conditions leading to a 'functional short bowel' including long segment Hirschprung's disease and radiation enteritis.

After an extensive bowel resection there are many factors determining outcome. All these factors will have a bearing on the management of the individual patient.

Infants are born with a small bowel length of 250 ± 40 cm [39]. Loss of intestinal length results in loss of surface area for absorption and loss of digestive enzymes and transport carrier proteins leading to malabsorption. In general, loss of up to 50% of small bowel can be tolerated without any major nutritional problems and clinical features of SBS usually result when more than 75% of the small intestine has been resected. Although it is important, the length of remaining bowel is not the only factor determining outcome; the site of resection, presence or absence of the ileo-caecal valve, the primary diagnosis and any ensuing complications will also influence the prognosis.

The key to survival after an extensive small bowel resection is the ability of the remaining bowel to adapt and take over the functions of the resected segment of bowel. Adaptation begins within 24–48 hours after resection. The remaining small bowel hypertrophies, increasing the surface area and the absorptive function. The absorptive functions of the jejunum and ileum are given in Table 8.1.

Despite the jejunum being the site of absorption of the majority of nutrients, loss of jejunum is tolerated better than ileal resection. The reasons for this are as follow:

- The ileum has a greater capacity for adaptation than the jejunum. The ileum can adapt and compensate for the absorptive functions of the jejunum, but the jejunum does not have the same potential for adaptation and cannot develop the specialist functions of the ileum, namely bile salt and vitamin B_{12} absorption.
- Transit time in the ileum is slower than in the jejunum, allowing luminal contents to be in contact with the mucosa for longer periods of time.

Table 8.1   Absorptive functions of the jejunum and the ileum.

Jejunum	Ileum
Glucose	Vitamin B_{12}
Disaccharides	Bile salts
Protein	Fluid
Fat	Electrolytes
Calcium	
Magnesium	
Iron	
Water-soluble vitamins	
thiamin	
riboflavin	
pyridoxine	
folic acid	
ascorbic acid	
Fat-soluble vitamins	
vitamin A	
vitamin D	

- The ileum has the capacity to absorb fluid and nutrients against an osmotic gradient leading to favourable absorption compared to the jejunum.

Presence or absence of the ileo-caecal valve also has an important part to play in determining outcome in patients with SBS. The valve slows transit time, which increases the duration of contact of luminal nutrients with the mucosal surface and minimises fluid and electrolyte losses. It also serves as a barrier to prevent bacterial overgrowth, which can interfere with nutrient and fluid absorption.

Residual disease may worsen the prognosis of infants following small bowel resection (e.g. after resection for NEC the remaining bowel may not be of good quality). This may affect function and reduce the potential for adaptation. A diagnosis of gastroschisis may be associated with intestinal dysmotility resulting in poor feed tolerance even in infants with a good length of bowel.

Dependance on parenteral nutrition (PN) appears to be most governed by the remaining intestinal length and absence of the ileo-caecal valve. This was recognised by Wilmore [40] and has since been confirmed by other studies [41,42].

Nutritional support

The aims of management are to maintain nutritional status, facilitate adaptation of the remaining bowel, control diarrhoea and minimise complications. Nutritional therapy needs to be tailored to the individual child and is ideally managed by a multidisciplinary nutrition team comprising a paediatric gastroenterologist, dietitian, pharmacist, specialist nurse and biochemist.

The development of PN is the most significant factor in the improved survival of children with SBS. PN assures adequate balanced nutrition to maintain hydration and nutritional status and to give time for intestinal adaptation to occur. Although PN provides essential fluid and energy, prolonged exclusive PN can lead to complications and it is important to give PN in the longer term as nutritional support rather than as the total source of nutrition.

Enteral feeds may be nutritionally insignificant, but they are nevertheless very important and should be commenced as soon as post-surgical

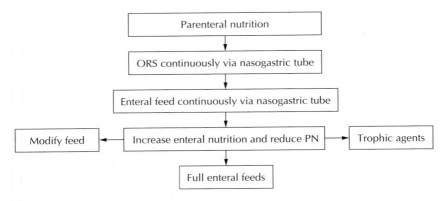

Figure 8.3   Progression from parenteral to enteral nutrition. ORS, oral rehydration solution; PN, parenteral nutrition.

ileus has resolved. Intraluminal nutrients are the single most important factor in promoting intestinal adaptation in SBS [43]. Enteral feeds:

- Promote pancreatic secretions, hormones and bile
- Are an important factor in preventing intestinal failure related liver disease [44]
- May also help to prevent bacterial translocation [45]

Although children with SBS may require PN for long periods there is potential for progression to full enteral nutrition. Figure 8.3 illustrates the progression from parenteral to enteral nutrition. Managing this transition is challenging as progression can be both prolonged and unpredictable. Initially, oral rehydration solutions (see Table 7.2) may be used, changing to a feed as tolerated. As feeds are increased PN can be reduced with the ultimate aim of independence from PN. The process may take months or even years to complete and can involve changing feeds and trials of trophic factors (see p. 137).

The ability to advance enteral feeds results from the process of intestinal adaptation. There are various strategies that can help this process. It is important to put some feed into the bowel and this should include feeding into a distal stoma, if present, to maintain function.

Choice of feed

The choice of nutrients may be important. Complex nutrients, especially long chain triglycerides (LCT), stimulate adaptation better than simple nutrients,

the hypothesis being that the more work the bowel has to do to digest a nutrient, the greater the stimulus to adapt [46]. There is no consensus regarding the best formula for infants with SBS. There is a lack of randomised trials and most human data on the nutritional management of SBS are derived from retrospective analysis of case series. As a result, in individual centres, practices depend more on years of personal experience than on research.

Protein
Infants with SBS might be expected to benefit from an extensively hydrolysed protein feed because of the insufficient luminal surface area for digestion and absorption, but protein digestion and absorption is completed in the upper small gut and is generally not a significant problem in SBS. There is probably little absorptive benefit from using amino acids or hydrolysed protein feeds [47] and complex proteins may in fact be superior in stimulating adaptation. Cow's milk protein intolerance can occur in surgical neonates and has also been reported in SBS so there may be a role for amino acid based feeds when inflammation is present [48].

Fat
A similar compromise is needed when considering dietary fat. LCT has the greatest potential for stimulating adaptation, may be a source of long chain polyunsaturated fatty acids and essential fatty acids and has a lower osmolarity than medium chain triglycerides (MCT). However, many children with SBS have significant fat malabsorption and feeds with a high content of LCT may result in steatorrhoea. In contrast, MCT is water soluble and

therefore efficiently absorbed. The disadvantage of MCT is its higher osmolarity and experimental evidence has shown that formulas containing MCT stimulate less intestinal adaptation than those containing LCT [49]. A mixture of LCT and MCT to combine the physiological advantage of MCT and the positive effects of gut adaptation from LCT may be the best compromise.

Carbohydrate

Carbohydrate has the greatest intraluminal osmotic effect, but potentially can be well absorbed as brush border enzyme activity can be induced according to the composition of the feed. Feeds containing sucrose will induce sucrase and those containing glucose polymer will induce isomaltase [50]. The exception to this is lactose.

Monosaccharides need no digestion but have a higher osmotic load than polysaccharides. Just as with protein and fat, it is suspected that polysaccharides may stimulate intestinal adaptation better than monosaccharides. Intact starch can also be fermented to short chain fatty acids in the colon, stimulating sodium and water absorption and providing a primary energy source for the colonocytes.

Breast milk

Breast milk may not seem the ideal feed as it contains intact protein and lactose. However, breast milk is associated with good gastrointestinal tolerance. As well as the psychological benefits for the mother of using breast milk, it contains high levels of immunoglobulin A (IgA), nucleotides and leucocytes. Glutamine, LCT and growth hormone in breast milk may have a role in intestinal adaptation and there may also be benefits associated with protective colonic bacteria. Importantly, in 2001, studies showed that the use of breast milk correlated highly with a shorter duration of PN and that highly specialised formulas conferred no advantage over breast feeding [51]. It is the practice in most centres managing infants with SBS to use mother's EBM in the initial stages of feeding.

Formula feeding

It is important to have a flexible approach to feeding and knowledge of gut anatomy and physiology allows informed decisions about nutritional management to be made. In the absence of EBM, or when there is intolerance of EBM, the most appropriate feed to try would be a protein hydrolysate feed with approximately 50% of the fat as MCT. Suitable feeds would be Pepti-Junior and Pregestimil (see Table 7.7).

As feed volumes are advanced, malabsorption frequently occurs. It is helpful then to formulate a feed to suit the individual child with a choice of ingredients not predetermined by the composition of a commercial formula. A modular feeding system allows this flexibility giving a choice of protein, fat and carbohydrate and the ability to manipulate ingredients separately to find a feed composition that is tolerated.

Tables 7.21–7.23 show some of the available components of a modular feed that may be used. The protein source can be a whole protein, hydrolysed protein or amino acids. The carbohydrate source may be polysaccharides, disaccharides (sucrose, lactose) or monosaccharides and in practice a combination of carbohydrate sources may be beneficial so as not to saturate the capacity of a single brush border enzyme. The ratio of LCT : MCT can also be manipulated to tolerance. Electrolytes and micronutrients are added to make the feed nutritionally complete (see Table 7.24). An example modular feed is shown in Table 7.26.

Establishing a modular feed involves systematic stepwise changes to feed concentration and volume. Information about the volume and consistency of stools needs to be documented carefully and serial analysis of stool or stoma fluid for reducing sugars, pH and fat is crucial to make informed decisions about feed composition.

Trophic agents

There are few studies conducted in infants and children regarding any trophic factors and, like other aspects of managing SBS, requires more controlled studies to justify their widespread use. Their current use is based on trial and error but as a non-invasive inexpensive intervention, a trial of pectin or glutamine may be useful.

Pectin (available as Pectigel) is a water-soluble fibre. In animal experiments pectin has been shown to slow gastric emptying, slow transit through the small bowel and enhance adaptation. Following fermentation to short chain fatty acids by colonic bacteria pectin may also improve colonic absorptive function [52–54]. Slower transit allows a longer nutrient contact time with the intestinal mucosa and in children with a preserved colon pectin may also stimulate water and sodium absorption [55]. A dose of 1 g/100 mL feed has been suggested [56].

Glutamine (available as Adamin G) is considered to be an important energy source for rapidly dividing cells such as the cells of the intestinal mucosa. The benefit is unclear but glutamine supplements may enhance adaptation, have an anabolic effect on body tissues and improve enterocyte glucose absorption [57]. Ideal dosage is unclear but animal studies suggest that increasing the glutamine content of feeds to 25% total amino acids may enhance adaptation [56].

Continuous tube feeding

Infants and children with SBS frequently tolerate continuous enteral feeds better than bottle or bolus enteral feeds. A slow infusion of feed allows constant saturation of brush border enzymes and carrier proteins leading to improved absorption. Luminal nutrients are the single most important stimulus for adaptation so maximising the time during which nutrients are in contact with the intestine will optimise the potential for adaptation.

Oral feeding

Continuous feeding allows for maximum nutrient absorption, but infants need to learn to suck, swallow and chew. Small intermittent breast or bottle feeds should be initiated to maintain oral feeding skills and to lessen the likelihood of feeding difficulties commonly seen in children who are tube fed for extended periods [58]. Oral feeding will also stimulate gallbladder contraction and gastrointestinal secretions and perhaps therefore contribute to a reduced risk of intestinal failure associated liver disease.

Solids should be introduced at the appropriate time around 6 months of age. There is no consensus on the type of solids offered, but it seems sensible when infants are receiving a special formula that they are cow's milk protein and lactose free. There is no evidence to support the avoidance of other foods such as egg, gluten, wheat or disaccharides but in individual cases it may be necessary to exclude other foods if intolerance is suspected.

Pharmacological agents

H$_2$ receptor antagonists and proton pump inhibitors

Gastric hypersecretion frequently occurs after massive bowel resection. This will increase gastric aspirates and stool and stoma output, but more importantly can impair absorption by inactivation of pancreatic enzymes. Treatment with antacids is commonly required.

Anti-diarrhoeal agents

Loperamide and codeine can be used to slow transit time and control diarrhoea.

Colestyramine

Resection of the terminal ileum can result in bile salt malabsorption. Bile salts are conjugated to bile acids by colonic bacteria leading to diarrhoea. Colestyramine may help to bind the bile salts.

Short bowel syndrome in older children

Intestinal adaptation begins 24–48 hours after resection but can continue for up to 3 years. As children get older their feeds need to be reviewed regularly. Feeds need to be age appropriate and always given at the maximum level of tolerance. Children often have voracious appetites, particularly after PN is stopped and will consume vast amounts of food to compensate for malabsorption. For this reason, overnight tube feeds are often continued to provide additional nutritional support.

Weaning from parenteral nutrition

The transition to full enteral nutrition may take many months or years to complete but many children with SBS can eventually be weaned from PN. As feed tolerance improves PN can be reduced. Initially, the number of hours on PN and the volume infused are reduced and, with time, it is usually possible to reduce the number of nights children receive their PN. Careful monitoring is required during the period of transition to ensure both optimal growth and to prevent micronutrient deficiencies.

Intestinal failure related liver disease

Parenteral nutrition has improved the outcome for children with SBS but paradoxically it is associated with many potentially fatal complications. These complications include intestinal failure related liver disease (IFRLD) which is seen in 40–60% of children on long term PN [59]. The cause of liver disease in children on PN is multifactorial with risk factors including: prematurity [60], nutrient excess, bacterial infection [61], failure to tolerate enteral feeds [62] and failure to establish continuity of the gut. Prevention and management of IFRLD involves aggressive use of enteral nutrition, prevention of line sepsis, the use of ursodeoxycholic acid and 'cycling' of PN to reduce the number of hours, or days, that a child receives parenteral nutrition.

Monitoring

Monitoring is an important part of management of children with SBS receiving PN and is even more important as they are weaned from PN. Assessment of stool output is crucial to monitor feed tolerance. This is the best indicator to assess the potential to increase enteral feeds and reduce PN.

Serial anthropometric measurements are useful to evaluate nutritional status and track progress. These should include not just weight and length but head circumference, mid upper arm circumference and skinfold measurements.

Nutritional bloods are also needed. Micronutrients may be poorly absorbed and deficiencies are commonly seen in children who are weaning from PN and in those who are exclusively enterally fed. The most common deficiencies seen are fat-soluble vitamins, calcium, magnesium, zinc, iron and selenium. Oral supplements should be started to avoid clinical signs of deficiency.

Vitamin B_{12} receptors are restricted to the terminal ileum and if this has been removed in the resection children will require life-long injections of B_{12} to prevent deficiency. Regular monitoring is needed to assess the appropriate time for commencement of vitamin B_{12}.

Sodium depletion can also occur in children with either high stoma output or watery diarrhoea and is a common cause of poor weight gain. Urinary electrolytes are a good indicator of sodium status and should be measured regularly, aiming to maintain a urinary sodium : potassium ratio of approximately 2 : 1.

Home parenteral nutrition

Many children with SBS can eventually be weaned from PN. However, if PN is required for extended periods of time it is appropriate to continue the treatment in the home environment and there is good evidence that catheter sepsis is reduced when children are discharged home [63].

Surgery

A number of surgical interventions have been tried to alter intestinal transit and promote adaptation in children with SBS. These include plication of the intestine and bowel lengthening procedures [64,65]. Some children who develop end-stage liver disease as a result of IFRLD, but have the potential to eventually achieve independence from PN, may benefit from isolated liver transplantation [66]. Small bowel transplantation has developed over the past 20 years to become a life-saving option for children with SBS who develop the complications of intestinal failure. For children with an extremely short bowel permanent intestinal failure is almost inevitable. Long term PN remains the treatment of choice for this group, but intestinal transplantation may be indicated for those children who develop irreversible liver disease or impaired venous access. Advances in surgical techniques and immunosuppression have improved the outcome of intestinal transplantation, but the survival rate does not yet justify transplantation for children who can be safely managed on parenteral nutrition [67].

References

1 Goyal A, Jones MO, Couriel JM, Losty PD Oesophageal atresia and tracheo-oesophageal fistula. *Arch Dis Child Fetal Neonatal Ed*, 2006, **91** F381–4.

2 Spitz L, Kiely EM, Morecroft JA *et al*. Oesophageal atresia: at-risk groups for the 1990s. *J Pediatr Surg*, 1994, **29** 723–5.

3   Myers NA *et al.* Oesophageal atresia and associated anomalies: a plea for uniform documentation. *Pediatr Surg Int*, 1992, **7** 97–100.

4   Chittmittrapap S *et al.* Oesophageal atresia and associated anomalies. *Arch Dis Child*, 1989, **64** 364–8.

5   Spitz L *et al.* Esophageal atresia: five year experience with 148 cases. *J Pediatr Surg*, 1987, **22** 103–8.

6   Spitz L Esophageal atresia and tracheo-esophageal malformations. In: Ashcraft KW, Holcomb GW, Murphy JP (eds) *Pediatric Surgery*, 4th edn. Amsterdam: Elsevier Saunders, 2005, pp. 352–70.

7   Puntis JWL, Ritson DG, Holden CE, Buick RG Growth and feeding problems after repair of oesophageal atresia. *Arch Dis Child*, 1990, **65** 84–8.

8   Patel SB, Ade-Ajayi N, Kiely EM Oesophageal atresia: a simplified approach to early management. *Pediatr Surg Int*, 2002, **18** 87–9.

9   Cimador M, Carta M, Di Pace MR *et al.* Primary repair in oesophageal atresia: The results of long term follow-up. *Minerva Pediatr*, 2006, **58** 9–13.

10 Spitz L Oesophageal substitution procedures. In: Martin V (ed) *The TOF Child*. Nottingham: TOFS, 1999.

11 Spitz L, Kiely EM, Sparnon T Gastric transposition for esophageal replacement in children. *Ann Surg*, 1987, **206** 69–73.

12 Hirschl RB, Yardeni D, Oldham K *et al.* Gastric transposition for esophageal replacement in children. *Ann Surg*, 2002, **236** 531–41.

13 Spitz L Esophageal atresia and tracheoesophageal fistula in children. *Curr Opin Pediatr*, 1993, **5** 347–52.

14 Curci MR, Dibbins AW Problems associated with a Nissen fundoplication following tracheoesophageal fistula and esophageal atresia repair. *Arch Surg*, 1988, **123** 618–20.

15 Anderson KD *et al.* Long-term follow-up of children with colon and gastric tube interposition for esophageal atresia. *Surgery*, 1992, **111** 131–6.

16 Davenport M *et al.* Long term effects of gastric transposition in children: a physiological study. *J Pediatr Surg*, 1996, **31** 588–93.

17 Chetcuti P *et al.* Adults who survived repair of congenital oesophageal atresia and tracheo-oesophageal fistula. *Br Med J*, 1988, **297** 344–6.

18 Little DC, Rescoria FJ, Grosfeld JL *et al.* Long-term analysis of children with esophageal atresia and tracheoesophageal fistula. *J Pediatr Surg*, 2003, **38** 852–6.

19 Spitz L Gastric transposition for esophageal substitution in children. *J Pediatr Surg*, 1992, **27** 252–9.

20 Ravelli AM *et al.* Gastric emptying in children with gastric transposition. *J Pediatr Gastroenterol Nutr*, 1994, **19** 403–9.

21 Rivkees SA *et al.* Hypoglycaemic pathogenesis in children with dumping syndrome. *Pediatrics*, 1987, **80** 937–42.

22 Samuk I *et al.* Dumping syndrome following Nissen fundoplication, diagnosis and treatment. *J Pediatr Gastroenterol Nutr*, 1996, **23** 235–40.

23 Khoshoo V *et al.* Nutritional manipulation in the management of dumping syndrome. *Arch Dis Child*, 1991, **66** 1447–8.

24 Veit F *et al.* Dumping syndrome after Nissen fundoplication. *J Paediatr Child Health*, 1994, **30** 182–5.

25 De Vries TW *et al.* Dumping syndrome in a young child. *Eur J Pediatr*, 1995, **154** 624–6.

26 Borovoy J *et al.* Benefit of uncooked starch in the management of children with dumping syndrome fed exclusively by gastrostomy. *Am J Gastroenterol*, 1998, **93** 14–18.

27 Mooney D *et al.* Newborn duodenal atresia: an improving outlook. *Am J Surg*, 1987, **153** 347–9.

28 Suri S, Eradi B, Chowdhary SK *et al.* Early postoperative feeding and outcome in neonates. *Nutrition*, 2002, **18** 380–2.

29 Kleinhaus S, Boley SJ, Sheran M, Sieber WK Hirschprung's disease: a survey of members of the surgical section of the American Academy of Pediatrics. *J Pediatr Surg*, 1979, **14** 588–97.

30 Rankin J, Pattenden SW, Abramsky L *et al.* Prevalence of congenital anomalies in five British regions. *Arch Dis Child Fetal Neonatal Ed*, 2005, **5** F374–9.

31 Randolph J Omphalocele and gastroschisis: different entities, similar therapeutic goals. *South Med J*, 1982, **75** 1517–19.

32 Sauter ER *et al.* Is primary repair of gastroschisis and omphalocele always the best operation? *Ann Surg*, 1991, **57** 142–4.

33 Sharp M, Bulsara M, Gollow I, Pemberton P Gastroschisis: Early enteral feeds may improve outcome. *J Paediatr Child Health*, 2000, **36** 472–6.

34 Kitchanan S, Patole SK, Muller R, Whitehall JS Neonatal outcome of gastroschisis and exomphalos: A 10-year review. *J Paediatr Child Health*, 2000, **36** 428–30.

35 Hoffman P *et al.* Omphalocele and gastroschisis: problems in intensive treatment. *Zentralb Chir*, 1986, **111** 448–56.

36 Adam AS *et al.* Evaluation of conservative therapy for exomphalos. *Surg Gynecol Obstet*, 1991, **172** 395–6.

37 Stringer MD *et al.* Controversies in the management of gastroschisis: a study of 40 patients. *Arch Dis Child*, 1991, **66** 34–6.

38 Davies BW, Stringer MD The survivors of gastroschisis. *Arch Dis Child*, 1997, **77** 158–60.

39 Bryant J Observations upon the growth and length of the human intestine. *Am J Med Sci*, 1924, **167** 499–520.

40 Wilmore DW Factors correlating with a successful outcome following extensive intestinal resection in newborn infants. *J Pediatr*, 1972, **80** 88.

41 Goulet O, Baglin-Gobet S, Talbotec C *et al*. Outcome and long-term growth after extensive small bowel resection in the neonatal period: a survey of 87 children. *Eur J Pediatr Surg*, 2005, **15** 95–101.

42 Spencer A, Neaga A, West B *et al*. Paediatric short bowel syndrome. Redefining predictors of success. *Ann Surg*, 2005, **242** 403–12.

43 Tappenden KA Mechanisms of enteral nutrient enhanced intestinal adaptation. *Gastroenterol*, 2006, **130** S93–9.

44 Goulet O Irreversible intestinal failure. *J Paediatr Gastroenterol Nutr*, 2004, **38** 250–69.

45 Alverdy JC, Aoys E, Moss GS Total parenteral nutrition promotes bacterial translocation from the gut. *Surgery*, 1988, **104** 185–90.

46 Warner BW, Vanderhoof JA, Reyes JD What's new in the management of short gut syndrome in children? *J Am Coll Surg*, 2000, **190** 725–36.

47 Ksiazyk J, Piena M, Kierkus J, Lyszkowska M Hydrolysed versus non hydrolysed protein diet in short bowel syndrome in children. *J Paediatr Gastroenterol Nutr*, 2002, **35** 615–18.

48 Taylor SF, Sonheimer JM, Sokol RJ *et al*. Noninfectious colitis associated with short gut syndrome in infants. *J Paediatr*, 1991, **119** 24–8.

49 Vanderhoof JA, Grandjean CJ, Kaufman SS *et al*. Effect of high percentage medium chain triglyceride diet on mucosal adaptation following massive bowel resection in rats. *J Parenter Enteral Nutr*, 1984, **8** 685–9.

50 Bochenek WJ, Narkzewska B, Grzebieluch M Effect of massive proximal small bowel resection on intestinal sucrase and lactase activity in the rat. *Digestion*, 1973, **9** 224–30.

51 Andorsky DJ, Lund DP, Lillehei CW Nutritional and other postoperative management of neonates with short bowel syndrome correlates with clinical outcomes. *J Paediatr*, 2001, **139** 127–33.

52 Koruda MJ, Rolandelli RH, Settle RG *et al*. The effect of a pectin supplemented elemental diet on intestinal adaptation to major small bowel resection. *J Parenter Enteral Nutr*, 1986, **10** 343–50.

53 Koruda MJ Rolandelli RH, Settle RG *et al*. Small bowel disaccharidase activity in the rat as affected by intestinal resection and pectin feeding. *Am J Clin Nutr*, 1988, **47** 448–53.

54 Roth JA, Frankel WL, Zhang W *et al*. Pectin improves colonic function in rat short bowel syndrome. *J Surg Res*, 1995, **58** 240–6.

55 Kles KA, Chang EB Short chain fatty acids impact on intestinal adaptation, inflammation, carcinoma and failure. *Gastroenterol*, 2006, **130** S100–5.

56 Booth IW Enteral nutrition as primary therapy in short bowel syndrome. *Gut*, 1994, **Suppl** S69–72.

57 Byrne TA, Persinger RL, Young LS *et al*. A new treatment for patients with short bowel syndrome. Growth hormone, glutamine and a modified diet. *Ann Surg*, 1996, **222** 243–54.

58 Mason SJ, Harris G, Blissett J Tube feeding in infancy: implications for the development of normal eating and drinking skills. *Dysphagia*, 2005, **20** 46–61.

59 Kelly DA Liver complications of paediatric parenteral nutrition – epidemiology. *Nutrition*, 1998, **14** 153–7.

60 Merritt RJ Cholestasis associated with total parenteral nutrition. *J Paediatr Gastroenterol Nutr*, 1986, **5** 9–22.

61 Sondheimer J, Asturias E, Cadnapaphornchai M Infection and cholestasis in neonates with intestinal resection and long term parenteral nutrition. *J Paediatr Gastroenterol Nutr*, 1998, **27** 131–7.

62 Kelly DA Intestinal failure associated liver disease: what do we know today? *Gastroenterol*, 2006, **130** S70–7.

63 Knafelz D, Gambarara M, Diamanti A *et al*. Complications of home parenteral nutrition in a large pediatric series. *Transplant Proc*, 2003, **35** 3050–1.

64 Bianci A Experience with longitudinal intestinal lengthening and tailoring. *Eur J Pediatr Surg*, 1999, **9** 256–9.

65 Kim HB, Fauza D, Garza J *et al*. Serial transverse enteroplasty (STEP): a novel bowel lengthening procedure. *J Pediatr Surg*, 2003, **38** 425–9.

66 Horslen SP Isolated liver transplantation in infants with end stage liver disease associated with short bowel syndrome. *Ann Surg*, 2002, **235** 435–9.

67 Gupte GL, Beath SV, Kelly DA *et al*. Current issues in the management of intestinal failure. *Arch Dis Child*, 2006, **91** 259–64.

Useful addresses

The Tracheo-Oesophageal Fistula Support Group (TOFS)
St George's Centre, 91 Victoria Road, Netherfield, Nottingham, NG4 2NN
www.tofs.org.uk

Gut Motility Disorders Support Network
Westcott Farm, Oakford, Tiverton, EX16 9EZ

GEEPS (support group for families of children with abdominal wall defects)
104 Riverside Road, Romford, RM5 2NS
www.geeps.co.uk

9 The Liver and Pancreas

Stephanie France

The liver

Liver disease in children differs greatly from that in adults. Klein *et al.* [1] have summarised the differences:

- Liver disease in paediatric patients is rare
- The causes of disease are more diverse
- There is a greater prevalence of inborn errors of metabolism, biliary tract disease, primary infections and auto-immune disorders
- The higher anabolic needs for growth plus catabolic effects of liver disease may result in more nutritional deficiencies

The nutritional management of an infant or child will depend on whether the liver disease is acute, chronic or metabolic. Potential problems warranting nutritional attention occur when there is a disturbance in the usual metabolic functions of the liver. These include glucose homoeostasis, protein synthesis, bile salt production, lipid metabolism and vitamin storage.

Dietary therapy is usually aimed at the presenting symptoms including:

- Hypoglycaemia from poor glycogen storage
- Fat malabsorption as a result of poor bile production or flow
- Reduction in protein synthesis especially albumin, exacerbating ascites (Fig. 9.1)

Specific inherited metabolic disorders (IMD) within the liver, however, require more specific dietary treatment. These include tyrosinaemia, fatty acid oxidation disorders, urea cycle defects, glycogen storage disease, galactosaemia and fructosaemia (Chapters 17–19).

Infants tend to present with symptoms of biliary tract disorders that can progress to a chronic condition. Acute presentations are usually caused by poisoning, or as a result of an IMD. An acute presentation in an older child may be caused by hepatitis infection, ingestion of a toxic substance or to decompensation of an underlying chronic liver disease that has been 'silently' progressing over time, such as Wilson's disease or auto-immune liver disease.

Mechanisms for malnutrition

Potential causes of malnutrition in liver disease can be summarised as:

Inadequate intake:
- anorexia, nausea, vomiting associated with liver disease
- early satiety as a result of tense ascites, enlarged liver/spleen
- behavioural feeding problems
- hospitalisation related depression
- unpalatable diet/feeds

Facial telanglectasia

Spider naevi

Splenomegaly

Hepatomegaly

Jaundice

Large abdomen

Vasodilatation

↑ Cardiac output

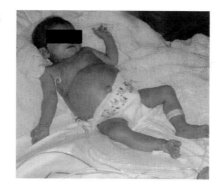

↑ Aldosterone

Ascites

Oedema

↓ Muscle bulk

↓ Skinfold thickness

Cutaneous shunts

Clubbing

Palmar erythema

Figure 9.1   Liver disease in children.

Impaired nutrient digestion and absorption:
- bile salt deficiency
- pancreatic insufficiency
- portal hypertension related enteropathy
- malnutrition related villous atrophy

Increased nutritional requirements:
- hypermetabolism (during stress such as infection)
- accelerated protein breakdown
- insufficient protein synthesis

Nutritional assessment

Routine nutritional assessment is the basis for identification and management of malnutrition in liver disease. Difficulty arises as the severity of malnutrition does not always correlate with measurable biochemical markers such as liver function tests or vitamin and mineral status [2]. Plotting length/height can indicate chronic malnutrition over long time periods [3] but is not a very sensitive marker in the short term. Weight measures can be useful initially but become meaningless with organomegaly and ascites [4]. Many other measures, biochemical in particular, are not useful in liver disease [5]. Serial measures of upper arm muscle circumference and triceps skinfold thickness are essential parameters [6] on which to rely for assessment of body fat and muscle stores [7,8]. However, there is a lack of reference data upon which to compare these measurements, particularly in the infant.

Data available are old, and not representative of the current population [9].

As well as serial anthropometric measures, assessment should include observation of physical signs of vitamin deficiences, dietary intake, degree of early satiety and any self-imposed restrictions. It is important to consider any nutrition related problems such as nausea, vomiting, diarrhoea or anorexia.

Nutritional requirements

Nutritional requirements are summarised in Table 9.1.

Acute liver disease

Acute liver failure describes severe impairment of liver function in association with hepatocellular necrosis, where there is no underlying chronic liver disease. The term fulminant is usually used when acute liver disease is associated with encephalopathy [11]. However, children often do not exhibit encephalopathy.

Causes of acute liver disease

- Infective (e.g. viral)
- IMD including haemochromatosis
- Toxins/drugs including chemotherapy

Table 9.1 Nutritional requirements in liver disease.

Cholestasis

Energy
Infants: 100–150 kcal (420–625 kJ)/kg/day depending on degree of malabsorption
150–180 mL/kg/day fluid usually as MCT based formula
Children: 100–120% EAR for age

Protein
10% energy from protein

Essential fatty acids
Additional depending on degree of malabsorption (walnut oil supplements)

Vitamins
Additional A, D, E, K given orally or IM if necessary

Chronic liver disease
Energy
Infants: 130–180 kcal (545–750 kJ)/kg/day
Children: 120–150% EAR for age

Protein
Infants: 3–6 g/kg/day
Children: 2 g/kg/day

Fluid
May be restricted if ascites

Sodium
No added salt where possible

Vitamins
Additional vitamins needed especially A, B, D, E, K

Minerals
Additional iron if blood losses; zinc in malabsorption
All requirements increased in generalised malabsorption associated with portal hypertension

Acute liver failure
Energy
120–150% EAR for age
Protein
100–120% RNI – may be gradually introduced if IMD suspected. Excessive amounts avoided

EAR, estimated average requirement; IM, intramuscular; IMD, inherited metabolic disorder; RNI, reference nutrient intake [10].

- Irradiation
- Ischaemic (e.g. Budd–Chiari syndrome)
- Infiltrative such as leukaemia
- Auto-immune
- Trauma from abuse or seat belt laceration in a road traffic accident

If presentation is rapid, infants and children are often well nourished, so management is based on maintaining nutritional status until there is some improvement. If onset is dramatic there is a possibility of the critical life-threatening complication of cerebral oedema, so patients are often treated in intensive care. If the child survives, liver function should return to near normal.

If the definition of fulminant hepatic failure is strictly adhered to, a problem arises. It is difficult to distinguish between disease that is actually acute and that which is (undiagnosed) chronic disease, manifesting as acute. The two conditions can appear the same. A thorough investigation of all possible causes is necessary. In particular, mitochondrial disorders of metabolism should be excluded.

Developments in treatment

Developments in the treatment of extreme cases of acute liver disease include auxiliary liver transplantation. A live donor may be used, but this is rarely necessary. A lobe of liver is transplanted and used in addition to the child's native liver. This can provide a temporary back-up in the acute situation. The obvious benefits are that the native liver is not removed, but allowed to get better. If this happens the transplanted liver is removed by surgery or destroyed by weaning down the immunosuppressive drugs. The immediate disadvantage is that the child may have a longer crisis and convalescence period because of the presence of the necrotic native liver and the addition of immunosuppression.

Auxiliary transplantation is also useful in the case of an IMD that originates from a defective enzyme in the liver, in that it provides a source of the required enzyme. It may be that genetic engineering will eventually supercede the need for transplantation so that the transplanted auxiliary liver could be removed, negating the need for lifelong immunosuppression. However, mitochondrial based defects are not organ specific and will eventually result in multisystem failure. There is no cure at present for these disorders and liver transplantation is not indicated.

Hepatocyte transplantation is an innovative treatment [12]. As with auxiliary transplant, the native liver remains, but instead cells are transplanted from a donor liver. This method is time dependent as the cells need to multiply sufficiently to take on the functions of the liver. So far, the technique has been advantageous in providing support to a failing liver, perhaps while a suitable organ is found, but has not yet been used in isolation. It does mean, if successful in the future, that a donor liver can be used for many more recipients and that live related donation is less risk associated for the donor.

Molecular adsorbents recycling system (MARS) is a form of dialysis technique for temporary liver support. Although results are promising in arresting fulminant liver failure in adults, research is lacking. Its use in children is anecdotal at present [13].

Liver directed gene therapy is awaited and considered to be on the threshold of human application [14].

Dietetic management in acute liver failure

The dietetic management of acute liver failure lacks consensus [15]. While several aspects of treatment remain controversial, current practice is to provide maximum nutritional support. For infants in particular, there is a difficulty surrounding the potential diagnosis. Metabolic disorders can be responsible for acute liver failure, the diagnosis of which can present a major challenge particularly if the liver is sufficiently damaged to produce secondary biochemical abnormalities [16]. Without a diagnosis a suitable feed choice is hindered and nutritional adequacy is therefore delayed.

Older children and adolescents in particular are less likely to have an undiagnosed IMD than are infants, with the exception of Wilson's disease. A standard enteral feed may be introduced for these patients and hence full nutritional requirements will be rapidly met.

Dietetic management in acute liver failure in infancy

On presentation a liver related IMD may be suspected (e.g. galactosaemia, fatty acid oxidation defect).

Initial treatment – emergency regimen
An emergency type regimen should be started as soon as possible, as intravenous (IV) dextrose (and saline) with additional potassium if the child is having diuretic therapy. Enteral feeding should be

established by the addition of glucose polymer (i.e. a lactose and fructose free source of carbohydrate) to either oral rehydration solution or water. Additional sodium/potassium supplements are necessary. The child should be fed continuously over 24 hours.

The aim of treatment initially is to meet glucose oxidation rates to prevent protein/fat catabolism. Guidelines for glucose requirements (see p. 392):

- Infants 8–9 mg/kg/min
- Toddlers 7 mg/kg/min
- Adolescents 4 mg/kg/min

The amount of glucose given can be increased slowly according to tolerance. Infants often tolerate 18 g glucose/kg/day (i.e. 12.5 mg/kg/min). A modular feed is then developed. Energivit is a useful feed if fatty acid oxidation defects have been excluded.

Addition of protein
Protein should be added to the feed as soon as possible. The protein source should be lactose free if galactosaemia has not yet been excluded, and fat free if fatty acid oxidation defects have not been excluded. Essential Amino Acid Mix is a suitable lactose and fat free source of protein. A child with any IMD, including those of protein metabolism, should tolerate some protein which contains all amino acids (providing the plasma ammonia level is not excessive).

Infants should be given 1.5–1.9 g protein/kg dry weight/day and children 0.8–1.0 g protein/kg dry weight/day, based on the minimum protein requirements (World Health Organization) [17].

If tyrosinaemia has not been ruled out, and depending on plasma amino acid levels, a tyrosine, methionine, phenylalanine free amino acid mix, XPTM Tyrosidon (fat free and lactose free) could be used until a diagnosis of tyrosinaemia is excluded.

It is important not to over-restrict protein, which could result in endogenous ammoniagenesis from protein catabolism. If a diagnosis of galactosaemia is excluded Vitapro, which contains traces of lactose, may be used as the protein source.

Addition of fat
Small quantities of walnut oil (p. 427) are needed to provide essential fatty acids (EFAs): 1 mL/100 kcal

(420 kJ) is recommended in the treatment of liver disease. However, additional fat will be necessary to meet energy requirements.

Long chain triglyceride (LCT) and/or medium chain triglyceride (MCT) fat emulsion, as Calogen and/or Liquigen, can be added to the feed as the condition of the child is monitored. Increments of 1 g fat/kg/day are recommended. A complete vitamin and mineral supplement will be necessary, such as Paediatric Seravit. It is essential to meet basal protein and energy requirements as soon as possible to prevent catabolism and the build-up of lethal metabolites as well as to preserve muscle and fat stores.

Usually, diagnoses of galactosaemia and tyrosinaemia are excluded quickly. Other conditions are likely to be ruled out from the presentation details. Hence the above is theoretical and, usually, following the use of the emergency regimen, a suitable formula can be used for the suspected condition.

Branched chain amino acids

Abnormal amino acid profiles are seen in liver disease. Plasma concentrations of aromatic amino acids increase and the branched chain amino acids (BCAAs) valine, leucine and isoleucine rapidly decrease [18]. The extent of these changes is thought to correlate with the degree of encephalopathy [19]. A Cochrane review by Als-Nielson *et al.* [20] concludes that the use of BCAAs as a supplement is ineffective as a treatment for encephalopathy. However, BCAAs are preferentially used in catabolism and, as a result, supplementation may allow a higher protein intake without deterioration in mental state [21]. Unfortunately, there have been no randomised controlled trials in children on the use of BCAAs in acute liver failure.

BCAA supplements can be provided by Generaid powder, Hepatamine, Generaid Plus, Heparon Junior and Hepatical.

Chronic liver disease

There are many causes of chronic liver disease, some of which are more likely than others to have an early presentation. Some diseases may not be recognised until the child is in adolesence.

Disorders presenting in infancy

- Inherited metabolic disorders including progressive familial intrahepatic cholestasis (PFIC), bile salt export pump (BSEP) deficiency
- Infections
- Biliary malformations including atresia
- Vascular lesions
- Toxic and nutritional disorders including hypervitaminosis A and total parenteral nutrition (TPN)
- Cryptogenic disorders (e.g. neonatal hepatitis)

Disorders presenting in children and adolescents

- Inherited disorders (e.g. cystic fibrosis; CF)
- Infections and inflammatory (e.g. sclerosing cholangitis)
- Biliary malformations such as choledochal cyst
- Toxic, nutritional, cryptogenic including malnutrition, non-alcoholic steatohepatitis (NASH)

Cirrhosis

This represents the end-stage of any chronic liver disease. The chronic disease may initiate a repetitive sequence of cell injury and repair. The consequence of this is cyclical necrosis and fibrogenesis which can lead to irreversible damage superimposed onto the original disease process [22]. The liver can compensate for the damage such that the cirrhosis is asymptomatic. Decompensated cirrhosis occurs when damage within the liver causes blood flow to be impaired resulting in symptoms such as portal hypertension, ascites and varices.

Symptoms that can necessitate nutritional intervention

Jaundice

Jaundice is classified as either conjugated or unconjugated. Conjugated bilirubin is made water soluble by the addition of glucuronide in the liver and enters the bile. If bile flow from the liver is reduced the stools will lack pigment. In this case the (conjugated) bilirubin glucuronide passes into the serum and is then excreted in urine. Conjugated hyperbilirubinaemia occurs when the total serum bilirubin is raised and more than 20% of the bilirubin is conjugated (normally <5% is conjugated). This type of jaundice, with pale stools and dark urine, represents significant hepatobiliary disease and is described as cholestatic liver disease.

Unconjugated hyperbilirubinaemia is characterised clinically by jaundice without bile in the urine. This may be physiological in the newborn and is not usually an indication for dietetic intervention. Many of the infants seen in a specialist liver centre present with conjugated hyperbilirubinaemia and the diagnosis of its cause is made later. Most of the possible diagnoses for conjugated hyperbilirubinaemia are given later (see p. 154). Dietetic management is summarised in Table 9.2.

If the bile flow from the liver into the gut is limited, fat emulsification and digestion is reduced. This leads to malabsorption of fat, fat-soluble vitamins and some minerals. Steatorrhoea, growth failure and rickets are common clinical consequences [23–25].

Fat malabsorption

To ensure an energy-dense diet is given, fat should not be restricted but given to tolerance. In infants, for whom fat is a more significant energy source, a proportion of fat should be given as MCT [26,27], which is independent of bile acids for absorption. Many infants compensate for the loss of energy resulting from fat malabsorption by taking increased volumes of formula. Intakes can be as much as 2–3 times normal fluid requirements. For this reason, an MCT rich formula (containing adequate amounts of EFAs; e.g. Caprilon) should be introduced to provide a form of fat and energy that can be absorbed and hence feed volume can be reduced to normal fluid requirements of 150–180 mL/kg (Table 9.2).

Breast fed babies with cholestasis tend to demand huge quantities of milk without thriving as a result of fat malabsorption. A significant proportion of their requirements should be met by an MCT rich formula (100–120 mL/kg), with breast feeds used as a top-up, at least until bile flow recovers. Beware of giving an energy supplement of MCT oil or Liquigen (combined with glucose polymer, e.g. Maxijul, if better tolerated) before each breast feed: care is needed to ensure adequate amounts of breast milk are still being taken to provide all other nutrients necessary for growth. All infants should be given some fat containing LCT,

Table 9.2   Summary of dietetic management for infantile conjugated hyperbilirubinaemia/cholestatic jaundice.

1   *Is galactosaemia suspected?*
No, change formula to Caprilon with or without breast feeds (or MCT Pepdite if protein hydrolysate is required)
Yes, change formula to MCT Pepdite or Pregestimil without breast feeds

2   *Is galactosaemia diagnosed?*
No, change to Caprilon with or without breast feeds
Yes, change to suitable lactose free formula

3   *Is infant breast fed?*
No, use 150–180 mL/kg Caprilon
Yes, use 100–120 mL/kg Caprilon, usually divided between each feed and given at the beginning with top-ups at the breast. If cholestasis is resolving, growth and intake adequate, continue exclusive breast feeds and monitor

4   *Are blood sugars maintained?*
No, consider adding glucose polymer (e.g. Maxijul) up to 3% initially, minimum 3-hourly feeds day and night, may need 2-hourly or continuous if necessary
Yes, continue management

5   *If infant is failing to thrive, is intake adequate?*
No, consider NG feeding
Yes, consider concentrating feeds, e.g. up to 20% Caprilon. Beware that adding energy supplements reduces the ratio of protein and EFAs to energy unless adequate supplied from solids

6   *At weaning*
Encourage as normal from around 6 months
Encourage rapid progression in texture if possible
Add Caprilon when making up dried baby foods instead of water
Alternatively, add household foods (cream, butter, cheese) and/or Duocal to supplement energy content of home cooked purée foods or commercial baby foods

7   *Continue to review and monitor*

NG, nasogastric.

either as breast milk or prescribed formula, to provide a source of EFAs.

It is possible to manage cholestatic babies solely on breast milk, particularly if cholestasis is resolving and there is no definitive diagnosis, which more frequently occurs in ex-premature babies. Growth and intake of the baby and the health of the mother should be monitored closely.

The amount of EFAs needed, as a percentage of total energy intake, is unclear in children with liver disease as deficiency may still occur in those who have received supplementation [28].

Table 9.3   Specialised products containing medium chain triglyceride (MCT) fats and their essential fatty acid (EFA) content.

| Product | % fat as MCT | EFAs as percentage energy | | |
		Linoleic acid	α-linolenic acid	Ratio
Caprilon (SHS)	75	5.6	0.8	7.5
Pregestimil (Mead Johnson)	55	10.1	0.6	16.8
MCT Pepdite (SHS)	75	5.1	0.8	6.4
Pepti-Junior (Cow & Gate)	50	12.8	0.2	64
Monogen (SHS)	90	1	0.2	4.6
MCT Step 1 (Vitaflo)	90	1.4	0.2	7
Calogen (SHS)*	0	24	4.7	5
Solagen (SHS)*	–	51	7.2	7
Liquigen (SHS)*	98	0	0	0
Duocal (SHS)*	35	4.4	1.1	4
Liquid Duocal (SHS)*	30	16.7	0.3	60
MCT Duocal (SHS)*	75	6.3	0.9	7
15% Caprilon + 5% Duocal	68	5.5	0.1	55
Generaid Plus (SHS)†	32	3.7	1.0	4
Heparon Junior (SHS)	49	9.3	1.3	7.1
Emsogen (SHS)†	83	3.4	0.1	47
Nutrison MCT (Nutricia)†	67	5.3	0.7	7.6
ESPGAN [29] recommendations		4.5–10.8		5–15

* These are energy supplements not infant formulas.
† Products used as comparison but are not infant formulas.

Recommendations from the European Society for Paediatric Gastroenterology and Nutrition (ESPGAN) [29] are that infant formulas (including those used for malabsorption) should contain 4.5–10.8% energy as linoleic acid and that the ratio of linoleic : α-linolenic acids is 5–15 (Table 9.3). It may be assumed that the aim should be to meet the upper limit as a significantly greater amount will be required in a state of fat malabsorption.

Older children are encouraged to consume an energy dense diet to meet the necessary increased requirements. Glucose polymers are useful energy supplements when a maximum fat intake is reached. There are MCT rich feeds that are suitable for older children (e.g. Emsogen, and Nutrison MCT). Some products do not contain a suitable proportion of EFAs, supported by clinical data [30], unless taken with an additional source of fat from solids or walnut oil. Up to 2 mL walnut oil per 100 kcal (420 kJ) may need to be added to meet the upper limit of EFAs depending on the levels already provided by the feed.

Pancreatic enzyme insufficiency
Some types of liver disease, including Alagille's syndrome, progressive intrahepatic cholestasis and choledochal cysts, may be accompanied by pancreatic enzyme deficiency which aggravates malabsorption. Because bile salts are required to activate pancreatic lipase a functional deficiency may be present in cholestasis. Finding a low stool elastase may support a deficiency. In these cases, pancreatic enzymes should be started and continued if a clinical benefit is seen. It is unwise to use doses above 10 000 units lipase/kg/day.

Hypoglycaemia
The liver is essential for glucose homoeostasis. It stores glycogen and during fasting mobilises glucose. Infants and children with liver disease commonly become hypoglycaemic as a result of impairment of this function. Muscle glycogen homoeostasis is also disrupted in liver disease. In infants, more frequent feeds may need to be offered, as well as ensuring an adequate volume is taken. Overnight continuous feeds may be indicated if the infant does not wake for feeds during the night. It may be necessary to add carbohydrate in the form of a glucose polymer to the infant formula feeds. Initially, 1–3 g/100 mL feed is added

and may be gradually increased to 6 g/100 mL if needed. Caution is necessary when feeds contain large amounts of glucose as hypoglycaemia may result from a rebound effect, particularly as the feed is discontinued.

In children, regular complex carbohydrate in meals and snacks is encouraged. Sugary foods and glucose drinks can also be encouraged as long as the intake is divided into regular portions to avoid the rebound effect. It may be necessary to provide a continuous overnight feed, or evening doses of uncooked cornstarch (see p. 395) to ensure blood glucose is maintained throughout the night. An IV infusion of dextrose may be the only way of controlling blood sugar initially while a feeding routine is established and is a more accurate way of determining the quantity of glucose required to maintain adequate blood sugar levels.

Failure to thrive

Failure to thrive is very common in children with liver disease as energy requirements are increased [31–33] and intake is unlikely to be adequate without intervention. A diet high in energy and protein is encouraged but utilisation of nutrients may be poor [34]. Additional supplements may be necessary but often, if appetite is poor, nasogastric (NG) feeding during the day or overnight is indicated.

As liver function diminishes, muscle wasting increases in decompensated liver disease. The value of BCAAs as a protein source is a subject of discussion. Chin et al. [35] showed an improvement in height and weight in children with end-stage liver disease when supplemented with a BCAA formula compared with an isocaloric, isonitrogenous standard formula. This is possibly because BCAAs are metabolised outside the liver and are preferentially utilised by skeletal muscle.

Generaid Plus, a formula containing BCAAs (37% of the protein) is sometimes used, though palatability is poor. Flavourings can be successfully added, or NG tube feeding may be required. Although Generaid Plus is not a complete feed and is not prescribable for children under 1 year, it has been successfully used in infants from 4–6 months when mixed solids would start to be introduced; adequate monitoring is necessary. Table 9.4 summarises a suggested strength administration. Generaid Plus has a lower level of some micronutrients and to meet the requirements of an infant

Table 9.4 Suggested initiation of Generaid Plus feeds.

Initiate at energy density of feed already being tolerated **or**
0–6 months initiate at 17% concentration, i.e. 0.75 kcal (3 kJ)/mL (supplement with calcium, phosphorus, magnesium)
6–12 months initiate at 22–34% concentration, i.e. 1.0–1.5 kcal (4.2–6.3 kJ)/mL
>12 months initiate at 22–44% concentration, i.e. 1.0–2.0 kcal (4.2–8.4 kJ)/mL
Ensure sodium intake is adequate
Ensure adequate calcium, phosphorous, magnesium, iron

throughout the first year an intake of 850 mL at 22% concentration is needed, which is rarely achieved in an infant less than 6 months of age. Supplements of calcium, phosphorous, magnesium and iron are needed at intakes below this level (Table 9.5).

Heparon Junior is soon to be made available in the UK and it awaits trials. It is designed for cholestatic infants and contains almost 50% fat as MCT and is supplemented with BCAAs (30% of the protein). It is fortified heavily with fat-soluble vitamins at a level that may not be justifiable in many cases.

Both Generaid Plus and Heparon Junior are low in sodium and do not meet the recommended levels for infant formulas. For this reason, care is needed to ensure an adequate intake of sodium and appropriate monitoring (Table 9.5). Conversely, Hepatamine and Hepatical, BCAA rich supplements designed for adults, contain high levels of sodium that limit their use in younger children.

Ascites and hepatomegaly

The greatest significance of ascites and hepatomegaly on nutritional status is the associated loss of appetite resulting from a reduced abdominal capacity for feeds and/or food. The aim is to give smaller, more frequent and nutrient dense meals and snacks. Supplementary NG feeding is often required. Ascites is a feature of decompensated liver disease and is managed aggressively with restriction of sodium and fluid intake. Diuretics are used in preference to restricting fluids to allow an adequate nutritional intake; however, resistant ascites may warrant a fluid restriction of 60–80% normal requirements. In extreme cases it may be that the infant self-restricts fluid intake to a greater extent than that imposed. A reduction in fluid volume will necessitate the need for a concentrated

Table 9.5 Examples of feeds suitable for infants with chronic liver disease.

	Energy (kcal)	(kJ)	Protein (g)	Fat (g)	MCT %	CHO (g)	Sodium (mmol)	Potassium (mmol)	Calcium (mmol)
Modular feed									
25 g Vitapro (Vitaflo)	98	408	19	1.5		2.3	3.3	4.5	2.5
125 g Maxijul (SHS)	475	2019				119	1.1	0.2	
25 mL Calogen (SHS)	113	463		12.5			0.1		
40 mL Liquigen (SHS)	180	740		20			0.5		
14 g Paediatric Seravit (SHS)	42	179				10.5	0.1		9.0
0.8 mL 30% Sodium chloride (50 mmol in 10 mL)							4.0		
5 mL Potassium chloride (20 mmol in 10 mL)								10.0	
Sterile water up to a total of 900 mL									
Total	908	3809	19	34		142.3	9.1	14.7	11.5
Per 100 mL	101	423	2.1	3.8	57	15.8	1.0	1.6	1.3
Concentrated Caprilon									
20 g Caprilon (SHS)									
Sterile water up to a total of 100 mL									
Per 100 mL	104	437	2.4	5.6	75	11.1	1.3	2.7	2.1
*Generaid Plus**									
22 g Generaid Plus (SHS)									
Sterile water up to a total of 100 mL									
Per 100 mL	102	428	2.4	4.2	32	13.6	0.7	2.6	1.7

NB. Per 850 mL calcium 14.6 mmol (RNI infant 0–12 mths 13.1 mmol); phosphorus 14.2 mmol (13.1 mmol); magnesium 80 mg (55–80 mg); iron 7.7 mg (1.7–7.8 mg).

	Energy (kcal)	(kJ)	Protein (g)	Fat (g)	MCT %	CHO (g)	Sodium (mmol)	Potassium (mmol)	Calcium (mmol)
*Heparon Junior**									
21 g Heparon Junior (SHS)									
Sterile water up to a total of 100 mL									
Per 100 mL	101	423	2.3	4.2	49	13.5	0.7	2.3	2.6

* Feeds do not meet sodium recommendations for infant formulas but used with caution when fluid volume is restricted in older infants and when sodium balance can be monitored.

feed, preferably with a low sodium content providing 1.2–1.5 mmol/kg/day. Generaid Plus can be used and concentrated to as much as 2 kcal (8.4 kJ)/ml (44% dilution) if this is done slowly and to tolerance. An MCT based infant formula such as Caprilon can be concentrated to as much as 1 kcal (4.2 kJ)/ml (20% dilution); in addition an energy supplement (e.g. Duocal) can be used added although sodium intakes may then be too high and protein intake inadequate.

A modular feed system based on Vitapro, glucose polymer and LCT and MCT fat emulsions may be used to meet all specific requirements. Sodium content can then be altered by the addition of sodium chloride. Such a modular feed will need vitamin and mineral supplementation. Examples of suitable feeds are given in Table 9.5 for comparison.

Modular feeds can be patient specific allowing flexibility in energy and protein contents, MCT : LCT ratio, electrolyte concentration and fluid volume. If increased cautiously, modular feeds can be given at a density of 2 kcal/mL (8.4 kJ/mL) (as with Generaid Plus), which is advantageous if nutritional requirements are high or fluid tolerance is poor. Care is needed when teaching parents to prepare feeds, particularly when more than two ingredients are used. At home parents will always need to ensure that they have an adequate supply of each ingredient.

All fluids given within the daily allowance should be nutritious, with proprietary supplements used if necessary. The discouragement of salty foods (see p. 210) can help to reduce natural thirst as well as enforcing a sodium restriction A rigid sodium restriction is difficult to impose in children and often results in a corresponding reduction in appetite and energy intake and should therefore be avoided.

Portal hypertension and malabsorption

Cirrhosis can obstruct blood flow to the liver causing portal hypertension associated with an enteropathy and malabsorption, possibly secondary to increased pressure in the mesenteric venous system (i.e. oedema of the mucosa of the small intestine). However, studies have failed to show a direct relationship between the degree of portal hypertension and extent of malabsorption [36,37]. The presenting malabsorption that clinically appears can be very difficult to control. Dietary treatment is not universal and depends on the extent of malabsorption. More frequent (if not continuous) feeds may increase absorption. Hydrolysed protein feeds may be required (see p. 97). However, in extreme cases TPN (preferably with some minimal enteral feeding to preserve a functioning gut mucosa) may be necessary.

Oesophageal varices

The presence of varices is not normally a contraindication to NG tube feeding, or to continuing a normal diet. Occasionally in end-stage liver disease, the huge varices that frequently bleed give rise to a high level of caution such that TPN has been warranted. Clear fluids and progression onto a soft diet are introduced only 16–24 hours after sclero-therapy.

Chronic encephalopathy

Restriction of protein is an accepted method of initially treating encephalopathy and reducing ammonia producing gut flora [11]. This can have a deleterious effect on the nutritional status of the child. The degree of encephalopathy must be assessed to determine the level of restriction. Ideally, energy intake should be increased to decrease the protein : energy ratio and prevent protein breakdown for energy. Sodium benzoate may permit tolerance of a higher protein intake. The use of BCAAs in encephalopathy has been discussed elsewhere (see p. 149). Dietetic management in chronic liver disease is summarised in Table 9.6.

Table 9.6 Summary of dietetic management in chronic liver disease.

Failure to thrive
Ensure adequate intake
Concentrate feeds
Advise protein and energy dense solids/food/snacks
Ensure an adequate protein : energy ratio (i.e. 2.5 g protein/100 kcal [420 kJ] or 10%)
Add energy supplement if overall protein : energy ratio maintained e.g. from solids
Use higher protein feed or supplements, consider Generaid Plus
Consider NG feeding
Consider continuous feeds for enhanced absorption

Hypoglycaemia
Optimise feed volume
Change to more frequent feeds/meals/snacks
Increase carbohydrate content of feeds
Consider NG feeding, continuous if necessary

Ascites
Change to smaller, more frequent feeds
Consider NG and continuous feeds
Optimise nutritional content of feeds if fluid restricted
Limit sodium intake (in feeds and advise on avoiding salty foods)
Consider Generaid Plus or an alternate lower sodium feed

Encephalopathy
Initiate emergency regimen if necessary
Introduce protein ideally within 24 hours, at a minimum level if necessary
Maximise protein provision as soon as possible
Ensure adequate energy intake
Consider supplementing with BCAAs
Monitor urea, ammonia and anthropometry to ensure optimum protein provision
Assess if sodium benzoate has been used, but may exacerbate ascites
Concentrate feeds and add energy supplements
Maxijul liquid or equivalent glucose drink can be useful supplement in older children if adequate protein consumed elsewhere

Portal hypertension and malabsorption
Initiate nutritional support
Consider hydrolysed protein feeds
Consider continuous feeds rather than bolus feeds
Assess the need for pancreatic enzyme replacement therapy
Consider parenteral nutrition preferably in addition to enteral nutrition

BCAA, branched chain amino acid; NG, nasogastric.

Additional factors to consider in assessing a child with chronic liver disease

- Weight can be an unreliable indicator of nutritional status.
- Organomegaly and the hepatic artery resistance index (HARI) can be assessed on ultrasound scan. An increase in liver size suggests worsening disease. An increase in spleen size can indicate worsening portal hypertension. A repeated HARI of >1 denotes reverse blood flow through the artery and indicates severe damage potentially warranting transplant. (All parameters can be temporarily worse in acute on chronic infection).
- A measure of prothrombin time or blood clotting (international normalised ratio, INR) can suggest poor synthetic liver function. If the INR is repeatedly >2 it can indicate transplantation is imminent.
- Repeatedly low albumin (Alb) denotes worsening liver function in chronic liver disease.
- Worsening liver function tests (LFTs) also show a declining synthetic function.
- All the above parameters can be temporarily worse in acute on chronic disease or infection.
- In the presence of ongoing jaundice with pale stools, the significant cholestatic liver disease will usually result in cirrhosis. However, cirrhosis may still occur in the absence or improvement of jaundice as hepatocyte damage can continue. This may not present as cholestatic disease and MCT fats may not be necessary.
- Fat malabsorption can still occur in some conditions (e.g. PFIC) where the bilirubin level is not significantly elevated. This is because of the inability to produce bile salts in the first place. Hence, there is an inability to emulsify and digest fat, but without the presence of significant jaundice. In these cases the diagnosis is an important consideration alongside the symptoms.

Enteral feeding

Nasogastric tube feeding

NG feeding improves body composition in paediatric liver disease [38]. The use of fine bore polyurethane/silicone tubes is well tolerated and is associated with low risk of variceal haemorrhage [39]. Feeds may be administered as boluses, top-up feeds, continuous feeds over 24 hours or overnight infusion via a pump. Overnight feeds are particularly useful as an addition to the usual daytime regimen. The continuous delivery of feeds is often the only route tolerated in cases of extreme malabsorption or hypoglycaemia.

Gastrostomy feeding

The placement of gastrostomies is contraindicated in liver disease, particularly if the child has ascites. It may also create potential problems with access to the abdominal cavity (because of adhesions) during liver transplantation. There is also a possibility of variceal formation at the stoma site. The enlarged liver and/or spleen creates a greater risk of puncture if undergoing endoscopic placement of gastrostomy. However, gastrostomies have been successfully placed in exceptional circumstances (Alagille's, CF) when portal hypertension is not too advanced [40].

Weaning

Weaning is encouraged as normal from about 6 months, with progression to nutrient dense foods. Dried baby foods can be mixed with infant formula, otherwise extra energy can be added in the form of household ingredients (butter, oil, cheese) or prescribed energy supplements.

Progression in texture should be encouraged as quickly as possible. Failure to give solids regularly during the normal stage of development when chewing is learned may have profound effects in terms of feeding behaviour later. Advice from speech and language therapists, play therapists, psychologists and health visitors can help, particularly if they are involved at an early stage.

Vitamins, minerals and essential fatty acids

All infants and children with cholestatic liver disease require additional fat-soluble vitamins [27]. Good levels may be achieved with a complete vitamin supplement daily (e.g. 5 mL Ketovite liquid, three Ketovite tablets and a separate vitamin K supplement; 1 mg IV preparation given orally), at least until cholestasis resolves. There are no studies to assess whether these children are deficient in water-soluble vitamins, but it is likely that there is a greater need for B vitamins with their increased energy requirements.

Fat-soluble vitamin deficiencies are a feature of cholestatic and long-standing severe liver disease. Colestyramine is prescribed to increase gallbladder contraction and impairs absorption of fat-soluble vitamins. The general supplement is continued in these cases. Adequate monitoring of fat-soluble vitamin levels is essential and separate oral vitamin doses should be given and adjusted accordingly if necessary. In severe malabsorption, adequate levels become difficult to achieve and this can highlight the need for the vitamins to be given as intramuscular (IM) injections.

Increased mineral requirements may include iron if bleeding has been a problem; zinc if vitamin A deficiency occurs; and calcium and phosphate if vitamin D deficient rickets is found. Selenium deficiency is associated with EFA deficiency.

EFA deficiencies may be seen in children with chronic cholestasis [41] and resulting severe fat malabsorption or those who have been on very low fat diets for long periods. Additional supplements of these may also be required. Walnut oil provides the ideal ratio of linoleic : α-linolenic acid (see p. 427). The extent to which a different pre- and post-transplant intake of EFAs can prevent deficiency and hasten recovery of EFA status remains to be determined [42].

Nutritional support pre-transplantation

As decompensation occurs, a good nutritional state becomes more and more difficult to maintain in the child with chronic liver disease. Fortunately, earlier liver transplantation offers a future for the majority at this stage. Although donor matching is based on blood type only, waiting time on the list is unpredictable. The advancement in live related transplantation is likely to lead to fewer fatalities while waiting.

A decline in nutritional status despite maximal nutritional support often highlights the need for transplantation, as malnutrition adversely affects the outcome of liver transplantation [43]. Improving nutritional status prior to transplant can help to reduce complications [44]. With transplantation as the particular aim, both patients and carers show increased willingness for aggressive nutritional support. Sometimes the struggle to maintain nutritional status necessitates a combination of enteral and parenteral nutrition.

Dietetic management pre-transplantation is summarised in Table 9.6.

Prescribing parenteral nutrition

Parenteral nutrition (PN) has been successfully used in the provision of adequate nutrition in children with chronic liver disease, although ideally enteral nutrition is maximised in the first instance. Prescriptions for PN must consider fluid and sodium restrictions. Fat is usually provided as LCT directly into the circulation, with due monitoring of lipid clearance by measuring plasma triglycerides. Fan *et al.* [45] demonstrated that lipid clearance can improve when using an LCT/MCT blend.

BCAAs have been given intravenously, although as with enteral administration, the evidence that they are beneficial is controversial. There may be a benefit in avoiding preterm amino acid solutions (e.g. Primene) as they contain higher levels of aromatic amino acids which are already elevated in liver disease. Manganese should be avoided as it is not cleared from the liver when bile flow is impeded and as such is toxic to hepatocytes. Manganese may also be deposited in the brain.

Nutritional support post-orthotopic liver transplantation

Immediately post-transplantation

Liver transplantation in children is technically more difficult than in adults. The liver is cut down to size match, sometimes just using the right or left, or part of the left lobe. As a result of the higher incidence of biliary tract disease as an indication for transplant in children, and the increased use of cutdown donor livers, it is unusual for the bile duct to remain intact. In a child who has not previously required a Kasai operation (see p. 155), a Roux loop will be fashioned from the intestine, through which the bile will drain from the transplanted liver. This reconstruction delays enteral feeding for 4–5 days.

For children who have had a previous Kasai procedure, enteral feeds may start on the third day. Feeds are gradually increased thereafter as tolerated. TPN should be considered when enteral feeds are delayed, but is not routine and depends on the nutritional status of the child. Double lumen enteral tubes are used in adults for gastric aspiration alongside jejunal feeding. However, such tubes are not available for children because of the variation in size requirements. It is not usual practice to insert two tubes; hence, adequate enteral nutrition may be delayed until gastric stasis resolves. Normal age appropriate feeding is introduced gradually over a couple of days. A good nutritional intake can be expected 7 days post-transplantation.

Generally, children with nutritional problems pre-transplantation continue to have problems post-transplantation. NG tube feeding is extremely common pre- and post-transplant especially in infants, and may be needed for up to a further 2 months after discharge post-transplant. However, intake of solids can rapidly improve and a normal diet for age is expected 6 months post-transplant [46].

The clearing of long-standing jaundice and the introduction of high dose steroids (as anti-rejection treatment) have an important role in promoting a good appetite post-transplant. It can be surprising how many children begin to eat well, including those previously reliant on tube feeds with little solid intake. Taste preferences can alter dramatically post-transplantation, possibly because of taste perception altered by ciclosporin (an anti-rejection drug). Parents are encouraged to offer new foods and to expect taste changes alongside an increased willingness to eat.

Possible complications

Chylous ascites may develop as a result of damage to lymph vessels during transplant surgery. This resolves but needs treatment for up to 2 weeks on a low LCT diet, using an MCT based formula to provide energy (e.g. Monogen, MCT Step 1 or Emsogen; see p. 148).

During periods of sepsis or rejection, bile flow may temporarily become limited, again necessitating the use of an MCT formula. Hepatic artery thrombosis may require retransplantation. Intestinal perforation will require gut rest. In both situations enteral feeds are further delayed and TPN may be needed.

Immunosuppression

Basic food hygiene rules using common sense should be encouraged. The commonly used anti-rejection drugs, tacrolimus and ciclosporin, present nutritional challenges. Tacrolimus absorption is affected by food and should ideally be given 1 hour before or after food. This can substantially reduce the hours available for feeding an infant and in practice this aim is overruled. Both ciclosporin and tacrolimus cause low serum magnesium. Levels need to be monitored and extra magnesium given, as much as 0.5–1.0 mmol/kg/day. These supplements are not well tolerated and can cause diarrhoea. Grapefruit (including juice) needs to be avoided when on tacrolimus as it may induce toxicity.

Liver diseases in young children requiring nutritional management

Infantile conjugated hyperbilirubinaemia is the most common presentation for an infant with hepatobiliary disease. The dietetic management is summarised in Table 9.2. It is not a diagnosis but a symptom and needs further investigation. Several tests (e.g. blood tests, ultrasound, biopsy report) will be required to find the diagnosis and at this stage an IMD may be considered. Galactosaemia needs to be excluded (in some parts of the UK screening for galactosaemia is routinely performed on the Guthrie card at birth).

Galactosaemia

The urine is tested for reducing substances using a Clinitest tablet and for glucose using a dip stick. Galactosaemia is unlikely if the urine is negative for reducing substances and negative for glucose. There can be a false negative result if the infant has not been fed lactose recently. Confirmation is via the measurement of blood galactose-1-phosphate uridyl transferase level (see p. 402). If there is any doubt while awaiting confirmation, a lactose free formula should be started and breast feeding discontinued (mothers should be encouraged to express their breast milk). MCT Pepdite and Pregestimil are suitable formulas as they also contain MCT fat.

Biliary atresia

Biliary atresia (BA) is a progressive disease which is defined as the complete inability to excrete bile because of obstruction, destruction or absence of the extrahepatic bile ducts. This leads to bile stasis in the liver with progressive inflammation and subsequent fibrosis. Bile drainage can be restored by the Kasai operation which bypasses the blocked ducts. It should be performed as soon as possible after birth. Late Kasai operations (i.e. after 8 weeks of age) are associated with a poor prognosis [47].

Prior to giving feeds with a high MCT content post-Kasai, the majority of children did not thrive [26]. It is now routine practice to advise a feed high in MCT, preferably up to 1 year of age. However, a recent audit [48] found poor growth in infants on a standard MCT formula and concluded that a greater macronutrient dense MCT feed is needed. Rarely, infants do well on breast feeding alone but a walnut oil supplement is recommended to ensure adequate EFAs (see p. 147). Additional vitamins orally and IM are prescribed. As BA is a progressive condition, despite having the Kasai procedure a large proportion of children will require liver transplantation at some point in the future. Hence, nutritional monitoring is essential and further intervention may well be necessary.

α₁-Antitrypsin deficiency

The genetic deficiency of the glycoprotein α_1-antitrypsin can cause various degrees of liver disease in infancy and can present with cholestasis. The exact physiological role of α_1-antitrypsin is not known. The liver disease is thought to be secondary to the uninhibited action of proteases which are critical in the inflammatory response (although the explanation is unlikely to be as simple as this). The severity of this condition, degree of liver involvement and nutritional management vary significantly. Some children require no nutritional intervention and are clinically well whereas others will need intense nutritional support and may come to transplantation before the age of 1 year. Initially, fat malabsorption is the main problem but as damage

progresses other symptoms of decompensated liver disease will require other dietary therapy.

Alagille's syndrome

This syndrome is diagnosed on a collection of features including intrahepatic biliary hypoplasia (paucity of the intrahepatic bile ducts) and cardiovascular, skeletal, facial and ocular abnormalities. It is a rare condition. Chronic cholestasis predominates clinically [49], although some have cyanotic heart disease as their main problem. Conjugated hyperbilirubinaemia presents followed by pruritus and finally, if severely affected, xanthelasma which usually appears by 2 years of age. This is possibly the most challenging condition in terms of nutritional management. Frequent problems include:

- Poor growth and failure to thrive
- Appalling appetite
- Pancreatic insufficiency and malabsorption
- Vomiting
- Severe itching thought to be exacerbated by improved nutrition

In those severely affected children who suffer with xanthelasma there is no evidence at present that restricting dietary cholesterol and saturated fats helps reduce their cholesterol levels. The majority that are severely affected are NG fed and warrant all possible nutritional intervention. Indeed, malnutrition and severe itching may be the main considerations for the need for transplantation, providing that the associated heart disease is not a compounding factor.

Choledochal cysts

Choledochal cysts are dilatations of all or part of the extrahepatic biliary tract. They may occur in infants (and can be detected *in utero*) and children. They may remain undiagnosed for years. Ursodeoxycholic acid is a drug used in this situation to improve bile flow and may enable a small cyst to disappear requiring no further treatment. However, cysts often require surgical removal. Indeed, some are so large and invasive that the extrahepatic bile ducts have to be removed and a Kasai procedure is performed (see above). Dietetic intervention is indicated when bile flow is affected and fat malabsorption occurs. Post-surgery, any required catch-up growth should occur quickly negating further nutritional intervention.

Haemangioma

These are benign vascular tumours of the liver and there are two types: they may undergo spontaneous regression by thrombosis and scarring, or they may grow rapidly. If large the tumours are supplied by wide blood vessels taking a large proportion of the cardiac output. Initially, spontaneous regression will be awaited. However, if cardiac failure develops in a young infant, hepatic artery ligation is essential to cut off the blood supply to the tumour. Nutritional intervention is often not needed at all.

In rare cases the child may require liver transplantation if for some reason ligation cannot be performed. These cases are dramatic, presenting with a huge liver, worsening cardiac function and a very small capacity for feeds. Continuous NG feeds will almost certainly be needed with restricted volume and sodium. A modular type feed or Generaid Plus may be the most useful formula (Table 9.5).

Cystic fibrosis

Cystic fibrosis can present in the newborn as conjugated hyperbilirubinaemia.

Neonatal hepatitis

The cause of the hepatitis is unknown. The severity varies and rarely results in cirrhosis. Usually, bile flow resolves in time. In these cases fat malabsorption is treated with dietary intervention until bile flow and adequate growth resume.

Inspissated bile syndrome

This is conjugated jaundice caused by a plug of thick bile blocking the bile duct and hence affecting bile flow. Resolution may occur naturally with time, or with the help of ursodeoxycholic acid (enhancing bile flow), or under percutaneous transhepatic cholangiography (PTC), or in rare cases it requires surgical excision. Nutritional intervention with an MCT containing formula may be necessary until this time. The syndrome often occurs in infants who have been nil by mouth (e.g. after surgery and long courses of TPN).

TPN induced cholestasis

The exact pathogenesis is unknown. The aetiology is multifactorial [50] and while components of the TPN can act as a direct insult to the liver, equally the damage to the immature liver can be caused by infections from lines and sepsis from gut bacterial translocation. There are several suggested measures [51–53] that appear to minimise effects on liver function. These include:

- Starting minimal enteral feeds if possible, preferably with some bolus feeds to stimulate bile flow
- Starting ursodeoxycholic acid to improve bile flow
- Minimising sepsis through line care
- Rotational antibiotics to prevent gut bacterial overgrowth
- Reducing the number of hours or days on TPN where possible

Minimising lipids is possibly helpful but only when adequate alternative energy can be provided.

TPN induced cholestasis is often associated with infants with short guts. The difficulty is providing adequate nutrition while the gut is given time to grow without necessitating a liver transplant from irreversible damage from TPN. Desperate measures have included gut lengthening surgery to decrease gut adaptation time [54], use of novel substrates (glutamine, growth hormone, fish oils, probiotics, e.g. Yakult), as well as continuous enteral feeding of adequate volumes to promote gut adaptation (see p. 137).

Isolated liver transplant has a role in selected children with intestinal failure, particularly those with a short but normally functioning gut who have progressive satisfactory intestinal adaptation, but developing liver disease. Those children with TPN related liver disease and unadapted gut or irreversible intestinal disease need combined liver and small bowel transplantation [55].

Progressive familial intrahepatic cholestasis

PFIC is a group of liver diseases involving membrane transport proteins involved in formation of bile. There are three types: PFIC 1, familial intrahepatic cholestasis (Byler's disease); PFIC 2, bile salt export pump (BSEP) deficiency; PFIC 3, multidrug resistance 3 (MDR3) disease. Children with MDR3 may have normal bilirubin levels but, because of low concentrations of phospholipids in bile, require MCT based formula.

PFIC 1 and BSEP have similar symptoms. Unlike other causes of cholestasis, the gamma-glutamyl transpeptidase is low. Average age of onset is 3 months (but in some not until later childhood). It can progress quickly to cirrhosis in the first year of life. Few survive beyond 20 years without treatment. Pruritus is a major symptom, out of proportion to the level of jaundice. Biliary diversion and liver transplantation are treatment options.

Growth is a major problem and most children are short in stature and thin. Malabsorption is considerable and poses a challenge to the dietitian. Apart from requiring MCT fat, a hydrolysed protein or amino acid based feed is often best tolerated (e.g. MCT Pepdite). NG feeds are commonly used; however, because of considerable scratching as a result of pruritus and general irritability, the tube often becomes dislodged. Gastrostomies have been considered more frequently in this group.

In PFIC 1 the success of liver transplantation is questionable, particularly as the severity of the condition is so diverse. Growth may not be improved and diarrhoea remains a problem as the defective gene, which is responsible for bile acid re-absorption, is also expressd in the intestine. Colestyramine has been used to treat the diarrhoea with some success, by binding the bile acids. However, fat and vitamin malabsorption is an associated side effect. Dietary therapy using hydrolysed protein feeds with a high MCT content continues post-transplant. Research is needed in this disease.

Common presentations of liver disease in older children

Auto-immune hepatitis

This rarely necessitates dietetic intervention, unless associated with inflammatory bowel disease (IBD). If dietetic input is required management of the presenting symptoms will be needed, which may range from failure to thrive and malabsorption, to obesity aggravated by steroid therapy.

Wilson's disease

This is an IMD resulting in defective copper metabolism. It leads to an accumulation of copper in the liver, brain, kidney and cornea. Accumulation can take years and hence presentation is delayed. Oral chelating agents (e.g. penicillamine) bind dietary copper and have negated the need for a strict low copper diet although avoiding foods with a high copper content is sensible: offal, particularly liver, and animals/fish eaten whole which thus contain the liver (e.g. shellfish). Other foods with a high copper content include cocoa and mushrooms but these are unlikely to be eaten in the quantity required to warrant a restriction. In advanced disease, or acute onset, liver transplant may be the only option because of the poisonous nature of copper.

Cystic fibrosis related liver disease

Significant portal hypertension and associated malnutrition are characteristics of the liver disease related to CF. Jaundice is rarely seen. Liver function tests are not reliable markers for disease severity. Assessment and treatment needs to take into account:

- Usual weight for height percentages used in the nutritional assessment of CF are not useful as a result of ascites and organomegaly (see p. 143). Anthropometry of the upper arm is more reliable.
- An increase in malabsorption with progressive liver disease in CF is most likely to be as a result of portal hypertension enteropathy. Increases in pancreatic enzyme replacement therapy above 10 000 units lipase/kg are thus unlikely to be helpful.
- Large volumes of feeds are not tolerated well because of organomegaly and ascites.
- Restrictions in sodium may not be needed as requirements are greater in CF.

An amino acid based feed containing MCT fat (e.g. Emsogen) may be beneficial and does not require an increase in the dose of enzyme supplements. The feed may be concentrated into small volumes and fed overnight. Hyperosmolar feeds tend to be well tolerated in CF. Data suggests that aggressive nutritional support providing 50% estimated average requirement (EAR) for energy for age [10], via overnight NG feeding, improves nutritional status prior to transplantation, using mid upper arm anthropometry as a measure [56].

Liver tumours

These tumours rapidly infiltrate the liver whether benign or malignant. Medical management includes the use of steroids and chemotherapy to reduce the tumour size. Resection may then be possible allowing the liver to regenerate, otherwise transplant may be the only option. Nutritional support and monitoring will be required throughout the course of treatment.

Bone marrow transplantation – immunodeficiency disorders

Immunodeficiency causing liver destruction has led to a need for bone marrow transplantation followed by liver transplantation in some cases. The main nutritional complications have included severe vomiting and diarrhoea, requiring nutritional support in the form of enteral and parenteral nutrition throughout the critical course of treatment.

Non-alcoholic steatohepatitis

This condition is an inflammation of the liver associated with the accumulation of fat in the liver. The inflammation causes damage, cirrhosis and eventually end-stage liver failure. There are no known causes but it is associated with obesity, diabetes mellitus and hyperlipidaemia [57]. It is becoming more common in children as a result of the increasing incidence of obesity in childhood and most frequently presents between the ages of 9 and 16 years. Most children with NASH are overweight.

There is no specific treatment, but improvement is seen on dietary change and weight loss, diabetic control and lowering of lipid levels. It must be stressed to children and their carers how important dietary compliance is as the consequence of cirrhosis at such a young age is life threatening.

The pancreas

Congenital anomalies

The incidence of congenital anomalies is uncertain. Children are often asymptomatic and anomalies are found incidentally. They include annular ectopic pancreas, pancreatic agenesis, hypoplasia and dysplasia, and ductal abnormalities. Some anomalies are complicated (e.g. the common channel syndrome) whereby the common bile duct and pancreatic duct are seen together for a longer segment than usual, and is implicated in the pathogenesis of choledochal cysts and development of pancreatitis [58]. In childhood this can present with jaundice, cholangitis and pancreatitis and may well require surgery. Abnormalities can be so severe that they result in pancreatic insufficiency and require enzyme replacement therapy.

Hereditary disorders

These include:

- CF (see Chapter 11)
- Schwachman's syndrome
- Johanson–Blizzard syndrome
- Exocrine pancreatic insufficiency with refractory sideroblastic anaemia
- Isolated enzyme deficiencies

Many inherited disorders result in pancreatic insufficiency and fat malabsorption necessitating enzyme replacement therapy. Required dosage is usually the greatest in CF.

Acquired disorders

Malnutrition has been associated with decreased pancreatic enzyme production [59] although enzyme activity usually returns with adequate nutrition [60]. Surgical resection of the pancreas (e.g. in the treatment of nesidioblastosis, which is a cause of hyperinsulinaemia and hypoglycaemia in infancy) may result in insufficient pancreatic function. Tumours are rare in children, but if found may also require surgical resection. Enteropathies (e.g. coeliac disease) are associated with pancreatic insufficiency [61]. Enzyme replacement therapy will be required.

Acute pancreatitis

Injury to the liver and pancreas is the most common cause of acute pancreatitis. Abdominal trauma may be as a result of child abuse, handlebars on bicycles and seatbelts in road traffic accidents, or sporting injuries from ball games, contact sports or even horse riding. Infections, gallstones and vasculitis are also possible causes. Hereditary forms of recurrent acute pancreatitis are recognised. Acute pancreatitis of childhood, although considered sometimes as a minor disorder, carries significant morbidity and mortality [62].

Goals of nutritional support

- Cover increased metabolic demands:
  catabolism and increased proteolysis of skeletal muscle
  gluconeogenesis increases glucose clearance and reduces oxidation. Insulin may be required
  lipid clearance from the blood can be reduced
- Prevent stimulation of pancreatic secretion
- Prevent further complications such as infection

Hence, nutritional requirements can be markedly increased and malnutrition rapidly occurs.

Diagnosis and severity

A UK working party on acute pancreatitis has concluded the diagnosis can be made by measuring serum amylase levels, which is widely available and provides accuracy of diagnosis [63]. Lipase estimation, if available, is preferred in acute pancreatitis. When there is doubt in the diagnosis, imaging via contrast enhanced computerised tomography (CT) is the most useful. Severity is defined as mild, moderate or severe.

Nutritional management

Management has traditionally been based on the concept of resting the pancreas. The fasting state results in a decrease in pancreatic enzymes, while gastric secretions are removed via an NG tube. However, the need for gut rest needs revising as it is now thought that stimulation of pancreatic enzymes occurs in the fasting state and with PN. The necessity for gut rest also depends on the severity of the pancreatitis. If symptoms include vomiting and paralytic ileus, little argument can be made against gastric decompression. The nutritional management of acute pancreatitis is controversial and there are very few published data for nutritional management in childhood. There is also a

lack of controlled clinical trials in adults. While Pitchumori et al. [64] recommend the prompt use of enteral nutrition, Dejong et al. [65] conclude that early TPN is advantageous with enteral nutrition introduced as soon as tolerated.

The controversies include:

- The use of the enteral or parenteral route. Traditionally, PN has been given.
- The route via which enteral feeds should be given. Feeding via the jejunum rather than the gastric or duodenal routes reduces the secretory response.
- The substrates used. Elemental feeds are thought to reduce pancreatic stimulation though polymeric and peptide based feeds, and low fat diets have also been used.

To date the European Society for Parenteral and Enteral Nutrition (ESPEN) guidelines on nutrition in acute pancreatitis (in adults) are [66] as follows:

Mild–moderate acute pancreatitis
- No evidence that either enteral or parenteral nutrition has a beneficial effect on clinical outcome in patients with mild–moderate disease.
- Caution is required with pre-existing malnutrition.
- Nutritional therapy has to be considered earlier if re-feeding is delayed.
- Diet rich in carbohydrates and moderate protein and fat should be initiated, prior to normal diet.

Severe acute pancreatitis
- Nutritional support is essential in patients with severe pancreatitis.
- The route of nutritional delivery (parenteral/ enteral) should be determined by tolerance. Many will require a combination.
- Start early with an elemental diet given via a jejunal feeding tube. When the energy goal cannot be reached, give additional PN.
- When enteral feeding is not possible (e.g. paralytic ileus) combine PN with a small amount of elemental or immuno-enhancing diet continuously perfused into the jejunum.
- While IV lipids have been associated with pancreatitis [67], their use as part of PN is safe when hypertriglyceridaemia is avoided.

Published randomised trials in adults [68,69] and

a recent meta-analysis [70] have also concluded that enteral feeding is beneficial compared with PN in acute pancreatitis. However, a systematic review [71] summarises that although there is a trend towards reductions in the adverse outcomes of acute pancreatitis after administration of enteral nutrition, there are insufficient data to draw firm conclusions about the effectiveness and safety of enteral nutrition versus PN. Further trials are required with sufficient size to account for clinical heterogeneity and to measure all relevant outcomes. There are no patient controlled randomised trials that have evaluated potential benefits of nutritional therapy for acute pancreatitis in children.

Additional problems in management in children are:

- Malnutrition occurs more quickly and adversely affects growth. An assessment of nutritional status and growth history is essential for designing treatment in all severities of pancreatic disease.
- Treatment options may vary widely depending on the age of the child.
- While double lumen tubes are useful for combined feeding via the jejunum and gastric decompression, to date there are no such tubes designed for children.

Experience in the author's centre (King's College Hospital) is limited. While encouraged to initiate nasojejunal feeding in the first instance, Hart et al. [72] report on our lack of success in children with acute pancreatitis. The majority of cases have required TPN. From a review of our prescriptions we conclude that energy requirements in this group are on average above the EAR [10]. Recommendations are 110% EAR for the initiation of non-nitrogen energy provision, and 120% EAR when there is severe sepsis [73].

Chronic pancreatitis

This condition is characterised by the recurrence of abdominal pain with development of pancreatic insufficiency and/or diabetes mellitus. This may be the result of inherited pancreatic conditions, or anomalies within the pancreas or associated with metabolic disease (α_1-antitrypsin deficiency, Wilson's disease).

Malnutrition and growth failure may result from food avoidance, abdominal pain, nausea, vomiting and increased losses of fat. A high energy diet, with adequate fat intake, is required to achieve normal growth. Enteric coated pancreatic enzymes should be used and the dose tailored to the individual child. Additional fat-soluble vitamins may be necessary. When diabetes mellitus is a feature, control of associated symptoms is not easily achieved on diet therapy alone. This is particularly hard to achieve when trying to improve energy intake. Treatment with insulin may be necessary but the amounts needed are often low.

References

1 Klein S et al. Nutritional support in clinical practice. Review of published data and recommendations for future research directions. J Parenter Enteral Nutr, 1997, **21** 133–54.

2 Chin SE et al. The nature of malnutrition in the children with end stage liver disease awaiting orthotopic liver transplantation. Am J Clin Nutr, 1992, **56** 164.

3 Goulet OJ et al. Preoperative nutritional evaluation and support for liver transplant in children. Transplant Proc, 1987, **4** 3249.

4 Sokol RJ, Stall C Anthropometric evaluation of children with chronic liver disease. Am J Clin Nutr, 1990, **52** 203.

5 Novy MA, Schwarz KB Nutritional considerations and management of the child with liver disease. Nutrition, 1997, **13** 177–84.

6 Hehir DJ et al. Nutrition in patients undergoing orthotopic liver transplant. J Parenter Enteral Nutr, 1985, **9** 695–700.

7 Frisancho AR Triceps skinfold and upper arm muscle size norms for assessment of nutritional status. Am J Clin Nutr, 1974, **27** 1052.

8 Frisancho AR New norms of upper limb fat and muscle areas for assessment of nutritional status. Am J Clin Nutr, 1981, **34** 2540–5.

9 Paul AA et al. The need for revised standards for skinfold thickness in infancy. Arch Dis Child, 1998, **78** 354–8.

10 Department of Health Report on Health and Social Subjects No. 41, Dietary Reference Values for Food Energy and Nutrients for the United Kingdom. London: The Stationery Office, 1991.

11 Mowat AP Liver Disorders in Childhood, 3rd edn. London: Butterworths, 1994.

12 Walker JP, Bumgardner GL Hepatocyte immunology and transplantation: current status and future potential. Curr Opin Organ Transplant, 2005, **10** 67–76.

13 Tissieres PMD *et al.* Liver support for fulminant hepatic failure: Is it time to use the molecular adsorbents recycling system in children? *Pediatr Crit Care Med*, 2005, **6** 585–91.

14 Thompson R Pediatric liver disease. *Curr Opin Gastroenterol*, 1999, **15** 249–52.

15 Cabre E, Gassull MA Nutrition in liver disease. *Curr Opin Clin Nutr Metab Care*, 2005, **8** 545–51.

16 Clayton P Diagnosis of inherited metabolic disease. *J Inherit Metab Dis*, 2003, **26** 135–46.

17 World Health Organization *Energy and protein requirements*. Report of a Joint FAO/WHO/UNU Meeting. Geneva. WHO Technical Report Series, 1985, p. 724.

18 Weisdorf SA *et al.* Amino acid abnormalities in infants with extrahepatic biliary atresia and cirrhosis. *J Pediatr Gastroenterol Nutr*, 1987, **6** 860.

19 Morgan MY, Milsom JP, Sherlock S Plasma ratio valine, leucine, and isoleucine to phenylalanine and tyrosine in liver disease. *Gut*, 1978, **19** 1068.

20 Als-Nielson B *et al.* Branched chain amino acids for hepatic encephalopathy. *Cochrane Database Syst Rev*, 2003, **1**.

21 Keohane PP *et al.* Enteral nutrition in malnourished patients with hepatic cirrhosis and acute encephalopathy. *J Parenter Enteral Nutr*, 1987, **7** 346–50.

22 Walker WA, Drurie PR, Hamilton JR, Walker-Smith JA, Watkins JB *Pediatric Gastrointestinal Disease – Pathophysiology, Diagnosis, Management*, 1st edn, vol. 2, Philadelphia/Toronto: BC Decker Inc, 1991.

23 Glasgow JFT *et al.* Fat absorption in congenital obstructive liver disease. *Arch Dis Child*, 1973, **48** 601.

24 Gourley GR *et al.* Essential fatty acid deficiency after hepatic portoenterostomy for biliary atresia. *Am J Clin Nutr*, 1982, **36** 1194.

25 Andrews WS *et al.* Fat soluble vitamin deficiency in biliary atresia. *J Pediatr Surg*, 1981, **16** 284.

26 Cohen MI, Gartner LM The use of medium chain triglycerides in the management of biliary atresia. *J Pediatr*, 1971, **79** 379–84.

27 Francavilla R *et al.* Hepatitis and cholestasis in infancy: clinical and nutritional aspects. *Acta Paediatr Suppl*, 2003, **92** 101–4.

28 Yamashiro Y *et al.* Docosahexaenoic acid status of patients with extrahepatic biliary atresia. *J Pediatr Surg*, 1994, **29** 1455.

29 Aggett PJ *et al.* ESPGAN Committee Report on Nutrition; Comment on the content and composition of lipids in infant formulas. *Acta Paediatr Scand*, 1991, **80** 887–96.

30 Kaufmann SS *et al.* Influence of Portagen and Pregestimil on essential fatty acid status in infantile liver disease. *Pediatrics*, 1992, **89** 151–4.

31 Pierro A *et al.* Resting energy expenditure is increased in infants and children with extrahepatic biliary atresia. *J Pediatr Surg*, 1989, **24** 534.

32 Dolz C *et al.* Ascites increases the resting energy expenditure in liver cirrhosis. *Gastroenterology*, 1991, **100** 738–44.

33 Greer R *et al.* Body composition and components of energy expenditure in children with end stage liver disease. *J Pediatr Gastroenterol Nutr*, 2003, **36** 358–63.

34 Schneeweiss B *et al.* Energy metabolism in patients with acute and chronic liver disease. *Hepatology*, 1990, **11** 387.

35 Chin SE *et al.* Nutritional support in children with end stage liver disease: a randomised crossover trial of a branched chain amino acid supplement. *Am J Clin Nutr*, 1992, **56** 1–6.

36 Taylor R *et al.* Intestinal absorption in children with portal hypertension. *Arch Dis Child*, 1999, **80** 21.

37 Taylor R *et al* Combined sugar absorption test in children with portal hypertension. *J Pediatr Gastroenterol Nutr*, 1999, **28** 585.

38 Holt R *et al.* Nasogastric feeding enhances nutritional status in paediatric liver disease but does not alter circulating levels of IGF-I and IGF binding proteins. *Clin Endocrinol*, 2000, **52** 217–24.

39 Chin SE *et al.* Pre-operative nutritional support in children with end-stage liver disease accepted for liver transplantation: an approach to management. *J Gastroenterol Hepatol*, 1990, **5** 566.

40 Duche M *et al.* Percutaneous endoscopic gastrostomy for continuous feeding in children with chronic cholestasis. *J Pediatr Gastroenterol Nutr*, 1999, **29** 42–5.

41 Socha PM *et al.* Essential fatty acid status in children with cholestasis, in relation to serum bilirubin concentration. *J Pediatr*, 1997, **131** 700–6.

42 Lapillonne A *et al.* Effects of liver transplantation on long-chain polyunsaturated fatty acid status in infants with biliary atresia. *J Pediatr Gastroenterol Nutr*, 2000, **30** 528–32.

43 Shepherd RW Pre- and post-operative nutritional care in liver transplantation in children. *J Gastroenterol Hepatol*, 1996, **11** S7–10.

44 Lochs H, Plauth M Liver cirrhosis: rationale and modalities for nutritional support. *Curr Opin Clin Nutr Metab Care*, 1999, **2** 345–49.

45 Fan ST *et al.* Metabolic clearance of fat emulsion containing medium chain triglycerides in cirrhotic patients. *J Parenter Enteral Nutr*, 1992, **16** 279–83.

46 France S, Jundt R Feeding patterns in infants post liver transplant. *J Pediatr Gastroenterol Nutr*, 2004, **39** S94.

47 Mieli-Vergani G *et al.* Late referral for biliary atresia: missed opportunities for effective surgery. *Lancet*, 1989, **1** 421–3.

48 Stevenson R Nutritional intervention and growth in infants with biliary atresia in the first year. Proceedings of BSPGHAN Annual Conference of Associate Members and Trainees – abstracts (presented), London, October 2005.

49   Alagille D Management of paucity of interlobular bile ducts. *J Hepatol*, 1985, **1** 561.

50   Heine RG, Bines JE New approaches to parenteral nutrition in infants and children. *J Paediatr Child Health*, 2002, **38** 433–7.

51   Meadows N Monitoring and complications of parenteral nutrition. *Nutrition*, 1998, **14** 806–8.

52   Narkewicz M *et al.* Effect of ursodeoxycholic acid therapy on hepatic function in children with intrahepatic cholestatic liver disease. *J Pediatr Gastroenterol Nutr*, 1998, **26** 49–55.

53   Kaufman SS Prevention of parenteral nutrition-associated liver disease in children. *Pediatr Transplant*, 2002, **6** 37–42.

54   Goulet O *et al.* Irreversible intestinal failure. *J Pediatric Gastroenterol Nutr*, 2004, **38** 250–69.

55   Muiesan P *et al.* Isolated liver transplant and sequential small bowel transplantation for intestinal failure and related liver disease in children. *Transplantation*, 2000, **69** 2323–6.

56   Bartlett FM *et al.* Enteral feeding improves nutritional status in cystic fibrosis patients, with liver disease. *Neth J Med*, 1999, **54** S66.

57   Chitturi SM *et al.* Etiopathogenesis of nonalcoholic steatohepatitis. *Semin Liver Dis*, 2001, **21** 27–41.

58   Kato O, Hattori K, Suzuki T *et al.* Clinical significance of anomalous pancreaticobiliary union. *Gastrointest Endosc*, 1983, **29** 94–8.

59   Pitchumoni CS Pancreas in primary malnutrition disorders. *Am J Clin Nutr*, 1973, **26** 374–9.

60   Barbezat GO, Hansen JDL The exocrine pancreas and protein energy malnutrition. *Pediatrics*, 1968, **42** 77–92.

61   Bustos Fernanez L *et al.* Exocrine pancreas insufficiency secondary to gluten enteropathy. *Am J Gastroenterol*, 1970, **53** 564–9.

62   Benifla M, Weizman Z Acute pancreatitis in childhood: analysis of literature data. *J Clin Gastroenterol*, 2003, **37** 100–2.

63   Johnson CD *et al.* UK working party on acute pancreatitis. UK guidelines for the management of acute pancreatitis. *Gut*, 2005, **54** 1–9.

64   Pitchumoni CS *et al.* Factors influencing mortality in acute pancreatitis: can we alter them? *J Clin Gastroenterol*, 2005, **39** 798–814.

65   Dejong C *et al.* Nutrition in patients with acute pancreatitis. *Curr Opin Crit Care*, 2001, **7** 251–6.

66   Meier R *et al.* ESPEN guidelines on nutrition in acute pancreatitis. *Clin Nutr*, 2002, **21** 173–83.

67   Lashner BA, Kirsner JB, Hanauer SB Acute pancreatitis associated with high concentrated lipid emulsion during total parenteral nutrition therapy for Crohn's disease. *Gastroenterology*, 1986, **90** 1039.

68   Windsor AC *et al.* Compared with parenteral nutrition, enteral feeding attenuates the acute phase response and improves disease severity in acute pancreatitis. *Gut*, 1998, **42** 431–5.

69   Kalfarentzos F *et al.* Enteral nutrition is superior to parenteral nutrition in severe acute pancreatitis: results of a randomized prospective trial. *Br J Surg*, 1997, **84** 1665–9.

70   Marik P, Zaloga GP Meta-analysis of parenteral nutrition versus enteral nutrition in patients with acute pancreatitis. *Br Med J*, 2005, **328** 1407–12.

71   Al-Omran M *et al.* Enteral versus parenteral nutrition for acute pancreatitis. *Cochrane Database Syst Rev*, 2003, **1**.

72   Hart CM *et al.* Experience of nasojejunal feeding in a cohort of children with acute pancreatitis. *J Pediatr Gastroenterol Nutr*, 2004, **39** S165.

73   France S, Jundt R Energy requirements in acute pancreatitis in children. *J Pediatr Gastroenterol Nutr*, 2004, **39** S90.

Useful address

Children's Liver Disease Foundation
AXA Equity & Law House, 35–37 Great Charles Street, Queensway, Birmingham, B3 3JY.
Tel: 0121 212 3839
www.childliverdisease.org
e-mail: info@childliverdisease.org

10 Diabetes Mellitus

Alison Johnston

Introduction

There is a marked geographical variation in the incidence of type 1 diabetes mellitus (onset 0–14 years) throughout Europe ranging from <10 cases to >30 per 100 000. The incidence of type 1 diabetes in children is increasing at the rate of 2% per annum and in Scotland stands at 26 per 100 000 population per year in the under 15-year-old age group [1]. The prevalence of childhood onset type 1 diabetes has increased in most western countries [2]. It is primarily a hormone deficiency disease, caused by auto-immune destruction of the pancreatic islet β cells. Ideally, children with diabetes should attend a specialist children's diabetes clinic and be cared for by a paediatric multidisciplinary diabetes team [3–5]. This team should include a paediatrician, a diabetes nurse specialist and a paediatric dietitian, and should have access to psychological services and social workers in addition to services offered in primary care. The team should work collaboratively to educate and support the child and their families, while empowering them to manage diabetes on a day-to-day basis.

The parents of a child who is diagnosed as having a chronic disease (including a newly diagnosed diabetic child) are initially shocked and devastated. Parents can also feel a sense of guilt: they may feel that their child has developed diabetes because they have permitted him or her to eat sweets excessively. Because diabetes is partly genetic, parents feel guilty about passing on 'bad genes', a feeling enhanced if there is a family history.

The dietitian's role is to balance the necessity of strict glycaemic control within the family diet and to convert the scientific theory about food into practical and sensible advice. An effective, family based dietary education programme which will result in the modification of a child's eating habits can only begin when parents are allowed to grieve and come to terms with the diagnosis of diabetes in their child. It is vital to develop a rapport with the family so that a high quality of consistent dietetic care can be provided. Frequent and short teaching sessions are preferable, with the entire family if appropriate. Conducting the teaching sessions in the family's own home has many advantages: less disruption, familiar surroundings and the child's usual food and exercise pattern is maintained. First hand knowledge of the domestic set up enables teaching to become more learner centred. The disadvantages are that these sessions are costly in terms of travelling time and resources.

The eating plan for a child with diabetes

Aims of the eating plan

1 To meet the child's nutritional requirements. Children with diabetes have the same basic nutritional needs as their non-diabetic

counterparts. It can be emphasised that the eating plan recommended is 'healthy eating' for the entire family.

2   To contribute towards optimising blood sugar levels and hence ideal HbA1c (glycosylated haemoglobin) results of <7.5%, avoiding swings between hyper- and hypoglycaemia. Children should be offered the most appropriate insulin preparation for the individual. The dietary advice should relate to the chosen insulin regimen. The amounts and timing of carbohydrate containing foods eaten are significant and should balance the effects of the injected insulin. A preprandial blood glucose of 4–6 mmol/L is ideal; however, a target of obtaining 80% of the blood sugars in the range 4–10 mmol/L is probably more realistic. It is imperative to aim to maintain blood glucose concentrations close to the normal range to decrease the frequency and severity of long term microvascular and cardiovascular complications [6]. Recurrent episodes of hypoglycaemia are undesirable, particularly in young children where the developing brain may be particularly susceptible.

3   To promote normal growth and development. Dietary energy should be sufficient for growth and allow for variable exercise patterns, but should not provoke obesity. Growth should be plotted at regular intervals using standard height and weight charts. Growth velocity charts and body mass index are useful for anticipating the onset of obesity or stunting. Growth can be a useful indicator of diabetic control, as poor physical development may be a consequence of inadequate diabetic management. Obesity is less of a problem in diabetic children than in diabetic adults, but if children do gain weight disproportionately to their height, suitable dietetic advice should be given at a very early stage. Particular care should be taken to monitor the weight of adolescent girls, as this group is most prone to obesity [7] because they reach adult stature before their peers and generally take less exercise than boys.

4   The diet should minimise the development of diabetic complications such as cardiovascular and microvascular disease. If insufficient carbohydrate is allowed then children will tend to compensate by eating more protein and fat containing foods, which is undesirable.

5   To inculcate good dietary habits for optimum health.

Recommendations

There are published recommendations for people with diabetes: the British Diabetic Association's 1980 document [8], updated in 1992, *Dietary Recommendations for People with Diabetes: An Update for the 1990s* [9]; *Dietary Recommendations for Children and Adolescents with Diabetes* published in 1989 by the British Diabetic Association [10]; *The Implementation of Nutritional Advice for People with Diabetes* published in 2003 [11]. The latter outlines the most recent consensus based recommendations for people with diabetes and there are significant changes from the earlier guidelines: greater flexibility in the proportions of energy derived from carbohydrate and monosaturated fat, relaxation in the amount of sucrose permitted and promotion of foods with a low glycaemic index.

Dietary carbohydrate should never be restricted below the usual family intake and should ideally provide 45–60% of the total energy intake. The recommendations recognise that the energy distribution between carbohydrate, fat and protein will differ depending on age: breast fed infants will obtain approximately 55% energy from fat, 7% from protein and 40% from carbohydrate, whereas a 5-year-old may derive 35% energy from fat, 15% from protein and 50% from carbohydrate. Traditional dietary regimens have emphasised only the carbohydrate component. Present day practice adopts a more holistic dietary approach.

An increase in carbohydrate, particularly from high fibre sources, and a reduction in saturated and polyunsaturated fat are recommended. In addition, the energy content of the diet should be tailored to the individual. This is of major importance in order to minimise the risk of chronic degenerative disease such as obesity and coronary heart disease.

Carbohydrate

The current recommendation for the child with diabetes is that carbohydrate provides more than 45% energy. The formula: 120 g carbohydrate plus 10 g for every year of life reflects current thinking and provides a baseline of daily carbohydrate that should provide at least 40% energy from carbohydrate. For example, this formula suggests that a 2-year-old boy should have $120\,g + 20\,g$ $(140\,g)$ carbohydrate daily. His estimated average energy requirement is 1190 kcal; hence a minimum of 47% energy will be derived from carbohydrate.

It should be noted, however, that the dietary reference values for food energy [12] were not designed for the individual but for groups. Allowance should be made for the child's body weight and activity. A 5-year-old boy growing along the second centile will weigh 15 kg, while a boy growing along the 98th centile will weigh 24 kg. Both are growing within normal limits, yet their weights vary by 9 kg. These two boys will require different energy and carbohydrate intakes.

The amount of carbohydrate eaten has a greater influence on glycaemia than the source or type [13], nevertheless, many factors affect the glycaemic response to food: the amount of carbohydrate eaten, the composition of the carbohydrate, the effects of cooking or processing, and other foods eaten along with the carbohydrate.

The type of carbohydrate is relevant and attempts have been made to quantify the glycaemic effect of different foods by means of the Glycaemic Index (GI). There are practical limitations to this system although it can be used as a guide to food choices by dividing the carbohydrate containing foods into low, medium and high GI groups.

Sugar

It is now accepted that up to 10% of daily energy may be provided from sucrose with the stipulation that it is eaten within the context of a healthy diet.

The use of sugar taken as part of a mixed meal does not have a detrimental effect on blood sugar control in well-controlled insulin dependent diabetics who are not obese [14,15]. It is also recognised that the rate of absorption of carbohydrates depends on a great many factors, and the idea that sucrose always causes a rapid rise in blood sugar is perhaps too simplistic. Rapidly absorbed carbohydrate such as a chocolate biscuit can be included in the dietary allowance at the end of a main meal, when the glycaemic response will be lower. The

inclusion of a controlled amount of 'sugary' foods has a number of benefits:

- It makes the child feel that his or her diet is not too different from that of peers
- It may increase dietary compliance
- It increases palatability and variety
- It discourages the use of diabetic products

Fibre (non-starch polysaccharide)

Dietary fibre is an integral part of any healthy diet. Diabetes UK makes no quantitive recommendation. Foods containing soluble fibre should be encouraged as they have beneficial effects on carbohydrate and lipid metabolism. Insoluble fibrous foods, although they have no such effects, are advantageous to gastrointestinal health and have a high satiety factor and may benefit those trying to lose weight. Gradual changes in fibre intake are necessary to minimise colic, flatulence and abdominal distension. High intakes can impair the absorption of calcium, iron and zinc because of the high level of phytate in high fibre foods, although it can be argued that these foods themselves, being less refined, have a higher vitamin and mineral content than lower fibre foods.

High fibre foods are less energy dense than those containing refined carbohydrate therefore the young child's total energy intake may be compromised if the diet contains large quantities of fibre. However, children can safely include a number of high fibre foods in their diet (e.g. wholemeal bread, high fibre breakfast cereals, baked beans and high fibre baked goods). A large proportion of children will eat at least two portions of fruit each day; many do not like vegetables, but will take them when included in soups and stews. Often raw vegetables will be taken in preference to those that are cooked. The five portions of fruit and vegetables per day that is recommended for all should be particularly endorsed.

Fat

Fat is necessary in children's diets to provide adequate energy, fat-soluble vitamins and essential fatty acids. Fish, especially oily fish, containing n-3 polyunsaturated fat should be eaten once or twice per week. If an older child's fat intake is higher than 35% energy, or rapid weight gain is a problem at any age, the following advice can be given to reduce dietary fat:

- Eat grilled and oven-baked foods in preference to fried foods
- Cut off visible fat on meat
- Take fish and poultry instead of red meat
- Cut down on the quantity of crisps eaten to 2–3 bags per week (often a compromise of a maximum of one bag per day has to be conceded); use reduced fat crisp varieties
- Take reduced fat cheeses or varieties that are lower in fat (cottage cheese is not popular with children, so it is more realistic to limit the amount of high fat cheese and encourage lower fat varieties such as Edam or half-fat hard cheese)
- Use semi-skimmed or skimmed milk. This advice should only be given to children with a high fat intake or a high weight gain. A supplement of vitamins A and D should be considered for children under the age of 5 years who are taking skimmed milk

Identifying any family history of coronary heart disease is important. Patients with diabetes are prone to dyslipidaemia so attention to dietary fat intake is as important as good metabolic control.

Protein

Children with diabetes should have protein intakes no higher than those taken by other children. In the diets of most children protein provides 15% of dietary energy, although actual requirements are considerably lower than this [12].

Low sugar and diabetic products

Low calorie drinks are extremely valuable in the diet of a child with diabetes. Other low sugar products marketed for the general population can also be useful, for instance reduced sugar jams, fruit canned in natural juice, low sugar desserts. Diabetic products, however, have no place in the diet for the child with diabetes. They are expensive, can be unpalatable and in addition may contain

sorbitol. The child should be encouraged to regard the diet as one of 'sensible eating' and not one that relies on the need to eat different or 'special' foods.

Sweeteners

Nutritive sweeteners have no proven advantage over sucrose. Fructose has no taste benefit and gives less satisfactory results in baking. Although it does not require insulin for its metabolism it has a glucose sparing effect in the body and causes a rise in blood sugar if large quantities are taken. Sorbitol and other sugar alcohols have a similar energy value to carbohydrate. They are poorly absorbed and can cause osmotic diarrhoea, particularly in children, who have a lower body mass than that of the adult, for whom the products are designed.

Non-nutritive sweeteners can be useful in drinks and desserts and to sprinkle on breakfast cereals. However, many people find that saccharin has a bitter aftertaste. Aspartame (Canderel brand sweetener), which many find more palatable, has a limited use because sweetening power is lost when it is subjected to prolonged heating. Sucralose (SPLENDA brand sweetener) has been shown to have no effect on blood glucose control or insulin levels and retains sweetness under the high heat of cooking and baking, does not lose its sweetness with low pH foods and remains sweet even with prolonged storage.

Recommending an eating plan

A dietary assessment is essential on diagnosis, so that the child's normal intake and meal pattern can be ascertained. The carbohydrate or energy allowance and distribution can then be tailored to the home situation and most appropriate insulin regimen. Providing the child is not overweight, the usual energy intake prior to the onset of diabetic symptoms can be used as a basis for deciding the diet. Carbohydrate should provide 45–60% of energy, and fat should be kept as low as practical, depending on the child's age.

Recommendations for dietary management must take into consideration the child's current insulin regimen to achieve the best possible glycaemic control without provoking disabling hypoglycaemia. Regimens include:

- Single isophane insulin injection daily (no longer commonly used)
- Twice daily injections (one before breakfast and one before evening meal) of mixed soluble and isophane insulin or analogue mixture insulin
- Split evening insulin (three injections per day): mixed soluble and isophane insulin or analogue mixture insulin before breakfast, soluble or rapid acting analogue before dinner and isophane before bed
- Basal bolus (four or more injections per day): soluble insulin or rapid acting analogue is given as a bolus before meals and snacks containing >20 g carbohydrate and isophane or long acting analogue insulin once or twice daily as basal insulin before breakfast and/or before dinner or bedtime
- Pump therapy, continuous subcutaneous insulin infusion (CSII)

Twice daily insulin

It is important for children to take carbohydrate at regular intervals so that hypoglycaemia may be avoided and hyperglycaemia prevented. Meals should be consumed 30 minutes after an insulin injection of mixed soluble and isophane insulin (unless low blood sugar dictates otherwise) in order to optimise postprandial blood sugar profiles. Meals should be eaten directly following analogue mixture insulin. Carbohydrate in excess of 50–60 g given at any one time may also produce an inappropriately raised postprandial blood sugar. A meal pattern of three meals and three snacks each day is appropriate for most children, although very young children and adolescents may need more snacks. Carbohydrate should be distributed throughout the day taking account of the peak periods of insulin action.

Split evening insulin

The above applies, except that giving a dose of analogue or soluble insulin before the evening meal allows more flexibility. If more or less carbohydrate than usual is desired the insulin dose can be adjusted accordingly. The timing of the evening meal may also be adjusted, the soluble insulin given 30 minutes prior to food and the analogue directly before food. The insulin dose can be reduced if an active evening is anticipated.

Basal bolus

This offers even greater flexibility with regard to mealtimes – there is no need to adhere to rigid meal and snack times as a bolus of insulin is injected prior to food. Many families prefer using rapid acting analogue insulin in conjunction with long acting analogue insulin. There is no requirement to wait 30 minutes between injecting and eating because of the fast onset of analogue action, and most children appreciate this. The additional advantage of insulin analogue is that, because of its short period of action, snacks between meals are not always necessary. This is useful for teenagers trying to lose weight (especially girls) and those who find eating snacks tedious.

Children who prefer to eat snacks (especially at bedtime) may prefer soluble insulin to cover the meal and snack rather than have an additional injection.

Carbohydrate counting is increasingly more common amongst those on a basal bolus regimen. The family learn about the relationship of carbohydrate and insulin doses and therefore calculate the carbohydrate : insulin ratio. For example, if 4 units of insulin are given before a 40 g carbohydrate lunch and the resulting blood glucose level is satisfactory the family can assume that the child needs 1 unit of insulin per 10 g of carbohydrate. However, they must be prepared to use trial and error and to interpret the blood glucose results.

Pump therapy

Carbohydrate counting is essential for children on pumps. The children are given around half of their required daily insulin as a total basal dose over the 24-hour period and the remainder is given as bolus doses before each meal and snack. The amount of insulin given as the bolus is dependent on the amount of carbohydrate consumed and the carbohydrate : insulin ratio.

Table 10.1 shows a typical day's diet with carbohydrate distributed according to insulin regimen, and peak action times are shown (Fig. 10.1).

Table 10.1   A 10-year-old girl is on a split evening regimen of premixed 30% soluble and 70% isophane insulin before breakfast, soluble insulin before dinner and isophane before bed and has a daily allowance of 220 g carbohydrate (see Fig. 10.1c).

7 am	Insulin injection		
7.30 am	Breakfast: 40 g CHO	2 Weetabix	20 g
		200 mL semi-skimmed milk	10 g
		1/2 large slice of wholemeal toast and polyunsaturated spread	10 g
10.30 am	Mid morning: 20 g CHO	Apple	10 g
		1 small box raisins	10 g
1 pm	Lunch: 50 g CHO	2 wholemeal rolls with chicken and salad	40 g
		1 carton of diet fruit yoghurt	10 g
		Low calorie drink	
3.30 pm	Mid afternoon: 30 g CHO	Wholemeal scone and reduced sugar jam	20 g
		1 small packet crisps	10 g
		Low calorie drink	
5 pm	Insulin injection		
5.30 pm	Dinner: 50 g CHO	Bowl of lentil soup	10 g
		Wholemeal pasta, bolognaise sauce, side salad	30 g
		1 scoop of ice cream	10 g
		Low calorie drink	
7.30 pm	Mid evening snack: 10 g CHO	1 banana	10 g
9 pm	Bedtime: 20 g CHO	1 large slice wholemeal toast with polyunsaturated spread	20 g
9.30 pm	Insulin injection		

CHO, carbohydrate.

Teaching approaches

It is important to give the family practical dietary advice that is age appropriate and children should be involved as soon as they are old enough. The information should be delivered at a rate that considers the social, intellectual and cultural background of the child. Verbal instructions should be reinforced with appropriate written information and other resources should be used where possible (e.g. DVD, website; see further reading, p.177).

Whether quantitative or qualitative methods should be adopted continues to be a controversial subject. Limited evidence is available concerning the optimal type of diet therapy [16] and there is a lack of evidence to recommend either a qualitative or quantitative approach as the most effective. Most dietitians (88%) who provide a service to children with diabetes use quantitative methods [17].

Quantitative method – carbohydrate counting

The child, parents and carers must have an understanding of the nutritional content of foods. At present the 10 g carbohydrate system (using handy measures) offers the best system for children, where a daily allowance of carbohydrate is given along with a suggested distribution at each meal and snack time for those on twice daily or split evening regimens. Children on basal bolus or pump therapy can use their knowledge of food and carbohydrate : insulin ratio to establish how much insulin to take for each meal and snack. See Table 10.2 for a brief list of 10 g carbohydrate portions.

Qualitative diet

Alternative methods of dietary advice which do not

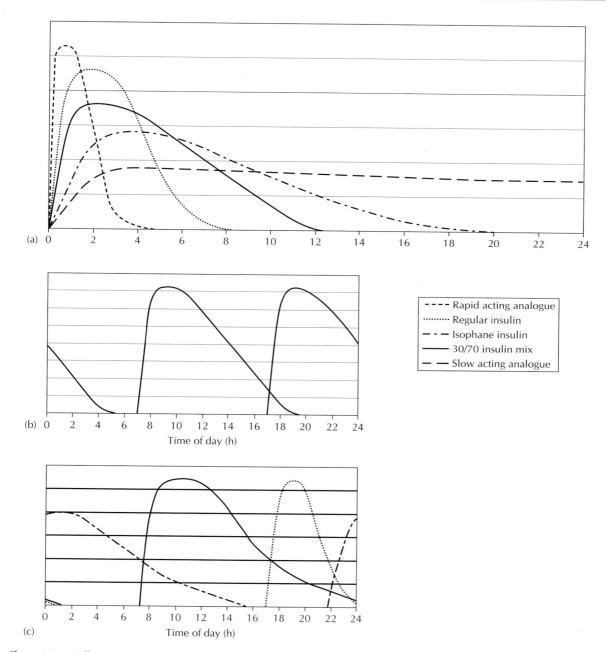

Figure 10.1   Differing insulin action profiles. (a) Insulin action profiles. (b) Twice daily mixed insulin. (c) Split evening insulin – regular. (d) Split evening insulin – analogue. (e) Basal/bolus insulin – isophane. (f) Basal-bolus insulin – long acting analogue. (g) Continuous subcutaneous insulin infusion. *Continued on p. 170.*

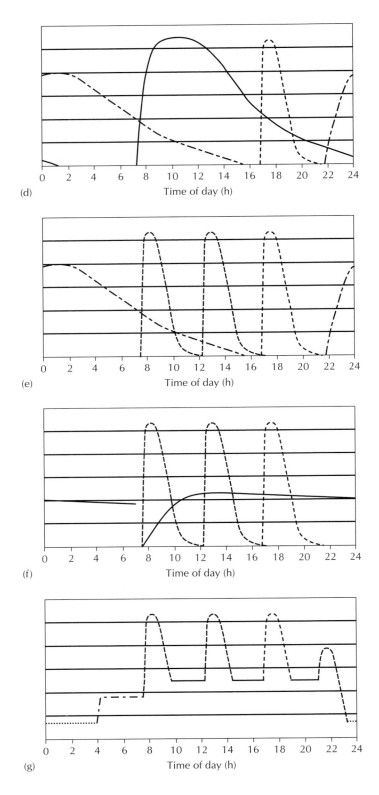

(d)

Time of day (h)

(e)

Time of day (h)

(f)

Time of day (h)

(g)

Time of day (h)

Figure 10.1 (Cont't).

Table 10.2 A brief list of 10 g carbohydrate exchanges.

Bread

Wholemeal or white	¹/₂ large slice/1 small slice
Rolls, baps	¹/₂ roll

Breakfast cereals

All Bran, Branflakes	5 tablespoons
Cornflakes	5 tablespoons
Weetabix	1 biscuit
Porridge	7 tablespoons

Rice and pasta

Brown or white rice cooked	3 tablespoons
Spaghetti	10 long strands
Pasta (e.g. macaroni)	3 tablespoons
Spaghetti – tinned	¹/₃ small tin

Biscuits

Oatcakes	1 large
Crackers	2
Crispbread (wholewheat rye)	2
Digestive	1

Potatoes

Boiled	1 small
Baked	1 medium
Chips	5 average sized
Crisps	1 small packet

Beans

Baked in tomato sauce	5 tablespoons
Dried uncooked	2 tablespoons

Fruit

Apple	1
Banana	1
Grapes	10
Orange	1
Pear	1

Milk

Semi-skimmed, whole, skimmed	1 glass (200 mL)
Natural/diet fruit yoghurt	1 carton
Fruit sweetened yoghurt	¹/₂ carton

Others

Soup	1 ladle (180 mL)
Ice cream	1 scoop (30 g)

NB All tablespoon measures are level.

involve measuring or estimating the carbohydrate value of individual foods include the 'plate model', where a meal or snack of approximately equal carbohydrate content is given at regular intervals; the meal as a whole is assessed by eye and no attempt is made to quantify individual foods. The exact amount of carbohydrate is less important than the type, and the diet is high in fibre which slows the absorption of carbohydrate from the gut. This method is widely used in the treatment of adult diabetes but there is controversy over its use in childhood, particularly for very young children who may be erratic eaters and who may not accept or tolerate a high fibre diet [18]. A compromise may be to teach a measured diet initially on diagnosis, as many parents feel more secure using the 10 g exchange system, then to move onto an unmeasured diet when appropriate.

Dose Adjustment for Normal Eating (DAFNE)

The DAFNE Project [19] teaches adults to make insulin adjustments to match the carbohydrate in a free diet on a meal-by-meal basis. Encouraging results have lead to the project being extended to children and young people.

Hypoglycaemia

Causes of hypoglycaemia include:

- Exercise, without additional food or reduction in insulin dose
- Insufficient carbohydrate eaten, or being late for or missing a meal or snack
- Too much insulin or dose given at the wrong time
- Food not absorbed (e.g. vomiting and diarrhoea)
- Alcohol

Symptoms are similar to those seen in the adult and mild hypoglycaemia symptoms include pallor, mood swings, irritability, headache, hunger and fatigue. Children often find it difficult to describe their own symptoms, but might experience shaky or wobbly legs or a 'funny' feeling. If the hypoglycaemia is moderate, the child may be unaware of it, but may appear confused and unco-operative. In severe hypoglycaemia, the child is unconscious and may have seizures. Regular hypoglycaemic episodes indicate that the diet and insulin are out of balance and that the whole regimen needs assessing. The possibility of surreptitious extra insulin administration should also be considered. Treatment depends on the severity of the hypoglycaemic episode.

Mild hypoglycaemia

For mild hypoglycaemia, 10 g of rapidly absorbed carbohydrate should be sufficient to alleviate the symptoms. Examples include three glucose tablets, 50 mL glucose drink such as Lucozade, or two teaspoons of ordinary jam, honey or syrup. If the response is not adequate, more can be administered after 10–15 minutes. Ordinary sweets and sweet drinks should be used with caution as a routine treatment because children may fake hypoglycaemia in order to have these 'forbidden foods'. The suggestion of performing additional blood sugar testing at the time of a suspected hypoglycaemia is often enough to act as a deterrent. If hypoglycaemia occurs just prior to a meal, then sufficient quick acting carbohydrate should be given to alleviate symptoms and the meal or snack given soon after. If the next food is not due for an hour or more it is important to use a back-up of slower acting carbohydrate such as a digestive biscuit or piece of fruit in order to prevent blood levels dropping before the next meal.

Moderate hypoglycaemia

At the stage of moderate hypoglycaemia, the child will need help to take a sugary drink or food and Glucogel (formerly known as Hypostop) can be most useful. Glucogel, which is available on prescription, is a rapidly absorbed glucose gel in a tube packaging, which can be squeezed into the mouth if the child is unco-operative. This should be followed up with starchy carbohydrate once the child has recovered.

Severe hypoglycaemia

Most centres advise that parents keep an emergency supply of a GlucaGen HypoKit for severe hypoglycaemia. This is a glucagon injection to use at home if the child is unconscious or having seizures or if they are unable to resolve hypoglycaemic symptoms.

Exercise

Exercise improves insulin resistance and lipid profile and lowers blood pressures. It can also contribute toward maintaining ideal body weight and daily exercise should be promoted to children with diabetes. Advice must be given on prevention of hypoglycaemia during and after additional activity. Exercise has the effect of lowering blood glucose levels by increasing the non-insulin dependent uptake of glucose by cells and increasing insulin sensitivity. Insulin doses can be reduced before periods of heavy exercise, but a child's energy expenditure is so variable from day to day and hour to hour that it is more practical (except for those on an insulin pump or basal bolus therapy) to cover additional activity with extra carbohydrate. Additional carbohydrate given need not be in the form of simple sugars, although the child often favours these. Sugar based refined carbohydrate (e.g. a fun size bar) should be given prior to exercise to minimise the risk of hypoglycaemia. If more than 10 g carbohydrate is required the sugary carbohydrate should be mixed with a more unrefined source (e.g. a chocolate wheaten biscuit). The amount required varies from individual to individual and is also dependent on the amount and type of 'work' done and the insulin regimen.

If exercise is prolonged or strenuous it will be necessary to 'top-up' blood sugar during the exercise period, and this is most practically achieved by using rapidly absorbed simple sugars such as a glucose drink or sweet food. It is particularly important to avoid hypoglycaemia during potentially hazardous activities such as swimming or skiing, where altered concentration or consciousness could have serious consequences. Families need to be made aware that post-exercise hypoglycaemia may occur several hours after strenuous exercise, even during the night, and extra unrefined carbohydrate should be eaten at bedtime following an active day. Families and children themselves become the experts on how much and what type of carbohydrate to have. This comes with experience after trial and error, and with frequent blood sugar monitoring.

Illness

Children often do not wish to eat during periods of illness and infection. Blood sugars are likely to be high at these times, so it is important that insulin injections are continued. A change in the insulin regimen to several doses of rapid acting insulin may be advised. Carbohydrate must be given to prevent the body using fat reserves as a source of fuel and producing ketones. Carbohydrate intake must not be cut to control the blood sugars. Blood sugars should be controlled by the insulin therapy.

If the usual diet is refused it is not essential to completely replace all the carbohydrate. A realistic aim is to give 70–80% of the normal intake. Small frequent doses of rapidly absorbed carbohydrate, preferably as a liquid, are often best tolerated. For example, if the usual diet provides 180 g carbohydrate, distributed 40.20.40.20.40.20, then the aim would be to provide 35–40 g carbohydrate as hourly drinks between the usual breakfast and lunch times, 45–50 g between the usual lunch and evening meal and 50–55 g during the evening and night. In addition low calorie or sugar free drinks should be encouraged to prevent dehydration. During recovery the child should return gradually to foods normally eaten.

Diet throughout childhood

Regular and continued dietetic input is essential in order that the dietary advice is appropriate for the child's continuing and changing needs.

Babies

Adequate nutrition to promote growth is of major importance during the early months of life. Infants with diabetes should have their carbohydrate allowance based on requirement for milk feeds, which are the principal source of nutrition. The feeding pattern of infants is one of frequent and regular feeds and this is ideal for the diabetic regimen. If at the time of diagnosis the infant is breast fed the mother should be encouraged to continue. However, many mothers are anxious about hypoglycaemia if they are uncertain of the amount being consumed at each feed and will need reassurance. Whether breast or bottle fed, a baby's fluid requirement is 150–200 mL/kg/day; 150 mL breast or infant formula contains approximately 10 g carbohydrate. Providing growth and development is normal, the daily carbohydrate intake can be based on the baby's usual feeding pattern with the insulin

dose adjusted accordingly. As with all infants, breast milk or infant formula should be the milk of choice until the child is 12 months old.

Weaning

Weaning can start at the usual time at around 6 months of age. Non-carbohydrate foods may be used initially (e.g. 1–2 teaspoons puréed vegetables) as these will not alter the carbohydrate intake. This allows the baby to become accustomed to the different taste and texture of solids without any anxiety being generated by food refusal. Once the baby has become familiar with spoon feeding and the amount taken increased to 1–2 tablespoons, carbohydrate exchanges may be introduced. At first, 5 g carbohydrate exchanges are useful when only small quantities of food are being taken (e.g. half a rusk, 25 g potato, 5 g baby rice). The amount of mixed feeding will gradually increase and by the time babies are 1 year old they will probably be having about 90 g carbohydrate as solids, the remainder of the carbohydrate intake coming from milk. Water and dilute low sugar squashes can be given as an additional drink.

Weaning is an anxious time for any parent and this anxiety is heightened if a dietary modification has to be observed. Tension about food must be relieved as a baby may refuse solids completely if the mother is fussing or worrying.

The Department of Health recommendations for vitamin supplements for infants and young children [20] also apply to the child with diabetes. The first year of life is the period of most rapid growth. Dietary intake is constantly changing because of the child's progression through normal feeding and developmental milestones. It is essential that the dietitian is in frequent contact with the family to offer advice.

Hypoglycaemia is a real fear for parents and can be hard to recognise in babies. It may only be noted when parents are routinely checking blood sugars. Advice should be given on how to recognise and treat symptoms. Extra milk, with or without additional sugar, or Maxijul, Ribena or sweetened fruit juice may be used. Usually, 10 g carbohydrate given as 150 mL baby milk or 75 mL baby milk plus 1 teaspoon of Maxijul is sufficient to treat hypoglycaemia. It may be necessary to introduce a cereal based weaning food (e.g. baby rice) earlier than 6 months of age if there is a problem with regular hypoglycaemia. Nocturnal hypoglycaemia is a concern of parents, and milk and a cereal can be given before settling for the night if the baby is no longer having night feeds and blood sugars are dropping overnight.

Toddlers

After 1 year of age the child can drink cow's milk and from 2 years semi-skimmed milk can be introduced as long as the child is taking a nutritionally adequate diet. Fully skimmed milk, however, contains too little fat (and hence energy) for the under fives and is not usually recommended. The introduction of skimmed milk over the age of 5 is a useful way to reduce the overall fat content of the diet. There is little fibre in the diets of children in their first year of life, but this can gradually increase from weaning. Some forms of fibre, such as Weetabix, raisins, bananas, lentil soup and baked beans, are popular with children; vegetable fibre and wholemeal bread need to be encouraged.

Small children do not understand the importance of their diet, so parents and health professionals must be flexible and compromise as much as is practical. Food strikes are common in children between 2 and 4 years of age. Rigid meals and snacks often do not work and well-presented finger foods can be offered throughout the day. Most families manage to cope with the 'food refusal syndrome' without being manipulated, but the toddler with diabetes poses a real problem; with hypoglycaemia always a possibility, food refusal can become a powerful weapon. Parents are torn between maintaining good glycaemic control with the accompanying risk of hypoglycaemia, and allowing the blood sugars to be a little raised. Advice should be given not to force feed, nor to offer numerous alternatives, and to avoid fuss around mealtimes. The parents should rely on the child's falling blood sugar to cause hunger and a desire to eat. In a small minority of cases toddlers' food refusal can be a persistent and unremitting problem causing parents enormous worry about hypoglycaemia. One practical solution is to allow the child to eat meals with no fuss and when the meal is over to give an appropriate dose of insulin analogue to cover the amount of food consumed.

In addition to food strikes, some young children with diabetes complain of incessant hunger. This may occur if control is poor and sugar is being lost in the urine or if the child is using food as a means to seek attention. Measurements of height, weight and dietary intake should be carried out regularly to reassure parents that adequate nutrition is being maintained.

This can prove to be a challenging stage when it is often difficult to achieve good glycaemic control and the families need plenty of support from their diabetes team.

Schoolchildren

While at school the teacher becomes one of the child's main carers and must know about the condition and in particular how to recognise and treat hypoglycaemia. Written information which offers a good explanation should be given to each child's teacher. The dietitian and/or the diabetes nurse specialist may offer to visit the school to provide advice. Children with diabetes are advised to carry a hypo remedy (glucose tablets) at all times. The teacher should be equipped with glucose tablets and/or drink in case of hypoglycaemia.

Physical education teachers should be aware of the need for extra carbohydrate before exercise and to check that children are carrying extra carbohydrate during periods of prolonged exercise. School lunches can, but should not, present a problem; it is not always possible for children to go home and they may prefer to have a school lunch with their friends. Older children with a good grasp of their diet can choose their own meal and the cafeteria style canteen allows a flexible choice of food. The organisation and provision of school meals can vary from area to area; it is not desirable for the child to have a 'special diet' away from friends or at a different time from them. A normal main course should be suitable, with the dessert or pudding being replaced by fresh fruit or diet yoghurt. Discussion with the school cooks as well as teachers should help smooth problems. Advice can be given to parents about suitable packed lunches.

Children frequently eat sweets in the school playground and it is tempting for a child with diabetes to eat sweets also. Other less sweet snacks such as fruit, bread, low sugar cereal bars, raisins and sugar free chewing gum should be suggested as alternatives. The best attitude is to use positive reinforcement when the child is doing well and to recommend that the best time for sweets is prior to exercise or after a main meal. If habitual bingeing is causing a problem the services of a child psychologist may be needed; bingeing suggests underlying stress.

Adolescents

Adolescence is often a period of rebellion and diabetes treatment is one more thing to rebel about. Snacking and eating out in the evening are common. Advice about alcohol and its hypoglycaemic effect will be necessary for teenagers.

Adolescent girls have a tendency to become obese and appropriate advice is needed. Occasionally, weight control can be achieved by simply cutting out crisps and fried foods and exercising. The amount of carbohydrate in the diet should only be reduced after very careful examination of the diet as a whole, as this may cause an increase in consumption of fat and protein. In order to get the message across, it is useful to point out the energy content of some of the carbohydrate portions (e.g. one packet of crisps provides 10 g carbohydrate and 150 kcal; one apple also contains 10 g carbohydrate but only 50 kcal). Teenagers soon become aware of the fact that poor control can result in weight loss. A number will omit insulin as a method of weight control. The benefits of weight loss achieved by healthy lifestyle (eating and exercise) should be reinforced and the risks associated with poor control outlined.

Some teenagers, both male and female, can have a distorted view of their weight. Eating disorders such as bingeing, anorexia nervosa and bulimia can present just as in the non-diabetic population. Diabetes may increase the risks of eating disorders as there is a greater focus on food, on weight (weighing people at each clinic visit, rapid weight gain with insulin) and a fear of hypoglycaemia often coupled with low self-esteem. Young adults suffering from an eating disorder need careful monitoring and intervention by the diabetes team and the psychiatrist or psychologist.

Parties and eating out

Parties are highlights in a child's life and advice is required to ensure that children with diabetes can enjoy the party as much as everyone else. They can eat most of the party fare and it is important to ensure that sufficient carbohydrate is eaten to compensate for extra activity and excitement. The host can help by providing low calorie drinks for everyone.

Many of the fast food eating places publish the carbohydrate content of their foods. Children should be educated about their diet as soon as possible so that they are able to manage it independently, with support from parents as necessary. All children are different, but most children from the age of about 8 years should be actively encouraged to have a full understanding of their diet. Parents may need encouragement gradually to hand over responsibility of treatment to the child.

Travel

Travel should pose no problems with a little extra planning. Carbohydrate foods (e.g. sandwiches, fruit or biscuits) should be carried to cover inevitable delays, as should a hypo remedy. Activity holidays will mean that more food is required and possibly a reduction in the insulin dose too, in order to prevent hypoglycaemia. When travelling abroad advice should be given on how to avoid food poisoning and as always the children should wear some form of identification (e.g. SOS Talisman or Medicalert).

Injections

Children should be appropriately involved in all aspects of their care including blood glucose monitoring, injections and learning about diet from as early an age as possible and a balance struck between offering support and encouraging independence. If a child is over 10 years old and has difficulty doing their own injection this may start to impinge on their social life by restricting visits with friends, prohibiting staying overnight with friends and relatives and barring school trips. At this stage a psychologist or diabetes nurse specialist can be invaluable as they can teach the child coping mechanisms to reduce procedural anxiety.

Transition

The age of transition from paediatric to adult clinic varies widely across the UK depending on geographical location and resources available. There is general consensus that this is an area that requires improvement and that the transition from one clinic to another be as seamless as possible to encourage attendance and provide continuity of care while there are many other changes happening in the teenager's life.

Parents may feel isolated and need much support and reassurance from the diabetes team. Diabetes UK has a part to play by producing useful publications and updates about food, and organising children's holiday camps and parent–child weekends. A local parents' group allows families in a similar situation to meet. Young people with diabetes should have an optimal quality of life in which a suitably tailored eating plan is an essential part.

The dietitian has a unique role in the management of childhood diabetes, and nutritional assessment and support must be an integral part of initial and continuing education programmes. The diabetes team should strive for optimal glycaemic control; this is often far from ideal but does not detract from the importance of balanced nutrition in this serious chronic disease.

Non-type 1 diabetes

Although type 1 diabetes is most common in childhood there are a number of other forms of diabetes that can affect this age group. Both type 2 diabetes and monogenic forms such as maturity onset diabetes of the young (MODY) exist and are reported to be on the increase. They remain comparatively uncommon. In a UK survey of children with non-type 1 diabetes, 25 of the 112 children had type 2 diabetes and 20 of the 112 had MODY. The crude minimum UK prevalence of type 2 diabetes under 16 years is 0.21 per 100 000, and of MODY is 0.17 per 100 000. Children with type 2 diabetes are more likely to be female, overweight or obese and be of ethnic minority origin. The prevalence of type 2 diabetes is 0.10 per 100 000 in white UK children and 1.42 per 100 000 in children of Southern Asian origin. Children with MODY are generally not obese nor insulin resistant [21].

Management

Type 2 diabetes

Nutritional advice is essential for the prevention of type 2 diabetes in those at risk and for the effective management of the condition. Healthy eating, weight reduction and physical activity and exercise are advocated. Dietary management alone may be inadequate and children with type 2 diabetes commonly need prescription of an oral hypoglycaemic agent. Metformin is used because of its insulin sensitising effects and has the added advantage of reducing appetite (which may be beneficial to the obese child). Hypoglycaemia and weight gain is less likely with this than with sulphonylureas. Insulin is an appropriate treatment when oral therapy is unsuccessful but because of its anabolic nature progressive weight gain can be a problem. It may be possible to minimise this by using a combination of insulin and metformin.

MODY

Management options are governed by the genetic mutation responsible. Some types may be managed by diet alone whereas other may require treatment with a sulphonylurea and, very rarely, with insulin.

Acknowledgement

The author would like to thank Dr Ian Craigie for designing Fig. 10.1(a–g).

References

1   Rangasami JJ, Greenwood DG, McSporran B *et al.* Rising incidence of type 1 diabetes in Scottish children, 1984–93. *Arch Dis Child*, 1997, **77** 210–13.
2   Gale EA The rise of childhood type I diabetes in the 20th century. *Diabetes*, 2002, **51** 3353–61.

3   St Vincent Joint Task Force for Diabetes *The Report*. Department of Health/British Diabetic Association. 1995, **4.04** 10–11.

4   Publication No 55 *Management of Diabetes* The Scottish Intercollegiate Guidelines Network (SIGN). SIGN Executive, November 2001, **1** 1.1.

5   *Type 1 Diabetes Diagnosis and Management of Type 1 Diabetes in Children and Young People*. National Institute for Clinical Excellence, September 2004, 7 2.1.

6   The Diabetes Control and Complications Trial Research Group The effect of intensive treatment of diabetes on the development and progression of long–term complications in insulin-dependent diabetes mellitus. *N Engl J Med*, 1993, **329** 977–86.

7   Jackson R Growth and maturation of children with insulin dependent diabetes. *Pediatr Clin North Am*, 1984, **31** 545–67.

8   Report of the Nutrition Sub-committee of the Medical Advisory Committee of the British Diabetic Association Dietary Recommendations for diabetics for the 1980s. *Hum Nutr Appl Nutr*, 1982, **36A** 378–94.

9   Nutrition Subcommittee of the British Diabetic Association's Professional Advisory Committee. Dietary recommendations for people with diabetes: an update for the 1990s. *Diabet Med*, 1992, **9** 189–202.

10 Nutrition Subcommittee of the Professional Advisory Committee of the British Diabetic Association Dietary recommendations for children and adolescents with diabetes. *Diabet Med*, 1989, **6** 537–47.

11 Nutrition Subcommittee of the Diabetes Care Advisory Committee of Diabetes UK The Implementation of Nutritional Advice for People with Diabetes. *Diabet Med*, 2003, **20** 786–807.

12 Department of Health Report on Health and Social Subjects No 41 *Dietary Reference Values for Food Energy and Nutrients for the United Kingdom*. London: The Stationery Office, 1991.

13 Franz MJ, Bantle JP, Beebe CA *et al*. Evidence based nutrition principles and recommendations for the treatment and prevention of diabetes and related complications. *Diabetes Care*, 2002, **25** 148–98.

14 Mann J What carbohydrate foods should diabetics eat? *Br Med J*, 1984, **288** 1025–6.

15 Slama G, Haardt M, Joseph P *et al*. Sucrose taken during mixed meal has no additional hyperglycaemic action over isocaloric amounts of starch in well controlled diabetics. *Lancet*, 1984, **12 July** 122–4.

16 Waldron S Current controversies in the dietary management of diabetes in childhood and adolescence. *Br J Hosp Med*, 1996, **56** 450–5.

17 Waldron S, Swift P, Raymond N *et al*. A survey of the dietary management of children's diabetes. *Diabet Med*, 1997, **14** 698–702.

18 Taitz LS, Wardley BL *Handbook of Child Nutrition*. Oxford: Oxford University Press, 1990.

19 DAFNE Study Group Training in flexible, intensive insulin management to enable dietary freedom in people with type 1 diabetes: dose adjustment for normal eating (DAFNE) randomised controlled trial. *Br Med J*, 2002, **325** 746–9.

20 Department of Health and Social Security Report on Health and Social Subjects No 32 *Present Day Practice in Infant Feeding, Third Report*. London: The Stationery Office, 1988.

21 Ehtisham S, Hattersley AT, Dunger DB *et al*. First UK survey of paediatric type 2 diabetes and MODY. *Arch Dis Child*, 2004, **89** 526–9.

Further reading/information

Alison Johnston *Best Ideas for Diabetes – Dietary Information*. Available from Diabetes Service, Royal Hospital for Sick Children, Glasgow G3 8SJ, and on website www.diabetes-scotland.org

Childhood diabetes website www.diabetes-scotland.org

Childhood Diabetes The No Nonsense Guide. DVD sponsored by the Scottish Executive, available from the Small Video Company 0141 647 4857

Useful address

Diabetes UK (formerly British Diabetic Association) 10 Queen Anne Street, London, W1M 0BD

11 Cystic Fibrosis

Carolyn Patchell

Introduction

Cystic fibrosis (CF) is the most common recessively inherited genetic disease in Caucasian populations. It has an incidence of 1 in 2415 live births in the UK [1] and 1 in 25 of the population are carriers [2]. The incidence in non-Caucasians is lower, with estimates around 1 in 20 000 in black populations and 1 in 100 000 in Oriental populations [3]. It is almost unknown in Japan, China and black Africa [4].

There is widespread dysfunction of exocrine glands with disturbances of ion and fluid movement resulting in abnormally thick and dehydrated secretions. This leads to multiorgan obstructive lesions including:

- Chronic lung disease with predominant airway obstruction and recurrent, persistent infections
- Exocrine pancreatic insufficiency with steatorrhoea
- Intestinal obstruction in neonates and older patients
- Infertility, especially in males
- Abnormally high levels of sodium chloride in sweat, resulting from the failure of salt reabsorption in sweat gland ducts [5]

Gastrointestinal involvement is present in 85–95% of all cases and hepatobiliary complications in 5–15% (Table 11.1) [6]. Most patients develop initial symptoms before the age of 2 years, but occasionally if the disease is mild it may be undiagnosed for many years.

In 1989, the gene responsible for CF was localised to the long arm of chromosome 7 [7]. This gene encodes a protein called the CF transmembrane conductance regulator (CFTR). Its main role is as a cyclic adenosine monophosphate (cAMP) regulated chloride channel controlling secretions in sweat glands, respiratory, gastrointestinal and reproductive tracts [8]. More than 1000 mutations of the gene have been identified which are categorised into five classes on the basis of CFTR alterations [9]. The most predominant mutation, which accounts for approximately 70% of all the CFTR genes worldwide, is F508, but there is geographical variation and it is less common in non-white races.

The life expectancy of those with CF has increased in many countries, probably as the result of increased availability of medication, overall rigorous care with the development of specialist treatment centres and diagnosis of the milder forms of the disease [10]. Where previously this disease was considered lethal in childhood, recent data suggest that patients with CF born after 1998 have a median survival of 49.5 years for males and 47 years for females [11]. Survival is largely dependent on the severity and progression of lung disease and more than 90% of the mortality is brought about by chronic bronchial infections and their complications

Table 11.1 Clinical features of cystic fibrosis.

Intestine	Abdominal pain
	Rectal prolapse
	Distal intestinal obstruction syndrome
	Steatorrhoea/diarrhoea
	Abdominal distension
	Malabsorption
	Intussusception
	Gastrointestinal reflux
	Colonic strictures
	Digestive cancer
Pancreas	Pancreatic failure
	Pancreatitis
	Glucose intolerance
	Diabetes mellitus
Liver	Hepatomegaly
	Cirrhosis
	Portal hypertension
Gall bladder	Cholecystitis
	Cholelithiasis
	Obstructive jaundice
Lungs	Repeated respiratory infections
	Asthma/wheezing
	Nasal polyps
	Bronchiectasis
	Hyperinflation
	Clubbing of fingers
	Haemoptysis
	Pneumothorax
	Cor pulmonale
	Aspergillosis
	Sinusitis
Other	Growth failure/failure to thrive/weight loss
	Delayed puberty
	Salt depletion
	Male sterility
	Arthritis
	Fat-soluble vitamin deficiency
	Psychological (child and family)

[2]. Patients with pancreatic insufficiency have a worse prognosis in terms of growth, pulmonary function and long term survival. The mortality of females is generally greater than that of males [1,12]. As early as 1979 [13], an accelerated deterioration rate in pulmonary function was reported in females. This correlated with weight centiles and poorer survival. Even social class has been shown to be an important determinant of life expectancy in CF [14].

Clinical features

Chronic respiratory disease

The lungs are normal at birth, but may become affected within a few weeks of life. As a result of the abnormal secretions and resulting mucus there is obstruction in the small airways, with secondary infection which is progressive and destructive. The host inflammatory response also contributes to the lung disease. Common organisms cultured from the lung are *Staphylococcus aureus*, *Haemophilus influenzae* and subsequently *Pseudomonas* species. This leads to damage of the bronchial wall, bronchiectasis and abscess formation [15]. The child has a persistent, loose cough productive of purulent sputum. On examination there is hyperinflation of the chest because of air trapping, coarse crepitations or respiratory rhonchi.

A major objective of respiratory management is to control infection and remove thickened bronchial secretions, thereby maintaining respiratory function and delaying rate of lung damage. This is achieved by:

- Antibiotic therapy administered either intermittently or continuously (by aerosol, orally or intravenously)
- Regular chest physiotherapy
- Use of bronchodilators, other anti-asthma treatment and oral steroids

Frequent follow-up and routine bacterial surveillance are essential. General measures including avoidance of tobacco smoke, viral and other infections are important.

Gastrointestinal symptoms

Pancreatic insufficiency

This is the most common gastrointestinal defect in CF. It develops when >90% of acinar function is gone. Damage begins *in utero* with ongoing destruction and eventual replacement of the acini with fibrous tissue and fat [16]. As a result of pancreatic damage, the secretion of digestive enzymes and bicarbonate is disrupted, resulting in malabsorption of fat, protein, nitrogen, bile, fat-soluble vitamins and vitamin B_{12}.

It is estimated that up to 90% of CF patients have pancreatic insufficiency. In the other 10% of patients, although enzyme secretions are diminished, it is still adequate for digestion and absorption of nutrients without the necessity for pancreatic enzyme supplementation [17]. Pancreatic sufficiency is genetically determined by one or two mild CFTR mutations.

Meconium ileus

Meconium ileus can occur in up to 15% of infants with CF seen *in utero* with polyhydramnios, or within 48 hours of birth as abdominal obstruction [18]. This is caused by the blockage of the terminal ileum by highly proteinaceous meconium. 'Meconium ileus equivalent' or 'distal intestinal obstruction syndrome' (DIOS) may occur in childhood or adult life.

Abdominal pain

Abdominal pain has been reported in up to 11% of CF patients [19]. It is particularly common in children with poorly controlled malabsorption, but may be caused by many other disorders, which may or may not be related to CF including intussusception, appendicitis, constipation and Crohn's disease.

Gastro-oesophageal reflux

Gastro-oesophageal reflux (GOR) has been frequently reported in CF and it has been estimated that as many as 1 in 5 newly diagnosed infants with CF have pathological GOR [20]. Although the mechanism of GOR in CF is unclear, there is evidence that it is mainly caused by inappropriate relaxation of the gastro-oesophageal sphincter [21]. Postural drainage chest physiotherapy increases the risk of GOR [22]. GOR is more prevalent in young CF children, but improves with increasing age. It may adversely affect lung disease by aspiration and reflex bronchospasm [23].

Colonic strictures (fibrosing colonopathy)

The development of fibrotic strictures and ulceration of the ascending colon in some children with CF is known as fibrosing colonopathy. It is an irreversible lesion that usually requires surgery (frequently ileostomy and colectomy) for control. It was first reported in 1994 [24]. The pathogenesis of this disorder is unknown, but there is an association with high dose, enteric-coated pancreatic enzyme supplements [25] or the pancreatic enzyme coating [26].

Other gastrointestinal problems

Other problems include rectal prolapse, acute pancreatitis, duodenal ulcer, coeliac disease, Crohn's disease and cow's milk protein enteropathy. There is also evidence that the risk of cancer of the digestive tract is significantly elevated and incidence will increase with increased longevity [27].

Effect on growth

Chronic malnutrition, with significant weight retardation and linear growth failure, has long been recognised as a general problem among most CF populations. Patients have poor height and delayed puberty, and the eventual weight of those surviving to adulthood is commonly below average [28]. Bone age and onset of menarche may be delayed [6,29] and pubertal delay can occur despite good clinical state [6]. Nutritional impairment is noted at birth, with CF infants having an average birthweight of about 0.5 standard deviations (SD) lower than that of the normal populations [30]. Head circumference has also been shown to be 1.0 SD below normal at 4 years of age [31].

Reported growth patterns are similar. In a cross-sectional study of UK CF clinics, the mean body weight in boys was between −0.25 and −0.5 SD below the population mean until the age of 10 years. In girls, mean body weight was approximately −0.5 SD below the population mean during the same period. Body mass index (BMI) decreased from the age of 5 years. Post-pubertal stature and weight maintenance in the CF population shows substantial deficits [32]. In children 5 years and under, no differences have been noted between screened and non-screened patients [33].

In a further cross-sectional survey of 223 patients attending a CF centre in Denmark, BMI was approximately 98% of normal in the younger patients, but declined to 90% in adult men and 83%

in adult women with CF. All patients had a normal height, although the final height was achieved a little later than healthy controls [12]. In the USA, the heights and weights of 13 116 children with CF aged 0–18 years were reported; children had sub-normal growth at all ages. Mean and median height and weight for age were found to be at the 30th and 20th percentiles in children with CF. Malnutrition (height or weight for age <5th percentile) was par-ticularly pronounced in infants (47%) and adoles-cents (37%) and patients with newly diagnosed CF (47%) [34]. Comparison of growth data between Canada and the USA demonstrated suboptimal growth in both countries, although Canadian patients had better weight and height scores [35].

Growth hormone has been used to improve growth in small groups of patients with CF with some success [5,36].

Other clinical problems

Cystic fibrosis related diabetes

Prevalence and incidence of diabetes mellitus (DM) in CF patients is high, varies according to CF geno-type and increases with age. Progressive fibrosis and fatty infiltration of the exocrine pancreas lead to destruction of islet architecture, which in turn leads to loss of endocrine cells secreting insulin, glucagon and pancreatic polypeptide. Using the World Health Organization (WHO) criteria for the diagnosis of DM [37], the prevalence of impaired glucose tolerance and DM range from 14–36% and 5–24%, respectively, in three European centres [38–40]. The prevalence of DM in CF patients aged 10, 20 and 30 years is reported to be 1.5%, 13% and 50% [41]. Cystic fibrosis related diabetes (CFRD) is a distinct type, with features of both types 1 and 2 DM. The diabetes is usually non-ketotic and insulin dependent [42]. An insidious decline in clinical sta-tus often occurs before the diagnosis is made [43].

Although the diabetes is usually mild, it has an impact on survival rates, particularly for females. The median survival age is 47 years compared to 49 years for non-diabetic male patients with CF, and 30 years compared to 47 years for female patients with CF [11]. Diagnosis can be difficult, but early intervention can have an impact on patient wellbe-ing and protects against clinical deterioration. Oral glucose tolerance tests (OGTT) and serial glucose monitoring are the most specific tools for screening for CFRD.

The frequency of serious secondary complica-tions (e.g. microangiopathy and nephropathy) is increasing [44–46]. Careful control of diabetes is important; identifying patients who are at risk is desirable and it is recommended that annual screening with OGTT be carried out in all CF patients over the age of 12 years [47].

Liver disease

The prevalence of liver disease among CF patients ranges between 9% and 37%, depending on the definition of liver disease [48] and peaks during adolescence [49]. There is some evidence that it may occur more commonly in patients with pan-creatic insufficiency [50]. Children with CF exhibit a spectrum of liver abnormalities, with intermittent rises in serum transaminases a common early find-ing. Abnormalities range from hepatic steatosis to focal biliary cirrhosis and eventually multilobular cirrhosis with portal hypertension. Variceal bleed-ing may occur. Clinical signs of cirrhosis occur late even when the disease is advanced. Patients are also at increased risk of developing gallstones with complications of cholecystitis, cholangitis, pancre-atitis or complete obstruction of the biliary tree [49]. There is a 3.4% mortality rate from liver complica-tions [51]. Liver transplantation has been success-ful in patients with advanced liver disease [52]. Prompt recognition of liver disease is important as there is evidence that ursodeoxycholic acid, a bile acid found in very low concentrations in humans, may prevent progression of CF-related liver disease [53], but long term benefit has still to be determined.

Diagnosis

The sweat test remains the most reliable diagnostic laboratory test [54]. Sweat sodium, chloride and potassium concentrations are all raised but meas-urement of potassium is less reliable. When performed correctly, sweat testing has a low false negative rate of <2%. If possible, it should be car-ried out in combination with DNA analysis [55].

Neonatal screening for CF has been imple-mented in some areas for 25 years [56] and will be introduced across the UK within the next 2–3 years. Immunoreactive trypsin (IRT) is 2–5 times higher in neonates with CF and is measured from dried blood spots on Guthrie cards in the UK. It has a poor sensitivity and it should be used in combination with DNA analysis and sweat testing [15].

Nutritional management

In the past, weight loss and poor growth were considered to be inevitable in CF; however, in the 1970s the CF clinic in Toronto was able to demonstrate good nutritional status and improved survival in their patients if given a high fat, high energy diet. Corey et al. [3], in a comparative study between patients in Toronto and Boston, concluded that the longer survival of the patients in Toronto was a result mainly of the aggressive nutritional support given in this centre. Good survival figures have also been reported in other CF centres with aggressive nutritional support programmes [12].

A variety of complex organic and psychological factors contribute to malnutrition in CF and will vary considerably between patients depending on their disease expression, clinical state, age and sex. Malnutrition has several adverse effects including poor growth, impaired muscle function [57], decreased exercise tolerance, increased susceptibility to infection and decreased ventilatory drive. Studies indicate that BMI strongly correlates with lung function [58], but the exact mechanism of this relationship has not been fully determined. Achieving optimum nutrition and growth may minimise the progressive decline in pulmonary function commonly seen in CF.

Causes of malnutrition

The nutritional problems in CF are determined by three factors: energy losses, increased energy expenditure and low energy intake.

Energy losses

Malabsorption
Because pancreatic exocrine secretions contain less enzymes and bicarbonate, have a lower pH and are of a smaller volume, the physical properties of proteins and mucus within the lumen are affected. This results in obstruction to the small ducts and secondary damage to pancreatic digestive enzyme secretions causing malabsorption. Other problems such as gastric hypersecretion, reduced duodenal bicarbonate concentration and pH, disorders of bile salt metabolism, disordered intestinal motility and permeability, liver disease, and short bowel syndrome after intestinal resection in the neonatal period, may all contribute to malabsorption. The severity of malabsorption is variable; there can be significant malabsorption of protein and fat-soluble vitamins despite adequate use of enzyme supplements. Murphy et al. [59] have estimated that stool energy losses account for 11% of gross energy intake in CF patients, three times higher than normal.

Other losses
Energy may be lost as a result of vomiting following coughing, physiotherapy or GOR. Diabetes mellitus if undiagnosed or poorly controlled may increase energy losses resulting from glycosuria. Further substantial nutrient losses may occur in the sputum. Nitrogen losses in the sputum can reach 10 g/day during severe acute pulmonary exacerbation, especially from *Pseudomonas aeruginosa* [60]. Sputum is particularly rich in amino acids [61].

Increased energy expenditure

The increased energy needs of patients with CF vary widely and have been estimated at 120–150% of the requirements for healthy age- and sex-matched children [62].

Resting energy expenditure (REE), an estimate of basal metabolic rate, is 10–20% greater than in healthy controls and may contribute to energy imbalance [62,63]. Increased REE appears to be closely associated with declining pulmonary function [62,64] and subclinical infection [63]. Bronchial sepsis leads to local release of leukotrienes, free oxygen radicals and cytokines including tumour necrosis factor α (TNFα) [65]. Antibiotics have been shown to reduce energy requirements of moderately ill patients with chronic *Pseudomonas aeruginosa* [66].

Abnormal pulmonary mechanics may increase REE. Continuous injury to the lungs leads to progressive parenchymal fibrosis and airway obstruction with probable increased oxygen cost and work of breathing [65]. Even long term bronchodilator therapy with drugs such as salbutamol [67] and feeding has been shown to increase REE.

Controversy remains over the effect of genotype on REE. Patients homozygous for the mutation ∆F508 have been found to have a higher REE than those with other genotypes [68], whereas more recent studies have shown no genotype-dependent differences in REE in asymptomatic or pre-symptomatic CF infants, children and adults when confounding variables such as body composition, lung function and nutritional status are taken into account [64,69,70].

Data are also conflicting on total energy expenditure [69,71] with evidence that patients with moderate lung impairment adapt to an increased REE by reducing their activity levels, thereby maintaining total energy expenditure levels with controls [69]. The variability in energy requirements between patients emphasises the need for individual assessment.

Anorexia and low energy intake

Poor dietary intake is often a major contributory factor in growth failure of CF children. During pulmonary exacerbations, energy requirements increase yet appetite often reduces. This in turn leads to the familiar pattern of slow weight gain, punctuated by weight loss during exacerbations.

Although dietary assessments in CF children demonstrate that energy intake is greater than in controls, it rarely exceeds 111% of requirements and growth and weight gain is suboptimal (Table 11.2) [72–75]. Healthy controls tend to under-report their dietary intake whereas CF patients often overestimate theirs to be in agreement with the nutritional advice they are usually receiving [60].

Factors associated with a reduced appetite include:

- Chronic respiratory infection and other complications of CF such as DIOS, abdominal pain, GOR resulting in oesophagitis, pain and vomiting
- Behavioural feeding problems in pre-school and school age children
- Media pressure to eat a healthy low fat, low sugar diet
- Inappropriate concepts regarding body image
- Depression
- Eating disorders in teenagers
- Poor use of dietary supplements
- Dislike of high energy foods
- Poverty

Behavioural feeding difficulties and poor child–parent interactions at mealtimes are a particular problem and have received much attention. Mealtimes are the most frequently reported area of difficulty for parents of pre-school children. Abnormal eating behaviours in toddlers and school children include excessively long meals, delay tactics, food refusal and spitting out food [75,76]. Toddlers with more feeding difficulties have lower energy intakes [76].

Table 11.2 Energy intake and growth of cystic fibrosis patients.

	Stark et al. [74]	Kawchak et al. [72]				Stark et al. [75]	Anthony et al. [73]
		Year 0	Year 1	Year 2	Year 3		
Age (years)	2–5	7.8	8.9	9.8	10.7	6–13	7–12
No. of children with CF	32	24	18	23	16	28	25
Controls*	Peers	Peers	Peers	Peers	Peers	Peers	Siblings
Energy % RDA: CF	95%	107%	100%	101%	128%	100%	107%
Controls	84%	94%	93%	90%	86%	95%	92%
Height z score: CF		−0.3	−0.3	−0.4	−0.797	−0.33	−0.4
Controls		0.1	0.4	0.3	0.371	0.48	0.3
Weight z score: CF		−0.3	−0.3	−0.4	−0.811	−0.25	−0.4
Controls		0	0	−0.1	−0.528	0.36	−0.2

RDA, recommended daily allowance; CF, cystic fibrosis.
* Control peers and siblings were all healthy.

Abnormal adaptive response to malnutrition

The adaptive response to malnutrition may be abnormal in CF. In the unaffected child, the response to infection is an increase in protein synthesis. Some CF children have been shown to have a decrease in protein synthesis during pulmonary exacerbations. This may lead to stunting in children with chronic infections, despite adequate energy intake [77].

Assessment of growth and nutritional status

Weight, height and head circumference

Sequential measurements of weight and height in all children, and head circumference in children under 5 years, should be carried out. The measurements should be plotted on the appropriate centile charts. Patients with CF often show delayed puberty, which should be taken into account when interpreting progress. During adolescence, delayed puberty may lead to an over-estimation of malnutrition as children will show a drop from their growth centiles before demonstrating catch-up during their pubertal growth spurt. Assessment of pubertal stage is therefore important when interpreting growth data. Growth velocity is another useful measure and may provide a more sensitive assessment of poor growth.

Body mass index

Body mass index is a useful measurement in clinical practice and should be plotted on the appropriate centile charts. The results should be interpreted with care in children with short stature or delayed puberty.

Percentage weight for age, height for age and weight for height

The measurements may be calculated using a Cole assessment slide rule [78] or by calculation of the weight or height expressed as a percentage of that expected for age, or weight for expected height. Serial measurements are useful in assessment of growth progress and assesses whether weight is in proportion to height. Again, care should be taken in using this measurement in patients with delayed puberty and errors in calculation are common in clinical practice [79].

Arm anthropometry

Skinfold thickness and mid upper arm circumference are simple methods of interpreting lean body mass and body fatness. These measurements have poor reproducibility and are not recommended in routine clinical practice.

Bone age

Delays in bone maturity increases with age and disease progression; an estimation of bone age is useful in children with stunting or delayed puberty.

Bone mineral density

Osteopenia and osteoporosis have been reported in children with CF [80] and the long term consequences of this are of concern with increasing longevity. Bone mineral density is assessed by dual X-ray absorptiometry (DEXA) scans. This process is expensive but regular scans should be considered in patients over 10 years of age [81].

Frequency of assessment

Infants should be weighed and measured at each clinic visit, at least every 2 weeks until they are thriving. Older children should have their height and weight measured every 3 months as a minimum. All measurements should be plotted on the appropriate centile chart.

Definition of growth failure

Children <5 years of age:	weight/height <85% weight loss or plateau in weight gain over a 4-month period
Children 5–18 years of age:	weight/height <85% weight loss over a 6-month period plateau of weight over a 6-month period

Aims of nutritional management

There are three main aims of nutritional management:

- To achieve optimal nutritional status
- To achieve normal growth and development
- To maintain normal feeding behaviour

Energy

Crude estimates have suggested that patients may require 120–150% of the recommended daily allowance or estimated average requirement (EAR) for age and sex [62,63,81]. More specific recommendations for energy intake taking into account REE, physical activity and disease severity have been published by a North American Consensus Committee [82]. Reilly et al. [83] tested the accuracy of both these methods; errors in estimation of energy requirements for individuals were large.

The heterogeneity of these patients, including presence of respiratory infection, activity and nutritional status, make it difficult to give universal recommendations for energy requirements. Each individual's energy requirements will vary depending on clinical condition and activity levels. The only practical method to gauge adequate nutrition is by closely monitoring weight gain and growth. Some children will grow normally by consuming no more than the EAR for energy, whereas those with advanced pulmonary disease may need 50–60% more energy than for normal populations. A useful guideline to follow is to assess the existing energy intake and increase this value by a further 20–30% if weight gain or growth is poor.

Protein

Exact protein requirements are unclear; it is generally accepted that the protein intake should be increased beyond the reference nutrient intake (RNI) to compensate for excessive loss of nitrogen in the faeces and sputum and increased protein turnover in malnourished patients [84]. Protein should provide 15% of the total energy intake. In practice, the vast majority of CF patients have no difficulty in achieving this level of intake.

Fat

Fat is the most concentrated source of energy in the diet and the only source of essential fatty acids. It is widely accepted that fat should be encouraged liberally and should provide 35–40% of the total energy intake. Some clinics have developed novel techniques to improve fat intake, including setting targets for daily fat intake [85]. Perhaps with the exception of severe liver disease, medium chain triglyceride (MCT) replacement of dietary fat has little role in CF. Theoretically, with MCT oil there is less dependence on intraluminal mechanisms of digestion. However, MCT oil has not been shown to improve growth, may result in essential fatty acid deficiency and may indirectly increase energy requirements as it requires more oxygen than carbohydrate to be oxidised in the liver. There is some parental concern about the effects of a high fat diet on blood lipid levels but in studies on adults with pancreatic insufficiency total cholesterol and lipid levels are normal to low [86]. However, given the increasing longevity of patients with CF and increased availability of polyunsaturated and monounsaturated fats in the normal diet, it would seem prudent to encourage a high fat diet, incorporating a mix of saturated, poly- and monounsaturated fats.

Carbohydrate

A high carbohydrate intake should be encouraged to provide 45–50% of the total energy intake. Carbohydrates are well tolerated as pancreatic amylase deficiency is compensated for by salivary amylase and, to a lesser degree, intestinal glucoamylase [60]. However, antibiotics can reduce the ability of colonic flora to ferment carbohydrate and lead to a less salvageable energy. Starchy foods such as bread, potatoes and pasta as well as simple sugars should be encouraged, the latter providing a valuable energy source. Disaccharide intolerance may be a problem following surgery for meconium ileus.

Fibre

The traditional high fat, high sugar diet for children with CF is low in dietary fibre. Reports of fibre intake confirm this and there is evidence that children with low intakes of fibre suffer from more abdominal pain and take higher doses of pancreatic enzymes [87]. It is possible that lack of fibre may compromise colonic function, causing stasis of substrate, constipation and abdominal pain. Furthermore, fatty acids, derived from unabsorbed fibre, provide the colon with its major source of nutrition [25]. A malnourished colon may be at greater risk of developing complications such as DIOS and fibrosing colonopathy. Further work is needed on the role of fibre in CF. A common sense approach should be taken regarding the inclusion of fibre rich foods in the diet and if the appetite of the child allows for the incorporation of high fibre foods these should be encouraged; however, not at the expense of energy dense foods which will support normal growth.

Nutritional support

Three levels of nutritional support are provided in cystic fibrosis:

- A high energy, high protein diet
- Dietary supplements
- Enteral feeding

High energy, high protein diet

It is recommended that children are regularly reviewed by a dietitian experienced in CF and that individual assessment is made and advice given based on the changing clinical and psychosocial needs of the patient. Energy intake from ordinary foods should be maximised. A good variety of energy rich foods should be encouraged, such as full cream milk, cheese, meat, full cream yoghurt, milk puddings, cakes and biscuits. Extra butter or polyunsaturated or monounsaturated margarine can be added to bread, potatoes and vegetables. Frying foods or basting in oil will increase energy density. Extra milk or cream can be added to soups, cereal, desserts or mashed potatoes and used to top tinned or fresh fruit. Regular snacks are important and should be encouraged as long as the appetite for meals does not diminish as a result. Malnourished children achieve higher energy intake when more frequent meals are offered [88]. It is important for parents to establish a good routine for meals and snacks and not allow children to substitute sweets and chocolate for savoury food at mealtimes.

Although this advice is simple, dietetic input should be intensive and dietary goals must be achievable and agreed in consultation with the child and parents at each clinic visit. Attention should be given to psychological, social, behavioural and developmental aspects of feeding. A meta-analysis of differing treatment interventions to promote weight gain in CF demonstrated that a behavioural approach was just as effective in promoting weight gain as invasive medical procedures [89].

Parents are encouraged to adopt normal feeding routines, limit meal times to a maximum of 30 minutes, develop consistent feeding strategies and, above all, remain positive if food is refused. If simple dietary advice and reassurance fails, enlisting the help of a psychologist with an interest in feeding problems is invaluable.

Dietary supplements

The role of dietary protein and energy supplements in the management of CF has been studied. The Calories in Cystic Fibrosis – Oral trial (CALICO) showed that moderately malnourished children with CF given protein and energy supplements in addition to standard dietetic advice over a 12-month period showed no benefit, in terms of BMI, over those given dietetic advice alone [80]. Rettammel et al. [90] studied a supplement designed for patients with CF which contained energy, fat, linoleic acid and fat-soluble vitamins. Mean adherence to the supplement was 69% (range 26–100%). Those who consistently took the supplement had an increased total energy intake, indicating that the supplement did not replace food intake. They also gained weight. However, weight and mean energy intake for the groups as a whole was unchanged before and after the intervention. In contrast, in a study on an energy–protein powder supplement (Scandishake), compliance was good and mean energy intake and weight gain improved in a group of 26 children and adults with CF [91].

The use of dietary supplements in the management of CF is therefore unclear; however, dietary supplements may be considered if dietetic counselling to improve energy and protein intake has been given and there is persistent:

- Weight loss
- Decline in height or weight centile position (providing weight centile is no more than one centile above height)
- Nutrient intake below dietary reference values

Guidelines for using dietary supplements in CF

The following is a useful guide:
1–3 years – 200 kcal (840 kJ)
4–5 years – 400 kcal (1680 kJ)
6–11 years – 600 kcal (2520 kJ)
over 12 years – 800 kcal (3360 kJ)

- Dietary supplements should be given 2–3 times daily after meals or at bedtime.
- No more than 20% of the EAR should be given as dietary supplements except during an acute infection or if the patient is being considered for enteral feeding. Excessive supplementation will impair appetite and decrease nutrient intake from normal foods.
- Dietary supplements should not be used to re-place food at mealtimes; they are best accepted if served cold.
- Parents or children should be encouraged to prepare their own homemade milk shakes.
- Care should be used when using high protein supplements (>6.0 g protein/100 mL) in children under 5 years. The nutrient profile of these products is not designed for young children.
- Pancreatic enzyme supplements are needed with milk shake supplements.

Suitable dietary supplements for children with CF are given in Table 11.3.

Enteral feeding

Approximately 5% of CF patients require enteral feeding [92]; the majority of these are teenagers reflecting the deterioration in nutritional status that occurs in adolescence. Enteral feeding should be considered if:

- Child is persistently less than 85% expected weight for height
- Child has failed to gain weight over a 3–6 month period
- Height and weight are below the second percentile

Table 11.3 Useful dietary supplements in cystic fibrosis suitable for children aged 1–16 years.

	Energy		Protein	Fibre
	(kcal)	(kJ)	(g)	(g)
Fortified milk shakes (per 100 mL)				
Paediasure	100	422	2.8	–
Paediasure with fibre	100	422	2.8	0.5
Paediasure Plus	150	630	4.2	–
Fortini	150	630	3.4	–
Fortini Multifibre	150	630	3.4	1.5
Fresubin	100	422	3.8	–
Clinutren 1.5	150	630	5.5	–
Clinutren ISO	100	420	3.8	–
Fortisip	150	630	6.0	–
Fortisip Multifibre	150	630	6.0	2.25
Resource Junior	150	630	3.0	–
Resource Shake	174	714	5.1	–
Fortified juice drinks (per 100 mL)				
Enlive Plus	150	630	4.8	–
Fortijuce	150	630	4.0	–
Provide Xtra	125	525	3.75	–
Fortified semi-solid supplements (per 100 g)				
Formance	147	622	3.5	–
Glucose polymer powders (per 100 g)				
Super soluble Maxijul	380	1596	–	–
Caloreen	390	1680	–	–
Polycal	380	1596	–	–
Vitajoule	380	1596	–	–
Glucose polymer drinks (per 100 mL)				
Liquid Polycal	247	1037	–	–
Liquid Maxijul	200	840	–	–

Enteral feeding is associated with improvements in body fat, height, lean body mass and muscle mass, increased total body nitrogen, improved strength and development of secondary sexual characteristics. Improvement in weight precedes improvement in height [93]. If pulmonary function is poor (i.e. forced expired volume in less than 1 second, FEV_1, is less than 40% predicted) at the start of enteral feeding, there may be little improvement in nutritional status [94]. Some studies have documented stabilisation [95] or improvement in pulmonary function in CF with enteral feeding [94,96].

To produce lasting benefit, numerous studies have demonstrated that enteral feeding should be continued long term [95–97]. However, Dalzell *et al.* [98] demonstrated significantly greater height and weight scores in a group of 10 CF children 4 years after cessation of tube feeding of only 1 year duration.

Types of enteral feed

Many types of preparations have been used for enteral feeding in CF. These include elemental (amino acid), semi-elemental (protein hydrolysate) and polymeric feeds. There are few published data comparing the efficacy of these feeds.

Polymeric feeds

Polymeric feeds are tolerated by most patients with CF and are the first feed of choice in most CF centres. Patients over 1 year will usually tolerate a 1.5 kcal/mL (6.3 kJ/mL) paediatric or adult (dependent on age or weight) standard feed. They have several advantages: they are cheap, prescribable (Advisory Committee on Borderline Substances, ACBS), have a low osmolality and are available in ready-to-hang packs. No difference in fat malabsorption, nitrogen absorption and weight gain has been observed when polymeric feeds, together with enzyme replacement therapy, and semi-elemental feeds have been compared [99].

Elemental feeds

Little work has been carried out comparing the efficacy of elemental feeds with polymeric feeds. Some centres in the UK prefer to routinely use an elemental formula for enteral feeding in CF. In theory, elemental feeds have a good buffering effect on gastric acidity at night and are low in fat. Some centres do not give pancreatic enzymes with elemental feeds, but this could be disputed as they contain a mixture of long chain as well as medium chain triglyceride fats. They are expensive, have a high osmolality and a low energy density. In adult practice it is common to supplement elemental formulas with glucose polymer and an MCT fat emulsion and concentrations of 2.6 kcal/mL (11 kJ/mL) have been tolerated [100].

High fat feeds

The role of high fat feeds in CF is uncertain. Fitting's [101] work has suggested that low carbohydrate, high fat feeds are not necessary for nutritional support in patients with chronic obstructive lung disease. However, Kane *et al.* [102] have demonstrated that giving the high fat feed Pulmocare resulted in lower CO_2 production (VCO_2) and respiratory quotient in CF patients with moderate to severe pulmonary disease, than did feeding with a high carbohydrate feed.

High carbohydrate feeds have been shown to cause hyperglycaemia in glucose-intolerant adult CF patients [103] and high fat, low carbohydrate feeds may be preferable. There is only one high fat feed available in the UK, Pulmocare. It is not prescribable on ACBS.

Administration of feed

The route used for feed will be influenced by the duration of feeding and by the preference of the patient, relatives and physician. Nasogastric, gastrostomy and jejunostomy feeds have all been used in CF and each method has merits and drawbacks (Table 11.4).

Percutaneous endoscopic gastrostomy (PEG) is the preferred route in children for long term

Table 11.4 Problems with enteral feeding in cystic fibrosis.

Nasogastric feeding
Nasogastric tube displacement
Gastro-oesophageal reflux
Nasal irritation
Insertion of nasogastric tube with nasal polyps

Gastrostomy feeding
Gastrostomy tube blockage
Leakage around gastrostomy site
Dislodgement of gastrostomy catheter

Gastrointestinal and tolerance
Nausea
Abdominal distention
Diarrhoea
Feed intolerance during pulmonary exacerbations
Feed aspiration
Hyperglycaemia

Growth and body image
Inhibition of oral feeding
Slow improvements in linear growth
Failure to improve body image in adolescent girls

feeding and can be replaced by a gastrostomy button after 2–3 months. Gastrostomy feeding improves weight gain, presumably because of better compliance and less loss of feeding time as a result of complications [104]. Problems associated with the nasogastric route in CF include difficulties inserting the tube (particularly if the child has nasal polyps), nasal irritation, tube displacement with coughing or vomiting and the potential risk of aspiration. Other complications include nasopharyngeal sepsis and oesophageal erosion [100].

It is common practice to give enteral feeding for 8–10 hours overnight with a 1 or 2 hour break before the first physiotherapy session in the morning. Allowing teenagers to have one or two nights off the feed each week helps compliance. At least 40–50% of the EAR for energy is usually given via the tube, with weight and growth being regularly reviewed. Hyperglycaemia is a potential problem and blood glucose should be monitored.

It is not known how best to give pancreatic enzymes with tube feeds and practices vary widely. There is some suggestion that it may be better to give them at the beginning of the feed and just before the child goes to sleep [105]. Dosage of pancreatic enzymes with enteral feeds is arbitrary but can be estimated by using the amount of pancreatic enzymes required for a normal meal and adjusting the quantity in accordance with the fat composition of the feed.

Vitamin and mineral supplements

Fat-soluble vitamins

Malabsorption of fat-soluble vitamins is likely in patients with CF, particularly in those who have pancreatic insufficiency. Biochemical evidence of deficiency of fat-soluble vitamins is well documented. Low fat-soluble vitamin status is associated with poor clinical status and reduced lung function, possibly related to the role of vitamin A as an antioxidant. Clinical symptoms of fat-soluble vitamin deficiency is rarely seen since the introduction of pancreatic enzyme replacement therapy (PERT) and routine supplementation; however, there is a risk in those patients with poorly controlled malabsorption, late diagnosis, bowel resection and those with poor adherence to treatment.

Vitamin A

Low serum vitamin A levels are commonly reported in CF and documented clinical features of vitamin A deficiency include night blindness, conjunctival and corneal xerosis, dry thickened skin and abnormalities of bronchial mucosal epithelialisation. Low vitamin A status may be multifactorial and studies have suggested a defect in the handling of retinol by the gastrointestinal tract [106]. Vitamin A status is difficult to assess, owing to lack of a reliable marker, and serum levels of retinol do not adequately mirror the concentration of vitamin A in the liver and may be a reflection of low retinol binding protein. Plasma retinol concentrations are also reduced during infection so levels should be checked at a time of clinical stability. Some researchers found liver stores of vitamin A in CF to be 2.5 times higher than those in control subjects, despite lower serum levels of retinol and retinol binding protein [107]. This has not been supported by other studies [108].

Vitamin E

A neuropathy resulting from vitamin E deficiency has been widely reported in adult CF patients. Symptoms and signs include absent deep tendon reflexes, loss of position sense and vibration sense in lower limbs, dysarthria, tremor, ataxia and decreased visual activity. Vitamin E may also be important in controlling the progression of lung disease in CF. The antioxidant function of vitamin E and the scavenger role of both vitamins A and E may protect the lungs from oxygen-radical damage during the inflammatory response to infection. Both water miscible and fat-soluble preparations of vitamin E are effective in achieving normal serum levels [109]. In one case report, ursodeoxycholic acid appears to aid absorption in the presence of liver disease and pancreatic insufficiency [110]. Serum or plasma vitamin E levels represent only a small proportion of the total body stores. Levels also vary depending on carrier lipoprotein so vitamin E : fasting lipid ratio should ideally be measured.

Vitamin D

Clinical evidence of vitamin D deficiency is rare in CF; however, reduced levels of 25-hydroxyvitamin

D have been described and osteopenia and osteoporosis have been seen in children with CF [111,112]. This may be related to poor nutritional status [113] and delayed puberty [114]. Rickets is rarely seen. Shaw *et al.* [114] demonstrated that 16 of 24 individuals with CF, aged 3–29 years, had a bone mineral density below the mean, with six individuals having values more than 2 SD below the mean. Only four patients had evidence of suboptimal vitamin D status. In contrast, in well-nourished patients with CF, bone mineral content has been shown to be normal [115]. The aetiology of reduced bone mineral density is probably multi-factorial and related to poor nutritional status and overall clinical status; however, every effort should be made to optimise vitamin D and calcium intake. Plasma 25-hydroxyvitamin D is a good indication of status, but seasonal variations are well recognised [116]. It is therefore recommended that vitamin D levels should be maintained at the upper end of the normal range [117].

Vitamin K

The true prevalence of vitamin K deficiency is unknown and there is no consensus on routine vitamin K supplementation. Studies of vitamin K status in CF patients have produced conflicting and inconclusive results, but recent evidence suggests it is as high as 78% in pancreatic insufficient patients [118]. There is now a suggestion that routine vitamin K supplementation should be considered in all patients with pancreatic insufficiency and particularly for patients with severe non-cholestatic and cholestatic liver disease, major small bowel resection and following prolonged antibiotic treatment. More studies are needed on the dosage and frequency of vitamin K supplementation in CF [118,119].

Dosage of fat-soluble vitamin supplementation

Fat-soluble vitamin supplements should be started on diagnosis in all pancreatic insufficient patients. Levels should be checked annually for all pancreatic sufficient patients and supplements started when low levels are detected. The ideal dosage of each vitamin has not been adequately established and there is considerable variation in the amount given worldwide [92,120,121]. Current dosage of vitamin supplementation are given in Table 11.5 and brands are given in Table 11.6. Regimens

Table 11.5 Vitamin supplementation commonly given in cystic fibrosis.

Vitamin	Dose per day
A	5000–10 000 IU
D	400–800 IU
E	10–200 mg

Table 11.6 Composition of vitamin preparations used in cystic fibrosis.

Multivitamin preparations		Vitamin A (IU)	Vitamin D (IU)	Vitamin E (mg)
Abidec liquid (Chefaro UK)	0.6 mL	4000	400	–
Dalivit liquid (LPC Medical UK Ltd)	0.6 mL	5000	400	–
Multivitamins BPC capsule or tablet	1	2500	300	–
A and D capsule	1	4000	400	
Forceval Caps	1	2500	400	10
Forceval Junior Caps (Alliance Pharmaceuticals Ltd)	1	1250	200	5
Vitamin E gelcaps	1	–	–	75
Vitamin E Susp	1 mL	–	–	100
Ketovite Tablets	3	–	–	5
Ketovite Liquid (Paines & Byrne Ltd)	5 mL	2500	400	–

combine a preparation containing vitamins A and D and an additional vitamin E supplement.

Compliance with vitamin therapy in CF is poor. A multivitamin preparation specially formulated for CF containing vitamins A, D, E and K (ADEK) was found to improve plasma vitamin A and E concentrations in children over 10 years. However, in children 7–10 years old, vitamin E concentrations were too high [122].

Monitoring levels of fat-soluble vitamins

Fat-soluble vitamin levels should be checked annually and adjustments made to the dosage as appropriate. The effects of alterations in dosage should be rechecked after 3–6 months. Combined vitamin supplements are routinely used, but it may be necessary to give separate vitamin A, D or E supplements to optimise plasma levels of individual vitamins in some patients.

Minerals

Sodium

There is a lack of consensus regarding the routine supplementation of sodium and practices vary across CF centres in the UK. Salt depletion can occur in hot weather through physical exercise causing increased sweating, and in infancy when a normal low electrolyte formula such as SMA Gold or Cow & Gate Premium is fed. Anorexia and poor growth may result from chronic salt depletion. Significant hyponatraemia may be accompanied by vomiting. Sodium deficiency can be confirmed by a spot urine analysis (sodium <10 mmol/L) and measurement of serum sodium. Some centres routinely supplement sodium in infants under 12 months of age and in older children during the summer months and if they visit hot countries; other centres choose to supplement only those children with evidence of sodium depletion. The amount given is arbitrary, but the following guidelines may be useful:

0–1 year   2 mmol/kg sodium in the form of sodium chloride solution (1 mL = 1 mmol sodium)

1–5 years   2 × 300 mg sodium chloride tablets (10 mmol sodium)

6–10 years   2 × 600 mg sodium chloride tablets (20 mmol sodium)

11 years +   (3–4) × 600 mg sodium chloride tablets (30–40 mmol sodium)

Essential fatty acid deficiency

Essential fatty acid deficiency is frequently reported in CF, particularly in infancy before a diagnosis is made [123]. Clinical features include increased water permeability of the skin, increased susceptibility to infection, impaired wound healing [124], growth retardation [125], thrombocytopenia and reduced platelet aggregation. It is characterised by a deficiency of linoleic acid with either low or normal arachidonic acid concentrations and increased concentrations of saturates and monounsaturates (such as palmitic, palmitoleic acid and eicosatrienoic acid).

The cause of essential fatty acid deficiency is debatable and has been demonstrated in both well-nourished young CF patients and undernourished patients [126]. It has been linked to both underlying defects of fatty acid metabolism, low fat diets and increased metabolic usage in undernourished patients. Possible causes include increased lipid turnover in cell membranes, defects in desaturase activity, increased oxidation of fatty acids for energy source, increased production of eicosanoids, increased peroxidation of polyunsaturated fatty acids or disorders of lipoprotein metabolism. Although linoleic acid supplements have been shown to be beneficial in CF and for children with recurrent respiratory infections [127], routine supplementation is not advocated and essential fatty acids are usually provided in adequate amounts from the CF diet.

Infant feeding in cystic fibrosis

Screened and non-screened infants have been shown to have nutritional problems at diagnosis. Failure to thrive, anaemia, tocopherol deficiency [128], hypoalbuminaemia [129] and even kwashiorkor [130] are seen in unscreened infants. Nutritional deficits in screened infants are more subtle, but include reduced body mass, length, total body fat, total body potassium and low levels of linoleic acid [131], serum retinol, 25-hydroxyvitamin D [132] and plasma carnitine [133]. Delayed catch-up growth following diagnosis has been seen in screened [134] and non-screened infants [135].

Energy requirements

The energy requirements depend on age and clinical and nutritional state at the time of diagnosis. There is some evidence that infants with CF have increased energy expenditure compared with normal infants of the same age [71,136]. Most infants with pancreatic insufficiency will thrive on a normal energy intake of 100–130 kcal/kg (420–540 kJ/kg) in conjunction with PERT. If weight gain is less than expected or if a meconium ileus has resulted in surgery and bowel resection, the energy requirements may be as high as 150–200 kcal/kg/day (630–836 kJ/kg/day).

Breast milk

Breast milk in conjunction with PERT is widely advocated for the baby with CF [137,138]. Infants on breast milk and PERT grow and gain weight appropriately with near zero z scores [139]. Breast milk has several theoretical advantages over formula:

- An optimal fatty acid profile may improve essential fatty acid status
- It provides immunological protection against infection
- It contains taurine which is necessary for bile salt synthesis
- It contains optimal essential amino acids and bioavailability of iron, calcium and protein
- Breast feeding is better psychologically for the mother

There are two concerns with breast feeding:

1 *Electrolyte depletion* Breast milk is low in sodium. Breast fed infants should be routinely supplemented with sodium. Urinary and sodium electrolytes should be checked if a breast fed baby has poor weight gain.
2 *Successful establishment of breastfeeding* A review

of feeding practices of CF infants in the UK suggests that only a small proportion of infants are breast fed by 3 months of age. The distress and anxiety associated with the diagnosis may lead to initial difficulties in production of breast milk and the pressure of time to undertake treatment and stresses associated with the diagnosis may be responsible for the early cessation of breast feeding. However, with good advice, encouragement and patience from health professionals, these will usually be resolved.

Formula feeding

Standard infant formulas

Women who choose not to breast feed should be supported in their decision. Infants with CF have been shown to thrive satisfactorily on infant whey or casein based formula and pancreatic enzymes. Artificial formula feeds are low in sodium and sodium supplementation may be needed [140].

High energy formulas

High energy formulas (Infatrini, SMA High Energy) are necessary if there is failure of catch-up weight, weight loss or decline in weight for height. High energy formulas are preferable to giving energy supplemented standard infant formulas as they have a better protein : energy ratio and a more concentrated micronutrient profile.

Protein hydrolysate formulas

Although protein hydrolysate formulas are commonly favoured in the USA, no advantages have been proven for their use in the routine care of newly diagnosed infants with CF [135]. They are also less palatable, more expensive and still need PERT administered with them. They should only be used in CF if an infant develops temporary disaccharide intolerance after surgery for meconium ileus.

Cow's milk protein intolerance

Persistent gastrointestinal symptoms despite adequate PERT may indicate cow's milk protein intolerance or lactose intolerance. A protein hydro-lysate formula should be used (Table 7.7).

Pancreatic enzyme replacement therapy: administration in infants

Pancreatic enzyme replacement therapy should be started once there is evidence of malabsorption. Signs may include fatty stools and poor weight gain despite an adequate nutritional intake. Pancreatic insufficiency can be confirmed by measurement of faecal pancreatic elastase-1 on a single stool sample; levels <100 µg/L are indicative of pancreatic insufficiency [141].

Pancreatin powders

Pancreatin powders are rarely used. They have several disadvantages: they taste unpleasant and enzyme on the outside of the infant's lips causes local skin irritation in the infant and of the breast feeding mother's nipples. Pancreatin powders should be mixed with a little expressed breast milk or infant formula and given from a spoon. If the powder is added to a bottle of formula milk it will start digesting the milk and the powder may also get stuck in the hole of the teat.

Enteric-coated microsphere enzyme preparations

The enteric-coated microspheres can be mixed with a little expressed breast milk or formula and then given to a baby from a spoon, but there is a tendency for granules to become lodged in the gums or cause choking. The most practical method of administering these enzymes is to mix them with a small amount of fruit purée (which will hold the enzymes in a gel) and give them from a spoon at the beginning of each feed. This method of enzyme administration can be started at the time of diagnosis and does not need to be delayed until weaning onto solids has begun.

Weaning

Solids should be introduced around the age of 6 months, but not before 17 weeks of age according to the Department of Health recommendations (see p. 525). Early weaning may significantly decrease the volume of breast milk or infant formula taken so there is little benefit in this practice. Parents are encouraged to introduce home-cooked or commercial weaning foods in the normal way. If dried commercial baby foods are used, they can be made up with infant formula instead of water. From 6 months, normal yoghurt and milk puddings can be introduced, although cow's milk should not replace infant formula milk or breast milk for the first year of life.

It is important that parents are encouraged to persist with trying to introduce more texture into the diet as weaning progresses. Often CF infants, like normal infants, will refuse to take lumpy or mashed weaning foods but will readily accept strained or puréed food. Parents will tend to continue with the strained consistencies as they feel that at least their infant is eating something. Failure to introduce more texture and encourage chewing may lead to later feeding problems.

Toddlers and behavioural feeding problems

Excessive focus on food, feeding and weight gain can lead to abnormal feeding patterns and negative feeding behaviour in children with CF. Many factors may precipitate food refusal including parental anxiety about food, acute infections, frequent disruptions because of hospital admissions, and vomiting and gagging associated with coughing spasms. Reports of prolonged mealtimes, vomiting and gagging, constant parental nagging and force feeding indicate that additional support on feeding behaviour management is needed.

The following simple guidelines are helpful when advising parents:

- Encourage parents to sit down at the table and eat together as a family so that mealtime becomes a social event. A lack of structure to mealtimes can lead to both poor routine and poor eating habits. Offer small regular meals.
- Advise parents not to make a fuss or push their child to eat food. If children are forced to eat, they will soon learn how to control the situation by being even more difficult.

- Initially, offer foods that the child will readily accept and gradually increase the variety. A microwave oven is useful to prepare small amounts of favourite food quickly. Favourite foods can be stored in a freezer so they are readily available.
- Remind parents to praise children if they eat anything, even if it is only a small amount. Uneaten food should be taken away without comment.
- Encourage parents to offer small portions of food. Second helpings can easily be given. Desserts served in small containers are particularly helpful.
- Remind parents that likes and dislikes may change from day to day and to keep offering foods even if they were previously refused. Avoid food for which the child has an obvious strong dislike.
- Advise parents not to rush children when eating – but do not let mealtimes drag on, otherwise one meal quickly runs into the next. It may be helpful to set a time limit of no more than 30 minutes.
- Ask parents not to use sweet foods as a bribe and keep these out of sight until savoury foods have been eaten at mealtimes.
- Ask parents not to discuss the child's feeding behaviour in front of them.
- If problems persist the involvement of a psychologist with an interest in feeding problems is indicated.

Pancreatic enzyme replacement therapy

Most CF centres predominantly use enteric-coated microspheres for all infants and children. The most common preparations include Creon Micro, Creon 10000 and Pancrease. These comprise pH sensitive enteric-coated microspheres contained within a gelatine capsule or as a granule preparation. The enteric coating protects the enzymes from stomach acid inactivation, disintegrating to release the enzyme only when pH rises above 5.5 in the duodenum [121]. The administration of enteric-coated microspheres should achieve at least 90% fat absorption if given in appropriate doses. Studies have demonstrated that enteric-coated microspheres are more effective than conventional

Table 11.7   Pancreatic enzyme preparations available in the UK.

Product (manufacturer)	Composition (per g powder/granules or per capsule/tablet BP units)		
	Lipase	Protease	Amylase
Powder			
Pancrex V (Paines & Byrne)	25 000	1400	30 000
Capsules			
Pancrex V (Paines & Byrne)	8000	430	9000
Pancrex V 125mg (Paines & Byrne)	2950	160	3300
Tablets			
Enteric-coated tablets			
Pancrex V (Paines & Byrne)	1900	110	1700
Pancrex V Forte (Paines & Byrne)	5600	330	5000
Enteric-coated microspheres			
Pancrease (Janssen-Cilag)	5000	330	2900
Creon 10000 (Solvay)	10 000	600	8000
Creon 25000 (Solvay)	25 000	1000	18 000
Creon 40000 (Solvay)	40 000	1600	25 000
Enteric-coated minitablets			
Pancrease HL (Cilag)	25 000	1250	22 500
Nutrizym 10 (Merck)	10 000	500	9000
Nutrizym 22 (Merck)	22 000	1100	19 800
Granule microspheres (per scoop)			
Creon⁾ Micro (Solvay)	5000	200	3600

pancreatic powder and enteric-coated capsules [142]. The composition of common pancreatic enzymes available in the UK is given in Table 11.7.

Several factors may influence the effectiveness of pancreatic enzymes: the buffering action of food may cause premature dissolution within the stomach leading to the destruction of the released enzyme; duodenal pH may be abnormally acid because pancreatic bicarbonate production is low and gastric hypersecretion is high [143].

High lipase pancreatic enzymes

In 1993, the UK Committee on Safety of Medicines recommended that Pancrease HL, Nutrizym 22 and

Panzytrat 25000 were contraindicated in CF for children aged 15 years and under. Most high lipase pancreatic enzymes containing 22 000–25 000 units of lipase per capsule are associated with the development of fibrosing colonopathy, although its precise aetiology remains uncertain. After the first reports in Liverpool similar cases were reported elsewhere in the UK [144–146], Ireland [147], Denmark [148] and the USA [149].

Fibrosing colonopathy should be considered in patients with CF who have evidence of obstruction, bloody diarrhoea or chylous ascites, or a combination of abdominal pain, distention with continuing diarrhoea and/or poor weight gain. Patients at higher risk include those less than 12 years of age, on high dosages of pancreatic lipase [150,151], who have a history of meconium ileus [152] or DIOS, and those who have had any intestinal surgery or have a diagnosis of inflammatory bowel disease [153]. However, not all high strength products (i.e. Creon 25000), have been found to be associated with colonic strictures. Preparations linked with colonic strictures in the UK are all minitablets which contain Eudragit-L, a co-polymer based on methylacrylic acid and ethyl acrylate, in their coating (e.g. Pancrease HL and Nutrizym 22). These compounds have been shown to have a toxic effect on the gut of experimental animals and may be a causal factor in the aetiology of fibrosing colonopathy [26]. This theory is supported by the observation of two cases of two younger children developing fibrosing colonopathy on the lower strength preparation, Nutrizym GR, which contains the methylacrylic co-polymer [154]. The USA has found no relationship between coating and fibrosing colonopathy, although their interpretation of statistics has been criticised [155].

Dose of pancreatic enzymes

Patients with CF vary in their degree of pancreatic insufficiency and individual PERT requirements differ. On average, infants and young children have a higher requirement for lipase per kilogram body weight than older children. This reflects the higher fat intake of their diet which is 5 g fat/kg/day for infants compared with 2 g fat/kg/day for adults. The dose should be titrated against the fat content of the meal or snack consumed with most patients

requiring between 50–100 IU lipase/g dietary fat/kg/day [156].

It is recommended by the Committee on Safety of Medicines (CSM) that a maximum of 10000 IU lipase/kg/day is given from pancreatic enzyme preparations, irrespective of formulation [157]. The dosage depends on residual pancreatic function, enzyme supplement properties, amount of fat and protein consumed and pathophysiological factors [121]. Dosage is often determined by stool output (frequency/colour/consistency), presence of abdominal pain and by faecal fat studies. Before the recommendations by the CSM, it was not uncommon for many patients to be on much higher doses of PERT. It has been demonstrated that dosage can be reduced to acceptable intakes for many patients without deterioration in growth and acceptable coefficient of fat absorption [158,159].

Parents and older children should receive education on the fat content of foods and should be taught to titrate their enzymes to correspond with the foods eaten. This education is essential if symptoms of malabsorption are to be minimised and should be ongoing. A variety of approaches can be taken including the use of fat exchanges in some centres, although a more general approach is to educate patients to identify high, medium and low fat foods, thus allowing them to titrate their enzyme dosage with sufficient accuracy.

A guideline for the maximum number of pancreatic enzymes, using standard preparation per kilogram body weight, is given in Table 11.8.

Administration of pancreatic enzymes

Pancreatic enzymes should be administered with all meals and protein and fat-containing snacks

Table 11.8 Maximum daily dosage of pancreatic enzyme preparation to provide 10 000 units lipase/kg/day.

Weight (kg)	Creon 10000	Pancrease
5	5	10
10	10	20
15	15	30
20	20	40
25	25	50
30	30	60
35	35	70

Table 11.9 General guidelines for the use of pancreatic enzyme preparations.

Give with every meal at the beginning and during the meal rather than all before or after

It may be necessary to give extra enzymes with fatty meals

Give enzymes with snacks (e.g. milk, crisps and chocolate biscuits). There is no need to give with squash, lemonade, fruit, boiled or jelly sweets

Give enzymes with supplemented milk shake drinks

Creon 10 000 and Pancrease capsules can be swallowed whole. Where swallowing is difficult, they may be opened and the contents taken with liquids or mixed with jam or honey (do not use honey in infants under 1 year of age). They should not be crushed or chewed

Do not mix with hot food or food with a pH of more than 5.5

(Table 11.9). There is evidence that PERT should be spread throughout the meal to optimise mixing and minimise partitioning of the pancreatin with the liquid phase of the meal, which empties more rapidly than the solid phase [160]. Young children should be encouraged to swallow the whole capsules as soon as possible, usually from 4–5 years of age. Until then, there is little option but to give the granules out of the capsule. However, some toddlers may chew the granules or hold them in their mouth for considerable periods of time, thus releasing the enzymes and predisposing to mouth ulcers. Toddlers often refuse their enzymes and coughing, choking and even vomiting is common. As the amount of food eaten by toddlers will vary from meal to meal, it is recommended to spread the pancreatic enzymes throughout the meal.

Adjunctive therapy to pancreatic enzymes

Histamine (H_2) receptor antagonists such as cimetidine have been used as an adjunct to PERT. They aim to reduce both the volume and the acid concentration of gastric secretion and thereby prevent acid/peptic inactivation of the enzymes. They may help increase efficiency of enteric-coated enzymes and are worth considering if patients have uncontrolled symptoms on large doses of pancreatic enzymes. Alternatives are proton pump inhibitors (e.g. omeprazole) which suppress gastric acid secretions.

Dietary management of diabetes in children with CF

There are conflicts between the dietary therapy of CF and diabetes mellitus and these should usually be resolved in favour of the CF diet; however, advice should be tailored according to the severity of the CF. Although the aim is to achieve normoglycaemia, the provision of optimal nutrition is still of paramount importance and any dietary restriction should be minimised. It is recommended that a CF specialist dietitian should advise the patient on an individualised dietary plan. In most instances, medical management should be tailored to the patient's needs rather than the diet being tailored to the insulin regimen [47].

Guidelines

- Encourage a high energy intake of 120–150% EAR
- Aim to give 40% of total energy as fat; consider the use of mono- and polyunsaturated fats
- Refined carbohydrates should not be routinely restricted, but there needs to be a balance between the timing, hypoglycaemic medication and activity levels; if possible, refined carbohydrates should be consumed after meals or with snacks containing complex carbohydrates, but not at the expense of nutritional intake
- Encourage regular meals and snacks containing complex carbohydrate
- A moderate fibre intake should be given to well-nourished patients
- Salt should not be restricted
- Dietary supplements should be used as necessary; milk based supplements are preferable to glucose polymers
- Nutritional status and blood glucose should be monitored closely

Poor diabetic control should be improved by alterations in insulin therapy rather than imposing dietary restrictions that may adversely affect nutritional status. When treating the child with CF and diabetes it is necessary to involve the expertise of the diabetic team who need to fully understand and support the rationale for the different dietary approach.

References

1 Dodge JA, Morison S, Lewis PA *et al.* (the UK Cystic Fibrosis Survey Management Committee) Incidence, population, and survival of cystic fibrosis in the UK, 1968–1995. *Arch Dis Child*, 1997, **77** 493–6.

2 Jackson A Clinical guidelines for cystic fibrosis care. *J Roy Coll Physicians*, 1996, **30** 305–8.

3 Corey M, McLaughlin FJ, Williams M, Levinson H A comparison of survival, growth and pulmonary function in patients with cystic fibrosis. *J Clin Epidemiol*, 1988, **41** 583–91.

4 Forstner G, Durie P Nutrition in cystic fibrosis. In: Grand RJ, Sutphen JL, Dietz WH (eds) *Pediatric Nutrition. Theory and Practice.* Boston: Butterworths, 1987.

5 Alemzadeh R, Upchurch L, McCarthy V Anabolic effects of growth hormone treatment in young children with cystic fibrosis. *J Am Coll Nutr*, 1998, **17** 419–24.

6 Johannesson M, Gottlieb C, Hjelte L Delayed puberty in girls with cystic fibrosis despite good clinical outcome. *Pediatrics*, 1997, **99** 29–34.

7 Kerem B-S, Rommens JM, Buchanan JA *et al.* Identification of the cystic fibrosis gene: genetic analysis. *Science*, 1989, **245** 1073–80.

8 Anthony H, Paxton S, Catto-Smith A, Phelan P Physiological and psychological contributors to malnutrition in children with cystic fibrosis: review. *Clin Nutr*, 1999, **18** 327–35.

9 Jaffé A, Bush A, Geddes DM, Alton EWFW Prospects for gene therapy in cystic fibrosis. *Arch Dis Child*, 1999, **80** 286–9.

10 WHO/ICF (M) A Therapeutic approaches to cystic fibrosis: Memorandum from a joint WHO/ICF (M) A meeting. *Bull World Health Organ*, 1994, **72** 341–52.

11 Carlos E, Milla MD, Billings J, Moran A. Diabetes is associated with dramatically reduced survival in females but not male subjects with Cystic Fibrosis. *Diabetes Care*, 2005, **28** 2141–4.

12 Nir M, Lanng S, Johansen HK, Koch C Long term survival and nutritional data in patients with cystic fibrosis treated in a Danish centre. *Thorax*, 1996, **51** 1023–7.

13 Guritz D, Francis P, Crozier M, Levison H Perspectives in cystic fibrosis. *Pediatr Clin North Am*, 1979, **26** 603–15.

14 Schechter MS, Margolis PA Relationship between socioeconomic status and disease severity in cystic fibrosis. *J Pediatr*, 1997, **132** 260–4.

15 Couriel J Respiratory disorders. In: Lissauer T, Clayden G (eds) *Illustrated Textbook of Paediatrics.* London: Mosby, 1997, pp. 157–71.

16 Kopito LE, Shwachman H, Vawter GF, Edlow J The pancreas in cystic fibrosis: chemical composition and comparative morphology. *Pediatr Res*, 1976, **10** 742–9.

17 Sokol RJ The GI system and nutrition in cystic fibrosis. *Pediatr Pulmonol*, 1990, **Suppl 5** 81–3.

18 Littlewood JM Gastrointestinal investigations in cystic fibrosis. *J Roy Soc Med*, 1992, **85** (Suppl 18) 13–19.

19 Littlewood JM Abdominal pain in cystic fibrosis. *J R Soc Med*, 1996, (Suppl 25) **88** 9–17.

20 Heine RG, Button BM, Olinsky A *et al.* Gastrointestinal reflux in infants under 6 months with cystic fibrosis. *Arch Dis Child*, 1998, **78** 44–8.

21 Cucchiara S, Santamaria F, Andreotti MR *et al.* Mechanisms of gastro-oesophageal reflux in cystic fibrosis. *Arch Dis Child*, 1991, **66** 617–22.

22 Button BM, Heine RG, Catto-Smith AG *et al.* Postural drainage and gastro-oesophageal reflux in infants with cystic fibrosis. *Arch Dis Child*, 1997, **76** 148–50.

23 Stringer DA, Sprigg A, Juodis E *et al.* The association of cystic fibrosis, gastro-esophageal reflux, and reduced pulmonary function. *Can Assoc Radiol J*, 1988, **39** 100–2.

24 Smith RL, van Velzen D, Smyth AR *et al.* Strictures of ascending colon in cystic fibrosis and high strength pancreatic enzymes. *Lancet*, 1994, **343** 85–6.

25 Dodge JA The aetiology of fibrosing colonopathy. *Postgrad Med J*, 1996, **72** (Suppl 2) S52–5.

26 Van Velzan D, Ball LM, Dezfulian AR *et al.* Comparative and experimental pathology of fibrosing colonopathy. *Postgrad Med J*, 1996, **72** (Suppl 2) 39–48.

27 Schoni MH, Maisonneuve P, Schöni-Affolter F, Lowenfels AB Cancer risk in patients with cystic fibrosis. *J Roy Soc Med*, 1996, **89** (Suppl 27) 38–47.

28 Bell SC, Bowerman AR, Davies CA *et al.* Nutrition in adults with cystic fibrosis. *Clin Nutr*, 1998, **17** 211–15.

29 Dodge JA The nutritional state and nutrition. *Acta Paediatr Scand*, 1985, **Suppl 317** 31–7.

30 Goodchild MC Nutritional management of cystic fibrosis. *Digestion*, 1987, **37** (Suppl 1) 61–7.

31 Ghosal S, Taylor CJ, Pickering M, McGaw J Head growth in cystic fibrosis following early diagnosis by neonatal screening. *Arch Dis Child*, 1996, **75** 191–3.

32 Morison S, Dodge JA, Cole TJ *et al.* Height and weight in cystic fibrosis: a cross sectional study. *Arch Dis Child*, 1997, **77** 497–500.

33 Chatfield S, Owen G, Ryley HC *et al.* Neonatal screening for cystic fibrosis in Wales and the West Midlands: clinical assessment after 5 years of screening. *Arch Dis Child*, 1991, **66** 29–33.

34 Lai H-C, Kosorok MR, Sondel SA *et al.* Growth status in children with cystic fibrosis based on the

national cystic fibrosis patient registry data: evaluation of various criteria used to identify malnutrition. *J Pediatr*, 1998, **132** 478–5.

35   Lai H-C, Corey M, FitzSimmons S *et al*. Comparison of growth status of patients with cystic fibrosis between the United States and Canada. *Am J Clin Nutr*, 1999, **69** 531–58.

36   Huseman CA, Colombo JL, Brooks MA *et al*. Anabolic effect of biosynthetic growth hormone in cystic fibrosis patients. *Pediatr Pulmonol*, 1996, **22** 90–5.

37   WHO Study Group Diabetes mellitus. *World Health Organ Tech Rep Ser*, 1985, **727** 1–113.

38   Lanng S, Hansen A, Thorsteinsson B *et al*. Glucose tolerance in patients with cystic fibrosis: 5 year prospective study. *Br Med J*, 1995, **311** 655–9.

39   Robert JJ, Grasset E, de Montalembert M *et al*. Research of factors for glucose intolerance in mucoviscidosis (in French). *Arch Fr Pediatr*, 1992, **49** 17–22.

40   De Luca F, Arigo T, Nibali SC *et al*. Insulin secretion, glycosylated haemoglobin and islet cell antibodies in cystic fibrosis children and adolescents with different degrees of glucose tolerance. *Horm Metab Res*, 1991, **23** 495–8.

41   Lanng S, Thorsteinsson B, Lund-Andersen C *et al*. Diabetes mellitus in Danish cystic fibrosis patients: prevalence and late diabetic complications. *Acta Paediatr*, 1994, **83** 72–7.

42   Cucinotta D, Arrigo T, De Luca F *et al*. Metabolic and clinical events preceding diabetes mellitus onset in cystic fibrosis. *Eur J Endocrinol*, 1996, **134** 731–6.

43   Lanng S, Thorsteinsson B, Nerup J, Koch C Influence of the development of diabetes mellitus on clinical status in patients with cystic fibrosis. *Eur J Pediatr*, 1992, **151** 684–7.

44   Sullivan MM, Denning CR Diabetic microangiography in patients with cystic fibrosis. *Pediatrics*, 1989, **84** 642–7.

45   Allen JL Progressive nephropathy in a patient with cystic fibrosis and diabetes. *N Engl J Med*, 1986, **315** 764.

46   Dolan TF Microangiography in a young adult with cystic fibrosis and diabetes mellitus. *N Engl J Med*, 1986, **314** 991–2.

47   Report of the UK Cystic Fibrosis Trust Diabetes Working Group *Management of Cystic Fibrosis Related Diabetes Mellitus*. CF Trust, Kent, 2004.

48   Wilschanski M, Rivlin J, Cohen S *et al*. Clinical and genetic risk factors for cystic fibrosis-related liver disease. *Pediatrics*, 1999, **103** 52–7.

49   Sharp HL Cystic fibrosis liver disease and transplantation. *J Pediatr*, 1995, **127** 944–6.

50   Colombo C, Apostolo MG, Ferrari M *et al*. Analysis of risk factors in the development of liver disease in CF. *J Pediatr*, 1994, **124** 393–6.

51   FitzSimmons SC The changing epidemiology of cystic fibrosis. *J Pediatr*, 1993, **122** 1–9.

52   Mack DR, Traystman MD, Colombo C *et al*. Clinical denouement and mutation analysis of patients with cystic fibrosis undergoing liver transplantation for biliary cirrhosis. *J Pediatr*, 1995, **127** 881–7.

53   Colombo C, Battezzati PM, Podda M, Bettinardi N, Giunta A & Italian Group for the study of ursodeoxycholic acid in cystic fibrosis Ursodeoxycholic acid for liver disease associated with cystic fibrosis: a double-blind multicentre trial. *Hepatology*, 1996, **23** 1484–90.

54   Gibson LE, Cooke RE A test for concentration of electrolytes in sweat in cystic fibrosis of the pancreas utilising pilocarpine by iontophoresis. *Pediatrics*, 1959, **23** 545–9.

55   Hill CM *Practical Guidelines for Cystic Fibrosis Care*. London: Churchill Livingstone, 1998.

56   Waters DL, Wilken B, Irwig L *et al*. Clinical outcomes of newborn screening for cystic fibrosis. *Arch Dis Child Fetal Neonatal Ed*, 1999, **80** F1–7.

57   De Meer K, Gulmans AM, van der Laag J Peripheral muscle weakness and exercise capacity in children with cystic fibrosis. *Am J Respir Crit Care Med*, 1998, **159** 748–54.

58   Thomson MA, Quirk P, Swanson CE *et al*. Nutritional growth retardation is associated with defective lung growth in cystic fibrosis: a preventable determinant of progressive pulmonary dysfunction. *Nutrition*, 1995, **11** 350–4.

59   Murphy JL, Wootton SA, Bond SA, Jackson AA Energy content of stools in normal healthy controls and patients with cystic fibrosis. *Arch Dis Child*, 1991, **66** 495–500.

60   Turck D, Michaud L Cystic fibrosis: nutritional consequences and management. *Baillière's Clin Gastroenterol*, 1998, **12** 805–22.

61   Barth AL, Pitt TL The high amino-acid content of sputum from cystic fibrosis patients promotes growth of auxotrophic *Pseudomonas aeruginosa*. *J Med Microbiol*, 1996, **45** 110–19.

62   Vaisman N, Pencharz PB, Corey M *et al*. Energy expenditure of patients with cystic fibrosis. *J Pediatr*, 1987, **111** 496–500.

63   Buchdahl RM, Cox M, Fulleylove C *et al*. Increased resting energy expenditure in cystic fibrosis. *J App Phys*, 1988, **64** 1810–16.

64   Fried MD, Durie PR, Tsui L-C *et al*. The cystic fibrosis gene and resting energy expenditure. *J Pediatr*, 1991, **119** 913–16.

65   Bell SC, Saunder MJ, Elborn JS, Shale DJ Resting energy expenditure and oxygen cost of breathing in patients with cystic fibrosis. *Thorax*, 1996, **51** 126–31.

66 Steinkamp G, Drommer A, von der Hardt H Resting energy expenditure before and after treatment for *Pseudomonas aeruginosa* infection in patients with cystic fibrosis. *Am J Clin Nutr*, 1993, **57** 685–9.

67 Vaisman N, Levy LD, Pencharz PB *et al*. Effect of salbutamol on resting energy expenditure in patients with cystic fibrosis. *J Pediatr*, 1987, **111** 137–9.

68 O'Rawe A, McIntosh J, Dodge JA *et al*. Increased energy expenditure in cystic fibrosis is associated with specific mutations. *Clin Sci*, 1990, **82** 71–6.

69 Spicher V, Roulet M, Schutz Y Assessment of total energy expenditure in free living patients with cystic fibrosis. *J Pediatr*, 1991, **118** 865–72.

70 Zemel BS, Kawchak DA, Cnaan A *et al*. Prospective evaluation of resting energy expenditure, nutritional status, pulmonary function, and genotype in children with cystic fibrosis. *Pediatr Res*, 1996, **40** 578–86.

71 Shepherd RW, Holt TL, Vasquez-Velasquez L, Prentice AM Increased energy expenditure in young children with CF. *Lancet*, 1988, **i** 1300–3.

72 Kawchak DA, Zhao H, Scanlin MF *et al*. Longitudinal, prospective analysis of dietary intake in children with cystic fibrosis. *J Pediatr*, 1996, **129** 119–29.

73 Anthony H, Bines J, Phelan P, Paxton S Relation between dietary intake and nutritional status in cystic fibrosis. *Arch Dis Child*, 1998, **78** 443–7.

74 Stark LJ, Jelalian E, Mulvihill MM *et al*. Eating in preschool children with cystic fibrosis and healthy peers: behavioral analysis. *Pediatrics*, 1995, **95** 210–15.

75 Stark LJ, Mulvihill MM, Jelalian E *et al*. Descriptive analysis of eating behavior in school-age children with cystic fibrosis and healthy control children. *Pediatrics*, 1997, **99** 665–71.

76 Crist W, McDonnell P, Beck M *et al*. Behavior at mealtimes and nutritional intake in the young child with cystic fibrosis. *Dev Behav Pediatr*, 1994, **15** 157–61.

77 Miller M, Ward L, Thomas BJ *et al*. Altered body composition and muscle protein degradation in nutritionally growth retarded children with cystic fibrosis. *Am J Clin Nutr*, 1982, **36** 492–9.

78 Cole TJ, Donnett ML, Stanfield JP Weight for height indices to assess nutritional status – a new index on a slide rule. *Am J Clin Nutr*, 1981, **34** 1935–43.

79 Poustie VJ, Watling RM, Ashby D, Smyth RL Reliability of percentage ideal weight for height. *Arch Dis Child*, 2000, **83** 183–4.

80 Poustie VJ, Russell JE, Watling RM *et al*. Oral protein energy supplements for children with cystic fibrosis; CALICO multicentre randomised controlled trial. *Br Med J*, 2006, **10** 1136.

81 CF Trust *Nutritional Management of Cystic Fibrosis*. UK CF Trust Nutrition Working Group, April 2002.

82 Ramsey BW, Farrell PM, Pancharz P & Consensus Committee Nutritional assessment and management in cystic fibrosis. *Am J Clin Nutr*, 1992, **55** 108–16.

83 Reilly JJ, Evans TJ, Wilkinson J, Paton JY Adequacy of clinical formulae for estimation of energy requirements in children with cystic fibrosis. *Arch Dis Child*, 1999, **81** 120–4.

84 Shepherd RW, Holt TL, Johnson LP *et al*. Leucine metabolism and body cell mass in cystic fibrosis. *Nutrition*, 1995, **11** 138–41.

85 Collins CE, O'Loughlin EV, Henry RL Fat gram target to achieve high intake in cystic fibrosis. *J Paediatr Child Health*, 1997, **33** 142–7.

86 Slesinski MJ, Gloninger MF, Costantino JP, Orenstein DM Lipid levels in adults with cystic fibrosis. *J Am Diet Assoc*, 1994, **94** 402–8.

87 Gavin J, Ellis J, Dewar AL, *et al*. Dietary fibre and the occurrence of gut symptoms in cystic fibrosis. *Arch Dis Child*, 1997, **76** 35–7.

88 Brown KH, Sanchez-Grinan M, Perez F *et al*. Effects of dietary energy density and feeding frequency on total daily energy intakes of recovering malnourished children. *Am J Clin Nutr*, 1995, **62** 13–18.

89 Jelalaian E, Stark LJ, Reynolds L, Seifer R Nutrition intervention for weight gain in cystic fibrosis: a meta analysis. *J Pediatr*, 1998, **132** 486–92.

90 Rettammel AL, Marcus MS, Farrell PM *et al*. Oral supplementation with a high-fat, high-energy product improves nutritional status and alters serum lipids in patients with cystic fibrosis. *J Am Diet Assoc*, 1995, **95** 454–9.

91 Skypala IJ, Ashworth FA, Hodson ME *et al*. Oral nutritional supplements promote significant weight gain in cystic fibrosis patients. *J Hum Nutr Diet*, 1998, **11** 95–104.

92 MacDonald A Nutritional management of cystic fibrosis: personal practice. *Arch Dis Child*, 1996, **74** 81–7.

93 Rosenfield M, Casey S, Pepe M, Ramsey BW Nutritional effects of long-term gastrostomy feedings in children with cystic fibrosis. *J Am Diet Assoc*, 1999, **99** 191–4.

94 Walker SA, Gozal D Pulmonary function correlates in the prediction of long-term weight gain in cystic fibrosis patients with gastrostomy tube feedings. *J Pediatr Gastroenterol Nutr*, 1998, **27** 53–6.

95 Boland MP, Stoski DS, MacDonald NE *et al*. Chronic jejunostomy feeding with a non-elemental formula in undernourished patients with cystic fibrosis. *Lancet*, 1986, **1** 232–4.

96 Shepherd RW, Holt TL, Thomas BJ *et al.* Nutritional rehabilitation in cystic fibrosis: controlled studies of effects of nutritional growth retardation, body protein turnover and cause of pulmonary disease. *J Pediatr*, 1986, **109** 788–94.

97 Steinkamp G, von der Hardt H Improvement of nutritional status and lung function after long-term nocturnal gastrostomy feeding in cystic fibrosis. *J Pediatr*, 1994, **106** 223–7.

98 Dalzell AM, Shepherd RW, Dean B *et al.* Nutritional rehabilitation in cystic fibrosis: a 5 year follow-up study. *J Pediatr Gastroenter Nutr*, 1992, **15** 141–5.

99 Erskine JM, Lingard CD, Sontag MK, Accurso FJ Enteral nutrition for patients with cystic fibrosis: comparison of a semi-elemental and non-elemental formula. *J Pediatr*, 1998, **132** 265–9.

100 Williams SGJ, Ashworth F, McAlweenie A *et al.* Percutaneous endoscopic gastrostomy feeding in patients with cystic fibrosis. *Gut*, 1999, **44** 87–90.

101 Fitting JW Nutritional support in chronic obstructive lung disease. *Thorax*, 1992, **47** 141–3.

102 Kane RE, Hobbs PJ, Black P Comparison of low, medium and high carbohydrate formulas for night time enteral feedings in cystic fibrosis patients. *J Parenter Enteral Nutr*, 1990, **14** 47–52.

103 Milla C, Doherty L, Raatz S *et al.* Glycemic response to dietary supplement in cystic fibrosis is dependent on the carbohydrate content of the formula. *J Parenter Enteral Nutr*, 1996, **20** 182–6.

104 Morton A, Conway S Enteral feeding by gastrostomy is more effective than by nasogastric route in patients with cystic fibrosis. XIIth International Cystic Fibrosis Congress – I.C.F. (M)A, Jerusalem (abstract), 1996.

105 Patchell CJ, Desai M, Smyth RC *et al.* Creon 10000 vs Creon 8000 – a preference study (abstract). Presented at 23rd European CF Conference, The Hague, The Netherlands, 1999.

106 Ahmed F, Ellis J, Murphy J *et al.* Excessive faecal losses of vitamin A (retinol) in cystic fibrosis. *Arch Dis Child*, 1990, **65** 589–93.

107 Smith FR, Underwood BA, Denning CR *et al.* Depressed plasma retinol-binding protein levels in cystic fibrosis. *J Lab Clin Med*, 1972, **80** 423–33.

108 Lindblad A, Diczfalusy U, Hultcrantz R *et al.* Vitamin A concentration in liver decreases with age in patients with cystic fibrosis. *J Pediatr Gastroenterol Nutr*, 1997, **24** 264–70.

109 Winklhofer-Roob BM, van't Hof MA, Shmerling DH Long-term oral vitamin E supplementation in cystic fibrosis patients: *RRR*-α-tocopherol compared with all-*rac*-α-tocopheryl acetate preparations. *Am J Clin Nutr*, 1996, **63** 722–8.

110 Thomas PS, Bellamy M, Geddes D Malabsorption of vitamin E in cystic fibrosis improved after ursodeoxycholic acid. *Lancet*, 1995, **346** 1230–1.

111 Henderson RC, Madsen CD Bone density in children and adolescents with cystic fibrosis. *J Pediatr*, 1996, **128** 28–34.

112 Donovan DS Jr, Papdopoulos A, Staron RB *et al.* Bone mass and vitamin D deficiency in adults with advanced cystic fibrosis lung disease. *Am J Respir Crit Care Med*, 1998, **157** 1892–9.

113 Laursem E, Mølgaard C, Michaelsen KF *et al.* Bone mineral status in 134 patients with cystic fibrosis. *Arch Dis Child*, 1999, **81** 235–40.

114 Shaw N, Bedford C, Heaf D, Carty H Osteopenia in adults with cystic fibrosis. *Am J Med*, 1995, **99** 690–1.

115 Salamoni F, Roulet M, Gudinchet F *et al.* Bone mineral content in cystic fibrosis patients: correlation with fat-free mass. *Arch Dis Child*, 1996, **74** 314–18.

116 Wolfe SP, Conway SP, Brownlee KG Seasonal variation in vitamin D levels in children with CF in the United Kingdom. 14th European CF Conference. Vienna 2001. (abstract)

117 Elkin SL, Fairney A, Burnett S *et al.* Vertebral deformities and low bone mineral density in adults with cystic fibrosis: a cross sectional study. *Osteoporosis International*, 2001, **12** 366–72.

118 Rashid M, Durie P, Andrew M *et al.* Prevalence of vitamin K deficiency in cystic fibrosis. *Am J Clin Nutr*, 1999, **70** 378–82.

119 Beker LT, Ahrens RA, Fink RJ *et al.* Effect of vitamin K_1 supplementation on vitamin K status in cystic fibrosis patients. *J Pediatr Gastroenterol Nutr*, 1997, **24** 512–17.

120 Peters SA, Rolles CJ Vitamin therapy in cystic fibrosis – a review and rationale. *J Clin Pharm Ther*, 1993, **18** 33–8.

121 Leonard CH, Knox AJ Pancreatic enzyme supplements and vitamins in cystic fibrosis. *J Hum Nutr Diet*, 1997, **10** 3–16.

122 Leonard CH, Ross-Wilson C, Smyth AR *et al.* A study of a single high potency multivitamin preparation in the management of cystic fibrosis. *J Hum Nutr Diet*, 1998, **11** 493–500.

123 Pencharz PB, Durie PR Nutritional management of cystic fibrosis. *Ann Rev Nutr*, 1993, **13** 111–36.

124 Jeppesen PB, Christensen MS, Høy CE, Mortensen PB Essential fatty acid deficiency in patients with severe fat malabsorption. *Am J Clin Nutr*, 1997, **65** 837–43.

125 van Egmond AWA, Kosorok MR, Koscik R *et al.* Effect of linoleic acid intake on growth of infants with cystic fibrosis. *Am J Clin Nutr*, 1996, **63** 746–52.

126 Parsons HG, Oloughlin EV, Forbes D *et al.* Supplemental calories improve essential fatty acid deficiency in cystic fibrosis patients. *Pediatr Res*, 1998, **24** 353–6.

127   Venuta A, Spano C, Laudizi L et al. Essential fatty acids: the effects of dietary supplementation among children with recurrent respiratory infections. J Int Med Res, 1996, **24** 325–30.

128   Swann IL, Kendra JR Case Report. Anaemia, vitamin E deficiency and failure to thrive in an infant. Clin Lab Haematol, 1998, **20** 61–3.

129   Bines JE, Israel EJ Hypoproteinemia, anemia and failure to thrive in an infant. Gastroenterology, 1991, **101** 848–56.

130   Phillips RJ, Crock CM, Dillon MJ et al. Cystic fibrosis presenting as kwashiorkor with florid skin rash. Arch Dis Child, 1993, **69** 446–8.

131   Marcus MS, Sondel SA, Farrell PM et al. Nutritional status of infants with cystic fibrosis associated with early diagnosis and intervention. Am J Clin Nutr, 1991, **54** 578–85.

132   Sokol RJ, Reardon MC, Accurso FJ et al. Fat-soluble vitamin status during the first year of life in infants with cystic fibrosis identified by screening of newborns (1989). Am J Clin Nutr, 1989, **50** 1064–71.

133   Lloyd-Still JD, Powers C Carnitine metabolites in infants with cystic fibrosis. Acta Univ Carol [Med] (Praha), 1990, **36** 78–80.

134   Greer R, Shepherd R, Cleghorn G et al. Evaluation of growth and changes in body composition following neonatal diagnosis of cystic fibrosis. J Pediatr Gastroenterol Nutr, 1991, **13** 52–8.

135   Ellis L, Kalnins D, Corey M et al. Do infants with cystic fibrosis need a protein hydrolysate formula? A prospective, randomized, comparative study. J Pediatr, 1998, **132** 270–6.

136   Girardet JP, Tounian P, Sardet A et al. Resting energy expenditure in infants with cystic fibrosis. J Pediatr Gastroenterol Nutr, 1994, **18** 214–19.

137   Green MR, Buchanan E, Weaver LT Nutritional management of the infant with cystic fibrosis. Arch Dis Child, 1995, **72** 452–6.

138   Anthony H, Catto-Smith A, Phelan P, Paxton S Current approaches to the nutritional management of cystic fibrosis in Australia. J Pediatr Child Health, 1998, **34** 170–4.

139   Holliday KE, Allen KJ, Walters DL et al. Growth of human milk-fed and formula fed infants with cystic fibrosis. J Pediatr, 1991, **118** 77–9.

140   Laughlin JJ, Brady MS, Eigen H Changing feeding trends as a cause of electrolyte depletion in infants with cystic fibrosis. J Am Diet Assoc, 1981, **87** 1353–6.

141   Cade A, Walters MP, McGinley N et al. Evaluation of faecal pancreatic elastase–1 as a measure of exocrine pancreatic function in children with cystic fibrosis. Pediatr Pulmonol, 2000, **29** 172–6.

142   Patchell CJ, MacDonald A, Weller PW Pancreatic enzymes with enteral feeds – how should we give them? 22nd European CF Conference, Berlin, Germany (abstract), 1998.

143   Barraclough M, Taylor CJ Twenty-four hour ambulatory gastric and duodenal pH profiles in cystic fibrosis: effect of duodenal hyperacidity on pancreatic enzyme function and fat absorption. J Pediatr Gastroenterol Nutr, 1996, **23** 45–50.

144   Oades PJ, Bush A, Ong PS, Breton RJ High-strength pancreatic enzyme supplements and large-bowel stricture in cystic fibrosis (letter). Lancet, 1994, **343** 109.

145   Campbell CA, Forrest J, Musgrove C High-strength pancreatic enzyme supplements and large-bowel stricture in cystic fibrosis (letter). Lancet, 1994, **343** 109.

146   Briars GL, Griffiths DM, Moore IE et al. High-strength pancreatic enzymes. Lancet, 1994, **343** 600.

147   Mahoney MJ, Corcoran M High-strength pancreatic enzymes. Lancet, 1994, **343** 599–600.

148   Knabe N, Zak M, Hanson A et al. Extensive pathologic changes of the colon in cystic fibrosis and high-strength pancreatic enzymes. Lancet, 1994, **343** 1230.

149   Frieman JP, FitzSimmons SC Colonic strictures in patients with cystic fibrosis: results of a survey of 114 cystic fibrosis care centers in the United States. J Pediatr Gastroenterol Nutr, 1996, **22** 153–6.

150   Smyth RL, Ashby D, O'Hea U et al. Fibrosing colonopathy in cystic fibrosis: results of a case-control study. Lancet, 1995, **346** 1247–51.

151   FitzSimmons SC, Burkhart GA, Borowitz D et al. High-dose pancreatic-enzyme supplements and fibrosing colonopathy in children with cystic fibrosis. N Engl J Med, 1997, **336** 1283–9.

152   Stevens JC, Maguiness KM, Hollingsworth J et al. Pancreatic enzyme supplementation in cystic fibrosis patients before and after fibrosing colonopathy. J Pediatr Gastroenterol Nutr, 1998, **26** 80–4.

153   Borowitz DS, Grand RJ, Durie PR & Consensus Committee Use of pancreatic enzyme supplements for patients with cystic fibrosis in the context of fibrosing colonopathy. J Pediatr, 1995, **127** 681–4.

154   Jones R, Franklin K, Spicer R et al. Colonic strictures in children with cystic fibrosis on low-strength pancreatic enzymes. Lancet, 1995, **346** 499–500.

155   Prescott P Pancreatic enzymes and fibrosing colonopathy. Correspondence. Lancet, 1999, **354** 250.

156   Durie P, Kalnins D, Ellis L Uses and abuses of enzyme therapy in cystic fibrosis. J Roy Soc Med, 1998, **91** (Suppl 34) 2–13.

157   Committee on the Safety of Medicines Report of the Pancreatic Enzymes Working Party. London.

Committee on the Safety of Medicines: Medicines Control Agency, 1995.

158   Lowden J, Goodchild MC, Ryley HC, Doull IJM Maintenance of growth in cystic fibrosis despite reduction in pancreatic enzyme supplementation. *Arch Dis Child*, 1998, **78** 377–8.

159   Beckles-Wilson N, Taylor CJ, Ghosal S, Pickering M Reducing pancreatic enzyme dose does not compromise growth in cystic fibrosis. *J Hum Nutr Diet*, 1998, **11** 487–92.

160   Taylor CJ, Hillel PG, Ghosal S *et al.* Gastric emptying and intestinal transit of pancreatic supplements in cystic fibrosis. *Arch Dis Child*, 1999, **80** 149–52.

Useful address

Cystic Fibrosis Trust
11 London Road, Bromley, Kent, BR1 1B7

12 The Kidney

Julie Royle

Introduction

The kidneys have an essential role in the maintenance of normal homoeostasis. A variety of diseases can affect the kidneys leading to a sudden deterioration in renal function (acute renal failure) or a progressive loss of nephrons (chronic renal failure). Impairment of excretory, regulatory and endocrine function is seen as kidney function deteriorates.

Acute renal failure

Acute renal failure (ARF) is characterised by a sudden and sustained decline in renal function leading to an increase in the blood concentration of urea and creatinine and the inability of the kidney to regulate fluid and electrolyte balance effectively. In childhood, ARF may be associated with anuria (urine output <1 mL/kg/day), oliguria (urine output <0.5–1 mL/kg/hour), a normal urine output or high urine output. The causes of ARF in children are classified as pre-renal, intrinsic renal or post-renal (Table 12.1) [1].

ARF occurs in 1–3% of admissions to neonatal units with half of these cases responding to a fluid challenge [2]. Up to 10% of children presenting acutely will have chronic renal disease. In pre-school children, diarrhoea associated haemolytic uraemic syndrome (HUS) remains the most common cause of intrinsic ARF. HUS is most commonly associated with verocytotoxin producing *Escherichia coli* (VTEC), usually of the serotype 0157:H7 [3]. Foods of bovine origin, including beef-burgers and unpasteurised milk, are major sources for human infection, although VTEC has been recovered from many retail foods. HUS is characterised by the sudden onset of haemolytic anaemia and the development of ARF after acute gastroenteritis, often with bloody diarrhoea.

Management of ARF

The management of ARF requires the correction of blood pressure, fluid and biochemical abnormalities. Transfer to a tertiary renal centre is indicated in children requiring renal replacement therapy (RRT). Such indications for RRT include:

- Persistent hyperkalaemia
- Fluid overload
- Severe uraemia
- Metabolic abnormalities including acidosis, hypo- or hypernatraemia, hypocalcaemia, hyperphosphataemia
- Creating 'space' for improved nutrition intake
- Removal of a dialysable drug or toxin

Table 12.1   Causes of acute renal failure in children.

Pre-renal failure	Intrinsic renal failure	Post-renal failure
Hypovolaemia (gastroenteritis, haemorrhage) Peripheral vasodilation (sepsis, antihypertensive medications) Impaired cardiac output Bilateral renal vessel occlusion Drugs (ciclosporin, diuretics)	Diseases of kidney or vessels (acute glomerulonephritis, acute tubular necrosis, haemolytic uraemic syndrome, vasculitis) Myoglobinuria Intratubular obstruction (uric acid) Iatrogenic factors (removal of solitary kidney) Tumour infiltrate Nephrotoxic drugs (antimicrobials, heavy metals, insecticides, cytotoxic agents)	Obstruction (posterior uretheral valves, calculi, tumours, trauma)

Choice of renal replacement therapy

The selection of RRT in critically ill children depends upon the availability of treatment modalities and ventilatory support, the patient's requirements for fluid and solute removal and haemodynamic stability. The choice is between acute peritoneal dialysis (PD), continuous veno-venous haemofiltration (CVVH), continuous veno-venous haemofiltration and dialysis (CVVHD), and acute haemodialysis (HD). Factors determining the choice of RRT include the desired outcome of therapy and clinical condition of the child as indicated in Table 12.2 [1].

Table 12.2   Indications for choice of renal replacement therapy in acute renal failure.

Indication for dialysis	Clinical condition	Modality indicated
Solute removal	Stable	HD
	Unstable	CVVH, CVVHD, PD
Fluid removal	Stable	PD, isolated ultrafiltration on HD
	Unstable	CVVH, CVVHD
Solute and fluid removal	Stable/Unstable	HD, PD, CVVHD
Tumour lysis syndrome	Stable/Unstable	HD followed by CVVH/CVVHD
Toxin or drug removal	Stable/Unstable	HD or CVVH

CVVH, continuous veno-venous haemofiltration;
CVVHD, continuous veno-venous haemofiltration and dialysis; HD, haemodialysis; PD, peritoneal dialysis.

Nutritional management of ARF

Children in ARF are highly catabolic. This is usually multifactorial manifesting as anorexia, the catabolic nature of the underlying disorder, increased breakdown and reduced synthesis of muscle protein, increased hepatic gluconeogenesis, nutrient losses in drainage fluids or dialysis and impaired access to food. Input from a paediatric dietitian with experience in renal disease is essential from the onset as the dietary prescription varies with clinical management and the stage of the illness [4].

Nutritional support aims to provide sufficient energy to avoid catabolism, starvation and ketoacidosis, and to control metabolic abnormalities; it is also believed to improve survival [5,6]. The provision of nutrition is often easier after the initiation of dialysis because the fluid removed by ultrafiltration permits more adequate volumes of feed to be given. Nutritional intervention for children with ARF depends on:

- *Clinical management:* conservative vs. RRT
- *Biochemical assessment:* plasma levels of sodium, potassium, bicarbonate, urea, creatinine, albumin, glucose, calcium, magnesium and phosphate should be regularly monitored and reviewed (Table 12.3a,b)
- *Cause of ARF* ± involvement of other organs
- *Gastrointestinal functioning*
- *Growth parameters:* height (if available) and weight plotted on a growth chart [7]; weight recordings prior to the onset of ARF will help determine a more accurate estimation of dry weight
- *Dietary history:* if the child is eating

Table 12.3 Biochemistry reference values. (a) Reference range: guidelines for normal plasma values (Manchester Children's Hospital NHS Trust).

Sodium (mmol/L)		135–145
Potassium* (mmol/L)	<1 month	3.5–6.0
	>1 month	3.0–5.0
Bicarbonate (mmol/L)		20–26
Urea (mmol/L)		2.5–6.5
Albumin (g/L)		30–45
Calcium* (mmol/L)	<2 weeks	1.9–2.8
	>2 weeks	2.2–2.7
Phosphate* (mmol/L)	<1 month	1.4–2.8
	5 weeks–1 year	1.2–2.2
	1–3 years	1.1–2.0
	4–12 years	1.0–1.8
	15	0.95–1.5
	Adult	0.8–1.4
PTH (pg/mL)		12–81
Magnesium (mmol/L)		0.65–1.0
Ferritin (µg/L)		30–275
Alkaline phosphatase* (IU/L)	<1 month	150–600
	>1 month–2 years	150–1100
	3–8 years	150–900
	Puberty	200–1200
Glucose (mmol/L)		3–6.5

PTH, parathyroid hormone.
* Age related.

(b) Reference range: guidelines for normal plasma creatinine values (Manchester Children's Hospital NHS Trust).

Age	Plasma creatinine (µmol/L)
1 week	40–125
2 weeks	35–105
3 weeks	25–90
4 weeks	20–80
6 months	20–50
2 years	25–60
6 years	30–70
10 years	30–80
Adult male	65–120
Adult female	50–110

Ketones interfere positively.
Bilirubin interferes negatively.

Methods of feeding

Enteral feeding

The child with ARF may initially take oral fluids willingly, driven by thirst. However, vomiting is common. Most children fail to achieve nutritional goals through diet alone. As the duration of the acute illness can be prolonged, the passing of a fine bore nasogastric tube is recommended. The tube can be passed at the time of sedation or when anaesthetised for other procedures including insertion of a peritoneal dialysis catheter or arterial line [4]. This allows the provision of early nutritional support because anorexia, vomiting or food refusal can impair management and may increase parental anxiety.

A continuous 24-hour feeding regimen using an enteral feeding pump at a slow rate (10–20 mL/hour) is advantageous in the initial stages of treatment when vomiting is present. As oral intake improves, the transition from continuous to overnight feeding provides the remaining nutritional prescription until appetite improves sufficiently to allow tube feeding to be discontinued. Those children with persistent diarrhoea may tolerate a hydrolysed protein feed (see p. 97) before considering parenteral nutrition.

Parenteral nutrition

The parenteral route is only considered when enteral nutrition is not tolerated. Standard hospital parenteral nutrition (PN) regimens are often unsuitable for the child with ARF because of their electrolyte composition and the amount of fluid that they provide. An appropriate daily nutritional prescription to meet individual requirements should be agreed by the dietitian, pharmacist and medical staff. When formulating PN, nitrogen and electrolyte modified solutions together with increased energy from carbohydrate and fat solutions where fluid allowance is limited need to be considered. On CVVH and CVVHD, the loss of nutrients through filtration and dialysis needs to be compensated for in the replacement fluids (see p. 209); levels need to be greater than those found in standard PN regimens. For many children PN is temporary and the enteral route is re-established as soon as gut function returns.

Nutritional considerations

There are few data on the nutritional requirements of critically ill patients in ARF and on RRT in the

Table 12.4   Nutritional guidelines for the child in acute renal failure.

	Energy* (kcal/kg body weight/day)	Protein (g/kg body weight/day)
Conservative management		
0–1 year	95–120 (400–500 kJ)	1.5–2.1
Children/adolescents	EAR for chronological age	1.0
Peritoneal dialysis		
0–1 year	95–120 (400–500 kJ)	2.2–2.5[†]
Children/adolescents	EAR for chronological age	1.5–2.0
Haemodialysis		
0–1 year	95–120 (400–500 kJ)	1.9–2.5
Children/adolescents	EAR for chronological age	1.2–1.5
Haemofiltration		
0–1 year	95–120 (400–500 kJ)	2.5–3.0
Children/adolescents	EAR for chronological age	2.5

EAR, estimated average requirement (Dietary Reference Values, 1991 [9]).
* These guidelines are rarely achieved in the acute stage because of fluid restriction.
[†] If dialysis is prolonged, increased protein may be required.

paediatric population. Most of the information is derived from adult data.

Energy

Little is known about the energy requirements of infants and children with ARF [8]. A minimum of the estimated average requirement (EAR) for energy (DRV 1991) [9] for healthy children of the same chronological age provides a guide as shown in Table 12.4. These recommendations are difficult to achieve during acute treatment and it is important to provide the maximum energy intake tolerated within the prescribed fluid allowance. The early addition of glucose polymers to water (flavoured with squash or cordial if desired) or to drinks of choice is recommended. It is wise to start at a concentration of 0.5 kcal/mL (2 kJ/mL), building up to a concentration of 1 kcal/mL (4 kJ/mL), or 25% carbohydrate (CHO) concentration, depending on individual tolerance. Liquid glucose polymer preparations can also be used, but require dilution with water to be tolerated by children. It is recommended to start with a 1 : 5 dilution of liquid glucose polymer, building up to a final 1 : 3 dilution. The neutral preparations can be flavoured with squash. When fluid is severely restricted, ice cubes and lollies can be prepared with energy-dense solutions and offered at frequent intervals.

Energy rich carbohydrate drinks including original bottled Lucozade Energy (0.73 kcal/mL, (3 kJ/mL or 18% CHO concentration) and Tesco Alive (0.74 kcal/mL, 3kJ/mL or 18.4% CHO concentration) can be useful alternatives for those children who refuse to drink prescribed energy supplements.

A list of energy supplements that can be considered are given in Table 12.5. These can be successfully added to infant formulas to increase energy density:

- in infants up to 6 months of age: 0.85–1.0 kcal/mL (3.6–4 kJ/mL) is usually tolerated
- infants 6–12 months of age: 1.0–1.5 kcal/mL (4–6 kJ/mL) should be tolerated

In children over 12 months of age or whose weight is >8 kg a nutritionally complete paediatric feed can be considered and modified as necessary to meet individual requirements (Table 12.5). Fat emulsions can be given as a prescribed medicine during the day.

A few children develop insulin resistance and hyperglycaemia can occur. This is exacerbated by the absorption of glucose from the peritoneal dialysis fluid and the intake of high carbohydrate supplements. Insulin infusions should be considered to control blood glucose levels before the reduction of dietary carbohydrate.

Table 12.5   Nutritional supplements.

Supplement	Suggested use
Energy	
Glucose polymers	
Powder, e.g. Polycal, Polycose, Super Soluble Maxijul, Vitajoule	Add to infant formula, baby juice, cow's milk, squash, fizzy drinks, tea, milk shake, ice cubes and lollies
Liquid, e.g. Polycal, Maxijul	Dilute with soda water, fizzy drinks of choice (unless fluid restricted), add to jelly
Fat emulsion e.g. Calogen, Liquigen	Add to infant formula, cow's milk, nutritionally complete supplements
Combined fat and carbohydrate e.g. Super Soluble Duocal Powder, Liquid Duocal, QuickCal	Add to infant formula, cow's milk, nutritionally complete supplements
Protein	
Protein powders e.g. Protifar, Vitapro, ProMod, Renapro	Add to infant formula, Liquid Duocal, modular feed components
Renal specific infant formula	
Kindergen	
Powder per 100 g: 7.5 g protein, 503 kcal (2104 kJ), 93 mg phosphate, 3 mmol potassium, 10 mmol sodium	For infants with chronic renal failure or conservatively managed acute renal failure
20 g powder made up to 100 mL with water: 1.5 g protein, 101 kcal (421 kJ), 18.6 mg phosphate, 0.6 mmol potassium, 2 mmol sodium	
Nutritionally complete feeds	
Nutrini per 100 mL: 2.8 g protein, 100 kcal (420 kJ), 50 mg phosphate, 2.8 mmol potassium, 2.6 mmol sodium	For oral or supplementary tube feed in infants/children >1 year and weight >8 kg
Paediasure per 100 mL: 2.8 g protein, 101 kcal (422 kJ), 53 mg phosphate, 2.8 mmol potassium, 2.6 mmol sodium	Can be combined with energy supplements
Nutrini Energy per 100 mL: 4.2 g protein, 150 kcal (632 kJ), 75 mg phosphate, 4.2 mmol potassium, 3.9 mmol sodium	Consider micronutrient contribution in younger children
Paediasure Plus per 100 mL: 4.2 g protein, 151 kcal (632 kJ), 80 mg phosphate, 3.5 mmol potassium, 2.6 mmol sodium	
Suplena per 100 mL: 3 g protein, 200 kcal (840 kJ), 74 mg phosphate, 2.9 mmol potassium, 3.4 mmol sodium	
Nepro per 100 mL: 7 g protein, 200 kcal (838 kJ), 69 mg phosphate, 2.7 mmol potassium, 3.7 mmol sodium	
Low electrolyte supplements (not nutritionally complete)	
Fortijuce per 100 mL: 4 g protein, 150 kcal (630 kJ), 13 mg phosphate, 0.5 mmol potassium, 0.7 mmol sodium	Can be diluted with water or fizzy drinks
Enlive Plus per 100 mL: 4.8 g protein, 150 kcal (683kJ), 11 mg phosphate, 0.4 mmol potassium, 0.5 mmol sodium	
Renilon 7.5 per 100 mL: 7.5g protein, 200 kcal (840 kJ), 6 mg phosphate, 0.3 mmol potassium, 2.6 mmol sodium	
Vita-Bite per 25 g bar: 0 g protein, 137 kcal (572 kJ), <1 mg phosphate, 0.1 mmol potassium, 0 mmol sodium	Confectionary bar
Low protein milk substitute	
Sno-Pro per 100 mL: 0.2 g protein, 65 kcal (273 kJ), <30 mg phosphate, <1.3 mmol potassium, <3.3 mmol sodium, <15 mg calcium	Use as a substitute for cow's milk to reduce protein and phosphate intakes
Renamil per 100 g: 4.6 g protein, 477 kcal (2003 kJ), 11 mg phosphate, 0.1 mmol potassium, 1.0 mmol sodium	

When PN is initiated, a high concentration dextrose solution up to 25% is indicated with lipids providing 10–20% of non-protein energy in addition.

Protein

In children with ARF who are being managed conservatively, protein should be limited to the reference nutrient intake (RNI) level to minimise uraemic symptoms. This needs to be gradually increased if RRT is started with its associated increased solute removal and possible protein losses. The RNI values for protein (DRV 1991) [9] are not appropriate for the child with ARF on RRT, and requirements should be individually determined. The age and weight of the child, the biochemistry and RRT, when implemented, all need to be considered. Nutritional guidelines are shown in Table 12.4.

Once RRT is established, the following increments can be used as a guide to increase protein intake to the levels in Table 12.4:

- increase by 0.2 g protein/kg/day increments if serum urea 10 mmol/L or below
- increase by 0.1 g protein/kg/day increments if serum urea is >10.1 mmol/L and <20 mmol/L

CVVH and CVVHD allow the nutritional support of highly catabolic states, but contribute to the nitrogen loss through filtration of free amino acids and small peptides across the haemofilters. Maxvold et al. [10] demonstrated that at similar blood and dialysate/prefiltered replacement fluid flow rates, there is equivalent urea clearance with CVVH and CVVHD. A negative nitrogen balance occurred in children with ARF on PN containing 1.5 g/kg/day protein and a caloric intake 20–30% above resting energy expenditure. An 11–12% loss of dietary amino acids was found on both modalities. A significant daily accumulative glutamine loss may potentiate nitrogen imbalance. A dose adjustment of amino acid formulation may be needed to overcome negative nitrogen balance in children with ARF on CVVH and CVVHD. An adult study by Scheinkestel et al. [11] showed that a protein intake of 2.5 g/kg/day and meeting energy requirements increased the likelihood of achieving a positive nitrogen balance and improving survival.

Nutritional supplements using the nasogastric route are frequently used to meet protein requirements in the initial stages of treatment. For infants, the commercially available standard whey based formulas which are low in electrolytes and phosphate are recommended; these can be modified as required. Kindergen, a renal specific, low phosphate, low potassium infant formula (Table 12.5) can be beneficial in infants not receiving RRT or receiving intermittent haemodialysis when serum biochemistry levels are unstable. The nutritionally complete, high energy feeds available for infants (Infatrini, SMA High Energy) can be useful if blood biochemistry allows when on RRT. The phosphate content of these feeds is higher than in standard infant formulas and serum phosphate levels should be regularly reviewed. For the older child a number of nutritionally complete supplements are available. These can be used solely or in combinations with their protein, phosphate and potassium contents assessed prior to use (Table 12.5). If protein hydrolysate formulas are indicated (usually when the diarrhoeal phase is prolonged in HUS) they should be modified to meet individual requirements. Introduction should be gradual and delivery is usually by the nasogastric route. Once the child's appetite improves and protein intake is met by their diet, energy supplemented drinks can then replace protein-containing supplements.

Fluid

The volume of fluid prescribed during conservative treatment is based on insensible fluid requirements of 400 mL/m^2 body surface area/day or approximately 20 mL/kg body weight/day, with a 12% increase for each °C above normal body temperature, and a reduction if the child is ventilated. Insensible losses should be added to the previous day's urine output to give the total daily fluid allowance. On dialysis, the fluid prescription is determined by monitoring the volume of fluid removed by ultrafiltration plus insensible losses. Ideally, fluid removal on dialysis should be flexibly managed to allow the maximum space for increased nutritional fluids. Maximal nutrient intakes using supplements should be provided within the fluid allowance and divided as evenly as possible throughout the day. A written prescription plan should be provided for the ward nurses and families.

Table 12.6   Potassium-rich foods and suggested alternatives.

Potassium-rich foods*	Suggested alternatives
Bananas, apricots, kiwi fruit, cherries, avocado, citrus fruits, e.g. oranges, grapefruit; dried fruit, e.g. raisins; tinned fruit in fruit juice; melon, plums, rhubarb, blackcurrants	Apples, pears, tinned fruit in syrup
Hi juice squash, fruit juices, e.g. orange, apple, tomato Instant coffee and coffee essence Malted drinks, e.g. Horlicks Cocoa, drinking chocolate	Squash, cordials, Lucozade, lemonade and fizzy pop, tea
Potato crisps and potato type snacks, nuts, peanut butter, salt substitutes, Bovril, Marmite	Corn or rice snacks (take account of sodium content), sweetened popcorn, jam, honey, marmalade, syrup
Jacket potatoes, chips (oven and frozen), roast potatoes	Rice (boiled or fried), spaghetti, pasta, noodles, bread, chapatti, nan, crackers
Mushrooms, spinach, tomatoes, spaghetti in tomato sauce, baked beans, pulses and hummus, soups	Carrots, cauliflower, swede, broccoli, cabbage
Chocolate and all foods containing it, toffee, fudge, marzipan, liquorice	Boiled sweets, jellies, mints, marshmallows
Chocolate biscuits	Biscuits – plain, sandwich, jam filled, wafer
Chocolate cake, fruit cake	Cake – plain sponge filled with cream and/or jam, jam tarts, apple pie, doughnuts, plain scones
Milk, yoghurt, evaporated and condensed milk	Low protein milk substitutes, e.g. Sno-Pro, Renamil

* Allowance will depend on individual assessment.

Electrolytes

The intake of electrolytes, especially potassium, is likely to be restricted in conservative management. Plasma levels and the use of RRT will dictate requirements thereafter.

Potassium rich foods including citrus fruits and fruit juices, bananas, potato crisps and chocolate are commonly brought into hospital by relatives. All carers should be advised about potassium restriction so that rich food sources are withdrawn and lower potassium alternatives given (Table 12.6). Phosphate restriction can partly be achieved when protein intake, particularly that of dairy products, is modified (Table 12.7). Cow's milk is generally restricted or eliminated from the diet during the acute phase because of its high protein, phosphate and potassium content. Avoidance of cow's milk also reduces the potential cow's milk protein or lactose intolerance which may follow the diarrhoeal prodrome in patients with HUS. If milk restriction proves difficult for some children, the use of a low protein milk substitute, such as Sno-Pro or Renamil, can be advised (Table 12.5). Reduction

of sodium can be achieved by the avoidance of salted snacks and no added salt (Table 12.8). The level of the above restrictions depends on each individual child and clinical condition; they should be frequently monitored to avoid unnecessary restrictions and compromising the overall diet.

Micronutrients

Vitamin supplementation should be considered if the dialysis treatment is prolonged. A general paediatric vitamin supplement of water-soluble vitamins should be adequate for the majority of children as appetite improves. Iron supplementation may be indicated in some children during the recovery phase, particularly in those who had a poor diet history prior to the onset of ARF.

When on CVVH and CVVHD water-soluble vitamins, especially folic acid, thiamine and vitamin C are eliminated. Actual requirements are unknown and a minimum of the RNI should be achieved.

Patients receiving CVVH and CVVHD have a loss of magnesium and calcium; this often leads to

Table 12.7   Phosphate-rich foods and suggested alternatives.

Phosphate-rich foods*	Suggested alternatives
Cow's milk (full cream, semi-skimmed, skimmed) Dried milk powder and other milk products	*Infants* Whey-based infant formula, e.g. Farley's First, Cow and Gate Premium, SMA Gold, Aptamil First for at least 1–2 years *Children* Reduced intake, consider low protein milk substitute
Yoghurt, fromage frais, mousse, ice cream, custard made with milk	Reduce intake Custard made with milk substitute
Evaporated milk, condensed milk, single cream	Double cream†
Cheese, e.g. Cheddar, Edam, processed cheese and cheese spread	Limit intake and/or encourage use of cottage cheese or full fat cream cheese
Egg yolk	Meringues
Cocoa, chocolate and chocolate-containing foods, toffee, fudge	Boiled sweets, mints, dolly mixtures
Sardines, pilchards, tuna	
Baked beans, pulses	
Nuts, peanut butter, marzipan	Jam, honey, marmalade, syrup
Coca Cola, and other cola drinks, Dr Pepper and any others containing phosphoric acid	Squash, cordials, lemonade, Lucozade

* Allowance will depend on individual assessment.
† Caution: vitamin A content (p. 224).

Table 12.8   Sodium-rich foods and suggested alternatives.

Sodium-rich foods	Suggested alternatives
Salted crisps, nuts and savoury snacks	Unsalted crisps, unsalted nuts
Tinned and packet soups	Homemade soups
Pot savouries	Sweet snacks instead of savoury
Other tinned foods with added salt	*Lower salt tinned products, e.g. reduced salt baked beans
Smoked meats and fish	Fresh meats and fish
Bacon, sausages and other processed meats, cheese	Fresh and home-made foods
Marmite, Bovril, pickles, sauces and chutneys	Herbs and spices instead of salt
Ready made meals and take away meals	Homemade meals using fresh ingredients

* Many processed/manufactured foods contain high amounts of salt and even lower salt varieties can have a high salt content.

negative balances requiring additional supplementation. Zinc is also abnormally lost but serum levels do not generally fall [12,13].

Recovery phase

As native renal function improves and urine output increases, RRT is stopped. Dietary restrictions, where instigated, can gradually be reduced. Serum electrolytes and dietary intake should be monitored as major losses of, for example, potassium during the diuretic phase can occur and dietary advice must be tailored accordingly.

Prior to discharge, advice should be given on normalising the diet while renal function continues to improve. The opportunity to educate the child and family about the principles of a well-balanced diet can also be taken if poor eating patterns were highlighted during the admission. Some children may need to continue energy and vitamin supplements for a short time, with monitoring of their progress in clinic.

Outcome of ARF

The prognosis for children with ARF depends on the underlying cause of the ARF. In isolated renal failure, the immediate results of treatment are good, but with other organ involvement, mortality increases. A small percentage of children with HUS and other causes of ARF will have albuminuria and impaired renal function leading to chronic renal failure. These children will require ongoing dietary advice.

Chronic renal failure

Renal failure is a continuum extending from mild renal insufficiency to end-stage renal failure (Table 12.9) [14]. Published UK data reveals a take-on rate for RRT of 88 per annum in 2002 for patients under 16 years of age, or 7.7 per million age-adjusted population [15]. The causes of chronic renal failure (CRF) in children are different from adults and are shown in Table 12.10 [16].

Management of progressive CRF

The management of children with progressive CRF is based on a multidisciplinary team approach in

Table 12.10 Causes of chronic renal failure in childhood in the UK [16].

	Percentage
Renal dysplasia and related conditions	28
Obstructive uropathy	20
Glomerular disease	17
Reflux nephropathy	9
Primary tubular and interstitial disorders	7
Congenital nephrotic syndrome	7
Renal vascular disorders	5
Metabolic disease	3
Polycystic disease	2
Malignant and related disorders	2

a specialist centre where the dietitian is a key member of the team. The aim of the team is to optimise the quality of life of the child and family both in childhood and adult life, while treating the complications of the disease and delaying the progression to end-stage renal failure. The fundamental management for children with CRF addresses:

- Nutrition
- Growth
- Fluid and electrolyte balance
- Acid–base abnormalities
- Renal bone disease
- Hypertension
- Preservation of renal function
- Anaemia
- Cardiovascular disease
- Education and psychosocial support
- Medication

A good knowledge of biochemical and haematological parameters is essential to identify variations from normal age specific reference ranges

Table 12.9 Stages of renal failure [14].

Stage	GFR (mL/min/1.73 m^2)	Residual functioning renal mass (%)	Comments
Mild renal insufficiency	80–50	50–25	Asymptomatic
Moderate renal insufficiency	50–30	25–15	Metabolic abnormalities, impaired
Severe renal insufficiency	30–10	15–5	growth, progressive renal failure
End-stage renal failure	<10	<5	RRT indicated

GFR, glomerular filtration rate; RRT, renal replacement therapy.

(Table 12.3a,b) when producing dietary management plans.

The plasma values of particular relevance include: urea, creatinine, sodium, potassium, bicarbonate, albumin, calcium, phosphate, alkaline phosphatase, parathyroid hormone (PTH), glucose, cholesterol and triglycerides. Haemoglobin, ferritin and percent hypochromic cells (<10%) can be used to assess iron status in combination with serum iron and total iron binding capacity (TIBC) to calculate the percentage transferrin saturation (TSAT = serum iron × 100 divided by TIBC) which should be maintained at >20%.

Assessment of glomuerlar filtration rate (GFR) provides an indication of overall level of renal function. GFR estimation by Cr51 EDTA clearance is used by the nephrologist to predict when RRT is likely to be required. GFR should not be measured before 1 year of age as kidney function may continue to mature during the first year of life. The nephrologist will often estimate GFR using the Haycock–Schwartz formula: predicted GFR = 40 × height (cm)/plasma creatinine (µmol/L).

Nutrition

Untreated renal failure results in malnutrition and growth retardation in children. Nutritional therapy can improve both the effects of renal failure and growth and may have a role in slowing the rate of progression of renal failure [17]. Individualised dietary prescriptions must be practical if targets are to be achieved and compliance maintained.

Dietary assessment

A 24-hour dietary recall in clinic plus twice yearly recording of a 3-day food diary (inclusive of one weekend day) are invaluable tools when estimating nutritional intakes and individual baseline requirements. The information on prescribed medications, presence or absence of nausea, vomiting, diarrhoea, constipation and energy levels can be helpful in the child's nutritional and medical assessments. Dietary intake should be computer analysed and a written report to the nephrologist and renal nurse, where appropriate, can reinforce discussions and recommendations made with the child and family.

Growth charts are used to assist in determining the child's nutritional requirements:

- Where the child is within normal percentile ranges for height (over second percentile), energy and micronutrient requirements can be based on the recommendations for children of the same chronological age (DRV 1991) [9].
- Where the child falls below the normal percentile ranges for height (under second percentile), the child's height age is used to determine acceptable baseline energy and micronutrient requirements when compared with recommended intakes [9] and adjusted accordingly thereafter.

Dietary principles in CRF

The dietary aims in managing children with CRF require attention to:

- Adequacy of energy intake
- Regulation of protein intake
- Fluid balance and electrolytes
- Regulation of calcium and phosphate intakes
- Adequacy of micronutrient and iron intakes

Dietary recommendations depend upon age, stage of management and nutritional assessment. The recommended intakes of energy and protein in conservatively managed children are given in Table 12.11. Children with CRF are typically anorexic and have spontaneous energy intakes below the EAR for age. To achieve the EAR for energy, most children with CRF require energy supplements (Table 12.5). The majority of infants and many young children need to have a feed delivered by a nasogastric or gastrostomy tube to optimise nutrition [18].

Energy

The provision of adequate energy is essential to promote growth in all children with CRF, but is particularly important during the conservative stage of treatment when protein intake may be modified to minimise uraemia. The EAR for energy for either height age (if the child's height is less than second percentile) or chronological age if the child falls

Table 12.11 Nutritional guidelines for the child with chronic renal failure.

Age	Energy (per kg body wt/day)		Protein (per kg body wt/day)
	(kcal)	(kJ)	(g)
Conservative Management			
Infants			
Preterm	120–180	500–750	2.5–3.0
0–3 months	115–150	480–630	2.1
4–12 months	95–120	400–500	1.5–1.6
1–3 years	95–120	400–500	1.1
Children/adolescents	Minimum of EAR for		1.0–1.1
4 years–puberty	chronological age (use height age		0.9–1.0
pubertal	if <2nd percentile for height)		0.8–0.9
post-pubertal			
Peritoneal dialysis (CCPD/CAPD)			
Infants			
Preterm	120–180	500–750	3.0–4.0
0–3 months	115–150	480–630	2.8–2.9
4–12 months	95–120	400–500	2.2–2.3
1–3 years	95–120	400–500	1.8–1.9
Children/adolescents			
4 years–puberty	Minimum of EAR for		1.7–1.9
pubertal	chronological age (use height age		1.6–1.8
post-pubertal	if <2nd percentile for height)		1.4–1.5
Haemodialysis			
Infants			
Preterm	120–180	500–750	3.0
0–3 months	115–150	480–630	2.5
4–12 months	95–120	400–500	1.9
1–3 years	95–120	400–500	1.5
Children/adolescents			
4 years–puberty	Minimum of EAR for		1.4–1.5
pubertal	chronological age (use height age		1.3–1.4
post-pubertal	if <2nd percentile for height)		1.2–1.3

These guidelines are for the initiation of management and require adjustments based on individual nutritional assessment.
Protein intakes reflect the reference nutrient intake (RNI) in the UK [9] plus an increment to achieve positive nitrogen balance including any transperitoneal losses [40].
EAR, estimated average requirement (Dietary Reference Values, 1991 [9]).

within percentile ranges, can be used as baseline guidelines as shown in Table 12.11. Raised serum urea levels in combination with increased serum potassium levels can be suggestive of catabolism and the need to increase non-protein energy intake.

High energy, low protein foods
These should be encouraged where possible and include sugar, glucose, jam, marmalade, honey, syrup. The liberal use of poly- or monounsaturated oils in cooking or margarine spread on bread, toast or added to vegetables can contribute significantly to the child's energy intake.

Energy supplements
Anorexia, protein modification and, in some instances, fluid restriction contribute to reduced energy intake. Energy supplements are helpful in

meeting this deficit. A number of supplements are available and enable a flexible approach (Table 12.5). Combined fat and carbohydrate supplements, including Duocal powder, or glucose polymer alone if additional fat is not tolerated, can be successfully added to infant formulas and supplementary tube feeds. The concentrations should be increased gradually to establish tolerance. Assuming normal gut function, the following upper limits for carbohydrate and fat can be worked towards:

- *Infants under 6 months:* 12% CHO and 5% fat
- *Infants over 6 months to 1 year:* 15% CHO and 6% fat
- *Toddlers aged 1–2 years:* 20% CHO and 7% fat
- *Older children:* 32% CHO and 9% fat

Liquid glucose polymers are useful when diluted with a fizzy drink or diluted squash and the volume used will depend on the fluid allowance. Powdered glucose polymers are useful in children who drink plenty of water, squash or baby juice. A target amount to use each day should be negotiated and a personalised record chart can help with compliance. Any prescription for energy supplements initiated at the outpatient clinic must be continued should the child be admitted as an inpatient.

Protein

Children have a high requirement for protein per kilogram body weight because of the demands of growth. Protein restriction has been of no advantage in delaying progression of renal failure [17] and in a short term study in infants was associated with inferior growth [19].

In order to optimise growth, children with CRF should receive at least the RNI for protein for their chronological age (or height age if less than second percentile) and no more than 3 g protein/kg. If dairy proteins have been limited to restrict phosphate intake, and adequate energy intake has been ensured to promote anabolism, further protein modification is rarely needed. However, when a child's blood urea remains >20 mmol/L, a gradual protein reduction based on the child's 3-day dietary assessment should be initiated to reduce the blood urea below 20 mmol/L. Protein of a high biological value should comprise 65–70% of the total dietary protein intake.

Growth

Growth is the most responsive marker of adequacy of CRF treatment. At each clinic visit accurate measurements of height or supine length, weight and, for children under 2 years of age, head circumference should be obtained and plotted for chronological age on appropriate percentile charts. Height velocity can be useful when calculated annually. Fall-off in growth velocity or weight can be used as early indicators of growth failure and potential causes must be explored.

Body mass index (BMI) can also form part of the nutritional assessment when calculated and plotted on a BMI chart [20]. Mid arm circumference (MAC) can be measured 6 monthly and compared to norms for age. X-rays of hands and wrists may be measured annually to determine bone age. Skinfold thickness (triceps and subscapular) may assist in assessing body protein and fat stores when compared with normal values. Such measurements should be carried out under a standard protocol, preferably by the same individual [21], but in practice children are reluctant to participate and it tends to be used more for research purposes. Standard deviation scores relative to age, sex and height, in the case of severe growth retardation, must always be used when calculating height, weight, height velocity, BMI, MAC and skinfold thickness.

Potential causes of growth retardation in CRF include inadequate energy intake, inappropriate protein intake, metabolic acidosis, sodium chloride deficiency, renal osteodystrophy, anaemia, infection, hormonal abnormalities, corticosteroid therapy and psychosocial effects. The paediatric dietitian, as part of the multidisciplinary renal team, contributes to optimising the management of these where appropriate. The pattern of growth in a child with CRF is determined by their age, the age at onset of CRF and their treatment [22]. Growth in childhood occurs in three phases. During the first 2 years of life rapid growth is nutritionally dependent. This is followed by a slowing of growth velocity during mid-childhood when growth is mainly dependent on growth hormone. At puberty, which is typically delayed in CRF, there is a rapid increase in growth velocity in response to sex steroids.

The importance of adequate nutrition and electrolyte balance in infancy to optimise growth is well recognised [23]. Supplementary feeding using the enteral route is invariably indicated in this group. Ongoing debate exists as to whether older children with renal failure are able to follow their growth percentiles with the provision of adequate nutrition alone. An improvement in height standard deviation scores (SDS) has been observed in a small group study [23]. For children with a height or height velocity for chronological age below –2 SDS, growth hormone therapy following the optimisation of nutritional management has been shown to increase height velocity and final adult height [24].

Fluid and electrolyte balance

Several causes of CRF in infancy, including obstructive uropathy and renal dysplasia, result in excessive sodium wasting. Sodium depletion results in contraction of the extracellular fluid volume and further impairment in renal function as well as impairing growth [25]. Sodium chloride supplements can be added to infant feeds or be given as a medicine. The amount should be increased until an improvement in growth is seen without the development of hypertension, peripheral oedema or hypernatraemia. Such infants typically require up to 4–6 mmol sodium/kg/day. These infants are usually polyuric and require free access to water or fluids in the form of supplemented feed.

In contrast, children with primary renal diseases resulting in hypertension may benefit from a reduction in sodium intake to a 'no added salt' diet avoiding salted snacks and encouraging fresh foods (Table 12.8).

Fluid restrictions are only instituted once urine output diminishes or oedema develops, usually when the GFR falls to <15 mL/min/1.73 m^2. Fluid prescriptions are individualised to take account of insensible losses and a typical day's urine output.

The majority of children with mild and moderate renal insufficiencies maintain potassium homoeostasis. If hyperkalaemia occurs, other correctable causes including drugs such as angiotensin-converting enzyme (ACE) inhibitors, metabolic acidosis and catabolism should be excluded before initiating a potassium modified diet (Table 12.6). A haemolysed blood sample will show a falsely high serum potassium level. In severe renal insufficiency, hyperkalaemia necessitates a potassium modified diet.

Hypokalaemia is seen in renal tubular disorders such as cystinosis and Bartter's syndrome. Potassium supplements are usually indicated together with medication (indometacin) that reduces renal salt, potassium and water losses [26]. Hypokalaemia can also result from the use of some diuretics as well as diarrhoea and vomiting.

Acid–base abnormalities

Maintenance of acid–base status is important in infants and children. Failure to thrive in infancy can be associated with persistent metabolic acidosis, as can bone demineralisation and hyperkalaemia. Extracellular potassium shifts occur with metabolic acidosis as bicarbonate is lost through the kidney. Acidosis is corrected with the administration of sodium bicarbonate. Sodium bicarbonate supplements do not usually cause sodium retention until renal failure is advanced and, as such, have little effect on blood pressure control and do not usually need to be included in an assessment of sodium intake.

In older children, an excess protein intake, and hence sulphur-containing amino acids, can increase endogenous acid production. Protein intake should be modified in such instances.

Renal bone disease

Excess dietary phosphate is excreted by the kidneys or stored in bone tissue. As renal function declines, accumulation of phosphate in the blood adversely affects mineral homoeostasis and bone turnover. This imbalance results in secondary hyperthyroidism and renal bone disease (renal osteodystrophy).

The effects of renal insufficiency on bone metabolism are seen from mild renal insufficiency (GFR 50–80 mL/min/1.73 m^2), with an increase in PTH level and reduction in 1,25-vitamin D level. The key to the successful management of renal bone disease is adequate control of plasma phosphate levels by a combination of limitation of dietary phosphate intake and the use of oral phosphate binders. Raised plasma phosphate is central in the pathogenesis of hyperparathyroidism. PTH levels are a sensitive marker of abnormalities in bone mineral metabolism and levels should be regularly monitored with an aim of maintaining levels within or less than twice the normal range [27].

Dietary phosphate restriction

Phosphate is present in most foods and gastro-intestinal absorption is very efficient (80–90%). Phosphate restriction should begin once the GFR indicates mild renal insufficiency and will continue into the management of end-stage renal failure (ESRF) (Table 12.7). In infants, standard whey-based infant formulas are used for at least 1–2 years because of their low phosphate content. Kindergen, usually in combination with a standard whey-based infant formula, can be used to provide a lower phosphate intake, with consideration given to its lower calcium and potassium content (Table 12.5). In older children, cow's milk can be introduced in a controlled amount. Individualised targets should be given for cow's milk and cow's milk products to aid compliance. Nutritional supplements with a lower phosphate content should be chosen and be included within the dietary allowance. Guidelines for phosphate intake are as follows and are based on body weight:

- Infants <10 kg: <400 mg/day
- Children 10–20 kg: <600 mg/day
- Children 20–40 kg: <800 mg/day
- Children >40 kg: <1000 mg/day

Care needs to be taken not to compromise protein intake while restricting dietary phosphate. A guide to the phosphorus content of different foods per gram of protein is given in Table 12.12. Dietary strategies should enable children and their carers to choose foods with less phosphate but to maintain an adequate protein intake. Maintenance of the serum phosphate within the normal reference values for age is desirable (Table 12.3a). During conservative management and when on haemo-dialysis, phosphate intake will be reduced with protein modification.

Calcium intake is compromised when phosphate is restricted in the diet and may need supplementation. An average of 20–30% of the calcium in calcium-based phosphate binders is absorbed and therefore supplements dietary calcium.

Hydroxylated vitamin D

Vitamin D is converted to the activated form in the healthy kidney. The decrease in activated vitamin D levels seen in CRF and the resultant hyper-parathyroidism may be addressed by a reduction in phosphate intake, but usually requires supplementation with hydroxylated vitamin D_3 in order to increase the absorption of calcium in the small intestine. The most common preparation used in the UK is 1α-hydroxycholecalciferol (alfacalcidol). The dose is based on serum calcium and PTH levels and is reduced or suspended if calcium levels are above the normal range (Table 12.3a).

Phosphate binders

When plasma phosphate remains above the reference values for age, oral phosphate binding drugs are prescribed to block intestinal phosphate absorption (Table 12.13). Currently, aluminium salts, although effective phosphate binders, have been abandoned because of their toxicity. Calcium carbonate is the first line phosphate binder in children. Tablets should be chewed and taken preferably just before meals or snacks as a lower pH improves binding capacity. Alternatively, tablets can be crushed to a fine powder or used in solution and then be added to feed bottles or to overnight or daytime bolus feeds. Regular shaking is recommended as the powder can settle out. Calcium carbonate impairs the absorption of iron; it should not be taken at the same time as oral iron supplements. Approximately 20–30% of the calcium contained in the phosphate binder will be absorbed and can result in hypercalcaemia. Calcium acetate achieves a similar control of serum phosphate at a lower dose of elemental calcium. It is taken during meals and swallowed whole. Calcium based binders can lead to an increase of the Ca × P ion product and the development of vascular and soft tissue calcification. Soft tissue calcification has been

Table 12.12   Guide to the phosphorus content of foods related to their protein content.

Type of food	Phosphorus (mg/g protein)
Poultry, meat and white fish	7–9
Pulses	12–18
Shell fish, oily fish, offal	15–20
Egg	18
Hard cheese	20
Milk, yoghurt	28
Peanuts	15
Almonds	26
Walnuts	48

Table 12.13   Phosphate binders.

	Elemental calcium mg (mmol) per tablet	Dosage	Flavour	Estimate of potential binding power
Calcium carbonate binders				
Setler's Tums tablets (500 mg)	200 (5.0)	1–3 tds	Spearmint, peppermint, various fruit flavours	Approx 39 mg P bound per 1 g calcium carbonate
Calcium carbonate (20% solution)	400 (10.0) per 5 mL	5–15 mL tds	–	
Rennie Tablets Digestif/Spearmint (680 mg)	272 (6.8)	1 tds	Peppermint/spearmint	
Remegel tablets (800 mg)	320 (8.0)	1–3 tds	Mint	
Calcichew tablets (1250 mg)	500 (12.6)	1 tds	Orange	
Adcal (1500 mg)	600 (15.0)	1 tds	Fruit flavour	
Calcium acetate binders				
Phosex Tablets (1000 mg)	250 (6.25)	1–3 tds	(swallow whole)	Approx 45 mg P bound per 1 g calcium acetate
Phosex Tablets (500 mg) named patient basis	125 (3.1)	2–4 tds	(swallow whole)	
Sevelamer				
Renagel (800 mg)	None	1–3 tds	(swallow whole)	Approx 80 mg P bound per 1 g sevelamer

Total intake of elemental calcium (including diet) should not be greater than 2000 mg/day calcium [40].

reported in 60% of autopsies of children with renal failure [28].

Sevelamer hydrochloride is a calcium free synthetic ion exchange polymer which binds phosphate and cholesterol. There is limited paediatric experience with this binder [29]. Its expense and the high dose needed to achieve target phosphate levels limits its use in children. Concerns have been raised that sevelamer may affect the absorption of fat-soluble vitamins [30]. Lanthanum carbonate has recently become available. It is also calcium free and trials have yet to be carried out in children.

Hypertension

Hypertension can arise from the primary renal disease or, in progressive renal failure, from sodium and water retention. Where there is evidence of fluid overload contributing to hypertension diuretics therapy and a salt restricted diet (Table 12.8) should be initiated.

Children readily exceed the adult daily recommendation for sodium intake of 100 mmol because of their high intake of processed foods. Dietary advice should take into account current lifestyles and the hidden salt in foods when devising targets to reduce salt intake. Advice needs to be given on interpreting food labels and giving ideas for lower salt snacks. The food industry needs to continue the policy of reducing the salt content of their products for the population at large. Poor compliance with salt restriction is a common observation. The Scientific Advisory Committee on Nutrition (SACN) [31] gives recommendations on salt intake for children throughout childhood which can be used as a guideline (Table 12.14).

In the absence of fluid overload, hypotensive therapy is started when the child's systolic or diastolic blood pressures are repeatedly greater than the 90th centile for age. The Dietary Approaches to Stop Hypertension (DASH) trial showed in adults that a salt reduction together with a healthy eating plan could reduce blood pressure by 11.5/5.7

Table 12.14 Recommendations on salt consumption in children [31].

Age range	Suggested daily salt intake	
	g	mmol
0–6 months	<1	17
7–12 months	1	17
1–6 years	2	34
7–14 years	5	85
15 years – adults	6	100

mmHg in hypertensive subjects and 7.1/3.7 mmHg in normotensives [32]. It would be prudent to avoid excessive sodium intakes in this group of children.

Preservation of renal function

In most children with CRF renal function continues to decline. This is associated with progressive glomerulosclerosis, interstitial fibrosis and vascular sclerosis. Control of proteinuria and hypertension has proven to be the strongest independent predictor for progression of renal disease [33]. Proteinuria is associated with inflammatory factors in the urine which contribute to renal disease progression. ACE inhibitors have a renoprotective benefit independent of their antihypertensive effects and are prescribed in some children with proteinuria [34].

The unconfirmed benefit of protein restriction in children was considered earlier (see p. 214). There is reluctance to recommend dietary modification in an attempt to delay the progression of chronic renal insufficiency in early renal failure [35]. Similarly, there is currently lack of evidence in the paediatric literature supporting the effects of addressing hyperlipidaemia and hyperhomocysteinaemia [16].

Anaemia

Anaemia is seen in children when their GFR is <35 mL/min/1.73 m². The blood film is a normochromic, normocytic anaemia as a consequence of inadequate erythropoietin production by the damaged kidneys. The aetiology of anaemia in CRF is multifactoral with iron and folate deficiency, reduced red cell survival, hyperparathyroidism induced bone marrow suppression and gastrointestinal loss. Serum ferritin is used to assess iron status (Table 12.3a) and should be >100 µg/L.

Management aims are to prevent the development of iron deficiency anaemia and the maintenance of adequate iron stores. Haematology results are frequently monitored and multidisciplinary working between nephrologists, dietitians, renal nurses and pharmacists is important.

Dietary assessment
Foods rich in iron, folic acid and vitamins C and B$_{12}$ should be advised to ensure children are achieving recommended intakes for age and sex (DRV) [9]. Sources of haem iron are to be recommended together with advice about non-haem iron and its potential inhibition by phytates in cereal grains and legumes; polyphenols including tannin in tea, coffee and cocoa; and calcium in milk and dairy products.

Oral iron supplements
Oral iron supplements are prescribed when dietary iron intake is insufficient to maintain adequate iron stores. As the child progresses to ESRF intravenous iron therapy is used.

Iron preparations can be prescribed as liquid, tablet or capsule to aid compliance. Vitamin C enhances the absorption of non-haem iron. It is important to avoid over supplementation. Oral iron is prescribed at a daily dose of 2–3 mg of elemental iron/kg body weight/day and given in two to three divided daily doses. Iron is best absorbed in the absence of medications (antacids or phosphate binders), food, infant formulas, milk or nutritional supplements. Ideally, it should be taken 1 hour before or 2 hours following a feed or meal and be taken with a micronutrient supplement where prescribed. Problems with compliance are common, particularly with the potential side effects including nausea, vomiting and constipation. The ideal prescription often tends to be impractical. A flexible approach that is conducive to the child's feed or diet, school and family should be advised.

Cardiovascular disease

Cardiovascular disease is the most common cause of death in patients with renal failure and is seen in the paediatric population [36]. Recognised risk factors in renal insufficiency include a pro-atherogenic state with left ventricular hypertrophy, hyperlipidaemia, hypoalbuminaemia, hypertension and elevated calcium : phosphate product. Published studies implying a benefit in childhood of therapeutic interventions against cardiovascular disease are lacking. Nevertheless, the lifelong nature of renal insufficiency would indicate dietetic involvement in connection with addressing dietary factors relating to cardiovascular disease and the aggressive treatment of hypertension and fluid overload.

Education and psychosocial support

The conservative stage of CRF management is a time for ongoing education and preparation for the child and family by all members of the renal team in preparation for ESRF management. Progressive renal failure is disruptive to a child's schooling, social life and family life. To many families nutrition is one of the more stressful parts of management. An understanding of the psychosocial effects of feeding such children is as important as the nutritional advice [37]. Many families travel long distances to their renal unit and continuity of the dietetic education is essential on the ward or at clinic visits. Regular telephone contact and visits to the home, nursery and school can be invaluable supportive measures. Good communication is essential with other team members to help develop practice, management strategies and share team philosophies which ultimately lead to better patient care. Adequate dietetic time is crucial to provide the close and frequent supervision that is required to monitor and maintain qualitative standards of care for each child, due to the changing needs for growth and development. Attendance on ward rounds, outpatients clinics and psychosocial team meetings are essential [38].

Medication

Many of the prescribed medications are nutrition related (e.g. phosphate binders, oral iron, sodium supplements, vitamins) and should be periodically reviewed by the dietitian as part of the dietary assessment. Children and their families should be advised on the correct administration and timing of medications to ensure compliance, optimal absorption and minimal potential side effects. Ongoing discussion with education and information about each medication should be routine with each dietetic review. The practicalities of taking medications, including at school, should be identified and regimens adjusted accordingly following medical and team discussion.

Management of end-stage renal failure

The aim for management of ESRF in children is to sustain life and enable a good quality of life. For many children the treatment can be cyclical between dialysis and transplantation. The treatment of choice for all children with ESRF is a successful renal transplant with pre-emptive transplantation occurring before dialysis is required. Children are usually activated on the national waiting list for cadaveric renal transplantation at UK Transplant when their GFR falls to approximately 10 mL/min/1.73 m^2. Living donor transplantation is the choice for an increasing number of families.

Pre-emptive transplantation is not always possible and may indeed be unsuitable for certain renal diseases or if the child is already in ESRF when they present. Dialysis is started once patients become symptomatic and biochemical abnormalities and fluid overload are unresponsive to conservative management alone. Dialysis in children can be by HD or PD. In the UK, PD is the preferred dialysis modality for children [39].

Chronic dialysis

PD is preferable for young and small patients. Its advantages are that it can be performed at home and allows regular school attendance, but gives a high level of responsibility to the child's carer. HD has the disadvantage of being a hospital based treatment which disrupts the home routine, but it can relieve the family of a great responsibility and may be used to give the carer some respite. Children will need to transfer to HD if there is a loss of peritoneal access or function.

PD uses the child's peritoneal membrane as an exchange mechanism for small solutes and water. Peritoneal membrane transport capacity can be estimated using a standardised peritoneal equilibration test (PET) which is used in determining PD prescription. PD can be performed intermittently (usually overnight) using an automated cycling machine. This continuous cycling peritoneal dialysis (CCPD) is the preferred option in children, combining five or six overnight exchanges with a long daytime dwell. Alternatively, the child may have continuous ambulatory peritoneal dialysis (CAPD) where the child or carer performs three or four exchanges of dialysate during the day with a long overnight dwell. In 2000 only 11.6% of children treated with PD were on CAPD [39]. Peritonitis is the single most common complication of PD.

HD is an intermittent process lasting 4–6 hours typically three times a week. Small molecular weight solutes are removed from the blood by diffusion through a semi-permeable membrane. HD provides a greater level of small molecule mass transfer than PD. Access to the circulation is usually through a central venous catheter in younger children and an arterio-venous fistula is created in older children when blood vessels allow. Central venous catheters pose an infection risk.

Nutrition and chronic dialysis

Children treated by dialysis require a nutritional prescription dependent on their age and treatment modality. This prescription requires regular dietetic review and includes all the points listed in the management of progressive CRF (see p. 211), together with consideration of the efficiency and demands of dialysis. Evidence based clinical practice guidelines for dialysis prescription produced by the National Kidney Foundation – Dialysis Outcomes Quality Initiative (NKF-DOQI) [40] can be used as a basis in paediatric patients. Currently, practice guidelines vary amongst UK units [38] and there is insufficient evidence to make definitive recommendations. Nutritional guidelines for the child on dialysis are found in Table 12.11.

The monitoring of dialysis prescriptions (dose of dialysis, solution(s), ultrafiltration) and urine output should be carried out by the nephrologist, renal nurse and dietitian and used when formulating a nutritional prescription. Dialysis dose affects growth and nutritional status in children. Dialysis adequacy is monitored by urea kinetic modelling, in particular by calculation of Kt/V (normalised whole body urea clearance) and PNA (protein nitrogen appearance). It is termed as the minimally

acceptable dose of dialysis and refers to the dose of dialysis below which a significant increase in morbidity and mortality would occur. The target Kt/V is >2.1. In contrast to adult patients, it is difficult to define in children and, as a consequence, published data on delivered dialysis doses, peritoneal transport characteristics and correlations in clinical outcome are limited [41], although in a recent longitudinal analysis of 51 children both the peritoneal properties and the intensity of dialysis were shown to independently affect the physical development of children on PD [42].

Energy

The EAR for energy is used as a guideline for requirements. This is corrected for height age if the child is below the second percentile (Table 12.11). There is no consistent evidence that energy requirements are raised on dialysis, although recent evidence suggests that haemodialysis stimulates the release of cytokines and complement which have the direct effect of increasing resting metabolic rate [43].

During PD glucose is absorbed from the dialysis fluid and Edefonti et al. [44] reported a mean energy contribution of 9 kcal/kg (38 kJ/kg) body weight/day. Table 12.15 gives a guide to the energy from glucose absorbed from PD fluid. For those children on PD who require an additional energy intake it is best to consider a nutritionally complete supplement (Table 12.5) in preference to a refined carbohydrate supplement in view of the

Table 12.15   Glucose absorption from peritoneal dialysate (PD).

PD solution concentration (%)	Grams of anhydrous glucose per litre			Osmotic effect
	1 L	1.5 L	2 L	
1.36	13.6	20.5	27.2	Weak hypotonic solution
2.27	22.7	34.1	45.4	Intermediate
3.86	38.6	57.9	77.2	Strong hypertonic solution

Total the grams of glucose from all the exchanges.
Multiply by 3.7 kcal/g.
Multiply by 60–80% for calories absorbed.

recognised raised triglyceride levels of children on PD and the additional source of exogenous glucose derived from the PD fluid. These children will also have increased protein requirements and will benefit from complete supplements. The use of complex carbohydrate foods such as bread, potatoes, rice and cereals should be encouraged. The replacement of glucose in PD fluid by glucose polymers (7.5% icodextrin) has been used in adults to sustain ultrafiltration in long term dwells [45]. Significantly increased dialysis with an icodextin daytime dwell in children on overnight CCPD showed no effect on albumin homoeostasis in the short term [46] but longer term studies are awaited. Icodextrin is not absorbed from the dialysate and therefore is not a source of additional energy.

Protein

There are limited data to demonstrate the optimal amounts of protein for children on dialysis. The RNI for protein is inappropriate for children on dialysis because of losses of protein and amino acids across the dialysing membrane.

Dietary protein restriction has led to poor growth in children on HD. Druml *et al.* [47] demonstrated a loss of 0.2 g amino acid/L filtrate in a HD session. Protein intake on HD needs to be sufficient for growth, but moderated in order to minimise large variations in blood urea levels between dialysis sessions. The aim for pre-dialysis serum urea levels should be <20 mmol/L, provided the child is not catabolic.

The protein requirements of children on PD are higher than when on HD to allow for the greater reported losses of protein and amino acids, with greatest losses being seen in the smaller, younger child (Table 12.11) [48]. The use of high phosphate foods as a source of dietary protein, including cow's milk and dairy foods, need to be restricted if hyperphosphataemia is to be controlled (Table 12.7). Most infants and children require complete nutritional supplements either as sip or tube feeds (Table 12.5) to meet recommended protein intakes. An insufficient intake of protein will be reflected in falling serum albumin levels.

Alterations to protein intake should always be made in conjunction with ensuring an adequate energy intake. Attention to serum urea, albumin and phosphate levels will indicate the individual's protein requirements. Serum albumin is a classic marker of nutritional status correlating with anthropometric indices of nutritional status and subjective global assessment in adult patients [49]. However, rapid changes in albumin levels can be attributed to non-nutritional factors including PD loss of albumin, hydration status, the presence of systemic disease, liver function and a persistent nephrotic state [41]. Supplementary tube feeding should be considered for those children who fail to take sufficient nutrition by the oral route.

During episodes of peritonitis or other intercurrent infections the protein requirements of children are further increased. Serum albumin levels fall and increased intakes of nutritionally complete supplements should be prescribed and encouraged. Nutrineal (Baxter) PD dialysate contains a mixture of amino acids as the osmotic agent rather than glucose and these are absorbed from the dialysate. Nurtrineal was developed for use in adults with protein or protein-energy malnutrition and there is little experience of its use in children. It may have a place in the management of those children needing nutritional support, particularly a higher intake of protein, who because of compliance problems are not receiving adequate protein through diet or supplements.

Protein supplements for infants

Protein powders that are relatively low in phosphate can be added to normal infant formulas, in combination with energy supplements (Table 12.5). Alternatively, infant formulas can be concentrated gradually to provide an increased balance of all nutrients (see p. 16). Frequent monitoring of biochemistry will be required, particularly with respect to potassium, phosphate and urea. A combination of Kindergen (a renal specific low phosphate and potassium infant formula) and a standard infant formula can be used to design a feed to correct high serum phosphate and potassium levels. For infants older than 12 months of age, or whose weights are >8 kg, nutritionally complete supplements can be considered (Table 12.5). Combining supplements to achieve specific intakes of particular nutrients is a common practice to achieve nutritional and biochemical goals.

Worked example

An 8-month-old infant on CCPD: weight 8 kg;

Table 12.16   Sample feed to meet the requirements of an infant on CCPD.

Feed recipe	Energy kcal (kJ)	Protein (g)	CHO (g)	Fat (g)	Na⁺ (mmol)	K⁺ (mmol)	PO4 (mg)
120 g C&G Premium	595 (2487)	12.5	66.6	31.1	7.7	14.5	221
30 g Duocal	148 (619)	0.0	21.8	6.7	0.3	0.0	2
8 g Vitapro	29 (120)	6.0	0.7	0.5	1.0	1.4	26
3 mL 30% NaCl	0	0.0	0.0	0.0	15.0	0.0	0
+ water to 800 mL							
Total per 100 mL	97 (403)	2.3	11.1	4.8	3.0	2.0	31
Total per 800 mL	772 (3226)	18.5	89.1	38.3	24.0	15.9	249
Total per kg	97 (405)	2.3	11.1	4.8	3.0	2.0	31

Table 12.17   Modified sample feed to address PD drainage issues.

Feed recipe	Energy kcal (kJ)	Protein (g)	CHO (g)	Fat (g)	Na⁺ (mmol)	K⁺ (mmol)	PO4 (mg)
115 g Kindergen	578 (2416)	8.6	67.9	30.2	11.5	3.5	107
30 g C&G Premium	149 (623)	3.1	16.7	7.8	1.9	3.6	55
8 g Vitapro	29 (120)	6.0	0.7	0.5	1.0	1.4	26
2 mL 30% NaCl	0	0.0	0.0	0.0	10.0	0.0	0
+ water to 650 mL							
Total per 100 mL	116 (486)	2.7	13.1	5.9	3.8	1.3	29
Total per 650 mL	756 (3159)	17.7	85.3	38.5	24.4	8.5	188
Total per kg	95 (395)	2.2	10.7	4.8	3.1	1.1	24

fluid allowance 800 mL; energy requirement 95–120 kcal/kg (400–500 kJ/kg); protein requirement 2.2–2.3 g/kg (Table 12.16).

Feed needs to be modified following PD drainage issues (necessitating fluid restriction to 650 mL) and an increase in the infant's serum K (6.5 mmol/mL) and serum PO4 (2.4 mmol/mL) levels (Table 12.17).

This feed needs to be revised with ongoing biochemistry results. The calcium content of the feed is almost half the RNI and needs to be addressed if used over a prolonged period of time.

Protein supplements for children and adolescents
It is recommended that a nutritionally complete low phosphate protein supplement is routinely prescribed on the commencement of PD [50] as part of the overall nutritional and dialysis prescription (Table 12.5). These supplements may also be required for children on HD who fail to achieve recommended intakes. Prescribed supplements should be treated as a medication and if taken orally they are best taken in divided amounts (preferably after food) during the day or as a drink before bed.

Carnitine
Carnitine is an amino acid derivative which has an important role in lipid metabolism. Altered carnitine metabolism is seen in CRF and limited protein intake, impaired carnitine synthesis, malnutrition and PD or HD all play a part. A low serum free carnitine concentration is seen in dialysis patients [51]. Carnitine supplements have been proposed as a treatment for symptoms or complications of dialysis including intradialytic arrhythmias, skeletal muscle cramps, hypertriglyceridaemia and anaemia. In paediatric practice there is a lack of data to support routine supplementation. However, in adults there is some evidence supporting the treatment of erythropoietin-resistant anaemia with carnitine supplements [52].

Fluid and electrolytes

Fluid
Fluid allowance is prescribed for the individual depending on insensible losses, residual urine output and dialysis modality. Insensible fluid losses

Table 12.18   Sample feed to meet the requirements of a 6-year-old girl acutely unwell on HD.

Feed recipe	Energy kcal (kJ)	Protein (g)	CHO (g)	Fat (g)	Na⁺ (mmol)	K⁺ (mmol)	PO4 (mg)
237 mL Nepro*	474 (1981)	16.6	52.6	22.8	8.7	6.4	164
237 mL Suplena*	474 (1981)	7.1	60.4	22.8	8.0	6.8	175
115 g Maxijul	437 (1827)	0.0	109.3	0.0	1.0	0.1	6
35 mL Calogen + water to 700 mL	158 (660)	0.0	0.0	17.5	0.1	0.0	0
Total per 100 mL	220 (920)	3.4	31.8	9.0	2.6	1.9	49
Total per 700 mL	1543 (6449)	23.7	222.3	63.1	17.8	13.3	345
Total per kg	91 (380)	1.4	13.1	3.7	1.0	0.8	20

* Adult renal specific feeds may be useful to achieve energy and protein requirements in a restricted fluid volume, but care needs to be taken with their micronutrient profile (see p. 225).

are calculated as 400 mL/m² body surface area/ day or approximately 20 mL/kg body weight/day. On PD the fluid removed by ultrafiltration is also included. Fluid weight gain between HD sessions can be problematic especially if the child is anuric; the fluid allowance is based on insensible fluid losses and fluid removal between dialysis sessions. Ideally, interdialytic weight gain should not exceed 5% of the child's estimated dry weight. Prolonged fluid overload in HD can cause cardiac problems, including cardiomyopathy. Accurate weighing of patients with careful interpretation of the intake and output of fluids can help with the interpretation of fluid balance.

In children and infants receiving enteral feeds, the fluid allowance needs to be negotiated with the medical staff to allow space for nutrition and to avoid over-concentration of feeds in order to meet nutritional requirements in a small volume of fluid.

Education of children on fluid restrictions should include practical ways of reducing fluid intake (e.g. using tablet rather than liquid medicines and the judicious use of foods with a high water content such as jelly, gravy, sauces and yoghurt). Thirst prevention techniques, including reducing salt intake and good mouth care, should be considered. Involving younger children in devising fluid record charts can aid compliance. It is also better, psychologically, to talk about a fluid allowance rather than a fluid restriction.

Worked example

A 6-year-old girl established on HD becomes acutely unwell and requires an enteral feed: weight 17 kg; fluid allowance 800 mL with 700 mL reserved for the feed; requirements 1545 kcal (6.45 MJ) and 1.4–1.5 g protein/kg (Table 12.18).

Sodium

Children on PD can become hyponatraemic (serum sodium <130 mmol/L) as a result of sodium losses into the ultrafiltrate. To maintain sodium balance, medicinal salt supplements are prescribed if increasing dietary sodium does not correct levels. Conversely, some children on PD are hypertensive and oedematous and for these a 'no added salt' diet is of value (Table 12.8).

On HD hypertension and excess interdialytic weight gain invariably relate to salt and water overload. A 'no added salt' diet should be advocated to reduce thirst and fluid intake. An intake of 1–3 mmol/kg body weight/day is usually acceptable.

Potassium

A child with a good urine output can cope with a more liberal potassium intake. In anuric or anephric infants and children, dietary potassium restriction is indicated. CCPD and the large volumes of dialysate used in CAPD in adolescents generally allow a moderate intake of potassium. However, advice should be targeted at preventing overindulgence of potassium rich foods and drinks (e.g. crisps may be taken occasionally but corn snacks are preferable, squash should be drunk in preference to pure fruit juices).

Although HD is effective at clearing potassium, because of the intermittent nature of the treatment (typically three times a week), children on HD invariably require dietary potassium advice to minimise problems with hyperkalaemia (Table 12.6). Some units allow potassium treats such as crisps or chocolate while receiving HD; these should be eaten within the first 30 minutes of HD and given in controlled amounts so that the potassium can be cleared before the dialysis session is over.

Hyperkalaemia can result in fatal cardiac arrhythmias. When plasma levels are >6.5 mmol/L, there is a prolongation of the PR interval and peaking of the T wave on electrocardiogram (ECG). In such instances salbutamol is prescribed to enhance cellular potassium uptake. An ion exchange resin such as calcium resonium can be used as a crisis management strategy. It can take several HD sessions after a high serum potassium level to achieve an acceptable baseline level because of the movement of potassium from the intracellular fluid.

Advice about potassium intake needs to be tailored to each individual with involvement of both the child and carers. Intakes need to be reviewed at frequent intervals together with blood biochemistry results and dietary analysis. A photographic album of foods rich in potassium and food models can be useful educational tools. Older children need to be involved in decision making and discussion of serum potassium levels can be helpful.

Phosphate
Phosphate restrictions continue when on dialysis (Table 12.7). In adults, 800 mg phosphate is typically removed during each HD session and 300–400 mg/day on PD. Removal figures will be lower in children because of flow rates and the volume of dialysate used.

Micronutrients in CRF

Little is known about the essential micronutrient requirements of children with CRF. They vary with age, appetite, growth and stage of renal disease. Individual dietary assessment is essential, taking into account the intakes from diet, micronutrient supplements, infant formulas and nutritionally complete supplements, the latter often being the sole source of nutrition for many patients. Only then can supplementation be individually and safely prescribed, if indicated. The RNIs [9] for healthy children of the same age and sex provide guidelines [53].

Adult renal studies have shown that there are potential peritoneal dialysate losses of vitamins C, B_6 and folic acid [54]. Published adult recommendations for these vitamins are likely to be too high for the majority of paediatric patients. Recommended intakes based on the RNI and from the few paediatric PD studies available [55] would suggest daily intakes of:

- Vitamin C 15 mg (infants): 60 mg (children)
- Vitamin B_6 0.2 mg (infants): 1.5 mg (children)
- Folate 60 µg (infants): 400 µg (children)

Excessive intakes of vitamin C should be avoided as elevated oxalate levels can lead to the development of vascular complications [56]. Vitamin A supplementation should be avoided, because elevated levels have been associated with hypercalcaemia, anaemia and hyperlipidaemia [57]. Vitamin A intakes should not exceed 200% of the RNI value. Micronutrient supplements containing vitamin D should also be avoided because hydroxylated vitamin D_3 is prescribed to manage bone disease. Further research on the links between vitamin B status and homocysteine, an amino acid intermediate, with cardiovascular disease may affect recommendations in the future [58]. Homocysteine is an intermediary of methionine metabolism which, at raised levels, is a risk factor for cardiovascular disease. Hyperhomocysteinaemia is common among adult patients with chronic renal insufficiency and appears to relate to reduced clearance of plasma homocysteine. Supraphysiological folic acid treatment can normalise homocysteine levels in chronic renal insufficiency but not in ESRD [59].

Dietary assessments typically reveal zinc and copper intakes below recommended values. It is helpful to measure serum levels before starting supplementation as these trace elements have impaired clearance with reduced renal function.

Children most at risk of possible micronutrient deficiencies include those who are anorexic and not under the direct care of a specialist renal unit and dietitian. Children who have prolonged periods on restricted diets when conservatively managed or who have prolonged time on dialysis, complicated by peritonitis or other intercurrent infections, are also of concern. Infants and children receiving nutritional support from complete nutritional supplements, usually by the enteral tube feeding route, are less likely to require supplementation. Older children, with an inadequate diet and poor compliance with oral nutritional supplements, often benefit from micronutrient supplements.

Micronutrient intakes can be greater than the RNI when adult renal specific feeds are used solely or in combination for children. Some nutrients, such as folic acid, have minimal toxic effects at high intakes; however, other nutrients, including pyridoxine and magnesium, can have toxic effects. Dietary intake should be evaluated and serum levels measured where intake far exceeds the RNI.

To aid compliance and acceptability in children the taste and presentation of micronutrient supplements are important factors. Currently, Ketovite tablets, providing vitamins C, E and B complex (dose: 1–3/day) are most widely prescribed. A renal specific micronutrient supplement, Dialyvit, Paediatric containing recommended dietary reference intakes for B complex vitamins, plus vitamins C, E, K, copper and zinc is now available [60]. Approval by the Advisory Committee on Borderline Substances (ACBS) is awaited.

Nutritional considerations for infants with CRF

Improved clinical experience in dialysis techniques and renal transplantation has seen increasing numbers of infants taken onto renal failure management programmes. The ultimate goal is a renal transplant; this is technically more complex in the very small child. Most units prefer to promote the growth of the child to a bodyweight >10 kg before taking them onto the transplant programme. Optimal nutrition, with or without early dialysis, is therefore essential in the care of such infants and has been one of the most important factors responsible for the improved outcomes and improved growth seen in recent years [61,62]. Data on growth, without the use of growth hormone, and the dietetic contact necessary to manage and support children and their families receiving chronic PD and intensive nutritional support illustrates the essential role of paediatric renal dietitians in the management of such families [63]. The provision of adequate nutrition for growth requires frequent adjustments of nutritional prescriptions in accordance with blood biochemistry, especially in children receiving nutritional support and in pre-school children.

Once diagnosis is established, there may be a period of conservative management to determine if renal function improves or stabilises. Supplementary tube feeding is indicated early to achieve and maintain adequate nutrition for growth. For infants requiring dialysis, CCPD has become the preferred choice because of capacity for fluid removal; supplementary tube feeding programmes should be commenced at the initiation of dialysis. Nasogastric tubes, percutaneous endoscopic gastrostomy (PEG) tubes, and gastrostomy button devices are the methods available [64,65]. Coleman *et al.* [65] insert a gastrostomy button at the same time as insertion of a chronic dialysis catheter in children under 5 years of age and increasingly practise this in older children when it is anticipated that there will be a struggle to meet the nutritional prescription.

Tube feeding reduces some of the parental anxieties associated with oral feeding while assuring nutritional and medication prescriptions are met. It is preferable to force feeding, which can result in vomiting and/or refusal of formula or food as well as having a detrimental effect on normal oral feeding behaviour in the long term [66].

Vomiting can be an ongoing problem for some infants; feed prescriptions should be closely monitored and altered appropriately. Some infants are sensitive to changes in their fluid balance and this should be considered in relation to vomiting. This continual vomiting is stressful for families, particularly mothers, and close dietetic and team support is required in the long term [37]. Gastro-oesophageal reflux and disturbances in gastrointestinal motility can be evident in infants with CRF [67] and investigations to detect and treat appropriately are essential. Advice about appropriate positioning of the baby when feeding should be initially advised and a thickened feed can be tried (see p. 116). Gastroparesis, delayed gastric emptying, can be treated with prokinetic agents such as metoclopramide, erythromycin and domperidone. Some medications, including calcium-channel blockers and calcitonin, can delay gastric emptying and should be reviewed. Persistent reflux can respond to proton pump inhibitors such as omeprazole and lansoprazole [68]. In extreme cases, anti-reflux surgery may be indicated; in a review of their population of infants in ESRF, Kari *et al.* [18] found that 22% of those who received enteral nutrition to achieve nutritional adequacy required a Nissen fundoplication to manage their persistent vomiting. Vomiting of a psychogenic nature can be seen in some children, particularly those living in stressful family circumstances [69]. Carers, especially those of infants, need frequent reassurance that lack of interest in food and reduced appetite is symptomatic of renal failure.

Weaning should be encouraged from the normal recommended age to enable the development of oral feeding experiences and the reduction of sensitisation to food. The feeding problems seen in infants and young children with CRF are multifactorial: these babies commonly pass large volumes of dilute urine which creates a thirst and preference for water rather than formula; the large number and volume of unpleasant tasting medications that they must take contribute to refusal to take adequate formula by mouth; these babies have disordered taste perception and refuse energy-dense sweetened foods in preference for salty foods; they often find difficulty in swallowing lumpy foods and fail to progress from purée baby foods to more energy-dense family foods; in extreme circumstances even puréed foods may cause choking and retching [70]. Carers must be reassured that it is usual for their child to want to take only small amounts of food and drink and that the early introduction of enteral feeding is recommended before growth failure is evident. The use of pacifiers and oral feeding while receiving daytime enteral bolus feeds can be encouraged to help minimise feeding issues [71]. Enteral feeding regimens that provide a balanced fat and carbohydrate profile to meet energy requirements do not enhance hyperlipidaemia [72].

Nutritional support

The initiation of enteral nutritional support should be considered when the child's oral intake fails to meet recommended nutritional requirements and when growth velocity is not maintained. If oral supplementation is unsuccessful, supplementary tube feeding should be instigated early and not after significant nutritional deficits and aversive feeding interactions have developed between the child and family.

There needs to be a discussion with the family and team members as to the most appropriate feeding route for each child. Essentially, a shared team philosophy of early and sustained nutritional support is required [64]. Play preparation with the use of videos, photograph albums, booklets and dolls can assist in teaching, while some families find it helpful to talk to others with similar experiences.

Overnight supplementary tube feeding using an enteral feeding pump is preferred so that the child has some appetite for oral feeding during the day. In practice, the majority will require intermittent bolus feeds by day to maintain an adequate nutritional intake. Continuous feeds for 20–24 hours, ideally delivered by a portable feeding pump, should only be considered if the latter regimens are not tolerated.

Diet following renal transplantation

Renal transplantation is the treatment of choice for children with ESRF to restore normal or near normal physiology and metabolic function without dialysis and dietary restrictions. Nutritional management remains an important aspect of treatment and the dietitian continues to be involved with the ongoing management. Most children in the UK receive maintenance immunosuppression in the form of triple therapy with a calcineurin inhibitor (ciclosporin or tacrolimus), steroids and either azathioprine or mycophenolate.

Initial management

Feeding commences on the return of normal bowel sounds. If there are no complications, the child usually develops an appetite with improving renal function and previous dietary restrictions can be relaxed. Fluid balance is dependent on output and is assessed daily by medical staff. A high fluid intake is initially encouraged to perfuse the transplanted kidney. Serum phosphate levels typically fall below reference ranges as a result of large tubular and urinary losses, and dietary advice should include foods and drinks rich in phosphate. Invariably, phosphate supplements are prescribed in the early post-transplant days to keep up with urinary losses. Magnesium levels can also fall and require supplementation. Children who experience acute tubular necrosis following renal transplantation may require a period of conservative management or dialysis therapy, including dietary prescription, until adequate renal function is achieved.

There are concerns that there may be a prolonged transition to exclusive oral nutrition in infants and children who commenced nutritional support via an enteral tube feeding route early in their management [71]; others have shown that long term tube feeding does not preclude the transition to normal feeding and the majority of children will eat and drink after a successful renal transplant [62]. Feeding dysfunction and impaired oral motor development appear to be more evident in infants who received nasogastric feeding than in those who had gastrostomy buttons for feeding [73].

It is recommended to cease gastrostomy feeding whenever possible at the time of renal transplantation, in order to stimulate appetite as renal function is restored and higher doses of corticosteroids are prescribed. To do this successfully the medical staff, dietitian and team members need to provide ongoing support to families. Most children do well and resume normal eating and drinking post-transplant [62,73]. There will always be exceptions to this approach, with some children requiring short periods of nutritional support, particularly in the first few weeks post-transplantation. In such patients a planned and agreed strategy to wean off enteral tube feeding must be implemented. Common experience is that some young children take time to adapt to drinking more fluids. In such cases fluid boluses delivered via the enteral feeding tube are given short term. Severe eating difficulties present in a small number of children; these may benefit from a behaviour modification approach [74].

Although a renewed appetite is favourable in the initial stages of management, care must be taken to prevent excessive weight gain and to avoid obesity in the long term. Both the child and family should be reminded of this soon after transplant. The principles of a sensible, healthy eating, well balanced diet for all the family is advised prior to discharge from hospital. An adequate calcium intake is recommended because of prolonged steroid therapy.

All patients on immunosuppressive therapy need to take care with food hygiene and avoid foods that carry a high risk of food poisoning organisms such as *Listeria* and *Salmonella*; this needs to be discussed with each child and family in discharge planning.

Hypertension can present following transplantation and antihypertensive therapy is prescribed. Early post-transplantation systolic hypertension strongly and independently predicts poor long term graft survival in paediatric patients [75]. Arterial wall stiffness has been demonstrated in young adults with end-stage renal disease since childhood, with hypertension being the main determinant [76]. Weight control and advice regarding salt intake, as part of the healthy eating recommendations, should be encouraged.

Hyperlipidaemia is seen in many children following transplantation. Studies have identified that 40% of deaths in adult renal transplant patients are attributed to cardiovascular disease and they occur at a younger age than in the general population [77]. There is growing evidence that dyslipidaemia hastens the progression of renal disease itself. Disordered lipoprotein metabolism results from complex interactions among many factors including the primary disease process; use of medications such as corticosteroids; the presence of malnutrition or obesity; and diet [78]. The systematic treatment of dyslipidaemia in children with CRF is controversial as conclusive data as to the risks and benefits are needed. However, it is prudent to advise on a diet favouring mono- and polyunsaturated fats and oils in preference to saturated fats, together with encouraging regular consumption of omega-3 fatty acids and antioxidants from fruit and vegetable intake.

Ongoing management

Children still receiving nutritional support post-transplant should be regularly review in the outpatient clinic. A transition period to encourage the oral route of feeding should be agreed with families. To stimulate the appetite, bolus feeds should be avoided during the day with minimal feed delivered overnight. Vitamin and/or trace mineral preparations may be required in those children whose micronutrient intakes are poor. Iron status should also be monitored.

Transplantation restores the conditions of normal growth. However, the use of corticosteroids and low GFR in the graft kidney both have growth suppressive effects. Steroids suppress growth mainly by interacting with the growth hormone and insulin-like growth factor 1 axis and affecting the growth plate [79]. An adequate balanced diet should be established to sustain normal growth while guarding against overnutrition.

The prevention of rapid weight gain leading to obesity can be a difficult problem particularly for adolescents where body image is important. The patient who was anorexic prior to transplantation may not engage in discussions to modify food intake to control body weight. Adolescents who experience rapid weight gain and change of body image can be susceptible to crash dieting and possible fasting to lose weight. Healthy eating and exercise should always be encouraged, including information on the health risks of alcohol and smoking. Adolescents need to be included in setting their dietary targets.

A small number of children develop steroid induced diabetes mellitus post-transplant which requires insulin therapy and appropriate dietary advice. Hyperglycaemia is also seen in a small number of children when acute rejection episodes are treated with pulses of methyl-prednisolone; this effect is often transitory.

Chronic rejection of the transplanted kidney will eventually result in the child returning to a dialysis programme with appropriate dietary intervention as for chronic renal failure.

Nephrotic syndrome

Nephrotic syndrome (NS) is characterised by heavy proteinuria (>100 mg/hour/m^2 body surface area or a urine protein : creatinine ratio of >600 mg/mmol) leading to hypoalbuminaemia (<25 g/L) and oedema. Hyperlipidaemia is invariably present. The syndrome can be subdivided into congenital, idiopathic (primary) and secondary types.

Idiopathic nephrotic syndrome is the most common in childhood with a reported incidence of 2–7 cases per 100 000 children. It is more common in males (2 : 1) and in Arabic and Asian children. The peak incidence is in the age range 2–5 years. Minimal change nephrotic syndrome (MCNS) is the most common variant, although the incidence of focal segmental glomerulosclerosis (FSGS) is

reportedly increasing [80]. Indirect evidence implicates a genetic component in its causation which alters the permselectivity barrier of the glomerular capillary wall so that albumin and other proteins are lost in the urine. The salt and water retention leading to oedema is determined by the effect on the plasma albumin concentration. The majority of children under the age of 10 years respond to corticosteroid treatment within 8 weeks and are classified as having steroid sensitive nephrotic syndrome (SSNS) [81]. Their prognosis is generally good with the likelihood of few long term dietary problems. However, children who relapse frequently and are steroid dependent usually require ongoing dietary intervention to monitor and maintain nutritional status and to prevent obesity [5]. Growth failure, disfigurement of facial and body appearance as well as behavioural changes remain important issues in their long term management [5,82].

Children with steroid resistant nephrotic syndrome have a poorer prognosis. Immunosuppressive drugs of various types are used to try and induce remission. Children whose proteinuria cannot be suppressed have a high risk of progression to end-stage renal disease [81] requiring management under the direction of a paediatric nephrologist and dietetic advice.

Complications of NS can be divided into acute, relating to infections and thromboembolic disease, and long term, especially the effects on bones, growth and the cardiovascular system [80]. Despite theoretical risks of bone density reduction with corticosteroid use, the prevalence of bone disease in children with NS is unclear. In children with long term NS, cardiovascular disease can be attributed to the use of corticosteroids, hyperlipidaemia, oxidant stress and hypertension. Hyperlipdiaemia results from complex interactions between disordered lipoprotein metabolism, medications and dietary factors. Increased hepatic lipoprotein synthesis in response to low plasma oncotic pressures have a key role. Whether or not to treat hyperlidipaemia in NS has been a source of controversy, especially because most children have treatable renal disease [83]. A small case series showing reduced serum lipids with the use of statins has been reported [84] but adequate long term safety and efficacy data for HMG-CoA-reductase inhibitors in children are not available.

Nutritional issues

Historically, both high and low protein diets have been advised. Studies have shown that albumin synthesis is limited by the capacity of the liver to synthesis albumin and is not increased with protein augmentation. There is no significant benefit on plasma albumin concentration or growth from a high protein intake [85,86]. Although a decrease in albuminuria has been shown with low protein diets in animal studies [87], a low protein diet in children carries the risk of malnutrition and poor growth, especially in early childhood. High and low protein diets can be impractical, resulting in dietary imbalances and additional family anxieties.

Nutritional assessment

The dietitian should be involved following diagnosis and should obtain a detailed dietary history and chart growth parameters for both weight and height [7], including those available prior to diagnosis. These can both help in the prediction of the child's acceptable dry weight and approximate nutritional requirements. Attention to fluid balance and plasma electrolytes is also important.

Nutritional management

Energy and protein

A balanced diet, adequate in both energy (EAR for children of the same chronological age) and protein (RNI for chronological age) [9] is adequate for most children. Energy intake needs to be reduced if the child gains excessive weight on corticosteroid therapy. Children with severe and prolonged oedema need to be evaluated for malabsorption as the gut and surrounding tissues may also be oedematous and therefore not function properly. The subsequent malnutrition will require intensive nutritional support with the possibility of supplementary feeding. Protein hydrolysate feeds may be indicated in this situation (see p. 97).

Sodium

Sodium intake is a major contributor to thirst and weight gain through fluid retention in children with NS [88]. A 'no added salt' diet (NAS) avoiding salted snacks, such as crisps, with advice about the high sodium content of manufactured foods (e.g. tinned and packet soups and pot savouries) is recommended (Table 12.8). Very low sodium diets and the use of specialist products are rarely necessary. A relaxed NAS diet is encouraged for the long term, in line with healthy eating advice, when the child is in remission.

Fluid

Restriction of fluid is combined with a NAS diet in the initial oedematous phase. Fluid restriction is determined by the medical staff.

Fats/oils

Diet is unlikely to significantly reduce the elevated lipid levels commonly seen in nephrotic patients. However, as part of the initial general healthy eating advice, the use of mono- and polyunsaturated margarines and oils with a reduction of saturated fat intake should be advocated. Such advice should be given with care so as not to compromise total energy intake [84].

Ongoing management

For most children the introduction of steroid therapy can greatly stimulate appetite. In practice the common dietary problem is the prevention of excessive weight gain. Early dietary advice to reduce the child's energy intake is recommended if obesity is to be prevented. Children will often feel hungry while on steroids and a reduction of energy-dense between-meal snacks such as biscuits, crisps, sweets, chocolate and sugar containing drinks should be encouraged, with the substitution of suitable low energy alternatives. Healthy eating advice for all the family should be reinforced and a leaflet/booklet on healthy eating can be helpful to aid compliance [89].

Nutritional support may be required in children who have prolonged anorexia or where there is evidence of malnutrition. Nutritional supplements taken orally or administered via a nasogastric tube should be considered (Table 12.5). An adequate calcium intake meeting RNI values [9] should be advised in children on long term corticosteroid therapy, together with the regular consumption of dietary sources of antioxidants.

Food allergy

A small number of reports have suggested that food hypersensitivity, particularly to milk and dairy products, may be involved in the aetiology of glomerular damage of both young and adult patients with NS [90,91]. Some parents become anxious about the possibility of allergies and a trial of a few foods diet may need to be considered, under close dietetic supervision (see p. 264). This situation arises infrequently. A small number of families may seek advice from alternative medicine practitioners.

Follow-up

It is recommended that the dietitian should see all nephrotic patients at least once in clinic following discharge, to monitor their clinical progress and nutritional intake. Healthy eating guidelines should be reinforced to ensure that the diet is practical for all family members and not unnecessarily restrictive.

Psychosocial support

Naturally, parents are anxious and concerned when they learn that their child has a chronic illness. Family friendly information about the management and treatment of NS is recommended. A parents' support group enables the sharing of experiences and can be of great benefit to parents who feel isolated.

Congenital nephrotic syndrome

Congenital nephrotic syndrome (CNS) is a rare inherited disorder. Infants present at birth or within the first few months of life with heavy proteinuria, hypoalbuminaemia and oedema. The two main causes of this syndrome are congenital nephrotic syndrome of the Finnish type and diffuse mesangial sclerosis. Marked lipid disturbances are seen. Proteinuria of up to 20 g/L is unresponsive to treatment. Daily albumin infusions are necessary to maintain the plasma albumin and support the circulation. Treatment is initially supportive with the aim of optimising nutrition and growth until the child is able to have renal replacement therapy. Unilateral or bilateral nephrectomies are performed to reduce the proteinuria and dialysis is established until kidney transplantation is possible. These patients require intensive dietetic support and intervention.

Nutritional management

It is the loss of proteins (90% of which is albumin with other protein losses including IgG, transferrin and ceruloplasmin) that is the main problem for infants with CNS [92]. This leads to protein malnutrition, reduced growth and a depressed immune system. Intensive nutritional therapy is required as malnutrition increases the incidence of mortality. Energy intake should be maximised to 130–150 kcal/kg (545–630 kJ/kg) estimated dry body weight with a protein intake of 3–4 g protein/kg. Albumin infusions are also required. The additional dietary protein is given as a casein based product added to the infant formula with additional energy given as glucose polymers (Table 12.5). Fluid allowance should be negotiated with medical staff to allow for adequate nutrition, but is usually restricted to 100–130 mL/kg. Sodium intake is minimised and can be achieved with the use of standard whey-based infant formulas. Many infants require early enteral feeding to ensure their nutritional requirements are met, but this may be difficult to achieve on a very restricted fluid allowance, despite concentrating the feed and adding energy supplements. Breast fed infants are unlikely to meet dietary requirements. Expressed breast milk can be supplemented with protein and energy supplements as described above. Normal weaning practice is encouraged. Complete paediatric nutritional supplements can be used for infants over 8 kg (estimated dry weight).

Patients usually require activated vitamin D, alfacalcidol, to enhance calcium absorption. Vitamin and micronutrient intakes should meet dietary reference values [9].

Some units have given rape seed oil (10–15 mL) and fish oil (2 mL) to patients with CNS to increase the P : S ratio of the diet [92], but the fatty acid profile of current infant formulas and paediatric enteral feeds has made this practice largely redundant. Thyroxine supplements are routinely given to compensate losses of thyroid-binding globulin.

Renal function declines with time and dietary prescriptions need to be modified to accommodate the metabolic consequences of chronic renal failure. Bilateral nephrectomies are performed when the infant reaches a target weight (typically 7–8 kg) which halts the protein losses in the urine and hence the nephrotic state. Dialysis is obligatory and dietary management is altered accordingly until the child receives a successful kidney transplant.

Nephrogenic diabetes insipidus

Nephrogenic diabetes insipidus (NDI) is a rare inherited disorder in which the kidney fails to respond to arginine vasopressin, the antidiuretic hormone (ADH). The infant with NDI is unable to concentrate urine above 100 mOsm/kg H_2O and presents in the first weeks of life with polyuria, polydipsia, dehydration and hypernatraemia.

The excessive fluid intake needed to excrete a normal renal solute load leads to a preference for water intake with consequent failure to thrive, exacerbated by anorexia and vomiting. Diagnosis is based on finding a low urine osmolality which is unresponsive to a water deprivation test or antidiuretic hormone replacement therapy. Decreasing the renal solute load of the feed reduces the volume of urine required for its excretion. Drug treatment is also initiated with a combination of a diuretic (e.g. chlorothiazide) which has an antidiuretic

effect and can reduce the polyuria by as much as 50%, and a non-steroidal anti-inflammatory drug, indometacin, which also reduces urinary output [93]. Parents should be advised that indometacin can cause gastroduodenal ulceration and so must be given with a feed.

Nutritional management

Infancy

A feed presenting a renal solute load of 15 mOsm/kg H_2O/kg body weight requires a fluid intake of >200 mL/kg body weight for excretion. Fluid intakes above this are hard to achieve consistently in young infants and may cause vomiting. The nutritional management of NDI is to provide adequate fluid intake from a low solute feed while providing the EAR for energy and the RNI for protein for height age [9]. The renal solute load of the feed should therefore be reduced to 15 mOsm/kg H_2O/kg body weight or less to reduce obligatory urine excretion. An estimate of the renal solute load of a feed can be made using the following formula:

Ion/protein	Contributory solute load (mOsm/kg H_2O)
1 mmol Na	1
1 mmol K	1
anions	$2 \times (Na + K)$
1 g protein	4

Worked example
A 6-month-old boy weighing 6.8 kg taking 700 mL feed with additional 700 mL water, offered after each feed (Table 12.19).

Table 12.19 Sample calculation of the renal solute load of an energy supplemented infant feed.

	Energy kcal (kJ)	Protein (g)	Sodium (mmol)	Potassium (mmol)
90 g SMA Gold	472 (1973)	10.8	4.9	12.7
45 g Maxijul + water to 700 mL	171 (723)	0	0.4	0.1
Total	643 (2696)	10.8	5.3	12.8
Per kg	95 (396)	1.6	0.8	1.9
Req/kg	95 (396)	1.6		

Renal solute load = Na + K + (2 × [Na + K]) + (4 × protein)
            = 5.3 + 12.8 + (2 × [5.3 + 12.8]) + (4 × 10.8)
            = 97.5 mOsm/kg H_2O
            = 14.3 mOsm/kg H_2O/kg body weight

Feed volume: 100 mL/kg
Water volume: 100 mL/kg
Total fluid volume: 200 mL/kg

Energy supplements are routinely used to meet energy requirements as the amount of formula must be limited to control renal solute load. Water should be offered after each feed. Maxijul can be added to the water to provide extra energy and will marginally increase the renal solute load. It is important to check that the feed provides the RNI for protein, vitamins and micronutrients, although this may not be achieved in the first few days after diagnosis when more dilute feeds with a lower renal solute load may need to be given while blood osmolality falls to an acceptable level. Low sodium weaning solids should be started at the usual age of around 6 months.

Childhood

Some authors suggest a sodium restriction of 1 mmol/kg/day [94] to control the craving for fluids while others consider a NAS diet to be adequate [93] provided the child is on long term medication. It is usual to liberalise the diet from low salt (0.6–1.0 mmol Na/kg) to NAS (1.5–2.0 mol Na/kg) as the child enters toddlerhood. However, if an increase in dietary salt leads to an increase in obligatory fluid intake that then inhibits the child's appetite for food, salt intake must be reduced to a level where the child no longer craves a large intake of water. Regular dietary assessment is necessary throughout childhood to ensure that recommended intakes for energy, protein and micronutrients (DRV) [9] are still being met. A high energy diet based on fats and sugars should be encouraged; glucose polymers can be added to the free water to improve energy intake. Most infants and children take adequate nutrition orally but if growth falters, enteral feeding should be considered. The child must have free access to fluid day and night.

Renal stones

In the UK, the incidence of renal stones in children is low. Presentation is generally between 6 and 15 years of age with boys being affected twice as frequently as girls. The formation of stones requires a supersaturated urine; the greater concentration of ions, the more likely they are to precipitate. The concentration of ions in the urine depends on the pH of the urine, the solute concentration and ionic strength. Urinary infection accounts for 60–80% of renal stones; the infective organisms produce an alkaline medium which favours the precipitation of calcium phosphate and magnesium ammonium phosphate. Congenital abnormalities of the urinary system cause urinary stasis and predispose to stone formation as the solute concentration of the retained urine increases. With metabolic stones the most common abnormality is hypercalciuria [95]. Calcium stones are found where there is hypercalciuria, hyperoxaluria and hypocitraturia.

Hypercalciuria

Hypercalciuria in childhood is defined as a 24-hour urinary calcium above 4 mg/kg/day. Urinary calcium excretion is influenced by many factors including diet, ethnicity, age and geography. Most children have normal serum calcium levels.

A diet history should be taken to determine fluid, sodium, calcium, animal protein, vitamin C and vitamin D intakes; all of these can contribute to an increase in urinary calcium excretion. Urinary sodium excretion correlates with calcium excretion so a diet high in sodium increases the excretion of calcium and hence the likelihood of calcium stone formation. In the majority of children an NAS restriction (Table 12.8) to reduce calcium excretion, together with a good fluid intake (2–3 L) to reduce the concentration of ions in the urine, is sufficient to prevent further stone formation. Restricting dietary sodium has the added benefit of increasing bone mineral density. It is important to give advice about fluids – water or reduced sugar drinks – to promote good dental health [96].

Dietary calcium restriction or the administration of sodium cellulose phosphate (which reduces calcium absorption) is not recommended for children with normocalcaemic hypercalciuria because of the potential effect on reducing bone mineralisation [95]. However, excessive calcium intakes should be avoided with the recommended calcium intake for chronological age (DRV) [9] being advised. Excessive intakes of vitamin D and vitamin C should be avoided as these can contribute to hypercalciuria and hyperoxaluria [97].

Oxalosis and hyperoxaluria

Oxalosis or primary hyperoxaluria is a rare autosomal recessive disorder where there is wide-

Table 12.20   Dietary sources of oxalate.

High oxalate content	Moderate oxalate content	Low oxalate content
Rhubarb and strawberries	Apples, apricots, oranges	Banana, grapefruit, green grapes
Blackberries, raspberries, blueberries and their juices	Peaches, pears, pineapples, plums Orange juice	Melon Apple juice
Beans in tomato sauce	Tomatoes	Cabbage, cauliflower, onions and peas
Beetroot	Asparagus, broccoli, carrots	
Celery, spinach and sweet potatoes		
Chocolate, cocoa, tea	Coffee, cola	Lemonade, jelly
Nuts		Beef, lamb, poultry, pork, seafood, cheese, eggs, milk and yoghurt Noodles, pasta, rice and oil

Also encourage a calcium intake to meet reference nutrient intake (RNI), increase fluid intake and avoid excess vitamin C intake.

spread deposition of calcium oxalate crystals in the kidneys, bones, heart and other organs. There is increased urinary excretion of oxalate. Treatment aims to keep urinary oxalate excretion below 0.4 mmol/L through a high fluid intake of >2 L/m^2/day [95]. Oral citrate can reduce calcium oxalate precipitation by making the urine more alkaline. Restriction of dietary oxalate has little influence on the disease as only 10–15% of urinary oxalate is derived from dietary intake; 60% of urinary oxalate is produced from the endogenous metabolism of glycine, glycolate and hydroxyproline. Pyridoxine sensitivity is seen in 10–40% of patients.

Secondary hyperoxaluria can be seen in patients with malabsorption syndromes. When there is less available calcium to bind oxalate, the absorption of oxalate increases [95]. The reduction of dietary oxalate and vitamin C, which is a precursor of oxalate, can be beneficial (Table 12.20).

Cystine stones

The formation of cystine stones is caused by a defect of renal transport and is a very rare autosomal recessive genetic disorder. Dietary treatment is described elsewhere: an NAS diet may be beneficial in lowering cystine excretion, but other dietary treatments such as a low methionine diet should only be used when all other treatments have failed [96].

Hypercalcaemia

When the rate of calcium entry into the extracellular fluid is greater than calcium excretion by the kidneys, hypercalcaemia results. This can be brought about by increased absorption of calcium from the intestinal tract as in William's syndrome and idiopathic infantile hypercalcaemia; increased release of calcium from the skeleton seen during immobilisation and malignancy; or reduced excretion of calcium from the kidney as in primary hyperparathyroidism. Infants presenting with hypercalcaemia have feeding difficulties, vomit and experience faltering growth [95]. Polydipsia and polyuria often result in a preference for water to milk feeds. In conditions where there is increased intestinal calcium absorption, dietary calcium and vitamin D intake should be reduced.

A dietary assessment to determine the child's intake should be performed. Calcium intake should be reduced so as not to exceed the RNI for age (DRV) [9]. A low calcium formula such as Locasol (0.2 mmol calcium/100 mL when reconstituted with deionised water) can be used and modified with energy supplements in the infant with faltering growth. The level of calcium in the local water supply should be checked as it may make a significant contribution to calcium intake (e.g. hard water may contain 0.3 mmol calcium/100 mL). Deionised (distilled, purified) water must be used if necessary and can be prescribed under ACBS for hypercalcaemia. Other rich sources of dietary calcium, including dairy produce, should be limited in the diet. In effect the infant and older child should follow a milk free diet with the additional advice to restrict foods with added vitamin D (e.g. fortified baby foods, breakfast cereals, margarine). A milk free diet will provide approximately 6–7 mmol/ day calcium. As serum calcium levels normalise, sources of calcium can be gradually introduced to the diet, depending on the individual child's response. This can be managed in portions of food containing approximately 3 mmol calcium (e.g. 100 mL cow's milk, 20 g cheese, 75 g fruit yoghurt). Vitamin supplements containing vitamin D must not be given.

Renal tubular disorders

The final regulation of the body's fluid, electrolyte and acid–base balance is the function of the renal tubule. Tubular dysfunction in childhood is rare, but when present can lead to severe electrolyte and volume disturbance. Children with hereditary tubular dysfunction typically present in the first year of life with non-specific symptoms including poor feeding, vomiting and poor growth. Biochemical analysis of both serum and urine are fundamental for diagnosis.

Bartter's syndrome

Bartter's syndrome describes a number of closely related renal tubular disorders characterised by hypokalaemic metabolic alkalosis, hypochloraemia, hyper-reninaemia and hyperaldosteronism with normal blood pressure. The underlying renal defect results in excessive urinary loss of sodium, chloride and potassium [26].

Treatment involves the correction of dehydration and electrolyte abnormalities. Indometacin, which reduces renal salt, potassium and water losses, is prescribed along with potassium supplements. It is difficult to restore serum potassium into the normal range and most patients tolerate a potassium concentration of 2.5 mmol/L without the expected associated problems [98]. Indometacin is given with food or milk. Side effects can include nausea, vomiting, abdominal pain and peptic ulcer. Nutritional supplements (Table 12.5)

are indicated where appetite remains poor and growth is impaired.

Cystinosis

Nephropathic cystinosis is a rare genetic storage disorder characterised by the intracellular storage of free cystine resulting from a defect in lysosomal cystine transport. It is the most common cause of Fanconi's syndrome in childhood. Cystine accumulation mainly affects the proximal tubules and presents in late infancy with poor feeding, excessive thirst, delayed growth, weakness and rickets. All ethnic groups are affected; Caucasians typically have blond hair and a fair complexion.

Treatment comprises rehydration and the administration of bicarbonate, electrolyte and vitamin D supplements. A cystine-depleting agent, cysteamine, is given to reduce progressive glomerular damage which if untreated leads to ESRF by 10 years of age. Renal transplantation is successful but does not correct the disorder. Cystine continues to accumulate in non-renal tissues causing multisystem dysfunction [98].

Poor growth in children with cystinosis can be caused by a combination of suboptimal nutritional intake, gastrointestinal dysfunction and multiple medications. Oral nutritional supplements should be used initially. Gastrostomy buttons can be used to improve nutritional intake as well as for the administration of medications. Overnight gastrostomy feeding has been shown to improve height and weight parameters [99].

Gastrointestinal symptoms are recognised. These were found to be common in a study undertaken on behalf of the Cystinosis Foundation [100] and occur at a younger age than was previously recognised. Functional abnormalities include gastro-oesphageal reflux, pseudo-obstruction and swallowing dysfunction. In extreme cases parenteral nutrition has been indicated.

Adults with cystinosis can show progressive neuromuscular dysfunction, with bulbar and upper extremity weakness. Feeding difficulties are common in children with cystinosis with many requiring gastrostomy feeds. A small study demonstrated oral motor dysfunction including hypotonia, abnormal gag reflex and congested voice [101]. Hypotonia, muscle weakness, gross and fine motor dysfunction and ataxia were seen on neurology examination. Long term information is needed to determine whether early oral motor problems predict the later development of progressive myopathy.

References

1 Fitzpatrick MM, Kerr SJ, Bradbury MG The child with acute renal failure. In: Webb N, Postlethwaite R (eds) *Clinical Paediatric Nephrology*, 3rd edn. Oxford: Oxford University Press, 2003, pp. 405–25.

2 Stapleton FB, Jones DB, Green RS Acute renal failure in neonates: incidence, aetiology and outcome. *Pediatr Nephrol*, 1987, **1** 314–20.

3 Milford DV, Taylor CM New insights into haemolytic uraemic syndrome. *Arch Dis Child*, 1990, **65** 713–15.

4 Coleman JE, Watson AR Nutritional support for the child with acute renal failure. *J Hum Nutr Diet*, 1992, **5** 99–105.

5 Haycock GB Renal disease. In: McLaren DS, Burman D, Belton NR, Williams AF (eds) *Textbook of Paediatric Nutrition*, 3rd edn. Edinburgh: Churchill Livingstone, 1991, pp. 240–2.

6 Bullock ML, Umen AJ, Finkelstein M, Keane WF The assessment of risk factors in 462 patients with acute renal failure. *Am J Kidney Dis*, 1985, **5** 97–103.

7 Freeman JV *et al*. Cross sectional and weight reference curves for the UK 1990. *Arch Dis Child*, 1995, **73** 17–24.

8 Grupe WE Nutritional issues in acute renal insufficiency. In: Grand RJ, Sutphen JL, Dietz WH (eds) *Paediatric Nutrition, Theory and Practice*, London: Butterworths, 1987, pp. 582–4.

9 Department of Health Report on Health and Social Subjects No 41. *Dietary Reference Values for Food, Energy and Nutrients for the United Kingdom*. London: The Stationery Office, 1991.

10 Maxvold NJ, Smoyer WE, Custer R, Bunchman TE Amino acid loss and nitrogen balance in critically ill children with acute renal failure: A prospective comparison between classic hemofiltration + hemofiltration with dialysis. *Crit Care Med*, 2000, **28** 1161–5.

11 Scheinkestel CD, Kar L, Marshal K, Bailey M *et al*. Prospective randomised trial to assess caloric and protein needs of critically ill, anuric, ventilated patients requiring continuous renal replacement therapy. *Nutrition*, 2003, **19** 909–16.

12 Klein C *et al*. Magnesium, calcium, zinc and nitrogen loss in trauma patients during continuous renal replacement therapy. *J Parenter Enteral Nutr*, 2002, **26** 77–93.

13 Berger M *et al*. Copper, selerium, zinc and thiamine balances during continuous venovenous hemodiafiltration in critically ill patients. *Am J Clin Nutr*, 2004, **80** 410–16.

14 Rigden S The management of chronic and end stage renal failure in children. In: Webb N, Postlethwaite R (eds) *Clinical Paediatric Nephrology*, 3rd edn. Oxford: Oxford University Press, 2003, pp. 427–45.

15 UK Renal Registry 6th Annual Report December 2003. Lewis M, Chapter 14 pp. 205–31.

16 Ramage IJ, Durkan AM Principles of management of chronic renal failure. *Curr Paediatr*, 2003, **13** 496–501.

17 Wingen AM, Fabian-Bach C, Schaefer F, Mehls O and the European Study Group for Nutritional Treatment of Chronic Renal failure in Childhood. Randomised multicentre study of a low protein diet on the progression of chronic renal failure in children. *Lancet*, 1997, **349** 1117–23.

18 Kari JA , Gonzalez C, Ledermann SE, Shaw V, Rees L Outcome and growth of infants with severe chronic renal failure *Kidney Int*, 2000, **57** 1681–7.

19 Uauy RD, Hogg RJ, Brewer ED, Reisch JS, Cunningham C, Holliday MA Dietary protein and growth in infants with chronic renal insufficiency: a report from the Southwest Paediatric Nephrology Study Group and the University of California, San Francisco. *Pediatr Nephrol*, 1994, **8** 45–50.

20 Cole TJ *et al*. BMI reference curves. *Arch Dis Child*, 1995, **73** 25–9.

21 Nelson P, Stover J Principles of nutritional assessment and management of the child with ESRD. In: Fine RN, Gruskin AB (eds) *End Stage Renal Disease in Children*. Philadelphia: WB Saunders, 1984, pp. 209–26.

22 Betts PR, McGrath G Growth pattern and dietary intake of children with chronic renal insufficiency. *Br Med J*, 1974, **2** 189–93.

23 Norman L, Macdonald I, Watson A Optimising nutrition in chronic renal insuffiency – growth. *Pediatr Nephrol*, 2004, **19** 1245–52.

24 Haffner D, Schaefer F, Nissel R, Wuhl E, Tonshoff B, Mehls O For the German study group for growth hormone treatment in chronic renal failure. Effect of growth hormone on the adult height of children with chronic renal failure. *N Engl J Med*, 2000, **343** 923–30.

25 Haycock GB The influence of sodium on growth in infancy. *Pediatr Nephrol*, 1993, **7** 871–5.

26 Dehourne J, Van't Hoff W Renal tubular disorders. *Curr Paediatr*, 2003, **13** 487–95.

27 Treatment of Adults and Children with Renal failure. Standards, Audit measure, 3rd edn, London: The Royal College of Physicians of London and The Renal Association, 2002.

28   Milliner DS, Zinsmaster AR, Lieberman E, Landing B Soft tissue calcification in pediatric patients with end stage renal disease. *Kidney Int*, 1990, **38** 931–6.

29   Mahdavi H, Kuizan BD, Gales B, Wang HJ, Elashoff RM, Salusky IB Sevelamer hydrochloride: an effective phosphate binder in dialysed children. *Pediatr Nephrol*, 2003, **18** 1260–4.

30   Ritz E The clinical management of hyperphosphatemia *J Nephrol*, 2005, **18** 221–8.

31   Salt and Health Scientific Advisory Committee on Nutrition 2003. London: The Stationery Office. Pub TS0 www.sacn.gov.yk

32   Sacks FM, Svetkey LP, Vollmer VVM, Appel LJ, Bray GA, Harsha D *et al*. Effects on blood pressure of reduced dietary sodium and the dietary approaches to stop hypertension (DASH) diet. *N Engl J Med*, 2001, **344** 3–10.

33   Khlar S, Levey AS, Beck GJ, Caggiula AW, Hunsicker L, Kusek JW, Striker G The effects of dietary protein restriction and blood pressure control on the progression of non-diabetic renal disease. *N Engl J Med*, 1994, **330** 877–84.

34   Taal MW, Brenner BM Renoprotective benefits of RAS inhibition: From ACEI to angiotensin II antagonists. *Kidney Int*, 2000, **57** 1803–17.

35   Wingen A-M, Mehls O Nutrition in children with preterminal chronic renal failure. Myth or important therapeutic aid? *Pediatr Nephrol*, 2002, **17** 111–20.

36   Chavers BM, Li S, Collins AJ, Herzog CA Cardiovascular disease in paediatric chronic dialysis patients. *Kidney Int*, 2002, **62** 648–53.

37   Norman LJ, Coleman JE, Watson AR Nutritional management in a child on chronic peritoneal dialysis: a team approach. *J Hum Nutr Diet*, 1995, **8** 209–13.

38   Review of Multi-Professional Paediatric Nephrology Services in the UK – Towards Standards and Equity of Care 2003. Report of a working party of the British Association for Paediatric Nephrology.

39   Lewis M, Shaw J Report of the Paediatric Renal Registry. In: Ansell D, Feest T (eds) *UK Renal Registry Report*, 2000. Bristol, UK Renal Registry, Chapter 15.

40   National Kidney Foundation Dialysis Outcome Quality Initiative Clinical practice guidelines; pediatric guidelines. *Am J Kidney Dis*, 2000, **35** 6 (Suppl 2) S105–36.

41   Shaefer F Adequacy of peritoneal dialysis in children. In: Fine RN, Alexander SR, Warady BA (Eds) *CAPD/CCPD in Children*, 2nd edn. Boston: Kluwer Academic Publishers, 1998, pp. 99–118.

42   Shaefer F, Klaus G, Mehls O and the Mid-European Paediatric Dialysis Study Group Peritoneal transport properties and dialysis dose affect growth and nutritional status in children on chronic peritoneal dialysis. *J Am Soc Nephrol*, 1999, **10** 1786–92.

43   Boxall MC, Goodship THJ Nutritional requirements in hemodialysis. In: Mitch WE, Klahr S (eds) *Handbook of Nutrition and the Kidney*, 5th edn. Philadelphia: Lippincott, Williams and Wilkins, 2005, pp. 218–27.

44   Edefonti A, Picca M, Damiani B *et al*. Dietary prescription based on estimated nitrogen balance during peritoneal dialysis. *Pediatr Nephrol*, 1999, **13:** 253–8.

45   Gokal R, Moberley J, Lindholm B, Salim M Metabolic and laboratory effects of icodextrin. *Kidney Int*, 2002, **62 (Suppl 81)** pp. 562–71.

46   Van Hoeck K, Rusthoven E, Vermeylen L, Vandesompel A, Marescoul B, Lilien M, Schroder C Nutritional effects of increasing dialysis dose by adding icodextrin daytime dwell to Nocturnal Intermittent Peritoneal Dialysis in Children. *Nephrol Dial Transplant*, 2003, **18** 1383–7.

47   Druml W, Fischer M, Liebisch B, Lenz K, Roth E Elimination of amino acids in renal failure. *Am J Clin Nutr*, 1994, **60** 418–23.

48   Quan A, Baum M Protein losses in children on continuous cyclic peritoneal dialysis. *Pediatr Nephrol*, 1996, **10** 728–31.

49   Churchill DN, Wayne Taylor D, Keshaviah PR *et al*. Adequacy of dialysis and nutrition in continuous peritoneal dialysis; association with clinical outcomes. *J Am Soc Nephrol*, 1996, **7** 198–207.

50   Coleman JE, Watson AR Vitamin, mineral and trace element supplementation of children on chronic peritoneal dialysis. *J Hum Nutr Diet*, 1991, **4** 13–17.

51   Sevgi M, Mehmet K, Mehmet Y *et al*. Effect of hemodialysis on carnitine levels in children with chronic renal failure. *Pediatrics International*, 2002, **44** 70–3.

52   Golper TA, Goral S, Becker BN, Langman CB L-carnitine treatment of anaemia. *Am J Kidney Dis*, 2003, **41 (Suppl 4)** S27–34.

53   Coleman JE Micronutrient supplements for children. *Br J Ren Med*, 1998, **3** 21–3.

54   Kopple JD, Blumenkrantz M Nutritional requirements for patients undergoing continuous ambulatory peritoneal dialysis. *Kidney Int*, 1989, **24** (Suppl 16) 295–302.

55   Warady BA, Kriley M, Uri SA *et al*. Vitamin status of infants receiving long-term peritoneal dialysis. *Pediatr Nephrol*, 1994, **8** 354–6.

56   Shah GM, Ross EA, Sabo A *et al*. Effects of ascorbic acid and pyridoxine supplementation on oxalate metabolism in peritoneal dialysis patients. *Am J Kidney Dis*, 1992, **20** 42–9.

57   Norman LJ, Coleman JE, Watson AR *et al*.

Nutritional supplements and elevated serum vitamin A levels in children on chronic dialysis. *J Hum Nutr Diet*, 1996, **9** 257–62.

58 Makoff RM, Dwyer J, Rocco MV Folic acid, pyridoxine, cobalamin and homocysteine and their relationship to cardiovascular disease in end stage renal disease. *J Ren Nutr*, 1996, **6** 2–11.

59 Friedman A, Bostom A, Selhub J, Levey A, Rosenberg I The kidney and homocysteine metabolism. *J Am Soc Nephrol*, 2001, **12** 2181–9.

60 Dixon P, Iurilli J, Watson A, Neill E, Foy J, Martin M Acceptability of a reformulated renal-specific micronutrient supplement. *Pediatr Nephrol*, 2004, **19** 1433–4.

61 Neu AM, Warady BA Special considerations in the care of the infant CAPD/CCPD patient. In: *CAPD/CCPD in Children*, 2nd edn. Boston: Kluwer Academic Publishers, 1998, pp. 281–301.

62 Ledermann SE, Shaw V, Trompeter RS. Long-term enteral nutrition in infants and young children with chronic renal failure. *Pediatr Nephrol*, 1999, **13** 870–5.

63 Coleman JE, Norman LJ, Watson AR Provision of dietetic care in children on chronic peritoneal dialysis. *J Ren Nutr*, 1999, **9** 145–8.

64 Watson AR, Coleman JE, Warady BA When and how to use nasogastric and gastrostomy feeding for nutritional support. In: Fine RN, Alexander SR, Warady BA (eds) *CAPD/CCPD in Children*, 2nd edn. Boston: Kluwer Academic Publishers, 1998, 281–301.

65 Coleman JE, Watson AR, Rance CH *et al.* Gastrostomy buttons for nutritional support on chronic renal dialysis. *Nephrol Dial Transpl*, 1998, **13** 2041–6.

66 Warady BA, Kriley M, Belden B *et al.* Nutritional and behavioural aspects of nasogastric tube feeding in infants receiving chronic peritoneal dialysis. In: Khanna R (ed) *Advances in Peritoneal Dialysis*. Toronto: University of Toronto Press, 1990, **6** 265–8.

67 Ravelli AM Gastrointestinal function in chronic renal failure. *Pediatr Nephrol*, 1995, **9** 756–62.

68 Hassall E Decisions in diagnosing and managing chronic gastroesophageal reflux disease in children. *J Pediatr*, 2005, **146** S4–12.

69 Gonzalez-Heydrich J, Kerner JA, Steiner H Testing the psychogenic vomiting diagnosis: four paediatric patients. *Am J Dis Child*, 1991, **145** 913–16.

70 Shaw V, Coleman J. Nutritional management of renal disease in childhood. *Annales Nestle*, 2003, **61** 21–31.

71 Strologo LD, Principato F, Sinibaldi D *et al.* Feeding dysfunction in infants with severe chronic renal failure after long-term nasogastric tube feeding. *Pediatr Nephrol*, 1997, **11** 84–6.

72 Kari JA, Shaw V, Valance DT *et al.* Effect of enteral feeding on lipid subfractions in children with chronic renal failure. *Pediatr Nephrol*, 1998, **12** 401–4.

73 Coleman JE, Watson AR Growth post-transplantation in children previously treated with chronic dialysis and gastrostomy feeding. In: Khanna R (ed.) *Advances in Peritoneal Dialysis*. Toronto: University of Toronto Press, 1990, **14**, 271–3.

74 Handen B, Mandell F, Russo D Feeding induction in children who refuse to eat. *Am J Dis Child*, 1986, **140** 52–4.

75 Mitsnefes M, Khoury P, McEnergy P Early post transplantation hypertension and poor long-term renal allograft survival in pediatric patients. *J Pediatr*, 2003, **143** 98–103.

76 Groothoff J, Gruppen M, Offringa M, de Groot E, Stok W, Bos W *et al.* Increased arterial stiffness in young adults with end-stage renal disease since childhood. *J Am Soc Nephrol*, 2002, **13** 2953–61.

77 Baigent C, Burbury K, Wheeler D Premature cardiovascular disease in chronic renal failure. *Lancet*, 2000, **356** 147–51.

78 Saland J, Ginsberg H, Fisher E Dyslipidemia in pediatric renal disease: epidemiology, pathophysiology and management. *Curr Opin Pediatr*, 2002, **14** 197–204.

79 Lombaerts R Children's growth after kidney transplantation. *Lancet*, 2005, **366** 103–4.

80 Eddy AA, Symons JM Nephrotic syndrome in childhood. *Lancet*, 2003, **362** 629–39.

81 Haycock G The child with idiopathic nephrotic syndrome. In: Webb N, Postlethwaite R (eds) *Clinical Paediatric Nephrology*, 3rd edn. Oxford: Oxford University Press 2003, pp. 341–66.

82 Rees L, Greene SA, Adlord P *et al.* Growth and endocrine function in steroid sensitive nephrotic syndrome. *Arch Dis Child*, 1988, **63** 484–90.

83 Querfeld U Should hyperlipidemia in children with the nephrotic syndrome be treated? *Pediatr Nephrol*, 1999, **13** 77–84.

84 Coleman JE, Watson AR Hyperlipidaemia, diet and simvastatin therapy in steroid resistant nephrotic syndrome of childhood. *Pediatr Nephrol*, 1995, **10** 171–4.

85 Al-Bander H, Kaysen GA Ineffectiveness of dietary protein augmentation in the management of nephrotic syndrome. *Pediatr Nephrol*, 1991, **5** 482–6.

86 Royle J, Postlethwaite RJ What protein intake is recommend for nephrotic children? *Pediatr Nephrol*, 1991, **5** 581.

87 Feehally J, Baker F, Walls J Dietary manipulation in experimental nephrotic syndrome. *Nephron*, 1988, **50** 247–52.

88 Grupe WE Nutritional issues in glomerular dam-

age. In: Grand RJ, Sutphen JL, Dietz WH (eds) *Paediatric Nutrition, Theory and Practice*, London: Butterworths, 1987, pp. 579–81.

89 Watson AR, Coleman JE Dietary management in nephrotic syndrome. *Arch Dis Child*, 1993, **69** 179–80.

90 Genova R *et al*. Food allergy in steroid resistant nephrotic syndrome. *Lancet*, 1987, 1315–16.

91 Lagrue G, Laurent J, Rostoker G, Lang D Food allergy in idiopathic nephrotic syndrome. *Lancet*, 1987, 277.

92 Holmberg C, Antikainen M, Ronnholom K, Ala-Houhala M, Jalanko H Management of congenital nephrotic syndrome of the Finnish type. *Pediatr Nephrol*, 1995, **9** 87–93.

93 Stern P Nephrogenic defects of urinary concentration. In: Edelman CM (ed) *Pediatric Kidney Disease*, 2nd edn. London: Little Brown, 1992.

94 Knoers N, Monnens L Nephrogenic diabetes insipidus. In: Holliday MA, Barratt TM, Avner ED (eds) *Pediatric Nephrology*, 3rd edn. Baltimore: Williams & Wilkins, 1994.

95 Jones C, Mughal Z Disorders of mineral metabolism and nephrolithiasis. In: Webb N, Postlethwaite R (eds) *Clinical Paediatric Nephrology*, 3rd edition. Oxford: Oxford University Press, 2003, pp. 87–101.

96 Thomas B (ed) *Manual of Dietetic Practice*, 3rd edn. Oxford: Blackwell Science, 2001, pp. 435–42.

97 Orson WM Kidney stones: pathophysiology and medical management. *Lancet*, 2006, **367** 333–44.

98 van't Hoff W Renal tubular disorders In: Webb N, Postlethwaite R (eds) *Clinical Paediatric Nephrology*, 3rd edn. Oxford: Oxford University Press, 2003, pp. 103–12.

99 Coleman JE, Watson AR Gastrostomy buttons for nutritional support in children with cystinosis. *Pediatr Nephrol*, 2000, **14** 833–6.

100 Elenberg E, Norling LL, Kleinman RE, Ingelfinger JR Feeding problems in cystinosis. *Pediatr Nephrol*, 1998, **12** 365–70.

101 Trauner DA, Fahmy RF, Mishler DA Oral motor dysfunction and feeding difficulties in nephropathic cystinosis. *Pediatr Neurol*, 2001, **24** 365–8.

13 The Cardiothoracic System

David Hopkins

Congenital heart disease

The incidence of congenital heart disease (CHD) is approximately 8 in every 1000 live births. It is the largest single group of congenital abnormalities and accounts for approximately 30% of the total. Eight lesions make up 80% of cases, the most common of which are ventricular septal defect, patent ductus arteriosus, atrial septal defect and tetralogy of Fallot. Children with certain syndromes have a higher incidence of congenital heart defects (e.g. 50% of infants with Down's syndrome have cardiac defects). This percentage is even higher in children with Noonan's syndrome, 80% presenting mainly with pulmonary stenosis or hypertrophic cardiomyopathy [1].

Congestive heart failure (CHF) describes a set of symptoms and clinical signs which show myocardial dysfunction with a cardiac output that is inadequate to meet the metabolic demands of the body. In infants and children it may be caused by increased cardiac workload. CHD is the cause of most CHF during infancy and childhood although severe anaemia may mimic signs of CHF at any age.

Both malnutrition and growth retardation are associated with complex congenital heart disease in infancy [2–10] and childhood [11]. Wynn Cameron *et al.* [12], defining acute malnutrition as <90% weight for height and chronic malnutrition as <90% of mean height for age, reported a prevalence of 33% and 64%, respectively, in hospitalised infants and children with CHD. Not all cardiac lesions result in failure to thrive; in isolated atrial septal defect (ASD) growth is usually adequate and primary repair is carried out later in childhood. Other defects such as coarctation of the aorta or transposition of the great arteries (TGA) usually require primary repair in the neonatal period and thereafter should not require long term dietetic intervention.

Causes of poor growth in infants and children with congenital heart disease

Underlying physiology

Congenital heart diseases can be divided into two main types, those that cause cyanosis and those that do not. Examples of a complex cyanotic and acyanotic lesion, and the complex lesion, tetralogy of Fallot, are shown in Figs 13.1–13.3. Children with cyanotic lesions appear to be at greatest risk of stunting [13]. The mechanism for this is uncertain but it is suggested that suboptimal tissue oxygenation may be a factor [13]. In contrast, complex acyanotic disease is associated more with wasting; pulmonary hypertension (high blood pressure in the lungs) appears to be a major causative factor [7,14]. In a normal circulation, blood pumped by the weaker right ventricle is under pressure that is less than one-third of that being pumped by the left

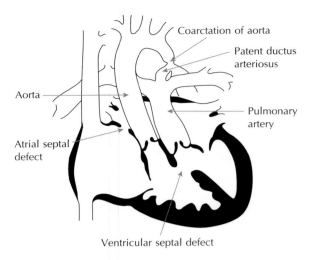

Figure 13.1   A complex cyanotic lesion.

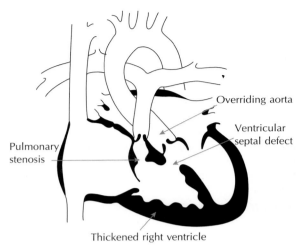

Figure 13.3   Tetralogy of Fallot.

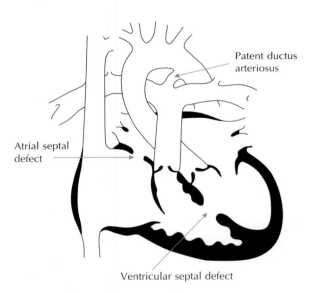

Figure 13.2   A complex acyanotic lesion.

ventricle. Any lesion that causes an excessive blood flow from the left to right circulation has a risk of causing increased pulmonary blood flow. This results in too much blood in the lungs for efficient oxygenation. As a result a disproportionate amount of energy is used up in the increased respiratory effort. These defects cause what is known as a 'left to right shunt'. An example would be a patient with a haemodynamically significant ventricular septal

defect (VSD), in which the hole between the two ventricles is large enough to cause excessive blood flow from the left to right pumping chamber. Varan *et al.* [7] have shown that children with complex cardiac defects that cause cyanosis as well as pulmonary hypertension are at the greatest risk of a combination of both stunting and wasting.

Energy expenditure and metabolism

Studies using doubly labelled water have been used to calculate energy expenditure in infants with various cardiac defects [15–18]. The average total daily energy expenditure (TEE) in normal infants appears to be 60–70 kcal kg/day (250–292 kJ/kg/day) [19]. Large VSDs, along with lesions that result in cyanosis, appear to elevate TEE to about 90 kcal/kg/day (376 kJ/kg/day) even though resting energy expenditure (REE) appears to be normal [16–18]. Increasing size of the 'left to right shunt' in patients with VSD has been shown to correlate with increasing TEE [17] and decreasing height standard deviation and body mass index (BMI) scores [20]. A TEE as high as 157 kcal/kg/day (656 kJ/kg/day) has been recorded [15]. Elevated TEE appears to be caused by an increase in the energy cost of physical activity [16–18]. Infants with lesions that do not result in CHF have a TEE between normal and those with CHF. Consequently, there is less energy available for growth. Malnutrition itself is known to reduce ventricular mass and cardiac output, which may further exacerbate a compromised circulation [21]. Energy expenditure depends on the type and severity of the cardiac lesion.

Lundell *et al.* [22] looked at lipid metabolism in two groups of infants with CHD. One group had VSD, the other group had cyanotic CHD. The cyanotic group all had transposition of the great arteries and their mean oxygen saturation was 68%. Both groups were given an intravenous (IV) lipid load. Severe growth retardation in infants in both groups was correlated to higher peak levels (after IV lipid load) of linoleic acid in the plasma free fatty acids. The peak levels of linoleic acid in the triglyceride fraction were positively correlated to weight standard deviation score. Peak glycerol levels were higher in the most growth retarded infants, indicating faster intravascular lipolysis. They concluded that their results supported the hypothesis that lipid metabolism is disturbed in infants with CHD [22].

Recent research indicates that hormone levels may also have a role in affecting the growth of children with cardiac abnormalities. Serum concentrations of insulin-like growth factor 1 (IGF1) are reduced in children with VSD. Reduced levels of IGF1 correlate with reduced BMI and increasing size of the 'left to right shunt'. It is postulated that hypermetabolism compromises nutritional status by reducing IGF1 synthesis, further slowing linear growth and weight gain [20].

Energy and nutrient intake

Increased breathlessness causes some cardiac patients to feed repeatedly for short periods of time. Energy intakes of 82–88% of those normally recommended have been demonstrated in children with CHD [15,23] and it has been suggested that this is the main reason for poor growth [24]. However, recent research findings indicate that energy intakes may actually be normal [16–18,20]. Vitamin and mineral intakes of young children with CHD may be lower than that of the normal population but appear to achieve the reference nutrient intake (RNI), with the exception of vitamin D [23]. A child with faltering growth whose diet history indicates a normal or above normal energy intake warrants a cardiac assessment as part of further clinical investigations.

Children who have a cardiac anatomy that results in pulmonary hypertension as well as cyanosis may have nutrient intakes significantly lower than those with pulmonary hypertension or cyanosis alone [7]. In addition, children with complex lesions needing palliative surgery, or a staged rather than single repair, may be at higher risk of poor growth and closer monitoring is required; for example, almost one-third of postoperative patients with hypoplastic left heart syndrome did not meet normal energy requirements during their hospital stay and almost 60% did not regain their birthweight by discharge following their first staged operation [25]. It is therefore important, wherever possible, to correct nutritional deficits and secondary growth disturbances that may ultimately put children at increased surgical risk [26].

Additional factors involved in poor growth are:

- Fatigue on feeding leading to low total intake
- Early satiety
- Anorexia
- Vomiting
- Frequent infections
- Frequent use of antibiotics affecting gut flora

Failure to thrive in CHD may therefore be multifactorial but it appears that raised energy expenditure affects the surplus available for growth. An understanding of the primary cardiac anatomy is important in order to identify those patients who are at risk. Table 13.1 categorises the various cardiac lesions in terms of potential nutritional risk. It is worth noting that although most patients have improved growth postoperatively, some continue to exhibit growth failure even after haemodynamic correction [27].

Gastrointestinal and hepatic function in infants and children with congenital heart disease

Gastro-oesophageal reflux

Infants with congenital cardiac defects have been found to have delayed gastric emptying [28] and are therefore more likely to have problems with gastro-oesophageal reflux (GOR). Positioning and feed thickeners may be used as a first line treatment if there is a suspicion of GOR (see p. 117). In the intensive care setting there is often a clear correla-

Table 13.1   Cardiac defects with 'high' or 'low' likelihood of needing dietetic intervention.

Low	Variable presentation/risk	High
Coarctation of aorta	Pulmonary atresia*	Ventricular septal defect (VSD) – moderate to large
Patent ductus arteriosus (PDA) – if early surgery performed	Tetralogy of Fallot*	Atrioventricular septal defect (AVSD)
Atrial septal defect (ASD)		Hypoplastic left heart*
Cor triatrium		Truncus arteriosus*
Transposition of the great arteries (TGA)*		Aorto pulmonary window
Total anomalous pulmonary venous drainage (TAPVD)*		PDA – if large
Pulmonary stenosis*		Tricuspid atresia*
		Ebstein's anomaly*
		Partial anomalous pulmonary venous drainage* (PAPVD)

* Cyanotic lesions.

tion between deterioration in cardiac function and reduced feed tolerance, which resolves if cardiac function improves. Additional drug treatment or a resort to naso jejunal feeding may be needed to control more severe vomiting. It is also worth considering other factors that may cause vomiting (e.g. cows' milk protein intolerance when a cow's milk free formula would be indicated) (see p. 97).

Necrotising enterocolitis

Some cardiac conditions may predispose infants to necrotising enterocolitis (NEC) even if they are born at term [29]. Hypoplastic left heart, truncus arteriosus and aortopulmonary window have all been identified as defects that increase the risk of the infant developing NEC [29] along with infants admitted in clinical shock. In addition, lesions requiring high doses of prostaglandin (>0.05 µg/kg/min) to keep the ductus arteriosus open, to ensure adequate blood flow to the lungs, may also place the patient at increased risk. The use of prostaglandin introduces a theoretical risk of blood being 'stolen' from the systemic circulation to the lungs, resulting in reduced mesenteric blood flow and perfusion of the associated gut tissue. Disturbed mesenteric artery blood flow in infants with such systemic to pulmonary circulatory shunts has been demonstrated [30]. However, in a separate

smaller study involving neonates with hypoplastic left heart, none developed NEC in spite of proven reduced mesenteric artery blood flow [31]. In none of the above studies has feeding *per se* been identified as an independent risk factor for NEC and it should therefore progress with caution. With the known benefits of breast milk in preventing NEC [32,33] it should be used as the feed of choice in this group of patients. If breast milk is not available then a normal infant formula may be used.

Coarctation of the aorta has not been identified as a predisposing factor for NEC in spite of the theoretical risks resulting from reduced systemic blood flow. Infants with coarctation of the aorta may be admitted with a history of taking feed volumes near the top of the normal range with no signs of intolerance. A number of cardiac units restrict feeding in these babies for the first few days post-operatively and if a baby has been admitted in clinical shock pre-operatively this may be prudent.

Protein-losing enteropathy

Children with a cardiac anatomy that gives them a single functional ventricle undergo a series of operations in which the venous return is eventually plumbed directly into the arteries of the lungs. This is known as a total cavo-pulmonary connection (TCPC) and has the benefit of improving oxygenation and reducing the load on the ventricle. Protein-losing enteropathy occurs in congestive heart failure [34] and there is a growing body of evidence that it occurs in 10–25% of patients who have undergone a TCPC procedure [35,36]. This may resolve as cardiac function improves following surgery or heart transplant [37]. Localised lesions have been treated by partial bowel resection [35]. There is limited evidence for the dietary treatment of protein-losing enteropathy but a useful starting point would be to follow that for intestinal lymphangiectasia (see p. 107). The diet should provide 5–10 g/day fat, be high in protein and use medium chain triglycerides (MCT) to improve overall energy intake.

Hepatic dysfunction

The TCPC operation is known to cause 'back pressure' on the liver, predisposing patients to hepatic dysfunction. Some go on to develop moderate to severe liver disease [38]. Prothrombin time becomes progressively deranged from the time of operation and it has been proposed that this, along with the ability to eliminate galactose, is used as a test of liver dysfunction in this population [38]. Dietary treatment will depend on the degree of liver failure and its progression.

Feeding the infant with cardiac abnormalities

Energy intake

Earlier studies have indicated that if sufficient energy is provided appropriate weight gain and linear growth can be achieved [39,40]. Yahav *et al.* [39] found a good correlation between energy intake and weight gain but a constant weight gain was observed only when energy intake exceeded 170 kcal/kg/day (710 kJ/kg/day). Below this the most severely nutritionally depleted infants continued to lose weight. Barton *et al.* have recommended intakes of 150 kcal/kg/day (627 kJ/kg/day) in order to achieve adequate growth [15]. Other studies measuring TEE seem to indicate that an intake of approximately 30 kcal/kg/day (125 kJ/kg/day) above the estimated average requirement (EAR) for energy should achieve adequate energy intake for growth in most infants [18–20]. A reason-

able starting point with an infant who is failing to thrive would therefore seem to be 120–130 kcal/kg/day (502–544 kJ/kg/day), with a proviso of increasing energy intake further should adequate weight gain not be achieved. The use of growth charts is essential to assess ongoing requirements.

Fluid restrictions after cardiac surgery

There is a need to limit the amount of fluid in the circulatory system postoperatively so that repaired tissue does not become subject to excessive circulatory pressure and strain. Keeping the lungs relatively dry also helps to wean the patient off the ventilator. The amount of fluid that a child is permitted to have in the days immediately following surgery varies between units but inevitably results in insufficient volume to achieve adequate nutrition. This fluid restriction is temporary and opportunities should be taken to improve nutritional intake over subsequent days as the fluid restriction is lifted. However, should the clinical condition and/or fluid balance of the patient result in fluid restrictions continuing beyond that normally expected, then steps need to be taken to ensure adequate nutrition. Rogers *et al.* [41] demonstrated that less than one-third of children undergoing cardiac surgery achieve their estimated energy requirement while on the intensive care ward and have significant falls in weight during their stay.

Fluid allowances on cardiac intensive care units are often expressed in terms of a percentage and is calculated cumulatively as follows:

- 4 mL/kg/hour for the first 10 kg in weight
- 2 mL/kg/hour for the second 10 kg in weight
- 1 mL/kg/hour for every kg above 20 kg

to give the patient a '100%' fluid allowance. Although a child may be having 100% fluid allowance this does not necessarily equate to normal fluid requirements and therefore nutrition will be compromised; for example, a baby weighing 6.2 kg on 100% fluid allowance would have $(6.2 \times 4 \times 24) = 595$ mL/day = 96 mL/kg/day (usual fluid requirement = 150 mL/kg/day). Table 13.2 illustrates how fluid allowances might be increased following surgery depending on whether the patient has had open heart surgery with cardiopulmonary bypass, or closed heart surgery (on

Table 13.2   Fluid allowance on paediatric intensive care unit after surgery.

Day post-surgery	Closed heart surgery (%)	Open heart surgery (%)
1	80	50
2	90–100	60
3	120	70
4	Free fluids	80
5		90
6		100
7		120–135
8		150

vessels surrounding the heart). Volumes of intravenous drug infusions are included in the total fluid allowance leaving limited room for feed in the days immediately after surgery.

Worked example of a 100% fluid allowance for a child weighing 30 kg

For the first 10 kg: $10 \times 4 = 40$ mL/hour
For the second 10 kg: $10 \times 2 = 20$ mL/hour
For the third 10 kg: $10 \times 1 = 10$ mL/hour
Total fluid allowance: 70 mL/hour

If the above child is on a 50% fluid restriction then he or she will receive only 50% of the calculated volume (i.e. 35 mL/hour).

Type of feed to use

Breast feeding or expressed breast milk (EBM), as with most infants, is the feed of choice for infants with CHD. The mechanism of breast feeding may cause less cardiorespiratory stress resulting in lower oxygen desaturation episodes [42] and has been attempted within 1 week of heart transplant [43]. If there is ongoing severe fluid restriction (<100 mL/kg) or inadequate weight gain, fortification of the breast milk is necessary. This may be done by adding 3–5% infant formula powder, or by using one of the commercially available breast milk fortifiers for the premature infant (see p. 15). Addition of a commercial fortifier has a negligible effect on delaying gastric emptying [44]. If breast milk is not available it will be necessary to use an infant formula. To meet the nutrient requirements for infants with CHD it is necessary to use a formula with a higher nutrient density than a standard infant formula. Two such formulas are available:

- SMA High Energy 91 kcal (380 kJ)/100 mL 2.0 g protein/100 mL
- Infatrini 100 kcal (420 kJ)/100 mL 2.6 g protein/100 mL

Table 13.3 shows a comparison of the energy and protein obtained from standard infant formula and nutrient-dense infant formula fed at increasing volumes, illustrating how the volumes and concentration of feed may be increased to facilitate growth in infants with CHD who have faltering growth.

A high to very high energy feed may be needed to achieve adequate weight gain and appropriate catch-up growth in some infants with CHD. If there are doubts regarding an infant's tolerance to higher energy feeds then standard infant formula should be used initially at a slightly increased concentration (15%) to provide approximately 80 kcal (334 kJ)/100 mL before progressing to a high energy formula (see p. 15). The strength and volume of feed can be increased as shown in Table 13.4. Pillo-Blocka *et al.* [45] demonstrated that if infants were provided with 80 kcal (334 kJ)/100 mL feed on day 1 of discharge from the intensive care unit, increasing to 100 kcal (420 kJ)/100 mL feed on day 3, there were significant improvements in weight gain at discharge compared with controls. Increases in the energy density of feeds are generally well tolerated.

If weight gain is unsatisfactory on Infatrini fed at 150 mL/kg and it is not possible to increase the volume of feed given, then a further gradual increase in energy density of the feed should be undertaken with the addition of Duocal in 1% daily increments up to a maximum of 4% until weight gain is achieved. At this level of fortification a reasonable protein : energy ratio of 9% is maintained. The final feed provides an energy density of 1.2 kcal/mL (5 kJ/mL). Alternatively, if the protein : energy ratio needs to be better preserved then addition of infant formula powder in 1% increments up to 4% may be considered, achieving a protein : energy ratio of approximately 10%. In some cases, a fine balance has to be made between giving a high enough energy density in the feed to achieve a nutritionally adequate intake yet not making the feed so concentrated that it causes large gastric aspirates, vomiting or diarrhoea.

Table 13.3 A 3-month-old infant with a congenital cardiac defect resulting in failure to thrive, weight 3.5 kg. Comparison of energy and protein intake from standard infant formula and Infatrini when fed at 100, 120 and 150 mL/kg.

		Energy		
		(kcal)	(kJ)	Protein (g)
Feeding 100 mL/kg				
Total fluid intake 360 mL				
Feeding 45 mL × 3 hourly × 8 feeds				
(a) 360 mL standard infant formula		245	1024	5
	per kg =	70	293	1.4
(b) 360 mL Infatrini		360	1505	9.4
	per kg =	100	418	2.6
DRV	per kg =	100 (EAR)*	418	2.1 (RNI)[†]
Suggested requirement per kg =		120+	502+	3+
Feeding 120 mL/kg				
Total fluid intake 440 mL				
Feeding 55 mL × 3 hourly × 8 feeds				
(a) 440 mL standard infant formula		299	1250	6.6
	per kg =	81	339	1.8
(b) 440 mL Infatrini		440	1848	11.4
	per kg =	120	505	3.1
DRV	per kg =	100	418	2.1
Suggested requirement per kg =		120+	502+	3–4.5
Feeding 150 mL/kg				
Total fluid intake 520 mL				
Feeding 65 mL × 3 hourly × 8 feeds				
(a) 520 mL standard infant formula		341	1432	7.8
	per kg =	97	405	2.2
(b) 520 mL Infatrini		520	2184	13.5
	per kg =	150	630	3.5
DRV	per kg =	100	418	2.1
Suggested requirement per kg =		120+	502+	3–4.5

* Estimated average requirement (Dietary Reference Values) [50].
[†] Reference nutrient intake (Dietary Reference Values) [50].

Methods of feed administration

By the time of discharge from hospital following surgery the majority of cardiac infants should be taking feeds orally but some will fail to complete feeds. This may be because of fatigue brought on by the effort of sucking, anorexia or early satiety. Factors that have been shown to have a detrimental effect on oral feeding capability are vocal chord injury, long postoperative ventilation and poor weight at surgery [46]. If an infant is regularly failing to complete feeds one of the following strategies should be employed:

- Offer smaller, more frequent feeds orally
- Complete feeds via nasogastric tube
- Give small frequent bolus feeds via nasogastric tube
- Top up small frequent daytime feeds with continuous feeds overnight via an enteral feeding pump

Table 13.4 Increasing feed strength and fluid volume using a staged approach.

	Fluid (mL/kg)	Feed	kcal/kg	kJ/kg
Day 1	100	15% Infant formula	78	326
Day 2	120	SMA High Energy	109	458
Day 3	120	Infatrini	120	502
Day 4	140	Infatrini	140	585
Day 5	150	Infatrini	150	627

- Give feeds continuously over 20–21 hours via an enteral pump, allowing the gut to rest for a short period and gastric pH to return to normal

There have been a number of studies looking at the efficacy of methods of feed administration in infants with CHD. Schwarz *et al.* [47] compared oral feeding, oral daytime feeds plus 12 hours continuous nasogastric feeding overnight, and 24 hours continuous nasogastric feeding in a group of infants with CHD and CHF. The feed used was fortified to an energy density of 1 kcal/mL (4 kJ/mL). During the 5 months of the study only the group of infants receiving 24-hour continuous nasogastric feeds achieved intakes in excess of 140 kcal/kg/day (585 kJ/kg/day). Others have demonstrated improvements in energy intake and body weight with nutritional counselling alone [40].

Vanderhoof *et al.* [26] studied a small group of children with complex congenital heart lesions who were all given feeds continuously via a nasogastric tube. These children had all failed to achieve adequate weight gain despite the use of orally administered fortified feeds. Continuous feeding was instigated using the same fortified feeds as had been offered orally. Energy intake and weight measurements were obtained at weekly or monthly intervals. Both mean daily energy intake and mean daily weight gain were greater after initiation of continuous nasogastric feeding. Heymsfield *et al.* [48] suggested that continuous feeding caused a smaller rise in basal metabolic rate and heart rate than occurs after bolus feeds.

A review by Ciotti *et al.* [49] of 37 children with cardiac disease who underwent percutaneous gastrostomy feeding showed improved standard deviation scores (SDS) for weight. However, comparison with nasogastric fed controls is difficult because of differences in starting SDS scores for weight. Patients who require long term tube feeding may benefit from this approach as it may have the added benefit of being less of an impediment to the development of oral feeding skills. The timing of weaning off gastrostomy feeds to allow for the development of independent feeding skills should be addressed for the individual child.

Sodium supplementation of infant feeds

Some infants with CHD may be failing to gain weight on an energy intake in excess of 140 kcal/kg (585 kJ/kg). Diuretic use in patients with CHD makes electrolyte depletion a possibility. These infants may need to have their feeds supplemented with sodium. A 24-hour urine sodium balance should be performed to establish urinary sodium losses. Once the level of sodium loss is known, sodium supplementation should be discussed with medical staff. It should be remembered that an infant feeding 150 mL/kg of a standard infant formula would be receiving 1.0–1.3 mmol Na$^+$/kg, depending on the formula. The RNI for sodium for an infant aged 0–3 months is 1.5 mmol Na$^+$/kg [50].

Anticoagulation and the vitamin K content of feeds

Children undergoing Blalock–Taussig shunts, Fontan or TCPC operations, pulmonary artery reconstruction and some operations requiring tissue homografts are given either aspirin or warfarin postoperatively for anticoagulation. Vitamin K has an antagonistic effect on some of the anticoagulation drugs and may be given in some instances to counter excessive anticoagulation, the dosage being 300 µg/kg/day. While most cardiac infants tolerate whole protein feeds there may occasionally be a need to use a protein hydrolysate formula, some of which have a high vitamin K content (e.g. Pregestimil). An infant weighing 5 kg who is feeding 150 mL/kg/day of such a formula may receive an additional 60 µg/day vitamin K. If a patient is anticoagulated the international normalised ratio (INR) should be monitored in the days following the introduction of such formula.

Chylothorax

Chylothorax is the accumulation of chyle in a pleural cavity from an internal lymphatic fistula. The origin of the fistula can be congenital, obstructive or traumatic [51]. Figure 13.4 shows the anatomy of the thoracic duct.

Constituents of chyle

Chyle contains fat from the intestinal lacteal system

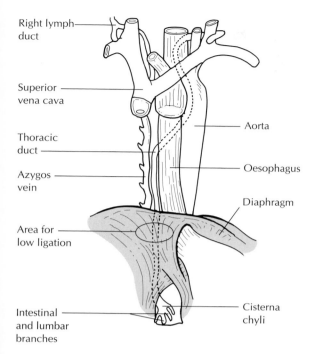

Right lymph duct

Superior vena cava

Thoracic duct

Azygos vein

Aorta

Oesophagus

Diaphragm

Area for low ligation

Intestinal and lumbar branches

Cisterna chyli

Figure 13.4   Anatomy of the thoracic duct. (Source: Merrigan *et al.* [52].)

which gives it a characteristically milky appearance. Sixty to seventy per cent of absorbed dietary fat passes through this system at a concentration of 5–30 g/L. Chyle contains lymphocytes, immunoglobulins, enzymes, triglycerides, cholesterol and fat-soluble vitamins the loss of which, if unchecked, would invariably lead to serious metabolic deficit. The concentration of triglycerides in chyle is higher than that of plasma, which can aid differentiation of chylous pleural effusions from those of other origin [52]. If chylothorax is suspected, the output from the chest drains at the patient's bedside can be checked. A sample with a triglyceride content of >1.1 mmol/L confirms diagnosis.

This condition can be treated conservatively using a minimal long chain triglyceride (LCT) diet [53,54] or with a surgical repair of the fistula [54,55]. A useful algorithm for the management of chylothorax has been produced by Cormack *et al.* [56] and is shown in Fig. 13.5.

The transport of ingested fats is the principal function of thoracic duct lymph. The flow of lymph in the thoracic duct can be increased by up to 10

times its resting volume following a high fat meal. A lesser but definite increase is seen after ingestion of a balanced meal containing protein, carbohydrate and fat [57]. The aim of conservative treatment is to reduce the lymph flow and so allow the fistula to heal. A minimal LCT diet greatly reduces the lymph flow. After hydrolysis in the intestinal lumen, dietary fats are absorbed as glycerol and fatty acids. In the mucosal cell, long chain fatty acids (12 or more carbon atoms) are re-esterified to triglyceride and pass into the lymph as chylomicra. The medium chain fatty acids (6–10 carbon atoms), however, do not undergo resynthesis and pass directly into the portal vein, where they are transported in the form of 'free fatty acids' bound to albumin (Fig. 13.6). In humans, dietary fat is mainly composed of LCT. MCT does not constitute more than a minor proportion of normal dietary fats.

Cardiac conditions predisposing to chylothorax

Chylothorax tends to occur in patients with right-sided obstructive cardiac lesions. With this group of patients longer term oxygenation is achieved by connecting the systemic veins directly to the pulmonary circulation in two operations known as the Glenn shunt and TCPC. A list of cardiac defects that may require these operations is shown in Table 13.5. The lymphatic system drains close to the superior vena cava and as it is moved during the operation the lymphatic drainage may be disturbed

Table 13.5   Conditions requiring Glenn and/or total cavo-pulmonary connection (TCPC) shunt operations (see Glossary for definitions).

Heart defect	Operation
Ebstein's anomaly	TCPC*
Pulmonary atresia with/without intact ventricular septum	Glenn shunt and TCPC
Tricuspid atresia	TCPC
Single ventricle physiology	Glenn shunt and TCPC
Hypoplastic left heart	Norwood stage 2 and 3[†]

* TCPC is one of a number of surgical options in Ebstein's anomaly.
[†] The second stage of the Norwood procedure may be similar to a Glenn shunt or TCPC and the third stage may be a TCPC operation.

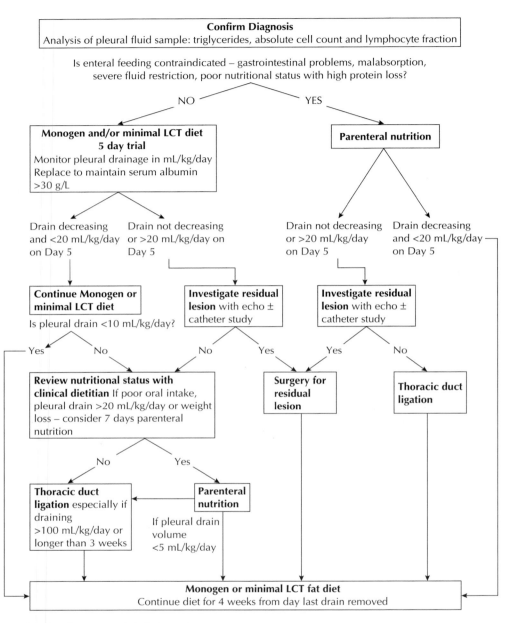

Figure 13.5   Algorithm for suspected chylothorax [56].

or damaged. This results in chyle accumulating in the thoracic cavity. An exacerbating factor may be the development of either a chest infection or a pleural effusion postoperatively. Under these circumstances the blood pressure in the lungs is increased resulting in 'back pressure' into the pul-monary arteries and the newly connected systemic veins. As a result the lymph does not drain well into the veins and the lymphatic vessels themselves become engorged and leaky, with chyle passing into the thoracic cavity. Chylothorax may therefore occur some days after operation.

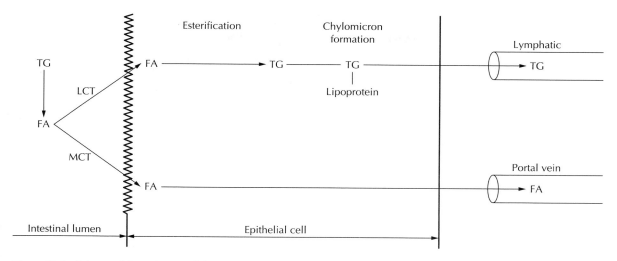

Figure 13.6   Scheme of the pathways of absorption of long chain triglyceride (LCT) and medium chain triglyceride (MCT). FA, fatty acid; TG, triglyceride.

Dietary treatment of chylothorax

- *Minimal LCT diet:* A general guide is to give not more than 1 g LCT per year of life up to a maximum of 4–5 g/day LCT
- *Addition of MCT:* The addition of MCT to the diet increases the energy value and palatability
- *Vitamin and mineral supplementation:* Because a wide range of foods must be either excluded from the diet or taken in reduced quantities, it is essential to check the vitamin and mineral content of the diet, giving supplements if needed

Minimal fat feed for the infant with chylothorax

- Monogen
- MCT Pepdite
- Minimal LCT modular feed based on Peptide Module 767

Monogen

Monogen is a minimal LCT, whole whey protein infant formula. The fat sources are fractionated coconut oil and walnut oil. Table 13.6 shows the nutritional composition of standard dilution

Monogen (17.5%). MCT Step 1 may also be used and has a very similar composition to Monogen.

If the infant has previously been tolerating normal or concentrated feeds prior to the development of chylothorax Monogen can usually be introduced at full strength without any intolerance in spite of the relatively high carbohydrate content (12%). If the baby has had limited enteral nutrition then, as a precaution, Monogen may be introduced at half strength (i.e. 9% dilution in the first 12–24 hours). Standard dilution provides 74 kcal (311 kJ)/100 mL. In cases of severe fluid restriction it will be necessary to gradually increase both concentration and energy density of the feed further in order to meet requirements. Feed concentration may be increased in 1–1.5% increments up to 22% dilution without causing large increases in the LCT content of the feed (Table 13.7). Additional carbohydrate or MCT

Table 13.6   Nutritional content of standard dilution Monogen per 100 mL.

Energy	74 kcal/313 kJ
Protein equivalent	2 g
Carbohydrate	12 g
Fat	2.1 g
MCT	1.9 g
LCT	0.21 g

Table 13.7   Plan for increasing concentration of Monogen.

Day	Monogen dilution (%)	Energy kcal/kJ per 100 mL	Protein (g/100 mL)	CHO (%)	Fat (%)	LCT (g)
1	17.5 (full strength)	74/313	2.0	12	2.1	0.21
2	19	80/337	2.2	13	2.3	0.23
3	20	85/355	2.3	13.7	2.4	0.24
4	21	89/373	2.4	14.4	2.5	0.25
5	22	93/391	2.5	15.1	2.6	0.26

CHO, carbohydrate; LCT, long chain triglyceride.

emulsion may then be added to increase energy density further if indicated. Monogen is a complete infant formula and does not need to be supplemented with essential fatty acids (EFAs).

In clinical practice, achieving adequate energy intake to facilitate growth may mean that the total LCT intake is marginally above the 1 g per year of life recommendation. As long as chest drain output is unaffected then this should be allowed to continue. If chest drains are not *in situ* then clinical signs, with increased respiratory effort and/or chest X-rays, can be used to monitor the tolerance of the increased LCT content of the feed.

There have been individual case reports of the hormone somatostatin or its analogue octreotide, both of which have anti-secretory and anti-diarrhoeal properties, being used in isolation or as an adjunct to a minimal LCT diet or parenteral nutrition to treat refractory chylothorax [58–61]. A dose of 1–4 µg/kg/hour is recommended. The exact mechanism of action remains unclear and attempts to use it regularly in a clinical setting on the author's unit have met with mixed results.

MCT Pepdite

If whole cow's milk protein is contraindicated (e.g. where the infant has a proven cow's milk protein intolerance) Monogen cannot be used. MCT Pepdite may be considered, but its recent reformulation to improve the essential fatty acid profile has resulted in an increase in LCT content: 0.68 g/100 mL, (25% of total fat) compared with 0.21 g/100 mL (10% of total fat) in Monogen. An infant weighing 3.5 kg feeding 150 mL/kg MCT Pepdite will receive in excess of 3.5 g/day LCT. This may not be low enough to reduce chyle flow adequately. Depending on the clinical condition of

the child, MCT Pepdite may be tried but it is most likely that a minimal LCT modular feed will need to be used.

Minimal LCT modular feed

This is a modular feed using Peptide Module 767 as a minimal fat protein source. It is free of cow's milk protein. To produce a nutritionally adequate infant feed it is necessary to add carbohydrate, a suitable fat source, electrolytes, minerals and vitamins. An example of this feed is shown in Table 13.8.

Once the full strength feed is tolerated, weight gain should be reviewed. It may be necessary to increase the energy density of the feed to facilitate weight gain. This should be done by the incremental addition of glucose polymer and MCT emulsion (e.g. Liquigen). A total of 12% carbohydrate as glucose polymer and 4% fat as MCT emulsion should be tolerated. If sufficient quantities of vitamin and mineral preparation are added to the modular feed, e.g. Paediatric Seravit, there should be no need for additional supplementation with the exception of sodium and potassium. If volumes taken are consistently <150 mL/kg then the need for supplementation would need to be assessed for the individual child.

Essential fatty acids

Essential fatty acids (EFAs) in phospholipids are important for maintaining the function and integrity of cellular and subcellular membranes. They also participate in the regulation of cholesterol metabolism, being involved in its transport, breakdown and ultimate excretion. A recent review of the literature indicates that long chain polyun-

Table 13.8   A modular feed for a 3-month-old infant who presents with or develops a chylothorax post-surgery and where whole cow's milk protein is contraindicated. Weight = 4 kg, fluid volume = 150 mL/kg.

	Na⁺ (mmol)	K⁺ (mmol)	Energy (kcal/kJ)	CHO (g)	Protein (g)	MCT (g)
16 g Peptide Module 767			55/231		13.8	
60 g Glucose polymer	0.5	neg	232/970	58		
24 mL Liquigen	0.3		108/451		12	11.8
17 g Paediatric Seravit	0.15		51/213	12.8		
5 mL KCl (2 mmol/mL)		10				
4 mL NaCl (1 mmol/mL)	4					
+ water to 600 mL						
Totals	4.9	10	446/1864	70.8	13.8	12
per 100 mL	0.8	1.6	74/311	11.8	2.3	2
per kg	1.2	2.5	111/464		3.4	

Day 1	Day 2	Day 3
4 g Peptide Module 767	8 g Peptide Module	12 g Peptide Module 767
15 g Glucose polymer	30 g Glucose polymer	45 g Glucose polymer
6 mL Liquigen	12 mL Liquigen	24 mL Liquigen
6 g Paediatric Seravit	12 g Paediatric Seravit	17 g Paediatric Seravit

Aims in constructing feed: 3+ g protein per kg; 74 kcal (239 kJ) per 100 mL; 12% carbohydrate concentration.
The feed concentration should be gradually increased daily as shown to achieve the full strength.

saturated fatty acids (LCPs) are important in the growth and development of term infants and that their addition to the diet in appropriate quantities is safe [62]. A deficiency state arising from an inadequate intake of linoleic acid has been demonstrated in children [63]. Although a specific deficiency state arising from inadequate dietary α-linolenic acid has not been demonstrated in healthy humans, it is regarded as a dietary essential [63]. It has been recommended that the neonate requires at least 1% of energy intake from linoleic acid (C18:2) and at least 0.2% of energy from α-linolenic acid (C18:3) [50]. Table 13.9 gives a comparison of EFA content of feeds used in the treatment of infants with chylothorax.

If EFAs need to be added to a feed this may be done using walnut oil. The fatty acid content of this oil will provide linoleic and α-linolenic in an acceptable quantity and ratio with a minimum of LCT. Walnut oil contains 58 g linoleic and 12 g α-linolenic acids per 100 mL (p. 427).

EFA supplementation of feeds

The addition of 0.15 mL of walnut oil to 100 mL of the minimal LCT Peptide Module 767 based feed will provide EFA (and at the same time contribute a minimum amount of LCT) to a minimum of 1% energy from linoleic acid and 0.2% energy from α-linolenic acid. As the energy content of the feed is increased it will be necessary to increase the EFA supplementation proportionately.

Minimal LCT weaning diet

The following foods contain minimal LCT and can be introduced as weaning solids:

- Puréed vegetables (e.g. potato, carrots, swede, green beans)
- Puréed fruit (e.g. pears, apples, banana, peaches)

Table 13.9   Percentage energy derived from linoleic and α-linolenic acids in current minimal LCT feeds.

	Energy from C18:2 (%)	Energy from C18:3 (%)
Monogen	1.0	0.21
MCT Pepdite	5.1	0.75
Minimal LCT modular feed	0	0

- Puréed boiled rice mixed with minimal fat milk
- Baby rice reconstituted with minimal fat milk
- Tins and jars of baby foods containing less than 0.2 g LCT per 100 g may be included in the diet – mainly the fruit based tins and jars. Other commercial baby foods may contain too much LCT and need to be avoided

Even when solids are introduced into the diet of the infant, a minimal LCT formula will continue to form a major part of the nutritional intake providing energy, protein, vitamins and minerals until at least 1 year of age. A sample day's menu for the toddler on a minimal LCT diet is given in Table 13.10. A minimal fat milk may replace the minimal fat formula from 1 year if nutritional intake is not compromised by doing so. This minimal fat milk can be flavoured with Nesquik powder, fruit Crusha syrups or low fat chocolate flavour topping. It can also be used on breakfast cereals, to make custard or in cereal puddings. The quantity of milk ingredients may be varied to taste if needed, to provide 70–90 kcal (292–376kJ)/100 mL. Extra energy can be added to the diet by increasing the concentration of glucose polymer in the milk or by using 10–15% solution of glucose polymer to make up fruit squash. Increased energy intake can be achieved by the addition of Liquigen to suitable foods such as mashed potatoes or other root vegetables.

Feeding the older child and adolescent with chylothorax

Keeping the LCT intake to a minimum necessitates the exclusion of many foods including animal and vegetable fats such as butter, lard, margarine and vegetable oils. It also makes it necessary to strictly limit or exclude the protein foods that also have a high fat content such as meat, fatty fish, full fat milk, cheese and eggs. All cakes, pastry and biscuits made with LCT fats must also be avoided. The diet relies on skimmed milk fortified with carbohydrate and MCT as a source of energy, protein, minerals and vitamins. MCT can be added to the diet in the form of MCT oil or MCT emulsion. The use of MCT oil allows fried foods to be included in the diet, such as fried fish, chips and crisps (p. 430). MCT

Table 13.10 Sample day's menu for a toddler on a minimal LCT diet.

Minimal fat milk (MFM)	
60g skimmed milk powder 35 mL Liquigen 30 g glucose polymer 8 g Paediatric Seravit + water to 600 mL Use throughout the day for drinks and mixed with appropriate foods	Provides 500 kcal (2090 kJ) 22 g protein 0.8 g LCT
Breakfast	10g Rice Krispies + 60 mL MFM Glass MFM (100 mL)
Mid morning	Glass MFM (100 mL) 2 MCT biscuits
Lunch	80 g baked beans + 50g MCT chips 50 g very low fat fromage frais Glass fruit squash + glucose polymer
Mid afternoon	Glass MFM (100 mL) Meringue or Rice Krispie cake
Supper	40 g white fish steak fried in MCT oil Fat free mashed potatoes plus 2 teaspoons Liquigen 40 g carrots 50 g very low fat ice cream Jelly
Bedtime	Glass MFM (100 mL)

Total LCT intake for the day = 2 g.

Table 13.11 Free foods for minimal LCT diet.

All fruits fresh, tinned or frozen (except olives and avocado pear)
All vegetables, fresh, tinned or frozen
Sugar, honey, golden syrup, treacle, jam, marmalade
Jelly and jellied sweets such as Jelly Tots, Jelly Babies, wine gums or fruit pastilles
Boiled sweets, mints (not butter mints)
Fruit sorbets, water ices, ice lollies
Meringue, egg white, Rite-Diet egg replacer
Spices and essences
Salt, pepper, vinegar, herbs, tomato ketchup, most chutney, Marmite, Oxo, Bovril
Fruit juices, fruit squashes, Crusha fruit flavouring syrups, Nesquik fruit flavouring powder, chocolate flavour topping, bottled fruit sauces
Fizzy drinks, lemonade, cola, Lucozade

oil and MCT emulsion can both be used in baking, cakes, biscuits, pastry; all these foods are valuable sources of energy and can greatly enhance the acceptability of the diet to the patient. Table 13.11 lists foods containing minimal LCT, which can be used freely in the diet.

The weights and fat contents of foods which can be used to construct a day's meals containing minimal fat for the child or adolescent with chylothorax are given in Table 13.12. A review of some suitable low fat foods indicates that there may be up to a threefold variation in fat content of some meat and fish products depending on the brand. To make the diet more manageable the family can be taught to calculate minimal LCT exchanges as shown below:

$$0.2 \text{ g fat exchange} = \frac{0.2}{\text{grams of fat}/100 \text{ g of food}} \times 100 \text{ g}$$

$$0.5 \text{ g fat exchange} = \frac{0.5}{\text{grams of fat}/100 \text{ g of food}} \times 100 \text{ g}$$

The final diet may contain 40–70 g MCT, depending on the age and energy requirement of the patient. This would be gradually introduced over a period of 7–10 days in order to avoid abdominal discomfort. A day's meals for a 14-year-old boy with chylothorax is shown in Table 13.13 and Table 13.14 gives a nutritional analysis of the diet.

Length of treatment period

The usual length of treatment on a minimal LCT diet is 4–6 weeks. Cormack *et al.* [56] have suggested a return to normal diet at 4 weeks when removal of the pleural drain did not result in recurrence of chylothorax. A chest X-ray at the end of the treatment period may help in deciding whether chylothorax has resolved.

If an older child with chylothorax requires tube feeding 'juice' sip feeds such as Enlive, Provide Xtra or Fortijuce may be used as the feed base as they do not contain any fat. These sip feeds require supplementation with some electrolytes and essential fatty acids from walnut oil to make them nutritionally complete (Table 13.15). They may be diluted if necessary should a 1.25–1.5 kcal/mL (5–6 kJ/mL) feed not be tolerated.

Glossary

Aorto-pulmonary window: A hole, 'window', is present between the aorta and the pulmonary artery. This results in higher pulmonary blood pressure with more blood than usual going to the lungs and less to the systemic circulation.

Atrial septal defect (ASD): A hole between the right and left atria. There is malformation of the septum between the two chambers. The defect may have anomalous pulmonary drainage associated with it, in which some of the venous return from the lungs enters the right atrium rather than the left.

Blalock–Taussig (BT) shunt: A procedure in which the subclavian artery is connected to the pulmonary artery in order to provide adequate blood flow to the lungs. Used when the defect results in no direct connection between the right ventricle and the pulmonary circulation (e.g. pulmonary atresia). A modified version of this procedure is to use a Gore-Tex graft between the subclavian and pulmonary arteries (modified BT shunt).

Coarctation of the aorta: A narrowing of the aortic arch near to where the ductus arteriosus connects in the fetal circulation. One of the signs is reduced or absent femoral pulses. Surgical repair is either with an end-to-end anastamosis, with the narrowed section being cut out, or by using a flap of subclavian artery.

Cor triatrium: A membrane divides the inside of the left atrium interfering with blood flow into the left ventricle.

DiGeorge syndrome (22Q11 micro-deletion): Cardiac defects that affect the pulmonary artery and aorta are associated with this syndrome. Parathyroid hormone is absent and infants often need calcium supplementation postoperatively. The thymus is also affected resulting in poor immune function and the need for irradiated blood products to be given if transfusion is required.

Double outlet right ventricle (DORV): Both aorta and pulmonary artery exit from the right ventricle. A VSD is present allowing blood to exit from the left ventricle.

Ductus arteriosus: This is a connecting vessel between the pulmonary artery and the aorta. Its function is to allow blood to bypass the lungs in the fetal circulation. If it remains open once the infant is born it is known as a 'patent ductus arteriosus'. This causes excess blood flow to the lungs.

Table 13.12 Long chain triglyceride (LCT) content of foods suitable for use in LCT diet.

Food	LCT per 100 g	Average portion size (g)	LCT per portion (g)
Breakfast cereals			
Branflakes	2.0	35	0.7
Cornflakes	0.9	25	0.2
Frosties	0.6	20	0.1
Sugar Puffs	1.6	25	0.4
Special K	1.0	20	0.2
Cocopops	2.0	20	0.4
Just Right	2.5	40	1.0
Rice Krispies	1.0	25	0.25
Ricicles	0.7	20	0.1
Weetabix	1.9	37.5 (2 biscuits)	0.7
Puffed Wheat	2.5	15	0.4
Frosted Shreddies	1.4	35	0.5
Weetaflakes	1.6	30	0.5
Bread			
White, large thin slice	1.6	35	0.4
Granary	1.7	35	0.6
Matzos	1.0	20	0.2
Crumpets, toasted	1.0	45 (1)	0.45
Dairy foods			
Reduced fat cottage cheese	1.4	50	0.7
Very low fat fromage frais	0.1	100	0.1
Condensed milk, skimmed sweetened	0.2–1.0	50	0.1–0.5
Very low fat yoghurt (Muller Light)	0.1	200	0.2
Very low fat ice cream	0.4	50	0.2
Fish			
White cod fillet, raw	0.1–0.7	100	0.7
White cod steak, raw	0.6	100	0.6
Grilled white haddock fillet	0.6	100	0.6
Steamed whiting	0.9	100	0.9
Steamed smoked haddock	0.9	100	0.9
Fish finger	7.2	25 (1 fish finger)	1.8
Tuna	0.2–0.6	100	0.2–0.6
Shell fish			
Prawns – peeled	0.5–1.7	80	0.4–1.4
Crabsticks	0.1	50	neg
Crab (canned)	0.9	50	0.4
Crab, (white meat only)	0.1	100	0.1
Shrimps (canned)	1.2	50	0.6
Cockles, boiled	0.3–3	50	0.1–1.5
Mussels	2–3	50	1.0–1.5
Meat, poultry and alternatives			
Roast turkey, light meat	1.4	70	1.0
Roast chicken, light meat	4.0	25	1.0
Roast lamb, lean	8.0	25	2.0
Roast beef, lean only topside	4.0	45	1.8
Silverside, lean only	4.9	40	2.0
Ham	2.3–7.0	40	1.2–2.8
Quorn mince	2.0	50	1.0
Legumes, pasta, rice			
Baked beans in tomato sauce	0.5	200	1.0
Tinned spaghetti in tomato sauce	0.1	200	0.2
White rice, boiled	0.3	150	0.4
White pasta, boiled	0.8	130	1.0

Table 13.13 Day's meals for a 14-year-boy with chylothorax. Aim: 4–5 g/day LCT.

Daily milk allowance

Fortified skimmed milk (FSM)	20% glucose polymer solution
100 g skimmed milk powder	40 g glucose polymer
100 g glucose polymer	+ water to 200 mL
50 mL Liquigen	
+ water to 1000 mL	

1000 mL FSM provides: 950 kcal (3971 kJ), 36 g protein, 1.3 g LCT

Breakfast	25 g cornflakes + FSM
	120 mL orange juice and glucose polymer
	Apple
Mid morning	Glass of FSM
	+ meringue + 2 MCT biscuits
Lunch	70 g roast turkey (light meat only)
	150g mashed potatoes + 15 mL Liquigen
	60 g carrots
	120 g tinned fruit
	+ 120 mL custard made with FSM
	Glass fruit squash made with glucose polymer solution
Mid afternoon	250 mL FSM + 1 sachet strawberry Build-up
	+ banana + 2 MCT biscuits
Supper	200 g baked beans + 100 g MCT chips
	Apple pie made with MCT pastry
	+ 100 g very low fat fromage frais
Bedtime	Glass of FSM

Table 13.14 Nutritional analysis of minimal LCT diet for a 14-year-old boy showing comparison with current dietary reference values.

		DRV*
Energy (kcal)	2700 (11.3 MJ)	2200 (9.2 MJ)
Protein (g)	87	42
LCT (g)	5	
Na (mmol)	100	70
K (mmol)	130	80
Ca (mmol)	42	25
Fe (μmol)	330	200
Vitamin D (μg)	13	10†
Vitamin A (RE μg)‡	1200	600
Vitamin C (mg)	165	35

* Dietary Reference Values [50].
† At risk individuals with little sunlight exposure.
‡ Retinol equivalent.

Table 13.15 Supplementation of 'juice' sip feeds to make them nutritionally complete for a 10-year-old boy.

Sip feed	Supplementation required
Enlive Plus	Sodium, potassium, calcium, magnesium, phosphorus
Fortijuce	Sodium, potassium, calcium*, magnesium, phosphorus
Provide Xtra	Sodium, potassium, chloride

All of the above require an essential fatty acid supplement.
* Small amount of additional calcium required.

Ebstein's anomaly: A deformed tricuspid valve, with missing leaflets, arises from the wall of the right ventricle lower than normal. This results in a small functional right ventricle with the pulmonary artery exiting from above the tricuspid valve. Poor pulmonary blood flow results.

Glenn shunt: A procedure in which the superior vena cava is disconnected from where it enters the right atrium and is attached to the right pulmonary artery. The venous return from the upper part of the body therefore flows directly into the pulmonary arteries.

Hypoplastic left heart: As a result of embryological defects the size of the left ventricle is severely reduced. The aortic and mitral valves are also defective or absent and the aorta is reduced in size.

Interrupted aortic arch: The aorta exits from the left ventricle but fails to continue round to form the usual arch. The descending part of the aortic arch remains connected to the pulmonary circulation via the ductus arteriosus.

Partial anomalous pulmonary venous drainage (PAPVD): As for TAPVD but fewer pulmonary veins are misdirected.

Patent ductus arteriosus (PDA): The hole that exists between the pulmonary artery and aorta in fetal circulation persists postnatally. Some cardiac lesions require this hole to remain open in order to get blood to the lungs and so be compatible with life. Prostaglandin E_1 is used to keep the duct patent.

Patent/persisting foramen ovale (PFO): The hole between the two atria that is normally present in the fetal circulation persists postnatally.

Pulmonary atresia: The outflow from the pulmonary artery is completely restricted either at the site of the pulmonary valve or the artery itself. A

VSD may or may not be present and this will affect the surgical course.

Pulmonary stenosis: The valve of the pulmonary artery is not formed correctly resulting in reduced blood flow to the lungs. There are three types with areas of tissue above or below the valve or the valve itself being affected.

Shunt: The redirection of blood flow from one area of the circulation to another via a 'short circuit'. This may be caused by a physiological defect as in the movement of blood from the left to right ventricle across a VSD or by an operation such as a BT shunt in which blood is redirected from the systemic to pulmonary circulation (see Blalock–Taussig shunt above).

Tetralogy of Fallot (see Figure 13.3): there are four aspects to this defect: a ventricular septal defect, pulmonary stenosis, right ventricular hypertrophy and an overriding aorta in which the aorta straddles the two ventricles.

Total anomalous pulmonary venous drainage (TAPVD): The four pulmonary veins usually return blood to the left atrium. In TAPVD all of these veins empty into a variety of other locations: the superior vena cava, the inferior vena cava, the hepatic vein, hepatic portal vein or the right atrium.

Total cavo-pulmonary connection (TCPC): An operation in which the inferior vena cava is connected directly to the right pulmonary artery. This operation follows on from a Glenn shunt (see above) and occurs when a child is older. These operations are used where there are right-sided obstructive cardiac lesions resulting in deoxygenated blood flowing from the body directly into the pulmonary circulation without going through the right side of the heart.

Transposition of the great arteries (TGA): The aorta exits from the right ventricle and the pulmonary artery exits from the left ventricle. Blood is able to mix because of a patent foramen ovale and patent ductus arteriosus. Initially, the PFO is enlarged, using a cardiac catheter in a procedure called a balloon atrial septostomy, to allow for better mixing of blood. Surgical repair in which the arteries are cut and switched over is carried out at about 2 weeks of age.

Tricuspid atresia: The tricuspid valve between the right atrium and right ventricle fails to form. A PFO or ASD along with a VSD ensures that this lesion is compatible with life.

Truncus arteriosus: A single large vessel exits from above the two ventricles as a result of the pulmonary artery and the aorta failing to divide in the embryo. There is only one single valve to this large vessel, having 3–6 leaflets. A VSD is also present just beneath where the vessel leaves the heart. Truncus arteriosus is classified into four types depending on where the right and left pulmonary arteries arise.

Ventricular septal defect (VSD): A hole between the two ventricles. There are various types. The most common is a perimembranous defect in which the hole is located at the 'top' of the ventricle near to where blood exits. Muscular VSDs are located near the 'bottom' or apex of the ventricle.

Acknowledgements

Dr Beverley Tsai, Consultant Cardiologist for checking medical details in text. Dr Alison Hayes, Consultant Cardiologist, for Figs 13.1–13.3. Miss Sarah Jorgensen, Paediatric Dietitian and Sheila Hopkins for proofreading.

References

1   Noonan J Noonan syndrome and related disorders. *Progress Pediatr Cardiol*, 2005, **20** 177–8.
2   Webb JG, Kiess MC, Chan Yan CC Malnutrition and the heart. *Can Med Assoc J*, 1986, **135** 753–9.
3   Bougle D *et al*. Nutritional treatment of congenital heart disease. *Arch Dis Child*, 1961, 799–801.
4   Naeye RL Organ and cellular development in congenital heart disease and in alimentary malnutrition. *J Pediatr*, 1965, Sept, 447–8.
5   Krieger I Growth failure and congenital heart disease: energy and nitrogen balance in infants. *Am J Dis Child*, 1970, **120** 497–504.
6   Pittman JG, Cohen P The pathogenesis of cardiac cachexia. *N Engl J Med*, 1964, **271** 403–9.
7   Varan B, Tokel K, Yilmaz G Malnutrition and growth failure in cyanotic acyanotic heart disease with and without pulmonary hypertension. *Arch Dis Child*, 1999, **81** 49–52.
8   Mehrizi A, Drash A Growth disturbance in congenital heart disease. *J Pediatr*, 1962, **61** 418–22.
9   Feldt R, Strictler G, Weidman W Growth of children with congenital heart disease. *Am J Dis Child*, 1969, **117** 573–9.
10 Huse D, Feldt RH, Nelson RA, Novak LP Infants with congenital heart disease food intake, body

weight and energy metabolism. *Am J Dis Child*, 1975, **129** 65–9.

11 De Staebel O Malnutrition in Belgian children with congenital heart disease on admission to hospital. *J Clin Nurs*, 2000, **9** 784–91.

12 Wynn Cameron J, Rosenthal MD, Olson AD Malnutrition in hospitalized children with congenital heart disease. *Arch Pediatr Adolesc Med*, 1995, **149** 1098–102.

13 Jacobs EGJ, Leung MP, Karlberg JP Postnatal growth in southern Chinese children with symptomatic congenital heart disease. *J Pediatr Endocrinol Metab*, 2000, **11** 195–202.

14 Rosenthal A, Castaneda A Growth and development after cardiovascular surgery in infants and children. *Progress Cardiovasc Dis* Vol. 18, **1** 27–37.

15 Barton J, Hindmarsh P, Scrimgeour C *et al.* Energy expenditure in congenital heart disease. *Arch Dis Child*, 1994, **70** 5–9.

16 Leitch CA, Karn CA, Peppard RJ *et al.* Increased energy expenditure in infants with cyanotic congenital heart disease. *J Pediatr*, 1998, **133** 755–60.

17 Farrell AG, Schamberger MS, Olson IL, Leitch CA Large left-to-right shunts and congestive heart failure increase total energy expenditure in infants with ventricular septal defect. *Am J Cardiol*, 2001, **87** 1128–31.

18 Ackerman IL, Karn CA, Denne SC *et al.* Total but not resting energy expenditure is increased in infants with ventricular septal defects. *Pediatrics*, 1998, **102** 1172–7.

19 Waterlow JC *Protein Energy Malnutrition*. London: Edward Arnold, 1992, pp. 231–2.

20 Soliman A, Madkour A, Abdel Galil M *et al.* Growth parameters and endocrine function in relation to echocardiographic parameters in children with ventricular septal defect without heart failure. *J Trop Pediatr*, 2001, **47** 146–52.

21 Ocal B, Unal S, Zorlu P *et al.* D Echocardiographic evaluation of cardiac function and left ventricular mass in children with malnutrition. *J Paediatr Child Health*, 2001, **37** 14–17.

22 Lundell KH, Sabel KG, Eriksson BO Plasma metabolites after lipid load in infants with congenital heart disease. *Acta Paediatr*, 1999, **88** 718–23.

23 Ronholt Hansen S, Dorup I Energy and nutrient intakes in congenital heart disease. *Acta Paediatrica*, 1993, **82** 166–72.

24 Thommessen M, Heiberg A, Kase B Feeding problems in children with congenital heart disease: the impact on energy intake and growth outcome. *Eur J Clin Nutr*, 1992, **46** 457–64.

25 Pillo-Blocka F, Miles C, Beghetti M *et al.* B Nutrition after surgery for hypoplastic left heart syndrome. *Nutr Clin Pract*, 1998, **12** 81–3.

26 Vanderhoof JA, Hofsschire PJ, Baluff M *et al.* Continuous enteral feedings: an important adjunct to the management of complex heart disease. *Am J Dis Child*, 1982, **136** 825–7.

27 Peterson RE, Wetzel GT Growth failure in congenital heart disease: where are we now? *Curr Opin Cardiol*, 2004, **19** 81–3.

28 Cavell B Gastric emptying in infants with congenital heart disease. *Acta Paediatr Scand*, 1981, **70** 517–20.

29 McElhinney D, Hedrick H, Bush D *et al.* Necrotising enterocolitis in neonates with congenital heart disease: risk factors and outcomes. *Pediatrics*, 2000, **106** 1080–7.

30 Cheung Y, Ho M, Cheng V Mesenteric blood flow response to feeding after systemic to pulmonary arterial shunt palliation. *Ann Thorac Surg*, 2003, **75** 947–51.

31 Harrison AM, Davis S, Reid J *et al.* Neonates with hypoplastic left heart syndrome have ultrasound evidence of abnormal superior mesenteric artery perfusion before and after modified Norwood procedure. *Paediatr Crit Care Med*, 2005, **6** 445–7.

32 Lucas A, Cole T Breast milk and neonatal necrotising enterocolitis. *Lancet*, 1990, **336** 1519–23.

33 La Gamma E, Ostertag S, Birenbaum H Failure of delayed oral feedings to prevent necrotising enterocolitis. *Am J Dis Child*, 1985, **139** 385–9.

34 Davidson JD *et al.* Protein-losing gastroenteropathy in congestive heart failure. *Lancet*, 1961, **1** 899.

35 Connor F, Angelides S, Gibson M *et al.* Successful resection of localized intestinal lymphangiectasia post Fontan: role of (99m) technetium dextran scintigraphy. *Pediatrics*, 2003, **112** 242–7.

36 Feldt R, Driscoll D, Offord K *et al.* Protein losing enteropathy after Fontan operation. *J Thorac Cardiovasc Surg*, 1996, **112** 672–80.

37 Brancaccio G, Adriano C, D'Argenio P *et al.* Protein losing enteropathy after Fontan surgery: resolution after cardiac transplantation. *J Heart Lung Transplant*, 2003, **22** 484–6.

38 Narkewicz M, Sondheimer H, Zeigler J *et al.* Hepatic dysfunction following the Fontan procedure. *J Pediatr Gastroenterol Nutr*, 2003, **36** 352–7.

39 Yahav J *et al.* Assessment of intestinal and cardiorespiratory function in children with congenital heart disease on high calorie formulas. *J Pediatr Gastroenterol Nutr*, 1985, **4** 778–85.

40 Unger R, DeKleermaeker M, Gidding S, Kaufer-Christoffel K Calories count: Improved weight gain with dietary intervention in congenital heart disease. *Am J Dis Child*, 1992, **146** 1078–84.

41 Rogers E, Gilbertson H, Heine R, Henning R Barriers to adequate nutrition in critically ill children. *Nutrition*, 2003, **19** 865–8.

42 Marino BL, O'Brien P, LoRe H Oxygen saturations

during breast and bottle feedings in infants with congenital heart disease. *J Pediatr Nurs*, 1995, **10** 360–4.

43 Owens B Breastfeeding an infant after heart transplant surgery (Case Report). *J Hum Lact*, 2002, **18** 53–5.

44 McClure RJ, Newell SJ Effect of fortifying breast milk on gastric emptying. *Arch Dis Child*, 1996, **74** F60–2.

45 Pillo-Blocka F, Adatia I, Sharieff W *et al*. Rapid advancement to more concentrated formula in infants after surgery for congenital heart disease reduces duration of hospital stay: a randomised clinical trial. *J Pediatr*, 2004, **145** 761–6.

46 Einarson KD, Arthur HM Predictors of oral feeding difficulty in cardiac surgical infants. *Pediatr Nurs*, 2003, **29** 315–19.

47 Schwarz SM *et al*. Enteral nutrition in infants with congenital heart disease and growth failure. *Pediatrics*, 1990, **86** 368–73.

48 Heymsfield SB, Hill JO, Evert M Energy expenditure during continuous intragastric infusion of fuel. *Am J Clin Nutr*, 1987, **45** 526–33.

49 Ciotti G, Holzer R, Pozzi M, Dalzell M Nutrition support via percutaneous endoscopic gastrostomy in children with cardiac disease experiencing difficulties with feeding. *Cardiol Young*, 2002, **12** 537–41.

50 Department of Health Report on Health and Social Subjects No. 14 *Dietary Reference Values for Food, Energy and Nutrients for the United Kingdom*. London: The Stationery Office, 1991.

51 Bessone LN, Ferguson TB, Burford TH Chylothorax collective review. *Ann Thorac Surg*, Nov 1971, **12** 527–45.

52 Merrigan BA, Winter DC, O'Sullivan GC Chylothorax. *Br J Surg*, 1997, **84** 15–20.

53 Cooper P, Paes ML Bilateral chylothorax. *Br J Anaesth*, 1991, **66** 387–90.

54 Puntis JWL, Roberts KD, Handy D How should chylothorax be managed? *Arch Dis Child*, 1987, **62** 593–6.

55 Stringer G, Mercer S, Bass J Surgical management of persistent postoperative chylothorax in children. *Can J Surg*, 1984, **27** 543–6.

56 Cormack B, Wilson N, Finucane K, West T Use of Monogen for pediatric postoperative chylothorax. *Ann Thorac Surg*, 2004, **77** 301–5.

57 Issalbacher KJ, Senior ED Mechanisms of absorption of long and medium chain triglycerides. In: *Medium Chain Triglyceride*. Philadelphia: University of Pennsylvania, 1968.

58 Cheung Y, Leung M, Yip M Octreotide for treatment of postoperative chylothorax. *J Pediatr*, 2001, **159** 157–9.

59 Pratap U, Slavik Z, Ofoe V *et al*. Octreotide to treat postoperative chylothorax after cardiac operations in children. *Ann Thorac Surg*, 2001, **72** 1740–2.

60 Pettit T, Caspi J, Bourne A Treatment of persistent chylothorax after Norwood procedure with somatostatin. *Ann Thorac Surg*, 2002, **73** 977–9.

61 Walther T, Theune P, Sullivan I, de Leval M Successful medical treatment of persistent pleural drainage after Fontan operation. *Interact Cardiovasc Thorac Surg*, 2003, **2** 348–9.

62 Fleith M, Clandinin M Dietary PUFA for preterm and term infants: Review of Clinical Studies. *Crit Rev Food Science Nutr*, 2005, **45** 205–29.

63 Hanson AE *et al*. Eczema and essential fatty acids. *Am J Dis Child*, 1947, **73** 1–18.

Further reading

Congenital heart disease

Krauss A, Auld A Metabolic rate of neonates with congenital heart disease. *Arch Dis Child*, 1975, **50** 539–41.

McDonnell N *The Paediatric Cardiac Surgical Patient*, 3rd edn. University of Brisbane, 2003. Copies available by e-mail: mcdonnem@ozemail.com.au.

Mitchell I, Davies P, Day J *et al*. Energy expenditure in congenital heart disease before and after cardiac surgery. *J Thorac Cardiovasc Surg*, 1994, **107** 374–80.

Chylothorax

Bond SJ, Guzzetta PC, Snyder ML, Randolph JG Management of paediatric postoperative chylothorax. *Ann Thorac Surg*, 1993, **56** 469–72.

Gracey M, Burke V, Anderson CM Medium chain triglycerides in paediatric practice. *Arch Dis Child*, 1970, **45** 445–52.

Hopkins, RL, Akingbola OA, Frieberg EM Chylothorax: Key References. *Ann Thorac Surg*, 1998, **66** 1845–6.

Kosloke AM, Martin LW, Schubert WK Management of chylothorax in children and medium chain triglyceride feedings. *J Pediatr Surg*, 1974, **9** 365–71.

Ramos W, Faintuch J Nutritional management of thoracic duct fistula. A comparative study of parenteral verus enteral nutrition. *J Parenter Enteral Nutr*, 1986, **10** 519–21.

14 Food Hypersensitivity

Kate Grimshaw

Introduction

Food hypersensitivity is a controversial diagnosis to which many symptoms have been attributed, and confusion over nomenclature has added to the controversy. In an effort to improve diagnosis, treatment and general understanding of allergic reactions the Nomenclature Review Committee of the World Allergy Organization issued a report proposing revised nomenclature for allergy [1]. This report states that any reaction to food that causes objectively reproducible symptoms or signs, even when the food is eaten unknowingly (blind), should be described as food hypersensitivity. If immunologic mechanisms can be demonstrated then the reaction can be described as a food allergy. If immunoglobulin E (IgE) is involved in the reaction then the term IgE mediated food allergy should be used. All other reactions should be described as non-allergic food hypersensitivity. These reactions have previously been described as food intolerance.

Important factors concerning food hypersensitivity reactions

- Some food hypersensitivity occurs as a result of enzyme deficiency such as lactase deficiency or disorders of amino acid or intermediary metabolism (e.g. phenylketonuria). These

reactions are non-allergic hypersensitivities, are well documented and are discussed elsewhere in this book.
- Some foods may cause unpleasant symptoms (e.g. caffeine in coffee and cola; vasoactive amines in cheese and wine; phenylethylamine in chocolate). These effects are pharmacological and are non-allergic.
- Some foods such as shellfish and strawberries contain histamine-releasing agents which may cause adverse reactions which appear to be IgE mediated food allergy but are not.
- A food hypersensitivity reaction is known as a food allergy where the immune system is involved. These reactions may involve IgE or may involve other immune mechanisms.

Food hypersensitivity is a large subject and this chapter can only provide an introduction. An effort has been made to concentrate on dietetic principles but it is essential to understand some of the mechanisms involved to ensure dietetic management is optimal. For more detail of the subject the reader is directed to the References and Further Reading sections at the end of this chapter. For information on prevention of food allergy see Chapter 32.

IgE mediated allergy

IgE is an immunoglobulin normally present at very low levels in the plasma of non-allergic individuals, but levels are raised in patients with allergic conditions such as asthma, atopic dermatitis and anaphylaxis. Production of allergen specific IgE is caused by class switching of B cells to produce this immunoglobulin isotype in preference to any other. Naïve B cells undergo class switching and affinity maturation when they become activated for the first time through antigens and T cells to produce IgE. IgE has a very short life in plasma ($t_{1/2}$ less than 1 day) but can remain fixed to mast cells in tissues for weeks or months. IgE antibodies exert their biological function via the high affinity receptor FcεR1 on mast cells and basophils and the low affinity receptor CD23 on macrophages, monocytes, lymphocytes, eosinophils and platelets. When food allergens penetrate mucosal barriers and reach IgE antibodies bound to mast cells or basophils, vasoactive and chemotactic mediators are released that induce vasodilation, smooth muscle contraction and mucus secretion, which result in symptoms of immediate food hypersensitivity.

Activated mast cells may also release a variety of cytokines, which may induce the IgE mediated late response. During the initial 4–8 hours, neutrophils and eosinophils invade the site of response. These infiltrating cells are activated and release a variety of mediators including platelet activating factor, peroxidase, eosinophil major basic protein and eosinophil cationic protein. In the subsequent 24–48 hours, lymphocytes and monocytes infiltrate the area and establish a more chronic inflammatory picture.

Clinical manifestation of IgE mediated food allergy

Symptoms generally appear within minutes after a very small amount of food has been consumed. Immediate symptoms may affect the gut, the skin and/or the lungs. They include vomiting, abdominal pain, urticaria, angioedema (swelling of the face/throat), erythema, pruritus, wheeze and cough.

Symptoms of upper airway obstruction (laryngeal oedema), lower airway obstruction (bronchoconstriction), hypotension, cardiac arrhythmias and even heart failure constitute the most severe and sometimes life-threatening reactions. This is known as anaphylactic shock. First symptoms may include sneezing and a tingling sensation on the lips, tongue and throat followed by pallor and feeling unwell, fearful, warm and lightheaded. The presentation of anaphylaxis is varied but the major causes of death are obstruction to the upper airway or shock, hypotension and cardiac arrhythmia [2].

The results of double blind placebo controlled food challenges (DBPCFC) from several studies in the USA have shown that the most common foods to provoke immediate reactions are peanuts, tree nuts, milk, egg, soy and wheat, fish and shellfish [3]. Seeds (e.g. sesame) may also cause this type of reaction.

Non-IgE mediated food allergy

These reactions are the classic delayed hypersensitivity reactions with symptoms appearing 24–48 hours after antigen exposure which have been implicated in food allergic disorders where the onset of symptoms is delayed. The mechanism involves sensitised T cells reacting with the antigen to produce cytokines, which mobilise non-sensitised cells to fight the antigen, causing inflammation, tissue damage and the formation of epitheloid and giant cells.

The importance of cell mediated hypersensitivity reactions in the pathogenesis of food allergy is not clear. It is widely held that the enteropathy of coeliac disease is caused by a local cell mediated immune response to dietary gluten and that a number of other gastrointestinal disorders are caused by cell mediated hypersensitivity reactions.

Clinical manifestation of non-IgE mediated food allergy

These reactions to foods may develop slowly after hours or days and only when a considerable amount of food has been consumed [4]. As with immediate symptoms, adverse reactions can affect the skin, gut or lungs. Symptoms include chronic diarrhoea, abdominal pain, failure to thrive, enteropathy, allergic eosinophilic oesophagitis, gastritis and gastroenteritis, allergic colitis, infantile colic, constipation, eczema and asthma. Gastrointestinal symptoms of food allergy are discussed in Chapter 7.

Non-allergic food hypersensitivity

In children, reactions to food that are not caused by

an immune reaction are often a result of enzyme deficiencies. More controversial problems which may be related to non-allergic food hypersensitivity are migraine, migraine with epilepsy, enuresis, and attention deficit hyperactivity disorder (ADHD). Dietary manipulation (elimination and challenge) is the mainstay for diagnosis and treatment of these conditions.

The many symptoms that have been attributed to food hypersensitivity are listed in Table 14.1. Some are more firmly established as being food related than others.

Table 14.1   Symptoms of food hypersensitivity.

	IgE mediated Immediate onset* Within 2 hours	Non-IgE mediated Delayed onset† Within a few hours to 3 days
Gastrointestinal	Swelling of lips, tongue and mouth Oral allergy syndrome Vomiting Colic Diarrhoea	Reflux Abdominal pain, bloating Enteropathy Failure to thrive Allergic colitis, rectal bleeding Diarrhoea Constipation
Cutaneous	Urticaria Angio-oedema Erythema, Pruritus	Eczema Urticaria (rarely)
Respiratory	Cough/wheeze/ sneeze Laryngeal oedema Bronchospasm	Asthma
Systemic	Cardiac arrhythmia Hypotension Anaphylaxis	
Controversial		Migraine Migraine with epilepsy ADHD Enuresis Rheumatoid arthritis Autism

ADHD, attention deficit hyperactivity disorder;
Ig, immunoglobulin.
* Occasionally immediate symptoms are not IgE mediated.
† 'Late phase' IgE mediated reactions may occur after 4–48 hours.

Tests for diagnosis of food hypersensitivity

IgE mediated allergy

Skin prick test

The skin prick test (SPT) indicates the presence of allergen specific IgE. Drops of food extract and positive (histamine) control and negative (saline) control are applied using skin pricks. Antihistamine treatment should be discontinued prior to the test. Food allergens eliciting wheals at least 3 mm larger than those induced by the negative control are considered positive. However, the positive predictive accuracy of SPTs is less than 50% (when compared with results from DBPCFC). Negative predictive accuracy is 95% [5]. This means that negative SPT responses are a worthwhile means of excluding IgE mediated allergies, but positive SPT responses only indicate an atopic individual and exclusion diets should not be based on these results alone.

Specific IgE test

Specific IgE is an *in vitro* assay for identifying food specific IgE antibodies from serum. It is more expensive than skin prick testing and the results are not available to the clinician immediately, possibly delaying diagnosis. This test may be preferred when patients have dermatographism, patients with severe skin disease and limited surface area for testing, and patients who have difficulty discontinuing antihistamines, or patients with exquisite sensitivity to certain foods [5]. Interpretation of results is as difficult as with SPTs. However, SPTs and specific IgE tests provide useful contributory information towards a diagnosis when added to the clinical history and interpreted by clinicians who are familiar with them. Sometimes the specific IgE values are put into bands or grades (I–IV) and these are used to classify the levels of specific IgE found in the blood. This is called a radio allergosorbent test (RAST).

Intradermal test

A report of the British Society for Allergy and Environmental Medicine (BSAEM) with the British Society for Nutritional Medicine (BSNM) does not recommend the use of intradermal tests and states that the significance of positive tests with foods is a matter of controversy [6]. Other medical authorities do not recommend them either because of the unacceptably high false positive rate and the fact that they can elicit systemic reactions [7].

Other diagnostic tests

To date there is no additional diagnostic procedure that can be recommended as a useful test in the diagnosis of IgE mediated food allergy. This includes tests determining specific IgG antibodies in serum, vega testing, hair analysis, cytotoxic test, kinesiology, iridology, electrodermal testing and sublingual provocative food testing [8].

Non-IgE mediated allergy

Results of non-specific laboratory tests may be abnormal in non-IgE mediated food allergy and for gastrointestinal allergies biopsies may provide much information. However, there are no tests that can identify foods responsible for the symptoms [9]. It has been suggested that atopy patch testing could be used to aid the diagnosis of non-IgE mediated food allergy but further studies are needed before its use can be widely advocated [10]. Currently, diagnosis can only be made by dietary manipulation (i.e. exclusion followed by challenge).

Non-allergic food hypersensitivity

As for food allergy, there is no proven test for the diagnosis of non-allergic food hypersensitivity. Advertised diagnostic methods such as applied kinesiology, hair tests or electrodermal tests were evaluated in a Consumer Association report [11]. The verdict was that known allergies in individuals were not picked up and the services exaggerated the number of allergies in the individual; this could result in unnecessarily restricted and inadequate diets. The report suggests that people should not waste their money on these tests. Vega testing has also been assessed in a double blind study and was shown to be unable to accurately diagnose food hypersensitivity of any mechanism [12].

Natural history of food allergy

The prevalence of food allergy is increasing [13,14]. It is most commonly acquired during the first year of life with peak incidence of 6–8% occurring at 1 year of age. The prevalence falls until late childhood where it plateaus at 1–2% through adulthood [15]. Eigenmann et al. [16] found one-third of children with eczema had associated food allergy. The picture is also the same for asthma [10]. Although the tendency to develop allergies clearly has a genetic component, it is strongly influenced by environment and lifestyle factors. These include air pollution, environmental tobacco smoke exposure, maternal and infant nutrition, environmental allergen exposure, family size, infections and hygiene [17].

The majority of reactions to foods in infants and young children are to egg and milk. It has long been established that most children grow out of these allergies [18]. It is commonly thought that peanut allergy does not resolve although Skolnick et al. [19] have shown that peanut allergy may be outgrown in 21.5% of patients. Tree nut, fish and shellfish allergies tend to develop in older children and are unlikely to be outgrown.

Although many children grow out of their food allergies it is evident that allergic disorders change and progress from eczema and food allergy to asthma and rhinitis. This phenomenon is referred to as the 'allergic march'. Allergen sensitisation is predominantly against foods in infancy but is largely replaced by inhalants such as house dust mite and pollen in later childhood [20,21].

Prevention of food allergy

Chapter 32 details strategies for the prevention of food allergy.

Dietary manipulation for food hypersensitivities

Currently, the only treatment for any food hypersensitivity is dietary avoidance of the causative allergen. This is called dietary elimination. An elimination diet may also be used in the diagnosis of food allergy. Whatever the reason for dietary restriction it is essential that the clinical symptoms are severe enough to warrant a diet as any type of dietary manipulation requires considerable effort on the part of the family.

Sometimes clinical history and diagnostic tests give a strong indication as to the food or foods that are causing the symptoms. In this case dietary exclusion advice is given to manage the symptoms, and reintroduction of these foods into the diet will not occur until there is an indication that the allergy may have been outgrown. However, in some cases (particularly for non-IgE mediated food allergy and non-allergic food hypersensitivities) it may not be clear which foods are causing the problems and it might be necessary to first devise an appropriate 'diagnostic' elimination diet which should be used for 3–6 weeks. The length of time will depend on frequency of symptoms, degree of restriction of diet and type of symptoms involved (improvement in gastrointestinal symptoms may occur within a day or two whereas improvement in eczema may take several weeks). If successful, the diet will result in significant relief of symptoms. There would then be a sequential open reintroduction of foods in an effort to identify provoking foods. Finally, a nutritionally adequate maintenance diet will be devised. Before a diagnostic elimination diet is embarked upon it is essential to consider whether the child and/or parent are sufficiently motivated and able to adhere to the diet as non-compliance renders the diet trial a waste of time.

Elimination diets for diagnosis

Throughout the period of the dietary manipulations and for at least a week before any diet starts it is extremely useful for the parent (or patient) to keep a symptom score diary. It is then possible to be reasonably objective about change in severity of symptoms. Physical symptoms can be listed at the end of each day and a numerical score can be given for each one (e.g. 0 for no symptoms, 1–3 for symptoms which are mild, moderate or severe). Where attention deficit and hyperactivity are concerned it is useful to use a shortened form of the Conners' Scale (Table 14.2) [22].

Phase 1: initial diagnostic diet

A full diet history is mandatory before embarking on a diet and may indicate possible provoking foods. It is often stated that parents' histories are notoriously unreliable. This may be true but they are a useful starting point. It is not uncommon for parents to be mistaken as to which foods affect their child and intolerance to staple foods eaten several times a day, such as milk and wheat, often go unnoticed. Keeping a food diary for some weeks before starting a diet may provide a baseline but seldom adds any useful information about suspect foods that has not been revealed by diet history. A diagnostic elimination diet should avoid disliked foods and foods that are craved or eaten in large amounts.

Table 14.2   Short form of Conners' Scale for hyperactivity.

Observation date	Degree of activity			
	Not at all	Just a little	Pretty much	Very much
Restless or overactive				
Excitable, impulsive				
Disturbs other children				
Short attention span				
Constantly fidgeting				
Inattentive, easily distracted				
Demands must be met immediately				
Cries often and easily				
Mood changes quickly and drastically				
Temper outbursts, explosive and unpredictable behaviour				

The initial diet may exclude one or a large number of foods. The choice of diet is a matter of clinical judgement taking into account age, severity of symptoms and whether diets have already been tried. There are broadly three levels of dietary restriction: an empirical diet, a few foods diet or an elemental diet.

Empirical diet

An empirical diet is used where food hypersensitivity is suspected and causative agents are not known. One or several of the most commonly provoking foods are avoided. Studies with children who have delayed reactions to food indicate anecdotally that the most common provoking foods are similar to those listed for immediate reactions to foods except that reactions to some food additives and chocolate appears more common and reactions to fish and nuts less common. In infants, the most frequent offender is cow's milk based infant formula so a cow's milk free diet is often used. A diet avoiding egg and milk, together with any known problem foods, is sometimes used for eczema. It is not unusual for paediatric gastroenterologists to use a diet free of milk, egg, wheat, (rye) and soya for children with gastrointestinal symptoms (p. 99). Several adult centres use a diet free of all grains (some include rice), egg, milk, chocolate and additives. This is sometimes known as a 'hunter gatherer' diet. A very similar diet was described by Rowe and Rowe [23] for the diagnosis and treatment of food induced asthma.

Additives that are most commonly cited as being potential problems are artificial colours (azo, coal tar and erythrosine dyes: E102–E219), benzoate preservatives (E210–E219), sulphur dioxide preservatives (E220–E224) and nitrite preservatives (E249–E252). However, there are reports of intolerance to some natural colours [24]. Foods containing the above additives usually also contain flavours which do not have E numbers and these cannot be assumed to be inert. Because most manufactured foods containing additives usually include several additives, it is difficult to get a picture of which ones give the most problems. An empirical additive free diet could be considered to avoid artificial colours, benzoate, sulphur dioxide, nitrite preservatives and food flavours where possible. This will automatically exclude major sources of natural colours.

There is some evidence that urticaria may sometimes be provoked by aspirin and this has been used as an argument for removing fruits and vegetables containing natural salicylates from the diet. A self-help group also suggests hyperactive children may be affected by these fruits and vegetables. The only available analysis of salicylate content of fruits and vegetables has been carried out by Swain et al. [25] and it is not clearcut which foods should be avoided on such a diet. Reactions to fruits should not be assumed to be caused by salicylate content. Many children with food hypersensitivity are affected adversely by some fruits but can tolerate others that contain salicylates.

Problems occur with empirical diets when excluded foods are inadvertently replaced by others that are equally capable of causing adverse reactions; for example, a child on a milk free diet may drink soya milk or orange juice instead and it is possible to be equally reactive to these foods. Failure to respond to an empirical diet does not rule out the possibility of food hypersensitivity.

Few foods diet

There are considerable difficulties in teaching people how to avoid a large number of foods. For very restricted diets it is easier to decide on which foods the child can eat and teach the diet in terms of which foods are allowed rather that concentrating on those that are forbidden. This is the basis for the few foods diet. Three to four weeks is the longest time one should consider using a very restricted diet, although improvement may occur in a shorter time.

The simplest few foods diet to have been described consists of lamb, pears and spring water only. Diets using one meat, one carbohydrate source, one fruit and one vegetable have been used [26]. If no improvement occurs a second diet containing a different set of foods can be used (Table 14.3) [27,28]. In extreme circumstances one could include rarely eaten foods such as rabbit, venison and sweet potatoes [29].

Because the above diets are extremely rigorous, slightly less restricted diets have been used which make adherence less of a problem (Table 14.4) [24,30–32]. It is much more difficult to find a completely different set of foods for a second attempt if the first is not helpful. However, it is possible to

Table 14.3 Two examples of few foods diets.
Children under 2 years require a nutritionally adequate milk substitute. This diet should not be used for longer than 4 weeks.

A	B
Turkey	Lamb
Cabbage, sprouts, broccoli, cauliflower	Carrots, parsnips
Potato, potato flour	Rice, rice flour
Banana	Pear
Soya oil	Sunflower oil
Calcium and vitamins (see Table 14.4)	Calcium and vitamins
Tap water	Tap water

Possible additions: milk free margarine, sugar for baking.
Possible variations: bottled water; rabbit instead of above meats; peaches and apricots, melon, pineapple instead of above fruits.

Table 14.4 Less restricted few foods diet.
This diet should be used for no more than 4 weeks. Children under 2 years require a nutritionally adequate substitute for milk. Choose two foods from each food group.

Meat	Lamb, rabbit, turkey, pork
Starchy food	Rice, potato, sweet potato
Vegetables	Broccoli, cauliflower, cabbage, sprouts (brassicas)
	Carrots, parsnips, celery
	Cucumber, marrow, courgettes, melon
	Leeks, onions, asparagus
Fruit	Pears, bananas, peaches and apricots, pineapple
Also included	Sunflower oil, milk free margarine
	Plain potato crisps
	Small amount of sugar for baking
	Tap or bottled water
	Juice and jam from allowed fruits
	Salt, pepper and herbs in cooking

A calcium (300–400 mg/day) and vitamin supplement is advisable: calcium gluconate effervescent 1 g × 3 daily; or calcium lactate 300 mg × 6 daily; or Sandocal 400 g × 1 tablet daily.
Abidec 0.6 mL/day.

monitor progress closely and change or further restrict the diet during the third or fourth week in an attempt to achieve eventual success.

The acceptability of the few foods diet depends greatly on the dietitian's advice as regards planning menus, giving ideas for meals and recipes for cooking with the foods allowed. Ideas for packed lunches should be given as school canteens cannot be expected to cope adequately with such a restricted diet. For vegetarians one would have to allow a larger range of vegetables, including pulses. The dietitian should keep in touch with the family and be available by telephone. Cost of the diet may be a problem and should be discussed with the family.

The few foods diet is most difficult to carry out in the toddler age group. Such children may still be very reliant on milk or formula. Ideally, they should take a hydrolysed protein formula but it may be refused. The diet can be altered to suit the individual. In some circumstances one can make it less restricted by including a larger range of meats, fruits and vegetables.

Few foods diets are generally carried out in the home environment. It is important that the child's lifestyle is not altered, otherwise changes in symptoms could be attributed to factors other than change in diet. Regular medication should not be altered before or during the diet trial for the same reason. Children on regular medication such as anticonvulsants should remain on these but be switched to a colour and preservative free version if possible. Attention should be paid to non-food items which may be consumed by small children such as toothpaste (a white toothpaste should be used), chalks and paints.

Elemental diet

Hypoallergenic or elemental diets based on amino acids (e.g. Neocate, Elemental 028) can occasionally be justified for those who have not responded to a restricted diet, but this treatment should be very much a last resort as suitable products are very unpalatable and tube feeding may be necessary to achieve adequate nutrition. This will involve a hospital admission. Suitable products are listed in Tables 7.9 and 7.12. These feeds have been used mainly for children with severe eczema and for gastrointestinal problems [33].

Phase 2: reintroduction of foods

The patient or the parent of a child who has experienced significant relief of symptoms on a diet will usually want to continue with it. Ineffective diets must be abandoned. Young infants who have done well on a cow's milk free formula should not be challenged with cow's milk too soon. Between 9 and 12 months may elapse before a trial of cow's milk. In the meantime the infant should be weaned on to milk free weaning foods (see Table 7.6).

In an older child, if the initial diet avoids several foods, these should be reintroduced singly in order to try and identify trigger foods. Each new food may be tried in a small test quantity, then given in normal amount every day for a week and then incorporated into the diet as desired. A guide to reintroduction of foods is given in Table 14.5. The order of reintroduction should depend on the child's or parent's preferences and the need for nutritional adequacy.

Sometimes a child may be seen whose parents have already put them on an exclusion diet and they come for advice because the diet is only partially successful or they are worried about nutritional adequacy. A full diet history is essential. The dietitian has an important role in ensuring provoking foods are completely avoided and in reintroducing foods in a sequential way to arrive at the broadest possible diet that is nutritionally adequate.

It is not unusual to find that children with multiple symptoms may react differently to different foods. Immediate and delayed reactions can occur in the same individual [34]. It is possible to have immediate reactions to one or more foods and slow onset reactions to others. Where there is a perceived risk of a severe reaction to a reintroduction then that food should either be avoided or given in hospital (see below).

Phase 3: maintenance diet

The maintenance diet is achieved when the introduction of all foods has been attempted and the child is having the widest possible variety of foods. Nutritional adequacy is paramount and supplements are sometimes necessary. Children without milk may need a calcium supplement (see Table 14.4) [35], which may need to be free of colours and preservatives. The dietitian has a vital role in ensuring that people know how to avoid the necessary foods, suggesting alternatives to avoided foods, giving recipes and meal plans where necessary and ensuring adequacy of the diet.

Because children often lose their reactivity over time, attempts should be made every 6–12 months to introduce the avoided foods (particularly if they are staples such as milk or wheat). This may happen in an unsupervised way as the result of an accidental or deliberate break in the diet. It is extremely important that introductions of food are performed at home only if there is no danger of a severe immediate reaction. If there is the possibility of a reaction then foods should be introduced in a hospital setting as part of a clinically supervised food challenge.

Food challenges

Food challenges are needed to either confirm or refute suspected food hypersensitivity. Children tend to grow out of some food allergies (e.g. milk, egg, wheat, soy) but are less likely to grow out of others (peanuts, tree nuts, fish, shellfish) and so food reintroductions will need to be considered from time to time. Some children may report to be allergic to certain foods, whereas others may show sensitisation (positive skin prick test or specific IgE) to a food that they have never knowingly eaten before.

Challenges can be performed as either open food challenges (OFC), single blind placebo controlled food challenges (SBPCFC) or double blind placebo controlled food challenges (DBPCFC).

Open food challenges

During open food challenges, both the clinician and patient (parent) is informed of the food being administered and these challenges should be sufficient to either confirm or refute most reported food hypersensitivities. However, many children are very reluctant to eat a food that they do not remember having eaten before, or that they have previously been told to avoid. Indeed, it is not uncommon for children who have had previous severe reactions to foods to exhibit some degree of food avoidance. It is therefore often advisable to provide the challenge in a 'single blind' form (culprit food mixed with another food acceptable to the child) simply to ensure that the child consumes it.

As OFCs are mainly used in the clinical setting,

Table 14.5   Open reintroduction of foods.
Each food should be given in normal quantities daily for a week before being allowed freely in the diet. A test dose may be recommended initially. The order of reintroduction depends on the patient's preference and on which foods were avoided initially.

Oats	Porridge oats, Scottish oatcakes, homemade flapjacks (if sugar is already allowed)
Corn	Sweetcorn, homemade popcorn, cornflour, maize flour, cornflakes if malt is tolerated
Meats	Try meats (including offal) singly, e.g. chicken, beef, pork
Wheat	Wholemeal or unbleached white flour for baking, egg free pasta, Shredded Wheat, Puffed Wheat, Weetabix
Yeast	Pitta bread; ordinary bread (this usually also contains soya)
Rye	Worth trying if wheat is not tolerated; pure rye crispbread; pumpernickel
Cow's milk	Fresh cow's milk, cream, butter, plain yoghurt, milk containing foods with tolerated ingredients, e.g. rice pudding. Try cheese separately later
Cow's milk substitute	If cow's milk is not tolerated try substitutes one by one Infant soya formula (if >6 months) or infant hydrolysate formula. Ewe's milk, goat's milk for >1-year-olds (boiled or pasteurised). Supermarket liquid soya/rice milk with additional calcium for >2-year-olds
Egg	Use one whole fresh egg per day for test period It may be preferred to begin with small amounts of egg in baking
Fish	Fresh or frozen (not smoked, battered etc.), e.g. cod, herring. If one type is not tolerated others may be Try shellfish separately later
Tomatoes	Fresh tomatoes, canned and puréed tomatoes, ketchup
Peas/beans	These include peas, green beans, kidney beans, lentils, baked beans in tomato sauce if tomato is tolerated
Orange	Pure orange juice, oranges, satsumas. If oranges are tolerated all citrus fruit probably are too
Sugar	Use ordinary sugar on cereal, in drinks and baking. Some parents comment that small amounts are tolerated whereas larger amounts are not
Chocolate	Try only if sugar is tolerated. If diet is milk free, use milk free chocolate Cocoa powder in drinks and cooking
Carob	Carob confectionery can be tried if chocolate is not tolerated. Check other ingredients – it may contain milk or soya
Tea/coffee	Add milk if this is already in the diet
Peanuts	Plain or salted peanuts (not for <4-year-olds) Peanut butter
Other nuts	Try singly or mixed
Malt	Malt/malt flavouring is present in most breakfast cereals. Try Rice Krispies if rice is tolerated
Nitrite/nitrate	Corned beef if beef is tolerated, ham and bacon if pork is tolerated
Sodium benzoate	Supermarket lemonade provided other ingredients are tolerated
Sodium glutamate	Stock cubes, gravy mixes, flavoured crisps, provided the other ingredients are tolerated
Sodium metabisulphite	Some squashes, sausages provided the other ingredients are tolerated, dried fruit
Vitamins and minerals	These may be given if needed to enhance nutritional adequacy and introduced singly to test tolerance

Other foods (e.g. fruit and vegetables) can be introduced gradually as desired. Manufactured foods such as ice cream, biscuits can be introduced taking into account known sensitivities. Many additives (e.g. colours, flavours) will be introduced as mixtures in manufactured foods such as sweets and canned/bottled drinks. For children with multiple cereal intolerances, flours such as buckwheat, soya, gram (chickpea), wheatstarch may be tried. Some of the special dietary products for gluten free and low protein diets may be suitable but other ingredients must be checked (they are not strictly prescribable for food hypersensitivity).

the main aim of the food challenge is to make a correct diagnosis. Although factors such as starting dose, dose increment and final dose may not be that critical, it is essential that the patient has consumed an adequate amount of food during the challenge to make a diagnosis accurate.

Single blind placebo controlled food challenges

During the SBPCFC, the health professionals involved know which food is the active and which is the placebo, but the patient does not. Sufficient masking of the challenge food is therefore very important and an active and placebo challenge will be used. SBPCFC are particularly useful when performing food challenges in children or adults who do not want to ingest a specific food.

Double blind placebo controlled food challenge

The gold standard for confirming or refuting food allergy is the DBPCFC [36]. Although the DBPCFC is necessary for research, in practice open challenges are more common. One of the strengths of the DBPCFC is that neither the patient nor the investigator knows when the active or the placebo challenge is performed. It therefore rules out reporting bias from the clinician and any psychological effect from the patient.

These challenges can be time consuming and difficult to manage. They need only be used in clinical practice where there is a possibility that any observed reaction could be caused by anxiety or in diagnosing subjective symptoms such as abdominal pain and nausea.

Considerations when performing food challenges

Elimination period

Prior to a food challenge, the identified food must be excluded from the diet. The length of time depends on the history of the patient; for example, chronic widespread eczema may take 2–4 weeks to clear up or improve a great deal; children with constipation may need up to 6 weeks for a definite improvement. Bock *et al.* [36] recommend an elimination period of 2–6 weeks for foods and 24 hours for additives. The elimination period should allow enough time for the symptoms to resolve.

Challenge dose

- *Starting dose* The patient's history should once again determine the amount of food used for the first dose, or a set protocol may be used in threshold studies [37]. Bock and Sampson have suggested that challenges should be performed in a graded fashion. The starting quantity should be about half of that estimated to be required to elicit a reaction [38]. However, some clinicians may prefer to start the challenge with a rub of the lip before commencing the oral challenge [39].
- *Dose given* For immediate type symptoms it has been suggested that the dose may be doubled at each interval, guided by the patient's history, or a logarithmic mean can also be used for increasing the challenge dose [37]. The interval between doses can be anything between 15 and 60 minutes but the timing between each dose should be dependent on the patient's history and sufficient to allow symptoms to develop.

Some researchers use a total of 8–10 g of the dried food for challenge purposes (mainly DBPCFC) [40,41] whereas others used 8 g as the final dose [42–47], thus giving about 18 g dried food in total. When using real food as opposed to dried food, it is recommended that 60–100 g of wet food should be used for challenge purposes.

The whole challenge should give enough food to elicit a reaction and should ultimately give the normal serving size of the food in question [37].

There are currently no specific recommendations regarding the dose or design to be used when performing food challenges to diagnose delayed symptoms such as constipation, apart from that the amount normally known to cause a reaction should be used [36]. This raises practical issues when the patient is a very vague historian. Another difficult issue is that some reactions only occur when the causative food is eaten in sufficient doses on consecutive days and this must be planned for when designing the food challenge. The advantage of these challenges is that the reactions are not life-threatening so the whole challenge can be completed at home.

Challenge duration

For immediate symptoms, if no reaction has occurred after all doses have been consumed, the child can go home after 1–2 hours with instructions to incorporate that food gradually into the diet [41,45]. A longer challenge period of 1–4 weeks is recommended when looking for delayed reactions [43,48,49].

Challenge food used
Dried, cooked or raw food, as indicated by the history, should be used in order to mimic the history as close as possible [37,50,51].

Challenge location
It is recommended to perform a food challenge in hospital if there is a history of immediate reactions or if the patient is sensitised to the offending food. In other words, if there is the slightest concern that the child may experience an immediate or IgE mediated reaction the challenge should be performed under professional supervision in experienced hospital units. All other challenges can be performed at home [52].

Considerations when performing double blind placebo controlled food challenges

Active and placebo challenges
Providing that the child does not react to the placebo challenge, one active and one placebo challenge should be sufficient when dealing with objective symptoms such as urticaria or angioedema [44,53–55]. However, in cases where patients present with subjective symptoms three active and three placebo dosages, or three plus two, may be used. This would be of particular importance if the patient reacts to placebo challenge (e.g. flare up of eczema) [56–58].

Time between active and placebo challenges
When dealing with immediate symptoms at least 2 hours, but ideally 3–4 hours, should be allowed between the active and placebo challenge. In the case of delayed symptoms 1 week between the active and placebo challenge should be allowed [36,37,59]. However, the patient's history will have a major role in the final decision.

Masking of the challenge food
The challenge food used should be blinded (masked) in terms of smell, flavour and texture. Ideally, the active and placebo challenges should be identical regarding taste, appearance, smell,

viscosity, texture, structure and volume, and blindness should also be assessed by standard tests [37,51]. Although this is paramount in performing food challenges for research purposes, it may not be necessary when performing DBPCFC for a clinical diagnosis.

There are a number of factors that should be taken into account when choosing a challenge vehicle or placebo:

- The fat content of the vehicle can influence the challenge outcome [60].
- The vehicle must also allow for enough challenge food to be used [36].
- Cooking, canning, roasting [61–66] can have different effects on the allergenicity of different foods. The food challenge should always conclude with consumption of a normal portion of the food, prepared according to the history to eliminate this issue [36,67].

A variety of foods can be used for blinding. It is often helpful to use foods that are readily accepted by children such as ice cream, yoghurt, milk shake, milky puddings, fruit purée, mashed potatoes, soup, chocolate pudding, fruit juice, cocoa/carob, peppermint [50,51,68]. Many commercial products such as egg free, milk free, wheat free cakes, biscuits or pastas can be used as placebo. Finding a suitable and acceptable vehicle or placebo is particularly difficult if children suffer from multiple symptoms of food hypersensitivity [50].

Capsules are not recommended to be used in DBPCFC, especially not in the case of oral allergy syndrome [37,69], when dealing with young children [50] or when performing home challenges [36].

Interpretation of food challenges

The final and most important part of the challenge is the interpretation of the symptoms during the challenge [57]. This is not always easy as there are some confounding effects such as disease patterns for eczema and chronic urticaria. Presence of aeroallergens, particularly during the hay fever season, may also affect the challenge outcome [50,70].

The outcome of the food challenge should either be documented on a food challenge chart (hospital challenge) or a food and symptom diary (home challenge). Any symptoms at home should be verified by the supervising clinician and dietitian [71], based on the child's history and the symptoms experienced. There are no clear guidelines with criteria for interpreting a challenge as positive or negative.

Dietary management of food hypersensitivities

The dietary management of food hypersensitivity consists primarily of educating patients and their families so they can avoid the causative food while still meeting all nutritional requirements. No dietary manipulation is easy so it is the role of the dietitian to not only give information on how to avoid the causative food, but also how to make the resultant diet as palatable as possible. Before any advice is given it is essential to consider how strict the diet needs to be. It is not necessary for a family to strive for complete avoidance of an allergen if reactions only occur when relatively large doses of the food are taken. On the other hand, when life-threatening reactions occur to tiny doses advice on complete avoidance is essential.

Advice on dietary avoidance

Information on the main sources of the food, foods that may contain the 'hidden' allergen and where the allergen may be contained in non-food items is the mainstay of any dietary avoidance advice. The new labelling laws that came into effect in November 2005 (Directive 2003/89/EC) aid dietary avoidance. In the past a label did not have to state the presence of an ingredient if it made up less than 25% of the final product. This allowed for many inadvertent dietary indiscretions and subsequent reactions. However, the new labelling laws require the presence of 12 food allergens, at any concentration, to be stated on the label. These foods are celery, cereals containing gluten (wheat, barley, rye and oats), crustaceans, eggs, fish, milk, mustard, tree nuts, peanuts, sesame seeds, soybeans, sulphur dioxide and sulphites (at levels above 10 mg/kg or litre). However, foods that are not prepacked are not covered by this legislation and it is important to ensure patients and their families are aware of this. Where life-threatening reactions are involved it is often the safest option if only prepacked foods are bought. Another labelling

issue that needs to be discussed, particularly when reactions to peanuts, tree nuts and seeds are involved, is the 'may contain' label. It needs to be stressed that this label is used to warn that a food allergen may be present. It causes confusion to patients and is often seen as defensive labelling, there to legally protect a food company. This is generally not the case and the warning should be taken seriously. The last issue that needs to be addressed when giving avoidance advice is to consider contamination issues. These are particularly relevant when buying loose foods from bakeries, delicatessens and eating out. Obviously, where reactions only occur to large doses it is important to stress that there is no need to worry about contamination issues and 'may contain' labelling.

Food manufacturers and supermarkets produce 'free from' lists for their products. These are very useful in managing avoidance diets and patients and carers should be encouraged to use these to identify alternative products that can be included in the diet.

Alternative foods

The choice of alternative foods that are now available can make dietary exclusion easier. Advice should be given on what products are available (e.g. milk substitutes, egg free cakes, wheat free pasta). Although children with wheat allergy cannot strictly have gluten free foods prescribed for them, some general practitioners will prescribe foods such as bread and pasta if requested. It is very helpful for parents to have lists of gluten free/ wheat starch free foods which are also egg, milk and soya free if necessary. They may choose to buy some of the items as well as obtain some on prescription (many are not prescribable). It is also useful to tell parents about wheat free items readily available in supermarkets (e.g. puffed rice cakes, Thai rice noodles). Most food manufacturers and supermarkets have a customer helpline and these telephone numbers can be given to parents so they can get information themselves.

Parents find recipes very useful. Some examples are cakes without egg, biscuits and cakes without wheat, and gravy and sauces without wheat. A general discussion about menu planning is helpful. Advice may include ideas for packed lunches and weaning foods. Other carers may need to be contacted (e.g. school caterers). Parents also appreciate tips on how to get a child to take a new food. For example, when introducing a milk substitute a covered mug may be preferred to an open cup and the use of flavouring (e.g. with Nesquik, if allowed) improves the taste considerably. Wheat free products are often better accepted initially if given with other flavours (e.g. jam on wheat free bread, sauce on wheat free pasta). A different carer other than the main carer is often able to persuade the child to take the new food.

Dietary supplements

Whenever a food is removed from the diet there is a likelihood that the diet will no longer meet nutritional requirements; the more foods that are cut out the greater the risk. It is always considered best if the diet itself can meet requirements by using fortified foods (e.g. breakfast cereals, calcium fortified milk substitute) but as this is not always possible dietary supplements may be required. Although a 24-hour recall can give a good indication of a child's intake often it is necessary to analyse a food diary kept by the family (for at least 3 days) to assess the adequacy of the diet.

If a dietary supplement is required it is important to assess the dose required and which would be best accepted by the child. Family doctors are generally happy to prescribe supplements but sometimes an over-the-counter supplement may be more readily accepted.

Follow-up

It is essential that children following an exclusion diet are followed up regularly. Children's diets vary enormously as they get older and nutritional requirements also change. There may also be advances in knowledge that may affect treatment strategies and it is also important to ensure that as the child gets older they themselves understand their diet.

Specific issues

Infant formulas for cow's milk allergic infants

Protein hydrolysate formulas

The hypoallergenic or protein hydrolysate (semi-elemental) infant formula is often the choice for an infant with immediate or delayed adverse reactions to cow's milk. There is a variety of such formulas where the protein has been extensively hydrolysed (Table 7.7). Casein hydrolysates have been in use for over 50 years, whey hydrolysates for rather less time and hydrolysates of pork/soya have been more recently introduced. All these products are regarded as extensively hydrolysed and are in regular use in the UK. However, there is some variation in the degree of hydrolysis, casein products being the most highly hydrolysed with more than 90% of the peptides being smaller than 1200 Da.

A major problem with these products is palatability: the infant will take them quite readily; the child over 1 year or so will not. Sweetening and flavourings improve the taste.

Much of the literature on the subject of the use of these formulas relates to IgE mediated allergy. As far as cow's milk sensitive enteropathy is concerned both casein and whey extensively hydrolysed formulas (eHF) have been shown to be satisfactory [72].

It should not be assumed that these formulas will always be tolerated. Anaphylactic reactions have been described with both casein and whey hydrolysates and this has been reviewed by Sampson et al. [73]. Also, late onset adverse reactions to eHF have been reported by Hill et al. [4]. However, the majority of cow's milk allergic infants will tolerate any of the eHF. The highly allergic infant may tolerate one and not another. It is possible that in such a situation, casein hydrolysate (being the most highly hydrolysed) will be most successful.

There are partially hydrolysed whey based formulas (pHF) available in some European countries, Canada and the USA, and one is available in the UK (NanHA). They are much more palatable than eHF and much cheaper but have a much larger proportion of peptides larger than 4000 Da. They are intended for prophylactic use and are not suitable for the treatment of cow's milk allergy because of the relatively high level of large peptides present which may cause an adverse reaction.

Amino acid based formulas

For those few cow's milk allergic children who cannot tolerate eHF an alternative must be found. Neocate (see Table 7.9), a formula where the protein source is pure synthetic amino acids, has been shown to be tolerated by infants and children with both slow onset and quick onset food hypersensitivity [4,73–76]. McLeish *et al.* [77] compared feed tolerance, palatability and growth in children randomised to receive a whey hydrolysate formula or an amino acid based formula and there was little difference between the two.

Formulas based on whole soy protein isolate

Infant formulas based on whole soy protein isolate have been available without prescription for many years and no doubt have been used inappropriately, without medical supervision, for vague symptoms. There is a difference of opinion among clinicians as to their usefulness.

Soy based formulas have in the past been used widely as an alternative to cow's milk formula in those infants who are milk allergic. However, in 2003 the Chief Medical Officer advised against the use of soy formula in infants under the age of 6 months unless there is a specific medical indication because of their high phytoestrogen content [78] (see p. 95). Soya formula can be given for the treatment of cow's milk allergy over the age of 1 year and can be given between 6 and 12 months of age if amino acid or extensively hydrolysed formulas are not taken because of palatability. Soya formulas taste better and are cheaper than hydrolysates. Soya containing products such as desserts enhance the variety in a cow's milk free diet and can be given from 6 months of age [79].

Sheep's and goat's milk

Sheep and goat milk are not suitable for infants with cow's milk protein allergy as their nutritional composition is unsuitable for infant feeding, there is sometimes concern about microbial content and their proteins can be as sensitising as cow's milk protein. Dean *et al.* [80] have shown that there is strong cross-reactivity *in vitro* between allergens in all mammalian milks (except human milk). Infant milks based on goat's milk are not available in the UK.

Human milk

Breast milk should be encouraged for all infants. Occasionally, infants exhibit allergic symptoms while being exclusively breast fed. It is known that allergens from the mother's diet can appear in breast milk [81]. Breast fed infants with multiple allergies have also been described [82]. The mother should be encouraged to avoid milk and egg and any other food that appears to upset the infant when she eats it. If symptoms cannot be controlled by maternal allergen avoidance, as a last resort breast feeding may have to be stopped. Isolauri *et al.* [83] recommend this particularly for infants with atopic dermatitis who have impaired growth. Breast feeding mothers on exclusion diets should be reviewed by a dietitian to check adequacy of their diets as they may need supplements, especially of calcium.

Discussion of specific symptoms

Autistic spectrum disorders

The dietary management of autistic spectrum disorders (ASD) is discussed in Chapter 26.

Migraine and epilepsy

Cheese, chocolate and red wine sometimes provoke migraine, allegedly owing to the presence of a pharmacologically active ingredient, tyramine.

However, children with severe migraine who have failed to benefit from avoidance of cheese and chocolate have been shown to respond to a few foods diet and the most common provoking foods on food reintroduction were those that are implicated in food hypersensitivity in general [28]. When migraine attacks are fewer than one per week it is difficult to use a diet approach. If symptoms are infrequent, 3 weeks of a few foods diet would not be long enough to assess change in rate of attacks and the reintroduction phase would be very muddled. However, for children with severe frequent migraine who have not responded to medication, a diet trial is a worthwhile procedure.

Sometimes, children with severe migraine have other symptoms and epilepsy may be one of these. A minority of children with epilepsy who also have migraine respond to diet whereas children with epilepsy alone do not [31]. As with migraine, the diet approach cannot be tried unless seizures are frequent. A trial of diet for such children who have not responded to conventional treatment is worth considering.

Attention deficit hyperactivity disorder

The question of diet and ADHD is very controversial. In 1975, Ben Feingold, an American allergist, claimed that hyperactive children would benefit from avoiding food containing salicylates together with artificial flavours and colours. Later, food preservatives were also excluded. The results of studies aimed at testing Feingold's hypothesis indicate that only a few hyperactive children respond to the elimination of food additives from their diets. Problems with methodology and interpretation of these studies have been discussed by Taylor [84]. Five studies [24,30,85–87] have looked at the relationship between food (not just additives) and behaviour. There are indications from this work that the idea that food can affect behaviour should be taken seriously, although the proportion of children who might benefit is not known. Although food additives may adversely affect hyperactive children [88], foods can also affect behaviour [89]. Unfortunately, it is not always possible to carry out a diet trial as many children (especially those over 7 or 8 years) may be completely out of control and non-compliant.

Many hyperactive children have cravings and bizarre eating habits and the first line of approach may be to enforce a more 'normal' diet. Any improvement may be the result of firmer parental control rather than anything else. An 'additive' free diet may serve the same purpose. However, to look into the possibility of food hypersensitivity properly one must use an empirical diet or few foods diet as described. This should only be attempted where the problems are severe as the difficulties of adhering to a diet can easily be worse than the behaviour problem itself. It must be stressed to parents that this is a little researched area and that dietary management might not be the answer for their child. Other treatments such as behaviour modification or stimulant medication may be more effective although some children may end up on a combination of these treatments. Parents of children with severe ADHD who wish to explore the dietary approach should be given the opportunity

to do so, otherwise they will be tempted to experiment with diet unsupervised.

Oral allergy syndrome

Oral allergy syndrome (OAS), described as itching or unpleasant sensation in the oral mucosa after eating certain fruits, is experienced by some children. Reactions are caused by cross-reactivity, usually with pollens, but occasionally to latex. Such cross-reactivity does not always indicate that avoidance of all these foods is necessary, and the clinical history will indicate which foods to avoid. The mucosal reactions are usually to raw fruit, so cooked or canned varieties can often be tolerated, and this advice is important in helping the child maintain their fruit intake.

Novel approaches in food hypersensitivity

Probiotics/prebiotics

Probiotics are live bacteria which, if taken orally, are said to improve intestinal microbial balance and exert beneficial effects on health. The intestinal microflora is an important constituent of the gut mucosal barrier [90]. Majamas and Isolauri [91] studied two groups of infants with eczema. One group took a hydrolysed formula and the other took the same formula and a probiotic (Lactobacillus GG). The group with lactobacillus showed significant skin improvement after 1 month whereas the other group did not. There were also some changes in markers of intestinal inflammation. Further work by this group has demonstrated that administering probiotics in the late stages of pregnancy and the first 6 months of life reduces the incidence of eczema up to 4 years of age [92]. Both these studies suggest that probiotic bacteria may act as a useful tool in the treatment of eczema and food allergy although further research is needed to clarify the mechanism involved.

Prebiotics are dietary substrates that stimulate the growth of beneficial bacteria already in the colon. They are oligosaccharides that are not digested in the small intestine such as fructo-oligosaccharides and inulin. They are intended as an additional (or alternative) approach to using probiotics.

It is to be hoped that further research will elucidate the role of both pre- and probiotics in the treatment of food hypersensitivity.

Problems with dietary treatment in food hypersensitivity

In this controversial area of medicine it is important to avoid giving inappropriate emphasis to dietary treatment. However, people who feel that diet has a role in their child's illness should have the opportunity to discuss in an unbiased fashion the possibilities of dietary treatment and, where appropriate, have the opportunity to try a diet. A lack of sympathetic approach may lead to self-imposed diets (likely to be inadequate) or self-referral to an unqualified practitioner. Whatever the prejudices of the professionals involved, the question of diet must be discussed as the child may be on an inadequate and inappropriate diet. Although some children may be on unhelpful diets, others benefit dramatically from the correct exclusion diet. The role of the dietitian is to assist in maintaining helpful diets and broaden the diet as much as possible. It is equally important to encourage people to abandon unhelpful diets. An open minded approach is necessary. Occasionally, parents will not take advice and in exceptional cases the restrictions imposed by the parent on the child may be regarded as a form of child abuse [93].

Acknowledgements

I would like to acknowledge Christine Carter, who wrote this chapter for the first and second editions. I have used much of her original text. I would also like to thank Carina Venter who provided information for the section on food challenges.

References

1   Johansson SGO, Bieber T, Dahl R *et al.* Revised nomenclature for allergy for global use: Report of the Nomenclature Review committee of the World Allergy Organization, October 2003. *J Allergy Clin Immunol*, 2004, **113** 832–6.
2   Patel L, Radivan FS, David TJ *et al.* Management of anaphylactic reactions to food. *Arch Dis Child*, 1994, **71** 370–5.
3   Bock SA, Sampson HA, Atkins FM *et al.* Double-blind placebo-controlled food challenge (DBPCFC) as an office procedure: a manual. *J Allergy Clin Immunol*, 1986, **82** 986–97.
4   Hill DJ, Hosking CS The cows milk allergy complex: overlapping disease profiles in infancy. *Eur J Clin Nutr*, 1995, **49** (Suppl 1) S1–12.
5   Sampson HA. Food Allergy. Part 2: Diagnosis and Management. *J Allergy Clin Immunol*, 1999, **103** 981–9.
6   British Society for Allergy and Environmental Medicine with the British Society for Nutritional Medicine. The First Report of the BSAEM/BSNM. Effective Allergy Practice. 1994. Report No: 1.
7   Sicherer SH Food allergy. *Lancet*, 2002, **360** 701–10.
8   Niggeman B, Gruber C Unproven diagnostic procedures in Ig-E mediated allergic diseases. *Allergy*, 2004, **59** 806–8.
9   Sampson HA Food allergy. *J Allergy Clin Immunol*, 2003, **111** S540–7.
10 Bock SA, Sampson HA Evaluation of food allergy. In: Leung DYM, Sampson HA, Geha RS, Szefler SJ (eds) *Pediatric Allergy. Principles and Practice.* St Louis: Mosby, 2003, pp. 478–87.
11 Health Which. Food allergy testing. *Health Which* 1998, **Dec** 12–15.
12 Lewith GT, Kenyon JN, Broomfield J *et al.* Is electrodermal testing as effective as skin prick tests for diagnosing allergies? A double blind randomised block design study. *Br Med J*, 2001, **322** 131–4.
13 Grundy J, Matthews S, Bateman B *et al.* Rising prevalence of allergy to peanut in children: Data from two sequential cohorts. *J Allergy Clin Immunol*, 2002, **110** 784–9.
14 Sicherer SH, Munoz-Furlong A, Sampson HA Prevalence of peanut and tree nut allergy in the United States determined by means of a random digit dial telephone survey: a five year follow-up. *J Allergy Clin Immunol*, 2003, **112** 1203–7.
15 Friedman NJ, Zeiger RS Prevention and natural history of food allergy. In: Leung DYM, Sampson HA, Geha RS, Szefler SJ (eds) *Pediatric Allergy. Principles and Practice.* St. Louis: Mosby, 2003, pp. 495–509.
16 Eigenmann PA, Sicherer SH, Borkowski TA *et al.* Prevalence of IgE mediated food allergy among children with atopic dermatitis. *Pediatrics*, 1998, **101** 3.
17 von Mutius E. Epidemiology of allergic diseases. In: Leung DYM, Sampson HA, Geha RS, Szefler SJ (eds) *Pediatric Allergy. Principles and Practice.* St. Louis: Mosby, 2003, pp. 1–9.
18 Sampson HA, Scanlon SM Natural history of food hypersensitivity in children with atopic dermatitis. *J Pediatr*, 1989, **115** 23–7.
19 Skolnick HS, Conover-Walker MK, Koerner CB *et al.* The natural history of peanut allergy. *J Allergy Clin Immunol*, 2001, **107** 367–74.

20 Kjellman NIM, Nilsson L From food allergy and atopic dermatitis to respiratory allergy. *Pediatr Allergy Immunol*, 1998, **9** (Suppl 1) 13–17.

21 Kulig M, Bergmann R, Klettke U *et al*. Natural course of sensitization to food and inhalant allergens during the first 6 years of life. *J Allergy Clin Immunol*, 1999, **103** 1173–9.

22 Conners CK, Barkley RA Rating scales and checklists for child psychopharmacology. *Psychopharmacol Bull*, 1985, **21** 809–43.

23 Rowe AH, Rowe A Bronchial asthma due to food allergy alone in ninety five patients. *J Am Med Assoc*, 1958, **169** 104–8.

24 Carter CM, Urbanowicz M, Hemsley R *et al*. Effects of a few food diet in attention deficit disorder. *Arch Dis Child*, 1993, **69** 564–8.

25 Swain AR, Dutton SP, Truswell AS Salicylates in foods. *J Am Diet Assoc*, 1985, **85** 950–60.

26 Minford AM, MacDonald A, Littlewood JM Food intolerance and food allergy in children: a review of 68 cases. *Arch Dis Child*, 1982, **57** 742–7.

27 Atherton DJ Dietary treatment in childhood atopic eczema. Proceedings of the second allergy workshop. Oxford: The Medicine Publ Foundation, 1983, pp. 109–10.

28 Egger J, Carter CM, Wilson J *et al*. Is migraine food allergy? A double-blind controlled trial of oligoantigenic diet treatment. *Lancet*, 1983, **2** (8355) 865–9.

29 Pike MG, Carter CM, Boulton P *et al*. Few food diets in the treatment of atopic eczema. *Arch Dis Child*, 1989, **64** 1691–8.

30 Egger J, Carter CM, Graham PJ *et al*. Controlled trial of oligoantigenic treatment in the hyperkinetic syndrome. *Lancet*, 1985, **1** (8428) 540–5.

31 Egger J, Carter CM, Soothill JF *et al*. Oligoantigenic diet treatment of children with epilepsy and migraine. *J Pediatr*, 1989, **114** 51–8.

32 Egger J, Carter CM Effect of diet treatment on enuresis in children with migraine or hyperkinetic behaviour. *Clin Pediatr*, 1992, **31** 302–7.

33 Devlin J, David TJ, Stanton RH Elemental diet for refractory atopic eczema. *Arch Dis Child*, 1991, **66** 93–9.

34 Bishop JM, Hill DJ, Hosking CS Natural history of cow milk allergy: clinical outcome. *J Pediatr*, 1990, **116** 862–7.

35 Devlin J, Stanton RH, David TJ Calcium intake and cows' milk free diets. *Arch Dis Child*, 1989, **64** 1183–4.

36 Bock SA, Sampson HA, Atkins FM *et al*. Double-blind, placebo-controlled food challenge (DBPCFC) as an office procedure: a manual. *J Allergy Clin Immunol*, 1988, **82** 986–97.

37 Bindslev-Jensen C, Ballmer-Weber BK, Bengtsson U *et al*. Standardization of food challenges in patients with immediate reactions to foods. Position paper from the European Academy of Allergology and Clinical Immunology. *Allergy*, 2004, **59** 690–7.

38 Bock SA, Sampson HA Evaluation of Food Allergy. In: Leung DYM, Sampson HA, Geha RS, Szefler SJ (eds) *Pediatric Allergy. Principles and Practice*. St Louis: Mosby, 2003, pp. 891–6.

39 Rance F, Dutau G Peanut hypersensitivity in children. *Pediatr Pulmonol Suppl*, 1999, **18** 165–7.

40 Sampson HA Utility of food-specific IgE concentrations in predicting symptomatic food allergy. *J Allergy Clin Immunol*, 2001, **107** 891–6.

41 Sicherer SH, Morrow EH, Sampson HA Dose–response in double-blind, placebo-controlled oral food challenges in children with atopic dermatitis. *J Allergy Clin Immunol*, 2000, **105** 582–6.

42 Eigenmann PA, Calza AM Diagnosis of IgE-mediated food allergy among Swiss children with atopic dermatitis. *Pediatr Allergy Immunol*, 2000, **11** 95–100.

43 Isolauri E, Turjanmaa K Combined skin prick and patch testing enhances identification of food allergy in infants with atopic dermatitis. *J Allergy Clin Immunol*, 1996, **97** 9–15.

44 Niggemann B, Sielaff B, Beyer K *et al*. Outcome of double-blind, placebo-controlled food challenge tests in 107 children with atopic dermatitis. *Clin Exp Allergy*, 1999, **29** 91–6.

45 Bock SA Prospective appraisal of complaints of adverse reactions to foods in children during the first 3 years of life. *Pediatrics*, 1987, **79** 683–8.

46 Bock SA, Atkins FM Patterns of food hypersensitivity during sixteen years of double-blind, placebo-controlled food challenges. *J Pediatr*, 1990, **117** 561–7.

47 May CD Objective clinical and laboratory studies of immediate hypersensitivity reactions to foods in asthmatic children. *J Allergy Clin Immunol*, 1976, **58** 500–15.

48 Baehler P, Chad Z, Gurbindo C *et al*. Distinct patterns of cow's milk allergy in infancy defined by prolonged, two-stage double-blind, placebo-controlled food challenges. *Clin Exp Allergy*, 1996, **26** 254–61.

49 Majamaa H, Moisio P, Holm K *et al*. Cow's milk allergy: diagnostic accuracy of skin prick and patch tests and specific IgE. *Allergy*, 1999, **54** 346–51.

50 Carter C Double-blind placebo controlled food challenges in children: a dietitian's perspective. *Allergy*, 1995, **4** 95–9.

51 Vlieg-Boerstra BJ, Bijleveld CM, van der HS *et al*. Development and validation of challenge materials for double-blind, placebo-controlled food challenges in children. *J Allergy Clin Immunol* 2004, **113** 341–6.

52 Venter C, Pereira B, Grundy J *et al*. Incidence of parentally reported and clinically diagnosed food hypersensitivity in the first year of life. *J Allergy Clin Immunol*, 2006, **117** 1118–24.

53   Zuberbier T, Edenharter G, Worm M *et al.* Prevalence of adverse reactions to food in Germany: a population study. *Allergy*, 2004, **59** 338–45.

54   Jansen JJ, Kardinaal AF, Huijbers G *et al.* Prevalence of food allergy and intolerance in the adult Dutch population. *J Allergy Clin Immunol*, 1994, **93** 446–56.

55   Hourihane JO, Bedwani SJ, Dean TP, Warner JO Randomised, double blind, crossover challenge study of allergenicity of peanut oils in subjects allergic to peanuts. *Br Med J*, 1997, **314** 1084–8.

56   Niggemann B Role of oral food challenges in the diagnostic work-up of food allergy in atopic eczema dermatitis syndrome. *Allergy*, 2004, **59** (Suppl 78) 32–4.

57   Gellerstedt M, Magnusson J, Grajo U *et al.* Interpretation of subjective symptoms in double-blind placebo-controlled food challenges: interobserver reliability. *Allergy*, 2004, **59** 354–6.

58   Briggs D, Aspinall L, Dickens A *et al.* Statistical model for assessing the proportion of subjects with subjective sensitisations in adverse reactions to foods. *Allergy*, 2001, **56** (Suppl 67) 83–5.

59   Muraro MA Diagnosis of food allergy: the oral provocation test. *Pediatr Allergy Immunol*, 2001, **12** (Suppl 14) 31–6.

60   Grimshaw KE, King RM, Nordlee JA *et al.* Presentation of allergen in different food preparations affects the nature of the allergic reaction: a case series. *Clin Exp Allergy*, 2003, **33** 1581–5.

61   Ballmer-Weber BK, Hoffmann A, Wuthrich B *et al.* Influence of food processing on the allergenicity of celery: DBPCFC with celery spice and cooked celery in patients with celery allergy. *Allergy*, 2002, **57** 228–35.

62   Simonato B, Pasini G, Giannattasio M *et al.* Food allergy to wheat products: the effect of bread baking and in vitro digestion on wheat allergenic proteins. A study with bread dough, crumb, and crust. *J Agric Food Chem*, 2001, **49** 5668–73.

63   Franck P, Moneret Vautrin DA *et al.* The allergenicity of soybean-based products is modified by food technologies. *Int Arch Allergy Immunol*, 2002, **128** 212–19.

64   Maleki SJ, Chung SY, Champagne ET *et al.* The effects of roasting on the allergenic properties of peanut proteins. *J Allergy Clin Immunol*, 2000, **106** 763–8.

65   Cooke SK, Sampson HA Allergenic properties of ovomucoid in man. *J Immunol*, 1997, **159** 2026–32.

66   Dreborg S, Foucard T Allergy to apple, carrot and potato in children with birch pollen allergy. *Allergy*, 1983, **38** 167–72.

67   Metcalfe DD, Sampson HA Workshop on Experimental Methodology for Clinical Studies of Adverse Reactions to Foods and Food Additives. *J Allergy Clin Immunol*, 1990, **86** 421–42.

68   Noe D, Bartemucci L, Mariani N *et al.* Practical aspects of preparation of foods for double-blind, placebo-controlled food challenge. *Allergy*, 1998, **53** (46 Suppl) 75–7.

69   Ortolani C, Bruijnzeel-Koomen C, Bengtsson U *et al.* Controversial aspects of adverse reactions to food. European Academy of Allergology and Clinical Immunology (EAACI) Reactions to Food Subcommittee. *Allergy*, 1999, **54** 27–45.

70   Reekers R, Busche M, Wittmann M *et al.* Birch pollen-related foods trigger atopic dermatitis in patients with specific cutaneous T-cell responses to birch pollen antigens. *J Allergy Clin Immunol*, 1999, **104** 466–72.

71   Pereira B, Venter C, Grundy J *et al.* Prevalence of sensitization to food allergens, reported adverse reaction to foods, food avoidance, and food hypersensitivity among teenagers. *J Allergy Clin Immunol*, 2005, **116** 884–92.

72   Walker-Smith JA, Digeon B, Phillips AD Evaluation of a casein and a whey hydrolysate for treatment of cow's-milk-sensitive enteropathy. *Eur J Pediatr*, 1989, **149** 68–71.

73   Sampson HA, James JM, Bernhisel-Broadbent J Safety of an amino acid-derived infant formula in children allergic to cow milk. *Pediatrics*, 1992, **90** 463–5.

74   Vanderhoof JA, Murray ND, Kaufman SS *et al.* Intolerance to protein hydrolysate infant formulas: an under recognized cause of gastrointestinal symptoms in infants. *J Pediatr*, 1997, **131** 741–4.

75   De BD, Dupont C Allergy to extensively hydrolyzed cow's milk proteins in infants: safety and duration of amino acid-based formula. *J Pediatr*, 2002, **141** 271–3.

76   Isolauri E, Sutas Y, Makinen-Kiljunen S *et al.* Efficacy and safety of hydrolyzed cow milk and amino acid-derived formulas in infants with cow milk allergy. *J Pediatr*, 1995, **127** 550–7.

77   McLeish CM, MacDonald A, Booth IW Comparison of an elemental with a hydrolysed whey formula in intolerance to cows' milk. *Arch Dis Child*, 1995, **73** 211–15.

78   Department of Health, London. Chief Medical Officer's Update 37, 2004.

79   Paediatric Group Position Statement on the use of soya protein for infants, British Dietetic Association, Birmingham, 2003.

80   Dean TP, Adler BR, Ruge F *et al. In vitro* allergenicity of cows' milk substitutes. *Clin Exp Allergy*, 1993, **23** 205–10.

81   Barau E, Dupont C Allergy to cow's milk proteins in mother's milk or in hydrolyzed cow's milk infant formulas as assessed by intestinal permeability measurements. *Allergy*, 1994, **49** 295–8.

82   De BD, Matarazzo P, Rocchiccioli F *et al.* Multiple food allergy: a possible diagnosis in breastfed infants. *Acta Paediatr*, 1997, **86** 1042–6.

83 Isolauri E, Tahvanainen A, Peltola T *et al*. Breast-feeding of allergic infants. *J Pediatr*, 1999, **134** 27–32.

84 Taylor E Toxins and allergens. In: Rutter M, Casaer P (eds) *Biological Risk Factors for Psychological Disorders*. New York: Academic Press, 1992.

85 Kaplan BJ, McNicol J, Conte RA *et al*. Dietary replacement in preschool-aged hyperactive boys. *Pediatrics*, 1989, **83** 7–17.

86 Boris M, Mandel FS Foods and additives are common causes of the attention deficit hyperactive disorder in children. *Ann Allergy*, 1994, **72** 462–8.

87 Schmidt MH, Mocks P, Lay B *et al*. Does oligoantigenic diet influence hyperactive/conduct-disordered children – a controlled trial. *Eur Child Adolesc Psychiatry*, 1997, **6** 88–95.

88 Schab DW, Trinh NT Do artificial colors promote hyperactivity in children with hyperactive syndromes? A meta-analysis of double blind placebo-controlled trials. *Develop Behav Pediatr*, 2004, **25** 423–33.

89 Bellisle F Effects of diet on behaviour and cognition in children. *Br J Nutr*, 2004, **92** S227–32.

90 Fuller R Probiotics in human medicine. *Gut*, 1991, **32** 439–42.

91 Majamas H, Isolauri E Probiotics: a novel approach in the management of food allergy. *J Allergy Clin Immunol*, 1997, **99** 179–85.

92 Kalliomaki M, Salminen S, Poussa T *et al*. Probiotics and prevention of atopic disease: 4-year follow-up of a randomised placebo-controlled trial. *Lancet*, 2003, **361** 1869–71.

93 Warner JO, Hathaway MJ Allergic form of Meadow's syndrome (Munchausen by proxy). *Arch Dis Child*, 1984, **59** 151–6.

Further reading

Committee on Toxicity of Chemicals in Food, Consumer Products and the Environment (COT) Adverse Reactions to Food and Food Ingredients. Department of Health, London, 2000.

Food allergy – getting move out of your skin prick tests. Editorial. *Clin Exp Allergy*, 2000, **30** 1495–8.

Holgate S, Church MK, Lichtenstein LM *Allergy*, 2nd edn. London: Mosby, 2002.

Joneja JV *Dietary Management of Food Allergies and Intolerances. A comprehensive guide*, 2nd edn. Vancouver: JA Hall, 1998.

Leung DYM, Sampson HA, Geha RS, Szefler SJ (eds) *Pediatric Allergy. Principles and Practice*. St Louis: Mosby, 2003.

Ortolani C, Bruijnzeel-Koomen C *et al*. Controversial aspects of adverse reactions to food. Position Paper. *Allergy*, 1999, **54** 27–45.

Sampson HA Update on food allergy. *J Allergy Clin Immunol*, 2004, **113** 805–19.

Sicherer SH Food allergy: when and how to perform oral food challenges. *Pediatr Allergy Immunol*, 1999, **10** 226–34.

Sicherer SH Food allergy. *Lancet*, 2002, **360** 701–10.

Useful addresses

Anaphylaxis Campaign

PO Box 275, Farnborough, Hampshire, GU14 6SX
Tel. 01252 373793
www.anaphylaxis.org.uk

Allergy UK

3 White Oak Square, Swanley, Kent, BR5 7AG
Tel. 01322 619898
www.allergyuk.org

Food Allergy Network

www.foodallergy.org

American Academy of Allergy Asthma and Immunology

www.aaaai.org

15 Immunodeficiency Syndromes, HIV and AIDS

Immunodeficiency Syndromes

Marian Sewell & Vivien Wigg

Introduction

The primary function of the immune system is to destroy pathogens and to minimise any damage they may cause. Inherent or innate immunity is the body's ability to fight some bacterial infections without requiring prior exposure to the pathogen or the production of antibodies. Adaptive immunity is the body's learned response as a result of exposure to pathogens and this involves the production of specific antibodies. Some pathogens, such as viruses, invade and replicate within individual cells. Others, including many bacteria, live and divide extracellularly within tissues, body fluids or body cavities. Defects or failures in the immune system may lead to immunopathological reactions and disease. This section looks at some of the disorders caused by immunodeficiency and the dietetic management of such disorders. Table 15.1 lists the components of the immune system.

Primary immune deficiency diseases are caused by inherent or genetic defects of the immune system. The two major types of lymphocytes involved in adaptive immune responses are the B and T cells. B lymphocytes develop from stem cells in the bone marrow and their main function is to produce antibodies: IgA, IgG, IgM, IgE. T lymphocytes are also derived from bone marrow and develop in the

Table 15.1 Cells of the immune system.

Cell type	Site of development	Function
B lymphocytes (B cells)	Bone marrow stem cells. B cells are found in bone marrow, spleen and lymph nodes	Production of antibodies (IgA, IgG, IgM, IgE)
T lymphocytes (T cells)	Bone marrow stem cells. T cells mature in the thymus and then migrate to the lymph nodes, blood, spleen and bone marrow	Attack viruses, fungi, and transplanted tissue Regulators of immune system
Complement system (18 serum proteins)	Some produced in liver, others by macrophages (phagocytic cells)	Defend against infection and promote inflammation
Phagocytes	Bone marrow stem cells. Phagocytes migrate to all tissues, particularly spleen, liver, lung, blood and lymph nodes	Ingest and destroy microorganisms such as bacteria and fungi

Ig, immunoglobulin.

Table 15.2   Immunodeficiency syndromes.

Immunodeficiency	Gastrointestinal complications
B lymphocytes defects	
IgA deficiency	Malabsorption, coeliac disease, gut infection
Transient IgA/IgG subclass deficiency of infancy	Malabsorption, food allergy
Hypogammaglobulinaemia (X-linked)	Malabsorption, steatorrhoea
Common variable immunodeficiency	Gut infection
T lymphocyte defects	
Autoimmune enteropathy	Chronic diarrhoea
DiGeorge's syndrome	Diarrhoea and intestinal infection
Class II MHC deficiency	Chronic diarrhoea
Wiskott–Aldrich syndrome	Malabsorption, food allergy
CD40 ligand deficiency	Gut infection, lymphoma of the small intestine, liver disease
T and B lymphocyte defects	
Severe combined immunodeficiency:	Infectious diarrhoea
Autosomal recessive	
X-linked	
Sporadic	
ADA, PNP deficiency	
Omenn's syndrome	
Phagocyte defects	
Chronic granulomatous disease	Diarrhoea, protein-losing enteropathy, pancolitis, small bowel obstruction [3]
Leucocyte adhesion deficiency	Mucosal infection and inflammation, appendicitis, perirectal abscesses [3]
HIV	Enteropathy, malabsorption

Source: Walker-Smith and Murch [2].
ADA, adenosine deaminase; HIV, human immunodeficiency virus; MHC, major histocompatibility complex; PNP, purine nucleoside phosphorylase deficiency.

thymus. There are three types of T cell: killer T cells which destroy cells infected with virus; helper T cells which co-ordinate immune responses; and suppressor T cells which switch off helper T-cell activity. Primary immunodeficiences include disorders of B cells where the differentiation or ability to produce antibody is compromised, T-cell defects, combined B and T cell defects, disorders of phagocytes and complement deficiencies. Approximately 100 diseases caused by primary immunodeficiency are recognised [1]. The most common disorders and the associated gastrointestinal complications are listed in Table 15.2.

B lymphocyte defects

Selective IgA deficiency

This is the most common of the primary immune deficiency diseases. Patients have severe deficiency or a total absence of IgA, but usually normal levels of the other immunoglobulins. IgA protects the mucosal surfaces from infections; deficiency therefore leads to recurrent or chronic infections such as sinusitis, pneumonia, bronchitis and gastrointestinal infections.

Selective IgA deficiency is associated with coeliac disease and the incidence of selective IgA deficiency in these patients is 10–16 times higher than in the general population [4]. The only difference between these and other children with coeliac disease is that IgA deficiency persists when on a gluten free diet despite the return of a normal mucosa. A gluten free diet is always indicated [5].

IgA deficiency is also associated with food allergy. It is estimated that 7% of atopic individuals have transient IgA deficiency [6].

IgG or IgG subclass deficiency

Children with low IgG or low IgG subclass deficiency also commonly have food allergy; it is estimated that 32% of patients with an IgG subclass deficiency are allergic to some foods [7]. The dietetic management of food allergy is described in Chapters 7 and 14.

T lymhphocyte defects

Autoimmune enteropathy

Autoimmune enteropathy is a condition of unknown aetiology in which there is persistent damage to the small intestinal mucosa, resulting from activation of mucosal T cells [8]. The disease may be confined to the small intestine, which shows severe inflammation and villous atrophy with crypt hyperplasia and increased mitosis, or it may be more widespread. These changes in the small intestinal mucosa may resemble those found in coeliac disease [2]. Such infants present with chronic diarrhoea and subsequent failure to thrive and may be unresponsive to nutritional interventions including parenteral nutrition (PN) [9]. Where infants have been maintained for extended periods on intravenous (IV) fluids alone their nutritional status is further compromised as malnutrition itself leads to worsening mucosal and pancreatic function. Early nutritional intervention is necessary to reverse this cycle of malnutrition. Most of these patients will require immunosuppressive therapy. For those patients where a primary immunodeficiency disease is identified, bone marrow transplantation may be a more appropriate treatment.

Dietetic management will follow that outlined for severe combined immune deficiency described below. When patients are able to start oral intake it is advisable to introduce foods slowly. Empirically, infants may be given weaning solids free from milk, egg, and wheat. Parents may be advised to give one new food at a time. For the older child the reintroduction of food could follow the few foods diet (p. 264).

Defects in phagocytes

Phagocytic cells, including neutrophils and monocytes, are important in host defence against pyogenic bacteria and other intracellular organisms. These cells leave the bone marrow and migrate to peripheral tissues, particularly at sites of infection or inflammation. Phagocytyes internalise pathogens and degrade them. Two genetic defects of phagocytes are clinically important in that they result in susceptibility to severe infections and may be fatal: chronic granulomatous disease and leucocyte adhesion defects. Some patients may present with gastrointestinal complications similar to those of inflammatory bowel disease [10]. Nutrition support may be indicated. The enteropathy associated with HIV infection is described later.

Defects of T and B lymphocytes

Severe combined immune deficiency

Infants with combined immune deficiency, including severe combined immunodeficiency (SCID), have a gene mutation characterised by profound deficiencies of T, B and natural killer cells. The condition is fatal if untreated. Infants present from birth with recurrent, severe infections which may be bacterial, fungal or viral. These infections may be very difficult to treat. There is frequently failure to thrive associated with malabsorption and persistent diarrhoea. There may be vomiting associated with gastro-oesophageal reflux [11]. Respiratory infections are common.

Gene therapy for SCID

Treatment has traditionally been bone marrow transplantation (BMT). It is now possible to correct the condition by *ex vivo* gene therapy. A working copy of the gene is inserted, by retrovirus carrier, into bone marrow stem cells from these children. Infusion of these stem cells has corrected the immunodeficiency in a number of patients with no adverse effects to date from the procedure [12]. Nutritional status may be compromised if chemotherapy such as melphalan is given for conditioning prior to gene therapy treatment. Dietetic management is similar to that outlined for BMT described below.

Dietetic management of infants with SCID

Infants with SCID frequently have a reduced oral intake and may be unable to meet their nutritional requirements. This may be because of frequent infections, diarrhoea or vomiting. Nutrition support may be needed to promote growth and weight gain.

The use of an energy dense formula (e.g. SMA High Energy) given orally or via a nasogastric tube is often indicated. In adenosine deaminase (ADA) deficient SCID, infants may fail to thrive, but their nutritional status will often improve with PEG-ADA enzyme replacement therapy which is given by intramuscular injection weekly.

Infants with SCID may be clinically very unwell and failing to thrive at presentation and unable to feed for some time while they are being stabilised. Parenteral hydration and nutrition may be necessary for extended periods while investigations are ongoing. However, nutrition is likely to be inadequate, particularly if the child has frequent infections and chronic diarrhoea. Parenteral nutrition (PN) may be required to maintain nutrition and, if possible, minimal enteral feeds (trophic feeds) should be continued as they may have a beneficial effect on gut mucosa. If the child is able to take feeds orally, the suck–swallow reflex may be maintained. If total gut rest is required, enteral feeds should be reintroduced as soon as possible. Oral rehydration solution such as Dioralyte may be given first; if this is tolerated then a suitable formula feed can be introduced.

Hydrolysed protein formulas such as Pepti-Junior or amino acid based formulas such as Neocate are likely to be better tolerated than a whole protein formula. Rarely, a modular feed will be tried (see p. 109). Reintroduction of feeds should be done slowly; frequently the child will tolerate only 5 mL/hour or less of feed to start with. Volumes should be increased very gradually as tolerated. Continuous feeding over 20–24 hours is recommended to begin with. Infants with SCID are likely to have increased requirements of nutrients, particularly if there is multiorgan involvement.

Hydrolysate and amino acid formulas have a higher osmolality than normal infant formulas and may be a cause of osmotic diarrhoea. A standard concentration of feed should be used until the child is tolerating a reasonable volume of formula (e.g. 50% of requirements). In order to maximise weight gain it may be necessary to increase the concentration of the formula slightly with or without the addition of energy supplements (e.g. Maxijul or Calogen) if tolerated. These changes should be made slowly, one at a time. The aim should be to give a 1 kcal/mL (4.2 kJ/mL) formula if possible.

The child may tolerate small amounts of normal infant formula orally while having enteral feeds of a hydrolysate formula. This may help to promote oral motor skills and avoid oral sensitisation. Such feeding can also be very valuable for the parent. Where a normal feeding experience is not possible, it should be replicated by cuddling and oral stimulation while an enteral feed is being given. These strategies are helpful in maintaining feeding skills and may reduce long term dependency on a tube for feeding.

Bone marrow transplantation

A number of children with immunodeficiency diseases and SCID can be successfully treated with BMT. In patients with SCID, BMT from a histocompatible sibling can result in 76% probability of disease free survival [13]. It is important to maintain a good nutritional intake in these patients as malnutrition can have a negative effect on the clinical outcome [14].

Children receiving an allogeneic haematopoietic BMT are given myeloablative immunosuppressive conditioning drugs for about 10 days prior to transplant depending on the individual protocol planned for each child.

'Mini' BMT is a relatively new treatment which is increasingly used; it has fewer potential side effects compared with standard BMT as a reduced conditioning protocol is used. This type of transplant may be used where there is a good matched sibling donor.

When children have co-existing organ damage, myeloablative conditioning therapy has been associated with increased treatment toxicity and morbidity. Low intensity conditioning regimens have been shown to be as effective in promoting engraftment and donor immune reconstitution, with minimal toxicity and improved survival [15].

Infection is one of the main threats to children having BMT and all patients are treated in a reverse isolation unit with high efficiency particulate air (HEPA) filter to keep out any airborne infections. Meals are provided following 'clean' meal precautions to reduce the risk of infection from foodborne organisms (see p. 27). Food restrictions will usually be continued for 3–6 months post-transplant. In hospital all formula feeds may be pasteurised as an additional precaution.

The majority of children will need nutrition support during the transplant and are usually unable to meet their nutritional requirements orally. PN has been the preferred method of nutrition support until recently, particularly because of concerns with mucositis, vomiting and diarrhoea. However, enteral feeding can be used successfully [16] and most children can be managed in this way, although some require PN for a short period of time if they develop severe gut problems. A suggested protocol is to pass a nasogastric tube at day +1, after conditioning drugs have been given and before mucositis may develop. Dietetic management will be similar to that outlined above for SCID patients. Hydrolysate formulas are generally better tolerated post-transplant than whole protein formulas. Most infants and older children will be fed overnight at first. Day bolus feeds are introduced, after solids are offered, if oral intake decreases. A normal 'clean' diet, including milk and milk-containing foods, is usually tolerated in small quantities and is to be encouraged.

Oral intake is often slow to recover and enteral feeds may be required for several months after discharge from hospital.

If PN is indicated it is important to ensure maximum energy is provided. It may not be possible to include lipid because of the risk of liver complications such as veno-occlusive disease. If it is not possible to give any enteral feeds it will be difficult to meet energy requirements. A supplement of walnut oil to meet essential fatty acid requirements should be considered (see p. 427).

In the early post-transplant period children may develop gastrointestinal problems such as diarrhoea and vomiting. This may be associated with viral load, infections or graft versus host disease (GVHD) of the gut. Enteral feeding will often be continued while oral intake is poor. Children with GVHD have green, watery diarrhoea often exacerbated by oral intake. These patients have a significant decrease in nutritional status [17]. Endoscopy may be carried out to confirm a diagnosis of GVHD. Total gut rest with PN is indicated until there is a significant reduction in stool output. Small volumes of an amino acid based formula will be used initially when enteral feeding is restarted and if tolerated, a simple diet of only a few foods (e.g. plain chicken with potato or rice) may be gradually reintroduced. It may be advisable to avoid milk, egg, and sometimes wheat and soya (see Table 7.11).

HIV and AIDS

Julie Lanigan

Introduction

Human immunodeficiency virus (HIV) is a retrovirus that attacks the human immune system. Acquired immunodeficiency syndrome (AIDS) is a disease complex occurring as a result of HIV induced cell-mediated immunodeficiency which may cause life-threatening opportunistic infections, tumours and other conditions.

The main source of HIV infection in young children is mother to child transmission (MTCT). The virus may be transmitted during pregnancy, labour and delivery, or by breast feeding. Improved antenatal testing, perinatal anti-retroviral therapy, planned vaginal or elective caesarean birth and safe infant formula feeding have dramatically reduced

MTCT to <1% in the UK [18]. In the UK, avoidance of all breast feeding by HIV infected women is recommended to prevent breast feeding transmission of HIV [19].

UK incidence and prevalence

National surveillance of paediatric HIV was established in 1986 and is carried out by the National Study of HIV in Pregnancy and Childhood (NSHPC) based at the Institute of Child Health, London. In total about 1750 individuals who were diagnosed with HIV under the age of 16 in the UK had been reported to the NSHPC by the end of 2005 and about 1000 children (under 16 years) were still living in the UK at that time (Pat Tookey, NSHPC, personal communication). Most children currently living with HIV in the UK are of African origin. The Collaborative HIV Paediatric Study (CHIPS) was set up in 2000 to monitor clinical, laboratory and treatment information on infected children on a regular basis [20]. CHIPS is a collaboration between the Clinical Trials Unit of the Medical Research Council, the paediatric centres looking after infected children and the NSHPC [21].

Breast feeding and HIV transmission

Breast feeding is a route of HIV transmission from mother to child and this poses a dilemma not least because of its importance in child development both biologically and emotionally. In developed societies women should follow the United Nations AIDS (UNAIDS) guidelines: when replacement feeding is acceptable, feasible, affordable, sustainable and safe, avoidance of all breast feeding by HIV infected mothers is recommended, otherwise, exclusive breast feeding is recommended [19]. In less developed societies this is problematic. In the first instance decisions about when conditions meet the above criteria can be complicated. Once the decision to breast feed has been made, however, adherence to exclusive breast feeding is recommended to help minimise the risk of transmission. There are many factors that influence the risk of transmission through breast feeding: high viral load, reduced CD4 count, breast pathology (e.g. mastitis), presence of infection and prolonged duration of breast feeding (>6 months) are all strongly related to increased transmission risk. Other related factors include non-exclusive breast feeding during the first 6 months of life, maternal vitamin deficiencies (B, C and E) and infant oral lesions [22]. Safer breast feeding can be achieved by encouraging:

- Exclusive breast feeding up to 6 months of age
- Good lactation management
- Abstaining from breast feeding during mastitis
- Prompt treatment of oral thrush in the baby
- Use of condoms

For mothers choosing to breast feed it is important that exclusivity is maintained to maximise the protective effect of breast feeding on the gut mucosa and thereby minimise the risk of viral transmission from breast milk. When new foods, including infant formula, are introduced breast feeding should cease immediately. This practice is termed 'abrupt weaning' and is aimed at reducing the risk of infection with pathogens such as rotavirus which may be transmitted from contaminated weaning foods. Gastrointestinal pathogens may compromise gut integrity and increase the likelihood of HIV transmission from breast milk.

Social problems

Many HIV infected children in the UK are born to mothers from high prevalence countries, particularly sub-Saharan Africa, and to a lesser extent intravenous drug using families. Associated poor or temporary housing facilities, isolation, physical and mental health of other family members may contribute to poor nutrition. Confidentiality and fears of disclosing the diagnosis of HIV can hinder liaison with appropriate health and social support providers. HIV is a disease with a great degree of social stigma attached and appropriate disclosure is an essential part of successful management. For many families the fear of friends and neighbours being made aware of the diagnosis can be greater than the fear of the disease itself and may lead to a loss of compliance with medication, diet and even to accessing treatment. For children this can be particularly distressing. In many cases parents are unwilling to disclose the diagnosis to the child and it is essential that the professional involved in the family's care is informed of the disclosure status within the family unit before attempting to give advice.

Diagnosis

The most available test worldwide (HIV-ELISA) detects antibodies to HIV rather than the virus itself. All babies born to infected women will have passively acquired antibodies to HIV which may persist, on average, to 10 months of age and in some cases up to 18 months. It is therefore not possible to diagnose infants reliably on the basis of antibody presence until beyond this age. In the UK a highly sensitive and specific test that can detect the presence of viral DNA, HIV DNA PCR (polymerase chain reaction) is available and can be used as a diagnostic test in infants from 4 weeks of age. Infection can be diagnosed in the majority of non-breast feeding infected infants by 1 month of age using this method. Testing should be carried out before the child is 48 hours old, repeated at 1–2 months and again at 3–6 months. Diagnoses in children over the age of 18 months can be reliably made on the presence of HIV antibody.

The Centers for Disease Control (CDC) in the USA revised the clinical classification system for HIV infection in children less than 13 years of age in 1994 [23]. A paediatric clinical and immunological staging system for HIV infection that includes age-related definitions of immune suppression was developed with the aim of guiding decisions to initiate treatment (Tables 15.3 and 15.4).

Disease progression

In children the course of disease has a more rapid progression to AIDS than in adults. Under the age of 5 years children have higher viral loads and are susceptible to more frequent recurrent bacterial infections than usual. Their immature immune system makes them more vulnerable to the opportunistic infections that are characteristic of HIV infection and these can take an aggressive course and be life threatening.

Diseases such as *Pneumocystis carinii* pneumonia (PCP) and cytomegalovirus (CMV) are common in children and PCP is the leading AIDS-defining cause of death in HIV infected babies undiagnosed at birth. Lymphocytic interstitial pneumonitis (LIP), a lung disease rarely seen in adults, occurs frequently in HIV infected children.

Paediatric HIV disease often presents as growth faltering that is diagnosed by a downward crossing of growth centiles and may be accompanied by frequent recurrent infections. In infants, neurodevelopment and motor skills such as crawling and walking may be delayed. There have been considerable advances in treatment of HIV infection in infants and children in the last 10 years following the introduction of highly active anti-retroviral therapy (HAART). Many trials have reported improvements in markers of disease progression, viral load (VL) and CD4 lymphocyte counts and infected children may remain healthy for many years. Cohort studies have reported that 40–50% of vertically infected children survive to around 10 years of age without anti-retroviral therapy [26]. Such children are referred to as long term non-progressors and do not require anti-retroviral treatment. They are also referred to as naïve, meaning that they have not yet received anti-retroviral therapy. It is important to preserve treatment options for all infected individuals and to minimise the risk of resistance. HAART is usually delayed until clinical symptoms develop or there is evidence of declining immune function. A broad spectrum antibiotic, co-trimoxazole (Septrin, GSK, Uxbridge, Middx), should be prescribed to all infected infants under the age of 1 year and to those at high risk of transmission. It is also used in HIV infected children of all ages who show signs of declining immune function. Adherence to treatment regimens is extremely important both to ensure maintenance of therapeutic levels and to prevent development of drug resistance.

A multidisciplinary approach to care planning is essential involving close liaison with doctors, nurses, dietitians, occupational therapists, physiotherapists, psychologist and social workers. Where possible, links with the community should also be made. Families with HIV need access to high quality medical care and a strategy to develop clinical networks for paediatric HIV treatment and care in London is currently under development [27]. The paediatric subgroup of the London HIV consortium aims to establish clinical networks employing lead clinicians who will develop common protocols and shared care guidelines in collaboration with the Children's HIV Association (CHIVA).

Nutritional considerations

HIV affects nutrition in many ways and a combination of increased energy expenditure, malabsorption and altered macronutrient metabolism can lead to negative energy balance and weight loss. Although studies among apparently healthy children infected with HIV show no difference in resting metabolic rate (RMR), studies among children with opportunistic infections do show they have raised energy expenditure [28]. Children infected with HIV may have increased energy requirements of around 10% and while recovering from illness this may increase by 50–100% above requirements of healthy uninfected children [29].

Table 15.3   Centers for Disease Control (CDC) classification for paediatric HIV infection.

Clinical category	Symptom severity	Type of symptoms
N	No Symptoms	Children who have no symptoms considered to be the result of HIV infection or only one of the symptoms listed in category A
A	Mildly Symptomatic: Children with 2 or more symptoms in category A, but none of the symptoms in category B/C	Lymphadenopathy; hepatomegaly; splenomegaly; dermatitis; parotitis; recurrent upper respiratory tract infection, sinusitis or otitis media
B	Moderately Symptomatic: Children have symptoms in category B	Anaemia, neutropenia or thrombocytopenia; single serious bacterial infection (e.g. pneumonia, bacteraemia); candidiasis, oropharyngeal (thrush); cardiomyopathy; cytomegalovirus infection; diarrhoea (recurrent or chronic); hepatitis; herpes stomatitis, recurrent; lymphoid interstitial pneumonia (LIP); nephropathy; persistent fever >1 month; varicella zoster (persistent or complicated primary chickenpox or shingles)
C	Severely Symptomatic: Examples of conditions in clinical category C include those listed, together with any condition listed in the 1987 surveillance case definition for AIDS, with the exception of LIP [6]. See link below for more details	1) Serious bacterial infections, multiple or recurrent 2) Opportunistic infections: Candidiasis (oesophageal, pulmonary); cytomegalovirus disease with onset of symptoms at age >1 month; cryptosporidiosis with diarrhoea persisting 1 month; *Mycobacterium* tuberculosis, disseminated or extrapulmonary; *Mycobacterium* avium complex or *M. kansasii*, disseminated; *Pneumocystis carinii* pneumonia (PCP); progressive multifocal leukoencephalopathy; toxoplasmosis of the brain with onset at age >1 month 3) Severe failure to thrive/wasting syndrome Crossing at least two percentile lines on the growth chart (e.g. 90th to 50th, or 50th to 10th) or less than the 3rd percentile and continuing to deviate downwards from it over a 3-month period, or more than 10% loss of body weight in older child *plus* a) chronic diarrhoea >30 days OR b) documented intermittent or constant fever >30 days 4) HIV encephalopathy At least one of the following progressive findings for at least 2 months in the absence of a concurrent illness other than HIV infection that could explain the findings: a) Failure to attain or loss of developmental milestones or loss of intellectual ability, verified by standard developmental scale or neuropsychological tests b) Impaired brain growth or acquired microcephaly demonstrated by head circumference measurements or by brain atrophy demonstrated by computerised tomography or magnetic resonance imaging (serial imaging for children <2 years of age) c) Acquired symmetric motor deficit manifested by two or more of the following: paresis, pathologic reflexes, ataxia or gait disturbance 5) Malignancy

Source: Adapted from MMWR, 1994 [24].
www.cdc.gov/mmwr/PDF/rr/rr4312.pdf

Table 15.4   1994 Revised human immunodeficiency virus paediatric classification system: immune categories based on age-specific CD4$^+$ T-cell count and percentage.

Immune category	<12 months		1–5 year		6–12 year	
	No/mm^3	(%)	No/mm^3	(%)	No/mm^3	(%)
Category 1: No suppression	≥1500	(≥25%)	≥1000	(≥25%)	≥500	(≥25%)
Category 2: Moderate suppression	750–1499	(15–24%)	500–999	(15–24%)	200–499	(15–24%)
Category 3: Severe suppression	<750	(<15%)	<500	(<15%)	<200	(<15%)

Source: After BHIVA guidelines, 2004 [25].

Providing optimal nutrition to children with HIV is critical for two reasons: it provides the greatest opportunity for normal growth and development and supports the optimal functioning of the immune system [30].

When planning nutritional advice for HIV infected children, several related aspects also need to be considered such as disease state, growth and development and social factors. Side effects of treatment regimens and their interactions with foods should be taken into consideration (Table 15.5).

Nutritional requirements

Increased RMR is an important contributor to energy imbalance in HIV infected patients [32]. Energy requirements of children with HIV are best estimated to meet 100% of the estimated average requirement (EAR) for age, with adjustments made for mobility, infection, weight loss and malabsorption. When assessing requirements these should be based on the child's actual size rather than expected weight/length for age, i.e. the child's height age (see p. 4). This provides a better estimate for achievable food intake.

HIV infection is associated with a loss of lean body mass and it is well established that this depletion has adverse effects on morbidity and mortality [33]. Loss of body protein is the result of decreased dietary intake, malabsorption and metabolic change. During energy restriction fat stores are depleted first, but in HIV infection several studies have shown that there is a preferential loss of body protein [34]. Evidence suggests that the metabolic mechanisms underlying changes in body composition that occur during HIV infection differ from those present during chronic food restriction and other diseases associated with rapid weight loss. Protein requirements for HIV infected children are not yet established and although these have been estimated to be 150–200% of the recommended daily allowance [35], there is insufficient evidence at present to suggest that additional protein can prevent loss of stores during the acute phase of infection. Moreover, clinical status may deteriorate if overfeeding occurs during sepsis [36]. Overall, existing evidence suggests that protein intake should be increased by about 10% to maintain body stores during the chronic asymptomatic phase of infection. During opportunistic infections, requirements for both energy and protein are likely to increase to about 30–50% above usual requirements, but it is unlikely that an unwell child will be capable of achieving increased intake above an additional 10%. Once the acute infection is resolved, further increases can be encouraged to help achieve nutritional recovery.

Vitamin and mineral requirements of HIV infected children are not known for certain. To date, with the exception of vitamin A supplementation in developing countries, no randomised controlled trials have investigated the effects of micronutrient supplementation in children and these should therefore be given with caution [37]. Evidence from randomised controlled trials suggest that regular megadose vitamin A supplementation may reduce diarrhoeal disease and mortality and all-cause morbidity and mortality in children under 5 years [38]. Supplements for individual nutrients are not prescribed unless there are

Table 15.5 Highly active anti-retroviral therapy (HAART): food restrictions, drug interactions and side effects.

Drug	Food interactions	More common side effects	Drug interactions	More severe/rare side effects
Nucleoside reverse transcriptase inhibitors (NRTIs)				
Lamivudine (3TC, Epivir) liquid and tablets	May be taken with or without food	Nausea or vomiting, abdominal pain, diarrhoea or constipation, headache, fatigue	None known	Pancreatitis MT
Zidovudine (ZDV, AZT, Retrovir) liquid and capsules	May be taken with or without food, pre-dose meal may reduce nausea	Nausea, vomiting, headache, muscular pain, sleep disturbance	Not to be prescribed with stavudine	MT Liver toxicity Myopathy Myositis
Stavudine (D4T, Zerit) liquid and capsules	None – pre-dose meal may reduce nausea	Peripheral neuropathy, headache, nausea or vomiting, diarrhoea or constipation	Not to be prescribed with AZT	LDS MT Raised liver enzymes
Abacavir (ABC, Ziagen) liquid or tablets	May be taken with or without food			Hypersensitvity (fever, fatigue, nausea, vomiting diarrhoea and abdominal pain or respiratory symptoms) Raised LFTs Raised CPK Lymphopenia MT
Didanosine (ddI, Videx) liquid and capsules	Essential that it is taken on an empty stomach, i.e. at least 1 hour before or 2 hours after food	Diarrhoea, nausea, stomach cramps, vomiting, rash	All foods – must be taken on an empty stomach H_2 antagonists	Peripheral neuropathy Electrolyte disturbances Retinal depigmentation Hyperuricaemia Raised liver enzymes
Non-nucleoside reverse transcriptase inhibitors (NNRTIs)				
Efavirenz (Sustiva) liquid, capsules, tablets	May be taken with or without foods. Taking with food may increase drug levels in some people. High fat meals may improve absorption and increase risk of side effects. Take with food with caution when initiating treatment	Skin rash. CNS disturbance (insomnia, nightmares, agitation)		Continuing CNS disturbance Liver toxicity
Nevirapine (Viramune) liquid and tablets	May be taken with or without food	Associated with skin rash, possibly life threatening (fever, nausea, headache)		Hepatitis, possibly life threatening (liver damage/failure)
Emtricitabine (Emtriva) liquid, capsules	May be taken with or without food	Headache, nausea, raised creatine kinase	Not known	Not known
Tenofovir (Viread) tablets	Preferably taken with food. High fat foods may increase absorption	GI disturbance Renal disturbance (hypophosphataemia, increased serum creatinine, glyosuria, proteinuria, calciuria, phosphaturia)	Lactic acidosis, hepatomegaly and steatosis seen with use of nucleoside analogues	Based on animal studies, at high doses there is a risk of osteomalacia (none reported in children)

continued on p. 288

Table 15.5 *(Cont'd)*

Drug	Food interactions	More common side effects	Drug interactions	More severe/rare side effects
Protease inhibitors (PIs)				
Amprenavir (APV, Agenerase) liquid and capsules	May be taken with or without food. Avoid taking with vitamin E supplements	Diarrhoea, vomiting, rash, perioral paresthesia (unusual feelings around the mouth)	None known	LDS DM Rash (possible sign of life threatening syndrome, Stevens–Johnson) Haemolytic anaemia
Nelfinavir (NFV, Viracept) tablets and powder	With or after food (helps absorption and reduces nausea)	Diarrhoea (can be controlled with loperamide), nausea	In adults – not to be recommended in conjunction with rifampicin	Persistent diarrhoea Abdominal pain LDS Hyperglycaemia, ketoacidosis and DM
Ritonavir (RTV, Norvir) liquid and capsules	Best with food (reduces GI side effects and increases absorption) Bitter tasting – can be disguised with strong tasting foods or fluids, e.g. blackcurrant cordial, peanut butter	Headache, nausea or vomiting, diarrhoea, tingling/numbness in mouth, tiredness	Ritonavir and ddI should be taken 2 hours apart from each other	LDS Renal disturbance DM Dyslipidaemia
Atazanavir (Reyataz) capsules	Take with food This is recommended as food increases drug concentrations	Raised unconjugated bilirubin. Headaches, fever, dizziness, nausea, vomiting, diarrhoea Sleep disturbances	Take at least 1 hour before or after antacid or ddI	LDS Hyperglycaemia DM Pancreatitis Ketoacidosis Hepatitis
Indinavir (IDV, Crixivan) Capsules	1 hour pre- or 2 hours post-food except when taken with RTV when a light low fat snack can help improve palatability. If given with ddI take 1 hour apart and on an empty stomach. Avoid grapefruit juice at the time of taking and increase fluid intake	Nausea, GI pain, headache, taste changes, dizziness Hyperbilirubinemia	NVP or EFV often decrease IDV levels	LDS Hyperglycaemia Ketoacidosis DM
Lopinavir+ Ritonavir (LPV/r, Kaletra) capsules + liquid	Take with food to maximise absorption Bitter tasting liquid – can be disguised with strong tasting foods or fluids, e.g. blackcurrant cordial, peanut butter	Mild to moderate diarrhoea, nausea, vomiting, GI disturbance	ddI 1 hour before or 2 hours after Increase dose if given with NNRTIs or previous PI exposure	Dyslipidaemia LDS Pancreatitis Hyperglycaemia Ketoacidosis DM Hepatitis
Saquinavir (SQV, Invirase, Fortovase) capsules	Take within 2 hours after a substantial meal	Diarrhoea, nausea, rash, fatigue, headache, peripheral neuropathy, numbness, dizziness		LDS Photosensitivity (use UV protection) Hyperglycaemia Ketoacidosis DM
Fusion inhibitors (FIs)				
Enfuvirtide (T20, Fuzeon) powder	Administered by injection	Not known	Not known	Not known

Source: Adapted from PENTA guidelines, 2004 [31]. CNS, central nervous system; CPK, creatine phosphokinase; DM, diabetes mellitus; GI, gastrointestinal; LDS, lipodystrophy syndrome; LFTs, liver function tests; MT, mitochondrial toxicity; UV, ultraviolet.

concerns that the reference nutrient intake (RNI) is not being met. Following a dietary assessment, if requirements cannot be met by dietary intake alone, multivitamin/mineral supplementation in order to reach 100% RNI may be advisable.

Complications associated with HIV infection

Frequent bacterial infections can lead to complications such as fever, more severe secondary infections and protracted diarrhoea with dehydration which may result in nutritional problems and hospital admissions. HIV infected children often suffer from candidiasis, a yeast infection that can cause severe nappy rash in infants and infections in the mouth and throat in children of all ages, making eating difficult. HIV related enteropathies are common, leading to food intolerance and malabsorption. Any one of these complications may reduce appetite and dietary intake, thereby compromising growth and development in childhood.

Growth faltering

Maintaining adequate growth of HIV infected children should be a priority for clinicians working in this area. Growth is an important predictor of morbidity and mortality and impairment is associated with increased gastrointestinal and respiratory infections [39,40]. Energy intake is the main determinant of energy balance [41] and in HIV infected children reduced intake leads to growth failure [28].

Periods of decreased dietary intake associated with frequent episodes of infections are commonly reported by parents of children who lose weight between clinic visits. Where HAART is available and access to food is not compromised chronic growth failure is not common. However, when growth faltering is diagnosed the contributory factors are often complex and interventions difficult to manage. Children who display suboptimal growth may not meet diagnostic criteria for initiation of HAART, which can reverse growth failure. In the absence of treatment the onus is on the dietitian to maintain growth, development and nutritional status through appropriate nutritional intervention.

Growth assessment

Growth assessment is essential for the effective management of HIV infected children. In the absence of population specific reference data, it should be recognised that the cut-offs for under- and overweight based on the UK growth charts [42] may not be appropriate for children from certain ethnic groups. When assessing growth it is important to consider the child's genetic and environmental history. For example, a child who presents with low height and/or weight for age may be genetically predetermined to be small and assessment of mid-parental height and weight can help to clarify this. Using the UK growth charts it is possible to calculate the mid-parental centile (MPC) and identify a growth centile range that reflects normal growth for a child based on their genetic potential (see p. 4). In many cases an HIV infected child may not reach their genetic potential because of early growth faltering as a result of disease, malnutrition or a combination of the two. In all cases a realistic growth target should be set with the aim of maintaining growth along the centiles that have been accepted as appropriate for the individual child. Downward centile crossing of two major centiles is indicative of growth faltering. In general, height and weight should not differ by more than two major centiles. However, low height for weight is commonly reported and increased linear growth is not usually achievable beyond the age of 2 years when the growth trajectory has been established. Upward centile crossing of weight should be closely monitored as this may indicate obesity onset. Measurements of body composition allow monitoring of adiposity and should be taken if possible.

Gastrointestinal complications

Food intolerance, malabsorption, constipation and diarrhoea are all features of HIV infection and HAART. These are often transitory, resulting from HIV related enteropathies in undiagnosed children or side effects of treatment. Protein hydrolysate and/or amino acid based feeds may be required in the short term while the infection is stabilised and the treatment regimen is adjusted (see Tables 7.7, 7.9 and 7.12). Lactose intolerance is particularly prevalent in this group who are largely of sub-Saharan African origin (a region where this condition is more common). Carbohydrate malabsorption occurs often in HIV infected children, even in those who are free from gastrointestinal infections and can be especially severe among immunocompromised children [43]. Specific advice for food intolerance should be provided for these children who will need supporting guidance and information regarding how to obtain and prepare appropriate foods. Where nutritional needs cannot be met orally, supplementary tube feeding may be used as an adjunct to the normal diet, and where long term nutritional support is predicted, gastrostomy feeding may be considered. These steps are rare in the UK environment where food is plentiful and affordable and where nutritional supplements are available free on prescription.

Dyslipidaemia and the lipodystrophy syndrome

The HIV associated lipodystrophy sydrome (HIV-LDS) combines redistribution of fat mass with features of the metabolic syndrome such as insulin resistance, impaired glucose tolerance and dyslipidaemia. This syndrome is characterised by a redistribution of adipose tissue which can manifest as a marked loss of subcutaneous fat in the periphery (lipoatrophy) and/or increases in intra-abdominal fat (lipohypertrophy). Many children experience dyslipidaemia which usually presents as raised total plasma cholesterol and triglyceride levels and in some cases increased low density lipoprotein cholesterol (LDL-C) and/or reduced high density lipoprotein cholesterol (HDL-C). These derangements of the lipid profile are associated with increased risk of cardiovascular disease (CVD) and appropriate diagnosis and management of HIV associated dyslipidaemia should be an included in treatment protocols for HIV infected children. Dietary management of dyslipidaemias is given in Chapter 20. Diagnosis of HIV-LDS is difficult in the absence of widely accepted objective diagnostic criteria but it is nevertheless an important consideration in the treatment of these children who have been found to be at increased risk of CVD [44].

Rare complications

Mitochondrial toxicity (MT) may result from therapy with certain classes of anti-retroviral drugs (Table 15.5) and is implicated in a wide range of toxicities including neurological disease in infants, peripheral neuropathy and hepatic stenosis. Lactic acidosis is a rare but serious side effect of MT and is potentially fatal. However, this has rarely been reported in children. There have been increasing reports of osteonecrosis and abnormalities of bone mineral metabolism in patients receiving HAART [31].

Nutritional assessment

At baseline all children should receive a nutritional assessment including:

- Weight
- Length/height
- Head circumference (infants and children under 2 years)
- Waist, hip and mid-upper arm circumferences. Longitudinal measurements (6 monthly) will allow monitoring of changes in body composition
- Detailed diet history, with special attention to: food intolerance, feeding difficulties, use of supplements
- Medication history, with special attention to: drug interactions (Table 15.5), vitamin and mineral supplements, alternative therapies
- Biochemical assessment, with special attention: to cholesterol/triglycerides (non-fasting) and glucose/insulin

This assessment should be repeated annually (apart from circumferences) and to monitor effects of HAART regimens some measurements should be carried out more frequently. For example, blood lipid levels should be checked about 3 months after a change to therapy has been made. Biochemical monitoring is a routine aspect of HIV care and where possible dietetic surveillance should be used to help identify children at risk of metabolic abnormalities. A fasting lipid measurement should be obtained at each annual assessment and requested for children with raised non-fasting total cholesterol or triglycerides (>95th percentile) on more than two occasions.

Height and weight should be measured at each clinic visit (ideally 3 monthly) and plotted on UK growth charts [42]. Downward crossing of centiles indicates the need for nutritional assessment and possible dietetic intervention.

Dietary treatment for children

Based on disease severity children fall into two broad categories: asymptomatic and symptomatic. However, children will cross categories throughout the course of treatment; for example, a child once referred for growth faltering may present at a later stage in treatment with overweight/obesity and/or lipid abnormalities. There is a wide range of symptoms and disease severity within the symptomatic children and careful assessment is needed for accurate dietetic diagnosis. The aims of advice and treatment are to:

- Provide optimal nutrition
- Support regeneration of the immune system
- Maintain growth, development and activity
- Help adherence to medication
- Preserve lean body mass
- Prevent overweight and obesity
- Encourage cardioprotective diet
- Encourage healthy eating
- Provide advice on food safety and hygiene

In symptomatic children additional advice may be needed to alleviate symptoms and meet increased requirements of disease.

A full diet history should be taken, with particular attention being paid to traditional diet and cooking methods, and will give the best estimate of the quality of the diet and its nutritional adequacy. This method poses the least burden to families who are often having difficulties managing the disease and their lives.

Many families will be refugees or immigrants and may be living in temporary accommodation with limited cooking facilities. Furthermore, knowledge of foods available in the UK may be poor and the skills of the dietitian will be called upon to glean information relating to eating practices in the country of origin. Careful advice will be needed to enable families to make food choices that will result in a balanced diet that is affordable, culturally acceptable and palatable. Demonstrating knowledge and understanding of traditional foods and eating practices is central to the successful transmission of dietary advice for a specific population. Careful questioning should be aimed at collecting the following information:

- In infants and young children, intake of milk and solids
- Weaning practices, including timing and usual foods
- Quantity and variety of sources of protein, carbohydrate, fat, vitamins and minerals
- Textures managed (e.g. puréed, soft, hard foods)
- Meal pattern and time taken to eat main meals
- Type and timing of snacks and drinks
- Amount of food eaten outside the home (e.g. at nursery or school)
- Feeding problems
- Cooking facilities and equipment
- Financial status

Some children present with feeding problems that may affect their nutritional intake. Many of these require referral to, and discussion with, other members of the multidisciplinary team (speech and language therapist, psychologist, social workers who are invaluable in assessing the need for and accessing financial and practical aid) after which appropriate dietetic interventions can be implemented. Some common problems and suggested dietary interventions are given in Table 15.6. Delays in growth and development may occur and the infant/child's developmental age rather than the actual age should be used to assess the most appropriate textures, feeding position and utensils.

Advice should be food based wherever possible and where it is necessary to increase energy and nutrient intake, this should initially be aimed at using foods in the usual diet.

Convenient high energy snacks can be recommended in the short term, but it should be stressed that this diet is only for the duration of an acute infection or period of growth failure, and that healthy eating should be encouraged in the long term. For children with dyslipidaemia, advice should be tailored towards a cardioprotective diet

Table 15.6 Dietary interventions in paediatric HIV.

Problem	Assessment	Referral/discussion	Intervention
Delayed weaning	Diet history Milk and solids intake Meal pattern Sleep and activity pattern		Assess and advise on appropriate milk intake for age, e.g. excessive milk intake and timing of feeds may reduce appetite for other foods
	Medical history Oral health Gastrointestinal problems	Refer to medical team if problems are reported, e.g. sore mouth, reflux, diarrhoea, constipation	Consider medical conditions and advise appropriately Food intolerance – may need hydrolysed protein/amino acid based feed Diarrhoea – avoid spicy and fried foods; fibrous foods, e.g. wholegrain cereals and salad vegetables; caffeinated drinks, e.g. tea, coffee and cola. Foods high in lactose may also affect some people, i.e. foods containing milk. Bland foods, e.g. potatoes, white plain boiled rice, bread and pasta should be advised Assess fluid loss and intake Constipation – increase fibre and fluid if appropriate
	Social history Financial status Cultural beliefs Isolation	Refer to social work team if financial or social barriers to weaning	Provide weaning advice adapted to cultural needs Direct to support groups and aid sources, e.g. Food Chain
Neuro-developmental delay	Diet history Feeding techniques Meal pattern Behaviour	Refer to speech and language therapy	Modify food consistency Encourage finger foods Encourage daily routine Consider supplementary tube feeding/gastrostomy
Eating difficulties: swallowing and/or chewing; inflamed/sore mouth	Diet history Meal pattern Feeding techniques Medical history Oral health	Refer to speech and language therapy Dental problems Side effects of medicines	Modify food consistency Advise on meal pattern Soft, non-acidic foods Avoid spicy food and drink Use straw to bypass lesions Suck ice lollies
Growth faltering	Diet history Appetite changes Meal pattern Timing of snacks and drinks Fluid intake Eating away from the home Disease progression Effects of medicines Social/cultural influences Behavioural problems	Refer to medical team to identify/eliminate organic cause Refer to psychosocial team	Encourage energy and nutrient dense meals with small nutrient dense snacks in between: full cream milk, cheese, fats (include PUFA and MUFA and moderate SFA, use of omega 3), sauces, sugar, honey, jam Space drinks and snacks away from meals Discourage excessive fluid intake Use age-appropriate supplements if unable to meet requirements through usual diet and where child is severely immunodeficient and/or symptomatic and losing weight

MUFA, monounsaturated acids; PUFA, polyunsaturated fatty acids; SFA, saturated fatty acids.

and total fat consumption should be in line with current dietary recommendations. Inclusion of omega-3 fatty acids, found in oily fish, nuts, seeds and their oils, should be encouraged for their known beneficial properties in reducing plasma triglycerides. Intake of non-milk extrinsic sugars should also be kept within recommendations and fruit and vegetable intake encouraged. An unrefined diet is particularly important for these children because this helps to reduce intake of trans fatty acids (which are strongly associated with CVD) and provides soluble fibre (which may help to reduce plasma cholesterol) and antioxidants (which may protect vascular integrity). If short term nutritional support is required, age-appropriate sip feed supplements may be considered. Examples of fortified milk shakes are given in Table 11.3.

References

1 Fischer A Primary immunodeficiency diseases: an experimental model for molecular medicine. *Lancet*, 2001, **357** 1863–9.

2 Walker-Smith JA, Murch SH The immune system of the small intestine. In: *Diseases of the Small Intestine in Childhood*, 4th edn. Oxford: Isis Medical Media Ltd, 1999, pp. 45–61.

3 Klein N, Jack D Immunodeficiency and the gut: clues to the role of the immune system in gastrointestinal disease. *Ital J Gastroenterol Hepatol*, 1999, **31** 802–6.

4 Cataldo F, Marino V, Ventura A *et al.* Prevalence and clinical features of selective immunoglobulin A deficiency in coeliac disease: an Italian multicentre study. *Gut*, 1998, **42** 362–5.

5 Klemola T, Savilahti E, Arato A *et al.* Immunohistochemical findings in jejunal specimens from patients with IgA deficiency. *Gut*, 1995, **37** 519–23.

6 Kaufman HS, Hobbs JR Immunoglobulin deficiencies in an atopic population. *Lancet*, 1970, **2** 1061–3.

7 Goldblatt D, Morgan G, Seymour ND *et al.* The clinical manifestations of IgG subclass deficiency. In: Levinsky RJ (ed) *IgG Subclass Deficiencies*. London: Royal Society of Medicine Services, 1989.

8 Murch SH, Fertleman CR, Rodrigues C *et al.* Autoimmune enteropathy with distinct mucosal features in T-cell activation deficiency: the contribution of T cells to the mucosal lesion. *J Pediatr Gastroenterol Nutr*, 1999, **28** 393–9.

9 Unsworth DJ, Walker-Smith JA Autoimmunity in diarrhoeal disease. *J Pediatr Gastroenterol Nutr*, 1985, **4** 375–80.

10 Schappi MG, Klein NJ, Lindley KJ *et al.* The nature of colitis in chronic granulomatous disease. *J Pediatr Gastroenterol Nutr*, 2003, **36** 623–31.

11 Boeck A, Buckley RH, Schiff RI Gastroesophageal reflux and severe combined immunodeficiency. *J Allergy Clin Immunol*, 1997, **99** 420–3.

12 Gasper RH, Parsley K, Howe S *et al.* Gene therapy of X-linked severe combined immunodeficiency by use of a pseudotyped gamma retroviral vector. *Lancet*, 2004, **364** 2181.

13 Fischer A, Landais P, Friedrich W *et al.* European experience of bone marrow transplantation for severe combined immunodeficiency. *Lancet*, 1990, **336** 850–4.

14 Papadopoulou A Nutritional considerations in children undergoing bone marrow transplantation. *Europ J Clin Nutr*, 1998, **52** 863–71.

15 Rao K, Amrolia PJ, Jones A *et al.* Improved survival after unrelated donor bone marrow transplantation in children with primary immunodeficiency using a reduced-intensity conditioning regimen. *Blood*, 2005, **105** 879–85.

16 Langdana A, Tully N, Molloy E *et al.* Intensive enteral nutrition support in paediatric bone marrow transplantation. *Bone Marrow Transplant*, 2001, **27** 741–6.

17 Papadopoulou A, Lloyd DR, Williams MD *et al.* Gastrointestinal and nutritional sequelae of bone marrow transplantation. *Arch Dis Child*, 1996, **76** 208–13.

18 Foster C, Lyall H Current Guidelines for the management of UK Infants born to HIV-1 infected mothers. *Early Hum Dev* 2005, **81** 103–10.

19 Department of Health HIV and Infant Feeding. Guidance for the UK Chief Medical Officer's Expert Advisory Group on AIDS, 2004. www.advisorybodies.doh.gov.uk/eaga/pdfs/hivinfantSep04.pdf

20 Gibb DM, Duong T, Tookey PA *et al.* Decline in mortality, AIDS, and hospital admissions in perinatally HIV-1 infected children in the United Kingdom and Ireland. *Br Med J*, 2003, **327** 1019.

21 http://www.bhiva.org/chiva/

22 Coutsoudis A Infant feeding dilemmas created by HIV: South African experiences. *J Nutr*, 2005, **1315** 956–9.

23 CDC. Revision of the CDC surveillance case definition for acquired immunodeficiency syndrome. *MMWR Morb Mortal Wkly Rep*, 1987, **36** (Suppl) 1–15.

24 Morbidity and Mortality Weekly (MMWR) Revised classification system for human immunodeficiency virus infection codes and official guidelines for reporting ICD-9-CM. *MMWR Morb Mortal Wkly Rep*, 1994, **43** 1–12.

25 BHIVA Writing Committee on behalf of the BHIVA Executive Committee, British HIV Association (BHIVA) guidelines for the treatment of HIV-infected adults with antiretroviral therapy: An Update, April 2005.

26 European Collaborative Study Natural history of vertically acquired human immunodeficiency virus 1 infection. *Pediatrics*, 1994, **94** 815–19.

27 London HIV Consortium, Paediatric Sub-Group Developing clinical paediatric HIV treatment and care in London. http://www.bhiva.org/chiva/.

28 Arpadi SM, Cuff PA, Kotler DP *et al.* Growth velocity, fat-free mass and energy intake are inversely

related to viral load in HIV-infected children. *J Nutr*, 2000, **130** 2498–502.

29 *Nutrient requirements for people living with HIV/AIDS: Report of a technical consultation* World Health Organization, Geneva, 13–15 May 2003. Geneva, World Health Organization, 2003.

30 Tomkins A Malnutrition, morbidity and mortality in children and their mothers. *Proc Nutr Soc*, 2000, **59** 135–46.

31 Sharland M, Blanche S, Castelli, G *et al*. PENTA guidelines for the use of antiretroviral therapy. *HIV Med*, 2004, **5** (Suppl 2) 61–6.

32 Hommes M, Romijn J, Godfried M *et al*. Increased resting energy expenditure in human immunodeficiency infected men. *Metabolism*, 1990, **39** 1186–90.

33 Macallan DC, Noble C, Baldwin C *et al*. Energy expenditure and wasting in human immunodeficiency virus infection. *N Engl J Med*, 1995, **333** 83–8.

34 Polsky B, Kotler D, Steinheart C HIV-associated wasting in the HAART era: guidelines for assessment, diagnosis, and treatment. *AIDS Patient Care STDS*, 2001, **Aug 15** 411–23.

35 Heller LS Nutrition support for children with HIV/AIDS. *J Am Diet Assoc*, 1997, **97** 473–5.

36 Poindexter BB, Ehrenkranz RA, Stoll BJ *et al*. Parenteral glutamine supplementation does not reduce the risk of mortality or late-onset sepsis in extremely low birthweight infants. *Pediatrics*, 2004, **113** 1209–15.

37 Fawzi W Micronutrients and human immunodeficiency virus type 1 disease progression among adults and children. *Clin Infect Dis*, 2003, **37** (Suppl 2) S112–16.

38 Friis H Micronutrients and HIV/AIDS: a review of current evidence 2005. http://www.who.int/nutrition/topics/consultation_nutrition_and_hivaids/en/index.html

39 Thea DM, St Louis ME, Atido U *et al*. A prospective study of diarrhoea and HIV-1 infection among 429 Zairian infants. *N Engl J Med*, 1993, **329** 1696–702.

40 Ikeogu MO, Wolf B, Mathe S Pulmonary manifestations in HIV seropositivity and malnutrition in Zimbabwe. *Arch Dis Child*, 1997, **76** 124–8.

41 Macallan DC, Noble C, Baldwin C *et al*. Energy expenditure and wasting in human immunodeficiency virus infection. *N Engl J Med*, 1995, **333** 83–8.

42 Freeman JV, Cole TJ, Chinn S *et al*. Cross-sectional stature and weight reference curves for the UK, 1990. *Arch Dis Child*, 1995, **73** 17–24.

43 Hsu JWC, Pencharz PB, Macallan D *et al*. Macronutrients and HIV/AIDS: a review of current evidence. Consultation on Nutrition and HIV/AIDS in Africa: Evidence, lessons and recommendations for action. Durban, South Africa, 10–13 April 2005. http://www.who.int/nutrition/topics/consultation_nutrition_and_hivaids/en/index.html

44 Charakida M, Donald AE, Green H *et al*. Early structural and functional changes of the vasculature in HIV-infected children: impact of disease and antiretroviral therapy. *Circulation*, 2005, **112** 103–9.

Useful addresses

Immune Deficiency Foundation
email: idf@primaryimmune.org

Children's HIV Association (CHIVA)
www.bhiva.org/chiva/index.html

Avert
www.avert.org/

Nam
www.aidsmap.com/

Children with AIDS Charity (CWAC)
www.cwac.org/

The Food Chain
www.foodchain.org.uk/

16 Ketogenic Diets

Liz Neal & Gwynneth McGrath

Introduction

Epilepsy is the most prevalent of the serious neurological disorders, the highest incidence occurring in early childhood and old age. Seizure activity is caused by abnormal and excessive discharge from the neurons in the brain, which can present in a range of different seizure types. The International League Against Epilepsy provides detailed information on classification of seizures and syndromes [1].

Although anti-epileptic medication can be used to control seizures in most cases, a minority do not respond to drug therapy. The ketogenic diet is a high fat, restricted carbohydrate regimen that was first used to treat epilepsy in the 1920s [2]. Following observations that fasting decreased seizure frequency, the diet was designed to induce a similar metabolic response, with the ketone bodies acetoacetate and β-hydroxybutyrate becoming the primary energy source for the brain in the absence of adequate glucose supply. Use of the diet decreased when new anti-epileptic drugs were introduced in the 1950s; it has regained recent popularity with concerns about side effects of medications.

There are two main types of ketogenic diet. The classical diet is based on a ratio of fat to carbohydrate and protein. The fat component is long chain triglycerides (LCT), mainly provided from foods.

Protein is based on minimum requirements for growth, and carbohydrate is very restricted. A modification of this diet was introduced in the 1970s using medium chain triglycerides (MCT) as an alternative fat source [3]. MCT yield more ketones per kilocalorie of energy provided than their long chain counterparts; they are absorbed more efficiently and carried directly to the liver in the portal blood. This increased ketogenic potential means less total fat is needed in the MCT diet, thus allowing inclusion of more carbohydrate and protein.

Efficacy

Many studies have reported efficacy of the ketogenic diet. Freeman *et al.* [4] found approximately 30% of 150 children achieved >90% seizure reduction and 50% achieved >50% reduction. In a systematic review of 11 studies in 2000, Lefevre and Aronson [5] concluded there was sufficient evidence to determine that the diet is efficacious in children with refractory epilepsy, although they were concerned about the lack of randomised controlled studies. This problem is also noted in the Cochrane review on the diet [6]. One such trial is currently being undertaken [7].

The diet has traditionally been reported to be most successful in treating patients with myoclonic or atonic seizures, or the mixed seizures seen in Lennox–Gastaut syndrome, although Freeman *et al.* [4] found no significant difference in seizure control between different types of seizure or epilepsy syndrome.

Many children also show improvements in development and behaviour. Few studies have systematically reviewed these benefits, although one study reported significant improvements in development quotient, attention and social functioning while on the diet [8].

Anti-epileptic medication dosage is frequently reduced in children on the diet, many becoming drug free, with significant cost reduction [9]. The effects of the diet can be long-lasting and some children who have seen benefit can return to a normal diet after about 2 years without resumption of seizure activity.

Mode of action

The exact mechanism of action of the ketogenic diet has not been fully elucidated. A number of hypotheses have emerged:

1 *Effects on cerebral energy metabolism* Failure to meet brain energy needs may contribute to initiation and spread of epileptic activity [10]; the ketogenic diet increases brain energy reserves by bypassing less efficient glycolysis pathways and maximising tricarboxylic acid cycle function. This may influence seizure activity by increased production of inhibitory neurotransmitters, improved ability to buffer the extracellular milieu, or alteration of resting membrane potential [10].
2 *Alteration of brain amino acid handling* Utilisation of ketone bodies as a brain substrate will alter metabolism of glutamate, an important excitatory neurotransmitter. Reduced transamination of glutamate to aspartate increases glutamate availability for synthesis of the main inhibitory brain neurotransmitter, gamma amino butyric acid (GABA), both directly, and via glutamine production [11].
3 *Molecular regulation* Metabolic adaptations to the ketogenic diet will be mediated at the molecular level by sensor mechanisms. The fatty acid activated transcription factor, peroxisome proliferator-activated receptor a (PPARa), is activated by ketogenesis and may be important in the anti-epileptic effects of the diet by influencing neurotransmitter metabolism [12].
4 *Direct effect of ketone bodies* Animal models suggest that ketone bodies may exert direct anticonvulsant action with acetoacetate, and particularly acetone, having stronger effects than β-hydroxybutyrate [13].
5 *Role of neuropeptides and norepinephrine* Anticonvulsant neuropeptides, galanin and neuropeptide Y are regulated by energy states, and may mediate action of the ketognic diet [14], with increased levels being released in the brain [15]. Norepinephrine, an inhibitory neurotransmitter, may also contribute to the anticonvulsant mechanism of the diet [16].
6 *Calorie restriction* Calorie restriction may underlie the anticonvulsant mechanism of the diet; this alone has been shown to reduce seizure susceptibility in mice [17].

Indications and contraindications

The ketogenic diet is generally used to treat intractable epilepsy when at least two anti-epileptic medications have failed or produced unacceptable side effects. Although there are a few reports of successful use in adults [18], it is primarily used in childhood epilepsy.

The diet should not be considered as a treatment for children who have inborn errors of metabolism that require high dietary fat as part of their treatment, or who have a history of renal stones or hyperlipidaemia. It should be used with caution if a child is taking diuretics or medications that increase risk of acidosis. Concomitant steroid use will limit ketosis.

The diet has limited success in children with behavioural problems such as food refusal. Dietary restrictions and food allergy are not necessarily a reason to withhold it, although the restrictions of multiple food allergies may make it inadvisable in this group.

Implementation

Implementation of the ketogenic diet is difficult and success depends on a number of core staff with a multidisciplinary approach to the care of the child: a skilled paediatric dietitian; a paediatrician with experience of the diet, who is preferably also a neurologist; and a specialist nurse. This team must be able to advise and assist patients when they run into problems that are either caused or exacerbated by being on the diet. Community support and easy hospital access must be available at all times.

If the diet is initiated in hospital, the family will be taught how to provide and monitor it during the admission. It has been estimated that such an episode could take about 20 hours of dietetic time, including the pre-admission work-up.

If the diet is started at home, the family will need to have thorough teaching on its use prior to commencement; this should include the management of possible early side effects such as excess ketosis and hypoglycaemia. A ketogenic diet should only be started in the outpatient setting if there is good community support from the dietetic team; this should include daily telephone contact for at least the first week or two.

The dietitian will prepare the dietary prescription, and once the diet has been established, further dietetic time is required to support the family and adjust the diet. The success of the diet requires a high level of commitment and willingness to comply with the regimen and all that it entails on the part of the family and carers. They need to be aware of the extent of the restrictions and the need to weigh and measure all the food. A reasonable level of literacy is needed to understand and implement the menus. They will need to be capable of monitoring and recording urinary ketones, and possibly blood glucose and ketone levels. They need to keep a seizure diary and to understand how to detect and treat both hypoglycaemia and hyperketosis in their child. Families who wish to be more involved with planning meals, or who are using an exchange system, will need to be confident with simple mathematical calculations.

Calculating the diet

Energy prescription

Energy intake is carefully controlled on the ketogenic diet as excess may compromise ketosis and seizure control.

The energy prescription for a child on the ketogenic diet should always be individually calculated, taking into account current dietary intake (a 4-day dietary history for analysis is suggested), current weight and height, recent growth trends, activity and seizure level and any relevant medication.

The energy requirement necessary on the classical ketogenic diet is likely to be less than the estimated average requirement (EAR) for energy as advised by the UK Department of Health [19]. The Johns Hopkins Hospital, a major centre for the ketogenic diet in the USA, recommends that the energy be 75% of the USA Recommended Dietary Allowances for energy [20]. Reducing energy to less than requirements must be done with care; a conservative reduction initially of 10% of the EAR is recommended. This can be adjusted later if the desired ketosis is not achieved. The following points should be noted:

- Younger children have higher energy requirements per kilogram body weight
- Active children need a higher energy intake than those who are wheelchair bound
- The underweight child may need at least the normal energy requirement, overweight children less

Recommendations for energy intake in MCT ketogenic diets have often used the EAR for age and so been more generous than those for the classical diet. However, early studies on both diets do not report differences in calorie prescriptions between the two types of diet [3,21]. A useful starting point for estimating the energy requirements for the MCT diet may be to use an amount that is between EAR and current dietary intake.

The energy prescription on classical and MCT ketogenic diets will need regular review and fine tuning as the child grows and the diet becomes established (e.g. as seizure activity decreases, mobility may increase and with it energy needs).

All calculations for the ketogenic diet are expressed in calories as the unit of energy.

Calculating the classical diet

Protein

The recommendations of the Joint Report of the FAO/WHO/UNU in 1985 for children aged 1–3 years on a normal diet are 1.1 g protein/kg body weight and less for older children [22]. This assumes that the protein is from a source of high biological value such as egg and milk. In 1996, Dewey suggested that these safe levels of protein intakes for growth were set too high [23]. The standard advice for the classical ketogenic diet is 1 g protein/kg body weight for older children and 1.5 g/kg for rapidly growing younger children. However, this includes protein from fruit and vegetables as well as egg, meat and milk products. The dietary protein intake when on the classical diet is therefore less than recommendations for normal diet and will be minimal for optimal nutrition.

Diet ratio

The classical ketogenic diet is calculated in a ratio of grams of fat to grams of protein plus carbohydrate. The most common ratio is 4 g fat to 1 g protein plus carbohydrate. This means that 90% of the energy comes from fat and 10% from protein plus carbohydrate. In this instance the ratio is expressed as 4 : 1. However, it is necessary at times to provide the diet at a lower ratio, such as 3 g fat to 1 g protein plus carbohydrate (3 : 1), giving 87% of dietary energy as fat. This is good practice when treating younger patients who achieve good ketosis on a lower ratio, or for patients on a medication that enhances ketosis. Some centres start the diet at a ratio of 2 g fat to 1 g of protein plus carbohydrate (2 : 1), and build to a higher ratio as tolerated.

Diet prescription

The calculation of the classical diet is based on three factors:

- energy requirements
- protein requirements
- the diet ratio of fat to protein plus carbohydrate

The most straightforward and flexible formula for this calculation is the one outlined in Freeman et al.'s book The Ketogenic Diet (pp. 110–15) [20]. This uses dietary units (Table 16.1). Each dietary unit reflects the diet ratio required (e.g. the 4 : 1 ratio reflects the energy in 4 g fat plus 1 g protein and carbohydrate, which is 40 kcal). The energy in other diet ratios is calculated in a similar fashion as tabulated.

Table 16.1 Diet units [20].

Diet ratio	Energy value per diet unit	Fat per diet unit (g)	CHO + Protein per diet unit (g)
2 : 1	22	2	1
3 : 1	31	3	1
4 : 1	40	4	1
5 : 1	49	5	1

CHO, carbohydrate.

The energy in each diet unit is then divided into the total daily energy requirements to give the number of daily diet units. The number of daily diet units is multiplied by 4 (on a 4 : 1 ratio diet), to give the total daily amount of fat in grams. The number of daily diet units multiplied by 1 gives the grams of protein plus carbohydrate. The protein requirement is subtracted from this to give the grams of carbohydrate. An example calculation is given in Table 16.2.

Having arrived at the total daily prescription of fat, protein and carbohydrate as above these amounts are then equally divided into either three or four meals (and snacks if wanted). Each meal is therefore in the same required ratio of fat to protein plus carbohydrate.

The actual amounts may need to be rationalised so that the diet prescription can be translated into food. However, the amount of protein should not be reduced to do this (Table 16.3). The amounts of food are calculated using UK food tables. The food tables in Freeman et al.'s book relate to US foods and are not suitable for use in the UK. This part of the calculation is laborious and time consuming when performed using the food tables alone. A computer program has recently been developed that is of assistance (see p. 302). Some centres have devised a system of exchanges; these are not standardised, but are individual to each centre.

When considering food choices it should be noted that a classical diet containing large amounts of double cream is high in vitamin A. A vitamin supplement is essential to this diet and there are no suitable supplements that do not contain vitamin A. This being the case it is wise to try an alternative fat source such as Calogen, which is a versatile substitute and does not contain vitamin A.

Table 16.2 Sample calculation of the classical ketogenic diet ratio 4 : 1.

Girl aged 5 years, weight 18 kg (50th centile)
Protein requirement = 1.0 g/kg
EAR for energy 82 kcal/kg = 1476 kcal
Energy prescription = 80% of EAR for energy as she is not mobile and uses a wheelchair = 1180 kcal

Number of dietary units
Each diet unit = 4 g fat : 1 g protein + carbohydrate = 40 kcal
1180/40 = 29–30 diet units
Quantity of fat = 30 × 4 = 120 g/day
Quantity of protein + carbohydrate = 1 × 30 = 30 g/day
Quantity of protein 1 g/kg = 18 g/day
Quantity of carbohydrate = (30 − 18) = 12 g/day

Daily prescription ratio 4 : 1
120 g fat
18 g protein
12 g carbohydrate
Divide this equally between the number of meals required (normally three or four)

4 meals a day each meal will contain
30 g fat
4.5 g protein
3 g carbohydrate
Ratio 4 : 1

3 meals a day each meal will contain
40 g fat
6 g protein
4 g carbohydrate
Ratio 4 : 1

Calculating the MCT diet

MCT content of the diet

The traditional MCT diet comprises 60% energy derived from MCT. This level of MCT can cause gastrointestinal discomfort in some children, with reports of abdominal cramps, diarrhoea and vomiting [24]. For this reason, a modified MCT diet was developed [24] using 30% energy from MCT, with an additional 30% energy from long chain fat. In practice, a starting MCT level somewhere between the two (40–50% energy) is likely to be the best balance between gastrointestinal tolerance and good ketosis. This can be increased or decreased as necessary during fine tuning; many children will tolerate 60% energy from MCT and need this amount for optimum ketone levels and seizure control.

Table 16.3 (a) Sample meal on the classical ketogenic diet.

Aim	30 g fat, 4.5 g protein, 3 g carbohydrate, ratio 4 : 1		
	Fat (g)	Protein (g)	CHO (g)
20 g lamb, raw	1.8	4.2	–
23 g butter	18.8	0.1	Tr
10 g green beans, cooked	Tr	0.2	0.5
20 g tomato, raw	0.1	0.1	0.6
30 g strawberries	Tr	0.2	1.8
25 g double cream	12.0	0.4	0.7
Total	32.7	5.2	3.6
Ratio	32.7 g fat : 8.8 g protein + CHO = 3.7 : 1		

Source: Food values taken from Holland B, Welch AA, Unwin ID *et al. McCance and Widdowson's The Composition of Foods*, 5th edn. Royal Society of Chemistry and Ministry of Agriculture, Fisheries and Food. London: The Stationery Office, 1991.

It is very difficult to achieve the exact amounts of food to fit the prescription without compromising the protein or using amounts of food that are difficult to measure.

Table 16.3 (b) Sample of classical diet emergency ketogenic 'milk shake'. This can replace the meal shown in Table 16.3(a).

	Fat (g)	Protein (g)	Carbohydrate (g)
5 g Protifar	0.1	4.5	0.1
3 g Maxijul	–	–	3.0
60 mL Calogen + water to 300 mL	30	–	–
Total	30.1	4.5	3.1
Ratio	30.1 g fat : 7.4 g protein + CHO = 4 : 1		

Some of the Maxijul could be replaced with fruit to provide carbohydrate and flavour; liquidise to make a 'smoothie'.

Some of the Calogen could be replaced by double cream for flavour.

MCT can be given in the diet as oil or an emulsion (Liquigen). MCT should be included in all meals and snacks. Mixing Liquigen with milk is a good way to incorporate it into the diet (best with skimmed or semi-skimmed milk as full fat

Table 16.4   (a) Example calculation of MCT diet.

Boy age 3 years, weight 14.5 kg (approx 50th centile)
EAR 1380 kcal
Diet history approx 1220 kcal/day
Energy prescription = 1300 kcal (average of diet history and EAR)

Diet prescription
45% energy from MCT = 585 kcal = 70.5 mL MCT oil or
141 mL Liquigen
15% energy from carbohydrate = 195 kcal = 48.8 g
10% energy from protein = 130 kcal = 32.5 g
Remaining 30% energy from fat in foods = 390 kcal = 43.3 g

Diet calculation
1   Milk allowance = 240 mL semi-skimmed milk (2 × 120 mL)
    = 11.3 g carbohydrate, 8.2 g protein, 4.1 g fat
2   Carbohydrate (aiming for 48.8 g/day): subtract 11.3 g
    (from milk allowance) = 37.5 g = 4 × 10 g exchanges
    (rounded up for ease of use)
3   Protein (aiming for 32.5 g daily): subtract 8.2 g (from milk
    allowance) and subtract 6 g (4 × 1.5 g from carbohydrate
    exchanges) = 18.3 g = 3 × 6 g exchanges
4   Fat (aiming for 43.3 g/day): subtract 4.1 g (from milk
    allowance) and subtract 9 g (3 × 3 g from fat-adjusted
    protein exchanges) = 30.2 g = 6 × 5 g fat exchanges

Daily prescription
141 mL Liquigen
240 mL semi-skimmed milk
4 × 10 g carbohydrate exchanges
3 × 6 g fat-adjusted protein exchanges
6 × 5 g fat exchanges

Suggested meal plan over the day
Breakfast: 40 mL Liquigen, 120 mL semi-skimmed milk,
1 carbohydrate exchange, 1 protein exchange, 2 fat exchanges
Lunch and dinner: 40 mL Liquigen, 1^1/$_2$ carbohydrate
exchanges, 1 protein exchange, 2 fat exchanges
Before bed milk drink: 21 mL Liquigen with 120 mL semi-skimmed milk

---

milk causes the mixture to thicken excessively); it can also be used in sugar free jelly, added to soups, mashed potato or used to make a sauce. Both MCT oil and Liquigen can be used in baking. A milk and Liquigen drink before bed will help maintain ketosis overnight.

The exact energy content of the MCT fat is controversial. Original studies use 8.3 kcal/g [3,21,24], although more recent literature suggests that this may be nearer 7 kcal/g or lower [25]. European law [26] dictates that for labelling purposes a value for MCT fat that is in line with LCT (i.e. 9 kcal/g) is

Table 16.4   (b) Sample of MCT diet emergency ketogenic 'milk shake'. Milk shake to replace lunch or dinner meals. Each contain 40 mL Liquigen, 1^1/$_2$ carbohydrate exchanges, 1 protein exchange, 2 fat exchanges = 15 g carbohydrate, 8.2 g protein (amount from carbohydrate exchanges included) and 16 g fat (amount from protein exchanges included).

	Fat (g)	Protein (g)	Carbohydrate (g)
225 mL semi-skimmed milk	3.9	7.7	10.6
25 g double cream	12.0	0.4	0.7
16 g banana	0	0.2	3.7
Total	15.9	8.3	15.0

Add 40 mL Liquigen to above and blend.
NB This is not designed to provide full vitamins, minerals and trace elements so should therefore only be used for short periods.

used. This may be amended in the near future, but until this issue is resolved a figure of 8.3 kcal/g is recommended for calculations for the ketogenic diet.

Diet prescription

Having established the level of MCT to be used, the remaining energy will be given from foods. Separate exchanges for protein (usually 10% energy), carbohydrate (15–19% energy) and LCT (11–15% energy) can be used; or 50 or 100 kcal food exchanges can be used. The MCT diet will therefore allow considerably more protein than the classical diet.

Initially, the daily amount of milk that is to be included is estimated. The protein, carbohydrate and LCT (or energy if using calorie exchanges) provided from this can be subtracted from the daily totals; the remaining nutrients can be distributed over the day by using the exchanges. An example calculation is given in Table 16.4, based on a child's preference of three meals and a bedtime drink only. Other snacks could be included in the day if needed (e.g. biscuits cooked with MCT oil or Liquigen). Tables 16.5–16.7 give example exchanges for carbohydrate (10 g), protein (6 g) and fat (5 g). The carbohydrate exchanges provide an average of 1.5 g protein each, and the protein exchanges are adjusted to give an average of 3 g fat per exchange.

Table 16.5 Example of selected 10 g carbohydrate exchanges for MCT ketogenic diet (each provides an average of 1.5 g protein).

Rice and pasta
12 g rice (dry weight)
13 g pasta or noodles (dry weight)

Breads and crackers
24 g wholemeal bread
22 g white bread
19 g scones or teacakes
15 g cream crackers

Breakfast cereals
14 g Bran Flakes
11 g Corn Flakes
11 g Rice Krispies
13 g Weetabix
13 g porridge oats (dry weight)

Vegetables
58 g potato – without skin (raw or boiled weight)
39 g roast potato
38 g sweetcorn, canned and drained
80 g parsnip (raw or cooked weight)
130 g carrots (raw or boiled weight)
200 g cabbage, spring greens, cauliflower or broccoli (raw weights)
300 g leeks, runner beans or courgette (raw or boiled weight)

Fruits
150 g raspberries, strawberries or blackberries
100 g apple, orange, pear, peach or plum (no stones)
65 g grapes
43 g banana

Miscellaneous
70 g tinned spaghetti in tomato sauce
170 g tinned tomato soup
13 g flour (plain/self-raising)

Table 16.6 Example of selected 6 g protein exchanges for MCT ketogenic diet (fat-adjusted, each provide an average of 3 g fat).

Fish
22 g tuna, tinned in oil
30 g white fish (e.g. cod, coley, plaice, haddock, halibut, whiting) with an extra 3 g oil or 4 g butter, margarine or mayonnaise
30 g smoked mackerel
25 g sardines, tinned in oil

Meat
26 g raw beef
20 g roast beef
30 g raw lamb
21 g roast lamb
28 g raw pork with an extra 2 g oil or 3 g butter, margarine or mayonnaise
19 g roast pork with an extra 2 g oil or 3 g butter, margarine or mayonnaise
30 g raw mince (beef, lamb or pork)
27 g raw chicken meat with an extra 3 g oil or 4 g butter, margarine or mayonnaise
20 g roast chicken breast with an extra 2 g oil or 3 g butter, margarine or mayonnaise
33 g ham with an extra 2 g oil or 3 g butter, margarine or mayonnaise

Cheese
24 g cheddar

Other
1 small egg (approx 50 g)
43 g Quorn

Table 16.7 Example of selected 5 g fat exchanges for MCT ketogenic diet.

6 g butter
5 g oil
6 g mayonnaise
10 g double cream

When teaching parents or carers, exchanges can either be given in total daily numbers, or structured over the day by specifying how many to be given for each meal. The latter method will allow a more careful balance of fat (both MCT and LCT) to carbohydrate and protein over the whole day, and may therefore improve ketosis and efficacy.

Meal distribution

The ketogenic diet is usually planned around three or four meals a day, with extra snacks if necessary.

On the classical diet, each meal (and snack) must be calculated in the correct ketogenic ratio. On the MCT diet, the MCT source should be included with each meal (and snack) and evenly divided up over the day. It is also important to give the last meal or snack as late as practical to maintain the best possible overnight ketosis.

Free foods

Free foods are very limited on the diet. They include sugar free drinks such as water, diet fizzy drinks and low calorie squashes. Flavourings such as herbs, spices and vanilla essence can be incorporated into meals freely as can carbohydrate free sweeteners such as saccharine. Powdered sweeteners should be avoided as they contain maltodextrin. Diabetic foods are generally unsuitable as they contain sorbitol and bulk sweeteners.

Some centres allow a range of free vegetables, particularly on the MCT version of the diet. It is preferable to allow prescribed amounts of different groups of vegetables, using an exchange list if necessary, to ensure control over the carbohydrate content of the diet.

Recipes

Imaginative use of food combinations is important, particularly ways to incorporate the high fat content of the diet. A range of recipe ideas can be developed and examples can be found on a helpful UK parents' support group website (www.matthewsfriends.org), which provides ideas without prescribed amounts. Some foods can be kept as special (e.g. cheesecake made from cream cheese and cream, and 'ketogenic cakes' made with ground almonds).

A computer calculation tool, EKM (MicroMan 2000 Ltd.), has recently been developed for use with ketogenic diets to help reduce the time they take to calculate. It is available free for download at www.edm2000.com. Once a dietitian has calculated a dietary prescription for a child, EKM can be used to plan meal ideas. Parents can also use this tool, but only if working in conjunction with a dietitian who provides target figures for meal calculations (confirmation from the medical/dietetic team is needed before download is authorised). The program does not calculate MCT exchanges, only individual meal recipes, therefore may be more appropriate to use with the classical diet.

Vitamins and minerals

The ketogenic diet requires full vitamin and mineral supplementation. There is no ideal product available for use with this diet in the UK. Paediatric Seravit contains too much carbohydrate. Forceval Junior is frequently the supplement of choice, although this has high levels of vitamin A, so should be used with caution if the diet is already high in vitamin A. Calcium, magnesium and phosphorus supplementation will usually be required, although this will not be necessary with a MCT diet that allows sufficient milk to meet requirements. Intake of all vitamins and minerals should be closely monitored and it is the responsibility of the individual dietitian to recommend the most appropriate supplement available for each child to ensure nutritional adequacy.

Fluid requirements

Each child's usual intake of fluid should be assessed. On both classical and MCT diets normal amounts of fluids are allowed [27]; however, excessive fluid intake should be discouraged as it may reduce ketosis. Adequate fluid intake is essential wherever possible as renal stones may be one of the side effects of the diet.

Initiating the diet

Although fasting has traditionally been used to initiate the ketogenic diet, this has been shown to be unnecessary [28] and adequate ketosis can be achieved by commencing directly onto the full dietary prescription.

The depth of ketosis on the classical diet will depend on the diet ratio; this can be increased as tolerated to increase the desired ketosis. Some centres recommend starting with a 2 : 1 ratio prescription and building up to 3 : 1 or 4 : 1 ratio over a period of days or weeks as needed. It is unusual to start the diet on a 4 : 1 ratio; this should be carried out with caution and in hospital.

On commencing the MCT diet, the Liquigen or MCT oil needs to be introduced much more slowly than long chain fat (over about 5–10 days), as it may cause abdominal discomfort, vomiting or diarrhoea if introduced rapidly. During this introduction period the rest of the diet can be given as prescribed.

Short term complications during the first few

days of diet initiation can include dehydration, drowsiness, hypoglycaemia, nausea, vomiting and diarrhoea [24]. These symptoms usually resolve after a few days, but it is important to initiate the diet slowly in order to minimise early side effects. This is especially important in children taking topiramate because of increased risk of acidosis and excess ketosis. Hypoglycaemia can occur and some centres recommend blood sugar levels should be checked regularly during diet initiation. Many children on the diet have lower blood sugars than normal; this is not a problem unless symptoms develop. Symptoms of low blood sugar include sweating, pallor, dizziness, becoming cold and clammy, jittery, confused or aggressive. Such symptoms, or blood glucose levels of 2.5 mmol/L or less, should be treated immediately by giving a drink that contains carbohydrate, such as fruit juice. A doctor should be contacted; ongoing monitoring of blood sugars will be necessary and further treatment may be needed.

Excess ketosis can be a problem on diet initiation: the signs of this are rapid, panting breathing; increased heart rate; facial flushing; irritability; vomiting; unexpected lethargy. This should be treated by giving 1–2 tablespoons of fresh fruit juice or alternative carbohydrate containing drink. If symptoms have not improved after 15–20 minutes, this should be repeated and the local doctor contacted. It will be necessary to alter the diet ratio if excessive ketone levels persist.

Fine tuning the diet

Fine tuning and ongoing modification of a child's ketogenic diet are an essential part of the dietetic care. Regular weight checks will enable calorie modifications as needed. If weight is being gained too quickly, the energy intake should be decreased by 100 kcal/day initially. If weight gain is judged to be too slow, energy intake should be increased by 100 kcal/day initially.

The ketogenic ratio (classical diet) or percentage energy from MCT and/or carbohydrate (MCT diet) may need increasing or decreasing to influence ketosis, depending on the child's ketone levels and tolerance. If the amount of MCT is increased, the corresponding amount of LCT fat can be reduced to keep the same total percentage energy from fat in the diet.

As a child grows, the diet may need recalculating to increase protein intake in line with increases in body weight. Meal and/or snack distribution may also need changing to fit with changes in a child's lifestyle (e.g. the start of a new school). Vitamin and mineral intakes should always be checked if they are likely to be altered by dietary modifications and supplementation reviewed as necessary.

Management of illness

When the child is unwell the ketogenic diet takes second place to the necessary treatment needed.

Vomiting and diarrhoea

The diet should be stopped. Clear fluids that are low in carbohydrate should be offered (e.g. water or sugar free squash) to ensure there is adequate hydration. Low glucose oral rehydration fluids such as Dioralyte may be used if necessary, but can upset ketosis. Should intravenous fluids be required then saline is recommended (the strength appropriate to the child's age and requirements) to limit disruption to ketosis. It may be necessary to add dextrose to this if there are concerns about hypoglycaemia, or if intravenous fluids are needed for a significant length of time. Blood glucose levels should to be checked regularly throughout the day to ensure the child does not become hypoglycaemic and blood ketones should be monitored in case the child becomes hyperketotic. These blood tests should follow any time of fast (e.g. on waking in the morning or if meals have been missed or not completed because of illness). Hypoglycaemia and hyperketosis should be treated with a carbohydrate containing drink, as previously discussed.

When the vomiting has subsided the diet should be reintroduced gradually with half the usual meal amounts for the first day or two. If the child is unable to complete meals, the meal constituents should be mixed together so that any food eaten is in the correct ratio of fat to protein and carbohydrate. If full fat meals are not tolerated because of continued diarrhoea or vomiting, it may be necessary to temporally reduce the fat in the diet. The ratio of the classical diet can be lowered by using half the prescribed amount of cream, butter, oil and/or mayonnaise at each meal for a day; this can be slowly increased back to normal over the next couple of days as tolerated. The Liquigen in the MCT diet may also need to be reduced by half and then built back up to full strength over 2–3 days. If diarrhoea is a continuing problem, the Liquigen may need to be introduced at one-quarter strength and built up to the full amount over 4–5 days. When reintroducing gastrostomy or nasogastric ketogenic feeds, initially use half strength for 24–48 hours, then gradually build up to full strength as tolerated over a few days.

Other illness

Illness may cause loss of appetite and this can be treated in a similar way offering smaller more frequent meals containing less fat. All medications such as antibiotics or painkillers should be carbohydrate and calorie free. Pharmacists can supply this information and it is always useful for parents to have a list of suitable over-the-counter preparations needed to treat minor illness and infections. Infection can cause a drop in ketones but once the child has recovered the ketosis will usually return to normal.

A recipe for a meal replacement in the form of an emergency ketogenic 'milk shake' (Tables 16.3b and 16.4b) should be calculated and given to parents in case of illness and food refusal. This milk shake can be kept frozen so that it is always available. It is made using a fat source appropriate to the type of diet, and protein and carbohydrate sources, which could include milk or prescribable dietary products if necessary. The mixture should be initially diluted with water so there is no more than a 10% fat solution; a higher solution may cause nausea and vomiting in an ill child. However, this milk shake should not be used for any length of time as it contains inadequate electrolytes, vitamins and minerals.

Which ketogenic diet?

Practice in the USA predominantly uses the classical diet and much of their literature advocates this as more efficacious, although the evidence base for this is poor. Ketogenic diet practice is more varied in the UK and Europe. A postal survey of 250 British Dietetic Association Paediatric Group members [29] found that of 22 UK centres that were using the ketogenic diet, 13 followed the classical protocol and nine the MCT protocol.

Schwartz et al. [24] compared the clinical and metabolic effects of three types of ketogenic diet – the classical 4 : 1 diet, the traditional MCT diet (60% energy as MCT) and the modified MCT diet (30% energy as MCT). They found all diets equally effective in controlling seizures, but this was not a randomised trial.

Palatability and ease of use should also be considered. The MCT diet allows considerably more carbohydrate and protein, thus a more normal diet, which may be better suited to some children, especially those with limited food choices.

Enteral feeds

The ketogenic diet can be given by enteral tube feed if necessary [30]. Enteral feeds should be based on the same total and percentage nutrient content as the oral diet. A modular feed can be devised using the required amounts of fat, protein, carbohydrate, vitamins, minerals, electrolytes and fluids necessary to make it nutritionally adequate.

On the classical diet, a prescribable fat source such as Calogen will form the basis of the feed; it is recommended that the fat be introduced gradually over several days to ensure tolerance. Any fat source used must have an adequate supply of essential fatty acids; if it does not then these must be added as a supplement. Protein and carbohydrate should be provided by suitable prescribable sources such as Protifar and Maxijul. It is important that a complete vitamin, mineral and trace element supplement is included in the feed. This is likely to be Paediatric Seravit, which contains carbohydrate, so no other carbohydrate source may be needed. Electrolytes will need to be included in the feed formula.

There is a complete tube feed formula available, Ketocal, suitable for use on a classical ketogenic diet which is ideal for the purpose. At present it is not available on prescription.

A similar modular approach can be employed for the MCT diet, using Liquigen and prescribable sources of protein, LCT and carbohydrate. As with the classical diet, it is essential to ensure the feed is nutritionally complete, providing essential fatty acids, and meeting requirements of all vitamins, minerals, trace elements and electrolytes.

When changing to a ketogenic enteral feed, the daily feeding regimen should be kept as similar as possible to the child's previous regimen. It should be given as conveniently as possible for the child and the regimen manipulated if necessary to improve ketosis.

Monitoring the diet

Daily monitoring

- The family or carers should keep a seizure diary recording number and type of seizures.
- Urine should be tested for ketones (acetoacetate) using a dipstick, initially at least twice daily, in the morning before breakfast and before another meal later in the day. Once the diet is established and stabilised urine ketone testing may be performed once daily. Ideally, tests should then be carried out at a different time each day, before different meals, so that an overall pattern can be seen. The aim is to have moderate to high ketones in the urine in the range of 4–16 mmol/L. Urinary ketones are typically lower in the morning reflecting the overnight fast.
- Finger prick blood ketone (β-hydroxybutyrate) monitors have recently been developed; this method may be easier to use and be more accurate than urinary ketone testing. Blood ketones should be tested initially twice daily, or more often if clinically required, and then once daily before different meals as for urinary ketones. Levels should ideally be at least 2 mmol/L, although seizure control has been shown to be optimal when blood β-hydroxybutyrate levels are 4 mmol/L or above [31]. However, blood ketone levels >5 mmol/L should be monitored carefully as the patient may become hyperketotic. In this case the diet will require adjustment (e.g. the ratio in the classical ketogenic might need to be reduced).

This daily monitoring will provide essential information on which dietary manipulations and changes will be based.

Three-monthly monitoring

- Growth monitoring using height, weight and mid arm circumference measures. Head circumference can be included in younger children.
- Biochemical nutritional screening including plasma lipids, nutritional indices and carnitine. This should be carried out prior to commencing the diet, after 3 months and at 6-monthly intervals thereafter.
- Urine testing for haematuria; calcium : creatinine ratio for renal stones.

Dietary adjustments are made according to the result of these screens and monitoring measurements as necessary (e.g. as weight increases so must the protein allowance).

Six-monthly monitoring

The following assessments should be carried out prior to the child starting the diet and then repeated at 6-monthly intervals thereafter:

- Nutritional assessment carried out by the dietitian to ensure the diet remains nutritionally adequate
- A complete biochemical nutritional screening as discussed above
- Electroencephalogram (EEG) examination
- Renal ultrasound scan (may be necessary sooner if problems are detected in 3-monthly urine tests)

Some centres also recommend 6-monthly electrocardiogram (ECG) examinations.

Adverse effects

Haematological disturbances have been reported in children on the diet, both impaired neutrophil function [32] and alterations in platelet function, with increased tendency to bruising and bleeding [33]. Raised serum cholesterol and triglyceride levels are common [34,35]; this may be less of a problem on the MCT diet [21]. There is no evidence from case reports that the diet causes any adverse effects on cardiovascular function later in adulthood [36].

To minimise hyperlipidaemia polyunsaturated fats are recommended.

Renal stones occur in 5–8% of patients receiving a ketogenic diet [37–39] with increased risk in children undergoing concomitant topiramate treatment. Other reported problems include cardiac complications [40], pancreatitis [41], hypoproteinaemia [42] and potentiation of valproate toxicity [43]. Constipation is a common problem because of the high fat, low carbohydrate nature of the diet. An increase in fluid may be needed. Using a small amount of MCT oil to replace some LCT in the classical diet can be useful. It may be necessary to prescribe a sugar free laxative if problems continue.

Weight gain may be slower than prior to the diet, particularly during the first 6 months, and the weight centile may gradually drop. Many children on the diet show a reduction in growth velocity [43–46]; this should therefore be closely monitored. A reduction in bone density can occur without adequate calcium supplementation [47].

Serum carnitine levels (both free and total) should be regularly monitored. Carnitine is involved in transport of LCT into mitochondria for oxidation and requirements may increase when following a high fat diet. If deficiency is found, a supplement of 50–100 mg/kg/day should be given to children [48]. Although most children do not require supplementation [49] those most at risk of deficiency are in the younger age groups and those on valproate medication.

Duration and discontinuation of the diet

Generally, a trial of 3 months on the ketogenic diet is recommended. If there is no improvement by then it should be discontinued. When the diet is successful the usual recommendation is that the child remains on it for at least 2 years or until they have been seizure free without medication for 1 year. There are as yet no formal studies to give guidance on how or when to safely withdraw the diet.

Discontinuation must be carried out cautiously. The longer the child has been on the diet and the more successfully it has controlled seizures, the more gradual should be the change back to a normal diet.

When coming off the classical diet a gradual increase of protein and carbohydrate and lowering of fat may be achieved by lowering the diet ratios slowly until normal diet is achieved. Recommendations from the Johns Hopkins Hospital suggest that if the diet has been successful in treating seizures the ratio be reduced from 4 : 1 to 3 : 1 for 6 months and then to 2 : 1 for another 6 months, followed by a gradual normalisation of the diet [20]. Parents may not be prepared to undergo such a long return to normal if the diet has not been as effective as they had hoped and the process may therefore have to be performed more quickly. However, the whole change should take place over weeks rather than days, as if the diet has had some effect and is withdrawn too quickly there is the risk of an increase in the number and intensity of seizures. If at any point the seizures return or worsen then the diet must revert to the previous ratio.

Discontinuing the MCT diet should also follow a stepwise, gradual process. The amount of MCT fat should be slowly reduced and the protein and carbohydrate increased. This could be achieved by reducing MCT in the diet by 5 g/day. Alongside this reduction, protein is increased by one exchange daily until normal size protein portions are achieved, then the carbohydrate is increased by one carbohydrate exchange daily until normal size portions are reached.

For both diets, the reintroduction of concentrated sources of refined carbohydrates should only take place gradually once the child is established on an otherwise normal regimen without ill effects. Ketone levels should continue to be monitored until a normal diet is achieved. The dietitian should guide the family through the whole process. If at any point there is deterioration then the diet needs to revert to the stage at which seizure control was acceptable.

KetoPAG

Ketogenic diet Professional Advisory Group (KetoPAG) is a group of dietitians, doctors and nurses who are involved with the use of the ketogenic diet in the UK. They have produced simple explanatory leaflets on the diet and also advice and guidelines on how to treat patients on the ketogenic diet when unwell. They may be contacted via the website www.ketoPAG.org.

References

1 Engel JA Proposed diagnostic scheme for people with epileptic seizures and with epilepsy: Report of the ILAE task force on classification and terminology. *Epilepsia*, 2001, **42** 796–803.

2 Wilder RM The effects of ketonuria on the course of epilepsy. *Mayo Clin Bull*, 1921, **2** 307.

3 Huttenlocher PR, Wilbourn AJ, Signore JM Medium chain triglycerides as a therapy for intractable childhood epilepsy. *Neurology*, 1971, **21** 1097–103.

4 Freeman JM, Vining EP, Pilas DJ *et al.* The efficacy of the ketogenic diet: a prospective evaluation of intervention in 150 children. *Pediatrics*, 1998, **102** 1358–63.

5 Lefevre F, Aronson N Ketogenic diet for the treatment of refractory epilepsy in children. A systematic review of efficacy. *Pediatrics*, 2000, **105** E46 1–7.

6 Levy R, Cooper P Ketogenic diet for epilepsy (Cochrane Review). In: *The Cochrane Library*, Issue 3, 2004. Chichester, UK: John Wiley & Sons Ltd.

7 Neal EG, Chaffe HM, Lawson M *et al.* Use of the ketogenic diet to treat childhood epilepsy – a randomised controlled trial. *Arch Dis Child*, 2004, **89** (Suppl 1) A5.

8 Pulsifer MB, Gordon JM, Brandt J *et al.* Effects of the ketogenic diet on development and behaviour: preliminary report of a prospective study. *Dev Med Child Neurol*, 2001, **43** 301–6.

9 Gilbert DL, Pyzik PL, Vining EPG *et al.* Medication cost reduction in children on the ketogenic diet: data from a prospective study. *J Child Neurol*, 1999, **14** 469–71.

10 Nordli DR, De Vivo DC Effects of the ketogenic diet on cerebral energy metabolism. In: Stafstrom CE, Rho JM (eds) *Epilepsy and the Ketogenic Diet*. Totowa, NJ: Humana Press, 2004.

11 Yudkoff M, Daikhin Y, Nissim I *et al.* Ketogenic diet, brain glutamate metabolism and seizure control. *Prostagland Leukotr Ess Fatty Acids*, 2004, **70** 277–85.

12 Cullingford TE The ketogenic diet; fatty acids, fatty acid-activated receptors and neurological disorders. *Prostaglandins Leukotr Essent Fatty Acids*, 2004, **70** 253–64.

13 Likhodi SS, Burnham WM The effect of ketone bodies on neuronal excitability. In: Stafstrom CE, Rho JM (eds) *Epilepsy and the Ketogenic Diet*. Totowa, NJ: Humana Press, 2004.

14 Weinshenker D Galanin and neuropeptide Y: Orexigenic peptides link food intake, energy homeostasis, and seizure susceptibility. In: Stafstrom CE, Rho JM (eds) *Epilepsy and the Ketogenic Diet*. Totowa, NJ: Humana Press, 2004.

15 Tabb K, Szot P, White SS *et al.* The ketogenic diet does not alter brain expression of orexigenic neuropeptides. *Epilepsy Res*, 2004, **62** 35–9.

16 Szot P The role of norepinephrine in the anticonvulsant mechanism of action of the ketogenic diet. In: Stafstrom CE, Rho JM (eds) *Epilepsy and the Ketogenic Diet*. Totowa, NJ: Humana Press, 2004.

17 Greene AE, Todorova MT, Seyfield TN Perspectives on metabolic management of epilepsy through dietary reduction of glucose and elevation of ketone bodies. *J Neurochem*, 2003, **86** 529–37.

18 Sirven J, Whedon B, Caplan D *et al.* The ketogenic diet for intractable epilepsy in adults: preliminary results. *Epilepsia*, 1999, **40** 1721–6.

19 Department of Health Report on Health and Social Subjects No. 41. *Dietary Reference Values for Food Energy and Nutrients for the United Kingdom*. London: The Stationery Office, 1991.

20 Freeman JM, Freeman JB, Kelly MT. *The Ketogenic Diet: A treatment for epilepsy*, 3rd edn. New York: Demos Medical Publishing, 2000.

21 Huttenlocher P Ketonemia and seizures: metabolic and anticonvulsant effects of two ketogenic diets in childhood epilepsy. *Pediatr Res*, 1976, **10** 536–40.

22 World Health Organization. *Energy and Protein Requirements*. Reports of the Joint FAO/WHO/UNU Meeting. Geneva: World Health Organization 1985 (WHO Technical Report Series 724).

23 Dewy KG, Beaton G, Fjeld C *et al.* Protein requirements of infants and children. *Eur J Clin Nutr*, 1996, **Suppl 1** S119–50.

24 Schwartz RH, Eaton J, Bowyer BD *et al.* Ketogenic diets in the treatment of epilepsy: short-term clinical effects. *Dev Med Child Neurol*, 1989, **31** 145–51.

25 Ranhotra GS, Gelroth JA, Glaser BK Levels of medium-chain triglycerides and their energy value. *Cereal Chem*, 1995, **72** 365–7.

26 European Council Directive on Food Labelling. *Official Journal of the European Communities*, No. L276/41. 1990, pp. 27–31.

27 Vaisleib II, Buchalter JR, Zupanc ML Ketogenic diet: outpatient initiation, without fluid or caloric restrictions. *Pediatr Neurol*, 2004, **31** 198–202.

28 Wirrell EC, Darwish HZ, Williams-Dyjur C *et al.* Is a fast necessary when initiating the ketogenic diet? *J Child Neurol*, 2002, **17** 179–82.

29 Magrath G, MacDonald A, Whitehouse W Dietary practices and use of the ketogenic diet in the UK. *Seizure*, 2000, **9** 128–30.

30 Hosain SA, La Vega-Talbot M, Solomon GE Ketogenic diet in pediatric epilepsy patients with gastrostomy feeding. *Pediatr Neurol*, 2005, **32** 81–3.

31 Gilbert D, Pyzik P, Freeman JM The ketogenic diet: seizure control correlates better with serum beta-hydroxybutyrate than with urine ketone levels. *J Child Neurol*, 2000, **15** 787–90.

32 Woody RC, Steele RW, Knapple WL *et al.* Impaired neutrophil function in children with seizures treated with the ketogenic diet. *J Pediatr*, 1989, **115** 427–30.

33 Berry-Kravis E, Booth G, Taylor A *et al.* Bruising and the ketogenic diet: evidence for diet-induced changes in platelet function. *Ann Neurol*, 2001, **49** 98–103.

34 Delgado MR, Mills J, Sparagana S Hypercholesterolemia associated with the ketogenic diet. *Epilepsia*, 1996, **37** (Suppl 5) 108.

35 Kwiterovitch PO, Vining EP, Pyzik P *et al.* Effect of high fat ketogenic diet on plasma levels of lipids, lipoproteins, and apolipoproteins in children. *J Am Med Assoc*, 2003, **290** 12–20.

36 Livingstone S, Pauli LL, Pruce I Ketogenic diet in the treatment of childhood epilepsy. *Dev Med Child Neurol*, 1977, **19** 833–4.

37 Hertzberg GZ, Fivush BA, Kinsman SL *et al.* Urolithiasis associated with the ketogenic diet. *J Pediatr*, 1990, **117** 743–5.

38 Furth SL, Casey JC, Pyzik PL *et al.* Risk factors for urolithiasis in children on the ketogenic diet. *Pediatr Nephrol*, 2000, **15** 125–8.

39 Kleib S, Koo HP, Bloom DA *et al.* Nephrolithiasis associated with the ketogenic diet. *J Urol*, 2000, **164** 464–6.

40 Best TH, Franz DN, Gilbert DL *et al.* Cardiac complications in pediatric patients on the ketogenic diet. *Neurology*, 2000, **54** 2328–30.

41 Stewart WA, Gordon K, Camfield P Acute pancreatitis causing death in a child on the ketogenic diet. *J Child Neurol*, 2001, **16** 633–5.

42 Ballaban-Gill K, Callahan C, O'Dell C *et al.* Complications of the ketogenic diet. *Epilepsia*, 1998, **7** 744–8.

43 Couch SC, Schwarzman F, Carroll J *et al.* Growth and nutritional outcomes of children treated with the ketogenic diet. *J Am Diet Assoc*, 1999, **99** 1573–5.

44 Williams S, Basualdo-Hammond C, Curtis R *et al.* Growth retardation in children with epilepsy on the ketogenic diet: A retrospective chart review *J Am Diet Assoc*, 2002, **102** 405–7.

45 Vining EP, Pyzik P, Mc Grogan J *et al.* Growth of children on the ketogenic diet. *Dev Med Child Neurol*, 2002, **449** 796–802.

46 Peterson SJ, Tangey CC, Pimentel-Zablah EM *et al.* Changes in growth and seizure reduction in children on the ketogenic diet as a treatment for intractable epilepsy. *J Am Diet Assoc*, 2005, **105** 725–6.

47 Hahn TJ, Halstead LR, De Vivo DC Disordered mineral metabolism produced by ketogenic diet therapy. *Calcif Tissue Int*, 1979, **28** 17–22.

48 DeVivo DC, Bohan TP, Coulter DL *et al.* L-carnitine supplementation in childhood epilepsy: current perspectives. *Epilepsia*, 1998, **39** 1216–25.

49 Berry-Kravis E, Booth G, Sanchez AC *et al.* Carnitine levels and the ketogenic diet. *Epilepsia*, 2001, **42** 1445–51.

17 Disorders of Amino Acid Metabolism, Organic Acidaemias and Urea Cycle Defects

Phenylketonuria

Anita MacDonald

Phenylketonuria (PKU) is an autosomal recessive genetic disorder [1]. It is usually caused by a deficiency of the hepatic enzyme, phenylalanine hydroxylase (phenylalanine 4-mono-oxygenase, EC 1.14.16.1). This is a mixed function oxidase which catalyses the hydroxylation of phenylalanine to tyrosine, the rate limiting step in phenylalanine catabolism [2]. Deficiency of this enzyme leads to an increased production of phenylketones (hence phenylketonuria), accumulation of phenylalanine resulting in hyperphenylalaninaemia, and abnormalities in the metabolism of many compounds derived from aromatic amino acids. This high level of phenylalanine is possibly the chief cause of neurotoxicity by increasing brain phenylalanine concentrations and decreasing the concentration of large neutral amino acids. This in turn decreases brain protein synthesis, increases myelin turnover and inhibits neurotransmitter synthesis [3,4]. The enzyme deficiency varies from complete absence of detectable activity, up to a residual activity up to 25% or more [5]. There is a 1 in 4 incidence of PKU in siblings of index cases and there is an equal sex ratio. Treatment is by a strict low phenylalanine diet.

History

Asbjörn Fölling first recognized classic PKU in 1934. In 1947, Jervis [6] observed that the administration of phenylalanine to normal humans led to prompt elevation in serum tyrosine but this response was absent in patients with PKU. In 1952, the enzyme system that converts phenylalanine to tyrosine was identified [7]. Woolf and Vulliamy [8] first suggested a low phenylalanine diet for the treatment of PKU and this was given to a 2-year-old child with PKU in 1953 [9]. The child had severe developmental problems; was unable to stand, walk, or talk; and spent her time groaning, crying and head banging. During treatment she learnt to walk, crawl, stand, climb on chairs, ceased head banging and her hair grew darker. By the 1960s, a microbial inhibition assay was used for mass screening of newborn babies for PKU. In the 1980s, the human phenylalanine hydroxylase (PAH) gene was mapped and cloned and the first mutation identified. In the 1990s, the catalytic core of human PAH was crystallised [10] and has allowed for the construction of a composite structural model for full-length, tetrameric PAH and provided a structural basis for the numerous mutations resulting in deficient PAH activity [11].

Classification of PKU

There are several classification schemes for PKU

depending on residual enzyme activity [12,13]. The following is a useful working classification:

- *Classical or severe PKU.* This is usually characterised by high blood phenylalanine concentrations (an arbitrary level >1200 µmol/L) at presentation. There is almost a complete loss of enzyme activity [14] and in the liver PAH activity is 0.3% or less of normal [15]. Individuals only tolerate 200–300 mg/day dietary phenylalanine to keep plasma phenylalanine concentrations <360 µmol/L.
- *Moderate PKU.* Individuals with moderate PKU tolerate 350–500 mg/day dietary phenylalanine. They will have a PKU genotype associated with residual enzyme activity (an arbitrary level >600–1200 µmol/L).
- *Persistent hyperphenylalaninaemia or mild PKU.* This is a milder form of the disorder in that there is only a partial reduction in the activity of the PAH enzyme of 2–5% of normal [14]. On a normal diet plasma phenylalanine is in the range 120–600 µmol/L. In the UK, 21% of all patients who have elevated phenylalanine levels have mild hyperphenylalaninaemia [1]. It is recommended that all children who have phenylalanine concentrations of ≥400 µmol/L should follow a low phenylalanine diet at least in early childhood [16].

There are also rarer forms of hyperphenylalaninaemia brought about by a deficiency of reductase or other enzymes involved in the biosynthesis of tetrahydrobiopterin [17–19]. These tetrahydrobiopterin deficiency disorders are sometimes referred to collectively as malignant hyperphenylalaninaemias, but the clinical picture is variable and some patients are only moderately affected, presenting late with neurological dysfunction. A low phenylalanine diet is not effective. In Caucasian populations, only 1–2% of cases of hyperphenylalaninaemias have tetrahydrobiopterin deficiency defects [20].

Prevalence

PKU is prevalent in many human populations and there is wide ethnic and geographical variation. It is particularly common in Turkey, Ireland, Poland, the former Czechoslovakia and in Yemenite Jews.

Table 17.1   Prevalence of phenylketonuria (PKU).

Population	Prevalence	Carrier rate
Turkish	1/2600	1/26
Irish	1/4500	1/33
Caucasian	1/10 000	1/50
West Midlands (UK)	1/14 000	
USA (National Institutes of Health Consensus Development Conference Statement 2000 on PKU)	1/15 000	
Japanese	1/143 000	1/200
Finnish	1/200 000	1/225

Source: After Mitchell and Scriver [124].

Overall, the frequency among Caucasians is approximately 1 in 10 000, corresponding to a carrier frequency of about 1 in 50. In Asian populations, PKU is rare (Table 17.1).

Biochemistry

The hydroxylation of phenylalanine to tyrosine is a complex biochemical reaction. The overall reaction is the sum of three reactions; each catalysed by a separate enzyme. Phenylalanine hydroxylase catalyses the hydroxylation of phenylalanine to tyrosine in the presence of the co-factor tetrahydrobiopterin (BH_4). During this reaction the co-factor is oxidised to quinonoid dihydrobiopterin, which is subsequently reduced to the tetrahydro form by dihydropteridine reductase (DHPR) (Fig. 17.1). This co-factor must be regenerated by a separate system of enzymes for PAH action to continue.

Normally, hydroxylation of phenylalanine contributes up to 50% of the tyrosine that is incorporated into tissue protein [5]. In classical PKU, there is an inability to convert phenylalanine into tyrosine. Subsequently, patients with PKU tend to have low–normal or reduced concentrations of tyrosine unless they have specific supplementation. Tyrosine is essential for the synthesis of the catecholamine neurotransmitters such as dopamine and norepinephrine.

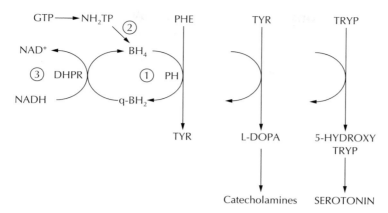

Figure 17.1   Hydroxylation of phenylalanine (phe), tyrosine (tyr) and tryptophan (tryp). Source: McLaren DS *et al.* (eds) *Textbook of Paediatric Nutrition*, 3rd edn. Edinburgh: Churchill Livingstone, 1991 with permission. 1 Classical PKU. 2 & 3 Defects in tetrahydrobiopterin metabolism. BH_4, tetrahydrobiopterin; DHPR, dihydropteridine reductase; GTP, guanosine triphosphate; NAD, nicotinamide adenine dinucleotide; NH_2 TP, dihydroneopterin triphosphate; PH, phenylalanine hydroxylase; q-BH_2, quinoid-dihydrobiopterin.

Genetics

PKU and related hyperphenylalaninaemia (HPA) are caused by mutations in the gene encoding phenylalanine hydroxylase enzyme. The gene is on the long arm of chromosome 12 in the band region of q22–q24.1 [21]. There is extensive mutant allelic hydroxylase heterogeneity. There are well over 400 disease causing mutations including deletions, insertions, missense mutations, splicing defects and nonsense mutations. The most prevalent mutations in the UK are R408W, IVS 12ntl and 165T. The first two of these are associated with a complete loss of enzyme activity so individuals who are homozygous or compound heterozygous for these mutant alleles exhibit the classical PKU phenotype. In some cases, mutations in PAH will result in the phenotypically mild form of PKU (HPA). In those cases where a patient is heterozygous for two mutations of PAH (i.e. each copy of the gene has a different mutation), the milder mutation will predominate.

Diagnosis

PKU is detected by routine neonatal screening. In the UK, the Newborn Screening Programme Centre policies and procedures for the Newborn Blood Spot Programme [22] state:

- Every newborn baby resident in the UK should be offered heelprick blood spot screening.
- Parents are entitled to choose whether to undergo screening, but need timely and written information about the process.
- The sample should be taken on day 5 of life (but between days 5 and 8 is acceptable). This should be irrespective of prematurity, illness, transfusion and milk feeding status.
- Babies with a phenylalanine level >240 µmol/L should be referred to a designated PKU team, with a paediatrician who has a case load of at least 20 patients with PKU, and should be seen within 24 hours of a positive screening result.
- Diet should commence on this visit and it is a standard that all infants should be on diet by 18 days of age.

The blood spot is commonly analysed by tandem mass spectrometry, but the Guthrie bacterial inhibition test, fluorimetry, thin layer or paper chromatography [18], or high pressure liquid chromatography may also be used.

Clinical outcome

Untreated PKU leads to mental retardation, hyperactive behaviour with autistic features, seizures, eczema and light pigmentation (eyes, hair and skin). If treatment is started within the first 3 weeks of life, irreversible mental retardation is prevented. Most early treated children who have started diet by 4 weeks of age fall within the broad normal range of general ability and attend mainstream schools [23,24], although some may need additional tutoring [25], may have to work harder than healthy controls to achieve the same results [24] or have variable school work performance [26]. Mildly depressed IQ is common in treated patients [27] and is about 0.5 standard deviations below population norms and unaffected siblings [28–30]. There is strong evidence to indicate that outcome is closely related to the quality of blood phenylalanine control [23]. For each 300 μmol/L increase in blood phenylalanine levels preschool, IQ decreases by about half a standard deviation [31]. In early and middle childhood, children with phenylalanine levels <400 μmol/L have near normal outcomes. The risk of intellectual deterioration declines dramatically in adolescence [32].

Some children exhibit problems in task orientated behaviour and may be more distractible [26]. Deficits have also been documented in information processing, abstract reasoning, high level problem solving and organisational skills, working memory, sustained attention and reduced performance speed [33–35]. Calculation tasks are performed more slowly and less well and a delayed linguistic ability and lack of autonomy and drive has been reported. Behavioural problems, including both internalising symptoms (e.g. solitary, unresponsive, anxious, depressed mood) [36] and externalising symptoms (e.g. hyperactivity, talkative, impulsive and restless) have also been identified [27]. Associations between behaviour problems, sustained attention and lower IQ with quality blood phenylalanine control are well documented [37]. Neurological signs (e.g. excessively brisk tendon jerks, ankle clonus and intention tremor) are common in children with early treated PKU with high blood phenylalanine concentrations [5,38]. Furthermore, white matter abnormalities of the brain have been observed in both inpatients with late onset neurological symptoms and in symptom-free patients remaining on diet [39–43].

In adults, good social outcome is associated with early treatment [44]. In a large group of 172 adults with PKU, 76% were in full-time employment, with some achieving higher degrees with university education. Only 31% obtained no educational qualifications. Agoraphobia, depression and anxiety have been reported following termination of treatment in young adult patients. Adults off diet have been shown to have more problems with eczema, headache, hyperactivity and lethargy [45]. Many report their quality of life improves when diet is restarted, even though their median phenylalanine concentrations may remain higher than treatment blood phenylalanine ranges [46].

There are a few patients with so called severe PKU mutations who have escaped mental retardation despite high blood phenylalanine levels and very poor dietary control. These patients appear to have near normal brain phenylalanine levels despite high blood phenylalanine levels.

Non-dietary treatments

Biopterin responsive phenylalanine hydroxylase deficiency

Since 1999 an increasing number of patients with mild or moderate PKU are reported to be able to decrease their plasma phenylalanine concentrations after a 6R-tetrahydrobiopterin (BH_4) challenge. It is estimated about two-thirds of all mild PKU patients are BH_4-responsive and thus can be potentially treated with BH_4 in pharmacological doses (up to 20 mg/kg/day in divided oral doses) instead of a low phenylalanine diet [47]. Large scale international trials on BH_4 supplementation in patients with PKU are being undertaken. In the future it may be recommended that BH_4 loading tests and mutation analysis is carried out routinely in all patients with PKU and that BH_4 is offered as an alternative treatment to diet in responsive patients.

Phenylalanine ammonia lyase enzyme substitution therapy

In 1980 it was shown that the plant enzyme phenylalanine ammonia lyase (PAL; EC 4.3.1.5) would survive in the gut long enough to degrade dietary phenylalanine in the gastrointestinal tract before being absorbed [48]. This enzyme converts phenylalanine to trans-cinnamic acid and a trace of ammonia. It does not require a co-factor. Currently, enzyme substitution therapy with PAL is under investigation. Subcutaneous administration of chemically modified PAL by pegylation results in a substantial lowering of plasma and significant reduction in brain phenylalanine levels in PKU mice [49]. It has not yet been tried in humans.

Genome targeted gene therapy

A novel technique for gene therapy has reduced blood phenylalanine concentrations to normal in PKU mice. A viral (bacteriophage) based procedure was used to deliver the functional mouse PAH gene to a specific region of the mouse genome After three applications, serum phenylalanine levels in all treated PKU mice were reduced to the normal range and remained stable thereafter. Their fur colour also changed from grey to black, indicating the reconstitution of melanin biosynthesis as a result of available tyrosine derived from reconstituted phenylalanine hydroxylation in the liver [50].

Dietary treatment

The aim of dietary treatment is to prevent excessive phenylalanine accumulation in the blood. Over the years, the duration of the diet has been the subject of much discussion and policy change. In the 1960s and 1970s, many PKU centres stopped diet as early as 4 or 8 years, when it was argued brain development would be substantially complete. A series of studies showing deterioration in IQ in children under 12 years of age [51,52] and neurological signs and neuropsychological deficits in problem solving in young adults has led to the recommendation of diet for life in the UK. There are still limited data on adult neurological functioning in PKU and controversy remains over the ideal blood phenylalanine concentration for individuals older than 12 years of age. Some countries' recommendations are more liberal than others. Some small studies suggest that relaxation of the strict diet in adolescence does not affect non-executive functions if blood phenylalanine concentrations remain <1200 µmol/L [27] whereas others demonstrate deterioration.

Principles of dietary management

The goals of dietary management in children are threefold:

- To prevent excessive phenylalanine accumulation by strict control of natural protein intake in combination with the administration of a phenylalanine free protein substitute
- To achieve normal growth and optimal nutritional status
- To ensure the diet is palatable, flexible and compatible with a modern day lifestyle

There are six key elements to dietary management:

1 Restriction of dietary phenylalanine to 25% or less of normal intakes to maintain blood phenylalanine concentrations within desirable PKU reference ranges in children. As phenylalanine comprises 4–6% of all dietary protein, high protein foods such as meat, fish, eggs, cheese, nuts and soya are not permitted in the diet of children with moderate or severe PKU.
2 Daily allocation of dietary phenylalanine from measured quantities of protein containing foods to provide phenylalanine requirements. These are given in the form of an exchange system, whereby one food can be exchanged or substituted for another of equivalent phenylalanine content.
3 Provision of a phenylalanine free protein substitute, with added tyrosine in order to meet nitrogen and tyrosine requirements.
4 Maintenance of a normal energy intake by encouraging liberal use of foods naturally low in phenylalanine and specially manufactured low protein foods such as bread, pasta and biscuits.
5 Provision of all vitamins and minerals to meet dietary requirements. These can either be added with the phenylalanine free protein substitute or as separate modules.
6 Attention to essential fatty acid status.

Phenylalanine exchanges

Phenylalanine tolerance is variable and depends on:

- Severity of disorder (genotype and residual enzyme activity)
- Target blood phenylalanine concentrations
- Compliance with protein substitute
- Energy intake
- Age and weight of the child

Children with moderate or severe PKU, maintaining blood phenylalanine within the target range of 120–360 µmol/L, usually tolerate 200–500 mg/day phenylalanine. Phenylalanine requirements are highest in early infancy. Acosta *et al.* [53] reported that to maintain blood phenylalanine concentrations at 60–324 µmol/L in infants, mean phenylalanine requirements were 0–3 months, 55 mg/kg/day; 4–6 months, 36 mg/kg/day; 7–9 months, 31 mg/kg/day; and 9–12 months, 27 mg/kg/day. Using indicator amino acid oxidation, Courtney-Martin *et al.* [54] suggested that mean phenylalanine requirement was 14 mg/kg/day for prepubertal children between the ages of 6–13 years with classical PKU. Generally, after the age of 1 year, there is a small continuous decline in phenylalanine intake per kg body weight per day in both males and females with PKU (Table 17.2). This parallels with decreasing growth rate and protein requirements. However, total daily phenylalanine requirements remain mainly unchanged on a strict diet [55].

In the UK, phenylalanine is given in the form of a 50-mg exchange system, whereby one food can be exchanged or substituted for another of equivalent phenylalanine content. This is quite different from systems used in other countries (e.g. in the USA and Australia a 15-mg phenylalanine exchange system is used and the phenylalanine content of all foods given in the diet is calculated) [56,57].

Table 17.2   Theoretical phenylalanine requirements.

Age	Approximate theoretical phenylalanine requirements (mg/kg/day)
0–3 months	50–60
4–6 months	40–50
7–12 months	30–40
1–2 years	25–30
2–3 years	20–25
4–6 years	15–25
7–8 years	15

Source: After Acosta *et al.* [53], Francis [125].

A 50-mg phenylalanine exchange is equivalent to about 1 g protein; when phenylalanine data analysis is not available it is acceptable to estimate phenylalanine content from protein analysis (with the exception of fruit and vegetables). It is useful to teach parents and patients to calculate 1-g protein exchanges directly from food packages and 'pocket size protein calculators' are helpful. Most fruit and vegetables only yield 30–40 mg phenylalanine per gram of protein so it is better to estimate exchange amounts directly from their phenylalanine analysis. The National Society for Phenylketonuria (NSPKU) Medical Advisory Panel have analysed and published the phenylalanine content of 172 foods, with an emphasis on fruit and vegetables [58].

The allocation of fruits and vegetables in the 50-mg phenylalanine exchange system has caused controversy and debate. Some, which contain between 50–100 mg/100 g phenylalanine (e.g. leeks, mushrooms and cauliflower), are allowed freely whereas others (broccoli, sprouts and yam) are counted as part of the phenylalanine exchange system (Table 17.3) [59]. There is evidence that all fruits and vegetables with a phenylalanine content <75 mg/100 g do not elevate plasma phenylalanine

Table 17.3   Protein and phenylalanine content of fruit and vegetables (51–100 mg phenylalanine/100 g).

Fruit and vegetables	Phenylalanine (mg/100 g) [58]	Protein (g/100 g) [126]	Current status
Phenylalanine 51–75 mg/100 g			
Raisins	51	2.1	Free
Banana	53	1.2	100 g/exchange
Leeks	53	0.7	Free
Sultanas	58	2.7	Free
Mushrooms	65	1.8	Free
Mange tout	66	3.2	30 g/exchange
Avocado	71	1.9	55 g/exchange
Mushrooms, fried	75	2.4	Free
Phenylalanine 76–100 mg/100 g			
Broccoli	76	3.1	30 g/exchange
Asparagus	84	3.4	1 serving/day
Cauliflower	89	2.9	Free
Brussels sprouts	92	2.9	35 g/exchange
Beansprouts	93	2.9	1 serving day
Yam	97	1.7	60 g/exchange

concentrations [60]. In addition, vegetables containing 76–100 mg/100 g phenylalanine do not increase plasma phenylalanine concentrations when eaten in small portions. However, the NSPKU Medical Advisory Committee does not yet advise that fruits and vegetables containing 51–100 mg/100 g phenylalanine be allowed as part of the free food system.

It is probably better to use foods such as potatoes, breakfast cereals, rice, baked beans and sweetcorn for phenylalanine exchanges for a child on a strict diet. Theoretically, any foods can be eaten as exchanges but high protein foods could only be accommodated in tiny amounts. Many young children do not understand phenylalanine exchanges and have difficulty in understanding why they cannot eat more of these foods. It may be unfair to accustom their taste to high protein foods and if they are used to eating ordinary bread, biscuits or chocolate for their phenylalanine allowances, low protein equivalent foods may appear less acceptable. A list of basic 50 mg phenylalanine exchanges is given in Table 17.4. Figures for the weight of food are rounded off to the nearest 5 g, although many families use electronic scales that are accurate to between 1 and 2 g. In the UK, dietitians have always recommended that all phenylalanine exchanges are weighed to ensure that natural protein allowance is not exceeded. However, many families find this an arduous and impractical recommendation. MacDonald *et al.* [61] reported it is possible with some foods to use validated household measures or photographs to determine phenylalanine exchanges instead of weighing (with an accuracy within 20% of the calculated weight of food for the exchanges), although further work is necessary to ensure it does not adversely affect blood phenylalanine control. Ideally, phenylalanine exchanges should be spread evenly throughout the day so that a load of dietary phenylalanine is not given at any one time. However, van Spronsen *et al.* [62] showed that plasma phenylalanine concentrations only increased above baseline by 10–18% when 50% of the total daily phenylalanine allowance was given at one time, and by 8–26% when 75% of the daily allowance was given at one time. This is in contrast to non-PKU individuals and may be because patients with PKU have a lower ratio of phenylalanine intake relative to plasma pool size [63].

Table 17.4   50 mg Phenylalanine food exchanges [59].

Dairy products	
Milk	30 mL
Single cream	40 mL
Double cream	60 mL
Soured cream	35 mL
Yoghurt	20 g
Vegetables	
Potatoes	
Boiled: boiled, mashed, jacket	80 g
Roast	55 g
Chips – frozen, fresh, oven, crinkle	45 g
Canned, new (drained weight)	100 g
Croquette	30 g
Instant mashed potato – dry powder	10 g
Baked beans	20 g
Bamboo shoots, raw	60 g
Peas – fresh, frozen and petit pois	25 g
Spinach, boiled	25 g
Sweetcorn kernels and baby corn – canned drained	35 g
Corn on the cob, raw or cooked weight	55 g
Length of cob	4 cm
Plain popped popcorn	10 g
Un-popped corn	10 g
Cereals	
Kellogg's Corn Flakes	15 g
Kellogg's Frosties	20 g
Kellogg's Rice Krispies	15 g
Sugar Puffs	15 g
Weetabix, Weetaflakes	10 g
Shredded Wheat	10 g
Ready Brek – Original	10 g
Puffed Wheat	5 g
Bran Flakes	10 g
Oatmeal (raw) and rolled oats	10 g
Rice (raw) white or brown	15 g
Rice (boiled) white or brown	45 g
Fruits	
Avocado pear, flesh only	55 g
Passion fruit	35 g

Protein substitutes

It is recommended that all children treated for PKU receive a protein substitute [16]. It supplies over 75% of protein requirements, usually in the form of L-amino acids and it also provides all tyrosine requirements. It was found as early as 1961 that protein substitute alone significantly decreased phenylalanine concentrations in three people with

PKU [64]. There is now evidence that the quantity, composition, diurnal distribution, acceptability and administration of the protein substitute could influence blood phenylalanine control.

Requirements

The optimal dose of protein substitute has been the subject of much international debate. In the UK, a high protein substitute intake is favoured and it is recommended that children under 2 years of age should take at least 3 g/kg body weight/day of amino acids; and those over 2 years take 2 g/kg body weight/day [16]. Although there is debate regarding protein substitute requirement, generous quantities of protein substitute should:

- Lead to increased nitrogen retention
- Improve phenylalanine tolerance
- Help prevent an imbalance of amino acid transport across the blood–brain barrier

MacDonald *et al.* [65] documented that higher doses of protein substitute were associated with better blood phenylalanine control although there was considerable variability between subjects. In addition, it has been demonstrated that when total protein intake from the protein substitute increases phenylalanine tolerance improves [66,67] and may also be important in optimising growth in head circumference [68].

Guidelines for the total protein requirements per kilogram body weight (i.e. protein from phenylalanine exchanges and protein substitute) are given in Table 17.5.

Table 17.5   Guidelines for total protein requirements in phenylketonuria (PKU) and other amino acid disorders.

Age (years)	Total protein* (g/kg body weight/day)
0–2	3.0
3–5	2.5
6–10	2.0
11–14	1.5
>14	1.0 (maximum 80 g/day)

* For example, in PKU total protein = protein equivalent is from protein substitute and phenylalanine exchanges (natural protein).

Timing of protein substitute intake

It is better to give protein substitute in small frequent doses, three to four times daily, spread evenly throughout the day, than once or twice daily [69]. Theoretically, it is better given with some of the phenylalanine allowance; carbohydrate added to the protein substitute may reduce leucine oxidation and increase net protein synthesis [70]. There is evidence that infrequent administration of large doses of protein substitute increases nitrogen excretion as well as oxidative utilisation of amino acids so this practice is not advocated. In nine patients with PKU and one with hyperphenylalaninaemia, protein substitute was taken in one or two doses on day 1, and on day 2 in three equal doses with meals. In eight patients excretion of nitrogen decreased from 6.3–12.4 g/day to 4.7–10.8 g/day when the total amount of amino acid mixture was given in smaller and frequent doses [71].

Types of protein substitute

Protein substitutes are presented as amino acid powders, capsules, tablets, bars and liquids and may contain added carbohydrate, fat, vitamins and minerals. The many types and features of these protein substitutes designed for children over the age of 1 year are given in Table 17.6. Compliance with protein substitutes has been a major issue [72,73] but the better range, taste, volume, presentation and convenience of current preparations has proved popular with patients and it is hoped there will be better acceptance and improved adherence. Clinical trials have proven the majority to be safe and efficacious.

Administration of protein substitute

Protein substitutes can be taken as a drink, paste, added to food, eaten like a chocolate bar or as tablets. There are several points that should be considered:

- Protein substitutes are hyperosmolar (e.g. XP Maxamaid in a 1 : 5 dilution has a osmolality of 968 mOsm/kg H_2O). If they are given in a small volume of water or as a paste they may cause abdominal pain, diarrhoea or constipation. An additional drink of water should always be

Table 17.6 Protein substitutes: presentation and composition.

Type	Amino acid (g/100 g)	Protein (g/100 g)	Energy (kcal/100 g)	Energy (kJ/100 g)	Added CHO (g/100 g)	Added fat (g/100 g)	Added Vits/mins	Advantages	Disadvantages	Presentation	Supporting research studies
L-amino acids											
PK Aid 4 (SHS)	93.2	77.8	326	1387	Nil	Nil	Nil	• Flexible • Low bulk • Easy to prepare	• No CHO • Poor palatability • Compliance with separate vitamin/mineral supplement poor	Powder (400 g tub)	
Aminogran Food Supplement (UCB Pharma)	97.2	–	400	1675	Nil	Nil	Nil			Powder (500 g tub)	
Phlexy 10 Drink Mix (SHS)	50	41.7	343	1456	44	Nil	Nil	• Flavoured • Palatable • Convenient • Moderate bulk • Flexible	• No added vitamins/Minerals	20 g sachets (powder) Available in apple and blackcurrant, citrus burst, tropical surprise	Shown to result in better compliance and improved phe control when compared with other protein substitutes [127, 128]
L-amino acids with added vitamins/minerals but minimal carbohydrate											
Milupa PKU2 (Milupa) Age >1 year	80.1	66.8	300	1275	8.2	Nil	Some	• Low bulk • Age specific • Easy to prepare	• Inflexible • Does not contain all vitamins/minerals • Minimal CHO • Poor palatability • Poor compliance • Unsuitable for all age groups	Powder (500 g)	
Milupa PKU 3 (Milupa) Age >8 years	81.6	68	288	1222	3.9	Nil	Some			Powder (500 g)	

continued on p. 318

Table 17.6 (Cont'd)

Type	Amino acid (g/100 g)	Protein (g/100 g)	Energy (kcal/100 g)	Energy (kJ/100 g)	Added CHO (g/100 g)	Added fat (g/100 g)	Added Vits/mins	Advantages	Disadvantages	Presentation	Supporting research studies
PKU Express (Vitaflo) Age >8 years	72	60	302	1260	15	<0.5	Yes	• Low bulk • Age specific • Easy to prepare	• Minimal CHO	25 g sachets (powder) Unflavoured, orange, lemon, tropical fruit	Acceptable, well tolerated, acceptable blood phe control, helped independence [129]
Lophlex (SHS) (unflavoured) Age >8 years		72	326	1384	9	0.2	Yes	• Low bulk • Age specific • Easy to prepare • No electrolytes	• Minimal CHO	28 g sachets Unflavoured, orange, berry	
L-amino acids with added CHO/vitamins/minerals											
XP Maxamaid (SHS) Age 1–8 years	30	25	300	1260	51	Nil	Yes	• Age specific • Easy to prepare • Contains all added vitamins/minerals	• Inflexible • Bulky • Poor palatability • Poor compliance • Unsuitable for all age groups	Powder (500 g)	Growth normal [130]
XP Maxamum (SHS) Age >8 years	47	39	290	1226	34	Nil	Yes			Powder (500 g)	XP Maxamaid associated with low ferritin concentrations [98]
PKU gel (Vitaflo) Age 1–10 years	50	42	342	1428	43	<0.5	Yes	• Age specific • Easy to prepare • Contains all added vitamins/minerals • Designed to be made as a paste • Moderate bulk	• Inflexible • Unsuitable for all age groups	20 g sachets Unflavoured, orange, raspberry	Produces normal growth, good phe control, normal nutritional biochemistry, reduces volume of protein substitute required [131]

Table 11.8 (cont.)

continued on p. 320

Type	Amino acid (g/100 g)	Protein (g/100 g)	Energy (kcal/100 g)	Energy (kJ/100 g)	Added CHO (g/100 g)	Added fat (g/100 g)	Added Vits/mins	Advantages	Disadvantages	Presentation	Supporting research studies
L-amino acids with added CHO/fat/vitamins/minerals											
Minaphlex (SHS) Age 1–10 years	35	29	390	1639	38	13.5	Yes	● Age specific ● Easy to prepare ● Contains all added vitamins/minerals	● Inflexible ● Bulky ● Poor palatability ● Poor compliance ● Unsuitable for all age groups	29 g sachets Unflavoured and pineapple/ Vanilla	Increases plasma and red cell ethrocyte α-linolenic acid levels [93]
Novel presentations											
Bars Phlexy 10 bar (SHS) Age > 8 years	23.8	19.8	371	1562	48.8	10.7	Nil	● Palatable ● Convenient	● Bulky ● No vitamins/minerals ● High energy ● Product fatigue	Bar (42 g)	Bars been shown to score highly on acceptability rating but did not improve compliance [73]
Capsules Phlexy 10 Capsules (SHS) Age > 8 years	50	16.7	176	747	2.3	Nil	Nil	● Convenient ● No mixing	● Need large numbers ● No vitamins/minerals	Capsules (0.5 g amino acid per capsule)	Acceptable to older patients Shown to decrease phe levels, increase tyrosine levels in patients with PKU [132, 133]
Tablets Aminogran PKU tablets (UCB Pharma) Age >8 years	97.2 per 100 tablets	– per 100 tablets	400 per 100 tablets	1675 per 100 tablets	Nil per 100 tabs	Nil per 100 tablets	Nil		● Suitable for older patients only ● No vitamins/minerals ● Need large numbers	Tablets (1.0 g amino acid per tablet)	
Tablets Phlexy 10 tablets (SHS) Age >8 years	100 per 100 tablets	83.3 per 100 tablets	380 per 100 tablets	1614 per 100 tablets	7.3 per 100 tabs	2 per 100 tablets	Nil	● No mixing ● Convenient	● Suitable for patients >8 years ● No vitamins/minerals ● Need large numbers	Tablets (1.0 g amino acid per tablet) (75 tablets per container)	As above

Table 17.6 (*Cont'd*)

Type	Amino acid (g/100 g)	Protein (g/100 g)	Energy (kcal/100 g)	Energy (kJ/100 g)	Added CHO (g/100 g)	Added fat (g/100 g)	Added Vits/mins	Advantages	Disadvantages	Presentation	Supporting research studies
Liquid Easiphen (SHS)	per 250 mL	per 250 mL	per 250 mL	per 250 mL	per 250 mL	per 250 mL		● Convenient ● No mixing	● Need large volume ● Quite viscous ● 1 carton = approx 17 g protein. Not easily compatible with adult protein substitute requirements	Available in 250 mL cartons Forest berries, grapefruit	
Age >8 years	20	16.8	163	688	12.8	5.0	Yes				
Liquid Orange or Purple PKU Cooler 15 (Vitaflo)	per 130 mL	per 130 mL	per 130 mL	per 130 mL	per 130 mL	per 130 mL		● No mixing ● Convenient	● Suitable for patients >8 years	Available in 130 mL pouches ACBS prescribable	Very acceptable and easy to take for older patients with PKU [122]
Age >8 years	18	15	92	386	7.8	Trace	Yes				
Lophlex LQ (SHS)	per 125 mL	per 125 mL	per 125 mL	per 125 mL	per 125 mL	per 125 mL		● No mixing ● Convenient	● Suitable for patients >8 years	Available in 125 mL pouches ACBS prescribable Orange, citrus, berry	
Age >8 years	25	20	115	490	8.8	Nil added	Yes				

CHO, carbohydrate; phe = phenylalanine; Vits/mins, vitamins and minerals.

given with protein substitute if it is diluted with less water than recommended.

- When powders are prepared in a drink format, the tyrosine is hydrophobic and so tends to form an insoluble layer. The children often refer to this as the 'froth' and either have it skimmed from the drink surface or leave it in the bottom of the cup. It is important to explain the importance of tyrosine to carers so they ensure all of the preparation is consumed.
- Protein substitute can be given as a paste. A small amount of water is added to each dose of protein substitute to make a thick paste or gel. Paste is a successful way of administering protein substitute but it needs to be introduced in this format early in a child's life. One to two teaspoons prior to solids is a useful way to accustom a young child to the taste in the weaning period. The contribution to overall nutrient intake should be considered.
- Ideally, all protein substitutes should be prepared immediately prior to use. It is important paste receives minimal handling, as excessive mixing may release sulphur containing amino acids.
- Giving protein substitute cold from a covered beaker will help disguise the smell.

Hints for taking protein substitute

- Always treat protein substitute as a medicine
- Establish a time routine – always give at the same time each day
- Always supervise
- Be firm, but give positive encouragement
- Do not allow excuses
- Be consistent
- If taken with meals, try and give before food to ensure it is taken

Large neutral amino acids

Large neutral amino acid (LNAA) supplementation has been found to reduce brain phenylalanine levels despite consistently high blood phenylalanine levels [74,75]. In non-compliant adults, this may help to protect the brain from acute toxic effects of phenylalanine. At the blood–brain barrier phenylalanine shares a transporter with other LNAAs (e.g. tyrosine, tryptophan, leucine, isoleucine, histidine, methionine, threonine) and they compete with phenylalanine for transport across the blood–brain barrier. A number of trials are currently underway to investigate this treatment for untreated adults and non-compliant adolescents. Although LNAAs have been used for patients aged 15 years and older in Denmark since 1985, further work is needed on the long term efficacy and safety of LNAAs in PKU.

Tyrosine

Tyrosine is an essential amino acid in PKU because of the limited hydroxylation of phenylalanine to tyrosine. It is important for the biosynthesis of the brain neurotransmitters epinephrine, norepinephrine and dopamine, although tyrosine supplementation has not consistently been found to improve neuropsychologic function in PKU [76]. Nevertheless, to ensure an adequate intake, the PKU MRC Working Group suggested that protein substitutes should supply 100–120 mg/kg/day tyrosine [16]. All Advisory Committee on Borderline Substances (ACBS) prescribable protein substitutes are supplemented with tyrosine and should supply this amount of tyrosine providing adequate protein substitute is given to meet protein requirements. Extra tyrosine may need to be given during pregnancy.

Diurnal variations in tyrosine concentrations are wide. Fasting blood tyrosine concentrations may be low but then high immediately following protein substitute intake [77]. Therefore, in PKU tyrosine supplementation produces marked but non-sustained increases in plasma tyrosine concentrations, with a calculated brain influx that often remains suboptimal. This could explain the lack of consistent neuropsychological benefit with tyrosine supplementation because of failure to achieve adequate levels of tyrosine in the brain [78]. There are suggestions that the recommended tyrosine intake in PKU may be over-estimated [77,79].

Low phenylalanine free foods

Energy requirements are normal in PKU [79]. Ensuring adequate energy intake is particularly important for children with severe PKU. The

Table 17.7   Fruits and vegetables allowed freely (phenylalanine content <50 mg/100 g).

Fruits
Most types (fresh, tinned, raw or cooked in sugar)
Apples, apricots, bilberries, blackberries, cherries, clementines, cranberries, currants (black, red and dried), damsons, figs (fresh *not* dried), gooseberries, grapes, grapefruit, greengages, guavas, lemons, limes, loganberries, lychees, kiwi fruit, kumquats, mandarins, mango, melon, water melon, medlars, mulberries, nectarines, olives, oranges, paw paw, peaches (*not* dried), pears, pineapple, plums, pomegranate, prunes, quince, raspberries, rhubarb, satsumas, strawberries, tangerines, mixed peel, angelica, glace cherries and ginger

Vegetables
Artichoke, aubergine, French beans, beetroot, cabbage, capers, carrots, cassava, celeriac, celery, chicory, courgettes, cucumber, endive, fennel, garlic, gherkin, karela, kohl rabi, lady's finger (okra), leek, lettuce, marrow, mooli, mustard and cress, onion, pickled onion, parsley and all herbs, pak choi, parsnip, peppers, pumpkin, radish, squash: acorn, butternut, spaghetti squash, swede, sweet potato, tomato, turnip, watercress, water chestnuts

effect of energy on protein utilisation and nitrogen balance is well recognised [80] and Illsinger *et al.* [81] demonstrated that phenylalanine concentrations decreased with energy supplementation in PKU. The majority of energy is provided in the form of carbohydrate with only 20–25% energy from fat [82].

There are a number of foods that are low in phenylalanine so can be eaten without restriction. These foods include:

- *Fruits and vegetables:* containing <50 mg phenylalanine/100 g (Table 17.7).
- *Fats:* butter, margarine, lard, dripping and vegetable oils.
- *Sugars and starches:* cornflour, custard powder, sago, tapioca, sugar, glucose, jam, honey, marmalade, golden syrup, treacle and sweets containing <0.3 g protein/100 g.
- *Miscellaneous:* vegetarian jelly, agar-agar, salt, pepper, herbs, spices and vinegar; tomato and brown sauce; baking powder, bicarbonate of soda and cream of tartar; food essences and colouring; gravy mixes containing <0.3 g

protein/100 mL; cook-in sauces containing <1.0 g protein/100 g.
- *Drinks:* squash, lemonade, cola drinks and fruit juice free of aspartame. Tea, coffee, tonic water, soda water and mineral water.
- *Low protein special foods:* a selection of low protein breads, flour mixes, pizza bases, pasta, biscuits, egg replacers and chocolate substitutes are available (see Appendix 17.1). Other low protein specialist products contain some phenylalanine (e.g. low protein cheese substitutes, snack pots, burger mixes, milk replacements) but can be incorporated into the diet as part of the 50-mg phenylalanine exchange system. The ACBS approves the vast majority for prescription on FP10.

It is important to introduce a variety of low phenylalanine foods into the diet as early as possible to give variety and adequate energy to meet estimated average requirements. The range of suitable foods that can be purchased either from supermarkets, health food stores, via the Internet or are available on ACBS prescription has greatly increased over recent years. The quality of specialist dietary products has improved and some of the newer low protein flours and cake mixes are simple to use and the cooking results are more consistent. From the day of diagnosis it is important to maintain a positive outlook with families. In recent years the diet has become easier to adhere to.

The following guidelines will maximise the use of low protein foods in the diet:

- Issue a picture book of all foods allowed so that parents, children, siblings and extended family can easily identify 'free' foods.
- Give extensive, but simple, snack and mealtime ideas.
- Teach parents and children how to interpret food labels so they can fully utilise all 'free' foods on the market.
- Issue families, schools and nurseries with PKU recipe books, recipe cards and cookery DVDs.
- Offer low protein cookery workshops, demonstrations and cookery helplines for parents, children and the wider family.
- Encourage parents and patients to support each other. They may recipe swap recipe ideas, cooking tips and practical issues.

Fat

Cholesterol

Many patients have low cholesterol levels [82–86] and there is a hypothesis that high plasma phenylalanine levels cause inhibition of cholesterogenesis. The low cholesterol content of the diet itself is likely to decrease serum cholesterol levels [86].

Essential fatty acids

Evidence suggests that children with PKU have reduced concentrations of arachidonic acid (AA) and docosahexaenoic acid (DHA) in plasma and membrane phospholipids when compared to controls. A strict low phenylalanine diet is also low in fat and α-linolenic acid [87], AA and devoid of any sources of eicosapentaenoic acid (EPA) and DHA. The extent to which long chain polyunsaturated fatty acids (LCPs) can be synthesised from the parent fatty acids (linoleic acid and α-linolenic acid) in PKU is debatable. Although many professionals would agree that fatty acid supplementation is desirable, it is unknown if this is better provided in the form of essential fatty acids (EFAs) or LCPs.

There have been various attempts to improve the fatty acid status of children with PKU and some studies have looked at the impact on visual function. In infants, a dietary supply of LCPs added to the phenylalanine free protein substitute is associated with lower reduction in DHA levels in later infancy [88]. In children aged 5–10 years, fish oil supplementation improves n-3 LCP status and visual function [89], although higher blood n-3 LCP concentrations than control groups have been documented [90]. Agostoni et al. [91] investigated the effects of a 12-month supplementation with LCPs. The daily dosage of the supplement was calculated to provide 0.3–0.5% of the daily energy requirements as LCPs. A balanced dietary supplementation with LCPs was associated with an increase of the DHA pool and improved visual function. However, a follow-up trial investigating this group of patients 3 years after the patients had stopped supplementation with LCPs found there were no differences in the concentrations of blood AA and DHA [92]. In a randomised controlled trial, Cleary et al. [93] described the use of a protein substitute containing EFAs rather than LCPs in 53 children aged 1–10 years, which resulted in higher increases in median DHA concentrations in erythrocyte phospholipids.

Vitamin and minerals

Reports of vitamin and mineral deficiency are common. They include selenium deficiency [94–96], low ferritin concentrations [97,98], low vitamin B_{12} concentrations [99,100] and decreased bone mineral density [101] brought about by the following:

- Failure of protein substitute or vitamin and mineral supplement to contain a specific micronutrient (e.g. selenium) leading to biochemical selenium deficiency [102,103]. The only reported clinical symptom is a dysrythmic ventricular tachycardia in a 9-month-old infant [104].
- Low bioavailability of micronutrients added to supplements (e.g. low ferritin concentrations despite normal haemoglobin and mean corpuscular concentrations) [60] and adequate dietary iron supplementation. Similar results were reported by Bohles et al. [105].
- Non-compliance with either protein substitute with added vitamin and minerals or separate vitamin and mineral supplement. Low vitamin B_{12} concentrations are commonly reported in older teenagers and young adults, attributed to failure to take prescribed supplements.

There is also a suggestion that elevated blood phenylalanine concentrations may alter the metabolism of iron, copper and zinc [106] and may adversely affect bone status in PKU mice [107].

Vitamin and mineral supplementation

Comprehensive vitamin and mineral supplementation is added to some protein substitutes (e.g. Minaphlex, PKU Gel); provided adequate quantities of protein substitute are taken no additional supplementation should be necessary. Other protein substitutes (e.g. PK Aid 4, Aminogran Food Supplement, Phlexy 10 drink mix), tablets and bars contain no vitamins and minerals so complete supplementation is necessary. Others contain only partial vitamin and mineral supplementation (e.g. PKU 2 and PKU 3). There are no ideal supplements so complete vitamin and mineral supplementation may be difficult to achieve. The most useful products are as follow.

Paediatric Seravit

A powdered vitamin, trace element and mineral mixture containing only trace amounts of sodium and potassium on a carbohydrate base; designed for infants and children; unflavoured and pineapple flavour; recommended dose dependent on age, body weight and dietary vitamin and mineral intake. Suggested daily dose:

- 0–6 months: 14 g
- 6–12 months: 17 g
- 1–7 years: 17–25 g
- 7–14 years: 25–35 g

Paediatric Seravit may be given as a drink (flavoured with suitable squashes, natural fruit juice or milk shake syrups) or as a paste with extra drinks given at the same time. It is better to give in 2–3 doses throughout the day. It is unpalatable.

Forceval Junior vitamin and mineral capsules (with additional calcium)

A hard, gelatin capsule containing 22 vitamins, minerals and trace minerals; does not contain calcium, sodium, potassium, chloride and only small quantities of magnesium; should not be taken on an empty stomach; not recommended for children <5 years of age because of difficulty in swallowing the hard capsules. Recommended daily dose for children >5 years of age is two capsules.

Although it is relatively easy to give an aspartame free calcium supplement it is difficult to supplement with extra magnesium and phosphorus. No extra sodium and potassium supplement should be necessary for older children, but intake of all nutrients should be carefully monitored. In older children, one adult Forceval vitamin and mineral capsule daily can be taken.

Phlexy-Vits

A comprehensive vitamin and mineral supplement designed for people 11 years of age and over, Phlexy-Vits does not contain sodium or potassium, is available in two presentations (powder and tablets). The powder can be mixed with water, fruit juice or aspartame free squashes; better to consume immediately after mixing. Recommended daily dose is one 7-g sachet or five tablets.

Monitoring of vitamin and mineral status

Annual testing of the biochemical and haematological vitamin and mineral status (e.g. haemoglobin, ferritin, selenium, zinc and vitamin A) together with a dietary assessment is recommended. In particular, vitamin B_{12} concentrations should be monitored in non-compliant teenagers and adults [108].

Aspartame

Aspartame (E951) is an artificial sweetener which is derived from a dipeptide composed of phenylalanine and the methyl ester of aspartic acid. It is commonly added to squashes, fizzy drinks, chewing gums, sweets, desserts, tabletop sweeteners and even some savoury snacks (e.g. flavoured crisps). It should be avoided in PKU. In addition, aspartame can also be found combined with another sweetener called acesulfame K and foods containing this will be identified as salt of aspartame and acesulfame K (E962) on food labels. This should also be avoided.

Monitoring the diet

Guidelines for desirable blood phenylalanine concentrations in PKU

Since the early 1960s it has been policy to maintain blood phenylalanine concentrations slightly above normal concentrations of 30–70 µmol/L [109–111] to avoid the risk of phenylalanine deficiency as there is evidence this is harmful to intellectual, neurological and nutritional status [28,112]. A MRC Working Group has published a set of UK monitoring guidelines [16]. Recommendations for treatment range blood phenylalanine concentrations (compared with recommendations from Germany and USA) are given in Table 17.8. Other recommendations are as follow:

- Frequency of blood phenylalanine monitoring:
  children 0–4 years: weekly
  children 5–10 years: fortnightly
  over 11 years: monthly
- Blood phenylalanine concentrations should be taken at a standard time each day, preferably before the first dose of protein substitute in the

Table 17.8   Target blood phenylalanine blood concentrations in phenylketonuria.

Age (years)	Target blood phenylalanine concentrations (μmol/L)		
	UK	Germany	USA
0–4	120–360	40–240	120–360
5–10	120–480	40–240	120–360
11–12	120–700	40–900	120–360
Adolescents/adults	120–700	40–1200	120–360

Source: Adapted from Blau and Burgard [134].

morning when blood phenylalanine concentrations are usually at their highest [113]. Blood levels may vary by 150 μmol/L/day.

Parents should be taught how to collect heel or thumb prick blood samples at home by a specialist nurse. Blood samples are posted to the hospital and analysed by tandem mass spectrometry, fluorimetry, high pressure liquid chromatography or, more rarely, the Guthrie bacterial inhibition technique. Ideally, the dietitian should contact the parents and patients with blood results to discuss their interpretation and instruct on any dietary changes.

Possible explanation for high phenylalanine concentrations

A high blood phenylalanine concentration should always be discussed with the parents or patient before reducing the phenylalanine intake as high phenylalanine concentrations may be brought about for many reasons:

- Inadequate intake of protein substitute either because of poor compliance or inadequate quantity prescribed
- Catabolism caused by infection, trauma or surgery
- Too much dietary phenylalanine: too much prescribed, excess eaten inadvertently or poor dietary compliance

Phenylalanine intake should be decreased by 25–50 mg/day if blood phenylalanine concentrations are consistently high and there appears no other explanation for this. Phenylalanine intake

should not be decreased below a total of three exchanges (150 mg) daily.

Possible explanation for low phenylalanine concentrations

- Inadequate prescription of dietary phenylalanine
- Failure to eat all phenylalanine exchanges
- Vomiting
- Anabolic phase, following an intercurrent infection

Prolonged inadequate intake of phenylalanine, especially in infants, may result in a skin rash (commonly seen around the nappy area) and growth failure. If the early morning blood concentration is <120 μmol/L, dietary phenylalanine should be increased by 25–50 mg/day.

Feeding different age groups with PKU

Infants

All infants with blood phenylalanine concentrations consistently >400 μmol/L are treated for PKU. However, the initial treatment will depend upon the diagnostic phenylalanine concentration.

Phenylalanine concentration >1000 μmol/L
Protein substitute (phenylalanine free formula) is given only. The phenylalanine source (breast or infant formula) is temporarily stopped. This is to achieve a rapid fall in plasma phenylalanine concentrations; a decrease of 300–600 μmol/L/day is normal during this period. The protein substitute should be given on demand and a minimal intake of 150 mL/kg/day should be encouraged. When concentrations are below 1000 μmol/L, either breast milk should be introduced or 50 mg/kg/day phenylalanine from formula feeds. It is important that the breast feeding mother is encouraged to regularly express breast milk when breast feeding is temporarily stopped. She should be supplied with a breast feeding pump and also needs good support by her midwife during this time. Ideally, plasma phenylalanine concentrations should be measured daily to monitor the rate of decrease and prevent possible phenylalanine deficiency.

Phenylalanine concentrations 600–1000 µmol/L
Not necessary to stop the phenylalanine source. From the time of diagnosis, either breast feeds are given in combination with a protein substitute or approximately 50 mg/kg/day phenylalanine from infant formula and a protein substitute.

Phenylalanine concentrations 400–600 µmol/L
Phenylalanine concentrations should be monitored weekly to ensure phenylalanine concentrations are consistently >400 µmol/L before dietary treatment is started. Minimal restriction of phenylalanine may be all that is necessary but depends on the individual baby. Dietary restriction of phenylalanine should always be given in combination with a protein substitute.

Breast feeding

Demand breast feeding was first reported in 1981 [114] and there is now wide experience. Successful breast feeding in 74 of 83 babies born with PKU in Norway has been reported [115]. Dietary treatment commenced between 5 and 33 days of age (mean 14 days). It took a mean of 8 days to normalise phenylalanine concentrations. Breast feeding duration was anything from 4 weeks to 16 months; growth was within normal parameters. In Turkey a further 86 breast fed babies with PKU has been reported [116].

Breast feeding is easy to maintain, should be always be encouraged and breast milk has several advantages:

- It is low in phenylalanine (46 mg/100 mL compared with approximately 60 mg/100 mL in whey based infant formula)
- It contains LCPs
- It is convenient and reduces the number of bottles that need to be given
- It helps establish good mother–infant bonding
- It gives the mother some control over the feeding process

Breast feeding the baby with PKU is based on the principle of giving a measured volume of a phenylalanine free infant formula before each feed, so reducing the baby's appetite and hence suckling, thus reducing the amount of breast milk taken and therefore phenylalanine intake. Babies can still feed on demand, varying the quantity of feeds from day to day provided the phenylalanine free formula (i.e. the protein substitute in this case) is always given first. Blood phenylalanine concentrations are used to determine the volume of phenylalanine free infant formula to be given. The quantity at each feed will vary according to plasma phenylalanine concentrations, age of diagnosis and frequency of breast feeds. In infants presenting with phenylalanine concentrations >1000 µmol/L, at each feed 40–60 mL phenylalanine free formula is usually given. Once blood phenylalanine concentrations are stabilised within target ranges, if phenylalanine concentrations then increase >360 µmol/L, the phenylalanine free formula is increased by 10 mL at each feed to decrease the volume of breast milk taken at that time. If phenylalanine concentrations are <120 µmol/L, the phenylalanine free formula is decreased by 10 mL per feed to increase the quantity of breast milk taken at each feed.

Initially, the mother will need much reassurance and support as she may feel the baby is taking little breast milk and may be slow to recommence suckling. Plasma phenylalanine concentrations should be checked twice weekly until they have stabilised and the baby weighed weekly. Breast feeding can continue as long as mother and baby desire.

Bottle feeding

Once phenylalanine concentrations are <1000 µmol/L, 50 mg/kg/day phenylalanine from normal infant formula should be introduced (Table 17.9). The total daily amount of calculated infant formula is divided between 6–7 feeds. Traditionally it is recommended that normal infant formula is given first, followed by the phenylalanine free infant formula (i.e. protein substitute) to ensure the entire phenylalanine source is given. The total volume provided by the two formulas should equate to a feed volume of 150–200 mL/kg/day (see worked example in Table 17.10). Providing the calculated volume of normal infant formula and infant protein substitute is consumed, the order of the feeds is not important. However, some infants may refuse the infant protein substitute, preferring the taste of normal infant formula. By giving the normal infant formula first it may be more difficult to ensure adequate volumes of protein substitute are taken. It is essential to give the infant protein substitute and the source of phenylalanine at the

Table 17.9 Phenylalanine content of whey based infant formulas.

Type	Amount equivalent to 50 mg phenylalanine exchange (mL)	Protein content per 100 mL (g)	Phenylalanine content per 100 mL (mg)
Premium (Cow & Gate)	90	1.4	53
Aptamil First (Milupa)	90	1.4	56
Farley's First (Farley's)	80	1.45	63
SMA Gold (SMA Nutrition)	90	1.5	59

Table 17.10 Worked example of daily feeding plan for 4 kg infant on infant formula having 50 mg phe/kg.

Total fluid intake 150 mL/kg/day (= 600 mL/day)
90 mL Cow & Gate Premium = 50 mg phenylalanine
Total number of feeds: 6 daily

Phenylalanine requirement
50 mg/kg = 4 × 50 mg = 200 mg phe/day
Daily formula intake from Cow & Gate Premium = 360 mL/day
= approximately 200 mg phe

Protein substitute
Total fluid requirement = 600 mL
Fluid from normal formula = 360 mL. Deficit = 240 mL
Therefore feed deficit made up with phenylalanine free protein substitute (e.g. XP Analog LCP = 240 mL/day)

Feeding plan
1st feed 60 mL × 6 feeds of Cow & Gate Premium
2nd feed 40 mL × 6 feeds of XP Analog LCP

phe, phenylalanine.

same feed to deliver the correct balance of all essential amino acids. The infant protein substitute is usually given in a separate bottle to the normal infant formula, but it is possible to mix them in the same bottle provided all the feed is taken.

When phenylalanine from food exchanges is introduced and the quantity of normal formula is reduced, the protein substitute may taste less acceptable and the infant may be reluctant to take it.

The quantity of infant formula is adjusted by 25–50 mg/day phenylalanine according to plasma phenylalanine concentrations. If plasma phenylalanine concentrations are <120 µmol/L the infant formula is increased. If the plasma phenylalanine is >360 µmol/L, the daily dietary phenylalanine is decreased by 25–50 mg, providing the infant is well and drinking adequate quantities of protein substitute. Initially, phenylalanine concentrations should be checked twice weekly until they have stabilised.

Infant protein substitutes

- *XP Analog LCP:* a phenylalanine free, otherwise nutritionally complete infant formula containing LCPs (AA and DHA); maintains DHA and AA concentrations in red blood cell membrane phospholipids closer to that of breast fed infants compared with non-supplemented formula [117]; 72 kcal (300 kJ)/100 mL and 1.95 g/100 mL of protein as L-amino acids; 1 scoop + 30 mL water.
- *XP Analog:* a phenylalanine free, otherwise nutritionally complete infant formula; 72 kcal (300 kJ)/100 mL and 1.95 g/100 mL of protein as L-amino acids; 1 scoop + 30 mL water.

Introduction of solids

Solids should be introduced around 17–26 weeks of age. It may be difficult to introduce variety and texture if weaning is delayed.

Start with 1–2 teaspoons low phenylalanine foods ('free' foods) such as homemade or commercial purée fruits or vegetables (protein content: 0.5 g/100 g or less). Useful first weaning foods include apple, pear, carrot, cauliflower, sweet potato. Encourage parents to introduce a wide variety of homemade weaning foods in the early weaning process.

Low phenylalanine weaning foods are usually offered after the breast or formula feeds so as not to inhibit appetite for the phenylalanine source and protein substitute. The intake of infant protein substitute should be carefully monitored to ensure this is not decreased.

Many low phenylalanine weaning foods have a low energy density so higher energy weaning foods should be encouraged including homemade low protein rusks or Aminex low protein rusks mixed with cooled boiled water to a smooth paste; low protein Promin Hot Breakfast cereal; low protein Promin pasta meal added to savoury foods; and custard made with diluted liquid Duocal or Calogen. Weaning foods are gradually increased to 3 times daily.

Once the infant is taking 8–12 teaspoons at a time, 50 mg phenylalanine exchanges from food are given instead of the equivalent quantity of infant formula or a breast feed. Introduce one 50-mg phenylalanine food exchange at a time, gradually replacing all breast or formula feeds with equivalent phenylalanine from solid food. Foods such as purée potato, peas, yoghurt, ordinary rusks, baby rice or vegetable-based weaning foods in jars or tins are useful phenylalanine exchange foods. Moderate protein powdered cheese or white sauce mixes can be introduced as part of the phenylalanine exchange allowance from the age of 6 months.

Gradually introduce more texture and lumpier food from 6 months. Introduce breakfast cereals such as Weetabix and Ready Brek for phenylalanine exchanges.

Finger foods such as low protein fingers of toast, soft fruits such as bananas, strawberries and peaches, soft vegetable sticks, fingers of low protein cheese (as phenylalanine exchanges), homemade low protein bread sticks, low protein rusks and biscuits can be given from 7 months of age. The infant protein substitute or a milk replacement such as diluted liquid Duocal can be given from a feeder beaker at 7 months of age.

From 9 months, introduce low pasta dishes, sandwiches made with low protein bread, chopped low protein burgers or sausages, finger exchange foods such as potato products (e.g. mini-waffles, 'Smiley faces' and other potato shapes) (Table 17.11).

Introduction of second stage protein substitute

As solids are introduced, the infant may be unable to drink more protein substitute so from the age of 5–6 months will struggle to meet total protein requirements from infant protein substitute and phenylalanine exchanges alone. It becomes necessary to introduce a more concentrated protein substitute in small quantities. This can be in the form of a non-supplemented L-amino acid mixture (e.g. PK Aid 4 or Aminogran Food Supplement powder) or a vitamin and mineral supplemented protein substitute such as unflavoured Minaphlex or PKU Gel. These can be mixed with a small quantity of water and given as paste before meals. These products are hyperosmolar and should be given with extra fluid. They should be cautiously introduced and the effect on stools closely monitored. Additional trace minerals and vitamins may need to be given with unsupplemented amino acid mixtures if the volume of infant protein substitute is <500 mL/day. The intake of vitamins and minerals from supplemented protein substitutes should be carefully monitored: 10 g Minaphlex provides 2.9 g protein equivalent, 3.0 mmol sodium, 2.5 mmol potassium and a vitamin and mineral profile that is slightly more concentrated than 100 mL XP Analog LCP or XP Analog. The entire infant protein substitute should not be replaced with the second stage protein substitute until infants are 1 year old. The infant protein substitute can be stopped at 1 year; if it is continued it is usually as a social drink perhaps given in the morning or evening.

Toddlers

Feeding problems are common in young children with PKU. MacDonald et al. [118] reported that 47% of mothers perceived their children to have at least three feeding difficulties. Principal problems were slowness to feed, a poor appetite, a dislike of sweet foods and a limited variety of foods consumed. Parents also perceived their children to have more gastrointestinal symptoms such as diarrhoea or constipation. Parents resorted to more mealtime coercive strategies to persuade children to eat, used less verbal encouragement at mealtimes and were more likely to feed their children in isolation. Particular difficulties were experienced with the administration of the protein substitute.

A number of reasons explain these feeding difficulties in PKU including:

- *Energy content of protein substitutes.* Some of the common protein substitutes contain a significant amount of energy; 100 g Minaphlex

Table 17.11   Sample menu for infant aged 9 months with classical phenylketonuria (PKU).

	Exchanges
Weight 8.4 kg	
On waking: phenylalanine free formula, e.g. XP Analog LCP	
Breakfast	
10 g PKU Gel as paste	
1 × 50 mg phe exchange, e.g. 10 g Weetabix plus diluted liquid Duocal	1
Low protein toast and butter	
Infant protein substitute, e.g. XP Analog LCP	
Midday	
10 g PKU Gel	
2 × 50 mg phe exchanges: 80 g mashed potato	1
Chopped, soft 'free' vegetables	
Homemade free vegetable sauce	
1 exchange yoghurt	1
Banana or soft fruit	
Fruit juice or diluted liquid Duocal	
Evening meal	
10 g PKU Gel	
1 × 50 g phe exchange, e.g. 50–60 g tinned spaghetti	1
Low protein toast	
Low protein custard and fruit	
XP Analog LCP	
	―――
	4
Bedtime	
XP Analog LCP	

Expected daily intake	*Protein intake (g)*
500 mL XP Analog LCP	9.8
30 g PKU Gel	12.6
4 phe exchanges	4
	26.4 g/day
	= 3.1 g/kg/day

phe, phenylalanine.

contains 374 kcal (1.56 MJ), providing 30% of a 1–3-year-old's energy requirements. Parents may be unaware of the energy contribution from protein substitutes and so have unrealistic expectations of how much food their children should eat and may try to coerce their children to eat when they are not hungry.

- *Refusal to eat phenylalanine exchanges*. Parents may become preoccupied in ensuring their children eat all phenylalanine exchanges. Repeated exchange refusal may cause parents to force feed resulting in unpleasant mealtimes.
- *Lack of verbal encouragement at mealtimes*. Parents may have to prepare two meals at mealtimes which may result in the child with PKU being fed first and given their meals alone. Lack of pleasant conversation and eating in isolation can only have a negative effect on appetite and feeding.
- *Difficulty in giving the protein substitute*. Crying, screaming, gagging, vomiting and deliberately spilling the protein substitute are common in this age group. Children are still teething in their second year and this can add to the difficulties of protein substitute administration.

Overcoming feeding difficulties in toddlers

Some feeding problems can be quite difficult to overcome, but if consistently applied the following tips may be helpful:

- Children with PKU should eat at the same time as everyone else in the family, even though the food offered may be different.
- Offer only small portions of food at mealtimes.
- Encourage parents to make mealtimes a positive experience so the child and family enjoy it. If a child is refusing to eat try to minimise negative communication such as 'hurry up', 'you are a naughty child' and bribery. Make up phenylalanine exchanges later in the day with yoghurt or milk.
- Encourage parents to offer a wide variety of low protein foods as early as possible and preferably during the weaning period. If a food is initially refused, try to persuade parents to try it again and again.
- Encourage children to start cooking with their foods as soon as possible. Perhaps they can put icing (made from icing sugar and water) onto low protein biscuits and decorate them with suitable low protein sweets. Alternatively, they can help to choose the toppings for their low protein pizza, or crush low protein biscuits to use as a biscuit base for a dessert. Young children may be encouraged to grow their own low protein vegetables in the family garden. All of this helps to create an interest in food and eating.
- At mealtimes encourage parents to prepare a similar dish for the child with PKU equivalent to that which the rest of the family is eating. For example, instead of spaghetti bolognese, a low protein pasta dish with tomatoes and mushroom sauce could be given; low protein burgers or vegefingers could be given instead of beefburgers or fish fingers.
- Encourage parents to make low protein dishes as colourful and interesting as possible. For example, adding ingredients such as tomato purée, custard powder and gravy browning improves the colour of low protein flour dishes.
- Suggest parents invite friends to low protein birthday parties, teas and picnics. If low protein food is eaten and enjoyed by peers, it will make the diet more acceptable.
- Try to persuade parents not to become angry, upset or frustrated if the protein substitute is refused. They should continue with encouragement, but at the same time discourage distractions (e.g. watching TV, playing) until the entire protein substitute is taken. Plenty of praise

should be given immediately afterwards. If the same routine is followed every day, a child will quickly learn this is the way it has to be, even though there may be a few protests from time to time. Parents should be encouraged to remember the 3 'P' rule when administering protein substitute to a defiant toddler: persistence, patience and positivity.

Eating in nurseries or other childcare centres

It is increasingly common for young children to spend part of their day in nurseries, other childcare centres or with child minders. Nursery teachers and other childcare workers should understand the basic principles of the PKU diet, foods permitted and forbidden, necessity for protein substitute and phenylalanine exchanges. Ideally, they should receive one-to-one verbal explanation from the dietitian or a specialist nurse working in PKU and the least they should expect is to receive written information about the diet. The NSPKU has a helpful guidance book for nursery teachers. Parents should be encouraged to supply aspartame free drinks or cartons of low protein milk substitute drinks (Sno-Pro or Loprofin PKU drink; each carton contains 25 mg phenylalanine), fruit or low protein biscuits for snacks, a small tin of suitable sweets for treats and a packed lunch. Parents should be encouraged to liaise closely with the nursery about cookery sessions or parties so alternative, suitable low protein food can be provided.

An example of a meal plan for a 4-year-old child is given in Table 17.12.

School children

By the time children are starting school, they spend increasingly more time away from their parents. Primary school teachers need basic information about PKU and any day-to-day practical implications of the special diet. Most parents give their children a packed lunch as most school dinner systems are only able to offer a limited choice of foods and are not usually able to prepare special dishes from low protein flour mixes. The NSPKU has a useful booklet on packed lunch ideas; a typical lunch box usually consists of low protein sandwiches (filled with low protein cheese, salad, or

Table 17.12 Menu plan for a 4-year-old girl on 5 × 50 mg phenylalanine exchanges.

	Exchanges
Breakfast	
Protein substitute	
1 × 50 mg phenylalanine exchange,	
e.g. 15 g cornflakes + protein free milk	
replacement	1
Low protein toast + fried mushrooms	
Fruit juice – aspartame free	
Midday	
Protein substitute	
Low protein bread + butter	
1 exchange of 'Cheezly' low protein vegan	
cheese	1
1 apple	
Fruit juice – aspartame free	
Mid-afternoon	
1 packet crisps	1
Evening meal	
Protein substitute	
45 g chips	1
20 g baked beans	1
Salad vegetables	
Low protein crumble + low protein custard	
Fruit juice – aspartame free	
Bedtime	
Protein free milk substitute	
	5 exchanges

jam), crisps, salad vegetables, fresh fruit, small packets of dried fruit, low protein biscuits and fruit juice. The packed lunch need not look any different from their peers' packed lunches.

Although the protein substitute should be given three times daily it is probably better not to give this at school. It may single out a child as being different and inadvertently lead to bullying. Instead, protein substitute may be given at breakfast, immediately after school and at bedtime, provided some of the daily phenylalanine is given with each dose.

School children spend time eating away from home (e.g. at friends' homes, parties and other events). It is important that PKU does not restrict social activities and parents and children need to be sensible in their approach to the diet. Children have to be trusted to eat the right things and it is helpful if they have a good knowledge of phenylalanine exchanges and portion sizes. They also need to

have a supply of appetising low phenylalanine/free foods with them so they are less tempted to cheat when they are eating out of the home and there are few suitable low protein foods available.

By the time a child is going to school it is important they are being educated about their condition. They need ongoing teaching about the foods they can eat, phenylalanine exchanges, why they take the protein substitute and the need for blood tests. The hospital PKU team may carry out one-to-one teaching or run group teaching sessions. Parents also need to take responsibility in ensuring their children become gradually involved in their own treatment to help aid future independence. The NSPKU produce a teaching skills guide 'Let's learn about PKU (7–11 years)'. It is designed to aid dietitians and nurse specialists.

Teenagers

Many teenagers who have closely adhered to their diet as children will still continue to maintain good control in their adolescent years. However, some teenagers regard PKU as a burden and poor dietary compliance and unsatisfactory blood phenylalanine control are persistent issues in older patients [119–121]. Many of these will have always struggled with their dietary treatment or have had a negative attitude towards PKU from the early days of treatment. If it is agreed that the diet is to be relaxed in teenage years to one aiming to maintain phenylalanine concentrations <700 µmol/L, the number of phenylalanine exchanges are gradually increased by one at a time. Plasma phenylalanine concentrations are monitored weekly or fortnightly until the new target is achieved and is stable.

Lack of compliance with vitamins and minerals or vitamin and mineral supplemented protein substitutes has compromised nutrient intake in teenage years. If patients are quite indifferent about their treatment, the daily discipline required in taking these often impedes compliance. Up until recently, most protein substitutes have required preparation that involves effort, causes inconvenience, embarrassment and there is a general unwillingness to consume protein substitutes in the presence of others. It is hoped the newer ready-to-drink preparations will be more effective in the long term. Short term studies are promising [122].

Monitoring of overall nutrient intake is particularly important during this vulnerable time and regular contact and communication with teenagers is essential. Health professionals should always remain helpful and supportive.

Teenage pregnancy

This is a particular concern in PKU. It is important that teenage girls and their families are educated and reminded about the potential risks of high maternal phenylalanine concentrations to the fetus, including facial dysmorphism, microcephaly, intrauterine growth retardation, developmental delay and congenital heart disease (CHD). Starting a strict maternal diet post-conception is associated with lower birth weight, smaller birth head circumference, lower developmental quotient, lower intelligence quotient and an incidence of CHD of 17% [123]. Women with PKU should start a strict diet maintaining phenylalanine concentrations at 100–250 µmol/L before conception, or as soon after as possible.

Management of illness

High blood phenylalanine concentrations are common during illness because of catabolism. Appetite may be poor and management can be quite difficult. In particular, children with no phenylalanine hydroxylase activity may experience more elevated blood phenylalanine concentrations during illness and be particularly sensitive to catabolism. There is little work defining the best management during illness in PKU, but the following guidelines may be helpful:

- Maintenance of protein substitute intake. This will support anabolism and help suppress phenylalanine concentrations. It may be better for this to be given in smaller, frequent doses throughout the day. Phenylalanine concentrations will quickly rise without protein substitute.
- Encouragement of frequent high carbohydrate drinks (e.g. Lucozade, Ribena or glucose polymer solution).
- It is sometimes recommended that phenylalanine exchanges should be omitted for 1 or 2 days. However, catabolism will probably increase blood phenylalanine concentrations more than allocated phenylalanine exchanges. Some children suffer from frequent intercurrent infections and run the risk of phenylalanine deficiency if exchanges are stopped during each illness episode. It is probably unnecessary to specifically omit dietary phenylalanine, but a sick child should not be forced to eat every phenylalanine exchange.
- Other low phenylalanine foods should be offered to appetite.
- Medications should be free of aspartame.

Maple Syrup Urine Disease

Marjorie Dixon

Maple syrup urine disease (MSUD) is caused by a deficiency of branched chain 2-oxo (keto) acid dehydrogenase enzyme complex (Fig. 17.2). This results in accumulation of the three essential branch chain amino acids (BCAA) leucine, isoleucine and valine and their respective ketoacids in plasma and urine. L-alloisoleucine is present in plasma and, as it is not normally found in significant amounts in plasma, is considered diagnostic for all forms of MSUD [135]. Leucine and 2-oxo-isocaproate are thought to be the main toxic metabolites and responsible for irreversible neurological impairment. MSUD varies considerably in clinical severity from severe classical to milder variant forms [136].

Classical MSUD

Babies usually present within the first 1–2 weeks of life with a progressive and overwhelming illness with poor feeding, lethargy and seizures leading to

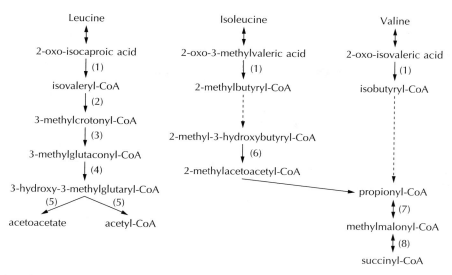

Figure 17.2   Selected inborn errors of the catabolic pathways of branch chain amino acids. 1 Maple syrup urine disease. 2 Isovaleric acidaemia. 3 3-Methylcrotonyl-CoA carboxylase deficiency. 4 3-Methylglutaconyl-CoA hydratase deficiency. 5 3-Hydroxy-3-methylglutaryl-CoA lyase deficiency. 6 2-Methylacetoacetyl-CoA thiolase deficiency. 7 Propionic acidaemia. 8 Methylmalonic acidaemia.

coma. The main problem is toxic encephalopathy with varied signs including irritability, changes in tone and full fontanelle. Marked metabolic acidosis is unusual. The characteristic smell of maple syrup in the urine may be present. Plasma leucine levels are grossly elevated, in the range 1000–5000 μmol/L (normal reference range 65–220 μmol/L). Plasma isoleucine and valine can also be markedly elevated but rarely to the same degree as leucine. Untreated, patients may die and survivors are severely mentally and physically retarded.

Variant MSUD

Babies who do not decompensate in the neonatal period may present later in infancy with developmental delay and neurological problems such as fits. Plasma BCAA are often chronically elevated. Other patients are normally well between acute episodes, which are usually precipitated by metabolic stress such as intercurrent infections or high dietary protein intake. Plasma BCAA levels are near normal between episodes and require only a modest or no restriction of dietary leucine intake.

Thiamin responsive MSUD

Thiamin is a co-factor in the branched chain 2-oxo (keto) acid dehydrogenase reaction and occasionally patients may respond to pharmacological doses of the vitamin. In general, presentation is less severe than in non-thiamin responders. Although dietary treatment is required in addition to thiamin supplementation, the degree of dietary restriction is less severe than in the child with classic MSUD. A restricted protein intake may be sufficient, although it may be beneficial or necessary for some patients to have supplements of BCAA (see below).

Dietary management of classical MSUD

Early diagnosis, combined with good long term metabolic control, is essential in minimising neurological impairment and poor intellectual outcome in MSUD [137–142]. Plasma leucine levels should, if possible, be maintained at the lower end of the recommended range as higher levels are associated with poorer intellectual outcome. However, it is also important to give sufficient to meet

Table 17.13　Recommendations for plasma branch chain amino acid levels in maple syrup urine disease.

	Aim (µmol/L)	Normal reference range (µmol/L)
Leucine	200–500	65–220
Isoleucine	100–200	26–100
Valine	100–300	90–300

normal requirements for protein synthesis and to avoid protein deficiency. Normal plasma reference ranges and the aims of treatment are given in Table 17.13.

Plasma leucine is generally elevated much more than isoleucine and valine. The diet is therefore related to leucine intake. The quantity given is adjusted according to plasma leucine levels. In the normal population, leucine requirements (per kilogram body weight) decrease with increasing age [143]. Isoleucine and valine requirements (per kilogram body weight) also decrease with age.

Considerable interindividual variations of BCAA requirements are reported during the first few months of life [144]. Personal experience has shown leucine requirements to be around 100–110 mg/kg body weight/day in 2–3-month-old infants, decreasing towards the age of 1 year to around 40–50 mg/kg body weight/day. Most children with well-controlled MSUD have total leucine intakes typically between 400 and 600 mg/day.

Once stabilised, there is relatively little variation in the total leucine intake irrespective of age – except during growth spurts or occasionally after prolonged infections when there has been a reduced intake of leucine.

Leucine intake is measured by an exchange system (i.e. the quantity of food providing 50 mg leucine is termed one leucine exchange). Leucine exchange foods need to be weighed carefully on digital scales which are accurate to 1 or 2-g increments. Leucine is usually provided by a variety of low biological value protein foods such as potato, vegetables, rice and cereals. Foods of high biological value protein are invariably avoided because their leucine content is high and energy contribution is low. The leucine allowance is spread throughout the day, ideally evenly distributed, between three and four meals, to reduce fluctuations in plasma BCAA levels. Table 17.14 provides a list of leucine exchange foods for use in MSUD.

The dietary requirements for isoleucine and valine are lower than for leucine, but the isoleucine and valine content of foods are also always lower than that of leucine content (Table 17.14). Often, the leucine exchanges will provide sufficient isoleucine and valine. If plasma concentrations of isoleucine and/or valine fall too low, a supplement of these amino acids is essential to prevent them becoming rate limiting for protein synthesis. An initial daily dose of 50–100 mg of isoleucine and/or valine, divided into two to three doses, is given with the amino acid supplement (see below) and leucine exchanges. If plasma isoleucine or valine levels remain low, the dosage is increased until concentrations fall within the recommended reference range (Table 17.13). Isoleucine and valine are added to the diet as either a powder or a solution of the pure L-amino acid. Vitaflo produce individual sachets of valine and isoleucine with a carbohydrate base. Each 4-g sachet provides 50 mg amino acid. These are available on FP10 prescription. Great care must be taken to ensure the correct amino acid is given. Alternatively, a 1% solution (1 g/100 mL) can be made, but this is more complicated for parents. In practice, parents make this solution at home. The amino acid is weighed accurately in pharmacy, the required amount of water is then added at home and the solution refrigerated. The medicine bottles are colour coded for the different amino acids to avoid confusion. The volume of solution required is measured in a syringe, 5 mL providing 50 mg amino acid.

Most patients require severe restriction of leucine in the diet, so the intake of natural protein is much less than that required for normal growth. It is therefore essential to give a supplement of amino acids free from BCAAs. Generous amounts of BCAA free amino acids are required because of their synthetic nature and lower bioavailability. This will also help minimise any disturbance of flux of amino acids across the blood–brain barrier [145]. No specific recommendations for intakes of amino acid supplements have been set for MSUD, so these are extrapolated from the PKU guidelines (p. 316) [16]. No recommendation is made for teenagers, but normal practice is to give around 1.0–1.5 g/kg/day. Table 17.5 gives guidelines for total

Table 17.14   Leucine exchanges for use in maple syrup urine disease.

Food	Weight (g)	Energy (kcal)	Energy (kJ)	Protein (g)*	Leucine (mg)[†]	Isoleucine (mg)[†]	Valine (mg)[†]
Milk							
SMA Gold	35 mL	23	96	0.5	[‡]	[‡]	[‡]
Cow & Gate Premium	35 mL	23	98	0.5	54	31	33
Cow's milk	15 mL	10	42	0.5	50	27	36
Single cream	20 mL	40	167	0.5	48	26	36
Double cream	35 mL	157	656	0.6	52	30	38
Yoghurt (natural/flavoured)	10	10	42	0.4	57	31	34
Custard	15 mL	18	75	0.5	57	31	42
Ice cream	15	25	105	0.4	53	28	36
Milk chocolate	5	26	109	0.4	46	27	30
Plain chocolate	15	79	330	0.7	45	27	40
Cereals							
Rice – raw	10	36	150	0.7	56	26	39
Rice – boiled	25	35	146	0.6	47	22	32
Pasta – raw	5	17	73	0.6	53	28	32
Pasta – cooked	15	16	66	0.5	50	27	30
Vegetables (boiled)							
Asparagus	35	9	36	1.2	50		
Baked beans (canned)	15	13	53	0.8	51		
Broccoli	45	10	45	1.4	51		
Brussels sprouts	35	12	54	1.0	53		
Cauliflower	40	11	47	1.2	53		
Mushrooms (fresh)	50	7	27	0.9	53		
Okra (fried in oil)	35	94	392	1.5	52		
Peas	15	12	50	1.0	45		
Petit pois	15	7	31	0.8	51		
Spinach	20	4	16	0.4	54		
Spring greens	25	5	20	0.5	51		
Sweetcorn (canned)	15	18	78	1.3	50		
Yams	45	60	255	0.8	49		
Potato[§]							
boiled, jacket	60	44	188	1.0	55		
roast	45	67	283	1.3	53		
chips	35	66	279	1.3	46		
Fruit (edible portion)							
Avocado	45	85	353	0.9	52		
Bananas	55	34	146	0.7	53		
Figs (green, raw)	90	39	166	1.2	51		
Kiwi fruit	90	44	186	1.0	51		
Dried fruits[¶]	60	162	693	1.4	56		

Sources:

* *McCance and Widdowson's The Composition of Foods*, 5th edn. Royal Society of Chemistry, Ministry of Agriculture, Fisheries and Food. London: HMSO, 1991 [126].

[†] Paul AA, Southgate DAT, Russell J *First supplement to McCance and Widdowson's The Composition of Foods*. London: HMSO, 1979 for milk and cereals; Leatherhead Food RA, Randalls Road, Leatherhead, Surrey, England, 1994 for fruits and vegetables. No data available for isoleucine and valine. Manufacturers' data for Premium.

[‡] Data available from manufacturer.

[§] Potatoes – the leucine content of potato varies between old, new and different varieties; an average figure has been used.

[¶] Dried fruits – the leucine content of different dried fruits is not too dissimilar, so an average figure has been used.

Table 17.15 Branch chain free amino acid products used in maple syrup urine disease.

Product*	Amino acids (g/100 g)	Protein equiv. (g/100 g)	Energy (kcal/100 g)	Energy (kJ/100 g)	Carbohydrate (g/100 g)	Fat (g/100 g)	Vitamins and minerals	Dilution	Osmolality mOsm/kg H₂O	Comment
MSUD Analog (SHS)	15.5	13	475	1990	54	23	Full range	15%	353	Infant formula, reconstituted 1 scoop to 30 mL
MSUD Maxamaid (SHS)	30	25	309	1311	51	<0.5	Full range	1 to 5	782	Suitable from 1 year of age, can be given as paste or drink
MSUD Maxamum (SHS)	47	39	297	1260	34	<0.5	Full range	1 to 5	1181	Suitable from 8 years of age, can be given as paste or drink
MSUD Aid III† (SHS)	93	77	326	1386	4.5	Nil	Calcium Phosphorus		332	Usually given as a paste from only 6 months
Mapleflex (SHS) Presentation – 29 g sachet	35	29	390	1639	38	13.5	Full range		1130	Suitable from 1 year of age, given as drink or paste
MSUD Gel (Vitaflo) Presentation – 20 g sachet	50	42	342	1428	43	Nil	Full range			Suitable from 1 year of age, given as a gel or low volume drink
MSUD Express Powder (Vitaflo) Presentation – 25 g sachet	72	60	302	1260	15	<0.5	Full range			Suitable from 8 years of age, given as a drink
MSUD Express Cooler (Vitaflo) Presentation – 130 mL foil pouch	18.2	15	92	386	7.8		Full range			Suitable from 8 years of age, ready to drink

All products are approved by the Advisory Committee Borderline Substances for prescription on FP10 (except MSUD Express Cooler which is about to be submitted for FP10 approval). Other MSUD products are manufactured by Milupa, Mead Johnson Nutritionals and Ross Laboratories, but are not currently available in the UK.
* All products are free from leucine, isoleucine and valine but otherwise contain all essential and non-essential amino acids.
† Requires complete vitamin and mineral supplementation.

protein intake expressed as protein equivalent from amino acid supplement (protein substitute) plus exchanges as natural protein. A number of prescribable BCAA free amino acid supplements (protein substitutes) of differing composition, suited to different age groups, are available. On reconstitution the physical format of the products vary: gels, pastes, juice or milk type drinks, infant feeds (Table 17.15). The supplement is given as an evenly divided dose ideally with natural protein (leucine), three times per day before meals in children, and more often in infants while they are still being demand fed.

To ensure adequate protein synthesis and normal growth, an adequate energy intake must be provided. Plasma BCAA levels will rise if sufficient energy is not given as this will precipitate catabolism. Most infants, if diagnosed early and not severely neurologically impaired, will eat well orally. However, if oral intake is inadequate, tube feeding is vital to prevent metabolic decompensation; both nasogastric and gastrostomy feeding have been successful. Long periods of fasting should be avoided, especially in infants, as plasma BCAA increase on fasting. Dietary energy is provided mainly by the following groups of foods which are allowed freely in the diet, although some is also provided by leucine exchanges and the amino acid supplement:

- Foods naturally very low in or free from leucine – most fruits and vegetables (Table 17.16); sugar and fats (Table 17.17).
- Specially manufactured low protein (low leucine) foods (e.g. bread, pasta, biscuits, cereals) (Appendix 17.1). The following low protein (low leucine) foods need to be counted as part of the leucine intake:
  Loprofin low protein snack pot – curry, tomato and basil
  1 pot = 40 mg leucine = 1 leucine exchange
  Promin low protein pasta in sauce – tomato, pepper and herb; cheese and broccoli
  1 sachet = 98 mg leucine = 2 leucine exchanges
  Promin low protein buger mix
  62 g sachet = 136 mg leucine (each sachet to make three small burgers, each burger = 1 leucine exchange)
- Energy supplements – glucose polymers, fat emulsions.

Table 17.16 Fruits and vegetables with low leucine content.

Fruits (<30 mg leucine/100 g [0.3–1.0 g protein/100 g])

Apple juice	Lemons	Passion fruit
Apples	Limes*	Peaches
Apricots	Lychees*	Pears
Blackberries*	Mandarins	Pineapples
Blackcurrants*	Mangoes*	Pineapple juice
Cherries	Melons	Plums
Cranberries	Mulberries*	Raspberries
Clementines	Nectarines	Rhubarb
Damsons	Olives	Satsumas
Gooseberries*	Orange juice	Strawberries
Grapefruits	Oranges	Tangerines
Grapes	Paw paw*	Tomato juice
Guavas		

Commercial baby fruit jars/tins which contain ≤0.5 g protein/100 g

Vegetables (<100 mg of leucine/100 g)

Aubergines	Fennel‡	Parsley‡
Artichokes‡	Garlic‡	Peppers
Beans (runner)†	Gherkins‡	Plantains†
Beans (French)†	Gourd‡	Pumpkins
Beansprouts†	Leeks†	Radishes
Beetroot	Lettuces†	Swedes
Cabbages†	Mange tout†	Sweet potatoes
Carrots	Marrows‡	Tomatoes
Celery	Onions	Tomato puree
Chicory	Onions (spring)	Turnips
Courgettes	Onions (pickled)	Watercress‡
Cucumbers	Parsnips†	

Source: Leatherhead Food RA, Randalls Road, Leatherhead, Surrey, England, 1994.

* No leucine data is available for these fruits. They are included on the free list because they contain <1 g protein/100 g and are consumed in small amounts, infrequently.

† These vegetables contain 50–100 mg leucine/100 g and could contibute significantly to leucine intake if eaten regularly in large quantities.

‡ No leucine data are available for these vegetables. They are included on the free list because they are usually consumed in small amounts, infrequently.

Supplements of all vitamins and minerals are necessary because of the limited range of foods that can be taken. Free fruits and vegetables may provide sufficient amounts of vitamins A and C. The source of the vitamins and minerals varies: they may be a constituent of the BCAA free amino acid supplement (Table 17.15), so no additional supplement is required; or a separate supplement will be needed if using pure amino acids (e.g. MSUD

Table 17.17 Foods with low protein content.

Fats	Butter, ghee, margarine, lard, dripping, solid vegetable fat, vegetable oils
Sugar and starches	Cornflour, custard powder (not instant), sago, tapioca, arrowroot
	Vegetarian jelly, agar agar
	Sugar, icing sugar, glucose
	Jam, marmalade, honey, golden syrup, maple syrup, treacle
Sweets	Sweets with ≤0.3 g protein/100 g
Desserts	Sorbet, ice lollies, ice cream wafers with ≤0.3 g protein/100 g
	Dessert sauces with ≤1.5 g protein/100 g
Drinks	Flavoured fizzy drinks, e.g. lemonade, cola, Lucozade, squash, cordials, Ribena
	Fruit juice
	Milk shake flavourings, e.g. Crusha syrup, Nesquik (not chocolate)
	Tonic water, soda water, mineral water
	Tea, fruit teas, coffee
Baking products	Baking powder, bicarbonate of soda, cream of tartar, food essences and colourings
Condiments and sauces	Salt, pepper, herbs, spices, pure mustard powder, vinegar
	Savoury sauces, vegetable spreads, chutney and pickles with ≤1.5 g protein/100 g
	Cook-in and pour-over sauces with ≤0.5 g protein/100 g
	Gravies (reconstituted) with ≤0.3 g protein/100 mL

Aid III). Paediatric Seravit is a comprehensive vitamin, mineral, trace element powder with a carbohydrate base but contains only trace amounts of sodium, potassium and chloride. It can be used for children of all ages, but palatability and quantity required may become a problem in older children. Phlexy-Vits (powder or tablets) is a comprehensive vitamin and mineral supplement suitable from 11 years of age. Forceval Junior Capsules (suitable from 5 years of age) are another good alternative but these contain no sodium, potassium, calcium, phosphate, chloride, inositol or choline and only a small amount of magnesium. A separate calcium supplement will be needed, but the diet may provide sufficient phosphate and magnesium from fruits and vegetables. Forceval Capsules are suitable from 12 years of age, they differ slightly in composition from the Junior Capsule; they contain small amounts of calcium, phosphorus and potassium but no vitamin K. An additional calcium supplement would still be required. A more comprehensive review of these vitamin and mineral supplement is given in the PKU section (see p. 323). The diet and supplement together should provide the reference nutrient intake (RNI) [146] for age for all vitamins and minerals.

Leucine content of foods

The only published UK data on amino acid content of foods is in the First Supplement to McCance and Widdowson's *The Composition of Foods*, The Stationery Office, London, 1979. As there were no plans to update or expand this very limited data, in 1994 the National Society for Phenylketonuria commissioned Leatherhead Food RA to analyse a range of fruits and vegetables for phenylalanine content. These were also analysed for leucine content. The analyses were performed at the Laboratory of the Government Chemist. At present the leucine data are unpublished and the author holds a copy of the leucine analyses. The leucine free and 50 mg leucine exchange lists for fruits and vegetables in the text are derived from these data (Tables 17.14 and 17.16).

Traditionally manufactured foods have been omitted from the MSUD diet because of lack of detail of their leucine content. The protein content of food alone is perceived to be a poor indicator of leucine content because it is too variable (e.g. a 50-mg leucine exchange of cereal, flour and milk all provide about 0.5 g protein whereas a 50-mg exchange of vegetables and fruit provides 1 g of protein or more). The exclusion of manufactured foods in the diet has made it extremely limited and boring for children with MSUD. Therefore, in 1999 a group of UK metabolic dietitians addressed this issue and decided that 0.5 g protein from manufactured foods could be taken to be equivalent to a 50-mg leucine exchange. Some specialist centres had already been using this value and maintaining good metabolic control. It was also reasoned that more manufactured foods were likely to have flour, milk or cereal as their main ingredient so there would be approximately 50 mg leucine per 0.5 g protein in a food. A 50-mg leucine exchange from a manufactured food is calculated as 50 ÷ (g protein per 100 g of food).

Management of the newly diagnosed infant

On presentation, the newly diagnosed baby with MSUD is usually acutely unwell, often encephalopathic and requiring intensive care. Plasma leucine level is usually greatly elevated and may be rapidly reduced with haemodialysis or haemofiltration [147–151], although this is not necessary in all cases. Apart from dialysis, the major route of removal of leucine from the plasma pool in MSUD is into protein synthesis [152] and this is best achieved by aggressive supplementation with branch chain free amino acids, a high energy intake and frequent 2–3 hourly feeding. Dietary treatment is therefore started as soon as possible, usually as nasogastric feeding. During the acute phase no dietary leucine is given until plasma leucine falls to around 800 μmol/L. This may take several days if the initial levels were high. Continuous feeding may be necessary in those patients who have problems with vomiting or hypoglycaemia. The infant is fed the branch chain free amino acid infant formula MSUD Analog, aiming to provide 3 g branch chain free amino acids/kg body weight/day and at least the normal energy requirement for age. This may take a few days to achieve in the very sick infant, commencing with a more dilute MSUD Analog solution supplemented with glucose polymer to a final concentration of 10% carbohydrate. As the plasma leucine level falls and the infant's clinical status improves, oral feeding can usually be established. The infant on dialysis is fed the same way with MSUD Analog, but dietary leucine will need to be reintroduced sooner because the rate of fall

of plasma leucine concentration level is usually more rapid on dialysis compared with dietary treatment alone [147]. Plasma leucine can fall to around normal levels in less than 24 hours. Rate of leucine clearance also varies with the mode of dialysis. However, with aggressive dietary treatment rapid improvement is also possible [153].

Plasma BCAA levels should be measured frequently, ideally daily. This is important not only to monitor plasma leucine concentrations but also isoleucine and valine which invariably drop to low levels as leucine falls from very high concentrations. If either the plasma isoleucine or valine levels drop below the lower end of the normal recommended reference range (100–150 μmol/L), a supplement (50–300 mg/day) is given to maintain plasma levels within the recommended reference range (Table 17.13). However, even earlier supplementation may be prudent particularly if leucine levels are high and the baby is not being dialysed. If these amino acids are not supplemented, plasma leucine level will remain high because they become rate-limiting for protein synthesis. Leucine is usually introduced as normal infant formula beginning with 50–100 mg/day (35–70 mL infant formula) divided between several feeds. The leucine intake is then increased according to plasma levels, aiming to maintain plasma leucine at 200–500 μmol/L. As leucine intake increases, the natural protein will also provide a source of the other BCAA and the individual supplements of these need to be adjusted, concomitantly. However, some patients do need to continue with a small daily dose of either or both isoleucine and valine indefinitely.

The infant with MSUD can be breast fed, although reports and experience of this are limited [154]. During the initial stabilisation period, when no dietary leucine is given, the mother needs to express breast milk to maintain a supply and the infant is fed MSUD Analog. Once the plasma leucine has fallen, measured volumes of breast milk are given to provide the source of leucine. Thereafter, similar to the management of the breast fed PKU infant (see p. 326), a measured quantity of MSUD Analog is given before breast feeds to suppress intake of breast milk. The infant is then breast fed on demand to provide the source of leucine. The amount of MSUD Analog given is adjusted according to plasma BCAA concentrations.

Table 17.18   Example of a feeding regimen for infant with maple syrup urine disease aged 2 months, weight 4.5 kg.

	Energy		Protein (g)	Amino acids (g)	Leucine (mg)	Isoleucine (mg)	Valine (mg)
	(kcal)	(kJ)					
300 mL Cow & Gate Premium 60 mL × 5 feeds	201	840	4.2		450	256	273
420 mL MSUD Analog 70 mL × 6 feeds	345	1442	9.4*	11.1	–	–	–
Totals	546	2282	13.6		450	256	273
Per kg	121	507	3.0		100	57	61
DRV per kg for 0–3 months	115–100	480–420	2.1				
Aim per kg (Table 17.5)			3.0				

DRV, dieteary reference value [146].
* Protein equivalent.

Feeding the infant and child with classical MSUD

The diet for the infant is provided by a combination of normal infant formula as the source of leucine and MSUD Analog. The leucine containing formula is given in evenly divided doses. The frequency of feeding will to an extent be dictated by how often the infant demands feeds. Initially this may be up to eight times per day, but with increasing age will decrease to five to six times per day. This is followed by a feed of MSUD Analog to appetite (Table 17.18). Weaning is commenced at the usual time of around 6 months. Normal weaning practices are followed; solids are introduced at one meal then two and three times per day and progressing from smooth purée to lumpier foods and finger foods during the first year. MSUD weaning is started with low leucine foods such as puréed apple, carrot, crushed low protein rusk, low protein cereal or commercial baby fruit desserts which contain ≤0.5 g protein/100 g. The low leucine food is given after the leucine containing formula and during or after the MSUD Analog feed. It does not matter therefore if solids are not completed as they do not affect total leucine intake. As the infant takes more solids, the amount of infant formula offered is reduced by one leucine exchange (approximately 35 mL) and replaced with one exchange (50 mg leucine) of food (e.g. 40 g cauliflower, 60 g potato or from a commercial baby food) (0.5 g protein from baby food provides one leucine exchange). The food exchange is given before the MSUD Analog.

This process is continued throughout the first year until all the leucine is provided by solids and is given divided between three main meals. As the intake of MSUD Analog decreases more energy is provided from low protein (low leucine) solids (Tables 17.16 and 17.17, Appendix 17.1).

MSUD Aid III (an amino acid supplement free from BCAA) is gradually introduced from around the time weaning to condition the infant to its flavour and texture and, in some, to maintain an adequate supply of branch chain free amino acids. The MSUD Aid III and vitamin and mineral supplement are mixed with water and milk shake flavouring, such as Nesquik or Crusha syrup, to form a paste. A teaspoon of fruit purée added to this mixture will make it less gritty and more palatable. A strong flavouring agent is essential to improve the taste of the product: in practice 10 g MSUD Aid III is mixed with 5 g Paediatric Seravit (a ratio of 2 : 1) plus 2–3 teaspoons water and Nesquik powder. Initially, one teaspoon of this paste is given at one meal per day before the measured leucine exchange. The MSUD Aid III mixture is gradually increased in quantity and is given before meals three times per day and will eventually replace the MSUD Analog. The infant's acceptance of the MSUD Aid III will determine how quickly the quantity offered can be increased; force feeding must be avoided. As the amount of paste taken increases it is important to give a drink of water after it because of its high osmolality. Flexibility is necessary when introducing the MSUD Aid III paste; a combination of both Analog and MSUD Aid III may be more acceptable throughout the toddler years. If MSUD Aid III is not taken well as a paste, it may need to be added to the MSUD Analog feed to maintain an adequate intake of branch chain free amino acids. Care must be taken as the feed will be hyperosmolar; 5 g MSUD Aid III can be safely added to 150 mL MSUD Analog.

If MSUD Aid III paste is not acceptable, the following branch chain free amino acid substitutes are recommended from 1 year of age, although it is often common practice to introduce small amounts before 1 year of age: MSUD Maxamaid, Mapleflex or MSUD Gel. More details on presentation and nutritional composition are given in Table 17.15. These products also contain a full range of vitamins and minerals. They are given three times per day, before meals. If taken as a low volume drink or paste it is important to follow with a drink of water because of their high osmolality.

- MSUD Maxamaid (contains glucose polymer) is given as a drink or paste. This product is not recommended for children under the age of 1 year because of its high osmolality. However, it can be introduced before 1 year of age as a diluted drink initially once per day, so the child can get used to the taste. The concentration is then gradually increased as tolerated to the recommended 1 in 5 dilution and the frequency to three times per day. These Maxamaid drinks are often taken in a greater concentration than 1 in 5 without a problem. Maxamaid can also be given as a paste with a drink to follow. Compared with MSUD Aid III paste mixture, this is much more bulky because of its carbohydrate (CHO) content. A strong flavouring agent needs to be added to MSUD Maxamaid. A ready flavoured orange version is available.
- MSUD Gel (contains glucose polymer) is given as either a gel or a low volume drink. Separate flavourpac sachets are available to help mask the taste of the amino acids.
- Mapleflex is given as either a drink or paste. It differs from the other products being milk based and containing fat, including the essential fatty acids.

From around 1 year the diet should have progressed so that all leucine exchanges come from food, MSUD Aid III paste is taken (or alternative

Table 17.19 Sample menu for child with MSUD age 4 years, weight 15 kg providing 450 mg leucine (nine exchanges per day).

	Leucine exchanges
Branch chain free amino acid supplement	
35 g MSUD Aid III (2 g amino acids/kg)	
20 g Paediatric Seravit	
Flavouring, e.g. strawberry Nesquik	
Add water to a paste ÷ 3	
or	
100 g MSUD Maxamaid (2 g amino acids/kg)	
Flavouring, e.g. blackcurrant juice	
Add water to 450 mL	
÷ 150 mL × 3 drinks	
Breakfast	
¹/₃ amino acid supplement	
3 × 50 mg leucine exchange	
18 g Weetabix	3
Protein free milk* + sugar	
Low protein bread + margarine + honey or jam	
Lunch	
¹/₃ amino acid supplement	
3 × 50 mg leucine exchange	
120 g potato	2
45 g broccoli tops	1
Low leucine vegetables and margarine	
Low protein apple crumble	
Low protein custard	
Supper	
¹/₃ amino acid supplement	
3 × 50 mg leucine exchange	
30 g peas	2
Low protein pasta + margarine + tomato	
Ketchup	
15 g ice cream	1
Fruit, fresh or tinned in syrup	
Snacks	
Low protein biscuits, cake or cereal	
Duobar high energy supplement, Vitabite or fruit	
Squash, fizzy drinks, protein free milkshake*	

* Protein free milks (Appendix 17.1).

supplement) and low leucine foods are taken to appetite. Table 17.19 provides a typical example of a child's daily diet. During childhood, the branch chain free amino acid supplement is increased to ensure an adequate intake of total protein (Table 17.5). From 8 years of age there are some alternative branch chain free amino acid supplements that can be used (Table 17.15). MSUD Maxamum is similar to MSUD Maxamaid but provides more amino acids and vitamins and minerals in a smaller dose. MSUD Express is a new amino acid substitute with a full range of vitamins and minerals for older children and adults. It consists of two interchangeable products: MSUD Express Cooler, an orange flavoured, ready to drink liquid available in foil pouches; MSUD Express powder, available in sachets of unflavoured powder. MSUD Express Cooler is a new product and not yet available on FP10 prescription. MSUD Express powder is reported to improve metabolic control in older MSUD patients and is a very acceptable product for adults being easy to prepare and take outside the home [155].

Monitoring branch chain amino acids

The concentrations of BCAAs in blood or plasma should be measured once a week in infants while growth is rapid, and every 1–2 weeks in 1–3 year olds. Thereafter, frequency varies between 2–8 weeks depending on the stability of the child. Ideally, the sample should be taken at the same time of the day. Diurnal changes in amino acids have been reported in MSUD, BCAA levels always being higher after an overnight fast than postprandially [156]. These factors need to be considered when interpreting BCAA concentrations. On analysis the parents are promptly advised of the results by the dietitian and any necessary changes to the diet are made. It is important to be aware that different acceptable BCAA reference ranges may be used for dried blood spot vs. plasma samples. Recommendations for acceptable plasma BCAA reference ranges are provided in Table 17.13.

Leucine intake is altered according to plasma BCAA levels. There are several reasons for high leucine levels, apart from intercurrent infections. These include inadequate energy intake with poor growth, insufficient branch chain free amino acid supplement, inadequate isoleucine and/or valine intakes, or poor compliance with diet (taking more leucine exchanges than the prescribed amount). It is also important to check the prescribed products as mistakes can occur; sometimes gluten free rather than low protein food products or the wrong amino acid substitute can be given. If the plasma leucine level is around 600–700 µmol/L leucine intake is decreased by 50–100 mg/day (one to two leucine

exchanges). If the plasma leucine level is less than 100–200 µmol/L, leucine intake is increased by 50–100 mg (one to two exchanges). Low leucine levels can also arise because of an inadequate leucine intake, a growth spurt such as puberty, or increased requirement post-illness. If either plasma isoleucine or valine level is less than 100 µmol/L, while the concentrations of the other amino acids are normal, a supplement of 50–100 mg of the relevant amino acid is given. Any dietary alteration is reviewed with a follow-up blood test within 1–2 weeks.

Hoffmann et al. [157] have recently reported the impact of longitudinal plasma leucine levels on intellectual outcome and recommend that plasma leucine levels should not exceed 200 µmol/L in infants and pre-school children to achieve best intellectual outcome. However, to achieve this would mean very severe dietary restriction which would have major implications for management of MSUD patients. The findings of this study need to be confirmed before instituting such major dietary changes.

Monitoring the diet

Clinical, biochemical and nutritional status is monitored specifically looking for signs of protein deficiency such as skin rashes. Protein, zinc and isoleucine deficiency have been seen in children with MSUD [158–160]. Periodic analysis of trace element status is important (see Table 1.7). The diet is assessed regularly to ensure all nutrients, particularly trace elements and minerals, provide the RNI for age [146].

Traditionally patients have been reviewed individually in the outpatient clinic. However, following on from the success of group PKU clinics [161] the author's centre has recently established group clinics for patients with MSUD. Groups of similarly aged children and their families attend together to undertake education on different topics. A pre-clinic questionnaire is completed on the telephone to collect information on the usual diet and to identify any dietary or other problems that need to be dealt with at the clinic.

Dietary management during illness

During intercurrent infections plasma BCAA

concentrations may rise rapidly, particularly that of leucine. This increase in leucine appears to be more attributable to inadequate energy intake than to the direct catabolic effect of the infection [162]. At the first sign of illness an emergency regimen (ER) is started to reduce the accumulation of leucine which can cause rapid neurological deterioration. If oral intake is poor, tube feeding should be started without delay. The usual leucine intake is stopped or substantially decreased. The standard ER (see p. 375) of a high CHO intake from glucose polymer and frequent 2–3 hourly feeding or even 24-hour continuous feeding are instituted. Furthermore, supplements of branch chain free amino acids are given to promote protein synthesis. This is the major route of removal of leucine from the plasma pool, as other losses (e.g. in the urine) are minimal. If branch chain free amino acids are not given, other amino acids will become rate-limiting for protein synthesis and plasma leucine concentrations will remain high. The aim is to provide the child's usual intake of branch chain free amino acids (using their normal product) and at least the normal energy requirement for age, although this can be difficult to achieve (e.g. the infant is given MSUD Analog with additional glucose polymer to a total concentration of 10–12% CHO) and the child either MSUD Maxamaid or Maxamum with glucose polymer added to 15–20% CHO. If the child is on MSUD Aid III or MSUD Gel this should continue to be given, but it may be more acceptable and better tolerated as smaller more frequent doses. This is combined with high CHO drinks according to the standard ER (see p. 375).

If the child normally has isoleucine and valine supplements these are continued, unless plasma levels become high. Plasma concentrations can fall to low levels during the recovery phase, particularly if plasma leucine levels have been high. Additional supplements in excess of the patients normal requirement may temporarily be required if the leucine levels are very high and the child has a prolonged illness.

Plasma BCAA levels should be measured frequently throughout illness, to monitor progress and determine when leucine can be reintroduced. Once the plasma leucine has fallen to around 600–700 µmol/L or the child is improving, dietary leucine can be gradually reintroduced, increasing to the usual intake over a few days according to plasma levels. It is important not to delay re-institution of the child's usual leucine intake because plasma leucine levels can fall to unacceptably low levels following illness. In milder illnesses, plasma leucine may not necessarily increase above 600–700 µmol/L if the ER has been instituted at an early stage. If the child does not tolerate the ER feeds, then intravenous (IV) fluids (10% dextrose) are given. There are no branch chain free parenteral amino acid solutions available in the UK but a solution can be obtained from a pharmacy in Munchen, Germany (e-mail contact: KMB.Apotheke@extern.Irz-muenchen). If needed, an alternative is to give IV fluids (dextrose and lipid) along with a continuous nasogastric feed of branch chain free amino acids such as MSUD Aid III, beginning with a small amount such as 0.5 g amino acids/kg and increasing as tolerated. Illness in variant and thiamin responsive MSUD also necessitates use of an ER similar to classical MSUD. If the child is not on branch chain free amino acids then the standard ER of high CHO feeds is used.

Tyrosinaemias

Marjorie Dixon

Tyrosinaemia type I

Tyrosinaemia type I is caused by reduced activity of fumarylacetoacetate hydrolyase which catalyses the final step of tyrosine degradation (Fig. 17.3). Fumarylacetoacetate and maleylacetoacetate accumulate and are further metabolised to succinylace-tone which is found in greatly increased quantities in plasma and urine. These metabolites are considered toxic and responsible for the clinical features of progressive liver failure with increased risk for hepatocellular carcinoma (HCC), renal tubular dysfunction with hypophosphataemic rickets and a porphyria-like syndrome [163,164]. Tyrosinaemia

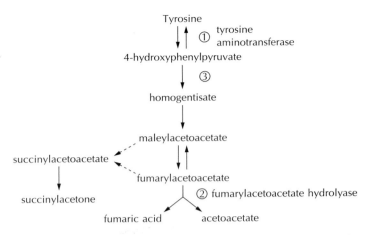

Figure 17.3 Pathway of tyrosine degradation. 1 Tyrosinaemia type II. 2 Tyrosinaemia type I. 3 4-Hydroxyphenylpyruvate dioxygenase (site of action of 2-(2-nitro-4-trifluoromethylbenzoyl)-1, 3-cyclohexanedione, NTBC).

type I can present at different ages with varying degrees of severity. In 1994 a new classification was proposed according to survival rate; this did not include data of patients treated with 2-(2-nitro-4-trifluoromethylbenzoyl)-1, 3-cyclohexanedione (NTBC, see below) (Table 17.20) [165].

At presentation, plasma tyrosine concentration is usually moderately increased (two to four times upper normal limit). Plasma methionine concentration can also be markedly increased. This is caused by secondary inhibition of S-adenosylmethionine synthetase [163]. High plasma methionine may affect normal liver function [166].

In the past, tyrosinaemia type I was treated with a low tyrosine, low phenylalanine diet to minimise formation of toxic metabolites. Initially, a reduced methionine intake was also used. Dietary treatment was shown to improve renal tubular dysfunction and growth. Liver function (in particular pro-thrombin time) sometimes improved a little but diet could not prevent the development of HCC and some patients developed progressive liver fail-

ure or had lethal porphyric crises. Until recently, liver transplantation was the only really effective treatment for tyrosinaemia type I. However, in 1992 Lindstedt *et al.* [167] described the use of NTBC as an alternative treatment. NTBC inhibits the enzyme 4-hydroxyphenylpyruvate dioxygenase and blocks the tyrosine degradation pathway at this level (Fig. 17.3). This prevents the formation of the hepato-toxic and nephrotoxic compounds and succiny-lacetone (which probably has an important role in neurotoxicity). NTBC treatment leads to rapid improvement in hepatic and renal problems and it prevents neurological dysfunction in most patients [168]. In those who have started on NTBC treat-ment early in life, the risk of early development of HCC is markedly reduced. However, in patients with late start of NTBC treatment, there remains a considerable risk for liver malignancy [169]. NTBC is now established as a very effective alternative to transplantation.

Plasma tyrosine concentrations increase with NTBC treatment because the tyrosine degradation pathway is blocked earlier, at the second step. In tyrosinaemia type II (see below) high plasma tyro-sine concentrations are the probable cause of the oculocutaneous manifestations and may also be associated with the mental retardation reported in some patients [163]. To reduce the risks linked with high plasma tyrosine concentrations, patients on NTBC are treated with a low tyrosine, low pheny-lalanine diet (in practice a low protein diet).

Table 17.20

Age of onset symptoms	1 and 2 year survival rates
Very early onset <2 months	38%, 29%
Early onset 2–6 months	74%, 74%
Late onset >6 months	96%, 96%

Dietary management for NTBC treated patients

The aim of dietary treatment is to maintain blood tyrosine concentrations below 600 µmol/L and above 200 µmol/L (normal reference range 30–120 µmol/L).

Natural protein intake is reduced, thereby limiting tyrosine and phenylalanine intakes. Intake is altered according to plasma tyrosine concentrations. The amount of natural protein tolerated varies between patients. It has been reported to decrease from a peak of 1.8–2.4 g protein/kg/day at 4–5 months to around 1 g protein/kg/day in late infancy (with mean plasma tyrosine levels in the range 322–497 µmol) [170]. This high peak of protein intake may have been related to catch-up growth following diagnosis. Thereafter, once the patient has stabilised, the total protein intake usually varies little irrespective of age, except during growth spurts. The natural protein intake is measured as 1 g protein exchanges (i.e. the weight of food which provides 1 g of protein) (Table 17.21).

Table 17.21 Basic list of 1 g protein exchange foods for low protein diets.

	Food	Weight (g) = 1 exchange
Infant formula	SMA Gold	65
	Premium	70
	Farley's First	65
	Aptamil First	65
Milk and dairy	Cow's milk	30 mL
	Single cream	40 mL
	Double cream	60 mL
	Yoghurt*	20
	Ice cream*	30
	Milk chocolate*	12
	Plain chocolate*	20
Potatoes and starchy vegetables[†]	Potato (boiled)	55
	Jacket potato (flesh only)	45
	Jacket potato (flesh and skin)	25
	Chips (fresh, frozen)	25
	Roast potato	35
	Crisps	15
	Sweet potato	90
	Plantain	125
	Yam	125

Table 17.21 (Cont'd)

	Food	Weight (g) = 1 exchange
Pulse vegetables	Baked beans*	20
	Beans aduki, broad, butter, haricot, black-eye, mung, red and white kidney	
	boiled	12
	raw	5
	Chick peas	
	boiled	12
	raw	5
	Lentils	
	boiled	12
	raw	5
	Peas	15
	Mange tout	30
	Sweetcorn	35
Vegetables[†]	Asparagus	30
	Brussels sprouts	35
	Broccoli tops	30
	Cauliflower	30
	Okra	40
	Spinach	45
Cereals	Cornflakes*	10
	Rice Krispies*	15
	Sugar Puffs*	20
	Weetabix*	10
	Oatmeal	10
	Rice	
	raw	15
	boiled	45
	Macaroni (white) (boiled)	35
	Spaghetti (white) (boiled)	30
	Semolina (raw)	10
	Flour (white)	10
	Flour (wholemeal)	8
Breads	White, wholemeal, brown*	12
	Rolls – soft, crusty*	10
	Nan*	12
	Pitta*	10

Source: Royal Society of Chemistry, Ministry of Agriculture, Fisheries and Food. *McCance and Widdowson's, The Composition of Foods*, 5th edn. London: The Stationery Office, 1991 [126].

* For manufacutered foods the weight for one exchange will be more accurate if calculated from the nutritional label on the food. The figures given can be used as a guide.

[†] The weight of one exchange is for cooked weight unless stated otherwise.

A supplement of tyrosine/phenylalanine free amino acids is usually given, even if the allowance of natural protein provides the safe level of protein intake for growth [144]. If plasma methionine is high then the supplement can also be methionine free. There are no set recommendations in the UK for amounts of amino acid supplement to give so these are either extrapolated from the PKU guidelines (see p. 316), no recommendation is made for teenagers, normal practice is to give 1.0–1.5 g/kg body weight/day or, together with natural protein intake, calculated to provide 10–12% of energy intake. Table 17.5 gives guidelines for total protein intake as protein equivalent from amino acid supplement plus exchanges as natural protein (phenylalanine exchanges). Generous intakes of the amino acid supplement should help minimise disturbance of flux of amino acids across the blood–brain barrier [145,171]. Several amino acid supplement (protein substitute) products of varying composition, appropriate for different age groups, are available for children with tyrosinaemia (Table 17.22). On reconstitution the physical format of the products vary: gels, pastes, juice drinks and infant formula. The supplement is given as a divided dose, preferably three times per day with natural protein at main meals in children and more frequently in infants while they are still being demand fed.

Low plasma phenylalanine concentrations have been observed in patients with tyrosinaemia type I on restricted tyrosine/phenylalanine intakes [172]. If plasma phenylalanine concentrations remain low they may become rate-limiting for protein synthesis and plasma tyrosine levels will remain high. It is therefore important to monitor phenylalanine levels and give supplements as necessary. Ideally, the phenylalanine supplement should be given as a divided dose along with the amino acid supplement. Phenylalanine can be added to the diet as either a powder or a solution of the pure L-amino acid as described for amino acid supplementation in MSUD (see p. 334).

An adequate energy intake must be supplied for normal growth and to prevent endogenous protein catabolism causing increased tyrosine concentrations. Energy comes from protein exchanges and the amino acid supplement; additional energy is provided by the following groups of foods which are allowed freely in the diet:

- Foods naturally low in or free of protein – fruits and some vegetables (Table 17.23); sugar and fats (Table 17.17)
- Manufactured low protein foods, e.g. bread, pasta, biscuits, cereals (Appendix 17.1). These products are ACBS approved and available on FP10 prescription in the UK
- Energy supplements such as glucose polymer and fat emulsions

Vitamin and mineral supplements are essential because of the limited intake of foods that would normally provide these. Additional vitamins and minerals can be supplied from either the amino acid product (e.g. XPhen Tyr Analog or Tyr Express) or, if using the pure amino acid mix, from a separate vitamin and mineral supplement as described for PKU and MSUD (see pp. 323, 337). The diet and supplements should together provide the RNI [147] for all vitamins and minerals.

Dietary management of the newly diagnosed infant

The newly diagnosed infant may be acutely unwell with liver failure. It may be necessary to decrease tyrosine and phenylalanine to a very low intake and give a generous amount of the amino acid supplement XPhen Tyr Analog for the first few days, to help reduce production of toxic metabolites. Natural protein can then be introduced as either breast milk or infant formula. The intake is determined by blood tyrosine levels, aiming to maintain these at 200–600 µmol/L. If breast feeding, a measured volume of XPhen Tyr Analog (and methionine free if desired) will be given before most breast feeds to suppress intake of breast milk and thus tyrosine/phenylalanine intake. The infant then breast feeds on demand to provide the required tyrosine intake. If infant formula is providing natural protein (tyrosine and phenylalanine), this is given as an evenly divided dose (usually six feeds), throughout the 24-hour period and followed by XPhen Tyr Analog on demand.

NTBC will be commenced at a dose of 1.0 mg/kg/day (usually as 0.5 mg/kg twice daily). Some patients may have a significant degree of cholestasis so an additional fat-soluble vitamin supplement such as Ketovite tablets and liquid may be required initially. Renal tubular dysfunction leads

Table 17.22 Manufactured products used in treatment of tyrosinaemia type I, II and III.

Product	Amino acids (g/100 g)	Protein equiv. (g/100 g)	Energy (kcal/100 g)	Energy (kJ/100 g)	Carbohydrate (g/100 g)	Fat (g/100 g)	Vitamins and minerals	Dilution	Osmolality (mOsm/kg)	Comments
XPhen, Tyr Analog* SHS	15.5	13	475	1990	54	23	Full range	15%	353	Infant formula, reconstituted 1 scoop to 30 mL
XPTM Analog† SHS	15.5	13	475	1990	54	23	Full range	15%	353	Infant formula, reconstituted 1 scoop to 30 mL
XPhen, Tyr Maxamaid* SHS	30	25	309	1311	51	<0.5	Full range	1 : 5	782	Suitable from 1 year of age, can be given as a drink or paste
XPTM Maxamaid† SHS	30	25	309	1311	51	<0.5	Full range	1 : 5	782	Suitable from 1 year of age, can be given as a drink or paste
XPhen, Tyr Maxamum* SHS	47	39	297	1260	34	<0.5	Full range	1 : 5	1181	Suitable from 8 years of age, can be given as a drink or paste
XPhen, Tyr Tyrosidon*‡ SHS	93	77	326	1386	4.5	0	Calcium and phosphorus only		363	Usually given as a paste
XPTM, Tyrosidon†‡ SHS	93	77	326	1386	4.5	0	Calcium and phosphorus only		365	Usually given as a paste
Tyroflex SHS In 29 g sachet	35	29	390	1639	38	13.5	Full range		1110	Suitable from 1–10 years. Given as a drink
Tyr Gel* Vitaflo In 20 g sachet	50	42	342	1428	43	<0.5	Full range			Given as a gel or low volume drink
Tyr Express* Vitaflo In 25 g sachet	72	60	302	1260	15	<0.5	Full range			Given as a low volume drink

* Contains a full range of essential and non-essential amino acids except phenylalanine and tyrosine.
† Contains a full range of essential and non-essential amino acids except phenylalanine, tyrosine and methionine.
‡ Requires complete vitamin and mineral supplementation.
XPhen, Tyr Maxamum and XTyr Maxamum are other formulations which can be produced if required.
Other products for tyrosinaemia are manufactured by Milupa and Ross Laboratories but are not currently available in the UK.

Table 17.23   Fruits and vegetables with a low protein content.

Fruit (protein content less than 1.0 g protein/100 g)

Apples	Grapes	Paw paw
Apricots (not dried)	Grapefruits	Passion fruit
Bananas (1 small daily)	Guavas	Peaches
Bilberries	Kiwi fruits	Pears
Blackberries	Lemons	Pineapple
Blackcurrants	Limes	Plums
Cherries	Lychees	Pomegranate
Clementines	Mandarins	Raisins
Cranberries	Mangoes	Raspberries
Currants	Melons (all types)	Rhubarb
Damsons	Mulberries	Satsumas
Figs (not dried)	Nectarines	Strawberries
Gooseberries	Olives	Sultanas
	Oranges	Tangerines

Commercial baby fruit jars/tins which contain ≤0.5 g protein/100 g – allow freely

Fruit juices usually contain around 0.5 g protein/100 mL

Vegetables (protein content of less than 1.0 g protein/100 g)

Artichokes	Cress	Parsley
Aubergines	Cucumber	Parsnip
Beans –	Fennel	Peppers
French/green/runner	Gherkins	Pumpkins
Beansprout	Gourd	Radishes
Beetroot	Leeks	Spring greens
Cabbage	Lettuces	Swedes
Carrots	Marrows	Tomatoes
Celeriac	Mushrooms	Turnips
Celery	Onions	Watercress
Chicory		
Courgettes		

Source: Royal Society of Chemistry, Ministry of Agriculture, Fisheries and Food. *McCance and Widdowson's, The Composition of Foods*, 5th edn. London: The Stationery Office, 1991.

to increased losses of phosphate, and prevention of rickets usually requires the administration of both a phosphate supplement and 1α-hydroxycholecalciferol (or 1,25-dihydroxycholecalciferol). There may also be increased losses of both bicarbonate and potassium in the urine, which necessitates supplements of these electrolytes. The renal problems will improve with NTBC so these supplements may only be needed in the early stages of treatment, and care should be taken to avoid vitamin D toxicity (e.g. hypercalcaemia).

Feeding the infant and child with tyrosinaemia type I

The diet for infants and children is provided by a measured intake of natural protein, the amino acid supplement (free from phenylalanine and tyrosine) and very low protein foods to appetite.

The guidelines given for the progression of the diet from infancy to and during childhood in MSUD (see p. 340) can be applied to tyrosinaemia but using 1-g protein exchanges and the phenylalanine/tyrosine free range of amino acid supplements (Table 17.22). The section on practical aspects of low protein diets later in this chapter also provides useful information (see p. 357).

Monitoring blood tyrosine and phenylalanine

The concentrations of tyrosine and phenylalanine in blood or plasma should be measured weekly in infants, because growth is rapid, and every 1–2 weeks in 1–3-year-olds; thereafter frequency will vary depending on the stability of the child. The aim is to maintain blood tyrosine concentrations below 600 µmol/L (because of the risks from high tyrosine concentrations of neurotoxicity and corneal opacities), and a normal blood phenylalanine concentration. A study of 11 patients treated with NTBC reported no ophthalmic side effects despite some patients in the group having consistently elevated concentrations of tyrosine. They suggest that corneal problems may only arise if plasma tyrosine approaches a much higher concentration of 2000 µmol/L [173]. Parents are taught how to collect blood samples at home for tyrosine and phenylalanine analysis. Blood samples are usually collected onto a Guthrie card and sent by first class post in a pre-addressed envelope to the chemical pathology department of the hospital.

The blood tyrosine concentration is used to determine natural protein intake. High tyrosine levels can occur for several reasons: catabolism caused by an inadequate energy intake or intercurrent illness; inadequate amino acid supplement or phenylalanine intake; or taking more than the prescribed amount of natural protein. Care must also be taken to ensure the correct amino acid supplement is being given and that low protein, not gluten free, products are being given. Low levels of tyrosine can occur because of inadequate natural protein intake or a growth spurt. If blood tyrosine is around 600–700 µmol/L protein intake is decreased by 1–2 g protein; if less than 200 µmol/L the diet is increased by 1 g protein. The plasma amino acid profile is also used to check that all other essential amino acids do not fall below the normal reference range, in particular phenylalanine. If blood phenylalanine levels are consistently <20 µmol/L, a phenylalanine supplement is given. In practice, the author has found an intake of around 10 mg/kg/day to normalise plasma phenylalanine level when plasma concentrations are low.

Monitoring the diet

The diet is monitored by clinical examination, biochemical assessment, anthropometric measurement and dietary assessment. The diet is reviewed regularly to ensure adequate intakes of all nutrients: total protein intake from amino acid supplement/protein substitute and natural protein (Table 17.5); vitamins, minerals and trace elements.

Dietary management during illness

A formal emergency regimen is not normally used in these patients when unwell. However, it would seem prudent to encourage the child to continue to take the amino acid supplement and/or a high energy intake from CHO drinks, to reduce catabolism and thus prevent plasma tyrosine concentrations from increasing to high levels. High tyrosine levels have been reported to cause eye lesions in tyrosinaemia type II during illness [174].

Tyrosinaemia type II: Richner–Hanhart syndrome

In tyrosinaemia type II there is accumulation of tyrosine resulting from deficiency of hepatic tyrosine aminotransferase (Fig. 17.3). Crystals of tyrosine are found intracellulary and these cause inflammation. The main clinical features are corneal erosions and plaques, palm and sole erosions and hyperkeratosis. Mental retardation has been reported in some patients [163]. At presentation plasma tyrosine concentrations are usually >1000 µmol/L (normal reference range 30–120 µmol/L).

Dietary management

Tyrosinaemia type II is treated with a low tyrosine, low phenylalanine diet to reduce high plasma tyrosine concentrations. A supplement of tyrosine/phenylalanine free amino acids is usually given. The principles of dietary management for type I tyrosinaemia can be applied to type II. Methionine restriction is not necessary. On institution of diet, the skin and eye problems usually improve rapidly. The optimum level for maintenance of plasma tyrosine remains unknown. Reported cases have maintained plasma levels at 500–1000 µmol/L [173,174]. The degree of dietary restriction is usually determined by the clinical response. Usually the oculocutaneous abnormalities resolve and do not recur provided the plasma tyrosine level is kept below 800 µmol/L. It is not certain whether this degree of restriction will completely prevent neurological complications. It is the author's practice to aim to keep blood tyrosine below 600 µmol/L. Regular monitoring of tyrosine and phenylalanine is therefore essential.

During intercurrent illness, although severe metabolic decompensation does not occur, it may be beneficial to give high CHO drinks similar to the standard emergency regimen drinks (see p. 375), to prevent large increases in plasma tyrosine concentrations which have been reported to cause eye lesions during illness [175].

Homocystinuria

Fiona White

Classical homocystinuria (HCU) is a disorder of methionine metabolism caused by deficiency of the enzyme cystathionine β-synthase (CBS). Methionine is initially converted into homocysteine by a series of enzyme dependant steps (Fig. 17.4).

Homocysteine is then normally converted to cystathionine by CBS in the transulfuration pathway. This step requires pyridoxal-5-phosphate (vitamin B_6) as a co-factor. A deficiency of CBS results in increased plasma concentrations of methionine,

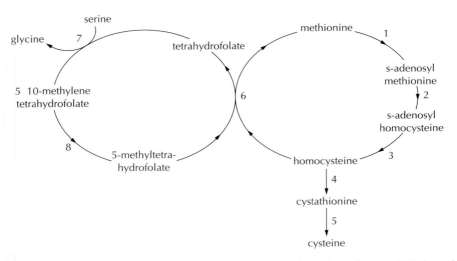

Figure 17.4   Metabolic pathways of homocysteine metabolism. 1 Methionine adenosyl transferase. 2 SAM dependent methyltransferase. 3 SAH hydrolase. 4 Cystathionine β-synthase. 5 γ-Cystathionase. 6 Methionine synthase. 7 Serine hydroxymethyltransferase. 8 Methylenetetrahydrofolate reductase.

homocysteine and other sulphur-containing metabolites (mixed disulphides) and low levels of plasma cysteine, cystathionine and serine. In addition, homocystine is present in large amounts in the urine (hence the condition being termed homocystinuria).

There are several other inherited metabolic disorders that also lead to homocystinuria with a raised plasma homocysteine, but with normal to low methionine levels. These are caused either by defects in the remethylation pathway by which homocysteine is normally converted to methionine (methionine synthase deficiency) or are caused by inherited disorders of the vitamins (B$_{12}$, folic acid) involved in the metabolic pathways of homocysteine metabolism (Fig. 17.4).

The most common cause of HCU is CBS deficiency (classical HCU) which can be classified into two types: pyridoxine responsive HCU and pyridoxine non-responsive HCU.

HCU was first described in 1962 [176]. It is inherited as an autosomal recessive trait. The defect found on chromosome 21 is in the CBS gene protein [177], and at least 130 mutations have been identified [178]. The worldwide incidence of HCU is approximately 1 in 344 000 [179], but there are large population differences with the incidence at least 1 in 65 000 in the Republic of Ireland [180]. The

incidence may be underestimated because of the infrequency of newborn screening for the disorder. DNA screening studies of newborn infants in a number of countries has shown that the incidence may be as high as 1 in 20 000 [178].

HCU may be diagnosed from screening in the neonatal period. However, few centres specifically screen for the disorder. Even in those infants with HCU screened in the newborn period, plasma methionine levels may not be significantly increased, particularly in pyridoxine responsive cases, or because of factors such as the increased trend to breast feed at least initially, so the baby has a lower methionine intake, and newborn screening being carried out earlier. Consequently, a significant proportion will only be diagnosed following the onset of clinical symptoms.

Individuals who have HCU are clinically normal at birth. Without early diagnosis and treatment there will be a gradual onset of the clinical features of HCU which are multisystemic [181] including:

- *Ocular system:* lens dislocation, iridodenesis, myopia, glaucoma
- *Skeletal system:* osteoporosis, scoliosis, elongation and thinning of the long bones, marfanoid appearance
- *Vascular system:* thromboembolisms, malar flush

- *Central nervous system:* developmental delay, learning difficulties, electroencephalogram changes, epilepsy, psychiatric disturbance

The complications of HCU are caused by the significantly raised plasma homocysteine levels [182].

In healthy normal subjects homocysteine is present in the plasma in several forms [183]:

- 10–20% as free, non-protein bound homocysteine comprising homocysteine (reduced form <2%), homocystine (disulphide of homocysteine) and mixed disulphide (homocysteine-cysteine)
- 80–90% as protein bound homocysteine

The plasma total homocysteine (tHcy) concentration is the sum of all the different forms. In plasma from normal subjects usually free homocysteine (fHcy) is undetectable and tHcy <15 µmol/L [184]. Free homocysteine only becomes detectable when total homocysteine exceeds 60 µmol/L [185]. At diagnosis, plasma tHcy in HCU patients will be significantly increased with levels often >200 µmol/L.

Pyridoxine responsive HCU

The enzyme CBS requires pyridoxal-5-phosphate, formed from pyridoxine (vitamin B_6), as its co-factor. A significant number of CBS deficient individuals show clinical and biochemical response to pharmacological doses of pyridoxine, up to 500 mg/day [186]. The defect in these cases is still within the CBS protein and is neither due to deficient pyridoxine status nor a disorder of pyridoxine metabolism. Pyridoxine is acting to increase residual CBS activity.

All individuals diagnosed as having classical HCU should be given a trial with pharmacological doses of pyridoxine. Worldwide up to 50% of cases of CBS deficiency HCU are pyridoxine responsive showing a decrease in plasma methionine and almost complete elimination of homocysteine from plasma (free homocysteine <5 mmol/L) and urine [180,187]. There are population differences with a much smaller percentage showing pyridoxine responsiveness in certain populations (e.g. Britain and Ireland). In CBS deficiency, folic acid requirements are probably increased because of an increased flux through the remethylation pathway

[188]. It is therefore essential to also give additional folic acid, 5 mg/day, and to ensure that plasma vitamin B_{12} levels (required for folate metabolism) are adequate. In those individuals with pyridoxine responsive HCU, treatment with pyridoxine and folic acid can prevent further deterioration in symptoms except for advanced eye disease [186].

Pyridoxine non-responsive HCU

In this group plasma homocysteine levels do not fall following pharmacological doses of pyridoxine. Treatment strategies aim at reducing homocysteine levels by:

- Decreasing the intake of the substrate methionine by use of a methionine restricted diet to reduce plasma methionine and homocysteine levels
- Utilising alternative pathways to remove homocysteine by giving betaine (a methyl donor) which remethylates homocysteine back to methionine and so reduces plasma homocysteine levels

Treatment aims and biochemical monitoring

Good long term biochemical control in HCU can prevent the onset of complications in early diagnosed individuals and can curtail further progression of the disorder in late diagnosed cases [186].

Formerly available methods of biochemical monitoring were only for the measurement of fHcy. More recently, measurement of tHcy has become more routine. From follow-up of patients treated over many years a lifelong median fHcy <11 µmol/L significantly reduces the probability of developing complications [180] and levels of fHcy <10 µmol/L indicates good biochemical control [186]. Data on acceptable tHcy levels in HCU is still limited and as yet data on lifelong tHcy and clinical outcome is not available.

In the normal population, tHcy levels are 5–15 µmol/L [184]. Free homocysteine is only detectable when tHcy >60 µmol/L. In those monitoring tHcy in HCU patients, levels of 80–120 µmol/L are being aimed for, with the lower levels more achievable in

Table 17.24   Biochemical monitoring in classical homocystinuria.

| | Plasma methionine | Plasma cysteine | Plasma homocysteine | |
			Free	Total
B$_6$ responsive	Normal range	Normal range	0–10 µmol/L	<50 µmol/L
B$_6$ non-responsive diet alone	Normal range	Normal range	<10 µmol/L	<80–120 µmol/L
B$_6$ non-responsive + betaine	High (up to 1000 µmol/L)	Normal range	<10 µmol/L	<80–120 µmol/L

pyridoxine responsive patients (personal communication). Until there are more data available on tHcy levels and clinical outcome, both plasma fHcy and tHcy need to be monitored.

Treatment aims will be dependent on the form of classical HCU and the treatment regimen in use (Table 17.24). In addition to the monitoring of plasma homocysteine, methionine and cysteine levels, vitamin B$_{12}$ and folate status should be assessed as low levels of these could cause inadequate response to treatment because of their intimate roles in homocysteine metabolism.

Dietary management of classical HCU

The principles of dietary management in common with other amino acid disorders are based on decreasing the load on the affected pathway and supplementing deficient products beyond the metabolic block. Early dietary treatments were described in 1966 [189,190] by Komorower in Manchester and Perry in Vancouver.

The aims of dietary treatment are to:

- Correct abnormal biochemistry (reduce plasma methionine levels to within or slightly above the normal age related reference range), decrease plasma homocysteine levels and increase plasma cysteine levels to within the normal range (Table 17.24)
- Ensure the diet is nutritionally adequate to achieve normal growth and micronutrient status
- Ensure the diet is palatable and flexible so as to fit in with modern lifestyles and thus help compliance

The principles of dietary management are as follows.

Reduce methionine intake by using a protein restricted diet

Because of their high methionine content, foods of a high biological protein value (e.g. meat, fish, eggs, dairy products, pulses, soya) are generally excluded from the diet. Methionine is an essential amino acid and thus an allowance, determined by individual tolerance to achieve target methionine and homocysteine levels, must be included in the diet. A methionine exchange system is used, predominantly consisting of foods of low biological protein value. One exchange contains 20 mg methionine, or approximately 1 g natural protein (Table 17.25). Where information on methionine content is not available (e.g. manufactured foods) the protein content is used.

Methionine intake varies between individuals. Amongst the author's patient group at the Willink Unit, Manchester, methionine tolerance, and hence allowance, falls within a range of 160–900 mg/day with a median value of 230 mg/day. The methionine allowance should ideally be evenly spread throughout the day to minimise fluctuations in plasma homocysteine levels.

Table 17.25   Methionine 20 mg exchanges (1 g protein) for use in homocystinuria.

Food	Weight*
Dairy products	
Cow's milk	20 mL
Aptamil First	65 mL[†]
Cow & Gate Premium	70 mL[†]
SMA Gold	55 mL[†]
Farley's First	55 mL[†]
Single cream	30 mL
Whipping cream	35 mL
Double cream	30 mL
Custard	20 mL
Yoghurt (natural/fruit/flavoured)	20 g

Table 17.25   *(Cont'd)*

Food	Weight*
Cereals	
All Bran	10 g
Cornflakes	10 g
Muesli	10 g
Oatmeal (raw)	10 g
Puffed Wheat	10 g
Ready Brek	10 g
Rice Krispies	15 g
Shredded Wheat	10 g
Sugar Puffs	20 g
Weetabix	10 g
Rice (raw)	15 g
Rice (boiled)	40 g
Potatoes	
Boiled, mashed (no milk)	85 g
Baked (flesh only)	50 g
Baked (flesh + skin)	60 g
Roast	45 g
Chips	35 g
Canned new	100 g
Instant mash (powder)	15 g
Crisps	20 g
Vegetables	
Baked beans (canned)	35 g
Broad beans (boiled)	75 g
Broccoli tops (boiled)	45 g
Brussels sprouts (boiled)	75 g
Cauliflower (boiled)	65 g
Mushrooms (raw)	35 g
Mushrooms (fried)	25 g
Peas (canned garden)	45 g
Peas (canned processed)	35 g
Spinach (boiled)	20 g
Sweetcorn (canned)	35 g
Yam (raw)	70 g
Yam (boiled)	85 g
Fruit	
Apricots (dried)	85 g
Avocado	30 g
Banana	100 g
Currants	35 g
Dates (dried)	75 g
Figs (dried)	70 g
Nectarine	55 g
Peach	85 g
Raisins	55 g
Sultanas	35 g

Source: Paul AA, Southgate DAT, Russell J First supplement to *McCance and Widdowson's, The Composition of Foods*, London: HMSO, 1979.
* Weight to nearest 5 g.
† Manufacturers' data, March 2006.

There can be periods of interindividual methione requirements, as also seen in other amino acid disorders (e.g. during growth spurts, or after prolonged infections).

Supplement intake of amino acids with a methionine free protein substitute

The dietary allowance of natural protein provides insufficient total protein for normal growth, therefore a protein substitute that is free from methionine is essential in ensuring an adequate total protein intake. The protein substitute used should contain cystine as this amino acid is normally formed from methionine but becomes deficient in HCU because of the metabolic block. A number of methionine free, cystine enriched protein substitutes are available (Table 17.26). Currently, the amino acid requirements recommended for PKU [191] are also used in HCU (Table 17.5). In this case the combined protein equivalent is from methionine exchanges (natural protein) and the protein substitute. These recommended protein intakes are high compared with normal recommended intakes for protein [192] to take into account the synthetic nature of the protein (as amino acids), the effect of this on their bioavailability and the aim of preventing protein catabolism and promoting protein synthesis. The protein substitute should be given in 3–4 divided doses throughout the day or more frequently in demand fed infants. It should be given together with the methionine exchanges at main meals, so as to provide the complete range of amino acids, to allow protein synthesis and prevent excessive rise in plasma homocysteine.

Achieve adequate energy intake to prevent protein catabolism and achieve normal growth

Dietary energy is provided from a number of sources, including:

- Foods naturally low or free from protein (methionine) – fruits and vegetables (Table 17.27), sugars and fats (Table 17.17)
- Specially manufactured low protein (low methionine) foods (e.g. flour, bread, breakfast cereals, pasta, biscuits) (see Appendix 17.1)

Table 17.26 Methionine free protein substitutes used in homocystinuria (per 100 g).

Product	Manufacturer	Amino acids (g)	Protein (equiv. g)	Energy kcal (kJ)	Carbohydrate (g)	Fat (g)	Vitamins and minerals	Age range	Presentation
XMet Analog[†]	SHS	15.5	13	475 (1986)	54	23	Full range	Infant formula	Tin
XMet Maxamaid[†]	SHS	30	25	309 (1292)	51	<0.5	Full range	From 1 year	Tin
XMet Maxamum[†]	SHS	47	39	297 (1241)	34	<0.5	Full range	From 8 years	Tin
XMet Homidom[†]	SHS	93	77	326 (1363)	4.5	Nil	Calcium and phosphorus*	Any age	Tin
HCU Gel[†]	Vitaflo	50.5	42	340 (1421)	43	0.14	Full range	From 1 year	Sachets
HCU Express[†]	Vitaflo	72	60	301 (1258)	15	0.1	Full range	From 8 years	Sachets
HCU LV	SHS	86	72	330 (1403)	9	1.0	Full range	From 8 years	Sachets

Products produced by Mead Johnson (HCY 1, HCY 2) and Ross (Hominex 1, Hominex 2) are also available in other countries, but not currently in the UK.
* Requires complete vitamin and mineral supplementation.
[†] All are ACBS approved and available on FP10 prescription in the UK.

- Energy supplements – glucose polymers, fat emulsions

Provide adequate vitamins, minerals and trace elements

Because of the limited range of foods allowed in the diet, it is essential to supplement the diet with the full range of vitamins, minerals and trace elements to achieve the RNI for age [192]. Many of the methionine free protein substitutes will provide these (Table 17.26). If the methionine free protein substitute does not contain vitamins, minerals or trace elements, a separate supplement is necessary (e.g. Paediatric Seravit, Phlexy-Vits or Forceval Junior capsules/Forceval capsules) together with separate calcium supplement).

Again, because of increased use of the remethylation pathway, an additional pharmacological dose of folic acid, 5 mg/day, is also prescribed to ensure adequate supply of folate.

Cysteine

Cysteine becomes an essential amino acid in HCU because of the metabolic block preventing cysteine being made from cystathionine (Fig. 17.4). Although all the methionine free protein substitutes are supplemented with cysteine plasma levels may still be low at times. Cysteine has poor solubility and care needs to be taken that it has not precipitated out of the protein substitute and left behind in the drinking vessel.

Cysteine and homocysteine-cysteine is present in plasma as free cysteine (cysteine and homocysteine-cysteine mixed disulphide) and protein bound cysteine. At increased concentrations of plasma homocysteine the amount of cysteine present, as the mixed disulphide homocysteine–cysteine, increases and cystine and protein bound cysteine decrease. When monitoring patients with HCU on dietary treatment cysteine status should ideally be assessed as total plasma cysteine (free and protein bound). As biochemical control improves with decreasing homocysteine levels, cysteine levels increase.

If total cysteine levels are very low the diet can be further supplemented with a cysteine supplement, starting at 1–2 g/day. Two products are currently available in the UK:

- L-cystine (SHS), a powder.
- Cystine AA Supplement (Vitaflo), a powder that forms a gel when mixed with water.

Management of the early diagnosed infant and child with HCU

Infants with HCU who fail to respond to a pharmacological dose of pyridoxine are commenced

Table 17.27 Low methionine fruits and vegetables.

Fruit
Fresh, frozen, or tinned in syrup (<15 mg methionine and/or <1 g protein/100 g)

Apple	Grapes	Pawpaw
Apricots	Guava	Pears
Blackberries	Kiwi fruit	Pineapple
Clementines	Lemon	Plums
Cherries	Lychees	Pomegranate
Cranberries	Mandarins	Raspberries
Damsons	Mango	Rhubarb
Fruit salad	Melon	Satsumas
Figs – green, raw	Olives	Strawberries
Gooseberries	Oranges	Tangerine
Grapefruit	Passion fruit	Water melon

Vegetables
Fresh, frozen or tinned (<20 mg methionine and/or <1 g protein/100 g)

Artichoke*	Endive*	Peppers
Asparagus	Garlic	Plantain
Aubergine	Gherkins	Pumpkin
Beans – French, green	Gourd*	Radish
Beansprouts*	Fennel	Spring greens
Beetroot*	Leeks*	Swede
Cabbage	Lettuce	Sweet potato
Carrots	Marrow	Tomatoes
Celery	Mustard and cress	Turnip
Chicory	Onions	Watercress*
Courgette*	Spring onion	
Cucumber	Parsley	

Source: Paul AA, Southgate DAT, Russell J First supplement to *McCance and Widdowson's The Composition of Foods* London: HMSO, 1979. Royal Society of Chemistry, Ministry of Agriculture, Fisheries and Food. *McCance and Widdowson's The Composition of Foods,* 5th edn. London: HMSO, 1991.
* These vegetables contain >20 mg methionine and/or 1 g protein/100 g but are generally eaten in small quantities.

on dietary therapy. Initially, all natural protein (methionine) intake is stopped and the infant is fed entirely on a methionine free infant formula, XMet Analog, aiming to give approximately 2.5 g methionine free protein (3 g amino acids)/kg body weight/day and normal energy requirements for age. After 48 hours a measured amount of natural protein as normal infant formula is reintroduced, usually initially to provide 120 mg methionine/day (personal practice). The normal infant formula is divided equally between several feeds (four to five times daily) with XMet Analog offered to appetite after each feed and at additional feeds as the infant demands. The quantity of normal infant formula is adjusted according to subsequent plasma methionine and homocysteine levels, aiming to keep within the desirable limits (Table 17.24).

As yet there has been no published practical experience of breast feeding an early diagnosed infant with classical HCU. In theory it should be possible for such an infant to be breast fed using the principles employed in the management of PKU. The infant would be given a measured amount of methionine free infant formula at the start of a feed and then breast fed on demand. The prescribed quantity of methionine free infant formula would be increased or decreased according to blood methionine/homocysteine levels in order to manipulate the amount of breast milk the infant takes.

Weaning

Solids are usually introduced at the normal recommended age for weaning. Initially, solids of a low protein content (free foods), e.g. fruits, some vegetables (Table 17.27), low protein rusk and commercial baby foods containing <0.5 g protein/100 g are used.

Once the infant is accepting low protein solids regularly then methionine (protein) containing solids are gradually introduced with a corresponding reduction in the normal infant formula allowance until protein containing solids make up all the methionine allowance. The protein containing methionine exchanges are given before the XMet Analog feeds. Once all the methionine allowance is provided from solids the exchanges are divided between the main meals.

Use of the manufactured low protein foods is encouraged as part of the weaning process to accustom the child to them as they will become important in providing variety and a source of energy in the diet.

From around 1 year of age a more concentrated methionine free protein substitute (e.g. HCU Gel or XMet Maxamaid) is introduced. These can be given as a drink or more concentrated as a paste. If there are concerns about achieving an adequate total protein intake before 1 year of age then HCU Gel or

XMet Maxamaid may be introduced earlier (from around 6 months of age) or additional methionine free amino acids (XMet Homidom a pure amino acid mix) is added into the XMet Analog.

Diet during childhood

During childhood the methionine allowance remains fairly constant. Periods of rapid growth may temporarily increase methionine tolerance. The intake of low protein foods gradually increases according to appetite to ensure an adequate energy intake. The quantity of the methionine free protein substitute prescribed should be reviewed regularly and increased to meet the protein requirements for age. From around 8 years of age HCU Express, HCU LV or XMet Maxamum, which are further concentrated in protein, can be introduced.

Dietary treatment must continue for life in order to prevent the development of late complications of HCU.

Management of illness

During intercurrent infections general advice is given to minimise protein catabolism and therefore prevention of an excessive rise in plasma homocysteine levels:

- Encouragement of the usual intake of methionine free protein substitute – without force feeding as this can lead to refusal once well
- Reduction of methionine exchanges – in practice a reduced appetite leads to reduced methionine intake
- Generous use of non-protein energy (e.g. high carbohydrate drinks)

A strict emergency regimen is not essential as acute metabolic decompensation does not occur.

Dietary management in later diagnosed cases

Individuals diagnosed late after the onset of clinical symptoms, or as a result of investigation following a sibling being diagnosed with classical HCU, are commenced on a methionine restricted diet. In the author's unit, the practice is to initiate a diet restricting methionine intake to 200 mg/day, together with an age appropriate methionine free protein substitute (Table 17.26) to make up the total protein requirement for age. If, from diet history, the normal dietary protein intake prior to diagnosis has been exceptionally high, a larger methionine allowance may be given. Subsequent methionine allowance is adjusted in the light of plasma methionine and homocysteine levels so as to achieve acceptable levels (Table 17.24).

Dietary compliance in this group can, in some cases, be difficult to achieve because they are used to a normal unrestricted diet. Most will have learning difficulties and so understanding the need for such a radical change in diet can be difficult to achieve. Individuals may cheat with high protein foods, take additional methionine exchanges or refuse the methionine free protein substitute. These problems need to be addressed. A positive family attitude and support from the multidisciplinary team, including clinical psychologist, are important if dietary treatment is to succeed. In some late diagnosed individuals in whom all attempts to give the methionine free protein substitutes have failed, a modified low protein diet using the minimum safe level of protein intake [193] (to minimise protein catabolism and poor growth) is used in conjunction with oral betaine therapy (see below).

Betaine therapy

Betaine is a methyl donor and promotes the remethylation reaction of homocysteine to methionine (Fig. 17.5). Use of betaine in HCU will normally result in plasma methionine levels being significantly increased, although this is not universal, and plasma homocysteine levels falling [194,195]. The use of oral betaine can be useful in improving biochemical control in circumstances where dietary compliance is poor (e.g. adolescents, adults and those late diagnosed). Compliance with betaine is not always good and it is unlikely to be able to replace dietary therapy [186].

Maternal HCU

CBS deficiency HCU in women appears to be

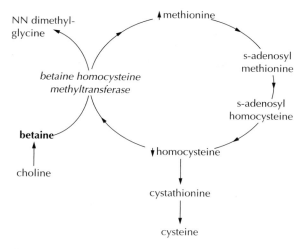

Figure 17.5   Methyl group donation by betaine.

associated with a higher incidence of spontaneous abortion. There is little evidence of other adverse effects on the fetus [187]. Betaine appears to be safe for use during pregnancy with infrequent reports of abnormalities being observed in offspring [196,197].

Both pregnancy and homocystinuria are risk factors for thromboembolism. Increased levels of homocysteine in the first few weeks postpartum have been reported which can be alleviated by anticoagulation therapy [196,197]. Current management of pregnancy in women with HCU would include good metabolic control and the use of anticoagulant therapy during the later stages of pregnancy and first 6 weeks postpartum to safeguard the mother's health.

Organic Acidaemias and Urea Cycle Disorders

Marjorie Dixon

Low protein diet for the management of urea cycle disorders and organic acidaemias

Protein requirements

Low protein diets must provide at least the minimum amount of protein, nitrogen and essential amino acids to meet requirements for normal growth. Safe levels of protein intakes (Table 17.28) and requirements for essential amino acid intake have been set by FAO/WHO/UNU Expert Committees since 1957, most recently in 1985 [193]. These safe levels are based on an intake of high biological value (HBV) protein foods, milk and hen's egg, with 100% digestibility, thus ensuring an adequate intake of all essential amino acids. It is important to be aware that the safe levels of protein intakes have been calculated as the mean requirement +2 standard deviations (SD) of the requirement, so as to meet or exceed the requirements of most individuals. However, for some individuals, a protein intake that is below the 'safe' intake may be adequate for their growth. These recommendations

were reviewed by Dewey *et al.* [198] and they suggested the safe levels of protein intakes have been set too high. Revised estimates are given (Table 17.28). These figures can certainly be used as a guide for very low protein diets. In 2007 the FAO/WHO/UNU will make available revised recommendations for protein and amino acid requirements of infants and children [143]. The new recommendations are reported to be comparable but uniformly lower than the earlier estimates for most ages, especially in the first 2 years of life.

Ideally, the protein source in low protein diets should be mainly from HBV protein, but this is not common practice because a greater variety of foods and a higher energy intake per gram of protein can be provided from low biological value (LBV) protein foods. Children on low protein diets who frequently consume a limited range of LBV protein foods may be at risk of one or more essential amino acids becoming rate-limiting for protein synthesis. It is therefore important that a variety of LBV protein foods (e.g. potato, cereals, rice, pasta, pulses) are taken to ensure an adequate intake of all essential amino acids. If the protein prescription is

Table 17.28 Safe level of protein intake for infants, children and adolescents.

Age	Safe level (g protein/kg/day) *	†
0–1 months	–	2.69
1–2	–	2.04
2–3	–	1.53
3–4	1.86	1.37
4–5	1.86	1.25
5–6	1.86	1.19
6–9	1.65	1.09
9–12	1.48	1.02
1–1.5 years	1.26	1.0
1.5–2	1.17	0.94
2–3	1.13	0.92
3–4	1.09	0.9
4–5	1.06	0.88
5–6	1.02	0.86
6–9	1.01	0.86
9–10	0.99	0.86
Girls		
10–11	1.0	0.87
11–12	0.98	0.86
12–13	0.96	0.85
13–14	0.9	0.84
14–15	0.9	0.81
15–16	0.87	0.81
16–17	0.83	0.78
17–18	0.8	0.7
Boys		
10–11	0.99	0.86
11–12	0.98	0.86
12–13	1.0	0.88
13–14	0.97	0.86
14–15	0.96	0.86
15–16	0.92	0.84
16–17	0.9	0.83
17–18	0.86	0.81

* Energy and protein requirements. Report of a joint FAO/WHO/UNU Expert Consultation [192].
† Dewey et al. [197].

generous enough, more HBV proteins should be included to improve the protein quality of the diet.

Protein tolerance will vary depending on residual enzyme activity of the specific disorder, growth rate, age and sex. During early infancy growth is at a maximum so protein requirements per kilogram body weight are greatest at this time. If the child has had a period of slow growth, protein intake may need to be temporarily increased during the following period of catch-up growth. Protein requirements may also be temporarily increased if a child has had repeated intercurrent infections with inadequate protein intakes.

Protein exchanges and free foods

Protein intake from LBV protein foods is measured by an exchange system (i.e. one exchange equals the amount of food that provides 1 g protein (Table 17.21). This allows greater variety in the diet as foods can be substituted for each other and still provide a similar protein content. Most manufactured foods have nutritional labelling with the protein content expressed as grams of protein/100 g and sometimes also grams of protein per portion. Parents should be taught how to interpret the food label and calculate exchanges.

For manufactured foods one exchange (1 g protein) is calculated as:

- 100 ÷ (g protein per 100 g food)
- If more than 1 g protein is desired this is multiplied by that number of exchanges

Ideally, the protein intake should be evenly distributed between main meals and some for snacks. Protein food exchanges should be weighed, at least initially. Digital scales which weigh in 1 or 2 g increments are recommended. If parents are unable to cope with the concept of protein exchanges or weighing, then a set menu with handy measures for foods is used.

The energy provided by exchange foods can range greatly; for example, an exchange of baked beans provides 20 kcal (84 kJ) and crisps 110 kcal (462 kJ). It may be helpful, particularly if the child has a poor appetite, to give parents advice on choosing protein exchanges that are more energy dense and provide more than 60 kcal (252 kJ) per exchange.

Energy

Low protein diets may not provide sufficient energy because the intake of many foods is restricted. This must be avoided as an inadequate energy intake causes poor growth and poor metabolic control with endogenous protein catabolism resulting in increased production of toxic metabolites (e.g. ammonia in urea cycle disorders). The aim is to provide around the normal energy requirement for age and sex. However, this may not be appropriate for all patients; some children with disorders of propionate metabolism may have reduced energy requirements and this will need to be adjusted for the individual.

Dietary energy can be provided by both the protein exchanges and the following groups of foods which are allowed without restriction in the diet:

- Foods naturally low in or free of protein – sugar, fats and a few commercial foods (Table 17.17), fruits and some vegetables (Table 17.23)
- Specially manufactured low protein foods (e.g. bread, pasta, biscuits; see Appendix 17.1)
- Energy supplements such as glucose polymer, fat emulsions

Manufactured low protein foods are not always popular with this group of patients. Children with urea cycle disorders (UCD) usually obtain sufficient energy from normal foods and prefer to eat these. Children with disorders of propionate metabolism often have poor appetite and are tube fed, hence they usually depend on energy supplements as their main energy source.

Vitamins, minerals and trace elements

Mineral deficiencies, particularly associated with low protein diets, have been reported in patients with organic acidaemias and UCD [199–201]. Vitamin and mineral supplements are almost always essential as intake will be severely limited. An adequate intake of vitamins A and C and folic acid could be provided from fruit and vegetables but iron, zinc, copper, calcium and B vitamins are most likely to be deficient. Together the diet and supplement should provide at least the RNI for vitamins and minerals [146]. The amount required will vary and needs to be assessed for the individual. The supplement is best given as a divided dose to enhance absorption.

Paediatric Seravit provides a comprehensive vitamin and mineral supplement (except for sodium, potassium and chloride). It can be added to the infant formula in the required dose. For older children it can be given as a drink or paste combined with a drink (because it is hyperosmolar). To mask the unpleasant flavour of Paediatric Seravit it can be added to fruit juice, squash, low protein milk with milk shake flavouring or mixed with honey, jam or fruit purée. It can be mixed with food such as breakfast cereal but it then becomes important that all the food is eaten. For older children Forceval Junior Capsules (suitable from 5 years of age) or Forceval Capsules (suitable from 12 years of age) can replace Paediatric Seravit as the vitamin and mineral supplement. It is important to be aware that Forceval Junior Capsules do not contain calcium, sodium, potassium, chloride, inositol and choline and contain only small quantities of magnesium. A separate calcium supplement will be needed. Forceval capsules differ slightly in composition from the Junior capsule; they contain small amounts of calcium, phosphorus and potassium but no vitamin K. An additional calcium supplement would still be needed. Phlexy-Vits (powder or tablets) is a comprehensive vitamin and mineral supplement suitable from 11 years of age. The powder is generally taken mixed with a strong flavoured drink. These and alternative vitamin and mineral supplements have been reviewed in the PKU and MSUD sections (see pp. 323, 337).

Essential fatty acids

Patients on therapeutic low protein diets may be at risk of inadequate intakes of EFA and their longer chain derivatives (DHA and AA) Sanjurjo et al. [202] reported a long chain polyunsaturated acid (LCPUFA) deficiency, specifically DHA in patients with UCDs and methylmalonic acidaemia, and recommended supplementation. More recently, Vlaardingerbroek et al. [203] also reported low plasma and red cell DHA concentrations in patients with UCDs and branched chain organic acidurias. The actual synthesis of LCPUFA in clinically stable patients with propionic acidaemia is reported to not be affected [204]. It is therefore important that low protein diets and modular feeds are assessed for EFA content and consideration should also be given to intakes of LCPUFA. At least 1% of energy intake from linoleic acid and 0.2% from α-linolenic acid should be provided in the diet [146]. If necessary, red cell and plasma fatty acid profiles should be measured.

Monitoring low protein diets

Protein and mineral deficiencies have been reported in patients with inborn errors of metabolism on restricted protein intakes [199–201]. This type of diet, comprising mainly LBV proteins, is often used in children with organic acidaemias and urea cycle disorders, therefore protein and amino acid intakes need to be carefully monitored. This should be carried out by clinical examination (skin and hair, looking specifically for signs of protein deficiency such as skin rashes), anthropometric measurements, biochemical assessment (quantitative amino acids, albumin and electrolytes) and regular dietary assessment. Periodic assessment of the following is important: plasma status of vitamins, minerals and trace elements (see Table 1.7); bone mineral density scans; plasma and red cell status of EFA and LCPUFA.

Low protein diets for infants and children

Infant feeding

Breast milk or a whey based infant formula should provide the main protein source for infants. Breast milk has many immunological and nutritional benefits. In the normal population breast fed babies produce significantly less propionic acid compared with bottle fed babies [205], so theoretically infants with disorders of propionate metabolism who are breast fed may have the additional benefit of reduced gut propionate production. However, there are few published reports of babies with these disorders being breast fed [155,206–208]. Demand breast feeding can be successful in UCDs and organic acidaemias provided there is regular monitoring of growth and metabolic status. During the initial stabilisation period when no protein is given the mother needs to express breast milk to maintain a supply and the infant is given a protein free feed. Once stabilised either expressed breast milk or breast feeding is gradually reintroduced. This is discussed in more detail in the sections on management of the newly diagnosed child. If demand breast feeding provides too much protein, intakes can be reduced by giving either a protein free, or precursor amino acid free (i.e. does not contain the amino acids that cannot be metabolised), supplementary bottle feed before some or all breast feeds of either:

- Energivit, a protein free otherwise nutritionally complete feed, containing CHO, fat, vitamins and minerals, suitable for UCDs and organic acidaemias
- A modular protein free feed for urea cycle disorders and organic acidaemias (Table 17.29)
- A specialised infant formula free from precursor amino acids (e.g. for disorders of propionate metabolism XMTVI Analog)

A protein free diet powder 80056 is produced by Mead Johnson Nutritionals; this can be made available on request, but it is not prescribable in the UK.

If a whey based infant formula is used, the amount is adjusted to provide at least the safe level of protein intake for age (Table 17.28) or more if

Table 17.29 Protein free modular feed.

	Energy						
	(kcal)	(kJ)	CHO (g)	Protein (g)	Fat (g)	Sodium (mmol)	Potassium (mmol)
55 g Maxijul	209	888	52	–	–	0.5	0.1
40 mL Calogen	180	756	–	–	20	0.2	–
12 g Paediatric Seravit	36	151	9	–	–	–	–
25 mL Normasol						3.9	
5.0 mL KCl solution							10.0
Plus water to 600 mL							
Totals	425	1785	61	–	20	4.6	10.1
Per 100 mL	71	298	10.2	–	3.3	0.8	1.7

Table 17.30   Low protein feed for 3-month-old male infant, weight 5 kg.

	Energy		CHO (g)	Protein (g)	Fat (g)	Sodium (mmol)	Potassium (mmol)
	(kcal)	(kJ)					
80 g SMA Gold	419	1760	45	9.6	23	4.4	11.3
40 g glucose polymer, e.g. Maxijul	152	638	38	–	–	0.4	<0.2
2 g Paediatric Seravit	6	25	1.5	–	–	–	–
Plus water to 750 mL							
Totals	577	2423	85	9.6	23	4.8[‡]	11.3[‡]
per 100 mL	77	323	11.3	1.3	3.1	0.6	1.5
per kg	115	485	–	1.9	–	1.0	2.3
DRV per kg 0–3 months*	115–100	480–420		2.1		2.0	3.4
Minimum protein requirement[†]				1.86			

* Dietary reference values [146].
[†] FAO/WHO/UNU safe level of protein intake (Table 17.28).
[‡] Additional sodium and potassium may be necessary (some medicines provide electrolytes).

clinically indicated. Additional fluid, energy, vitamins and minerals are added to make it a nutritionally adequate feed (Table 17.30). The aim is to produce a feed which gives the RNI for all vitamins and minerals [146] and is comparable to a normal infant formula. It is important to ensure the intake of sodium and potassium is adequate. Additional protein free feeds (see above) are given if the infant is still hungry. Alternatively, a combination of infant formula and Energivit is given: the infant formula provides the prescribed safe level of protein intake for age and Energivit provides the additional energy, fluid and vitamins and minerals. This is easier for parents than making a modular feed which has several ingredients.

Weaning

Weaning is started at the usual time around 6 months (26 weeks) of age. Normal weaning practices are followed: solids are introduced at one meal then two and three times per day and the infant progresses from smooth purées to lumpier foods and finger foods during the first year. The first solids given are 'protein free' such as fruit or low protein vegetable purées (Table 17.23), low protein rusk or low protein cereal (see Appendix 17.1), or commercial baby foods containing <0.5 g protein/100 g, so that if they are refused the total protein intake is not affected. Once these are accepted

protein containing solids are introduced from either commercial baby foods or home cooked foods such as potato, vegetables or cereals. The energy content of protein exchanges can be increased by adding butter or margarine to savoury foods and sugar to desserts. It is best to have a flexible approach as to when the protein food should be given; some infants may take this best before (if not too hungry) or between feeds.

One gram of protein from infant formula is replaced by 1 g protein from solids. This is less easy to regulate in the breast fed infant as the protein intake is not known. Therefore an aim for total protein intake (usually the safe level of intake) is set and as protein exchanges are introduced the number of breast feeds is reduced to compensate. It is important to ensure that an adequate energy intake is provided by exchanges and free foods, otherwise breast feeds will not be reduced sufficiently. In both the bottle and breast fed infant this process is continued throughout the first year of life or so and is dictated by what the infant can manage, until all the protein is provided by solid food. Ideally the protein exchanges should be evenly distributed between main meals. During this changeover period it is important to ensure that vitamin and mineral intakes are adequate. The vitamin and mineral supplement is increased and will need to be introduced to the breast fed infant with the progressive change to solids, as these foods are a poorer source of nutrients than infant formula and breast milk.

Diet in childhood

Throughout childhood the protein intake is increased to provide at least the safe level of protein intake (Table 17.28) for age or more if clinically indicated. This is given in conjunction with an adequate energy, vitamin and mineral intake for age. It is important to ensure the child consumes a variety of LBV protein foods. HBV foods can also provide some of the protein in the diet. Useful HBV foods include: thin sliced meats (ham, chicken or turkey), cheeses (Dairylea cheese triangles, Philadelphia cream cheese, Boursin), hot dog sausages, fish fingers, eggs, fromage frais and yoghurt (choosing the highest energy varieties). The energy content of the diet can be increased by frying foods, adding butter or oil, or double cream (1 g protein and 270 kcal [1080 kJ] per 60 mL) to savoury foods such as pasta, rice or potato. Sugar, glucose polymer or double cream can be added to desserts. High CHO drinks are encouraged, such as Lucozade or Ribena, and often glucose polymer is added to drinks to a final concentration of 15–25% CHO, depending on age. Low protein milks (Table 17.31) can be used to make milk shakes and desserts and can be poured on cereals. If the child does not consume all the daily protein allowance as food, it should be replaced with fluids; cow's milk with added glucose polymer to 15–20% CHO is often the simplest way to do this. Another useful alternative is to give a juice supplement such as Fortijuice which provides 1 g protein and 30 kcal (125 kJ) per 25 mL. Table 17.31 provides an example of a low protein diet.

Some children, particularly those with disorders of propionate metabolism, refuse to eat or have a very limited intake of solid food. They will depend on liquid feeds given by mouth or by tube to provide most of their low protein diet. A modular feed would be designed to meet the nutritional needs of the child and the specific disorder. An example of a low protein feed is shown in Table 17.32.

Disorders of propionate metabolism

The disorders of propionate metabolism, methylmalonic acidaemia (MMA) and propionic

Table 17.31 Low protein diet (20 g), for 6-year-old girl, weight 18 kg.

	Protein (g) (using 1 g protein exchanges)
Breakfast	
20 g cornflakes and sugar	2
Protein free milk*	
36 g (1 slice) bread	3
Butter, jam, honey, marmalade	
100 mL pure fruit juice + 10 g glucose polymer	
Mid morning	
15 g (1) chocolate digestive biscuit	1
1 can Lucozade	
Packed lunch	
36 g (1 slice) bread	3
Butter, tomato and mayonnaise	
30 g (1 packet) crisps	2
Portion fresh fruit	
200 mL carton Ribena	
Mid afternoon	
25 g milk chocolate	2
Squash + 150 mL water + 20 g glucose polymer	
Evening meal	
25 g (1) fried fish finger	3
50 g chips	2
15 g peas	1
Carrots and butter	
30 g ice cream	1
Tinned fruit	
Bedtime	
Protein-free milk shake	
or squash + 150 mL water + 20 g glucose polymer	
Daily	
10 g Paediatric Seravit	

* Protein free milk alternatives:
15 g Duocal and water to 100 mL
10 g glucose polymer or sugar, 10 mL Calogen + water to 100 mL
Low protein milks (see Appendix 17.1).

acidaemia (PA) share common biochemical and clinical features resulting from accumulation of propionyl-CoA and other metabolites (Fig. 17.2) which are formed from catabolism of the four essential amino acids, isoleucine, valine, threonine

Table 17.32 Low protein tube feed for a 4-year-old girl, weight 15 kg.

	Energy		CHO (g)	Protein (g)	Fat (g)	Sodium (mmol)	Potassium (mmol)
	(kcal)	(kJ)					
550 mL Paediasure	556	2335	60.5	15.4	27.5	14.3	15.4
170 g Maxijul	646	2713	161.5	–	–	1.5	0.2
60 mL Calogen	270	1134	–	–	30.0	0.2	–
8.0 g Paediatric Seravit	24	102	6.0	–	–	–	–
100 mL Normasol						15.4	
8.0 mL KCl solution							16.0
Plus water to 1200 mL							
Totals	1496	6283	228	15.4	57.5	31.4	31.6
Per 100 mL	125	524	19	1.3	4.8	2.6	2.6
Per kg	100	420		1.0		2.1	2.1
DRV 4–6 years*	1460	6120		1.1			
Safe level of protein intake†				1.0			

* Dietary reference values [146].
† FAO/WHO/UNU safe level of protein intake (Table 17.28).

and methionine, although about 50% is derived from other sources.

PA is caused by a defect of propionyl-CoA carboxylase which causes high plasma and urinary propionate levels and excretion of multiple organic compounds, including methylcitrate and 3-hydroxypropionate. MMA is caused by a defect of either methylmalonyl-CoA mutase-apoenzyme causing reduced (mut⁻) or absent (mut°) activity or alternatively a defect in the synthesis of its co-factor 5'-deoxyadenosylcobalamin. Impairment results in accumulation of methylmalonic acid and the compounds found in propionic acidaemia. These disorders vary widely in severity depending on the degree of enzyme deficiency. Some MMA patients are completely responsive to co-factor vitamin B_{12} and require no dietary treatment except for an emergency regimen during intercurrent illness.

Both disorders can present in the neonatal period or early infancy with a severe metabolic acidosis (although not always) [209], poor feeding, vomiting, lethargy, hypotonia and dehydration; or in early childhood with less severe symptoms including failure to thrive and developmental delay [210].

The prognosis of MMA and PA is generally not good [199,211–215]. The mechanisms of toxicity are complex and not well understood. Early onset of PA is associated with poor intellectual outcome and early death, while late onset may be complicated by a severe disabling movement disorder [216]. Others report a similar high mortality in both early and late onset patients, with better neurological outcome for late onset patients [214]. Severe MMA (mut°) is associated with developmental retardation and early death [211]. Cobalamin responsive patients have a much better long term outcome. In both early and late onset MMA patients, there is increased risk of developing new neurological symptoms with age; these normally develop following episodes of acute metabolic decompensation [217]. Other more recently recognised complications in both disorders include cardiomyopathy [218] and pancreatitis [219], and in MMA also chronic renal failure [212,220].

Although survival rate has improved, outcome on conventional therapy is still poor. Alternative forms of therapy are being used. There are a few reports of transplantation, either kidney, liver or combined liver and kidney transplants; however, these are associated with significant risk at the time of transplant and metabolic complications may still arise post-transplant such as metabolic stroke [221].

Sources of propionate

It is important to appreciate that propionate is formed from three main sources, not just from amino acid catabolism. Estimates of the contributions of these sources are:

- Around 50% is derived from the catabolism of the precursor amino acids, isoleucine, valine, threonine and methionine [222].
- Around 25% is produced from anaerobic bacterial fermentation in the gut [222]. Oral administration of the antibiotic metronidazole will reduce gut bacteria propionate production, but the long term efficacy and safety of this are still being studied [223].
- Probably around 25% is derived from the oxidation of odd-numbered long chain fatty acids (C15 and C17) [224] and other metabolites. These odd-chain fatty acids are synthesised by the normal pathway of fatty acid synthesis but propionyl-CoA acts as the primer instead of acetyl CoA, hence the additional odd number of carbons in the chain [225].

Dietary management

The aims of dietary treatment are to reduce production of propionate by both the restriction of precursor amino acids, using a low protein diet, and avoidance of fasting to limit oxidation of odd-chain fatty acids. The precursor amino acids (isoleucine, valine, threonine and methionine) do not accumulate in plasma in these disorders. It is therefore not possible to use the measurement of plasma levels of these amino acids to determine the intake of natural protein. Dietary protein intake can therefore only be restricted to the safe level of intake for growth (Table 17.28). Too low a protein intake can have serious effects, such as poor growth, skin rashes, hair loss, vomiting and metabolic decompensation. Dietary protein is increased according to age, weight, clinical condition and quantitative plasma amino acid concentrations, ensuring that diet always provides at least the 'safe level of protein intake'. However, it can be difficult to achieve a balance between provision of sufficient protein for growth but avoiding an excess of protein which precipitates illness. Practical aspects of low protein diets and feeds have been discussed above.

To improve the quality of low protein diets, some centres supplement the diet with synthetic amino acids which are free from the precursor amino acids. These can take the form of infant formula, drink mixes, gels, pure amino acids (e.g. XMTVI Analog, Maxamaid and Maxamum; MMA/PA gel; MMA/PA Express). However, the clinical value of these supplements remains controversial and no long term controlled studies have been published. Metabolic balance can be achieved without them, and they are unpalatable and difficult to administer to children unless they are tube fed. One study of two patients with MMA showed that although there was increased nitrogen retention when the low protein diet was supplemented with precursor free amino acids, there was no improvement in growth or decrease in methylmalonate excretion [226]. Touati et al. [227], in a retrospective review of 137 patients with either MMA or PA, concluded that amino acid mixture supplementation did not seem to have an important role in the long term nutritional and developmental outcome. Yanicelli et al. [228] reported improved growth and nutrition status in a short term study of children using a precursor free amino acid feed; however, energy intakes also increased in those patients whose growth in height improved.

It is recommended that long fasts are avoided to limit the production of propionate from the oxidation of odd-numbered long chain fats [229]. Mobilisation of fatty acids can be suppressed by the use of regular 3–4 hourly daytime feeding and overnight tube feeding. Currently, overnight tube feeding is used universally although many receive this because of feeding problems. In one patient with MMA, uncooked cornstarch was used to minimise lipolysis at night [230].

Impaired renal function is a common complication in the more severe variants of MMA, manifesting initially with a defect of urinary concentrating and acidification resulting from renal tubular dysfunction [231]. Glomerular failure develops later [232] with progression to chronic, then end-stage renal failure (ESRF). Supplements of sodium bicarbonate are often needed both to replace sodium losses and reduce acidosis. A generous fluid intake is often necessary to prevent dehydration. Increased urinary methylmalonate excretion also increases electrolyte losses.

The low protein diet used for MMA is also appropriate dietary treatment for those who develop chronic renal failure. It is also important to ensure a good energy intake and maintenance of adequate fluids. Further dietary manipulations may also be necessary with the progression towards ESRF, such as limiting the intake of phosphate and potassium and reducing protein intake further. Haemodialysis can cause symptomatic and biochemical improvement in ESRF [233]. Protein restriction remains necessary on dialysis, but the intake may be slightly increased compared with intake pre-dialysis (personal experience of two patients).

Gastrointestinal problems such as gastro-oesophageal reflux and vomiting are not uncommon in these patients. Treatment of these problems may require further dietary manipulation, such as the use of a hydrolysed protein feed.

Anorexia and feeding problems of varying degrees are almost invariably present in the children with more severe variants. The causative factors are unclear, but increased plasma propionate is a possibility [223]. Enteral feeding via nasogastric tube or gastrostomy is often essential to provide an adequate dietary intake, to prevent metabolic decompensation and to help the parents cope with a child who is difficult to feed. Food and fluid refusal is often acquired during the course of the disease and is frequently associated with repeated intercurrent infections. Many children have a poor appetite for solid food and often the diet is provided solely from oral fluids. Some will only eat a few selected foods, occasionally changing the type of foods that they will eat. Some are difficult feeders; parents complain of children being slow, fussy, retching or self-inducing vomiting with foods. Children with MMA have a preference for salty foods and may do so to compensate for increased urinary losses of sodium.

Resting energy expenditure (REE) has been measured in children with disorders of propionate metabolism and is reported to be decreased in some patients when they are well [234]. However, more recently, van Hagen et al. [235] reported increased REE and suggest this may be because of the higher body mass index (BMI) of their patients. Personal experience has shown that some children with disorders of propionate metabolism have reduced energy requirements resulting from impaired physical activity. Thus, energy intakes need to be adjusted individually to take account of the child's

metabolic state particularly during illness (see below) and growth.

Dietary management of illness

During intercurrent infections patients are at risk of developing metabolic acidosis and encephalopathy. Development of new neurological signs has been reported in MMA following episodes of acute metabolic decompensation [217].

To help prevent this, the standard ER (see p. 375) is given: a high CHO intake from glucose polymer is given orally and/or via a tube at frequent 2-hourly intervals both day and night or as a continuous tube feed. This will reduce protein catabolism and lipolysis and hence propionate production. The usual protein intake is stopped for the minimum time possible to prevent protein deficiency which could greatly exacerbate the effects of illness. Some protein is normally reintroduced early (within 2–3 days) and phased in over a period of 1–4 days depending on the clinical condition of the child. Obviously, a more rapid reintroduction of protein is beneficial. Practical advice on protein reintroduction is given in the section on ER below. Continuation of an adequate energy intake is important throughout this period.

Inadequate nutrition in these disorders leads to catabolism, making the metabolic disturbance worse. If a child is unable to be re-established on their normal diet and protein intake within a few days, or is experiencing repeated intercurrent infections with inadequate protein intake, then an early resort to parenteral nutrition becomes essential. Parenteral nutrition can reverse the catabolic spiral and improve the metabolic state. If parenteral nutrition is indicated a normal amino acid solution can be used, but the amount is limited to provide only the child's usual protein intake [236]. This may need to be increased further in a malnourished patient.

In addition to the standard ER, metronidazole is given to reduce gut propionate production, and carnitine (100 mg/kg/day) to increase the removal of propionyl groups as propionyl carnitine in the urine. In MMA a generous fluid intake and sodium bicarbonate are needed to prevent dehydration and reduce acidosis. This is extremely important in those with chronic renal disease who can rapidly become dehydrated. Additional potassium may also be necessary.

Treatment of the newly diagnosed patient

The newly diagnosed patient may be very sick in intensive care with severe acidosis and/or hyper-ammonaemia requiring ventilation and dialysis (to remove ammonia and toxic compounds). The aim of dietary treatment is to provide a high energy feed to reverse catabolism. Initially, a glucose polymer solution (10–15% CHO) is given and a fat emulsion is added in 1–2% increments as toler-ated. Provision of an adequate energy intake may initially be difficult because of fluid restrictions in the ventilated child. Intravenous fluids of 10% dextrose will contribute to the total energy intake. Electrolytes (sodium and potassium) are added to the feed to provide normal requirements for age, taking into account any contribution of these from intravenous fluids and medicines such as sodium bicarbonate and sodium benzoate (which is used for the treatment of hyperammonaemia in these disorders). However, in MMA electrolyte require-ments may be increased because of increased uri-nary losses. The feed is usually administered as frequent 2-hourly bolus feeds or continuous naso-gastric feeds. Energivit can be used to provide the protein free feed.

Protein is reintroduced with the minimum of delay once the acute metabolic derangement, including the acidosis, has been corrected and the plasma ammonia is ≤100 µmol/L (normal <40 µmol/L). Protein is usually commenced with 0.5 g protein/kg body weight/day from infant formula or expressed breast milk and increased to the final safe level of protein intake (Table 17.28) within a few days. Vitamins and minerals should be added to the feed if there is a delay in introducing or increasing protein intake. Paediatric Seravit can be used for this purpose. Table 17.30 provides an example of a nutritionally complete low protein infant feed.

If the baby is being breast fed the mother should be encouraged to express until the baby becomes more metabolically stable, then breast feeding can be reintroduced. Protein free feeds may need to be given in combination with breast feeds while metabolic control is being established, and even long term in some patients. Practical aspects of infant feeding have been discussed earlier (see p. 360).

Isovaleric acidaemia

Isovaleric acidaemia (IVA) is an inborn error of leucine metabolism caused by a deficiency of isovaleryl-CoA dehydrogenase resulting in accu-mulation of isovaleric acid and other metabolites (Fig. 17.2). IVA can present in neonates (acute form) with poor feeding, vomiting and lethargy progress-ing to coma, or in older children (chronic intermit-tent form) with non-specific failure to thrive and/or developmental delay. The neonate subsequently follows the chronic intermittent course. There is a wide spectrum of presentation with chronic and acute forms [237].

During remission the majority of isovaleryl-CoA is conjugated to isovalerylglycine which is not toxic and is excreted in large amounts in urine. Isovaleryl-CoA is also conjugated to carnitine to form isovaleryl carnitine which is also excreted in the urine. However, during acute episodes the natural capacity of this detoxification pathway is exceeded and isovaleryl-CoA is deacylated to pro-duce large amounts of toxic isovaleric acid which may cause an overwhelming illness [238]. The outcome of IVA is variable, ranging from normal psychomotor development to severe mental retar-dation [239].

Dietary management

The aim of dietary treatment is to limit dietary leucine intake and minimise formation of isovaleric acid. Sufficient leucine must be given for normal growth requirements. Leucine does not accumulate in plasma so it is not possible to use measurement of this to determine protein intake.

Usually a modest protein restriction (2 g/kg in infants and young children decreasing to 1.5–1.0 g/kg in older patients) combined with an adequate energy intake is sufficient to limit the production of isovaleric acid in the well child [237]. Higher protein intakes may be tolerated by some patients (personal experience). There are reports of dietary treatment with leucine free amino acids and protein intakes restricted to below 'safe levels'. However, in the author's experience this degree of restriction is not warranted. Although patients are not on very low protein diets it is still important to ensure that an adequate intake of all vitamins and minerals is provided. Practical management of low protein diets and feeds has been given above. Most children with IVA have a reasonable appetite but major feeding problems do occur in some.

In addition to diet, patients are treated with glycine (250 mg/kg/day) and carnitine (100 mg/kg/day) to increase conjugation and hence reduce isovaleric acid levels, particularly during periods of metabolic decompensation [238,240,241].

Clinical and dietary monitoring

The low protein diet is monitored as described on p. 360. There is no established laboratory marker for monitoring this disorder and therapeutic control. Plasma levels of leucine are not elevated in IVA. Plasma carnitine concentrations should be monitored.

Treatment of the newly diagnosed patient

The newly diagnosed infant with IVA may be very sick and in intensive care. The initial dietary management is similar to that described earlier for MMA and PA. A protein free feed is given while the infant is stabilised. Protein is then gradually introduced either from infant formula or expressed breast milk once the baby has improved. Introduction of protein should not be delayed. Gockay *et al.* [208] have reported successful long term demand breast feeding in one patient with IVA.

Dietary management during illness

During intercurrent infections protein catabolism will greatly increase production of isovaleric acid and patients are at risk of decompensation. To help prevent this, the standard ER (see p. 375) of frequent high CHO drinks day and night is given. Protein intake is stopped temporarily and reintroduced early within 1–3 days maximum and over a period of 1–4 days depending on the clinical condition of the child. Practical advice on protein reintroduction is provided in the ER section. Oral or intravenous glycine and carnitine should continue to be given as part of the ER and the doses may need to be increased temporarily.

Glutaric aciduria type 1

Glutaric aciduria type 1 (GA 1) is caused by a deficiency of the enzyme glutaryl-CoA dehydrogenase in the catabolic pathway of the amino acids L-lysine, L-hydroxylysine and L-tryptophan. Biochemically this results in the accumulation of glutaric acid, 3-hydroxyglutaric acid and (less frequently) glutaconic acids in body fluids and tissues [242]. Typically babies with GA 1 usually appear normal in the first months of life, although many will have macrocephaly. The majority of children typically present before 2 years of age with a median age of 9 months [243] following an intercurrent illness such as a respiratory or gastrointestinal illness which precipitates to an acute encephalopathic crisis. This characteristically results in striatal damage. Patients are consequently left with a severe dystonic–dyskinetic disorder that is similar to cerebral palsy and ranges from extreme hypotonia to choreathetosis to rigidity and spasticity [244]. Intellectual function is generally preserved initially. Morbidity and mortality is high in patients who have had a crisis. A minority of patients have a more insidious onset or later onset neurologic disease with no obvious encephalopathic episode preceeding the development of the movement disorder. Some patients with genetically proven GA 1 do not develop neurological disease at all [245].

Newborn screening programmes have been implemented in several countries around the world such as Australia, USA and Germany because early detection and presymptomatic initiation of treatment should in most, but not all, cases prevent the severe handicap which develops with the clinical presentation [246].

The Proceedings in Glutaryl-CoA dehydrogenase deficiency Report from the 3rd International Workshop on Glutaryl-CoA dehydrogenase deficiency and the 1st Guidelines meeting for Glutaryl-CoA dehydrogenase deficiency provide comprehensive information on: pathogenesis, diagnostic challenges, treatment strategies and monitoring and outlook [247].

Dietary management

The dietary manangement of GA 1 is controversial as the clinical value has not been proven; however, new evidence for benefits of dietary treatment in pre symptomatic patients is emerging (see below). The rationale for dietary treatment is to reduce production of glutaric acid and 3-hydroxyglutaric acid (which have toxic effects) by restriction of protein or more specifically by restriction of lysine, their precursor amino acid. Dietary practice varies around the world: low protein or low lysine diets plus supplements of lysine free, tryptophan reduced amino acids [247,248] are used in the treatment of both symptomatic and pre-symptomatic patients with GA 1; others (including the author's centre) use either a modest or no protein restriction and just recommend avoiding a high intake, but this has been for symptomatic rather than pre-symptomatic patients. It is known that protein restriction cannot reverse neurological damage that has already occurred and dietary protein restriction alone is not sufficient to prevent brain injury [245,249]. Dietary treatment in symptomatic patients is reported to be of no neurological benefit [243,247,250]. The rationale for use of a restricted lysine or protein diet in symptomatic patients appears limited. The efficacy of dietary treatment in patients with insidious or late-onset type disease is unclear.

In contrast, for pre symptomatic patients there is some evidence emerging that suggests dietary treatment may be of benefit. Naughten et al. [247] reported no striatal degeneration in their 10 high-risk screened patients and attributed this to their treatment protocol of a low protein diet supplemented with lysine, tryptophan free amino acids and an aggressive emergency regimen for illness. Strauss et al. [251] reported 20 patients diagnosed on newborn screening and treated with low protein diet and emergency regimen, 35% of whom developed basal ganglia disease. Kölker et al. [243], from an international cross-sectional study involving 35 metabolic centres (and including comparative data from Naughten and Strauss), have demonstrated that a lysine restricted diet is neuroprotective in pre symptomatic patients, but a protein restricted diet showed no beneficial effect. The actual protein or lysine intakes in these patients were not reported. Also the authors were not able to estimate the neuroprotective effect of emergency treatment for illness in pre symptomatic patients. This would have been of particular value because intercurrent illness generally precipitates neurological crisis. They have suggested that the low lysine diet rather than low protein is important as it reduces the accumulation of glutaric and 3-hydroxyglutaric acids in the brain but it remains to be proven. Supportive data for a low lysine diet also comes from studies in mice [252]. Greenberg et al. [253] report a less favourable outcome with three of four patients identified on newborn screening who experienced a neurological crisis following intercurrent illness and had been treated with diet and an illness plan. Francis et al. [254] reported that a diet providing 2.0–2.5 g protein/kg/day (so, only a moderate protein restriction) and rigorous management of intercurrent illness was associated with good outcome in four patients diagnosed on newborn screening. It is important to consider whether the better outcome in pre symptomatic patients is the result of aggressive management of intercurrent illness rather than the lysine restricted diet per se.

Low lysine, tryptophan reduced diet

The low lysine diet for GA 1 involves limiting the intake of the essential amino acid lysine to that required for normal growth for age. This will limit the intake of natural protein to below normal growth requirements and a supplement of lysine free, tryptophan reduced amino acids are needed. Lysine does not accumulate in plasma and can therefore not be used to accurately titrate against intake. The child is therefore at risk of inadequate intake of lysine and meticulous attention to other nutritional parameters, both clinical and biochemical, is needed to prevent a deficiency state. The principles and practical details of a low lysine diet have been described in greater detail by Kölker et al. [243] and Lindner et al. [254].

Feeding problems

Feeding problems are common in the group of patients with neurological disease and include chewing and swallowing difficulties resulting from dyskinesia, and reflux and vomiting resulting from truncal hypotonia. The extent of these feeding problems is related to the severity of the neurological disease, with acute onset being much worse than insidious onset. Dietary advice needs to be tailored to the individual child's needs: use of thickened fluids, energy dense foods of the correct consistency and energy supplements may be required to achieve an adequate nutrient and fluid intake. Tube feeding is often essential to maintain an adequate energy intake and to achieve satisfactory growth. Fundoplication (and insertion of gastrostomy) may be necessary in some patients for treatment of gastro-oesophageal reflux and vomiting.

Assessing energy requirements in this group of patients can be difficult; the worst affected patients cannot walk so should need less energy, but energy expenditure is reported to often be increased because of high muscle tone and dystonic movements and to disturbances in temperature control [244]. In the author's patient group provision of a near normal energy intake for age has resulted in satisfactory weight gain in most patients provided there were no problems with vomiting and gastro-oesophageal reflux. However, a small number still failed to thrive in early years. By contrast, in one patient with spasticity and rigidity, the energy requirement for normal growth was very low, around 50% of normal for age, thus emphasising the need for adjusting the diet to the requirements of the individual.

Additional fluids may be required in patients who have disturbances in temperature control with excessive sweating.

In addition to diet, carnitine supplementation (50–100 mg/kg/day) is given to enhance urinary excretion of glutaric acid as glutarylcarnitine and to avoid secondary carnitine deficiency.

Dietary management of illness

Prompt and aggressive management of intercurrent illness is critical in GA 1 to prevent neurological damage in pre-symptomatic patients and further injury in symptomatic patients. With increasing age and, in particular from 6 years of age, the risk of acute neurological insult appears to be much reduced; however, an emergency regimen (ER) is still important [243]. At the first sign of illness or loss of appetite (or usual feeds not being tolerated) the standard ER (see p. 375) of frequent high CHO drinks or tube feeds is given to minimise catabolism. If the child does not tolerate the ER it is crucial they are admitted to hospital without delay for intravenous therapy of 10% dextrose. Carnitine should also be given orally or if not tolerated, given intravenously. Once the child begins to improve, the usual diet is reintroduced and additional glucose polymer drinks/feeds are given particularly at night until the child has fully recovered and returned to the normal regimen. Parents will need guidance with written instructions on how to do this.

Urea cycle disorders

The urea cycle has two main functions: it converts waste nitrogen compounds generated from either dietary amino acids or from endogenous protein catabolism into urea (excreted by the kidney) and it is the biosynthetic pathway of arginine. The urea cycle consists of a series of six consecutive enzymatic reactions and inborn errors at each step of the pathway have been identified (Fig. 17.6). These disorders are inherited as autosomal traits apart from ornithine transcarbamoylase deficiency (OTC), which is an X-linked trait, and the most common of these disorders. Arginase deficiency is distinct from the other disorders and is discussed separately.

Deficiencies of these enzymes result in waste nitrogen accumulating as ammonia and glutamine, which are neurotoxic and may cause a severe encephalopathy. These disorders can present at any age from the neonatal period (neonatal onset) throughout childhood (late onset). The onset of symptoms in childhood may be chronic or acute, usually (but not always) precipitated by an intercurrent infection. Many of these children have had minor episodes before they present and self-select a low protein diet so that a diet history can be very revealing.

The clinical presentation varies depending on the age of onset. Loss of appetite, poor feeding and vomiting are common in all ages. In the newborn there is often respiratory distress with signs of hyperpnoea, seizures and collapse. In the later onset patients confusion, headache, disorientation, abnormal behaviour, ataxia, focal neurologial signs or coma can occur and in some there is also delayed physical growth and developmental delay [256].

The outlook for babies who present in the newborn period is very poor [257,258]. In late presenting patients many have some degree of learning

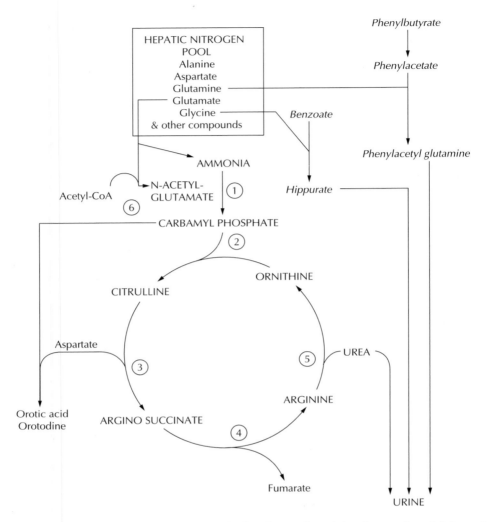

Figure 17.6 Hepatic nitrogen metabolism. Inherited metabolic disorder: 1 carbamyl phosphate synthase deficiency; 2 ornithine transcarbamoylase deficiency; 3 citrullinaemia; 4 argininosuccinic aciduria; 5 arginase deficiency; 6 N-acetyl glutamate synthase deficiency.

and neurological disability [258,259] and those with argininosuccinic aciduria are also prone to chronic hepatitis, potentially leading to cirrhosis. Patients who are treated prospectively generally have a much better outcome, although patients with argininosuccinic aciduria may still not do well.

Treatment

The urea cycle disorders are treated by:

- Medicines that utilise alternative pathways for the excretion of waste nitrogen
- Arginine supplements
- Restriction of dietary protein intake to decrease the need to excrete waste nitrogen

Medicines

Sodium benzoate and phenylbutyrate increase waste nitrogen excretion by using alternative pathways to the urea cycle (Fig. 17.6) [260]. Phenyl-butyrate is probably more effective than sodium benzoate as a vehicle for nitrogen excretion. Phenylbutyrate is metabolised *in vivo* to form phenylacetate which is conjugated with glutamine to form phenylacetylglutamine. If the reaction was complete then 2 moles of nitrogen would be excreted for each mole of phenylbutyrate given. However, recent studies indicate that only approximately 1 mole nitrogen is lost [261]. Sodium benzoate is conjugated with glycine to form hippurate so that 1 mole of nitrogen is excreted for each mole of sodium benzoate given. Both can be administered orally or IV and are usually prescribed in doses of up to 250 mg/kg body weight/day, divided between three or four doses. Parents are innovative in finding methods of masking the unpleasant flavour of these medicines. Some ideas are milk shake flavourings, jam, honey, yoghurt, peppermint essence and fruit purées. Sodium benzoate is available in powder, syrup or tablet form and phenylbutyrate as liquid, coated granules or tablets which are more readily taken.

In N-acetylglutamate synthase (NAGS) deficiency, N-acetylglutamate, the activator of carbamylphosphate synthase (CPS) is not formed. Patients are treated with carbamylglutamate which is an orally active form of N-acetylglutamate.

Arginine

Arginine becomes an essential or semi-essential amino acid in UCD because its synthesis is greatly reduced [262]. In OTC and CPS deficiency arginine supplements of 100–170 mg/kg body weight/day are given to replace that which would normally be formed. The aim is to maintain a normal plasma arginine concentration (normal reference range 40–120 μmol/L). Alternatively in OTC, in order to meet the arginine requirements, supplements of citrulline can be given as it is rapidly converted to arginine via the intact part of the urea cycle. Also, citrulline contains one less nitrogen atom than arginine, thereby reducing waste nitrogen production, but it is more expensive than arginine.

In citrullinaemia and arginosuccinic aciduria (ASA), large doses of arginine up to 700 mg/kg/day are given to replenish ornithine supply. The carbon skeleton of ornithine is needed for the formation of citrulline and arginosuccinic acid which accumulate and are excreted in citrullinaemia and ASA, respectively. Arginosuccinic acid is more effective than citrulline as it carries two waste nitrogen atoms and has a higher renal clearance. Arginine increases the concentrations of both citrulline and arginosuccinic acid, the full consequence of which is unknown; concerns have been expressed that high concentrations of arginosuccinic acid may have adverse effects on brain and liver [263,264]. These high doses of arginine may result in greatly increased plasma concentrations which may contribute to toxicity [265]. However, this appears to be less toxic than the accumulation of ammonia and glutamine. A plasma arginine concentration of up to 200 μmol/L is acceptable. Arginine can be administered orally or intravenously. It is available in liquid, powder or tablet form for oral use. It is given as a divided dose and usually in conjunction with the other medicines.

Dietary management – low protein diet

Urea cycle disorders are treated with a low protein diet. Urea production and excretion are linearly related to protein intake [266]. The load on the urea cycle can therefore be reduced by limiting protein intake. This will reduce the accumulation of waste nitrogen as glutamine and alanine. Even on the minimum protein intake for normal growth and maintenance there is always some flux through the urea cycle, as tissue protein is constantly being synthesised and broken down [267]. For those with severe defects the dietary protein intake is usually reduced to the safe level (Table 17.28), but patients with milder defects will tolerate a higher protein intake. Practical management of the low protein diet for infants and children is described on p. 357. In the author's patient group most manage to take their medicines, diet and essential amino acid supplements orally. If the child is unable to take sufficient orally, nasogastric or gastrostomy feeding must be used to prevent metabolic decompensation (most children will feed orally if metabolic control is good). A normal energy intake for age is provided to ensure normal growth and to prevent endogenous protein catabolism with consequent metabolic decompensation. Regular feeding and avoidance of prolonged fasts is recommended to help maintain good biochemical control as plasma glutamine and ammonia concentrations will increase with fasting and endogenous protein catabolism.

Essential amino acid supplements

For some children an essential amino acid (EAA) supplement is incorporated as part of the total protein intake. This is beneficial because, by limiting the intake of non-essential amino acids, waste nitrogen is utilised to synthesise these and hence nitrogen destined for excretion as urea will be reduced.

EAA supplements are often given first when the blood biochemistry cannot be corrected by altering the medicines because the child is either on maximum doses of medicines or refusing to take more. There is no set dose of EAA supplement. The amount prescribed usually varies between 0.2 and 0.5 g/kg/day, given as a divided dose between two or three meals. EAA supplements can also be used to improve the biological value of a low protein diet which may be lacking in one or more essential amino acids. This may occur if the protein is provided from a limited range of LBV protein foods.

EAA supplements are often used during the stabilisation period in newly diagnosed patients (see below). Details of EAA supplements are provided in Table 17.33.

Scaglia *et al.* [268] have observed selective BCAA deficiency despite adequate protein intake in patients treated with phenylbutyrate. The reasons for this are not yet clear, but may be related to a secondary effect of glutamine depletion. It is suggested that additional BCAA supplementation may be beneficial for some patients.

Monitoring the diet

Regular measurements of plasma ammonia and quantitative amino acids, including glutamine and arginine, are essential for the management of UCD. Monitoring 3–4 monthly is recommended for most patients who are stable but it may need to be carried out more frequently if the child is not well. A 24-hour profile of plasma ammonia and glutamine can be helpful in patients who are difficult to manage. Timing of the blood sample is also important as there are changes with meals and medicines. However, it is not always possible to collect samples under optimal conditions so the results need to be interpreted in the light of all the evidence. Plasma ammonia may be falsely elevated because of poor or difficult blood sample collection. Changes to dietary protein, essential amino acid intakes, arginine and medicines (sodium benzoate and phenylbutyrate, and arginine in ASA and citrullinaemia) are based on the results of these investigations and alterations will vary depending on the disorder (Table 17.34). High concentrations of glutamine

Table 17.33 Essential amino acid products used in urea cycle disorders.

Product	Amino acids (g/100 g)	Protein equivalent (g/100 g)	Energy (kcal (MJ)/100 g)	CHO (g/100 g)	Fat (g/100 g)	Vitamins and minerals	Comments
Dialamine*	30	25	360 (1.5)	65[†]	Nil	‡	Orange flavoured Suitable from 6 months Can be added to a feed, drink or given as a paste
Essential Amino Acid Mix*	94.5	79	316 (1.3)	Nil	Nil	Nil	Suitable for infants under 6 months

* A powdered mixture of essential amino acids (including cystine and histidine). Essential amino acid mix is Dialamine less CHO component.
† Contains a mixture of glucose polymer and sugar.
‡ Contains vitamin C and trace amounts of sodium, potassium, chloride, calcium, phosphorus and magnesium.
Both products are manufactured by Scientific Hospital Supplies. Other products are manufactured by Milupa and Ross Laboratories, but are not available in the UK.

Table 17.34 Outline of management decisions for urea cycle disorders (excluding arginase deficiency).

Ammonia (µmol/L) normal reference range <40	Glutamine (µmol/L) normal reference range 400–800	Quantitative plasma amino acids	Action
>80–100	>1000	Low	Increase medicines in OTC and CPS* Increase medicines in ASA and citrullinaemia† Increase natural protein or essential amino acids
>80–100	>1000	Normal	Increase medicines in OTC and CPS* Increase medicines in ASA and citrullinaemia† No change to diet
<80	<1000	Low	No change to medicines Increase natural protein
<80	<1000	Normal	No change to medicines No change to protein intake

* OTC and CPS – sodium benzoate and/or phenylbutyrate.
† ASA and citrullinaemia – arginine, sodium benzoate or phenylbutyrate. If plasma arginine is high (>200 µmol/L, normal reference range 40–120 µmol/L), arginine dose is not increased; sodium benzoate and/or phenylbutyrate would be increased instead. If plasma citrulline or arginosuccinic acid is too high, arginine is not increased; sodium benzoate and/or phenylbutyrate would be increased instead.

and ammonia in plasma may not only mean that protein intake is too high; similar results will be obtained during periods of chronic catabolism so growth and clinical status must always be considered when interpreting the results. Wilson et al. [269] have observed that patients with citrullinaemia tend to have higher plasma ammonia concentrations for a given plasma glutamine concentration compared with OTC deficiency.

Good biochemical control may be difficult to achieve during periods of slow growth before and particularly after puberty [270]. When the adolescent stops growing there may be a period of instability because protein is no longer needed for growth; protein intake and medicines may require adjustment to restore stability.

Glutamine
Poor appetite is observed in some children [271] with high glutamine levels implicated as a cause. It is thought that glutamine causes an increased influx of tryptophan (the precursor of serotonin) into the brain and promotes serotonin synthesis. Serotonin increases a feeling of satiety [270]. If plasma glutamine is maintained within the normal range then, in some children, appetite may improve.

Management of the newly diagnosed patient

Neonates with hyperammonaemia are almost invariably very sick, requiring ventilation and often haemofiltration or haemodialysis (to remove ammonia). The aim of dietary treatment is to provide a high energy feed to prevent catabolism. Initially a glucose polymer solution (10–15% CHO) is given; a fat emulsion may be added to this feed in 1–2% increments as tolerated. It is often difficult to provide sufficient energy because of restricted fluid intake in the ventilated child. Fluids are usually initially provided by intravenous 10% dextrose and medicines to control hyperammonaemia (sodium benzoate, phenylbutyrate and arginine). Enteral fluids will be gradually increased as 10% dextrose is decreased. Electrolytes, sodium and potassium are added to the feed to provide normal requirements for age, taking into account any contribution of these from intravenous fluids and medicines (e.g. sodium benzoate and phenylbutyrate). Energivit can be used to provide a protein free feed.

Protein needs to be introduced promptly to prevent protein catabolism with further metabolic decompensation. Once the plasma ammonia falls to ≤100 µmol/L, some natural protein is introduced from infant formula or expressed breast milk, usually 0.25–0.5 g/kg body weight/day and increased daily to the full allowance (around 2 g/kg/day) over a period of 3–4 days. Protein requirement is likely to be higher than this if the neonate has had no protein for several days and has been on haemodialysis. Plasma ammonia is monitored at least once per day during protein reintroduction. Guidelines for low protein feeds are given on p. 360. Occasionally it can be difficult to reintroduce protein without inducing hyperammonaemia; in these instances an essential amino acid supplement (e.g. Essential Amino Acid Mix; Table 17.33) is used and will be replaced with natural protein once the patient is more stable. It is also important to ensure sufficient energy is being provided to prevent hyperammonaemia and promote anabolism. Energy requirements will often be greater than normal because of low intakes both pre-diagnosis (poor feeding and vomiting) and during the initial days of stabilisation. If the baby is being breast fed the mother should be encouraged to express until the baby is more stable, then breast feeding can be reintroduced. Protein free feeds (see p. 360) may be required in combination with breast feeds to achieve good metabolic control.

For patients who present later in infancy or during childhood with hyperammonaemia the principles of initial dietary treatment are the same: a protein free, high energy diet and medicines are given initally and protein is reintroduced to the safe level of intake (Table 17.28) over 3–4 days once the plasma ammonia concentration has decreased and the patient is more stable.

Management of illness

During intercurrent illness, protein catabolism may cause rapid accumulation of ammonia and glutamine. The standard ER (see p. 375) is used to prevent these effects of illness. Protein intake is stopped temporarily and regular 2-hourly drinks of glucose polymer are given. The usual doses of sodium benzoate, phenylbutyrate and arginine are administered. If necessary during acute illness the dosage of both benzoate and phenylbutyrate can be temporarily increased to 500 mg/kg/day. Protein is usually reintroduced within 2–3 days and over a period of 1–4 days depending on the child's clinical condition. Practical advice on protein reintroduction is given in the ER section below.

If the child does not tolerate oral fluids and medicines, 10% dextrose and medicines are given intravenously. Oral fluids can usually be recommenced within 24–48 hours, with a gradual changeover from IV to oral, thus ensuring an adequate energy intake. Plasma ammonia and quantitative amino acids should be measured regularly. Once the plasma ammonia is less than 80–100 µmol/L, protein is gradually reintroduced over a period of 2–4 days. If hyperammonaemia is induced during protein reintroduction an essential amino acid supplement is used and energy intake is increased.

Arginase deficiency

Arginase deficiency (Fig. 17.6) is a rare disorder whose presentation is distinct from the other UCDs. It is characterised by a progressive spastic tetraplegia, seizures, developmental regression and poor growth [256]. Hyperargininaemia and a mild hyperammonaemia occur because of defective hydrolysis of arginine. The mechanisms responsible for the neurological damage are not yet completely understood, but arginine and its guanidino metabolites are possible neurotoxins [272,273]. Patients rarely present in the neonatal period but typically present with first symptoms at 2–4 years of age [274].

Dietary management – low protein diet

Arginase deficiency is treated with a low protein diet, sodium benzoate and phenylbutyrate. This treatment should prevent further neurological damage and may induce a partial recovery of skills over time [274]. Three patients treated from birth are reported to be largely asymptomatic [275].

All dietary nitrogen has the potential to be converted to arginine, this source being considerably greater than the small amount of arginine that is naturally present in protein. In the past, in order to restrict the nitrogen intake, diets comprised an EAA supplement with a very limited intake of natural protein. Nowadays, by giving sodium benzoate and phenylbutyrate a more generous intake of natural protein may be possible while still maintaining acceptable plasma arginine and ammonia levels. These medicines reduce available nitrogen destined for arginine synthesis by increasing its excretion via alternative pathways to the urea cycle (Fig. 17.6). Protein intake is restricted to the safe level (Table 17.28), and is provided by a combination of natural protein and an EAA supplement. The precise composition of protein intake must be determined by the balance of requirements for growth and the medicines necessary for good biochemical control. A combination of 50–75% as natural protein and 25–50% as EAA is suggested [274]. The practical management of the low protein diet and EAA supplementation are provided on pages 357 and 372, respectively.

The diet is monitored by regular measurements of plasma ammonia, plasma arginine and the other amino acids quantitatively. The aim is to maintain plasma arginine levels at <200 μmol/L (normal reference range 40–120 μmol/L) and a near normal plasma ammonia (normal range <40 μmol/L).

Management of illness

During intercurrent illness the standard ER (see p. 375) of a protein free high energy intake from frequent carbohydrate drinks is used to prevent hyperargininaemia and hyperammonaemia. This should be implemented promptly to prevent irreversible deterioration [272]. Hyperammonaemic crisis is rare and this may be because of the activity of a second arginase enzyme. However, deaths have been reported resulting from hyperammonaemic encephalopathy triggered by infection [274]. Sodium benzoate and phenylbutyrate should be given orally or intravenously.

Emergency Regimens

Marjorie Dixon

For some inborn errors of intermediary metabolism (Table 17.35) intercurrent infections, combined with a poor oral intake and fasting, will precipitate severe metabolic decompensation (accumulation of toxic metabolites, which is disorder specific, and causes metabolic encephalopathy). To help prevent this, the child's usual diet is stopped (although this often occurs naturally because of reduced appetite) and an emergency regimen (ER) is given. In some disorders the ER is combined with additional specific therapy (refer to respective disorders). Normally, the child's medicines are continued and may be increased in some disorders (refer to respective disorders).

The aim of the ER is to provide an exogenous energy source to:

- Reduce production of potentially toxic metabolites from either protein catabolism and/or lipolysis in disorders such as organic acidaemias (e.g. methylmalonic acidaemia, glutaric aciduria type I) and fatty acid oxidation defects (e.g. medium chain acyl-CoA dehydrogenase deficiency)
- Prevent hypoglycaemia in disorders such as ketotic hypoglycaemia or glycogen storage disease type I

Precise energy requirements for patients with inherited metabolic disorders during illness are not known, but are likely to be more than the estimated average requirement (EAR) for energy [146] for healthy children as requirements are known to increase during illness. Bodamer *et al.* [275] reported that resting energy expenditure (REE) was

Table 17.35 Inherited metabolic disorders at risk of metabolic decompensation.

Organic acidaemias, e.g. propionic acidaemia, methylmalonic acidaemia, isovaleric acidaemia, glutaric aciduria type I
Maple syrup urine disease
Urea cyle disorders, e.g. ornithine carbamoyl transferase deficiency
Fatty acid oxidation disorders, e.g. medium chain acyl-CoA dehydrogenase deficiency, long chain 3-hydroxy acyl-CoA dehydrogenase deficiency
Glycogen storage disorders type I, III and IX
Fructose 1, 6-bisphosphatase deficiency
Disorders of ketogenesis
Ketotic hypoglycaemia

Table 17.36   Emergency regimens.

Age	Glucose polymer concentration (% CHO)	Energy/100 mL		Osmolality* (mOsm/kg H$_2$O)	Suggested daily fluid volume†	Feeding frequency
		(kcal)	(kJ)			
up to 6 m	10	40	167	103	150 mL/kg	Initially 2–3 hourly,
7–12 m	12	48	202		120 mL/kg	night and day for
1 y	15	60	250	174	1200 mL	all ages
2–9 y	20	80	334	245	†	
>10 y	25	100	418	342	†	

* Data provided by Scientific Hospital Supplies International Limited.

† For children over 10 kg, normal fluid requirements can be calculated as follows:

11–20 kg	100 mL/kg for the first 10 kg, plus 50 mL/kg for the next 10 kg.
20 kg and above	100ml/kg for the first 10 kg, plus 50 mL/kg for the next 10 kg, plus 25 mL/kg thereafter, up to 2500 mL/day maximum.

increased by up to 30% in two children with MMA during acute illness. The basic ER is essentially the same for all disorders. A solution of glucose polymer is given as the main energy source because it is simple to administer and is usually well tolerated. These solutions alone will not provide the EAR for energy. Fat emulsions can be added as an additional energy source, but these may be less well tolerated, particularly in the child who is vomiting. Fat is contraindicated in disorders of fatty acid oxidation. The basic ER does not provide a source of electrolytes. The addition of these may be beneficial for some disorders such as methylmalonic acidaemia and are important during gastrointestinal illness (see below). Electrolytes can be added: 1 or 2 sachets of Dioralyte (oral rehdration soulution, ORS) added to the 24-hour ER. This is easily performed in hospital but may be more difficult at home. It is important to be aware that the child may obtain sodium from their standard medicines such as sodium benzoate in UCD and sodium bicarbonate in MMA.

The CHO concentration of the ER and fluid volumes given depend on the age of the child (Table 17.36). Too concentrated a solution of glucose polymer will be hyperosmolar, cause diarrhoea and exacerbate the effects of illness. To improve palatability the glucose polymer solution can be flavoured with squash, taking care not to exceed the recommended CHO concentration per 100 mL. Alternatively, glucose polymer powder can be added to fruit juice or carbonated drinks to the required concentration of CHO. Parents should be taught to make these drinks using handy scoop measurements. For children who are unfamiliar

with the taste of glucose polymer drinks it is worthwhile having a trial of different drinks when they are well to ascertain what they will take and to familiarise the parents with reconstitution of these in a non-emergency situation. Lucozade contains 17–18% CHO and Ribena in a carton 15% CHO; these drinks are convenient because they are ready to use, portable and can be stored for use in an emergency situation at nursery or school.

During gastrointestinal illness ORS supplemented with glucose polymer to provide extra energy, usually to a concentration of 10 g CHO per 100 mL (10%), is used. The osmolality of such feeds needs to be considered [277]; ORS with glucose polymer added to a final concentration of 10% has an osmolality around 320 mOsm/kg H$_2$O.

To reduce the period of fasting and optimise energy intake the ER is initially fed at frequent 2-hourly intervals night and day. In some circumstances (e.g. vomiting) it may be better to give small very frequent sips of the ER. Such frequent overnight feeding (2-hourly) can be difficult to achieve, particularly for patients without nasogastric tubes and more realistic targets should be considered.

The ER is normally commenced at home at the first signs of illness and is given orally or enterally. It is useful to teach the parents of patients who refuse to drink when they are unwell how to feed their child nasogastrically at home. If the child persistently vomits the ER or is obviously not recovering, then a hospital admission for stabilisation with IV therapy is usually necessary. Dextrose 10% is given by peripheral drip or more concentrated dextrose can be administered through a central line.

When oral fluids are reintroduced there is a gradual changeover from IV to oral feeding, thus ensuring an overall adequate energy intake. If oral or enteral feeds cannot be re-established then an early resort to parenteral nutrition is indicated for some disorders [278]; refer to specific disorders.

The basic ER of glucose polymer must not be continued for long periods of time because it does not provide adequate nutrition. If prolonged, malnutrition may develop surprisingly rapidly. Severe lactic acidosis caused by acute thiamin deficiency has been reported in two patients with propionic acidaemia who had high energy parenteral nutrition to restore anabolism, but no vitamins were given [279]. Poor growth and nutritional deficiencies will occur in patients on low protein diets who have repeated infections and are frequently on the ER. If so, it may be necessary to increase protein intake temporarily when the child is well to compensate for inadequate intakes of protein while on the ER.

As the child improves normal diet is reintroduced. With the exception of low protein diets the ER is often just replaced with the child's usual diet within 1–2 days. During the recovery phase if the child's appetite is reduced it is important to give additional ER drinks or feeds to maximise energy intake and prevent further metabolic decompensation.

For patients on low protein diets, the protein intake is stopped for the shortest time possible (1–3 days maximum). Protein, whether from feed or diet, is reintroduced by increasing the daily amount, providing one-quarter, half and three-quarters of the usual intake, resuming the normal allowance by the fourth day. If on diet, additional ER drinks are given throughout the reintroduction period (usually less frequently) to maximise energy intake. Vitamin and mineral supplements should be restarted promptly. If on feeds, additional glucose polymer is added to the infant formula or low protein tube feed to the same concentration as the ER. If the child's usual feed contains more CHO than the ER it will be increased up to this concentration (over the 4 days). If the feed normally contains fat and vitamins and minerals these too will be increased over the same 4 days. This reintroduction period will be performed more rapidly over fewer days if clinically indicated. In milder illnesses protein intake is generally not regraded. The child's usual feeding frequency is also gradually resumed as tolerated.

Instructions for parents

Treatment of intercurrent infections can be an anxious and difficult time for parents. To make this easier, parents should be taught a three-staged plan telling them what to do and when [280] and be encouraged to phone the metabolic team for advice at an early stage. This type of approach can also help reduce episodes of metabolic decompensation and hospital admissions.

1 If the parents are unsure whether their child is showing the first signs of illness (pallor, lethargy, irritability) then an ER drink is given as a precaution. Clinical observations are reported to be generally better than biochemical measurements for detecting decompensation; subtle changes in behaviour are usually the earliest signs of this and are most easily detected by parents [281]. The child's clinical state is then reviewed regularly within 1–2 hours.
2 If on reassessment the child has improved, the normal diet is resumed; however, if the child has deteriorated or shown no signs of improvement the full ER is commenced for a period of 24–48 hours. The parents are instructed how to reintroduce the usual diet.
3 If the child is not tolerating the ER (i.e. refusing ER drinks, vomiting or becoming encephalopathic) then the child is admitted to hospital.

The parents should be taught to recognise signs of encephalopathy such as disorientation and poor responsiveness, accompanied by a glazed look. Komaromy et al. [282] reported that monitoring of urinary ketones may be useful in deciding when to implement the ER. They observed that ketones were present during times of illness, but not in health. This tool would only be suitable for some patients as there is wide variation in how they respond so that each should be assessed individually. For obvious reasons, testing for ketones is not to be used in patients with disorders of fatty acid oxidation.

Parents should be given written instructions on practical aspects of the ER including recipes, suggested fluid volumes, feeding frequency and contact telephone numbers. Laminated 'parent-held guidelines' should also be given. These provide a basic explanation of the disorder, treatment required if a local hospital admission is necessary and contact telephone numbers for the specialist metabolic team. Open access to the local hospital's paediatric ward (avoiding the accident and emergency department) should be usually organised. These guidelines are also very useful for families when on holiday. Families can travel abroad, but it is best they go to countries that have expertise in the management of metabolic disorders should the child become unwell. Emergency regimen instructions and recipes need to be regularly reviewed and updated in accordance with the child's current dietary treatment, age and clinical condition. A Medic Alert bracelet may be useful for some children.

Acknowledgement

Marjorie Dixon thanks James V. Leonard, former Professor of Paediatric Metabolic Disease, Great Ormond Street Hospital for Children, NHS Trust and The Institite of Child Health, London for his invaluable contribution to this chapter.

Appendix 17.1

Manufactured low protein/low phenylalanine foods (ACBS approved, available on FP10 prescription in the UK)

Biscuits

Gluten Free Foods Limited (Tel: 0208 953 4444)

Aminex Low Protein Rusk	200 g
Aminex Low Protein Biscuits	200 g
Aminex Low Protein Cookies	150 g
PK Foods Low Protein Crispbread	76 g
PK Foods Low Protein Chocolate Chip Cookies	150 g
PK Foods Low Protein Orange Cookies	150 g
PK Foods Low Protein Cinnamon Cookies	150 g

SHS International Limited (Tel: 0151 228 8161)

Loprofin Low Protein Sweet Biscuits	150 g
Loprofin Low Protein Orange Cream Wafers	100 g
Loprofin Low Protein Vanilla Cream Wafers	100 g
Loprofin Low Protein Chocolate Cream Wafers	100 g
Loprofin Low Protein Cinnamon Cookies	100 g
Loprofin Low Protein Chocolate Chip Cookies	100 g
Loprofin Low Protein Chocolate Flavour Cream Biscuits	100 g
Juvela Low Protein Cinnamon Cookies	150 g
Juvela Low Protein Orange Flavour Cookies	150 g
Juvela Low Protein Chocolate Chip Cookies	130 g
Loprofin Low Protein Crackers (Savoury)	150 g
Loprofin Low Protein Herb Crackers	150 g

Ultrapharm Limited (Tel: 01491 578016)

Aproten Low Protein Biscuits	180 g
Aproten Crispbread	260 g
Ultra PKU Savoy Biscuits	150 g
Ultra PKU Cookies – Aniseed Flavour	250 g
Ultra PKU Biscuits	200 g
Harifen Low Protein Cracker Toast	200 g
Harifen White Chocolate Chip Cookies	200 g

Pasta

SHS International Limited

Loprofin Low Protein Pasta Spirals	500 g
Loprofin Low Protein Macaroni Penne	500 g
Loprofin Low Protein Vermicelli	250 g
Loprofin Low Protein Short Cut Spaghetti	500 g
Loprofin Low Protein Long Spaghetti	500 g
Loprofin Low Protein Lasagne	500 g
Loprofin Low Protein Rice	500 g
Loprofin Low Protein Snack Pot: Curry, Tomato and Basil	47 g
(1 pot = 23 mg phenylalanine)	

Firstplay Dietary Foods Limited (Tel: 0161 474 7576)

Promin Low Protein Pasta (six shapes)

Macaroni	500 g
Short Cut Spaghetti	500 g
Shells	500 g
Spirals	500 g
Alphabets	500 g
Elbows	500 g

Promin Low Protein Tricolour Pasta (four shapes)

Shells	500 g
Spirals	500 g
Alphabets	500 g
Elbows	500 g
Promin Low Protein Pastameal	500 g
Promin Low Protein Cous Cous	500 g
Promin Low Protein Imitation Rice	500 g
Promin Low Protein Pasta in Sauce: Tomato, pepper and herb	

(100 g made up pasta/sauce = 20 mg phenylalanine)
Promin Low Protein Pasta in Sauce:
Cheese and Broccoli
(100g made up pasta/sauce = 30 mg phenylalanine)

Ultrapharm Limited
Aproten Pastas:
Macaroni (Rigatini)	500 g
Flat Noodles (Tagliatelle)	250 g
Short Macaroni (Ditalini)	500 g
Spaghetti	500 g

Bread, flour and mixes

Fate Special Foods (Tel: 0121 5224434)
Fate Low Protein All-Purpose Mix	500 g
Fate Low Protein Cake Mix	2 × 250 g
Fate Low Protein Chocolate Flavour Cake Mix	2 × 250 g

General Dietary Limited (Tel: 0208 336 2323)
Ener-G Low Protein Rice Bread – sliced	600 g

Gluten Free Foods Limited
PK Foods Low Protein White Sliced Bread	550 g
PK Foods Low Protein Low Protein Flour Mix	750 g

SHS International Limited
Loprofin Low Protein Loaf – sliced and unsliced	400 g
Loprofin Bread White Rolls 6 × 4 rolls	
Loprofin Low Protein – Part Baked Bread Rolls 6 × 4 rolls	
Juvela Low Protein Loaf (vacuum packed, whole and sliced)	400 g
Juvela Low Protein Bread Rolls 5 × 70 g	
Rite-Diet Low Protein White Bread (unsliced) with Added Fibre	400 g
Loprofin Low Protein Mix	500 g
Rite-Diet Low Protein Flour Mix	500 g
Rite-Diet Low Protein Baking Mix	500 g
Juvela Low Protein Mix	500 g
Juvela Low Protein Pizza Bases	2 × 180 g

Ultrapharm
Aproten Low Protein Flour	500 g
Ultra PKU Flour Mix	500 g
Ultra PKU Fresh Bread	400 g
Ultra PKU Fresh Pizza Base 5 × 80 g	

(Not available through wholesalers, contact Ultrapharm directly to obtain these products)

Cereals

Firstplay Dietary Foods Limited
Promin Low Protein Hot Breakfast 6 × 57 g sachets
   Original
   Apple and Cinnamon Flavour
   Chocolate Flavour
   Banana Flavour

SHS International Limited
Loprofin Low Protein Breakfast Cereal Loops	375 g

Fat and carbohydrate products

SHS International Limited
Calogen LCT Emulsion –
plain, strawberry,
butterscotch	250 mL and 1 L bottles
Duocal – liquid	250 mL and 1 L bottles
Duocal – super soluble powder	400 g

Egg replacers

SHS International Limited
Loprofin Egg Replacer	250 g
Loprofin Egg White Replacer	100 g

General Dietary Limited
Ener-G Egg Replacer	454 g

Protein free high energy bar

SHS International Limited
Duobar – natural, strawberry,toffee	8 × 45 g bars
Loprofin Low Protein Crunch Bar	8 × 41 g bars

Vitaflo International Limited (Tel: 0151 709 9020)
Vita-bite	7 × 20 g bars

Jelly mixes and puddings

Gluten Free Foods Limited
PK Foods Low Protein Orange Jelly Mix (4 × 80 g)	320 g

PK Foods Low Protein Cherry Jelly Mix
(4 × 80 g)   320 g

Firstplay Dietary Foods Limited
Promin Low Protein Rice Pudding Mix
– original flavour (4 × 69 g sachets)   276 g

Low protein drinks

*These products contain some phenylalanine

Milupa (Tel: 08457 623 628)
*Milupa lp-drink   400 g
250 mL = half an exchange when made as
per instructions

SHS International Limited
*Loprofin PKU Long Life
Milk Drink   200 mL carton
Contains approximately half an
exchange per carton
*Sno-Pro Drink   200 mL carton
Contains half an exchange per carton

Burger mix

Firstplay Dietary Foods Limited
Promin Low Protein Burger Mix (2 × 62 g sachets)
1 sachet = 62 mg phenylalanine

References

1 Costello PM, Beasley MG, Tillotson S, Smith I Intelligence in mild atypical phenylketonuria. *Eur J Pediatr*, 1994, **153** 260–3.

2 Woo SL, DiLella AG, Marvit J, Ledley FD Molecular basis of phenylketonuria and potential somatic gene therapy. *Cold Spring Harb Symp Quant Biol*, 1986, **Pt I** 395–401.

3 Surtees R, Blau N The neurochemistry of phenylketonuria. *Eur J Pediatr*, 2000, **159** (Suppl 2) S109–13.

4 Scriver CR, Kaufman S Hyperphenylalaninemia: phenylalanine hydroxylase deficiency. In: Scriver CR, Beaudet AL, Sly WS, Valle D, Childs B, Kinzler KW, Vogelstein B (eds) *The Metabolic and Molecular Bases of Inherited Disease*, 8th edn. New York: McGraw Hill, 2001, pp. 1667–724.

5 Smith I The hyperphenylaninaemias. In: Lloyd JK and Scriver CR (eds) *Genetic and Metabolic Disease in Paediatrics*. London: Butterworths, 1985, pp. 166–210.

6 Jervis GA Studies on phenylpyruvic oligophrenia. The position of the metabolic error. *J Biol Chem*, 1947, **169** 651–6.

7 Udenfriend S, Cooper JR The enzymatic conversion of phenylalanine to tyrosine. *J Biol Chem*, 1952, **194** 503–11.

8 Woolf LI, Vulliamy DG Phenylketonuria with a study of the effect upon it of glutamic acid. *Arch Dis Child*, 1951, **26** 487–94.

9 Bickel H, Gerrard J, Hickmans E Influence of phenylalanine intake on phenylketonuria. *Lancet*, 1953, **2** 812.

10 Erlandsen H, Fusetti F, Martinez A *et al.* Crystal structure of the catalytic domain of human phenylalanine hydroxylase reveals the structural basis for phenylketonuria. *Nat Struct Biol*, 1997, **4** 995–1000.

11 Erlandsen H, Patch MG, Gamez A *et al.* Stuctural studies on phenylalanine hydroxylase and implications toward understanding and treating phenylketonuria. *Pediatrics*, 2003, **112** (6 Pt 2) 1557–65.

12 Guldberg P, Rey F, Zschocke J *et al.* A European multicenter study of phenylalanine hydroxylase deficiency: classification of 105 mutations and a general system for genotype-based prediction of metabolic phenotype. *Am J Hum Genet*, 1998, **63** 71–9. Erratum in: *Am J Hum Genet*, 1998, **63** 1252–3.

13 Kayaalp E, Treacy E, Waters PJ *et al.* Human phenylalanine hydroxylase mutations and hyperphenylalaninemia phenotypes: a metanalysis of genotypephenotype correlations. *Am J Hum Genet*, 1997, **61** 1309–17.

14 Ledley FD, Levy HL, Woo, SLC Molecular analysis of the inheritance of phenylketonuria and mild hyperphenylalaninemia in families with both disorders. *N Engl J Med*, 1986, **314** 1276–79.

15 Hilton MA, Sharpe JN, Hicks LG, Andrews BF A simple method for detection of heterozygous carriers of the gene for classical phenylketonuria. *J Pediatr*, 1986, **109** 601–4.

16 Medical Research Council Working Party on Phenylketonuria. Recommendations on the dietary management of phenylketonuria. *Arch Dis Child*, 1993b, **68** 426–7.

17 Kaufman S, Holtzman NA, Milstein S *et al.* Phenylketonuria due to a deficiency of dihydropteridine reductase. *N Engl J Med*, 1975, **293** 785–90.

18 Kaufman S, Berlow S, Summer GK *et al.* Hyperphenylalaninemia due to a deficiency of biopterin. A variant form of phenylketonuria. *N Engl J Med*, 1987, **299** 673–9.

19 Leeming RJ, Blair JA, Rey F Biopterin derivatives in atypical phenylketonuria. *Lancet*, 1976, **1** 99–100.

20 Pollitt RJ Amino acid disorders. In: Holton J (ed) *The Inherited Metabolic Diseases*. Edinburgh: Churchill Livingstone, 1994, pp. 67–113.

21 Kwok SC, Ledley FD, DiLella AG *et al.* Nucleotide sequence of a full-length complementary DNA clone and amino acid sequence of human phenylalanine hydroxylase. *Biochemistry*, 1985, **24** 556–61.

22 UK Newborn Screening Programme Centre. Policies and Standards for Newborn screening. Great Ormond Street Hospital for Children NHS Trust, 2005.

23 Medical Research Council Working Party on Phenylketonuria. Phenylketonuria due to phenylalanine hydroxylase deficiency: an unfolding story. *Br Med J*, 1993, **306** 115–19.

24 Weglage J, Fünders B, Wilken B *et al.* School performance and intellectual outcome in adolescents with phenylketonuria. *Acta Paediatr*, 1993, **81** 582–6.

25 Stemerdink BA, van der Meere JJ, van der Molen MW *et al.* Information processing in patients with early and continuously-treated phenylketonuria. *Eur J Pediatr*, 1995, **154** 739–46.

26 Stemerdink BA, Kalverboer AF, van der Meere JJ *et al.* Behaviour and school achievement in patients with early and continuously treated phenylketonuria. *J Inherit Metab Dis*, 2000, **23** 548–62.

27 Griffiths PV, Demellweek C, Fay N *et al.* Wechsler subscale IQ and subtest profile in early treated phenylketonuria. *Arch Dis Child*, 2000, **82** 209–15.

28 Smith I, Beasley MG, Ades AE Intelligence and quality of dietary treatment in phenylketonuria. *Arch Dis Child*, 1990, **65** 472–8.

29 Smith I, Beasley MG, Ades AE Effect on intelligence of relaxing the low phenylalanine diet in phenylketonuria. *Arch Dis Child*, 1991, **66** 311–16.

30 Holtzman NA, Kronmal RA, van Doorninck W *et al.* Effect of age at loss of dietary control on intellectual performance and behaviour of children with phenylketonuria. *N Engl J Med*, 1986, **314** 593–8.

31 Burgard P Development of intelligence in early treated phenylketonuria. *Eur J Pediatr*, 2000, **159** (Suppl 2) S74–9.

32 Weglage J, Pietsch M, Denecke J *et al.* Regression of neuropsychological deficits in early-treated phenylketonurics during adolescence. *J Inherit Metab Dis*, 1999, **22** 693–705.

33 Welsh MC, Pennington BF, Ozonoff S *et al.* Neuropsychology of early treated phenylketonuria: specific executive function deficits. *Child Dev*, 1990, **61** 1697–713.

34 Lou HC, Toft PB, Adresen J *et al.* An occipito-temporal syndrome in adolescents with optimally control led hyperphenylalaninaemia. *J Inherit Metab Dis*, 1992, **15** 687–95.

35 Pennington BF, van Doorninck WJ, McCabe LL *et al.* Neuropsychological phenylketonuric children. *Am J Ment Defic*, 1985, **5** 467–74.

36 Weglage J Comments on behavior in early treated phenylketonuria. *Eur J Pediatr*, 2000, **159** (Suppl 2) S94–5.

37 Huijbregts SC, de Sonneville LM, Licht R *et al.* Short-term dietary interventions in children and adolescents with treated phenylketonuria: effects on neuropsychological outcome of a well-controlled population. *J Inherit Metab Dis*, 2002, **25** 419–30.

38 Thompson AJ, Smith I, Brenton D *et al.* Neurological deterioration in young adults with phenylketonuria. *Lancet*, 1990, **336** 602–5.

39 Leuzzi V, Rinalduzzi S, Chiarotti F *et al.* Subclinical visual impairment in phenylketonuria. A neurophysiological study (VEP-P) with clinical, biochemical, and neuroradiological (MRI) correlations. *J Inherit Metab Dis*, 1998, **21** 351–64.

40 Bick U, Ullrich K, Stöber U *et al.* White matter abnormalities in patients with treated hyperphenylalaninaemia: magnetic resonance relaxometry and proton spectroscopy findings. *Eur J Pediatr*, 1993, **152** 1012–20.

41 Thompson AJ, Tillotson S, Smith I *et al.* Brain MRI changes in PKU. Associations with dietary status. *Brain*, 1993, **116** 811–21.

42 Toft PB, Lou HC, Krägeloh-Mann I *et al.* Brain magnetic resonance imaging in children with optimally controlled hyperphenylalaninaemia *J Inherit Metab Dis*, 1994, **17** 575–83.

43 Pietz J, Meyding-Lamandé UK, Schmidt H Magnetic resonance imaging of the brain in adolescents with phenylketonuria and in one case of 6-pyruvoyl tetrahydropteridine synthase deficiency. *Eur J Pediatr*, 1996, **155** S69–73.

44 Bhat M, Haase C, Lee PJ Social outcome in treated individuals with inherited metabolic disorders: UK study. *J Inherit Metab Dis*, 2005, **28** 825–30.

45 Koch R, Burton B, Hoganson G *et al.* Phenylketonuria in adulthood: a collaborative study. *J Inherit Metab Dis*, 2002, **25** 333–46.

46 Gassio R, Campistol J, Vilaseca MA *et al.* Do adult patients with phenylketonuria improve their quality of life after introduction/resumption of a phenylalaninerestricted diet? *Acta Paediatr*, 2003, **92** 1474–8.

47 Blau N, Erlandsen H The metabolic and molecular bases of tetrahydrobiopterin-responsive phenylalanine hydroxylase deficiency. *Mol Genet Metab*, 2004, **82** 101–11.

48 Hoskins JA, Jack G, Wade HE *et al.* Enzymatic control of phenylalanine intake in phenylketonuria. *Lancet*, 1980, **1** 392–4.

49 Sarkissian CN, Gamez A Phenylalanine ammonia lyase, enzyme substitution therapy for phenylketonuria, where are we now? *Mol Genet Metab*, 2005, **86** (Suppl 1) S22–6. Epub 2005 Sep 13.

50 Chen L, Woo SL Complete and persistent pheno-

typic correction of phenylketonuria in mice by site-specific genome integration of murine phenylalanine hydroxylase cDNA. *Proc Natl Acad Sci USA*, 2005, **102** 15581–6. Epub 2005 Oct 17.

51   Smith I, Lobascher ME, Stevenson JE *et al.* Effect of stopping low-phenylalanine diet on intellectual progress of children with phenylketonuria. *Br Med J*, 1978, **2** 723–6.

52   Hudson FP, Mordaunt VL, Leahy I Evaluation of treatment begun in first three months of life in 184 cases of phenylketonuria. *Arch Dis Child*, 1970, **45** 5–12.

53   Acosta PB, Wenz E, Williamson M Nutrient intake of treated infants with phenylketonuria. *Amer J Clin Nutr*, 1977, **30** 198–208.

54   Courtney-Martin G, Bross R, Raffi M *et al.* Phenylalanine requirement in children with classical PKU determined by indicator amino acid oxidation. *Am J Physiol Endocrinol Metab*, 2002, **283** E1249–56.

55   Wendel U, Ullrich K, Schmidt H, Batzler U Six year follow up of phenylalanine intakes and plasma phenylalanine concentrations. *Eur J Pediatr*, 1990, **149** S13–16.

56   Lyman FL, Lyman JK Dietary management of phenylketonuria with Lofenalac. *Arch Pediatr*, 1960, **77** 212.

57   Thompson S *Protocol for the use of XP Maxamaid in the Dietary Management of Phenylketonuria.* Liverpool: SHS, 1997.

58   Weetch E, MacDonald A The determination of phenylalanine content of foods suitable for phenylketonuria. *J Hum Nutr Diet*, 2006, **19** 229–36.

59   National Society for Phenylketonuria (NSPKU) Dietary information for the treatment of phenylketonuria. 2005/2006 revision. London: NSPKU, 2005.

60   MacDonald A, Rylance G, Davies P *et al.* Free use of fruits and vegetables in phenylketonuria. *J Inherit Metab Dis*, 2003, **26** 327–38.

61   MacDonald A, Gokmen Ozel H, Daly A *et al.* Phenylalanine exchanges in PKU: should they be weighed? Dietary management of inborn errors of metabolism. Royal College of Physicians, London. *Inborn Error Review Series*, 2006, **16** 12–13.

62   van Spronsen FJ, van Dijk T, Smit GPA *et al.* Phenylketonuria: Plasma responses to different distributions of the daily phenylalanine allowance over the day. *Pediatrics*, 1996, **97** 839–44.

63   van Spronsen FJ, van Rijn M, Van Dijk T *et al.* Plasma phenylalanine and tyrosine responses to different nutritional conditions (fasting/postprandial) in patients with phenylketonuria: effect of sample timing. *Pediatrics*, 1993, **92** 570–3.

64   O'Daly S Phenylketonuria treated with a high phenylalanine intake and casein-hydrolysate/amino acid mixtures. *Lancet*, 1961, **June 24** 1379–83.

65   Macdonald A, Chakrapani A, Hendriksz C *et al.* Protein substitute dosage in PKU: How much do young patients need? *Arch Dis Child*, 2006, **91** 588–93.

66   Acosta PB, Yannicelli S Protein intake affects phenylalanine requirements and growth of infants with phenylketonuria. *Acta Paediatr*, 1994, **83** (Suppl 407) 66–7.

67   Kindt E, Motzfeldt K, Halvorsen S, Lie SO Is phenylalanine requirement in infants and children related to protein intake? *Br J Nutr*, 1984, **51** 435–42.

68   Hoeksma M, Van Rijn M, Verkerk PH *et al.* The intake of total protein, natural protein and protein substitute and growth of height and head circumference in Dutch infants with phenylketonuria. *J Inherit Metab Dis*, 2005, **28** 845–54.

69   MacDonald A, Rylance G, Davies P *et al.* Administration of protein substitute and quality of control in phenylketonuria: a randomized study. *J Inherit Metab Dis*, 2003, **26** 319–26.

70   Motil KJ, Matthews DE, Bier DM *et al.* Whole body leucine and lysine metabolism: response to dietary protein intake in young men. *Am J Physiol*, 1981, **240** E712–21.

71   Schoeffer A, Herrmann M-E, Brösicke HG, Mönch E Influence of single dose amino acid mixtures on the nitrogen retention in patients with phenylketonuria. *J Nutr Med*, 1994, **4** 415–18.

72   MacDonald A Diet and compliance in phenylketonuria. *Eur J Pediatr*, 2000, **159** (Suppl 2) S136–41.

73   Prince AP, McMurry MP, Buist NRM Treatment products and approaches for phenylketonuria: improved palatability and flexibility demonstrate safety, efficacy and acceptance in US clinical trials. *J Inherit Metab Dis*, 1997, **20** 486–98.

74   Pietz J, Kreis R, Rupp A *et al.* Large neutral amino acids block phenylalanine transport into brain tissue in patients with phenylketonuria. *J Clin Invest*, 1999, **103** 1169–78.

75   Moats RA, Moseley KD, Koch R, Nelson M Jr Brain phenylalanine concentrations in phenylketonuria: research and treatment of adults. *Pediatrics*, 2003, **112** 1575–9.

76   Poustie VJ, Rutherford P Tyrosine supplementation for phenylketonuria. *Cochrane Database Syst Rev*, 2000, **2** CD001507.

77   van Spronsen FJ, Smit PG, Koch R Phenylketonuria: tyrosine beyond the phenylalanine-restricted diet. *J Inherit Metab Dis*, 2001, **24** 1–4.

78   Kalsner LR, Rohr FJ, Strauss KA *et al.* Tyrosine supplementation in phenylketonuria: diurnal blood tyrosine levels and presumptive brain influx of tyrosine and other large neutral amino acids. *J Pediatr*, 2001, **139** 421–7.

79   Allen JR, McCauley JC, Waters DL *et al.* Resting

energy expenditure in children with phenylketonuria. *Am J Clin Nutr*, 1995, **62** 797–801.

80 Millward DJ, Rivers JPW The nutritional role of indispensable amino acids and the metabolic basis for their requirements. *Eur J Clin Nutr*, 1988, **42** 367–93.

81 Illsinger S, Lucke T, Meyer U *et al.* Branched chain amino acids as a parameter for catabolism in treated phenylketonuria. *Amino Acids*, 2004, **28** 45–50.

82 Galli C, Agostoni C, Mosconi C *et al.* Reduced plasma C-20 and C-22 polyunsaturated fatty acids in children during dietary intervention. *J Pediatr*, 1991, **119** 562–7.

83 Schulpis KH, Scarpalezou A Triglycerides, cholesterol, HDL, LDL, and VLDL cholesterol in serum of phenylketonuric children under dietary control. *Clin Pediatr*, 1989, **28** 466–9.

84 Galluzzo CR, Ortisi MT, Castelli L *et al.* Plasma lipid concentrations in 42 treated phenylketonuric children. *J Inherit Metab Dis*, 1985, **8** (Suppl 2) 129.

85 Acosta PB, Alfin-Slater RB, Koch R Serum lipids in children with phenylketonuria (PKU). *J Am Diet Assoc*, 1973, **63** 631–5.

86 Colome C, Artuch R, Lambruschini N *et al.* Is there a relationship between plasma phenylalanine and cholesterol in phenylketonuric patients under dietary treatment? *Clin Biochem*, 2001, **34** 373–6.

87 Rose HJ, White F, MacDonald A *et al.* Fat intakes of children with PKU on low phenylalanine diets. *J Hum Nutr Diet*, 2005, **18** 395–400.

88 Agostoni C, Harvie A, McCulloch DL *et al.* Randomized trial of long-chain polyunsaturated fatty acid supplementation in infants with phenylketonuria. *Dev Med Child Neurol*, 2006, **48** 207–12.

89 Beblo S, Reinhardt H, Muntau AC *et al.* Fish oil supplementation improves visual evoked potentials in children with phenylketonuria. *Neurology*, 2001, **57** 1488–91.

90 Giovanni M, Biasucci G, Agostoni C *et al.* Lipid status and fatty acid metabolism in phenylketonuria. *J Inherit Metab Dis*, 1995, **18** 265–72.

91 Agostoni C, Massetto N, Biasucci G *et al.* Effects of long-chain polyunsaturated fatty acid supplementation on fatty acid status and visual function in treated children with hyperphenylalaninemia. *J Pediatr*, 2000, **137** 504–9.

92 Agostoni C, Verduci E, Massetto N *et al.* Long term effects of long chain polyunsaturated fats in hyperphenylalaninemic children. *Arch Dis Child*, 2003, **88** 582–3.

93 Cleary MA, Feillet F, White FJ *et al.* Randomised controlled trial of essential fatty acid supplementation in phenylketonuria. *Eur J Clin Nutr*, 2006, **60** 915–20.

94 van Bakel MM, Printzen G, Wermuth B, Wiesmann UN Antioxidant and thyroid hormone status in selenium-deficient phenylketonuric and hyperphenylalaninemic patients. *Am J Clin Nutr*, 2000, **72** 976–81.

95 Kauf E, Seidel J, Winnefeld K *et al.* Selenium in phenylketonuria patients. Effects of sodium selenite administration. *Med Klin*, 1997, **92** (Suppl 3) 31–4.

96 Jochum F, Terwolbeck K, Meinhold H *et al.* Effects of a low selenium state in patients with phenylketonuria. *Acta Paediatr*, 1997, **86** 775–7.

97 Arnold GL, Kirby R, Preston C, Blakely E Iron and protein sufficiency and red cell indices in phenylketonuria. *J Am Coll Nutr*, 2001, **20** 65–70.

98 Bodley JL, Austin VJ, Hanley WB *et al.* Low iron stores in infants and children with treated phenylketonuria: a population at risk for iron-deficiency anaemia and associated cognitive deficits. *Eur J Pediatr*, 1993, **152** 140–3.

99 Robinson M, White FJ, Cleary MA *et al.* Increased risk of vitamin B_{12} deficiency in patients with phenylketonuria on an unrestricted or relaxed diet. *J Pediatr*, 2000, **136** 545–7.

100 Hanley WB, Feigenbaum ASJ, Clarke JTR *et al.* Vitamin B12 deficiency in adolescents and young adults with phenylketonuria. *Eur J Pediatr*, 1996, **155** S145–7.

101 Zeman J, Bayer M, Stepan J Bone mineral density in patients with phenylketonuria. *Acta Paediatr*, 1999, **88** 1348–51.

102 Lipson A, Masters H, O'Halloran M *et al.* The selenium status of children with phenylketonuria: Results of selenium supplementation. *Aust Paediatr J*, 1988, **24** 128–31.

103 Wilke BC, Vidailhet M, Favier A *et al.* Selenium, glutathione peroxidase (GSH-Px) and lipid peroxidation products before and after selenium supplementation. *Clin Chim Acta*, 1992, **207** 137–42.

104 Greeves LG, Carson DJ, Craig BG, McMaster D Potentially life-threatening cardiac dysrhythmia in a child with selenium deficiency and phenylketonuria. *Acta Paediatr Scand*, 1990, **79** 1259–62.

105 Bohles H, Ullrich K, Endres W *et al.* Inadequate iron availability as a possible cause of low serum carnitine concentrations in patients with phenylketonuria. *Eur J Pediatr*, 1991, **150** 425–8.

106 Gropper SS, Yannicelli S, White BD, Medeiros DM Plasma phenylalanine concentrations are associated with hepatic iron content in a murine model for phenylketonuria. *Mol Genet Metab*, 2004, **82** 76–82.

107 Yannicelli S, Medeiros DM Elevated plasma phenylalanine concentrations may adversely affect bone status of phenylketonuric mice. *J Inherit Metab Dis*, 2002, **25** 347–61.

108 National Society for Phenylketonuria Medical Advisory Panel. Management of PKU. Gateshead: NSPKU, 1999.

109 Green A, Isherwood D Reference data excluding neonates. In: Clayton BE, Round JM (eds) *Clinical Biochemistry and the Sick Child*. Oxford: Blackwell Science, 1994, pp. 523–39.

110 Gregory DM, Sovetts D, Clow CL, Scriver CR Plasma free amino acid values in normal children and adolescents. *Metabolism*, 1986, **35** 967–9.

111 Scriver CR, Gregory DM, Sovetts D, Tissenbaum G Normal plasma-free amino acid values in adults: the influence of some common physiological variables. *Metabolism*, 1985, **34** 868–73.

112 Hanley WB, Linsao L, Davidson W, Moes CAF Malnutrition with early treatment of phenylketonuria. *Pediatr Res*, 1970, **4** 318–27.

113 MacDonald A, Rylance G, Hall SK *et al*. Does a single blood specimen predict quality of control in PKU? *Arch Dis Child*, 1997, **78** 122–6.

114 Francis DEM, Smith I Breast-feeding regime for the treatment of infants with phenylketonuria. In: Bateman C (ed) *Applied Nutrition*. London: John Libbey, 1981, pp. 82–3.

115 Motzfeldt K, Lilje R, Nylander G Breast-feeding in phenylketonuria. *Acta Paediatr Suppl*, 1999, **88** 25–7.

116 Dermirkol M, Huner G, Kuru N *et al*. Feasibility of breastfeeding in inborn errors of metabolism: experience in phenylketonuria. *Ann Nutr Metab*, 2001, **45** (Suppl 1) 497–98.

117 Biasucci G Randomised controlled trial of a long chain polyunsaturated fatty acid (LC-PUFA) supplemented phenylalanine free infant formula. International Metabolic Dietitians' Group, York: Society for the Study of Inborn Errors of Metabolism, 1999.

118 MacDonald A, Rylance G, Asplin D *et al*. Abnormal feeding behaviours in phenylketonuria. *J Hum Nutr Diet*, 1997, **10** 163–70.

119 Walter JH, White FJ Blood phenylalanine control in adolescents with phenylketonuria. *Int J Adolesc Med Health*, 2004, **16** 41–5.

120 Walter JH, White FJ, Hall SK *et al*. How practical are recommendations for dietary control in phenylketonuria? *Lancet*, 2002, **360** 55–7.

121 Mundy H, Lilburn M, Cousins A, Lee P Dietary control of phenylketonuria. *Lancet*, 2002, **360** 2076.

122 MacDonald A, Lilburn M, Davies P *et al*. 'Ready to drink' protein substitute is easier is for people with PKU. *J Inherit Metab Dis*, 2006, **29** 526–31.

123 Lee PJ, Ridout D, Walter JH, Cockburn F Maternal phenylketonuria: report from the United Kingdom Registry 1978–97. *Arch Dis Child*, 2005, **90** 143–6.

124 Mitchell JJ, Scriver CR Phenylalanine hydroxylase deficiency. *Gene reviews*, 2005. Funded by National Institute of Health, developed by University of Washington, Seattle, USA. www.genetests.org

125 Francis D *Diets for Sick Children*, 4th edn. Oxford: Blackwell Science, 1987, pp. 224–62.

126 Holland B, Welch AA, Unwin ID *et al*. *McCance and Widdowson's The Composition of Foods*, 5th edn. Royal Society of Chemistry and Ministry of Agriculture, Fisheries and Food. London: The Stationery Office, 1991.

127 Clark B, MacDonald A, Lilburn M, Watling R A novel approach for the prescription of protein substitutes for phenylketonuria. *Proceedings of the VI International Congress: Inborn Error of Metabolism*, Milano, Italy. Poster No 15, 1994.

128 Rohr FJ, Munier AW, Levy HL Acceptability of a new modular protein substitute for the dietary treatment of phenylketonuria. *J Inherit Metab Dis*, 2001, **24** 623–30.

129 MacDonald A, Lilburn M, Cochrane B *et al*. A new, low-volume protein substitute for teenagers and adults with phenylketonuria. *J Inherit Metab Dis*, 2004, **27** 127–35.

130 Wardley BL, Taitz LS Clinical trial of a concentrated amino acid formula for older patients with phenylketonuria (Maxamum XP). *Eur J Clin Nutr*, 1988, **42** 81–6.

131 MacDonald A, Daly A, Davies P *et al*. Protein substitutes for PKU: What's new? *J Inherit Metab Dis*, 2004, **27** 363–71.

132 MacDonald A, Cochrane B, Asplin D *et al*. Protein substitute tablets useful in PKU? Symposium on Phenylketonuria: Present knowledge and future challenges. Elsinore, Denmark, 2002, p. 56. (Abstract)

133 MacDonald A, Ferguson C, Rylance G *et al*. Are tablets a practical source of protein substitute in phenylketonuria? *Arch Dis Child*, 2003, **88** 327–9.

134 Blau N, Burgard P Disorders of phenylalanine and tetrahydrobiopterin metabolism. In: Blau N, Hoffmann GF, Leonard J, Clarke JTR (eds) *Physicians Guide to the Treatment and Follow-up of Metabolic Diseases*. Berlin: Springer–Verlag, 2006, pp. 25–34.

135 Schadewaldt P, Bodner-Leidecker A, Hammen HW *et al*. Significance of L-alloisoleucine in plasma for diagnosis of maple syrup urine disease. *Clin Chem*, 1999, **45** 1734–40.

136 Chung DT, Shih VE Maple syrup urine disease (branched-chain ketoaciduria). In: Scriver CR *et al*. (eds) *The Metabolic and Molecular Bases of Inherited Disease*, 8th edn. New York: McGraw-Hill, 2001.

137 Hilliges C, Awiszus D, Wendel U Intellectual performance of children with maple syrup urine disease. *Eur J Pediatr*, 1993, **152** 144–7.

138 Nord A, Doornick W, Greene C Developmental profile of patients with maple syrup urine disease. *J Inherit Metab Dis*, 1991, **14** 881–9.

139 Treacy E, Clow CL, Reade TR *et al*. Maple syrup urine disease: interrelations between branched-chain amino, oxo and hydroxy acids; implications for treatment; associations with CNS dysmyelination. *J Inherit Metab Dis*, 1992, **15** 121–35.

140 Kaplan P, Mazur A, Field M *et al*. Intellectual outcome in children with maple syrup urine disease. *J Pediatr*, 1991, **119** 46–50.

141 le Roux C, Murphy E, Hallam P *et al*. Neuropsychometric outcome predictors for adults with maple syrup urine disease. *J Inherit Metab Dis*, 2006, **29** 201–2.

142 Simon E, Wendel U, Schadewaldt P Maple syrup urine disease treatment and outcome in patients of Turkish descent in Germany. *Turk J Pediatr*, 2005, **47** 8–13.

143 Protein and amino acid requirements in human nutrition. Report of a Joint WHO/FAO/UNU Expert Consultation. Technical Report Series, No. 935. 2006, in press.

144 Wendel U Disorders of branched-chain amino acid metabolism. In: Fernandes J, Saudubray J, Tarda K (eds) *Inborn Metabolic Diseases, Diagnosis and Treatment*. Berlin: Springer-Verlag, 1990.

145 Pratt OE The needs of the brain for amino acids and how they are transported across the blood-brain barrier. In: Belton NR, Toothill C (eds) *Transport and Inherited Disease*. Boston: MTP Press, 1981, pp. 87–122.

146 Department of Health Report on Social Subjects No 41. *Dietary Reference Values for Food, Energy and Nutrients for the United Kingdom*. London: The Stationery Office, 1991.

147 Jouvet P, Poggi F, Rabier D *et al*. Continuous venovenous haemodiafiltration in the acute phase of neonatal maple syrup urine disease. *J Inherit Metab Dis*, 1997, **20** 463–72.

148 Schaefer F, Straube E, Oh J *et al*. Dialysis in neonates with inborn errors of metabolism. *Nephrol Dial Transplant*, 1999, **14** 910–18.

149 Puliyanda DP, Harmon WE, Peterschmitt MJ *et al*. Utility of hemodialysis in maple syrup urine disease. *Pediatr Nephrol*, 2002, **17** 239–42.

150 Hmiel SP, Martin RA, Landt M *et al*. Amino acid clearance during acute metabolic decompensation in maple syrup urine disease treated with continuous venovenous hemodialysis with filtration. *Pediatr Crit Care Med*, 2004, **5** 278–81.

151 Phan V, Clermont MJ, Merouani A *et al*. Duration of extracorporeal therapy in acute maple syrup urine disease: a kinetic model. *Pediatr Nephrol*, 2006, **21** 698–704.

152 Thompson G, Walter J, Bresson J *et al*. Protein and leucine metabolism in maple syrup urine disease. *Am J Physiol*, 1990, **258** 654–60.

153 Morton DH, Strauss KA, Robinson DL *et al*. Diagnosis and treatment of Maple Syrup Urine Disease a study of 36 patients. *Pediatrics*, 2002, **109** 999–1008.

154 Macdonald A, Depondt E, Evans S *et al*. Breast feeding in IMD. *J Inherit Metab Dis*, 2006, **29** 299–303.

155 Hallam P, Lilburn M, Lee PJ A new protein substitute for adolescents and adults with maple syrup urine disease. *J Inherit Metab Dis*, 2005, **28** 665–72.

156 Schwahn B, Wendel U, Schadewaldt P *et al*. Diurnal changes in plasma amino acids in maple syrup urine disease. *Acta Paediatr*, 1998, **87** 1245–6.

157 Hoffmann B, Helberg C, Schadewaldt P *et al*. Impact of longitudinal plasma leucine levels on the intellectual outcome in patients with classic MSUD. *Pediatr Res*, 2006, **59** 17–20.

158 Giarcoia GP, Berry GT Acrodermatitis enteropathica-like syndrome secondary to isoleucine deficiency during treatment of maple syrup urine disease. *Am J Dis Child*, 1993, **147** 954–6.

159 Puzenat E, Durbise E, Fromentin C *et al*. Iatrogenic acrodermatitis enteropathica-like syndrome in leucinosis. *Ann Dermatol Venereol*, 2004, **131** 801–4.

160 Templier I, Reymond Jl, Nguyen MA *et al*. Acrodermatitis enteropathica-like syndrome secondary to branched-chain amino acid deficiency during treatment of maple syrup urine disease. *Ann Dermatol Venereol*, 2006, **133** 375–9.

161 Stafford J, Cleary M, Mumford N *et al*. Group clinic model for management of PKU. *J Inherit Metab Dis*, 2005, **28** 40 (Abstract 079).

162 Thompson G, Francis D, Halliday D Acute illness in maple syrup urine disease: dynamics of protein metabolism and implications for management. *J Pediatr*, 1991, **119** 35–41.

163 Mitchell GA, Grompe M, Lambert M, Tanguay RM Hypertyrosinaemia. In: Scriver CR *et al*. (eds) *The Metabolic and Molecular Bases of Inherited Disease*, 8th edn. New York: McGraw-Hill, 2001, pp. 1777–805.

164 Mitchell G, Larochelle J, Lambert M *et al*. Neurologic crisis in hereditary tyrosinaemia. *N Engl J Med*, 1990, **322** 432–7.

165 van Spronsen FJ, Thomasse Y, Smit GP *et al*. Hereditary tyrosinaemia type I: a new clinical classification with difference in prognosis on dietary treatment. *Hepatology*, 1994, **20** 1187–91.

166 Michaels K, Matalon R, Wong K Dietary treatment of tyrosinaemia type I. *J Am Diet Assoc*, 1978, **73** 507–14.

167 Lindstedt S, Holme E, Lock EA *et al*. Treatment of hereditary tyrosinaemia type I by inhibition of 4-hydroxyphenylpyruvate dioxygenase. *Lancet*, 1992, **340** 813–17.

168 Lindstedt S, Holme E Tyrosinaemia type I and NTBC (2-(2-nitro-4-trifluoromethylbenzoyl)-1,3-cyclohexanedione). *J Inherit Metab Dis*, 1998, **21** 507–17.

169 Holme E, Lindstedt S Nontransplant treatment of tyrosinaemia. *Clin Liver Dis*, 2000, **4** 805–14.

170 van Wyk KG, Clayton PT Dietary management of tyrosinaemia type I. In: *International Metabolic Dietitians Group, 2nd dietitians meeting SSIEM*, Gothenberg, Sweden, 1997.

171 Fernstrom JD, Fernstrom MH Dietary effects on tyrosine availability and catecholamine synthesis in the central nervous system: possible relevance to the control of protein intake. *Proc Nut Soc*, 1994, **53** 419–29.

172 Wilson CJ, van Wyk KG, Leonard JV et al. Phenylalanine supplementation improves the phenylalanine profile in tyrosinaemia. *J Inherit Metab Dis*, 2000, **23** 677–83.

173 Gissen P, Preece MA, Willshaw HA et al. Ophthalmic follow-up of patients with tyrosinaemia type I on NTBC. *J Inherit Metab Dis*, 2003, **26** 13–16.

174 Barr D, Kirk J, Laing S Outcome in tyrosinaemia type II. *Arch Dis Child*, 1991, **66** 1249–50.

175 Halvorsen S Tyrosinemia. In: Fernandes J, Saudubray J, Tada K (eds) *Inborn Metabolic Disease: Diagnosis and Treatment*. Berlin: Springer-Verlag, 1990.

176 Carson NAJ and Neill DW Metabolic abnormalities detected in a survey of mentally backward individuals in Northern Ireland. *Arch Dis Child*, 1962, **37** 505.

177 Skovby F, Krassikoff N, Franke U Assignment of the gene for cystathionine β synthase to human chromosome 21 in somatic cell hybrids. *Hum Genet*, 1984, **65** 291–4.

178 Moat SJ, Bao L, Fowler B et al. The molecular basis of cystathionine β synthase deficiency in UK and US patients with homocystinuria. *Hum Mutat*, 2004, **23** 206–11.

179 Mudd SH, Levy HL, Skovby F Disorders of trans-sulferation. In: Scriver CR, Beaudet AL, Sly WS, Valle D (eds) *The Metabolic and Molecular Bases of Inherited Disease*, 7th edn. New York: McGraw-Hill, 1995, pp. 1279–368.

180 Yap S, Naughten E Homocystinuria due to cystathionine β synthase deficiency in Ireland: 25 years experience of a newborn screened and treated population with reference to clinical outcome and biochemical control. *J Inherit Metab Dis*, 1998, **21** 738–47.

181 Andria G, Sebastio G Homocystinuria due to cystathionine β synthase deficiency and related disorders. In: Fernandes J, Saudubray and van den Berghe G (eds) *Inborn Metabolic Disorders: Diagnosis and Treatment*, 2nd edn. Berlin: Springer-Verlag, 1996, pp. 177–82.

182 Grieco AJ Homocystinuria: pathogenic mechanisms. *Am J Med Sci*, 1977, **273** 120–32.

183 Mudd SH, Finkelstein JD, Refsum H et al. Homocysteine and its disulphide derivatives. A suggested consensus terminology. *Arterioscler Thromb Vasc Biol*, 2000, **20** 1704–6.

184 Ueland PM, Refsum H et al. Total homocysteine in plasma or serum, methods and clinical application. *Clin Chem*, 1993, **39** 1764–9.

185 Moat SJ, Bonham JR, Tanner MS Recommended approaches for the laboratory measurement of homocysteine in the diagnosis and monitoring of patients with hyperhomocysteinaemia. *Ann Clin Biochem*, 1999, **36** 372–9.

186 Walter JH, Wraith JE, White FJ et al. Strategies for the treatment of cystathionine β synthase deficiency: the experience of the Willink Biochemical Genetics Unit over the past 30 years. *Eur J Pediatr*, 1998, **157** (Suppl 2) S71–6.

187 Mudd SH, Skovby F, Levy HL et al. The natural history of homocystinuria due to cystathionine β synthase deficiency. *Am J Hum Genet*, 1985, **37** 1–31.

188 Wilcken B, Turner B Homocystinuria. Reduced folate levels during pyridoxine treatment. *Arch Dis Child*, 1973, **48** 58–62.

189 Komorower GM, Lambert AM, Cusworth DC, Westall RG Dietary treatment of homocystinuria *Arch Dis Child*, 1966, **41** 666–71.

190 Perry TL, Dunn HG, Hansen, S et al. Early diagnosis and treatment of homocystinuria. *Pediatrics*, 1996, **37** 502–5.

191 Smith I Recommendations on the dietary management of phenylketonuria. *Arch Dis Child*, 1993, **68** 426–7.

192 Department of Health Report on Health and Social Subjects No. 41. *Dietary Reference Values for Food Energy and Nutrients for the United Kingdom*. London: The Stationery Office 1991.

193 Energy and protein requirements. Report of a joint FAO/WHO/UNU Expert Consultation. Geneva: WHO 1985.

194 Smolin LA, Benevenga NJ, Berlow S The use of betaine for the treatment of homocystinuria. *J Pediatr*, 1981, **99** 467–72.

195 Wilcken DEL, Wilcken B, Dudman, NPB, Tyrrell, PA Homocystinuria – the effects of betaine in the treatment of patients not responsive to pyridoxine. *N Engl J Med*, 1983, **309** 448–53.

196 Yap S, Barry-Kinsella C, Naughten ER Maternal pyridoxine non-responsive homocystinuria: the role of dietary treatment and anticoagulation. *Br J Obstet Gynaecol*, 2001, **108** 425–8.

197 Levy HL, Vargas JE, Waisburn SE et al. Reproductive fitness in maternal homocystinuria due to

cystathionine beta-synthase deficiency. *J Inherit Metab Dis*, 2002, **25** 299–314.

198 Dewey KG, Beaton G, Fjeld C *et al.* Protein requirements of infants and children. *Eur J Clin Nutr*, 1996, **50** (Suppl 1) 119–50.

199 Lenhert W, Sperl W, Suormala T *et al.* Propionic acidaemia: clinical, biochemical and therapeutic aspects. Experience in 30 patients. *Eur J Pediatr*, 1994, **153** 68–80.

200 Bodemer C, DeProst Y, Bachollet B *et al.* Cutaneous manifestations of methylmalonic and propionic acidaemia: a description based on 38 cases. *Br J Dermatol*, 1994, **131** 93–8.

201 Yannicelli S, Hambidge KM, Picciano MF Decreased selenium intake and low plasma selenium concentrations leading to clinical symptoms in a child with propionic acidaemia. *J Inherit Metab Dis*, 1992, **15** 261–9.

202 Sanjurjo P, Ruiz JI, Montejo M Inborn errors of metabolism with a protein-restricted diet: effect on polyunsaturated fatty acids. *J Inherit Metab Dis*, 1997, **20** 783–9.

203 Vlaardingerbroek H, Hornstra G, de Koning TJ *et al.* Essential polyunsaturated fatty acids in plasma and erythrocytes of children with inborn errors of amino acids metabolism. *Mol Genet Metab*, 2006, **88** 159–65.

204 Desci T, Sperl W, Koletzko B Essential fatty acids in clinically stable children with propionic acidaemia. *J Inherit Metab Dis*, 1997 **20** 778–82.

205 Edwards CA, Parrett AM, Balmer SE *et al.* Faecal short chain fatty acids in breast-fed and formula fed babies. *Acta Paediatr*, 2004, **83** 459–62.

206 Dixon MA, White FJ, Leonard JV Breast feeding in metabolic disease: how successful is this? Compilation of papers presented at the Fifth Dietitians Meeting at the VIII International Congress of Inborn Errors of Metabolism, Cambridge, 2000, pp. 4–8.

207 Huner G, Baykal T, Demir F *et al.* Breastfeeding experience in inborn errors of metabolism other then phenylketonuria. *J Inherit Metab Dis*, 2005, **28** 457–65.

208 Gokcay G, Baykal T, Gokdemir Y *et al.* Breast feeding in organic acidaemias *J Inherit Metab Dis*, 2006, **29** 304–10.

209 Walter JH, Wraith JE, Cleary MA Abscence of acidosis in the initial presentation of propionic acidaemia. *Arch Dis Child*, 1995, **72** 197–9.

210 Fenton WA, Gravel RA, Rosenblatt DS Disorders of propionate and methylmalonate metabolism. In: Scriver CR *et al.* (eds) *The Metabolic and Molecular Bases of Inherited Disease*, 8th edn. New York: McGraw-Hill, 2001, pp. 2165–93.

211 Matsui S, Mahoney M, Rosenberg L The natural history of the inherited methylmalonic acidaemias. *N Engl J Med*, 1987, **38** 857–61.

212 Baumgarter ER, Viardot C Long-term follow-up of 77 patients with isolated methylmalonic acidaemia. *J Inherit Metab Dis*, 1995, **18** 138–42.

213 van der Meer SB, Poggi F, Spada M *et al.* Clinical outcome of long-term management of patients with vitamin B_{12} unresponsive methylmalonic acidaemia. *J Pediatr*, 1994, **125** 903–8.

214 van der Meer SB, Poggi F, Spada M *et al.* Clinical outcome and long-term management of 17 patients with propionic acidaemia. *Eur J Pediatr*, 1996, **155** 205–10.

215 Dionisi–Vici C, Deodato F, Röschinger *et al.* 'Classical' organic acidurias, propionic aciduria, methylmalonic acidaemia and isovaleric aciduria: Long-term outcome and effects of expanded newborn screening using tandem mass spectrometry. *J Inherit Metab Dis*, 2006, **29** 383–9.

216 Surtees R, Matthews E, Leonard J Neurologic outcome of propionic acidaemia. *Pediatr Neurol*, 1992, **8** 333–7.

217 Nicolaides P, Leonard JV, Surtees R Neurological outcome of methylmalonic acidaemia. *Arch Dis Child*, 1998, **78** 508–12.

218 Massoud A, Leonard J Cardiomyopathy in propionic acidaemia. *Eur J Pediatr*, 1993, **152** 441–5.

219 Kahler SG, Sherwood WG, Woolf D *et al.* Pancreatitis in patients with organic acidaemias. *J Pediatr*, 1994, **124** 239–43.

220 Molteni KH, Oberley TD, Wolff JA *et al.* Progressive renal insufficiency in methylmalonic acidaemia. *Pediatr Nephrol*, 1991, **5** 323–6.

221 Chakrapani A, Sivakumar P, McKiernan P *et al.* Metabolic stroke in methylmalonic acidaemia five years after liver transplantation. *J Pediatr* 2002, **140** 261–3.

222 Thompson G, Walter JH, Bresson JL *et al.* Sources of propionate in inborn errors of propionate. *Metabolism*, 1990, **39** 1133–7.

223 Thompson G, Chalmers RA, Walter JH *et al.* The use of metronidazole in management of methylmalonic and propionic acidaemias. *Eur J Pediatr*, 1990, **149** 792–6.

224 Sbai D *et al.* Possible contributions of odd-chain fatty acid oxidation to propionate production in methylmalonic and propionic acidaemia. *Pediatr Res*, 1992, **31** 188A.

225 Wendel U Abnormality of odd-numbered, long-chain fatty acids in erythrocyte membrane lipids from patients with disorders of propionate metabolism. *Pediatr Res*, 1989, **25** 147–50.

226 Ney D, Bay C, Saudubray JM *et al.* An evaluation of protein requirements in methylmalonic acidaemia. *J Inherit Metab Dis*, 1985, **8** 132–42.

227 Touati G, Valayannaopoulos V, Mention K *et al.* Methylmalonic acidaemia and propionic acidurias: Management without or with a few supplement of

specific amino acid mixture. *J Inherit Metab Dis*, 2006, **29** 288–98.

228 Yannicelli S, Acosta PB, Velazquez A *et al.* Improved growth and nutrition status in children with methylmalonic or propionic acidaemia fed an elemental medical food. *Mol Genet Metab*, 2003, **80** 181–8.

229 Sbai D, Narcy C, Thompson GN *et al.* Contribution of odd-chain fatty acid oxidation to propionate production in disorders of propionate metabolism. *Am J Clin Nutr*, 1994, **59** 1332–7.

230 Wasserstein MP, Gaddipati S, Snyderman SE *et al.* Successful pregnancy in severe methylmalonic acidaemia. *J Inherit Metab Dis*, 1999, **22** 788–94.

231 D'Angio C, Dillon M, Leonard J Renal tubular dysfunction in methylmalonic acidaemia. *Eur J Pediatr*, 1991, **150** 259–63.

232 Walter JH, Dillon MJ, Leonard JV *et al.* Chronic renal failure in methylmalonic acidaemia. *Eur J Pediatr*, 1989, **148** 344–8.

233 van't Hoff WG, Dixon M, Taylor J *et al.* Combined liver-kidney transplant in methylmalonic acidaemia. *J Pediatr*, 1998, **132** 1043–4.

234 Feillet F, Bodamer OA, Dixon MA *et al.* Resting energy expenditure in disorders of propionate metabolism. *J Pediatr*, 2000, **136** 659–63.

235 van Hagen CC, Carbasius Weber E, van den Hurk TA *et al.* Energy expenditure in patients with propionic acidaemia and methylmalonic acidaemias. *J Inherit Metab Dis*, 2004, **27** 111–12.

236 Sperl W, Skladal D, Endres W *et al.* Parenteral administration of amino acids in disorders of branched chain amino acid metabolism. *J Inher Metab Dis*, 1994, **17** 753–4.

237 Vockley J, Ensenauer R Isovaleric acidaemia: New aspects of genetic and phenotypic heterogeity. *Am J Med Genet C Semin Med Genet*, 2006, **142C** 95–103.

238 Sweetman L, Williams JC Branched chain organic acidurias. In: Scriver CR *et al.* (eds) *The Metabolic and Molecular Bases of Inherited Disease*, 8th edn. New York: McGraw-Hill, 2001, pp. 2125–63.

239 Berry G, Yudkoff M, Segal S Isovaleric acidaemia: medical and neurodevelopmental effects of long-term therapy. *J Pediatr*, 1988, **113** 58–63.

240 Naglak M, Salvo R, Madsen K *et al.* The treatment of isovaleric acidaemia with glycine supplement. *Pediatr Res*, 1988, **24** 9–13.

241 Fries MH, Rinaldo P, Schmidt-Sommerfeld E *et al.* Isovaleric acidaemia: response to a leucine load after 3 weeks of supplementation with glycine, l-carnitine, and combined glycine-carnitine therapy. *J Pediatr*, 1996, **129** 449–52.

242 Goodman SI, Frerman FE Organic acidaemias due to defects in lysine oxidation: 2-ketoadipic acidaemia and glutaric acidaemia. In: Scriver CR *et al.* (eds) *The Metabolic and Molecular Bases of Inherited Disease*, 8th edn. New York: McGraw-Hill, 2001, pp. 2195–204.

243 Kölker S, Garbade SF, Greenberg CR *et al.* Natural history, outcome and treatment efficacy in children and adults with Glutaryl-CoA dehydrogenase deficiency. *Pediatr Res*, 2006, **59** 840–7.

244 Baric I, Schocke J, Christensen E *et al.* Diagnosis and management of glutaric aciduria type I. *J Inherit Metab Dis*, 1998, **21** 326–40.

245 Superti-Furga A, Hoffman GF Glutaric aciduria type I (glutaryl-CoA-dehydrogenase deficiency): advances and unanswered questions. *Eur J Pediatr*, 1997, **156** 821–8.

246 Lindner M, Kölker S, Schulze A *et al.* Neonatal screening for glutaryl-CoA dehydrogenase deficiency. *J Inherit Metab Dis*, 2004, **27** 851–9.

247 Proceedings in Glutaryl-CoA dehydrogenase deficiency: Report from the 3rd International Workshop on Glutaryl-CoA dehydrogenase deficiency and the 1st Guidelines meeting for Glutaryl-CoA dehydrogenase deficiency. *J Inherit Metab Dis*, 2004, **27** 797–926.

248 Monavari AA, Naughten ER Prevention of cerebral palsy in glutaric aciduria type I by dietary management. *Arch Dis Child*, 2000, **82** 67–70.

249 Hoffman GF, Zschocke J Glutaric aciduria type I: from clinical diversity to successful therapy. *J Inherit Metab Dis*, 1999, **22** 381–91.

250 Kyllerman M, Skjeldal O, Christensen E *et al.* Long-term follow-up, neurological outcome and survivial rate in 28 Nordic patients with glutaric aciduria type 1. *Eur J Pediatr*, 2004, **8** 121–9.

251 Strauss KA, Puffenberger EK Robinson DL *et al.* Type I Glutaric aciduria, Part 1: Natural history of 77 patients. *Am J Med Genet*, 2003, **121C** 38–52.

252 Sauer SW, Okun JG, Fricker G *et al.* Intracerebral accumulation of glutaric and 3-hydroxyglutaric acids secondary to limited flux across the blood-brain barrier constitute a biochemical risk factor for neurodegeneration in glutaryl-CoA dehydrogenase deficiency. *J Neurochem*, 2006, **97** 899–910.

253 Greenberg CR, Prasad AN, Dilling LA *et al.* Outcome of the first 3-years of a DNA – Based Neonatal Screening Program for Glutaric Acidaemia Type 1 in Manitoba and Northwestern Ontario, Canada. *Mol Genet Metab*, 2002, **75** 70–8.

254 Francis D, Humphrey M, Boneh A Newborn screening for glutaric aciduria type 1: the dietary challenge. *J Inherit Metab Dis*, 2005, **28** (Suppl 1) Abstract 091-P.

255 Kölker S, Christensen E, Leonard JV *et al.* Guideline for the diagnosis and management of glutaryl-CoA dehydrogenase deficiency (glutaric aciduria type1). *J Inherit Metab Dis*, 2007, **30**(1) 5–22.

256 Brusilow S, Harwich A Urea cycle enzymes. In: Scriver CR *et al.* (eds) *The Metabolic and Molecular*

Bases of Inherited Disease, 8th edn. New York: McGraw-Hill, 2001, pp. 1909–63.

257 Leonard JV Urea cycle disorders In: Fernandes J, Saudubray JM, van den Berghe G (eds) *Inborn Metabolic Diseases, Diagnosis and Treatment*, 2nd edn. Berlin: Springer-Verlag, 1995, pp. 167–76.

258 Nassogne MC, Heron B, Touati G *et al.* Urea cycle defects: Management and outcome. *J Inherit Metab Dis*, 2005, **28** 407–14.

259 Feillet F, Leonard JV Alternative pathways for urea cycle disorders. *J Inherit Metab Dis*, 1998, **21** (Suppl 1) 101–11.

260 Brusilow S, Tinker J, Batshaw ML Amino acid acylation: a mechanism of nitrogen excretion in inborn errors of urea synthesis. *Science*, 1980, **207** 659–61.

261 Kasumov T, Brunengraber LL, Comte B *et al.* New secondary metabolites of phenylbutyrate in humans and rats. *Drug Metab Dispos*, 2004, **32** 10–19.

262 Brusilow S Arginine, an indispensable amino acid for patients with inborn errors of urea synthesis. *J Clin Invest*, 1984, **74** 2144–8.

263 Batshaw M, Mac Arthur RB, Tuchman M Alternative pathway therapy for urea cycle disorders: Twenty years later. *J Pediatr*, 2001 **138** 46–55.

264 Leonard JV Komrower lecture: Treatment of inborn errors of metabolism: A review. *J Inherit Metab Dis*, 2006, **29** 275–8.

265 Lee B, Singh R, Rhead WJ *et al.* Considerations in the difficult-to-manage urea cycle disorder patient. *Crit Care Clin*, 2005, **21** 19–25.

266 Young VR, El-Khoury AE, Raguso CA *et al.* Rates of urea production and hydrolysis and leucine oxidation change linearly over widely varying protein intakes in healthy adults. *J Nutr*, 2000, **130** 761–6.

267 Leonard JV The nutritional management of urea cycle disorders. *J Pediatr*, 2001, **138** 40–5.

268 Scaglia F, Lee B Effect of alternative pathway therapy on branched chain amino acid metabolism in urea cycle disorder patients. *Mol Genet Metab*, 2004, **81** 79–85.

269 Wilson CJ, Lee PJ, Leonard JV Plasma glutamine and ammonia concentrations in ornithine carbamoyltransferase deficiency and citrullinaemia. *J Inherit Metab Dis*, 2001, **24** 691–5.

270 Bachman C Ornithine carbamyl transferase deficiency: findings, models and problems. *J Inherit Metab Dis*, 1992, **15** 578–91.

271 Hyman S, Porter CA, Page TJ *et al.* Behaviour management of feeding disturbances in urea cycle and organic acid disorders. *J Pediatr*, 1987, **111** 558–62.

272 Lambert M, Marescau B, Desjardins M *et al.* Hyperargininaemia; intellectual and motor improvement related to changes in biochemical data. *J Pediatr*, 1991, **118** 420–4.

273 Prasad AN, Breen JC, Ampola MG *et al.* Argininemia: a treatable genetic cause of progressive spastic diplegia simulating cerebral palsy: case reports and literature review. *J Child Neurol*, 1997, **12**, 301–9.

274 Crombez EA, Cederbaum SD Hyperargininemia due to liver arginase deficiency. *Mol Genet Metab*, 2005, **84** 243–51.

275 Scaglia F Brendan L Clinical, Biochemical, and Molecular Spectrum of Hyperargininemia due to arginase I deficiency. *Am J Med Genet C Semin Med Genet*, 2006, **142C** 113–20.

276 Bodamer OAF, Hoffman GF, Visser GH *et al.* Assessment of energy expenditure in metabolic disorders. *Eur J Pediatr*, 1997, **156** 24–8.

277 Verber I, Bain M Glucose polymer regimens and hypernatraemia. *Arch Dis Child*, 1990, **65** 627–8.

278 Morris AAM, Dixon MA Parenteral nutrition for patients with inherited metabolic diseases. In: *British Inherited Metabolic Disease Group Newsletter*, 1997 Issue 13.

279 Matern D, Seydewitz HH, Lehnert W *et al.* Primary treatment of propionic acidaemia complicated by acute thiamine deficiency. *J Pediatr*, 1996, **129** 758–60.

280 Dixon M, Leonard J Intercurrent illness in inborn errors of intermediary metabolism. *Arch Dis Child*, 1992, **67** 1387–91.

281 Morris AAM, Leonard JV Early recognition of metabolic decompensation. *Arch Dis Child*, 1997, **76** 555–6.

282 Komaromy DC, Gick JA, Eardley JEL *et al.* When should families use the emergency regime – are urinary ketones a useful guide? *J Inherit Metab Dis*, 2005, **28** Abstract 095-P.

Useful addresses

British Inherited Metabolic Disease Group (BIMDG)
www.bimdg.org.uk

Society for the Study of Inborn Errors of Metabolism (SSIEM)
www.ssiem.org

National Society for PKU (NSPKU)
PO Box 26642, London, N14 4ZF
e-mail: nspku@ukonline.co.uk
www.nspku.org

PAH/PKU Knowledgebase
www.pahdb.mcgill.ca

Children Living with Inherited Metabolic Diseases (CLIMB)
Climb Building, 176 Nantwich Road, Crewe, CW2 6BG
e-mail: steve@climb.org.uk
www.climb.org.uk

18 Disorders of Carbohydrate Metabolism

Glycogen Storage Diseases

Marjorie Dixon

Glycogen storage disease type I

The enzyme glucose-6-phosphatase has a central role in glucose production, catalysing the final common pathway for endogenous glucose synthesis from glycogenolysis and gluconeogenesis (Fig. 18.1). It is normally expressed in liver, kidney and intestine. Glycogen storage disease type I (GSD I) is caused by either deficiency of glucose-6-phosphatase itself (type Ia) or of the glucose-6-phosphate transport system (type Ib) [1]. Glucose production is inadequate because of the deficiency and hypoglycaemia will occur after relatively short periods of fasting. The clinical manifestations also include growth retardation and hepatomegaly caused mainly by fatty infiltration of the liver. Increased glycolytic flux leads to lactic acidosis and hyperlipidaemia, with triglycerides more markedly elevated than cholesterol [2]. Additionally in type Ib, there is neutropenia and impaired neutrophil function which increases susceptibility to bacterial infections, particularly of the skin and respiratory tract [2]. A chronic inflammatory bowel disease similar histopathologically to Crohn's disease is also commonly seen [3].

Long term complications have been reported: renal disease (both glomerular and tubular dysfunction occur), hepatic tumours (mostly benign adenoma, but with the potential for malignant transformation), osteopenia and polycystic ovaries in females [4,5].

Dietary management

The aim of dietary treatment is to promote normal growth by maintaining a normal blood glucose level. This will also improve the secondary metabolic abnormalities, but it is recognised that these cannot be completely normalised [6]. Infants and children are administered a frequent supply of exogenous glucose both day and night at least until they have stopped growing. Glucose requirements are calculated from basal glucose production rates in normal children [7]. It is important to be aware that these requirements for glucose decrease with age (Table 18.1). Dietary energy is provided as follows: 60–70% from carbohydrate (CHO), 20–25% from fat and 10–15% from protein. Fat intake is decreased to compensate for increased carbohydrate intake.

Provision of carbohydrate to GSD I patients has altered over the years. Traditionally, frequent CHO feeding was given day and night. In 1976, Greene *et al.* [8] reported the intensive regimen of regular drinks of glucose polymer by day and continuous nasogastric feeding at night. In 1984, Chen *et al.* [9] introduced uncooked cornstarch to the diet to provide a source of slow release glucose. Most centres now use a combination of continuous overnight feeding and 2-hourly feeding using glucose polymers; or uncooked cornstarch during the daytime; or uncooked cornstarch throughout the 24-hour period (see p. 395). With this intensive dietary treatment growth has improved in children with GSD I.

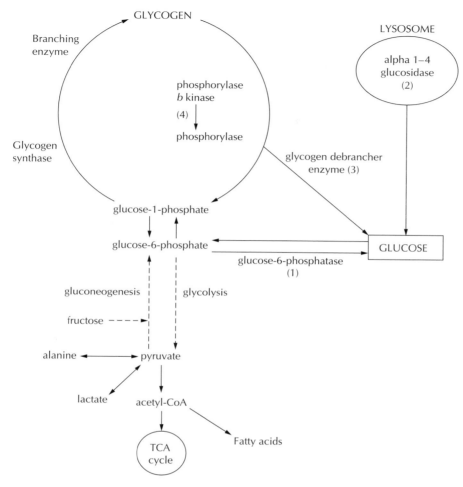

Figure 18.1 Pathway of liver glycogen metabolism. 1 Glycogen storage disease type I. 2 Glycogen storage disease type II. 3 Glycogen storage disease type III. 4 Phosphorylase system deficiencies. TCA, tricarboxylic acid.

Table 18.1 Glucose requirements based on glucose production rates [6].

Age	Glucose (mg/kg/min)	Glucose (g/kg/hour)	
		Day	Night
Infants	8–9	0.5	0.5
Toddlers and children	5–7	0.3–0.4	0.3–0.4
Adolescents and adults	2–4 at night		0.2–0.25

Some centres restrict fructose and galactose in the diet because these sugars are not converted to glucose via the gluconeogenic pathway but, instead, increase lactate production [5,10]. However, a mildly elevated blood lactate level of up to 4.0 mmol/L is considered acceptable because lactate provides an alternative source of energy to the brain and therefore has a protective effect against fuel depletion [11]. Indeed, Melis *et al.* [12] have highlighted the impact that this disorder has on brain function, which needs to be considered. Consequently, many feel that the restriction of these sugars is not essential and that regular provision of glucose is the more important dietary manoeuvre. The dietary management guidelines from the European Study on Glycogen Storage Disease Type I [13] recommends that lactose, fructose and sucrose is restricted, but no consensus exists on the degree of restriction required. The author's unit does not limit intake of these sugars.

Replacement of saturated fat with polyunsaturated fat is recommended by some in an attempt to improve the hyperlipidaemia [14], but this is less important than supplying a frequent CHO intake. Despite persistent hyperlipidaemia, no evidence of premature arteriosclerosis has yet been observed [15–18], as antioxidant status appears higher than normal in these patients [19].

Glucose requirements

Glucose intakes for children with GSD I are calculated to be similar to normal hepatic glucose production [8,20]. Glucose requirements (g/kg/hour or mg/kg/minute) decrease with age (Table 18.1). Although these figures can be used as a guide when planning the diet, it is the author's practice to use total CHO intake (g CHO/kg/hour), i.e. all sugars, not just glucose and starch, as the fuel source rather than just grams of glucose/kg/hour. It is important to ensure that only the required amount of glucose is administered at night and as 2-hourly daytime CHO drinks; large quantities of exogenous glucose will exacerbate swings in blood glucose levels and make patients more prone to rebound hypoglycaemia and will induce peripheral body fat storage [13,21]. Obesity is a problem for some GSD patients and hence another reason for avoiding excessive glucose intakes. Equally important is the need to provide adequate glucose as insufficient amounts will lead to high plasma lactate levels and growth retardation. Achieving optimum biochemical control is difficult. For some patients it may be beneficial to measure blood glucose at home; however, this is not perceived to be essential for daily management. Repeated continuous subcutaneous glucose monitoring has been suggested to be a possible useful tool for the assessment of long term management of GSD I patients [22], but this needs to be properly evaluated.

Nasogastric feeding

Continuous nasogastric feeding is used to provide glucose overnight. Careful management of this is necessary because it can render the patient more sensitive to hypoglycaemia [6]. Indeed, fatalities have been reported because of unplanned cessation in delivery of the glucose feed, and the pump feed not being switched on [23,24]. It is therefore essential that the paediatric feed pump accurately controls flow rate and alarms if there is electrical or mechanical pump failure. The tubing used for the delivery system and nasogastric tube needs to be secure [24]. Parents need thorough teaching and must be adept and confident with the enteral feeding system prior to home use. Gastrostomy feeding is a possible alternative to nasogastric feeding, but this requires careful consideration. Insertion of a gastrostomy is a surgical procedure requiring anaesthesia and GSD patients have increased risk factors for surgery, such as an increased bleeding tendency and hypoglycaemia. In patients with type Ib gastrostomy is contraindicated because of infection risk and poor wound healing [13].

When commencing the continuous overnight tube feed, an oral or bolus feed is given if the child has not been fed for 2 hours. On discontinuation of the night feed it is extremely important that the child is fed within 15 minutes to avoid hypoglycaemia [5]. In practice, usually a small bolus feed is given immediately on cessation of the night feed and then the child is fed again after 30 minutes.

Diet for infants

Most patients with GSD type I present before 1 year of age [5]. Infants need a frequent supply of exogenous glucose both day and night. Regular 2-hourly feeding during the day and continuous nasogastric feeds by night are needed to maintain normoglycaemia. Initially, CHO requirements (0.5 g CHO/kg/hour) can be provided by infant formula fed at normal fluid volumes of 150–200 mL/kg. Additional glucose polymer is not always necessary. During the daytime infants may demand feed and take more than 0.5 g CHO/kg/hour; however, the night feed should be maintained at the CHO requirement of 0.5 g CHO/kg/hour. At the beginning and end of the night feed, an oral or bolus feed providing sufficient glucose to last for 30 minutes is given. An example of an infant's feeding regimen is shown in Table 18.2. Breast feeding is a possibility but experience of this is limited.

Table 18.2   Example infant feeding regimen GSD type I. A 5-kg infant: aim 0.5 g carbohydrate/kg/hour.

	Fluid (mL)	Energy (kcal)	Energy (kJ)	CHO (g)	Protein (g)	Fat (g)
SMA Gold	840	546	2282	60	12.6	30
Amount/kg	170	110	456	12.0	2.5	
Amount/kg/hour				0.5		
Amount/hour				2.5		

Daily feed distribution:

Day: Oral feeds 70 mL
8.30 am, 10 am, 12 noon, 2 pm, 4 pm,
6 pm = 420 mL.

Night: Continuous nasogastric feeds 35 mL
every hour from 8 pm finishing at 8 am = 420 mL
Bolus nasogastric feeds – 20 mL at 8 pm and 8 am
(extra to calculated fluid requirement).

Weaning is commenced at the normal time around 6 months (26 weeks) of age. Establishing a feeding pattern for solids can be very difficult. Often, the infant is not hungry because of the frequent day and overnight feeding and consequently feeding problems are common. A regular intake of starchy foods is recommended (e.g. baby rice, rusk, potato). As the intake of starchy food increases it can replace the infant feed at main meals as the source of glucose for the following 2 hours. As relatively small quantities of food provide the glucose requirements, a complicated CHO food exchange system is not always necessary. It can sometimes be sufficient just to teach parents which foods provide CHO and to include these at main meals. However, if the introduction of solids is difficult, a list of quantities of foods that provide the necessary amount of CHO per meal can prove extremely useful. For example, an 8-kg infant requires 0.5 g CHO/kg/hour which equates to 8 g CHO for a 2-hour period; a list of weights of starchy foods that provide 8 g CHO would be given.

Invariably, it becomes commonplace for the parents of infants with feeding problems to rely on using the nasogastric tube to provide some or even all of the necessary daytime CHO. This practice also occurs in infants presenting later, who can already have feeding problems prior to diagnosis and then have difficulty in establishing a 2-hourly daytime regimen. Feeding problems often begin to improve when uncooked cornstarch is introduced as the interval between feeding times can be increased. As more energy is derived from solids, the infant should take smaller volumes of daytime feeds. To ensure adequate intake of CHO, glucose polymer is added to the infant feed to give a final concentration of 10–15% CHO. From 9 months onwards, some of the between meal infant feeds can be replaced by CHO drinks such as baby juices with added glucose polymer or glucose polymer solution, or starchy snacks. However, it is important that the daily intake of infant formula does not fall too low because it continues to provide a major source of nutrients in the older baby's diet. Care must be taken to avoid giving drinks that are too concentrated in CHO content because their osmolality may precipitate diarrhoea. Intermittent diarrhoea or loose stools occurs in some patients, but the cause is not completely understood [25–27]. A maximum concentration of 12–15% CHO is recommended in older infants. An example of a weaning diet is shown in Table 18.3.

Infant formula can continue to be given overnight, but for older infants large volumes would need to be given to provide the required amount of CHO which would compromise the daytime appetite. Therefore, the volume of infant formula is decreased and glucose polymer added to provide 0.5 g CHO/kg/hour, with the ultimate aim of providing all CHO as glucose polymer from about 1 year of age.

Diet for children

During the daytime a source of CHO continues to be given at 2-hourly intervals either from a meal or snack containing CHO or a CHO drink. The portion size of CHO foods (appropriate for age) will make the CHO content of main meals in excess of the specified requirement (0.3–0.5 g CHO/kg/hour). In between meal snacks or drinks should aim to provide only the specified requirement of CHO as excessive amounts may reduce appetite for main meals and cause excess weight gain. Parents are given information on different drinks and snacks that supply only the required amount of glucose. Starchy foods such as potato, rice, pasta, bread and

Table 18.3   Example of a diet for a 10-month-old infant with GSD type I. Weight 8 kg, providing 0.5 g carbohydrate/kg/hour (4 g CHO/hour).

Time	Food or drink	Total CHO (g)	CHO (g/kg/hour*)	Protein (g)	Energy (kcal)	Energy (kJ)
8.15 am	1 Weetabix	10.0	0.9	1.7	50	209
	100 mL SMA Gold	7.2		1.5	65	272
10.00 am	15 mL concentrated baby juice diluted to 100 mL	9.0	0.5	–	36	150
12.00 midday	Minced beef, vegetable	–		6.0	60	250
	Small potato	10.0	1.6	1.0	40	167
	100 g yoghurt	15.0		5.0	80	334
2.00 pm	90 mL SMA Gold + glucose polymer to 10% CHO	9.0	0.5	1.3	68	284
4.00 pm	1 slice bread + butter	12.0		2.2	70	292
	Ham filling	–	1.3	4.0	30	125
	Small banana	10.0		0.5	40	167
6.00 pm	90 mL SMA Gold + glucose polymer to 10% CHO	9.0	0.5	1.3	68	284
8.00 pm to 8.00 am finish	30 mL hourly for 12 hours SMA Gold + glucose polymer to 13% CHO	47.0	0.5	5.4	317	1325
8.00 pm and 8.00 am	15 mL bolus SMA Gold + glucose polymer to 13% CHO	3.9		1.0	26	109
Totals		142		30.0	950	3968
% Energy intake		60%		13%		

* The portion size of carbohydrate foods (appropriate for age) will make the carbohydrate content of main meals in excess of the specified requirement of 0.5 g/kg/hour.

cereals are encouraged in preference to sugary foods because these are more slowly digested to produce glucose.

From 1 year of age the night feed is often changed to a solution of glucose polymer, provided that the requirement for other nutrients is supplied by the daytime diet. As the child gets older more concentrated glucose polymer solutions are used: 15% CHO in 1–2-year-olds, 20% CHO in 2–6-year-olds, 25% up to a maximum of 30% CHO for older children. Occasionally, a paediatric enteral feed is administered at night in preference to glucose polymer alone, particularly when growth and nutrient intakes are inadequate. If the child has not eaten for 2 hours a bolus or oral feed will be given at the start of the night feed, providing sufficient glucose for 30 minutes. On cessation of the night feed a bolus feed (same as the pre-night feed) is given. As many children with GSD I find it very difficult to eat breakfast as a result of being fed overnight, a CHO drink (plus cornflour for some patients) is usually given 30 minutes after stopping the feed.

Children with GSD I can be at risk of vitamin and mineral deficiencies [28], particularly as a high percentage of the dietary energy intake may be provided as glucose polymer and pure starch. Inadequate calcium intakes have been reported in GSD I patients who were demonstrated to have reduced bone mineral density [29] although this also occurs in patients reported to have normal calcium intakes [30]. Vitamin and mineral intakes should be regularly assessed, in particular calcium and vitamin D, as these patients are known to be at risk of osteopenia. Supplements of vitamins and minerals are often necessary. Monitoring of bone density is recommended [13].

A major reduction in exercise capacity in adult patients with GSD I has been reported, with mean blood glucose levels for patients showing a progressive decrease throughout exercise and recovery [31]. Therefore, children are likely to require additional CHO when exercising; parents often report the need to give food or sugary drinks before or after exercise. Ideally, CHO should be given as starchy food in advance of the exercise.

Cornstarch therapy

Uncooked cornstarch (UCCS) as cornflour is slowly digested, primarily by pancreatic amylase to release glucose. When compared with glucose polymer feeding, a smoother blood glucose profile is produced and less glucose is required [32]. Satisfactory glycaemia has been reported to last 4–9 hours after ingestion [9,32]. However, the author's group has reported only achieving satisfactory glycaemia for a median of 4.25 hours (range 2.5–6.0) [33]. This variation in duration of response may, in some patients, be attributable to malabsorption [34]. New work from a trial of a novel starch has reported longer duration of euglycamia and better short term metabolic control compared with cornstarch [35].

UCCS can obviate the need for 2-hourly feeding. It is administered at regular intervals throughout the day (and night for some patients) in doses that approximate the basal glucose production rate. In practice, the amount of UCCS given per dose is 2 g/kg body weight in young children, decreasing to around 1.5 g/kg in older children and 1 g/kg in adolescents who have stopped growing. In obese children lower doses are given. Usually, a dose of UCCS is required every 4–6 hours but this is based on the results of the UCCS load test (see below). UCCS can be introduced around 2 years of age. In younger children it may not be adequately digested to maintain normal blood glucose because pancreatic amylase activity only reaches adult levels at 2–4 years of age, although its activity is reported to be induced by oral starch [14]. Success has been

reported with UCCS in children <2 years of age using smaller, more frequent doses [36–38].

Cornflour is given raw; cooking or heating disrupts the starch granules by hydrolysis and thus makes it much less effective. To increase palatability of UCCS it can be mixed with different drinks such as milk, squash, carbonated drinks or with cold food such as ice cream, yoghurt, fruit purée, thin cold custard, or mixed with milk then poured on cereal. If mixed with food it gives more bulk for the child to eat. Some studies have reported that mixing UCCS with sugary drinks makes it less effective because of increased insulin production [9,32,39].

When initiating UCCS treatment, a fasting 'UCCS load test' is performed in hospital to assess the child's metabolic response by serial measurement of blood glucose and lactate. These biochemical results are used to determine the frequency and quantity of UCCS given. Prior to this, UCCS will have been introduced at home to test its palatability and acceptance. The dose of UCCS is gradually increased to 2 g/kg at one meal, beginning with 5 g and increasing by 5 g every week to the required dose. Some patients may experience side effects such as diarrhoea, abdominal distention and flatulence but these are usually transient. The child's usual 2-hourly daytime feeding regimen will continue during this introductory period of UCCS. Some children will not take UCCS. Instead, it is given via the nasogastric tube, although it is important to continue to encourage the UCCS to be taken orally.

The dose and frequency of UCCS needs to be reviewed regularly taking into consideration growth velocity, frequency of hypoglycaemia and biochemical results. Ideally, patients should have a 24-hour glucose and lactate profile, and UCCS load test every 1–2 years. Common times for performing a UCCS load test are: on initiation of UCCS, increasing age, consideration of discontinuation of night feed, poor growth/biochemical indices and starting or changing school. An example of a diet incorporating UCCS is given in Table 18.4. When planning the regimen it is important to be aware that cornflour takes around 30 minutes to start releasing glucose. The diet usually comprises 2–3 doses of UCCS during the daytime. A lower dose may be given in the evening if there is a relatively short interval between this time, the evening meal and the night feed.

Table 18.4　Example of a diet for a 7 year old child with GSD type I. Weight 25 kg; aim 0.3 g carbohydrate/kg/hour overnight.

Time	Food or drink	
7.30 am	Breakfast including: CHO foods, e.g. breakfast cereal, bread, chapatti, pitta bread 50 g cornflour mixed with 100 mL water + squash	2 g/kg
12.30 pm	School dinner including: CHO foods, e.g. potato, rice, pulses, biscuits (crackers or semi-sweet), fruit 50 g cornflour mixed with 100 mL milk	2 g/kg
5.30 pm	Evening meal including: CHO foods, e.g. potato, pasta, bread, fruit, yoghurt 25 g cornflour mixed with 50 mL milk	1 g/kg
8.00 pm to 7.00 am	20% glucose polymer 40 mL hourly	Provides 0.3 g CHO/kg/hour overnight
8.00 pm and 7.00 am	20 mL bolus of 20% glucose polymer	

In children, continuous overnight nasogastric feeding is usually continued until they have stopped growing. However, some families prefer to use UCCS at night as it is less complicated and more socially acceptable than tube feeding, but the main disadvantage of this for young children is the need to wake at around 4–6-hourly intervals, thereby interrupting sleep. Parents will also need to wake up to give the UCCS and rely on an alarm clock to do so.

After puberty some form of nocturnal glucose therapy needs to continue to prevent fasting hypoglycaemia and biochemical abnormalities [40]. Adolescents should be reassessed at this time to determine their fasting tolerance. The recent experience of the author's unit is that discontinuing the overnight tube feed is difficult even when growth ceases, as UCCS does not maintain normoglycaemia for sufficiently long periods.

A comparative study of long term management of both forms of treatment, UCCS versus continuous nocturnal nasogastric glucose feeds, reported no significant differences in physical growth and biochemical parameters, but growth in height was still not optimal [41]. Inadequate growth in height has also been reported in a study of long term continuous glucose therapy with cornstarch begun in infancy [38]. Mundy et al. [42] have reported improved growth with intensive dietary treatment but there is a subset within their patient group who, despite therapy, has poor growth. These patients had measured endocrine responses similar to those reported for untreated patients but the reasons for this are not yet clear.

Obesity is a problem for some GSD I patients. Interestingly, in the study of Mundy et al. [42] the more obese patients were tallest, although as a group they were significantly shorter than average.

Cornflour and glucose polymer are approved by the Advisory Committee Borderline Substances (ACBS) for prescription on FP10.

Hypoglycaemia

It is inevitable that hypoglycaemia will occasionally occur. Parents need to recognise early warning signs such as sweating, irritability or drowsiness. They should respond to these by immediately giving a sugary drink and, on recovery, some starchy foods. Glucogel (see p. 172) is another extremely useful alternative for treatment of hypoglycaemia.

Cornflour is not a suitable treatment for hypoglycaemia because it releases glucose too slowly.

Illness

During intercurrent infections, the frequent supply of glucose must be maintained to prevent hypoglycaemia and lactic acidosis. Parents need to be aware of the different stages of metabolic decompensation from mild to more serious symptoms and the action needed [13]. At least the basal glucose requirement must be given (Table 18.1) and an adequate intake of fluids. Often a change in dietary regimen is needed because of loss of appetite. During the daytime, 2-hourly glucose polymer drinks or continuous tube feeds of glucose polymer will often replace either the usual 2-hourly dietary regimen, or UCCS. Parents are given glucose polymer based recipes for use during illness. If the child has diarrhoea and is vomiting, an oral rehydration solution supplemented with glucose polymer to a maximum of 10% CHO is given; it is important to ensure this also provides sufficient g CHO/kg/hour for age. If the child does not tolerate the intensive glucose polymer regimen then a hospital admission for intravenous therapy becomes essential. Severe, symptomatic hypoglycaemia can develop rapidly in this situation and intravenous treatment needs to start with minimal delay. The child's usual dietary regimen can be reintroduced during the recovery period.

Monitoring the diet

This intensive 24-hour feeding regimen is extremely demanding and time consuming for parents particularly when managing the young child. It requires constant watching of the clock and great attention to detail. Families need to be given continued support and dietary advice. The dietary guidelines from the European Study on Glycogen Storage Disease Type I recommend 2–3 monthly dietary reviews for children [13].

The child's dietary regimen needs to be regularly monitored and adjusted for age and growth needs to ensure:

- Adequate provision of CHO (g CHO/kg/hour) from the overnight feed and 2-hourly daytime feeds or UCCS (check dose size and frequency of administration)
- Nutritional adequacy of vitamin and mineral intake (specifically calcium and vitamin D)

It is important to regularly check the parents' understanding of:

- Illness management and that recipes for use during illness are updated regularly for age and weight
- Treatment of hypoglycaemia

Glycogen storage disease type Ib

The dietary treatment of patients with type Ib is the same as for GSD I. However, the additional problems seen in type Ib may necessitate further dietary manipulation. Mouth ulcers are a feature of type Ib and can make oral feeding difficult and painful. Meals and snacks may need to be temporarily replaced with nutritionally complete fluid supplements and if necessary these can be given via the nasogastric tube. The author's centre has occasionally used a

pepdite based feed if the bowel has been inflamed and bleeding. The initial trial results from a new nutritional therapy in four type Ib patients using a polymeric diet supplemented with transforming growth factor beta 2 (TGF-β2), reports a reduction in bowel inflammation in two patients [43].

Glycogen storage disease type III

Glycogen storage disease type III (GSD III) is characterised by abnormal activity of the glycogen debrancher enzyme in various tissues including liver and muscle (Fig. 18.1). This enzyme has two activities: it transfers three glucose residues to a neighbouring glycogen chain and hydrolyses the branch-point directly to glucose. The debrancher enzyme can be absent in liver and muscle (GSD type IIIa) or just in liver (GSD type IIIb) or have defects in its transferase activity in liver and muscle (GSD type IIId) [2]. The production of glucose from glycogenolysis is greatly limited as a result of debrancher deficiency. However, the gluconeogenic pathway is functional for endogenous glucose production and this prevents the development of profound hypoglycaemia during fasting, although it can still occur.

Patients can present either in infancy with symptoms similar to GSD I (hepatomegaly and hypoglycaemia), or later in childhood with poor growth and hepatomegaly resulting from both glycogen and fat accumulation. Secondary metabolic disturbances include ketosis and hyperlipidaemia. However, spontaneous catch-up growth does occur during puberty [44]. Type IIIa and IIId patients can also suffer from myopathy and develop cardiomyopathy but these are mainly problems found in adults, although many children do tire easily with exercise. The outlook for those with GSD IIIb appears to be good. Bone mineral density is markedly reduced in GSD III, with type IIIa patients being much more affected than IIIb [45].

Dietary management

The main aims of dietary treatment in GSD III are to promote normal growth and prevent hypoglycaemia. Controversy surrounds which dietary therapy is best for patients. Either CHO intake can be increased to provide a continuous supply of glucose (similar to GSD I) or protein intake can be increased to rely on gluconeogenesis as the main source of glucose. A high protein diet has been recommended because patients with GSD III may have increased gluconeogenic activity associated with decreased circulating levels of the gluconeogenic substrates alanine and lactate [46–48]. This increased demand for gluconeogenesis and loss of muscle amino acids may be a contributory factor to the myopathy seen in some patients with type IIIa. Use of a high protein diet and night feed has been reported to be beneficial in improving muscle strength in patients with a myopathy [45]. However, six of seven patients studied were not on any dietary treatment and so perhaps similar improvements could have been achieved with a high CHO diet and night feed. Whole body protein turnover has been shown not to be altered in a GSD IIIa patient and consequently questions the role of a high protein diet [49].

Alternatively, provision of a regular high CHO intake using uncooked cornflour can be used to maintain normoglycaemia and reduce the need for production of glucose via gluconeogenic substrates [50–52]. Hence, this treatment may be as effective as the high protein diet. One study has compared UCCS diet with a high protein diet and shown unchanged glycaemic control, liver function tests and lipid profiles in both regimens, but better growth and reduced liver spans when using UCCS. Two of the patients with muscle involvement showed increased creatine phosphate kinase levels on UCCS diet [53]. There are no long term data to determine which diet therapy is best for patients with myopathy.

From a practical viewpoint, UCCS is certainly easier to administer, less invasive and more economical than a high protein diet and night feed and long term compliance may be easier to achieve compared with taking a high protein diet. The choice of dietary management for children with GSD III will also vary depending on the severity of the disorder. The diet needs to be individually tailored to the child's specific requirement. The author's unit uses a high CHO diet.

High CHO diet

Infants who present early with hypoglycaemia and poor fasting tolerance require a more intensive dietary regimen with increased CHO, the same as for GSD I. At night, continuous nasogastric feeding is used and regular 2-hourly feeding or UCCS (from 2 years of age) during the daytime. There is greater emphasis on the inclusion of high protein foods in the diet compared with GSD I. Children with GSD III may be able to replace nocturnal feeds with UCCS before they have stopped growing if their fasting tolerance is >6 hours. This can happen at 4–9 years. It is important to monitor carefully the energy distribution of the diet because overtreatment with too high an energy intake from CHO can cause rebound hypoglycaemia [54].

Children who present later with short stature and hepatomegaly are treated with UCCS which is given to try and improve growth rate. Symptomatic hypoglycaemia is generally not a problem for these children. Regimens (1–2 g/kg/dose) will vary depending on age, growth rate and response. In general, a dose is given before bed, sometimes one during the night and 2–3 times during the day. Children should have regular meals that contain starchy foods and protein foods, and a starchy bedtime snack is also important. Fat intake should be decreased to compensate for the increased CHO intake. Guidelines for this diet are provided in Table 18.5. Overweight and obesity is a problem for some GSD III patients.

With both the intensive dietary regimen and UCCS a high percentage of the dietary energy intake is provided as pure starch or glucose polymer. The child will therefore be at risk of vitamin and mineral deficiencies, so intakes need to be regularly checked and supplements given as required.

High protein diet

If a high protein diet is used, it is recommended that this provides 20–25% energy intake from protein, 50–55% from CHO and 20–25% from fat [46,48]. No studies of high protein diets have been reported in infants or young children. Such a high protein intake may not be tolerated or warranted in this age group. A gradual increase in protein intake with age or if there is evidence of myopathy may be more appropriate, although there is no evidence to support this protecting muscle function.

Similar to the high CHO diet, the high protein diet needs to be individualised according to the

Table 18.5 High starch, normal protein, low fat diet or high protein, normal starch, low fat diet for glycogen storage disease type III.

Carbohydrate foods (starch and sugar)
Starch foods At least one serving at three main meals and include at bedtime snack, e.g. bread, chapatti, pitta, cereal, potato, rice, pasta, fruit, plain biscuits or crackers, tea cake, muffins, scones
Sugar These foods are allowed but should be kept to a minimum, e.g. table sugar, sweets, cakes, ice cream, preserves

High protein, low fat foods*
Milk	Semi-skimmed or skimmed milk, milk puddings, e.g. rice, custard, semolina, fromage frais + yoghurt (low fat)
Meat	Lean red meat (<10% fat content), trim off all visible fat
Poultry	White meat in preference to dark meat
Fish	White fish instead of oily
Cheese	Low fat cheese, e.g. cottage, Edam type, half fat Cheddar, quark
Pulses	Beans, lentils, peas, sweetcorn
Eggs	Egg white in preference to yolk
Meat alternatives	Tofu, Quorn

Fats
High fat foods should be used sparingly, e.g. butter, margarine, vegetable oil, animal fats, cream (double, whipping, single), imitation cream, mayonnaise, salad dressings
Avoid fried or roasted foods. Spread butter or margarine thinly on bread

Snack foods
Most children choose high fat or sugary snack foods, e.g. crisps, nuts, sweets, chocolate
Low fat, high protein or high carbohydrate snack foods should be used instead, e.g. yoghurt, fromage frais, crackers and cheese, glass of milk for high protein diet or sandwich, plain biscuits, crumpet, fruit for high starch diet

Number of servings depends on diet:
High protein diet for GSD III – at least one serving of high protein, low fat foods at three main meals and bedtime snack. Generous intakes of milk or high protein drinks should also be given.
High starch diet for GSD III – one serving of high protein, low fat foods at two meals. Include milk (or milky foods) in the daily diet.

child's clinical symptoms. The more intensive regimen, as described for GSD I, but with greater emphasis on protein intake, is required for infants or young children who have a poor fasting tolerance. Additional protein powders, such as Vitapro, could be added to the infant formula or cow's milk if essential. High protein foods at meals and snack times should be encouraged.

Children with milder disorders, who rarely experience hypoglycaemia, need regular meals and snacks (including a bedtime snack) that provide high protein and starchy foods and are limited in fat. Practical guidelines for this are given in Table 18.5. Children who have a good appetite and enjoy milk may possibly achieve a sufficiently high protein intake from protein rich foods, but protein supplements are likely to be necessary. A variety of high protein supplements are available. Protein powders, such as Vitapro, are versatile and can be fairly easily incorporated into drinks or food. Most high protein drinks or dessert supplements are often too high in energy intake to be very useful. An overnight tube feed may not always be needed. It may be sufficient just to provide a high protein, starchy bedtime snack or a dose of UCCS.

Alcohol

Adolescents and adults must be made aware that alcohol is a potent inhibitor of gluconeogenesis and even quite moderate amounts may reduce glucose production. Alcohol intake should be limited and must always be taken in combination with food [55].

Illness

Children with GSD III are at risk of hypoglycaemia and therefore during illness a frequent supply of glucose must be maintained. The guidelines given for management of intercurrent illness in GSD I can also be used for patients with GSD type III (see p. 396).

Glycogen storage disease type II

GSD II is a generalised lysosomal storage disorder caused by deficiency of acid maltase (alpha 1–4 glucosidase) (Fig. 18.1). Glycogen accumulates in the lysosomes which damages muscle cells and impairs muscle function. The infantile onset form (Pompe's disease) is associated with poor prognosis and early death resulting from cardiorespiratory failure. The later onset form is less severe and progresses more slowly. It is generally characterised by a slowly progressive muscle weakness and respiratory insufficiency. This form can present any time from childhood through adulthood. Life expectancy varies but death generally occurs from respiratory failure. At present there is no effective treatment for any form of GSD II although trials of enzyme replacement therapy are currently taking place in both infantile and later onset forms. Myozyme (Genzyme, Oxford) was approved in 2006 for long term enzyme replacement therapy in patients with a confirmed diagnosis of Pompe's disease.

Dietary treatments have been reported to delay progression in the later onset forms. A high protein diet providing 25% dietary energy from protein was reported to improve muscle strength by reducing protein catabolism, and hence delay the downward course of the childhood form [56,57]. Others have reported that not all patients benefited from this diet [58]. The long term value of this diet is not proven. L-alanine therapy has been reported to reduce protein degradation in late onset GSD II [59]. Two separate case reports of longer term use of L-alanine in clinical practice reported no functional improvement in an adult [60] but some functional benefits in a child [61].

Nutritional support with tube feeding is usually necessary in the infantile form because of severe muscle weakness and respiratory insufficiency. Later onset forms may also require nutritional support for the same reasons.

The phosphorylase system

Deficiencies of the phosphorylase system (Fig. 18.1), of which X-linked phosphorylase b-kinase is most prevalent, have similar symptomatology to, but are much milder than, GSD III [2]. In phosphorylase disorders glycogen degradation is reduced but gluconeogenesis is functional for endogenous glucose production. Children present with hepatomegaly and growth retardation but a late growth spurt and complete catch-up in final height does occur [62–64]. Hypoglycaemia is generally mild and usually only occurs after prolonged fasting or infection [14]. Most adults will be entirely asymptomatic with a normal life expectancy.

Many patients do not require specific dietary treatment. Nevertheless, general dietary advice on provision of increased intakes of protein and starch and avoidance of prolonged fasts, particularly during illness, would be appropriate. To reduce the period of overnight fasting a late night bedtime snack rich in protein and starch should be given. However, for some patients more aggressive treatment with UCCS (see p. 395), or even a more intensive regimen as in GSD I, may be necessary both to prevent low blood glucose levels and improve growth. Because alcohol is a potent inhibitor of gluconeogenesis, it is recommended that these patients only drink in moderation and preferably in combination with food [55].

Disorders of Galactose Metabolism

Anita MacDonald

There are three autosomal recessive disorders of galactose metabolism: deficiencies of the enzymes: (i) galactokinase; (ii) galactose-1-phosphate uridyl transferase (GALT); and (iii) uridine diphosphate galactose-4-epimerase (GALE) which result in the inability to metabolise the monosaccharide galactose (Fig. 18.2).

Galactosaemia

Classical galactosaemia is the most severe and common of these disorders with an incidence of 1 in 45 000 in the UK [65]. It is particularly common in the travelling population of the Republic of Ireland where incidence is estimated to be 1 in 480 [66]. Over 180 different mutations have been described worldwide and there is some genotype–phenotype correlation. The most common mutation in Europe and North America is Q188R [67,68]. Homozygosity for the Q188R mutation results in substantial or complete loss of GALT activity and is associated with a relatively poor cognitive outcome [68]. Several partial forms of

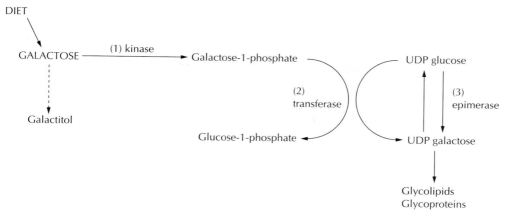

Figure 18.2 Pathways of galactose metabolism. 1 Galactokinase. 2 Galactose-1-phosphate uridyl transferase. 3 Uridine diphosphate (UDP) galactose-4-epimerase.

transferase deficiency have been reported of which Duarte is the best known [69]. These are all associated with some residual enzyme activity and a relatively good long term outcome.

Galactosaemia is caused by a deficiency of the GALT enzyme which catalyses the conversion of galactose-1-phosphate to glucose-1-phosphate and uridine diphosphate galactose (UDP-galactose) (Fig. 18.2). Direct biochemical consequences of GALT deficiency include accumulation of galactose-1-phosphate, which in turn is metabolised to galactitol and galactonate, both of which accumulate in abnormal quantities in tissues [70]. Galactitol is an osmotically active compound that causes cataracts by increasing the water content of the lens [71]. Galactonate is believed to have a role in acute hepatic and renal toxicity.

Classical galactosaemia presents in the neonatal period with life-threatening illness after galactose is introduced in the diet. Symptoms and signs include poor feeding, vomiting and diarrhoea, weight loss, jaundice, hypotonia, cataracts, hepatomegaly and encephalopathy [72]. Abnormal findings include abnormal liver function tests, abnormal clotting, hypoglycaemia, raised plasma amino acids and renal tubular dysfunction [73]. Rarely, patients may present after the newborn period.

Early diagnosis and treatment is essential. Rapid improvement occurs on stopping lactose containing feeds and a life-long lactose free diet is recommended to prevent any recurrence of severe toxicity. Normal growth usually occurs although decreased height z scores compared to mid-parental target height has been described [74]. Bone mineral density may be decreased in both sexes [75,76].

Even with early diagnosis and excellent dietary treatment, neuropsychological development is significantly impaired [77,78]. In most studies of cognitive development in older children and adults, mean IQ for patients has been in the range of 70–90, although normal and above average intelligence in individual patients has been described [69,79,80]. IQ levels may fall during childhood, although no consistent decline has been demonstrated in patients who have been tested repeatedly with the same IQ test [80].

Speech and language defects, particularly delayed vocabulary and verbal dyspraxia, are common [81,82]. Ataxia and intention tremor may occur in older children and adults. Interpersonal problems and bullying have been documented in children and older patients [83]. Adults may have shy and timid personalities being tense, over-anxious or over-sensitive with poor self-image. Ovarian dysfunction with hypergonadotrophic hypogonadism occurs in most girls [72,84,85]. Most women develop primary or secondary amenorrhoea [86] and premature menopause usually occurs in the third decade [69]. A few successful pregnancies have been reported [87,88]. Pubertal development and fertility are normal in boys.

Endogenous production of galactose

Endogenous galactose production has been suggested to be a major cause of late complications [89]. It is now known that significant amounts of endogenous galactose are formed in patients with galactosaemia with release rates being several-fold higher in infants than in adults [90]. It is estimated that adults produce approximately 13 mg/kg body weight/day compared with approximately 41 mg/kg body weight/day in newborns [91].

Diagnosis of galactosaemia

Galactosaemia is diagnosed by the Beutler test (a fluorescent spot test for galactose-1-phosphate uridyl transferase activity); a red blood cell galactose-1-phosphate uridyl transferase assay; red blood cell galactose-1-phosphate concentrations; and DNA analysis [65]. Neonatal screening is not routine in England and Wales, although it is well established in many other European countries. With national screening occurring at days 5–8, it is possible that the results of the assay would be available only after the onset of clinical illness. However, in Germany, newborn screening performed at day 5 is associated with reduced acute morbidity and mortality [92].

Biochemical monitoring of galactosaemia

Measurement of red cell galactose-1-phosphate has been widely used to monitor dietary compliance. This is high at diagnosis and falls progressively after the introduction of dietary treatment but it may still take up to 1 year to fall to an acceptable level. Levels do not decrease to the concentrations found in normal healthy individuals. The units used to express galactose-1-phosphate concentrations vary between different laboratories, usually according to methodology [65]. The upper limit of the acceptable range quoted in different units is as follows:

- 150 µmol/L red cells
- 50 µg/mL packed red cells
- 5 mg/100 mL red blood cells
- 0.5 µmol/g haemoglobin.

Table 18.6 Suggested frequency of measuring galactose-1-phosphate concentrations [64].

Age	Frequency of measuring galactose-1-phosphate concentrations
0–1 year	Every 3 months
1–14 years	Every 6 months
Over 14 years	Annually

Galactose-1-phosphate concentrations do not vary greatly in individual patients providing dietary compliance is reasonable so frequent monitoring is not indicated [65] (Table 18.6). No correlation with long term clinical outcome has been shown [65]. Urinary galactitol is also being investigated as a less invasive way of monitoring diet.

Dietary management

Life-long dietary restriction of galactose is the only effective treatment for galactosaemia. Even though there is no doubt that lactose must be avoided, a diet free of dairy products still contains some galactose from plant and animal sources. Free and bound galactose is found in many plant foods. Although safe amounts of dietary galactose have not been defined [93] it would be difficult to have a totally galactose free diet [94]. There is little evidence to suggest that avoiding galactose from plant and non-milk animal sources is beneficial; some UK centres have 25 years of experience avoiding milk and milk products only in a galactosaemia diet [95] without obvious adverse consequences. Therefore, in the UK only a lactose free diet is advocated and galactose from other sources is disregarded [65], but international practices vary [96].

Sources of galactose

Lactose
The main source of galactose in the diet is the disaccharide lactose (milk sugar) consisting of one glucose monomer and one galactose monomer. Once lactose is hydrolysed in the gut to form galactose and glucose, galactose is transported across the epithelial cells and enters the portal vein to undergo further metabolism in the liver. To

Table 18.7 Lactose and galactose content of foods [96].

Foog	Lactose content (g/100 mL or g/100 g)	Galactose content (g/100 mL or g/100 g)
Skimmed milk	4.4	2.2
Whole milk	4.5	2.3
Single cream	2.2	1.1
Fruit low fat yoghurt	4.4	2.2
Butter	0.6	0.3
Milk chocolate	10.1	5.1
Ice cream: dairy	5.2	2.6

exclude lactose from the diet all milk, milk products and manufactured foods containing milk need to be avoided. Lactose and galactose in milk based foods are shown in Table 18.7. Constituents of milk are also likely to be found in foods such as biscuits, some sweets and tinned and processed meats (Table 18.8). Many spreads (including reduced fat) now include milk components to improve their flavour. The lactose content of whey derivatives such as whey powder is high, comprising 70% of total solids. In contrast, the lactose content of casein is low, with the Casein and Caseinates Regulations (2002) stating the maximum anhydrous lactose content of casein should not exceed 1% by weight [97]. Butter oil and ghee contain only minimal lactose, but it is still recommended that these are avoided.

Table 18.8 Milk, milk products and milk derivatives.

Milk and milk products
Cow's milk, goat's milk, sheep's milk
Cheese, cream, butter
Ice cream, yoghurt, fromage frais, crème fraiche
Chocolate

Milk derivatives
Skimmed milk powder, milk solids, milk protein, non-fat milk solids, separate milk solids
Whey, hydrolysed whey protein, margarine or shortening containing whey, whey syrup sweetener, casein, hydrolysed casein, sodium caseinate, calcium caseinate
Lactose
Buttermilk, butterfat, butter oil, milk fat, animal fat (may be butter), ghee, artificial cream
Cheese powder

Lactose as a filler may be used in:
Flavourings
Table-top or tablet artificial sweeteners

Table 18.9 Non-milk derivatives.

Lactic acid E270, sodium lactate E325, potassium lactate E325, calcium lactate E327

Lactitol, lactalbumin, lactoglobulin, lycasin, stearoyl lactylates, glucona-delta-lactone, monosodium glutamate, cocoa butter, non-dairy cream

NB: Lactitol does not contain lactose but may contain some galactose and should be avoided.

Lactose powder is also added to a diverse range of food products including bakery goods, confectionery, dry mixes, dried vegetables and crisps. It is one-sixth as sweet as table sugar, so it is added to food as a slightly sweet source of carbohydrate. It is often added to prepared foods to prevent caking or as a coating. It may be used in bakery goods for enhancing browning and reducing sweetness. It is commonly used as a filler and flowing agent in seasoning mixes for foods such as instant pot noodles. It may also act as a carrier for flavours and seasonings. It may be added to some artificial table-top or tablet sweeteners. Non-milk derivatives that may be added to food products are shown in Table 18.9; these do not need to be avoided with the exception of lactitol. This is a polyol made from galactose. Some residual galactose is left after fermentation in the gut so is unsuitable in galactosaemia.

Galactosides
The α-galactosides are part of the oligosaccharides (raffinose, stachyose and verbacose) which are a potential source of galactose. Studies investigating the effects of galactosides in galactosaemia are few, limited in subject numbers, short term and inconclusive. Galactosides are found in foods such as peas, beans, lentils, cocoa and nuts (Table 18.10). There is also evidence that raffinose and stachyose are found in many cereals such as wheat, oat flour and vegetables [98]. The α-galactosidase linkage in oligosaccharides is not hydrolysable by the human small intestinal mucosa *in vitro* or *in vivo* [99]. Instead, the galactosides are rapidly degraded and fermented by the caecal microflora to produce volatile short chain fatty acids. However, this may not be the case when the small intestine is colonised by bacteria capable of releasing galactose during episodes of diarrhoea [100]. Galactoside avoidance is not advocated in the UK galactosaemia diet.

Table 18.10 Dietary sources of galactosides and nucleoproteins.

Galactosides	Peas, beans, lentils, legumes, chick peas, dhals, grams, spinach Texturised vegetable protein Soya (other than soya protein isolates), soya beans, soya flour Cocoa, chocolate Nuts
Nucleoproteins	Offal – liver, kidney, brain, sweetbreads, heart Eggs

Table 18.11 Free galactose in fruit and vegetables (mg/100 g).

Food	UK unpublished*	USA [103,104]
Tomato	10	23
Grape	<10	2.9
Cucumber	20	4.0
Banana	10	9.2
Water melon		14.7
Kiwi fruit		10

* Data analysed by UK Galactosaemia Support Group.

Galactose storage organs

Galactocerebrosides and gangliosides are found in offal [69]. There was a recommendation in 1963 [101] that offal such as liver, brain and pancreas (sweetbreads) should be avoided in galactosaemia. There appears to be limited information on the galactose content of these foods. Their specific effect has not been studied in galactosaemia, but they are not avoided in the UK diet.

Free and bound galactose

Free galactose has been reported in many fruits, vegetables and legumes [94]. Free galactose content may vary from <0.1 mg/100 g to 35 mg/100 g [102]. In addition, bound galactose is present in many plant foods and β-1-4 linked galactosyl residues in chloroplast membranes of green plant tissue (galactolipids). Galactose, in the form of β-1-4 linkage and as monogalactosydiacylglycerol, may be released by galactosidases in animal and plant tissues [94]. There has been a reluctance to restrict high galactose containing fruits and vegetables from the diet of children with galactosaemia and there is little scientific evidence to support the benefit of this. In one study, one patient was given a synthetic diet containing <8 mg/day of galactose and then challenged with 200 mg/day galactose for 3 weeks. This had little effect on metabolite concentrations and it was suggested that endogenous galactose production is primarily responsible for the elevated galactose metabolites in patients on lactose free diets [105]. Avoidance of free and bound galactose in fruit and vegetables is not advocated in the UK galactosaemia diet (Table 18.11).

Lactose free diet

There are several practical issues in managing a lactose free diet in galactosaemia (Table 18.12) including choice of milk substitute, calcium supplementation, use of hard mature cheese, interpretation of food labels and cross-contamination with milk in the manufacturing process. It is important to maintain a satisfactory intake of energy and all nutrients to ensure optimum nutrition and normal growth. Annual dietary assessments are recommended to monitor calcium intake in particular. Parents and carers should be encouraged to use a wide range of non-milk containing alternative foods (e.g. soya spread, soya yoghurt, soya cheese and carob chocolate) to help enhance energy and calcium intake. Labels of carob chocolate products need to be carefully checked as sometimes milk derivatives are added. The UK Galactosaemia Support Group produces a wide range of materials for parents and carers (developed by dietitians) including a biannual list of manufactured lactose free foods; a low lactose diet guide; picture books of lactose free foods which are particularly useful for carers who cannot read or speak English; and a glossary of food ingredient definitions.

Milk substitutes

Breast feeding and cow's milk based infant formulas are contraindicated for the infant with galactosaemia because they contain lactose. In the absence of milk it is important that infants and young children are provided with a nutritionally adequate formula. Several factors influence the choice of milk substitute including nutritional composition, evidence of satisfactory growth, nutritional status of the child, safety, palatability

Table 18.12 Lactose free diet. Lactose free foods are listed. Manufactured foods that contain or could contain milk or milk derivatives are shown in italics.

Milk, milk products and milk derivatives
These should all be avoided – refer to Table 18.8

Soya milk and soya products
Infant soya formula
Liquid soya milk – calcium enriched (not before 1 year of age)
Soya cheese, soya yoghurt, soya desserts

Fats and oils
Milk free margarine
Many margarines and low fat spreads contain milk – refer to GSG list
Vegetable oils
Lard, dripping, suet

Meat and fish
Meat, poultry, fish, shellfish (fresh or frozen)
Ham and bacon (lactose may occasionally be used as a flavour enhancer – see ingredient label)
Fish fingers
Quorn
Tofu
Many meat or fish products such as sausages, burgers, pies, breaded or battered foods or in sauce may not be suitable – refer to GSG list

Eggs

Cereal, flour, pasta
All grains; wheat, oats, corn, rice, barley, maize, sago, rye, tapioca
Pasta, spaghetti, macaroni, dried noodles, couscous
Tinned pasta such as spaghetti hoops may contain cheese, refer to GSG list
Flour; plain, self-raising, cornflour, rice flour, soya flour
Custard power, semolina
Carob

Breakfast cereals
Most are suitable, e.g. Weetabix, Corn Flakes, Rice Krispies
A few cereals may contain chocolate or milk derivatives – refer to GSG list

Bread and yeast products
Most bread is suitable
Milk bread and nan bread contain milk – avoid
Pitta, chapatti
Muffins, crumpets, teacakes may not be suitable – refer to GSG list

Cakes, biscuits, crackers
Many cakes, biscuits and crackers contain milk – refer to GSG list

Desserts
Sorbet, jelly, soya desserts, soya ice cream, soya yoghurt
Homemade soya milk custard or rice pudding
Most desserts contain milk in some form – refer to GSG list

Fruit
All fresh, frozen, tinned or dried fruit

Vegetables
All fresh, frozen, tinned or dried vegetables
Most dried and tinned pulses, e.g. red kidney beans, chick peas, lentils
Baked beans and ready made vegetable dishes such as coleslaw, potato salad – refer to GSG list

Savoury snacks
Plain crisps, poppodom
Nuts, peanut butter
Flavoured crisps may not be suitable because they contain cheese or lactose as a filler in the flavouring, low fat crisps may contain lactose – refer to GSG list for suitable flavoured crisps
Dry roasted nuts and popcorn – refer to GSG list

Seasonings, gravies
Pepper, salt, pure spices and herbs, mustard
Marmite, Bovril, Bisto
Gravy granules and stock cubes – refer to GSG list

Soups
Tinned, packet, carton soups – refer to GSG list

Sugar, sweet spreads
Sugar, glucose, fructose
Pure artificial sweeteners
Powdered and tablet artificial sweeteners may contain lactose – refer to GSG list
Jam, syrup, honey, marmalade, lemon curd

Confectionery
Boiled sweets, most mints, marshmallow, plain fruit lollies, chewing gum
Milk chocolate, most plain chocolate, butterscotch and fudge, toffee
Plain or carob chocolate – refer to GSG list

Drinks
Soya milk
Milk shake syrup or powders
Fizzy drinks, squash, fruit juice
Cocoa, tea, coffee
Drinking chocolate – refer to GSG list
Instant milk drinks and malted milk drinks – avoid

Miscellaneous – used in baking
Baking powder, yeast, gelatine, marzipan

Flavourings
Lactose may be used as a 'carrier' for flavourings particularly in crisps and similar snack foods. In sweets lactose is rarely used for this purpose except in some dairy flavours

Eating out
The GSG list provides information on lactose free foods for some popular restaurants

GSG, Galactosaemia Support Group.

of the product, ease of preparation, cost and availability.

Soya infant formula

Soya infant formulas (e.g. Farley's Soya Formula, InfaSoy, Wysoy) are lactose free and oligosaccharides are removed during manufacture (see nutritional profile Table 7.5). Despite the recommendation by the UK Department of Health [106] that soya based infant formula should not be used as the first choice formula for the management of infants with galactosaemia and galactokinase deficiency because of concerns regarding its phytoestrogen content [107] (see p. 95), it is believed by many working in galactosaemia that there is little other appropriate choice. Soya infant formula is therefore still widely used in infants with galactosaemia and it is also advocated by the European Society for Paediatric Gastroenterology, Hepatology and Nutrition (ESPGHAN) for infants with galactosaemia [108].

Low lactose and protein hydrolysate formula

Other alternative ACBS listed infant formulas include both low lactose formulas and protein hydrolysate formulas (Table 18.13). All formulas based on cow's milk protein will undoubtedly contain some residual lactose and the amounts vary between formulas. Manufacturers of casein based hydrolysates and some low lactose formulas declare their lactose content at 10 mg/100 mL or below. Therefore, a 5-kg infant taking 200 mL/kg of formula would have approximately 10 mg/kg/day of galactose from this source. Furthermore, it is estimated that endogenous galactose production is likely to be at its highest peak in infancy (calculated at 41 mg/kg body weight/day) [91]. The 5-kg infant taking a low lactose formula would receive 24% extra galactose from formula which is not insignificant.

Whey hydrolysate formulas are likely to contain a higher concentration of residual lactose and Pepti-Junior, for example, is likely to contain 100 mg/100 mL of lactose (personal communication, Cow & Gate, Nutrica). Pepti whey hydrolysate formula is only partly reduced in lactose and contains 2.6 g/100 mL. These formulas are unsuitable for infants with galactosaemia.

Formulas based on hydrolysed meat and soya should be free of lactose (see nutritional profile Table 7.7).

Table 18.13 Low lactose formulas and protein hydrolysate formulas.

Infant formula	Protein source	Lactose content (per 100 mL)
Low lactose		
Enfamil Lactofree (Mead Johnson)	Milk protein (isolate)	<7 mg
Galactomin 17 (SHS International)	Caseinate	<10 mg
SMA LF (SMA Nutrition)	60% whey, 40% casein	<10 mg
Casein hydrolysate		
Nutramigen 1 and 2 (Mead Johnson)	Enzymatically hydrolysed casein	<5 mg
Pregestimil (Mead Johnson)	Enzymatically hydrolysed casein	<5 mg
Whey hydrolysate		
Pepti-Junior (Cow & Gate)	Hydrolysed whey protein	0.1 g
Meat and soya hydrolysate		
Pepdite (SHS International)	Hydrolysed pork and soya amino acids	Nil
Prejomin (Milupa)	Porcine collagen, soya hydrolysate	Nil

Amino acid formula

This is a possible alternative suitable lactose free formula. There has been one recent successful case report of an infant whose erythrocyte galactose-1-phosphate levels decreased rapidly to within the treatment ranges on an infant elemental formula [109]. The main concern with using such a formula is the possibility that infants at a later stage would not establish a taste for useful soya based foods like yoghurt or soya cheese. However, the use of infant amino acid formula is worthy of further study in galactosaemia.

Unsafe milks

Animal milk (e.g. goat's and sheep's) contain lactose as their carbohydrate source and are unsuitable. Low lactose milks (e.g. Lactolite, Aral Foods), contain an added enzyme that may lower the lactose content by 95%. However, these milk formulas still contain significant quantities of lactose and are contraindicated in galactosaemia. Lactase enzymes drops that reduce the lactose content of milk are also unsuitable.

Inclusion of hard mature cheese

A small number of hard mature cheeses are allowed in the diet in galactoseamia. The basis of cheesemaking relies on the fermentation of lactose by bacteria. Lactose entrapped in the curd is trans-converted to lactic acid and other acids by bacterial action during curing. The lactose may be altered by the strain of bacteria used to treat cheese. Generally, the longer the cheese has matured the lower the lactose content.

Soft and processed cheeses are higher in lactose. Non-fat milk and cheese whey may be added to processed cheese products so this will increase their lactose content compared to natural cheese. Unfortunately, the analysis of lactose and galactose content are few and existing information is inconsistent and variable.

In European countries other than the UK, the most common hard cheeses permitted are Emmental, Gruyere and Tilsiter cheese. In the UK, Emmental, Gruyere and mature Cheddar cheese (matured for over 12 months) have been allowed since 2001. UK analysis indicated no detectable lactose or galactose in Emmental or Gruyere. West Country Farmhouse Mature Cheddar cheese had a median lactose content of <2.8 mg/100 g and no galactose [110]. Only the West Country Farmhouse Association's mature and very Mature Cheddar cheeses have been tested for their lactose and galactose content. Mature Cheddar cheese should only be used if it has the PDO (Protected Designation of Origin) seal on the label. Information regarding the availability of the suitable West Country Farmhouse mature Cheddar cheese and the PDO seal is available from www.farmhousecheesemakers.com.

Interpreting food labels

New European ingredient listing rules [111,112] applied across the EC are providing more comprehensive information about prepackaged foods that contain intentional milk, milk derivatives or lactose. The new law requires that milk and all milk containing derivatives have to be clearly identified on food ingredient labelling. Milk or lactose in carry-over additives or flavourings and any other substances used as processing aids are identified. Unfortunately, this only applies to prepackaged foods (e.g. canned and packet foods and alcoholic drinks), so foods sold loose (non-prepackaged), foods served in restaurants and certain fancy confectionery products are exempt.

The new rules remove the 25% compound ingredient listing exemption (or '25% rule') under which individual ingredients making up a compound ingredient in a food did not have to be listed if the compound ingredient made up less than 25% of the finished product. Therefore, under the new food labelling legislation all hidden milk components should be identified on food package ingredient lists.

Some manufacturers have voluntarily extended their information on food allergens and provide an additional 'contains' allergen box on food packaging (e.g. product contains 'milk' or 'gluten'). Although this may be helpful, any information should still be cross-referenced with the ingredients list in case of error.

The new law is undoubtedly helping families with galactosaemia to expand the range of foods eaten. However, guidance in identifying the milk source on the label is still required. They require particular help when dining in restaurants and popular fast food outlets and when eating foods that are not prepackaged.

Cross-contamination of manufactured foods with milk

Both milk free and milk containing foods may be manufactured in the same plant or even using the same machinery. Cross-contamination with milk is always possible and such foods may be voluntarily labelled 'may contain milk or milk products'. It is likely the quantity of milk that such a product would contain if cross-contaminated would be minute. The Galactosaemia Support Group Medical Advisory Panel has decided not to exclude foods that carry a risk of cross-contamination with milk only.

Calcium supplementation

Decreased bone mineralisation in both female

patients as a result of ovarian insufficiency and treated prepubertal children (boys and girls) with galactosaemia has been reported [74,113]. Decreased bone mineral density in childhood may increase the risk of osteoporosis and fractures in adult life. Optimum mineral intakes and vitamin D are important for bone metabolism. Vitamin K may also have an important role and supplements may be advocated in the future [114]. It acts as a co-factor in the post-translational carboxylation of osteocalcin which has a regulatory role in the mineralisation and remodelling of bone [75].

Reference nutrient intakes for calcium vary between 325 and 1000 mg/day in children [115]. Soya infant formula normally provides adequate calcium in the first 1–2 years if the child will take it, but it may be necessary to change to a calcium enriched soya drink or to give calcium supplements after the age of 1 year. Low calcium intake is commonly reported in patients with galactosaemia [113,116,117] and in other children on milk free diets [118,119]. Unfortunately, compliance with calcium supplementation is poor. Many are bulky and acceptability and compliance are major problems. There are few calcium preparations specifically designed for young children (Table 18.14).

Factors that need to be considered when choosing the supplement include its physical properties such as solubility, presentation, concomitant medications, adverse effects and palatability. Dose, timing, administration with food and vitamin D intake may all affect bioavailability.

Lactose in medications

Lactose is an established excipient with properties that make it ideal as a tablet filler or binder and is found in many medications. For most medications the amount of lactose is unlikely to be significant, particularly if the medication is being used for a short time period [69]. However, it is still important to check the quantity of lactose; for example, the common laxative lactulose contains high quantities of lactose (<7.5 g/100 mL) and galactose (<11 g/100 mL) and is contraindicated in galactosaemia [120].

Alcohol

There is no evidence to support the hypothesis that

Table 18.14 Suitable calcium preparations in galactosaemia.

Preparation	Available calcium
Sandocal 400 (Novartis) effervescent (calcium lactate gluconate, calcium carbonate) effervescent tablet	400 mg
Sandocal 1000 (Novartis) effervescent (calcium lactate gluconate, calcium carbonate) effervescent tablet	1000 mg
Adcal (Strakan) calcium carbonate chewable tablet	600 mg
Calcium gluconate (non-proprietary) effervescent tablet	89 mg
Calcichew (Shire) calcium carbonate chewable tablet	500 mg

NB Calcium Sandoz liquid (Alliance) is based on calcium lactobionate. It is contraindicated in galactosaemia because β-galactosidase in human intestinal mucosa hydrolyses lactobionate freeing galactose [93]. The amount of galactose released is unknown.

alcohol is more harmful to patients with galactosaemia than to the normal population [65].

Long term dietary treatment

Although a life-long lactose free diet is still recommended for galactosaemia there is debate about how strict the dietary treatment should be in teenage years and beyond. There have been at least two case reports of treated patients who discontinued diet at the age of 3 years (both with Q188R homozygosity and severely reduced erythrocyte galactose-1-phosphate uridyl transferase activity) with good long term outcome [121,122]. Bosch *et al.* [123] increased oral galactose intake to 600 mg/day for 6 weeks in three adolescent patients homozygous for the Q188R mutation. No significant changes were observed in clinical observations, ophthalmic examination and laboratory measurements of dietary control. Historically, even the early dietetic textbooks suggested that some relaxation could be considered in school age children as rigid dietary control did not appear to have a role in intellectual development [124]. However, it is important that the advice to patients and carers remains that a strict lactose free diet is followed until convincing evidence to either support or negate the need for life-long diet is available.

Pregnancy in women with classical galactosaemia

Apart from taking a nutritionally adequate lactose free diet, no additional treatment is required during pregnancy for women with classical galactosaemia. Normal healthy infant outcome is reported in the few pregnancies documented. Maternal galactose-1-phosphate concentrations increase towards the end of pregnancy and after delivery which may be related to endogenous breakdown and lactation. There are no reports of continued breast feeding in mothers with galactosaemia [69].

Galactokinase deficiency

Galactokinase deficiency is an autosomal disorder which results in the formation of nuclear cataracts. Galactokinase normally catalyses the phosphorylation of galactose with adenosine triphosphate (ATP) to form galactose-1-phosphate (Fig. 18.2). Consequently, most of the ingested galactose is excreted as such or as its reduced metabolite, galactitol, resulting in osmotic damage to the lens fibre. Hepatic and renal damage and neurological disturbances do not occur. Bosch *et al.* [125] reviewed the clinical features of galactokinase deficiency in 55 patients from 25 publications. Cataracts were reported in most patients. Clinical abnormalities other than cataract were reported in 15 of 43 (35%) cases on which information was available. However, all symptoms were reported infrequently and were more likely to be coincidental. Pseudotumour cerebri occurs by the same mechanism as for cataract formation. It has been suggested that this may be a rare complication of galactokinase deficiency. Growth in galactokinase deficiency is normal.

Treatment is a lactose free diet. When the diagnosis is quickly made and dietary management is prompt (i.e. during the first 2–3 weeks of life) cataracts can clear. When treatment is late and cataracts are dense they will not clear completely (or at all) and must be removed surgically.

The incidence of galactokinase deficiency is low and cannot be assessed with any accuracy [69]. In most parts of Europe, in the USA and in Japan, birth incidence is in the order of 1 in 150 000 to 1 million. It is higher in the Balkan countries, the former Yugoslavia, Rumania and Bulgaria, where it is common in travelling or Romany families [126].

UPD-galactose 4-epimerase deficiency

This is a very rare autosomal disorder and the prevalence varies amongst different ethnic groups. Epimerase deficiency galactosaemia results from the impairment of UDP-galactose-4-epimerase (GALE), the third enzyme in the Leloir pathway of galactose metabolism (Fig. 18.2). The majority of patients have a clinically benign condition (peripheral epimerase deficiency) with enzyme impairment principally in their erythrocytes [69]. Their growth and development is normal. A generalised, rare, severe form has also been described with enzyme impairment affecting a range of tissues. Isolated cases of clinically and/or biochemically intermediate cases of epimerase deficiency have also been reported [127].

The severe form of GALE deficiency resembles classical galactosaemia [72]. This form requires a galactose restricted diet. Epimerase forms UDP-galactose from UDP-glucose. Theoretically, a complete absence of galactose from the diet and lack of UDP-galactose formation would result in an inability to form glycoproteins and glycolipids. However, a narrow balance between dietary galactose requirements for biosynthesis (galactosylated compounds) and excess causing accumulation of galactose-1-phosphate should be aimed for [72].

It has been suggested that glycoprotein and glycolipid production may be sufficient, possibly because of some residual epimerase activity in the liver [128] so it may be unnecessary to give dietary galactose.

Disorders of Fructose Metabolism

Marjorie Dixon

Hereditary fructose intolerance

Hereditary fructose intolerance (HFI) is caused by a deficiency of the enzyme fructose-1,6-bisphosphate aldolase (aldolase B) in the liver, kidney and small intestine. This enzyme is an essential step in the metabolism of fructose (Fig. 18.3).

Symptoms will only develop when the child is given fructose. In the UK, exposure to fructose is uncommon prior to weaning as breast milk and infant formula are fructose free. During the introduction of solid food, sources of fructose become abundant from fruits, vegetables and commercial baby foods. While the clinical picture and dietary history should enable a diagnosis of HFI to be made in older patients, the diagnosis can be more difficult in young patients. However, even in older patients symptoms may be minimal because they develop an aversion to sweet tasting foods and self select a low fructose diet. Nevertheless, these children may still be given fructose from unexpected sources such as medicines.

In the infant and young child the main clinical symptoms include poor feeding, vomiting, abdominal distention and failure to thrive. Hypoglycaemia may develop after exposure to fructose. Continued exposure to fructose causes severe liver failure, proximal renal tubular dysfunction and specific metabolic disturbances [129]. None of these problems are specific and the key to diagnosis is a very accurate clinical and dietary history.

The main treatment of HFI is strict exclusion of fructose, sucrose and sorbitol from the diet. This results in a rapid improvement of symptoms. The long term prognosis is good although hepatomegaly and fatty changes in the liver may persist [130]. The diet needs to be continued for life without relaxation as even small amounts of fructose have been shown to be harmful [131]. Abdominal pain and vomiting can occur if a child on the diet is accidentally exposed to fructose.

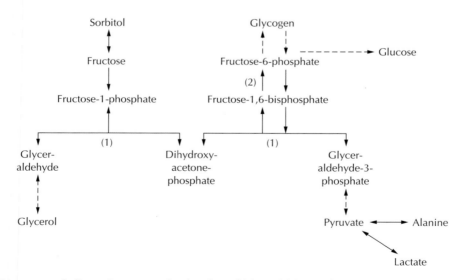

Figure 18.3 Fructose metabolism. 1 Fructose-1,6-bisphosphate aldolase (aldolase B) (hereditary fructose intolerance). 2 Fructose-1,6-bisphosphatase.

Sources of fructose

Fructose in the diet comes from fructose, sucrose and sorbitol. Fructose is absorbed by a carrier mediated process across the small intestine and then enters the liver to undergo further metabolism (Fig. 18.3). The disaccharide sucrose is cleaved in the small intestine by sucrase-isomaltase to form a molecule of both glucose and fructose. Sorbitol, a sugar alcohol, diffuses slowly across the intestinal absorptive surface with only 10–30% being absorbed. In the liver it is rapidly converted via sorbitol dehydrogenase to fructose. The trisaccharide raffinose and the tetrasaccharide stachyose are possible sources of fructose; however, it is thought unlikely that these are hydrolysed to any significant extent in the small intestine and therefore little of the fructose is absorbed. Fructans such as inulin are widespread in various plants (e.g. artichokes) [132]. Again these are not absorbed; instead they undergo bacterial fermentation in the colon.

Another potential source of fructose is from industrially manufactured polyols (polyhydric alcohols), produced by hydrogenation of selected sugars. Polyols are sugar free, low energy bulk sweeteners which are used in many foods and medicines. The most widely used are sorbitol, mannitol (derived from fructose) and malitol (which contains sorbitol). Absorption of polyols varies; most are slowly and incompletely absorbed from the intestine, and for others absorption is minimal. Nevertheless, they may remain a possible source of fructose. Oligofructose is obtained from inulin through enzymatic hydrolysis, producing a mixture of chains of fructose molecules of varying chain length (2–20 molecules). Commercial syrups of oligofructose contain small amounts of fructose and sucrose.

Minimal fructose, sucrose, sorbitol diet

The aim of dietary treatment of HFI is complete elimination of fructose, sucrose and sorbitol, but it is not possible to exclude these sugars completely (Table 18.15). In practice it is not possible to get the intake of fructose from all sources to be less than 1–2 g/day. The normal average daily intake of fructose (including contribution from sucrose) in unaffected infants has been reported as 20 g/day

Table 18.15 Minimal fructose, sucrose and sorbitol diet (<2 g/day).

Foods allowed	Foods to avoid
Sugars, sweeteners and preserves Glucose, glucose polymers, glucose syrup, dextrose, lactose, starch, maltose, maltodextrin, malt extract Saccharin, aspartame	Sugar or sucrose (cane or beet) – white, brown, caster, icing Fruit sugar, fructose, laevulose Honey, treacle, molasses Sorbitol, polyols (check suitability) Golden syrup, corn syrup, invert syrup, high fructose or isoglucose syrups, hydrogenated glucose syrup Jam, marmalade, lemon curd
Fruit Avocado, rhubarb (occasionally)	All other fruit and fruit products
Vegetables (cooked, boil and discard water) *Group 1 (<0.5 g fructose/100 g)** Celery, globe artichokes, mange tout, mushrooms, spinach, watercress Beans: haricot, mung, red kidney Dried split peas, lentils Potato: old potato, plain potato crisps, (potato waffle, potato croquette – check food label)	Beetroot, Brussels sprouts, carrots, gherkins, green beans, kohl rabi, okra, onion, parsnip, peas, pepper, plantain, shallots, spring onion, squash, sweetcorn, sweet potato, tomato, tomato purée Beans – green, French, runner Baked beans, tinned vegetables with added sugar, mayonnaise or salad cream, coleslaw Flavoured crisps

continued on p. 412

Table 18.15   *(Cont'd)*

Foods allowed	Foods to avoid
Group 2 (0.5–1.0 g fructose/100 g)* Aubergine, asparagus, beansprouts, broccoli, cabbage, cauliflower, courgette, cucumber, fennel, artichoke, leeks, lettuce, marrow, new potato, pumpkin, radish, spring greens, swede, turnip Beans: black-eye, broad, butter, soya Marrowfat peas, processed peas canned in water, chick peas	Pickles, chutney
Milk Infant formula milk, cow's milk, unsweetened evaporated milk, Original Coffeemate powder, dried milk powder Cream Cheese, plain cottage cheese Natural yoghurt	Flavoured milk, condensed milk, milk shake powders/syrups Liquid soya milk Aerosol cream Cheese with added ingredients, e.g. nuts, fruit Fruit and flavoured yoghurt, fromage frais Ice cream
Eggs Allowed	
Meat and poultry All fresh meat and poultry If processed read label to check for added sucrose, fructose or honey	Processed meats which have added sucrose, e.g. meat pastes, frankfurters, salami, paté, sausages, tinned meat Tendersweet meats, e.g. ham, Honey cured meats Ready-made meat meals – possible sources are the gravy, sauces, vegetables, breadcrumbs, batter, pastry
Meat substitutes Soya meat, tofu, Quorn	
Fish Fresh and frozen fish, shell fish, fish tinned in brine	Fish tinned in tomato sauce, fish paste, fish cakes, fish oil or water fingers Ready-made fish meals – possible sources are the sauce, vegetables, breadcrumb, batter, pastry
Flour and cereals Flour (white in preference to wholemeal), buckwheat, cornflour, custard powder, sago, semolina, tapioca, oatmeal, barley Flaky pastry, shortcrust pastry (not sweetened)	Bran, wheatgerm
Pasta and rice Spaghetti, macaroni, other pasta (white in preference to wholemeal) Noodles, egg noodles Rice (white in preference to brown)	Pasta tinned in tomato sauce Pot Noodle
Breakfast cereals Porridge, puffed wheat, Original Ready Brek, Shredded Wheat, (Kallo) puffed rice cereal	Most manufactured breakfast cereals
Bread and crackers White bread (prepacked)	Wholemeal bread, sweetened breads, e.g. malt bread, soda bread, currant bread

Table 18.15   (Cont'd)

Foods allowed	Foods to avoid
Bakers' bread – check if sugar is added to dough mixture Cream crackers, Matzo crackers, water crackers, original Ryvita (not sesame), plain rice cakes, crumpets	Savoury snack biscuits

Cakes, biscuits and pastries

Foods allowed	Foods to avoid
Home-made using permitted ingredients and sweeteners	All cakes, biscuits and pastries

Desserts

Foods allowed	Foods to avoid
Home-made using permitted ingredients, e.g. custard sweetened with glucose, choux pastry	Most desserts, e.g. jelly, meringue, mousse, gateaux, fruit pie or crumble, ice cream, yoghurts

Fats and oils

Butter, margarine, vegetable oils, lard, suet

Drinks

Foods allowed	Foods to avoid
Soda water, mineral water (without fruit flavour)	Fruit juices, vegetable juices, fruit squash, fizzy drinks, diabetic squash containing sorbitol or fructose, low calorie drinks, tonic water
Some low calorie drinks may be suitable (check the label for frutose, sucrose, sorbitol, polyols or comminuted fruits) Tea, coffee, cocoa	Drinking chocolate, malted milk drinks Instant tea mixes, coffee essence

Confectionery

Foods allowed	Foods to avoid
Unflavoured glucose tablets may be suitable	Sweets, chocolate, toffee, jelly, ice lollies, chewing gum Diabetic sweets (sweetened with fructose, sorbitol or other polyols) Glucose tablets, e.g. orange flavour Lucozade tablets

Gravies, sauces and soups

Foods allowed	Foods to avoid
Marmite, Bovril White or cheese sauce made with milk, flour, fat and cheese only	Gravy granules, stock cubes Bottled sauces and dressings, e.g. tomato ketchup, horseradish sauce, mint sauce, soy sauce Sauce mixes, e.g. sweet and sour, curry Mayonnaise, salad cream All soups (packet, tinned or fresh)

Herbs, spices, nuts and seeds

Foods allowed	Foods to avoid
Pure herbs, mustard and spices, salt, pepper Sesame seeds Pumpkin and sunflower seeds maximum of 10 g/day total	Nuts, peanut butter, marzipan

Baking products

Baking powder, bicarbonate of soda, yeast, arrowroot, food colourings, food essences, gelatine

* Total fructose content of vegetables is calculated as fructose plus $1/2$ sucrose.

NB

- Always read the label of manufactured food to check for sucrose, fructose, sorbitol or polyols (check suitability)
- Check toothpaste for sorbitol

Analysis of fructose and sucrose content of foods

1   *Cereals and Cereal Products – The Third Supplement to McCance and Widdowson's 'The Composition of Foods'* 4th edn, 1988.
2   *Milk and Milk Products and Eggs – The Fourth Supplement to McCance and Widdowson's 'The Composition of Foods'* 4th edn, 1989.
3   *Vegetables, Herbs and Spices – The Fifth Supplement to McCance and Widdowson's 'The Composition of Foods'* 4th edn, 1991.
4   *Fruit and Nuts – The First Supplement to McCance and Widdowson's 'The Composition of Foods'* 5th edn, 1992.

Publishers of above: Holland B, Unwin ID, Buss DH, The Royal Society of Chemistry and Ministry of Agriculture, Fisheries and Food, The Stationery Office.

[133]. Obviously, intakes in older children on normal diets would be much greater and could easily be of the order of 100 g/day.

Fructose is the natural sugar present in fruit, vegetables and honey. Sucrose is also found in fruit and vegetables but a much greater source is from sugar cane or beet. These are refined to produce table sugar which is used extensively in food manufacture as a sweetener and bulking agent. Sugar is a major ingredient in cakes, biscuits, desserts and soft drinks. Many other commercial foods (e.g. stock cubes, tinned meats, bottled sauces and savoury snack biscuits) contain sugar but are much less obvious sources. Indeed, very few manufactured foods are suitable for inclusion in the diet. Flavourings can be another potential source of sucrose and fructose as these sugars are sometimes used as carriers for flavouring compounds.

Only vegetables that have a very low fructose content and contain predominantly starch can be included in the diet, but in restricted amounts (Table 18.15). Fructose from vegetables should not exceed 1.0–1.5 g/day as small amounts of fructose from cereals will increase the total intake to the 2 g maximum. Permitted vegetables have been divided into two groups (with a fructose content of <0.5 g/100 g and 0.5–1.0 g/100 g) to give a wider choice. It is important to note the difference in fructose content between raw and cooked vegetables. Cooking causes a loss of free sugars, consequently cooked vegetables have a lower fructose content and are recommended in preference to raw. New potatoes have a higher fructose content than old (0.65 g/100 g vs. 0.25 g/100 g). Sucrose content of stored potatoes has previously been reported to both decrease and increase on storage [134,135]. More recent information from the Institute of Food Research, Norwich reports that potatoes in cold storage (<8°C) have a higher fructose content compared with those in warm temperatures (>15°C). Wholemeal flour contains more fructose than white because the germ and bran contain sucrose. Similarly, other wholegrain foods (e.g. brown rice, wholemeal pasta) contain more sucrose than the refined varieties. No accurate analysis for the fructose content of bread is available; however, it would appear prudent to choose white in preference to wholemeal. Bread has previously been restricted in the diets of children with HFI. Nowadays this restriction is probably unnecessary because most flour improvers for bread making do not contain sugar. If the bread does contain sugar it has to be declared on the ingredient label. If there is any doubt about suitability of a bread the manufacturer should be contacted. Caution should be applied where richer doughs are used (e.g. in soft rolls) because often the flour improver does contain sugar in these instances. Bread bought from craft bakers may also contain sugar and bakers are under no legal obligation to declare this information to the consumer.

Polyols, which are used as low energy bulk sweeteners, are potential sources of sorbitol and fructose. Foods and medicines that contain these need to be checked for suitability. Different proprietary brands of polyols exist (e.g. Lycasin, Neosorb, Roquette, Lestrem, France). Polyols should be declared on the food ingredient and nutritional labels in the UK, therefore making them relatively easy to identify. Parents need to check with a pharmacist about the suitability of medicines.

Intravenous fructose and sorbitol are potential lethal sources of fructose; these are rarely used in the UK, but are more commonly used in Europe [136].

Starch, glucose and lactose can be included in the diet. Glucose can be used as an alternative sweetener to sucrose and can also provide a useful source of energy. The relative sweetness of glucose is only half that of sucrose, so additional sweetening may be needed in baked goods. Some intense sweeteners (e.g. Sweetex) can be successfully added to cooked food; others (e.g. aspartame) decompose on heating and are therefore not suitable for baking. Extra sweetening may not be necessary or desirable as children with HFI dislike and avoid sweet tasting foods. Glucose is not prescribable on FP10 for treatment of HFI.

Nutritional problems

Children with HFI are at risk of vitamin C and possible folic acid deficiency because of the exclusion of the major dietary sources of these vitamins (i.e. fruits and vegetables). Pure vitamin C powders are available (e.g. Nature's Best Vitamin C powder, Tunbridge Wells, Kent) and should be prescribed to meet the reference nutrient intake (RNI) [115]. Lack of dietary fibre may also be a problem. This could be overcome by including pulses and oats, which contain only very small amounts of fructose, in the diet.

Fructose-1,6-bisphosphatase deficiency

In the fasting state, glycogen initially provides the major fuel source for glucose production. As the duration of fast extends and glycogen stores are depleted, glucose is synthesised via gluconeogenesis from lactate, glycerol and the gluconeogenic amino acids such as alanine. A deficiency of fructose-1,6-bisphosphatase (Fig. 18.3) blocks the gluconeogenic pathway and as a result, during fasting, patients develop hypoglycaemia and a marked lactic acidosis with ketosis.

Fructose-1,6-bisphosphatase deficiency may present in the newborn period or, in older children, during intercurrent infections associated with prolonged fasting [129]. Once diagnosed, these life-threatening acute episodes can be prevented with careful treatment. The prognosis is good, with normal growth and development.

Dietary treatment

The aims of the dietary management of fructose-1,6-bisphosphatase deficiency are to:

● Provide good glycogen reserves
● Prevent hypoglycaemia
● Reduce the need for gluconeogenesis

This can be achieved by avoidance of prolonged fasts and provision of regular meals, with a high intake of carbohydrate from starch. Patients should be carefully assessed for fasting tolerance, which should improve with age. The majority of children will be well controlled without the need for fructose restriction when they are well. Nevertheless, it is inadvisable for them to have a very high intake of fructose as this may cause hypoglycaemia and lactic acidosis. During illness fructose must be completely avoided.

Diet when well

The young infant is fed at 4-hourly intervals during the day and night. Even when weaning is well established, a late night and early morning feed is still given to reduce the duration of overnight fasting.

The older child is given regular meals containing a high carbohydrate intake from starch to provide a constant supply of 'slow release' glucose. Fasting overnight is not normally a problem provided a starchy bedtime snack and early breakfast is given. A high intake of fructose as sucrose in cakes, biscuits, confectionery and sugary drinks is discouraged.

Alcohol inhibits gluconeogenesis and if taken in excess in healthy adolescents can precipitate hypoglycaemia. Alcohol should therefore be taken in moderation and only with food.

Diet during illness

Poor appetite and fasting are common in the sick child. In the child with fructose-1,6-bisphosphatase deficiency it is critical to prevent such prolonged fasts because the gluconeogenic pathway for production of glucose is blocked. During intercurrent illnesses an exogenous source of glucose must be supplied. The standard emergency regimen (see p. 375) must be given during times of illness to reduce the risk of hypoglycaemia and lactic acidosis. Fructose, sucrose and sorbitol must be excluded because these will exacerbate the metabolic derangement. Fat should be avoided during decompensation as glycerol may exacerbate the illness. Emergency regimen drinks need to be restricted to glucose polymer. Fruit juice and squashes should not be added because they contain sucrose. Even most low calorie squashes will be unsuitable because invariably they contain fructose, sucrose or sorbitol or comminuted fruits. It is advisable to check these carefully for suitability. Unflavoured oral rehydration solutions can be given, but flavoured varities may contain sucrose or fructose and therefore not be suitable. Glucose polymer needs to be added to oral rehydration solutions to provide an adequate glucose intake (see p. 91). Medications must also be free of fructose, sucrose and sorbitol. Some patients may decompensate rapidly, becoming very ill with marked acidosis. The impact can be reduced by giving sodium bicarbonate up to 4 mmol/kg/day. If there are signs of metabolic acidosis the patient's condition must be assessed in hospital. Once the child improves, normal diet can be resumed, with a gradual reintroduction of fructose and sucrose containing foods. It is helpful to provide parents with a list of foods that are high in fructose and sucrose. During the recovery period extra glucose polymer drinks should continue to be given, particularly at night.

Acknowledgement

Marjorie Dixon thanks Dr Philip Lee, Reader in Inherited Metabolic Disease, The National Hospital for Neurology and Neurosurgery, London for his helpful review of glycogen storage diseases.

References

1   Burchell A, Waddell I Identification, purification and genetic deficiencies of the glucose-6-phosphatase system transport proteins. *Eur J Pediatr*, 1993, **152** (Suppl 1) 14–17.

2   Chen YT Glycogen storage diseases. In: Scriver CR *et al.* (eds) *The Metabolic and Molecular Bases of Inherited Disease*, 8th edn. New York: McGraw-Hill, 2001, pp. 1521–51.

3   Roe T, Thomas DW, Gilsanz V *et al.* Inflammatory bowel disease in glycogen storage disease type IB. *J Pediatr*, 1986, **109** 55–9.

4   Lee PJ, Leonard JV The hepatic glycogen storage diseases – problems beyond childhood. *J Inherit Metab Dis*, 1995, **18** 462–72.

5   Rake JP, Visser G, Labrune P *et al.* Glycogen storage disease type I: diagnosis, management, clinical course and outcome. Results of the European Study on Glycogen Storage Disease Type I (EGSD I). *Eur J Pediatr*, 2002, **161** 20–34.

6   Stanley CA, Mills J, Baker L Intragastric feeding in type I glycogen storage disease: factors affecting the control of lacticacidaemia. *Pediatr Res*, 1981, **15** 1504–8.

7   Bier D, Leake RD, Haymond MW *et al.* Measurement of true glucose production rates in infancy and childhood with 6,6-diodeuteroglucose. *Diabetes*, 1977, **26** 1016–23.

8   Green H, Slonim AE, O'Neill JA *et al.* Continuous nocturnal nasogastric feeding for management of type I GSD. *N Engl J Med*, 1976, **294** 423–5.

9   Chen Y, Cornblath M, Sidbury J Cornstarch therapy in type I glycogen storage disease. *N Engl J Med*, 1984, **310** 171–5.

10   Fernandes J The effect of disaccharides on the hyperlacticacidaemia of glucose-6-phosphatase-deficient children. *Acta Paediatr Scand*, 1974, **63** 695–8.

11   Fernandes J, Berger R, Smit P Lactate as a cerebral metabolic fuel for glucose-6-phosphatase deficient children. *Pediatr Res*, 1984, **18** 335–9.

12   Melis D, Parenti G, Della Casa R *et al.* Brain damage in glycogen storage disease type I. *J Pediatr*, 2004, **144** 637–42.

13   Rake PJ, Visser G, Labrune P *et al.* Guidelines for management of glycogen storage disease type I – European Study on Glycogen Storage Disease Type I (EGSD I). *Eur J Paediatr*, 2002, **161** 112–19.

14   Fernandes J The glycogen storage disease. In: Fernandes J, Saudubray JM, Tada K (eds) *Inborn Metabolic Diseases, Diagnosis and Treatment*. Berlin: Springer-Verlag, 1990.

15   Fernandes, J, Alaapovic P, Wit J Gastric drip feeding in patients with glycogen storage disease type I: its effects on growth and plasma lipids and apolipoproteins. *Pediatr Res*, 1989, **25** 327–31.

16   Schmitz G, Hohage H, Ullrich K Glucose-6-phosphate; a key compound in glycogenosis I and favism leading to hyper- or hypolipidaemia. *Eur J Pediatr*, 1993, **152** (Suppl 1) 77–84.

17   Lee PJ, Celermajer DS, Robinson J *et al.* Hyperlipidaemia does not impair vascular endothelial function in glycogen storage disease Ia. *Atherosclerosis*, 1994, **110** 95–100.

18   Ubels FL, Rake JP, Slaets JPJ *et al.* Is glycogen storage disease 1a associated with atherosclerosis? *Eur J Pediatr*, 2002, **161** 62–4.

19   Wittenstein B, Klein M, Finckh B *et al.* Plasma antioxidants in pediatric patients with glycogen storage disease, diabetes mellitus and hypercholesterolemia. *Free Radic Biol Med*, 2002, **33** 103–10.

20   Schwenk WF, Haymond WM Optimal rate of enteral glucose administration in children with glycogen storage disease type I. *N Engl J Med*, 1986, **314** 1257–8.

21   Collins J, Bartlett K, Leonard JV *et al.* Glucose production rates in type I glycogen storage disease. *J Inherit Metab Dis*, 1990, **13** 195–206.

22   Hershkovitz E, Rachmel A, Ben-Zaken H *et al.* Continuous glucose monitoring in children with glycogen storage disease type I. *J Inherit Metab Dis*, 2001, **24** 863–9.

23   Leonard J, Dunger D Hypoglycaemia complicating feeding regimens for glycogen storage disease. *Lancet*, 1978, **11** 1203–4.

24   Dunger DB, Sutton P, Leonard JV Hypoglycaemia complicating treatment regimens for glycogen storage disease (letter). *Arch Dis Child*, 1995, **72** 274–5.

25   Fine R, Kogut M, Donnell G Intestinal absorption in type I glycogen storage disease. *J Pediatr*, 1969, **75** 632–5.

26 Milla PJ, Atherton DA, Leonard JV *et al.* Disordered intestinal function in glycogen storage disease. *J Inherit Metab Dis*, 1978, **1** 155–7.

27 Visser G, Rake JP, Kokke FTM *et al.* Intestinal function in glycogen storage disease type I. *J Inherit Metab Dis*, 2002, **4** 261–7.

28 Kishnani PS, Boney A, Chen YT Nutritional deficiencies in a patient with glycogen storage disease type Ib. *J Inherit Metab Dis*, 1999, **22** 795–801.

29 Lee PJ, Patel JS, Fewtrell M *et al.* Bone mineralisation in type I glycogen storage disease. *Eur J Pediatr*, 1995, **154** 483–7.

30 Rake PJ, Visser G, Huismans D *et al.* Bone mineral density in children, adolescents and adults with glycogen storage disease type 1a: a cross sectional and longitudinal study. *J Inherit Metab Dis*, 2003, **26** 371–84.

31 Mundy H, Georgiadou P, Davies LL *et al.* Exercise Capacity and Biochemical Profile during Exercise in Patients with Glycogen Storage Disease Type I. *J Clin Endocrinol Metab*, 2005, **90** 2675–80.

32 Smit GPA, Berger R, Potasnick R *et al.* The dietary treatment of children with type I glycogen storage disease with slow release carbohydrate. *Pediatr Res*, 1984, **18** 879–81.

33 Lee PJ, Dixon MA, Leonard JV Uncooked cornstarch – efficacy in type I glycogenosis. *Arch Dis Child*, 1996, **74** 546–7.

34 Bodamer OA, Feillet F, Lane RE *et al.* Utilization of cornstarch in glycogen storage disease type 1a. *Eur J Gastroenterol Hepatol*, 2002, **14** 1251–6.

35 Bhattacharya K, Orton RC, Mundy H *et al.* Preliminary data on a starch to improve treatment of hepatic glycogen storage diseases. *J Inherit Metab Dis*, 2006, **29** (Suppl 1), Abstract 0-19-4.

36 Hayde M, Widhalm K Effects of cornstarch treatment in very young children with type I glycogen storage disease. *Eur J Pediatr*, 1990, **149** 630–3.

37 Ogata T, Matsuo N, Ishikawa K *et al.* Effect of cornstarch formula in an infant with type I glycogen storage disease. *Acta Paediatr Jpn*, 1988, **30** 547–52.

38 Wolfsdorf JI, Crigler JF Effect of continuous glucose therapy begun in infancy on the long-term clinical course of patients with type I glycogen storage disease. *J Pediatr Gastroenteral Nutr*, 1999, **29** 136–43.

39 Sidbury J, Chen Y, Roe L The role of raw starches in the treatment of type I glycogenosis. *Arch Intern Med*, 1986, **146** 370–3.

40 Wolfsdorf JI, Crigler JF Biochemical evidence for the requirement of continuous glucose therapy in young adults with type I glycogen storage disease. *J Inherit Metab Dis*, 1994, **17** 234–41.

41 Chen YT, Bazarre CH, Lee MM *et al.* Type I glycogen storage disease: nine years of management with cornstarch. *Eur J Pediatr*, 1993, **152** (Suppl 1) 56–9.

42 Mundy HR, Hindmarsh PC, Matthews DR *et al.* The regulation of growth in glycogen storage disease type I. *Clin Endocrinol (Oxf)*, 2003, **58** 332–9.

43 Mention K, Touati C, Elbim C *et al.* Digestive and hematological manifestations in glycogenosis type Ib. Beneficial effect of a new nutritional therapy. *J Inherit Metab Dis*, 2005, **28** (Suppl 1) Abstract 420.

44 Dunger DB, Leonard JV, Preece MA Patterns of growth in the hepatic glycogenoses. *Arch Dis Child*, 1984, **59** 657–60.

45 Mundy HR, Fewtrell M, Williams J *et al.* Bone mineral density in glycogen storage disease type III. *J Inherit Metab Dis*, 2004, **27** (Suppl 1) 206 Abstract 407.

46 Slonim A, Coleman R, Moses W Myopathy and growth failure in debrancher enzyme deficiency: improvement with high protein nocturnal enteral therapy. *J Pediatr*, 1984, **105** 906–11.

47 Slonim AE, Weisberg C, Benke P *et al.* Reversal of debrancher deficiency myopathy by use of high-protein nutrition. *Ann Neur*, 1982, **11** 420–2.

48 Slonim AE, Coleman RA, Shimon M *et al.* Amino acid disturbances in type III glycogenosis: differences from type I glycogenosis. *Metabolism*, 1983, **32** 70–4.

49 Bodamer OAF, Mayatepek E, Leonard JV Leucine and glucose kinetics in glycogen storage disease type IIIa. *J Inherit Metab Dis*, 1997, **20** 847.

50 Borowitz SM, Greene HL Cornstarch therapy in a patient with type III glycogen storage disease. *J Pediatr Gastroenterol Nutr*, 1987, **6** 631–4.

51 Ullrich K, Schmidt H, van Teeffelen-Heithoff A *et al.* Glycogen storage disease type I and III and pyruvate carboxylase deficiency: results of long-term treatment with uncooked cornstarch. *Acta Paediatr Scand*, 1998, **77** 531–6.

52 Gremse D, Bucuvalas J, Balisteri W Efficacy of cornstarch therapy in type III glycogen storage disease. *Am J Clin Nutr*, 1990, **52** 671–4.

53 McCallion N, Irranca N, Naughten E Uncooked cornflour (UCF) compared to high protein diet in the treatment of glycogen storage disease type III. *J Inherit Metab Dis*, 1998, **21** (Suppl 2) 93.

54 Lee PJ, Ferguson C, Alexander FW Symptomatic hyperinsulinism reversed by dietary manipulation in glycogenosis type III. *J Inherit Metab Dis*, 1997, **20** 612–13.

55 Collins JE, Bartlett K, Leonard JV *et al.* The effect of ethanol on glucose production in phosphorylase *b* kinase deficiency. *J Inherit Metab Dis*, 1989, **12** 312–22.

56 Slonim AE, Coleman RA, McElligot MA *et al.* Improvement of muscle function in acid maltase deficiency by high protein therapy. *Neurology*, 1983, **33** 34–8.

57   Umpleby M *et al.* Protein turnover in acid maltase deficiency before and after treatment with a high protein diet. *J Neurosurg Psych*, 1987, **50** 587–92.

58   Bodamer OA, Leonard JV, Halliday D *et al.* Dietary treatment in late-onset acid maltase deficiency. *Eur J Pediatr*, 1997, **156** (Supp 1) 39–42.

59   Bodamer OA, Halliday D, Leonard JV *et al.* The effects of l-alanine supplementation in late-onset glycogen storage disease type II. *Pediatr Neurol*, 2002, **27** 145–6.

60   Mundy HR, Williams JE, Cousins AJ *et al.* The effect of l-alanine therapy in a patient with adult-onset glycogen storage disease type II. *J Inherit Metab Dis*, 2006, **29** 226–9.

61   Bodamer OA, Haas D, Hermans MM *et al.* L-alanine supplementation in late infantile glycogen storage disease type II. *Pediatr Neurol*, 2002, **27** 145–6.

62   DiMauro S, Bruno C Glycogen storage diseases of muscle. *Curr Opin Neurol*, 1998, **11** 477–84.

63   Smit GPA, Fernandes J, Leonard JV *et al.* The long term outcome of patients with glycogen storage diseases. *J Inherit Metab Dis*, 1990, **13** 411–18.

64   Schippers HM, Smit GP, Rake JP *et al.* Characteristic growth pattern in male X-linked phosphorylase-b kinase deficiency (GSD IX). *J Inherit Metab Dis*, 2003, **26** 43–7.

65   Walter JH, Collins JE, Leonard JV Recommendations for the management of galactosaemia. *Arch Dis Child*, 1999, **80** 93–6.

66   Murphy M, McHugh B, Tighe O *et al.* Genetic basis of transferase-deficient galactosaemia in Ireland and the population history of the Irish Travellers. *Eur J Hum Genet*, 1999, **7** 549–54.

67   Tyfield L, Reichardt J, Fridovich-Keil J *et al.* Classical galactosemia and mutations at the galactose-1-phosphate uridyl transferase (GALT) gene. *Hum Mutat*, 1999, **13** 417–30.

68   Shield JP, Wadsworth EJ, MacDonald A *et al.* The relationship of genotype to cognitive outcome in galactosaemia. *Arch Dis Child*, 2000, **83** 248–50.

69   Holton JB, Walter JH, Tyfield LA Galactosaemia. In: Scriver CR, Beaudet AL, Sly W, Valle D, Childs B, Kinzler KW, Vogelstein B (eds) *The Metabolic and Molecular Bases of Inherited Disease*, 8th edn. New York: McGraw-Hill, 2001, pp. 1553–87.

70   Ridel KR, Leslie ND, Gilbert DL An updated review of the long-term neurological effects of galactosaemia. *Pediatr Neurol*, 2005, **33** 153–61.

71   Berry GT, Nissim I, Lin Z *et al.* Endogenous synthesis of galactose in normal men and patients with hereditary galactosaemia. *Lancet*, 1995, **346** 1073–4.

72   Rake JP, Visser G, Smit PA Disorders of carbohydrate and glycogen metabolism. In: Blau N, Hoffmann GF, Leonard J, Clarke JT (eds) *Physician's Guide to the Treatment and Follow-up of Metabolic Diseases*. Berlin: Springer-Verlag, 2006, pp. 161–80.

73   Roe TF, Ng WG, Smit PGA Disorders of carbohydrate and glycogen metabolism. In: Blau N, Duran M, Blaskovics ME, Gibson KM (eds) *Physician's Guide to the Laboratory Diagnosis of Metabolic Diseases*. Berlin: Springer-Verlag, 2003, pp. 335–56.

74   Panis B, Forget PP, van Kroonenburgh MJ *et al.* Bone metabolism in galactosaemia. *Bone*, 2004, **35** 982–7.

75   Rubio-Gozalbo ME, Hamming S, van Kroonenburgh MJ *et al.* Bone mineral density in patients with classic galactosaemia. *Arch Dis Child*, 2002, **87** 57–60.

76   Panis B, Forget PP, Nieman FH *et al.* Body composition in children with galactosaemia. *J Inherit Metab Dis*, 2005, **28** 931–7.

77   Antshel KM, Epstein IO, Waisbren SE Cognitive strengths and weaknesses in children and adolescents homozygous for the galactosemia Q188R mutation: a descriptive study. *Neuropsychology*, 2004, **18** 658–64.

78   Kaufman FR, McBride-Chang C, Manis FR *et al.* Cognitive functioning, neurologic status and brain imaging in classic galactosemia. *Eur J Pediatr*, 1995, **154** (Suppl 2) 2–5.

79   Schweitzer S, Shin Y, Jacobs C, Brodehl J Long-term outcome in 134 patients with galactosemia. *Eur J Pediatr*, 1993, **152** 36–43.

80   Waggoner DD, Buist NRM, Donnell GN Long-term prognosis in galactosemia: results of a survey of 350 cases. *J Inherit Metab Dis*, 1990, **13** 802–18.

81   Nelson D Verbal dyspraxia in children with galactosemia. *Eur J Pediatr*, 1995, **154** (Suppl 2) 6–7.

82   Leigh Webb A, Singh RH, Kennedy MJ, Elsas LJ Verbal Dyspraxia and Galactosaemia. *Pediatr Res*, 2003, **53** 396–402.

83   Lambert C, Boneh A The impact of galactosaemia on quality of life: a pilot study. *J Inherit Metab Dis*, 2004, **27** 601–8.

84   Gibson JB Gonadal function in galactosemics and in galactose-intoxicated animals. *Eur J Pediatr*, 1995, **54** (Suppl 2) 14–20.

85   Kaufman FR, Donnell GN, Roe TF, Kogut MD Gonadal function in patients with galactosaemia. *J Inherit Metab Dis*, 1986, **9** 140–6.

86   Kaufman FR, Reichardt JK, Ng WG *et al.* Correlation of cognitive, neurologic, and ovarian outcome with the Q188R mutation of the galactose-1-phosphate uridyltransferase gene. *J Pediatr*, 1994, **125** 225–7.

87   Menezo YJ, Lescaille M, Nicollet B, Servy EJ Pregnancy and delivery after stimulation with rFSH of a galatosemia patient suffering hypergonadotrophic hypogonadism: case report. *J Assist Reprod Genet*, 2004, **21** 89–90.

88   Kimonis V Increased fertility in a woman with classic galactosaemia. *J Inherit Metab Dis*, 2001, **24** 607–8.

89   Berry GT, Nissim I, Lin Z *et al*. Endogenous synthesis of galactose in normal men and patients with hereditary galactosemia. *Lancet*, 1995, **346** 1073–4.

90   Berry GT, Moate PJ, Reynolds RA *et al*. The rate of de novo galactose synthesis in patients with galactose-1-phosphate uridyltransferase deficiency. *Mol Genet Metab*, 2004, **81** 22–30.

91   Schadewaldt P, Kamalanathan L, Hammen HW, Wendel U Age dependence of endogenous galactose formation in Q188R homozygous galactosemic patients. *Mol Genet Metab*, 2004, **81** 31–44.

92   Schweitzer-Krantz S Early diagnosis of inherited metabolic disorders towards improving outcome: the controversial issue of galactosaemia. *Eur J Pediatr*, 2003, **162** (Suppl 1) S50–3. Epub 2003 Nov 12.

93   Gitzelmann R Disorders of galactosaemia. In: Fernandes J, Saudurbray J-M, van den Berghe G (eds) *Inborn Metabolic Diseases Diagnosis and Treatment*. Berlin: Springer-Verlag, 2000, pp. 103–11.

94   Acosta PB, Gross KC Hidden sources of galactose in the environment. *Eur J Pediatr*, 1995, **154** 7 (Suppl 2) S87–92.

95   Clothier CM, Davidson DC Galactosaemia workshop. Report of a workshop held at Alder Hey Children's Hospital, Liverpool on 30 April, 1982. *Hum Nutr Appl Nutr*, 1983, **37** 483–90.

96   MacDonald A, Portnoi P Galactosaemia: one diet for Europe? A compilation of papers from the sixth international dietitians meeting, Society for Study of Inborn Errors of Metabolism 2001, Prague, 2002, pp. 24–8.

97   Casein and Caseinate Regulations. 2002. Subsidiary Regulations 231.50. Legal notice 113 of 2002. 1 July, 2002.

98   Roe MA, Finglas PM, Church SM *McCance and Widdowson's 'The Composition of Foods'*, 6th summary edition. Cambridge: Royal Society of Chemistry, 2002.

99   Matthews, RH, Pehrsson PR, Farhat-Sabet M Sugar content of selected foods: individual and total sugars. United States Department of Agriculture, Human Nutrition Information Service. *Home Economics Research Report* **48** 1987.

100   Gitzelmann R, Auricchio S The handling of soya alphagalactosides by a normal and a galactosaemic child. *Pediatrics*, 1965, **36** 231–5.

101   Koch R, Acosta P, Ragsdale N, Donnell GN Nutrition in the treatment of galactosaemia. *J Am Diet Assoc*, 1963, **43** 216–22.

102   Gross KC, Acosta PB Fruits and vegetables are a source of galactose: implications in planning the diets of patients with galactosaemia. *J Inherit Metab Dis*, 1991, **14** 253–8.

103   Gropper SS, Gross KC, Olds SJ Galactose content of selected fruit and vegetable baby foods: implications for infants on galactose-restricted diets. *J Am Diet Assoc*, 1993, **93** 328–30.

104   Gropper SS, Weese JO, West PA, Gross KC Free galactose content of fresh fruits and strained fruit and vegetable baby foods: more foods to consider for the galactose-restricted diet. *J Am Diet Assoc*, 2000, **100** 573–5.

105   Berry GT, Palmieri M, Gross KC *et al*. The effect of dietary fruits and vegetables on urinary galactitol excretion in galactose-1-phosphate uridyltransferase deficiency. *J Inherit Metab Dis*, 1993, **16** 91–100.

106   CMO's Update 37. Department of Health, 2003. www.dh.gov.uk/assetRoot/04/07/01/76/040701 76.pdf

107   The Committee on Toxicity of Chemicals in Food, Consumer Products and the Environment (COT). *Phytoestrogens and health*. Food Standards Agency, 2003. www.foodstandards.gov.uk/multimedia/ pdfs/phtoreport0503

108   Agostoni C, Axelsson I, Goulet O *et al*. Soy protein infant formulae and follow-on formulae: a commentary by the ESPGHAN Committee on Nutrition. *J Pediatr Gastroenterol Nutr*, 2006, **42** 352–61.

109   Zlatunich CO, Packman S Galactosaemia: early treatment with an elemental formula. *J Inherit Metab Dis*, 2005, **28** 163–8.

110   Portnoi P, MacDonald A Analysis of mature cheese for lactose content. IX International Congress on Inborn Errors of Metabolism, Brisbane Australia, 2–6 September, 2003, p. 252 (abstract).

111   Directive 2003/89/EC amending Directive 2000/13/EC of the European Parliament and of the Council of 20 March on the approximation of the laws of the Member States relating to the labelling, presentation and advertising of foodstuffs.

112   The Food Labelling (Amendment) (England) (No. 2) Regulations 2004.

113   Kaufman FR, Loro ML, Azen C *et al*. Effect of hypogonadism and deficient calcium intake on bone density in patients with galactosemia. *J Pediatr*, 1993, **123** 365–70.

114   Panis B, Vermeer C, van Kroonenburgh MJ *et al*. Effect of calcium, vitamins K1 and D3 on bone in galactosemia. *Bone*, 2006, **39** 1123–9. E pub 2006 Jun 19.

115   Department of Health Report on Health and Social Subjects No. 41. *Dietary Reference Values for Food Energy and Nutrients for the United Kingdom*. London: The Stationery Office, 1991.

116   MacDonald A Calcium and Galactosaemia. A com-

pilation of papers presented at the 2nd Dietitians' meeting at the Society for Study of Inborn Errors of Metabolism. Gothenburg, Sweden, 1997, pp. 2–6.

117   Rutherford PJ, Davidson DC, Matthai SM Dietary calcium in galactosaemia. *J Hum Nutr Diet*, 2002, **15** 39–42.

118   Davidovits M, Levy Y, Avramovitz T, Eisenstein B Calcium-deficiency rickets in a four-year-old boy with milk allergy. *J Pediatr*, 1993, **122** 249–51.

119   Madsen CD, Henderson RC Calcium intake in children with positive IgG RAST to cow's milk. *J Paediatr Child Health*, 1997, **33** 209–12.

120   www.duphalac.com/professionals/productinformationpro/productdetails/0,998,10310-2-0,00.htm 2006.

121   Lee PJ, Lilburn M, Wendel U, Schadewaldt P A woman with untreated galactosaemia. *Lancet*, 2003, **362** 446.

122   Panis B, Bakker JA, Sels JP *et al.* Untreated classical galactosemia patient with mild phenotype. *Mol Genet Metab*, 2006, **89** 277–9.

123   Bosch AM, Bakker HD, Wenniger-Prick LJ *et al.* High tolerance for oral galactose in classical galactosaemia: dietary implications. *Arch Dis Child*, 2004, **89** 1034–6.

124   Francis DEM Galactosaemia. In: *Diets for Sick Children*, 3rd edn. Oxford: Blackwell Scientific Publications, 1974, pp. 227–32.

125   Bosch AM, Bakker HD, van Gennip AH *et al.* Clinical features of galactokinase deficiency: a review of the literature. *J Inherit Metab Dis*, 2002, **25** 629–34.

126   Hunter M, Heyer E, Austerlitz F *et al.* The P28T mutation in the GALK1 gene accounts for galactokinase deficiency in Roma (Gypsy) patients across Europe. *Pediatr Res*, 2002, **51** 602–6.

127   Openo KK, Schulz JM, Vargas CA *et al.* Epimerase-deficiency galactosemia is not a binary condition. *Am J Hum Genet*, 2006, **78** 89–102.

128   Kingsley DM, Krieger M, Holton JB Structure and function of low-density-lipoprotein receptors in epimerase-deficient galactosemia. *N Engl J Med*, 1986, **314** 1257–8.

129   Steinmann B, Gitzelmann R, Van den Berghe G Disorders of fructose metabolism. In: Scriver CR *et al.* (eds) *The Metabolic and Molecular Bases of Inherited Disease*, 8th edn. New York: McGraw-Hill, 2001, pp. 1489–520.

130   Odièvre M, Gentil C, Gautier M *et al.* Hereditary fructose intolerance in childhood: diagnosis, management and course in 55 patients. *Am J Dis Child*, 1978, **132** 605–8.

131   Oberhaensli R, rajagopalan B, Taylor DJ *et al.* Study of hereditary fructose intolerance by the use of 31P magnetic resonance spectroscopy. *Lancet*, 1987, (24 Oct) 931–4.

132   Rumessen J, Bode S, Hamberg O *et al.* Fructans of Jerusalem artichokes: intestinal transport, absorption, fermentation and influence on blood glucose, insulin and C-peptide responses in healthy subjects. *Am J Clin Nutr*, 1990, **52** 675–81.

133   Mills A, Tyler H *Food and Nutrient Intakes of British Infants aged 6 to 12 Months*. London: Ministry of Agriculture, Fisheries and Foods, The Stationery Office, 1992.

134   Francis D Galactosaemia, fructosaemia and favism: dietary management. In: *Diets for Sick Children*, 4th edn. Oxford: Blackwell Science, 1987, pp. 335–47.

135   Bell L, Sherwood W Current practices and improved recommendations for treating hereditary fructose intolerance. *J Am Diet Assoc*, 1987, **87** 721–31.

136   Collins J Metabolic disease, time for fructose solutions to go. *Lancet*, 1993, **341** 600.

Useful addresses

Association for Glycogen Storage Disease (UK)
9 Lindop Road, Hale, Altrincham, Cheshire, WA15 9DZ
www.agsd.org.uk
www.pompe.org.uk
www.worldpompe.org

European Galactosaemia Society (EGS)
c/o Jeroen and Maaike Kempen, Zandoogjelaan 4, NL-5691 RJ Son
www.galactosaemia.eu

UK Galactosaemia Support Group
c/o Sue Bevington
31 Cotysmore Road, Sutton Coldfield, West Midlands, B75 6BJ
www.galactosaemia.org

19 Disorders of Fatty Acid Oxidation and Ketogenesis

Marjorie Dixon

Introduction

Fatty acids are a major fuel source for most tissues of the body, especially during fasting. They are the principal energy source for cardiac muscle and for skeletal muscle in the resting state and during prolonged exercise. Fatty acid oxidation is also important for the production of ketone bodies; these are another important fuel, particularly for the brain during prolonged fasting. Fatty acids consist of a hydrocarbon chain with a carboxylic acid group at one end. Most naturally occurring fatty acids have a chain length of 16–18 carbon atoms and are referred to as long chain fatty acids. Fatty acids are stored as triglycerides, in which the carboxylic acid groups of three fatty acids are esterified to glycerol.

Fat metabolism begins in adipose tissue with the release of free fatty acids from triglycerides into the blood stream. The fatty acids are then transported to the tissues bound to albumin. In tissues where they are used, fatty acids enter the mitochondria bound to carnitine. This pathway is sometimes called the carnitine cycle and it includes the regulatory step for fatty acid oxidation (carnitine palmitoyl transferase I, CPT I). Within mitochondria, fatty acids are broken down by the spiral pathway of β-oxidation (Fig. 19.1). Every turn of the spiral involves four steps, catalysed by

several enzymes of different chain length specificities. The first step, for example, is catalysed by very long chain, medium chain and short chain acyl-CoA dehydrogenases (VLCAD, MCAD and SCAD). The third step in the β-oxidation spiral is another dehydrogenation reaction: both of these reactions release energy, which can be harnessed for use by the cell. This is achieved by passing electrons to the mitochondrial respiratory chain, either directly or via electron transfer flavoprotein (ETF) and ETF dehydrogenase. In addition to producing energy, each turn of the β-oxidation spiral releases a molecule of acetyl-CoA and shortens the fatty acid by two carbon atoms. Acetyl-CoA can be metabolised in the tricarboxylic acid cycle, but in the liver it is converted to ketone bodies. Ketone bodies are used by cardiac and skeletal muscle and during prolonged fasting they are a major fuel for the brain.

A number of disorders of the mitochondrial fatty acid oxidation pathway have now been described. These vary in severity and may present at any time from the neonatal period to adulthood [1]. The clinical features probably result from the accumulation of toxic intermediates and/or an energy deficit. The most common disorder is MCAD deficiency. Typically, this presents in early childhood with hypoglycaemia and acute encephalopathy brought on by fasting or an acute infection. The fatty acid

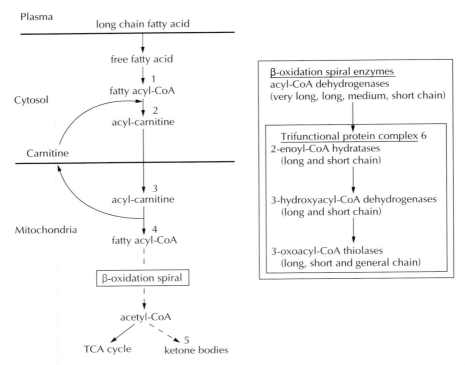

Figure 19.1 Pathway of mitochondrial fatty acid oxidation. Enzymes involved: 1 acyl-CoA synthase; 2 carnitine palmitoyl transferase I (CPT I); 3 carnitine acylcarnitine translocase (CAT); 4 carnitine palmitoyl transferase II (CPT II); 5 3-hydroxy-3-methylglutaryl-CoA (HMG-CoA) Synthase and lyase; 6 trifunctional protein complex is composed of long chain enoyl-CoA hydratases, long chain 3-hydroxyacyl-CoA dehydrogenases (LCHAD) and long chain 3-oxothiolases. TCA, tricarboxylic acid cycles.

oxidation defect impairs the production of ketone bodies and the hypoglycaemia is therefore 'hypoketotic'. Most other defects affect long chain fatty acid oxidation, either because they involve long chain specific β-oxidation enzymes or because they affect the carnitine mediated entry of long chain fatty acids into mitochondria. Defects of ETF and ETF dehydrogenase cause multiple acyl-CoA dehydrogenase deficiency (MADD); in this condition there is impaired oxidation of long chain, medium chain and short chain fatty acids and various other substrates. Patients with long chain fatty acid oxidation defects may present with hypoglycaemia and encephalopathy, as in MCAD deficiency. They may also have additional problems, such as cardiomyopathy, weakness or episodes of muscle breakdown (rhabdomyolysis).

The synthesis of ketone bodies occurs via the intermediate, 3-hydroxy-3-methylglutaryl-CoA (HMG-CoA), and depends primarily on the enzymes HMG-CoA synthase and HMG-CoA lyase. Deficiencies of these enzymes also present with hypoketotic hypoglycaemia.

Disorders of fatty acid oxidation and ketogenesis are treated primarily by diet. Some aspects of management are universal but other aspects vary with the underlying disorder. The main aim is to minimise the oxidation of fatty acids by using an emergency regimen during illness, avoiding fasting and in severe defects by limiting the intake of dietary fat. A number of countries worldwide now undertake newborn screening for fatty acid oxidation disorders, particularly MCAD deficiency. With the exception of MCAD deficiency, most disorders of fatty acid oxidation are rare and experience of dietary treatment is limited. Moreover, in the long chain defects, treatment needs to prevent long term complications. Proper evaluation of treatment requires long term controlled studies in which other aspects of management are unchanged – such studies are not being undertaken at present.

Medium chain acyl-CoA dehydrogenase deficiency

MCAD deficiency is the most common fatty acid oxidation defect with an estimated incidence of up to 1 in 10 000 in some regions of the UK [2]. It is also relatively common in some European populations. Newborn screening is undertaken in a number of countries and a trial of screening has recently taken place in the UK [3]. All newborn babies in England will be screened within two weeks of birth for MCAD deficiency in 2009.

MCAD deficiency usually presents clinically between 6 months and 4 years of age but neonatal onset can also occur. The typical picture is of encephalopathy with hypoketotic hypoglycaemia, precipitated by metabolic stress such as fasting, gastrointestinal illness or respiratory infections [4–6]. Without prompt treatment, there is a high morbidity and mortality; some patients die suddenly, probably from cardiac arrhythmias. Between episodes the patients are usually completely well.

Dietary management during illness

If a child with MCAD deficiency is unwell and has a reduced appetite, they should be given the standard emergency regimen (ER) of very frequent drinks containing glucose polymer, day and night. This will minimise fasting and provide a fat free source of energy (see p. 375). Fat should be excluded from the diet during the acute period. As the child improves, the normal diet can be resumed but extra ER drinks should be given, particularly during the night, until the child is fully recovered and eating well. If the ER is refused or vomited the child should have rapid access to their local paediatric services, avoiding a wait in the accident and emergency department, so there is no delay in starting an intravenous infusion containing glucose; 10% glucose 0.45% saline is generally suitable but electrolytes should be monitored. Management decisions should be based on the child's clinical state. Monitoring of blood glucose at home is not recommended because precision is poor at low concentrations and because hypoglycaemia is a relatively late finding during illness in MCAD deficiency [7].

Normal diet

Under basal conditions, the oxidation of medium chain fatty acids (MCFA) has been reported to be near normal in patients with MCAD deficiency caused by overlapping enzyme substrate specificity [8]. The well child can therefore have a normal diet without restriction of long chain fat. However, it is important to avoid prolonged fasts as fatty acid oxidation rates increase with fasting. In infants, fatty acid oxidation rates rise after a shorter duration of fasting and frequent feeding is therefore recommended. There are few published data on the safe duration of fasting in MCAD deficiency. Guidelines for the duration of fasting at different ages are available from the British Inherited Metabolic Disease Group (Table 19.1). There are also guidelines for other aspects of dietary management and information sheets for parents at www.BIMDG.org.uk.

Neonatal deaths have been reported in MCAD deficiency [9]. It is essential that infants at risk of MCAD deficiency receive adequate feeds during the first few days of life. The baby should be fed regularly, at least 3–4 hourly day and night, until a diagnosis of MCAD deficiency is confirmed or excluded. Breast fed babies are at particular risk because only small volumes of breast milk are available initially and top-ups of formula milk are may be necessary for the first 24–72 hours. If there are concerns about the baby, an intravenous infusion containing glucose should be started.

Table 19.1 Medium chain acyl-CoA dehydrogenase (MCAD) deficiency: guidelines for 'maximum safe fasting times' for the well child.

Age	Time in hours
Positive screening result* to 4 months of age	6
From 4 months	8
From 8 months	10
From 12 months onwards	12

* Around 2 weeks of age.

Children with MCAD deficiency need to avoid medium chain triglycerides (MCT). This is because MCFA can enter mitochondria without being bound to carnitine, bypassing the step at which fatty acid oxidation is normally regulated (CPT I). MCT ingestion could therefore lead to a more severe metabolic disturbance than for long chain fats. Normal diets contain predominantly fatty acids with a chain length of C16 and C18. MCFAs C8 and C10 occur in only a few foods and in small amounts (e.g. in butter, cow's milk) and these can be included in the diet. Coconut is the only exception where 5% of the fatty acids have a chain length of C8 or C10; for coconut oil the figure is 13%. Small amounts of coconut are acceptable in healthy children with MCAD deficiency but precautions should be taken in countries such as the Philippines, where coconut oil is used as the main cooking oil. Small amounts of MCFAs are present in the vegetable oils of normal infant formulas, but the quantities are not sufficient to cause a problem. MCT is added to some specialised dietetic feeds such as Pregestimil, Pepti-Junior, MCT Pepdite and Monogen, some low birthweight infant formulas and some paediatric enteral feeds. These should not be given.

The following guidelines should be followed when treating a child with MCAD deficiency.

Infants (under 1 year of age)

- Breast feeding or normal infant formula
- Avoidance of long fasts (Table 19.1)
- Demand feeding every 3–4 hours throughout the day
- Feeds given just before going to bed, once during the night and on waking in the morning
- Weaning is commenced at the normal time around 6 months (26 weeks) of age
- Weaning onto a normal diet and encouragement of regular starchy foods as weaning progresses
- Avoidance of specialised infant formulas that contain added MCT

NB: newborn infants at risk for MCAD deficiency must receive adequate feeds (as described above).

Children (from 1 year of age)

- Regular meals containing starch (three main meals daily, including breakfast, which must not be missed)

- A bedtime snack containing starchy foods such as bread, potato, pasta, rice, chapatti or cereals
- Missed meals should be replaced with a starchy snack or sugary drink (see p. 375)
- Avoidance of dietetic products that contain added MCT
- A maximum fasting interval of 12 hours overnight is recommended (Table 19.1)

Alcohol

Adolescents and adults need to know that an excessive alcohol intake is hazardous. Alcohol inhibits gluconeogenesis. Moreover, symptoms of hypoglycaemia might be attributed to intoxication. Vomiting and loss of appetite associated with excessive alcohol intake can be particularly dangerous. Alcohol intake should be limited and must always be taken in combination with food [10].

Carnitine

Plasma carnitine concentrations are often below the normal range in patients with MCAD deficiency, particularly after illness. Supplements are sometimes given but, in the author's experience, patients usually do well without this treatment. There is conflicting evidence concerning the effect on exercise tolerance [11,12]. No randomised controlled studies have been undertaken.

Long chain fatty acid oxidation disorders

The long chain fatty acid oxidation disorders include:

- *Defects of the carnitine cycle.* Carnitine palmitoyl transferases I and II (CPT I and II), carnitine acylcarnitine translocase (CAT) and the transporter for uptake of carnitine across the cell membrane (OCTN2)
- *Defects of β-oxidation.* Very long chain acyl-CoA dehydrogenase (VLCAD) and the trifunctional protein (TFP) complex, which includes the long chain 3-hydroxyacyl-CoA dehydrogenase enzyme (LCHAD) (Fig. 19.1)

Hypoglycaemic encephalopathy is common in long chain fatty acid oxidation disorders. This is the only problem in many patients with CPT I deficiency, but some patients also have renal tubular acidosis during infancy. Other long chain fatty acid oxidation disorders tend to cause additional problems, particularly affecting the heart or muscles. Many patients present with cardiomyopathy and arrhythmias in infancy, often in the neonatal period. Muscle weakness is common and so are episodes of muscle breakdown (rhabdomyolysis). Rhabdomyolysis may be induced by illness in early childhood, but episodes are more commonly precipitated by exercise in older children or adults. Indeed, patients with partial deficiency of CPT II usually present as adolescents or adults with exercise-induced myalgia and myoglobinuria [13]. LCHAD deficiency is associated with specific long term complications, particularly a pigmentary retinopathy and peripheral neuropathy.

Patients with defects of the transporter for cellular carnitine uptake (OCTN2) show an excellent response to carnitine (100 mg/kg/day divided into two or three doses); during illness an emergency regimen similar to that for MCAD deficiency is recommended, but most patients tolerate a normal diet when they are well. Treatment of other long chain fatty acid oxidation disorders is primarily by diet. The response to dietary treatment is usually good but a number of patients have long term problems.

Principles of dietary management

The main aim of dietary treatment is to minimise fatty acid oxidation. Because fatty acids for oxidation are derived from both dietary fat and adipose tissue, it is usual practice to restrict the intake of dietary fat and to institute frequent feeding with a high carbohydrate intake to reduce production of fatty acids from adipose tissue. The safe upper limit for long chain fat intake is unknown and will vary with the severity of the disorder.

In patients with VLCAD and TFP defects (including LCHAD deficiency), MCT provides a useful energy source and may have other beneficial effects [14]. Dietary MCT is absorbed through the hepatic portal vein and is rapidly converted to ketone bodies. These inhibit the mobilisation of fatty acids from adipose tissue and the oxidation of fatty acids by cardiac muscle. MCFAs may also suppress long chain fatty acid oxidation without being converted to ketone bodies; they have been

shown to inhibit the accumulation of potentially toxic long chain intermediates in cultured skin fibroblasts from LCHAD and TFP deficient patients [15]. It has therefore been suggested that patients should maintain a high intake of MCT throughout life (10–20% energy intake) [16].

The role of MCT is less clear in defects of the carnitine cycle. In several infants with CPT I deficiency, renal tubular acidosis has only resolved when they have been changed to an MCT based feed. MCT has also been used with apparent benefit in patients with mild CAT deficiency. In patients with severe CAT and CPT II deficiencies, however, use of MCT has sometimes been abandoned because it led to markedly abnormal blood acylcarnitines and dicarboxylic aciduria. This may be because commercially available MCT preparations contain large amounts of C10 fatty acids and under normal circumstances these enter mitochondria partly bound to carnitine.

Triheptanoin, an oil containing C7 fatty acids, has recently been substituted for conventional MCT in a number of patients with long chain fatty acid oxidation defects. Improved cardiac function and/or muscle weakness has been reported in three patients with VLCAD deficiency [17]. Use of MCT leads to the production of acetyl-CoA but it is hypothesised that a shortage of oxaloacetate prevents this from being oxidised in the citric acid cycle. Triheptanoin generates acetyl-CoA and also propionyl-CoA. The latter can be converted to oxaloacetate, which acts as an 'anaplerotic' substrate for the citric acid cycle. Care is needed to avoid excessive weight gain in patients on triheptanoin. Triheptanoin is not yet widely available outside the centre that has pioneered its use (Baylor University Medical Center, Texas, USA).

Frequent feeding is recommended to reduce lipolysis, with 3-hourly feeding during the day and continuous nasogastric or gastrostomy feeding overnight. If this is not possible, the child should be woken for feeds during the night. Uncooked cornstarch (UCCS) can provide a source of 'slow release glucose' and in older children it may replace continuous tube feeding overnight. It may also be useful for some children during the daytime to extend the interval between feeding times. Before use, the metabolic response to UCCS should be assessed because this varies between patients (p. 430). Patients with mild variants of the disorders may tolerate overnight fasting without problems.

Patients on minimal long chain fat diets require supplements of fat-soluble vitamins and essential fatty acids (EFA). At least 1% of total energy intake should come from linoleic acid and 0.2% from α-linolenic acid [18]. Most sources of EFA (such as walnut oil) do not provide long chain polyunsaturated fatty acids (LCPUFA), such as arachidonic, eicosapentaenoic and docosahexaenoic acids (DHA), but these are expected to be synthesised from the EFA that are provided. DHA deficiency has been reported in LCHAD deficient patients but, in the author's experience, this is rare if patients are receiving adequate EFA in the form of walnut oil [19].

It remains uncertain whether carnitine supplements should be given to patients with long chain fatty acid oxidation disorders. Plasma free carnitine concentrations are often below the normal range, particularly after episodes of illness, but not low enough to affect fatty acid oxidation. Supplements may facilitate the excretion of metabolites but, by increasing the level of long chain acylcarnitines, it is possible that they may increase the risk of arrhythmias. Creatine treatment is reported to have improved muscle strength in a few patients.

The following provides a guide to the typical energy distribution and long chain fat intake of the diet for long chain disorders (based on personal practice):

- 70–75% energy from carbohydrate
- 10–15% energy from protein
- Up to 20% energy from medium chain fat (depending on the disorder)
- 1.2–2% energy from EFAs

Long chain fat intake (including EFAs):

- Infants: <3 g/day
- 1–3 years: up to 6 g/day
- 4–8 years: up to 8 g/day
- 8–12 years: up to 12 g/day

Similar dietary practices are reported to be used by others [16].

Minimal long chain fat diet – practical aspects

Infants

Infants need a minimal long chain fat (LCT), high carbohydrate feed with frequent feeding. This can

Table 19.2   Nutritional content per 100 mL Monogen standard dilution (17.5%).

Energy	74.2 kcal (313 kJ)
Protein	2 g
Carbohydrate	12 g
Fat	2.1 g
MCT* (90%)	1.89 g
LCT (10%)	0.21 g
Ratio n6 : n3 fatty acids 4.6 : 1	
% energy from	
Linoleic acid	1.0
α-Linolenic acid	0.21

* 49 g of C8:0 and 36 g of C:10 fatty acids per 100 g fatty acids.
Reconstitution: 1 scoop (5 g) added to 25 mL or 1 oz water.

be provided by, e.g. Monogen, a nutritionally complete infant formula with minimal LCT (Table 19.2). Monogen contains MCT, so it is important to establish if MCT can be oxidised before using this feed. MCT Step 1 is very similar in composition to Monogen and is a suitable alternative. A modular feed without fat (long or medium chain) may need to be used until the diagnosis is established and subsequently, if MCT is considered inadvisable (as in, perhaps, severe CAT or CPT II deficiencies). Skimmed milk powder or a whey protein powder (e.g. Vitapro) can be used as the protein base with glucose polymer and additional minerals and vitamins to provide recommended intakes. EFAs should also be provided if the infant remains on a modular feed for several days. Scientific Hospital Supplies International Ltd produces a Low Fat Module feed (0.14 g fat/100 mL) which may also be useful during the initial stages of management.

The newly diagnosed infant is likely to be on intravenous (IV) 10% dextrose. While oral or nasogastric feeds are being introduced, IV fluids should be gradually reduced so that an adequate energy intake is maintained and further metabolic decompensation is prevented. The initial feeds given may vary depending on the clinical situation but should, if possible, provide 10 g carbohydrate/100 mL (10% CHO). Once the infant is well and established on full feeds of Monogen these should be given 3-hourly during the daytime and as a continuous feed overnight. The night feed can be commenced 2 hours after the last 3-hourly day feed was given and can probably be stopped 2 hours before the first oral feed in the morning. The amount of glucose required overnight to minimise lipolysis is not known. For older infants, current practice is to provide 0.5 g CHO/kg/hour which will equal basal glucose production rates (see p. 391) and should therefore minimise lipolysis. This amount will easily be exceeded in the young infant who is being fed Monogen throughout the day and night at normal fluid requirements.

Weaning is commenced at the normal time around 6 months (26 weeks) of age. Solids should have a minimal fat content (<3 g/day) and be high in CHO. Rice cereal, potato, fruit and vegetables are suitable as first weaning foods. Once these have been introduced, low fat, high protein foods can also be given (e.g. turkey, white fish, lentils and low fat yoghurt). Commercial baby foods can be included in the diet but need to be limited to those which have a low fat content. Wet baby foods with a fat content of <0.5 g/100 g and dried baby foods with a fat content of <2 g/100 g can be given freely (Table 19.3). Baby foods with a higher fat content need to be counted as part of the daily fat intake. Parents can be taught how to calculate the amount of fat a food provides from the nutritional labelling (discussed in more detail below). As the amount of starchy solid food increases, this should replace some of the 3-hourly Monogen day feeds. At least 1.5 g CHO/kg (or 0.5 g CHO/kg/hour) is needed to replace one of the 3-hourly Monogen feeds. Infants who eat well will easily exceed this amount of CHO in a meal but the amount of solids taken needs to be checked in those who feed poorly. MCT oil can be incorporated into the diet of older infants who are eating well. Use of MCT oil is described in more detail below. Table 19.3 provides a suggested menu plan for infants.

Monogen can continue to be given overnight, but large volumes are needed to provide the required amount of CHO and this may interfere with the daytime appetite or lead to excessive weight gain. By 1 year of age, the volume of Monogen has usually been decreased and glucose polymer added to provide the required amount of CHO (0.5 g CHO/kg/hour).

Fat-soluble vitamin supplements will be required once the daily intake of Monogen becomes <600 mL. Monogen will provide an adequate intake of EFAs when it is fed at 150 mL/kg and provides the sole source of nutrition. An additional source of

Table 19.3 Minimal long chain fat (<3 g) weaning diet: sample menu.

8 am Breakfast	*Commercial baby cereal mix with Monogen
11 am	Monogen feed
1 pm Lunch	Purée turkey, chicken (white only), white fish or lentils Purée potato Purée vegetables Commercial baby savoury foods*
4 pm Tea	Purée fruit and sugar or commercial baby fruit dessert* Very low fat yoghurt or fromage frais Milk pudding (custard, cornflour, ground rice) made with Monogen
7 pm	Monogen
9 pm to 6 am	Continuous overnight feed of Monogen 30 mL/hour provides 0.5 g CHO/kg/hour for a 7-kg infant

Extra feeds of Monogen or baby juice can be given with meals

* Commercial baby foods.
Allow freely: wet baby foods ≤0.5 g fat/100 g and dried baby foods ≤2 g fat/100 g.
Allow one serve per day: wet baby foods 0.5–1.0 g fat/100 g or dried baby foods 2–5 g fat/100 g.
Walnut oil – refer to text for dose.

EFAs is needed once solids are being taken and the volume of Monogen decreases. Walnut oil provides a good source of EFAs at an acceptable ratio and allows a minimum amount of LCT to be given (Table 19.4). To provide the suggested require-

Table 19.4 Walnut oil – essential fatty acid composition.

1 mL walnut oil provides:	
Energy	8.4 kcal
	35 kJ
Fat	0.93 g
Linoleic acid	0.58 g
α-Linolenic acid	0.12 g
Ratio n6 : n3 fatty acids	4.5

Analysis from: Fatty acids 7th Supplement to *McCance and Widdowson's 'The Composition of Foods'* 5th edn. The Royal Society of Chemistry, Cambridge and the Ministry of Agriculture, Fisheries and Food, London, 1992.

ment of EFAs the dose of walnut oil needed is 0.1 mL/56 kcal (235 kJ) of the estimated average requirement (EAR) for energy for age [18], subtracting the energy provided by Monogen feeds. It is administered as a single dose and given as a medicine from a spoon or via the feeding tube. In the UK, walnut oil can be purchased from most large supermarkets. It should be stored as recommended to avoid peroxidation.

Children

Children should remain on a minimal LCT, high CHO diet, with an energy distribution as previously outlined. Inevitably, daily intake of long chain fat increases with age. The figures quoted above are based on the lowest possible long chain fat intake that is practicably achievable for that age, as the safe upper limit for long chain fat intake is not known. Ideally, the high CHO intake should be derived from starchy foods (e.g. rice, pasta, potato, bread, cereals) because these are more slowly digested than sugary foods. It is recognised, however, that some children cannot manage such a bulky diet and sugar containing foods, such as jelly, low fat ice cream, cake or biscuits, should form part of their diet. The diet should contain very low fat sources of protein, such as white fish, white chicken or turkey meat, pulses (Table 19.5). Nowadays there

are many very low fat alternatives to regular high fat foods such as crisps, sauces, desserts, ice cream and cheeses, which can also be incorporated into the diet. To allow a greater variety of foods, parents need to be given guidance on interpreting food labels for fat content and on understanding the many and potentially misleading wording used to describe the fat content of food (e.g. reduced fat, low fat, virtually fat free, 90% fat free). The different types of fat (e.g. saturated, mono- and polyunsaturated) can cause confusion and it is helpful to explain that total fat should be used when calculating fat intake. Manufactured foods have nutritional labelling with the total fat content expressed as grams of fat per 100 g and sometimes also grams of fat per portion. Parents can be taught how to calculate the amount of food that provides 1 g fat, making it easier to monitor and calculate the daily fat intake. Manufactured foods which have a fat content of <0.5 g/100 g can generally be allowed in the diet freely, unless large amounts are being consumed.

MCT oil should be incorporated into the diet if possible because of the potential beneficial effects discussed above. Unless MCT oil is introduced, the intake of MCT will naturally fall as children get older and consume less of the MCT based infant formula. Use of MCT oil may also increase the palatability of the diet and some patients may profit

Table 19.5 Minimal long chain fat diet.

	Foods allowed	Foods to avoid
Milk	Skimmed milk, condensed skimmed milk Natural yoghurt, very low fat yoghurt and fromage frais Low fat cottage cheese 95% fat free cheeses* Quark (skimmed milk soft cheese) Low fat ice cream	Full fat and semi-skimmed milk. Cream Full fat yoghurt and fromage frais Full and half fat cheeses Ice cream†
Egg	Egg whites	Egg yolks
Fish	White fish (no skin), e.g. haddock, cod, sole, plaice Crab, crabsticks, tuna, prawns, shrimps, lobster	Oily fish, e.g. sardines, kippers, salmon, mackerel Fish in breadcrumbs, batter, sauces, pastry
Poultry	Chicken,* turkey* (white breast meat, no skin)	Chicken, turkey (dark meat and skin), basted poultry, duck Chicken in breadcrumbs, batter, sauces, pastry
Meat	Lean red meat* (<5% fat content)	Fatty meat, sausages (normal and low fat), burgers, meat paste, paté, salami, pies
Meat substitutes	Soya mince, Quorn,* tofu*	

Table 19.5   (Cont'd)

	Foods allowed	Foods to avoid
Pulses	Peas, e.g. chick peas, split peas, lentils Beans, e.g. red, white, borlotti, black-eyed	
Fats/oils	Medium chain triglyceride oil as permitted	Butter, margarine, low fat spread, vegetable oils, lard, dripping, suet, shortening
Pasta and rice	Spaghetti, macaroni, other pasta, noodles, cous cous, rice (white)	Wholemeal pasta, pasta in dishes, e.g. macaroni cheese, carbonara Brown rice, egg noodles
Flours and cereals	Flour (white), cornflour, custard powder, semolina, sago, tapioca	Flour (wholemeal), soya flour, oats, bran Foods made with flour which contain fat, e.g. pastry, sauces, cake, biscuits, batter, breadcrumb coatings
Breakfast cereals	Most are suitable Wholewheat cereals, e.g. Weetabix, bran flakes are higher in fat content than non-wholewheat cereals, e.g. Rice Krispies, cornflakes	Cereals with nuts, e.g. muesli All-bran, Ready Brek
Bread and crackers	White bread,* white pitta, crumpets, muffins Some crackers have a low fat content, e.g. rice cakes, Matzos, Ryvita (not sesame)	Wholemeal, wholegrain breads, nan bread, chapatti made with fat, croissant, oatcakes, cheese crackers, crackers[†]
Cakes and biscuits and pastry	Only those made from low fat ingredients 95% fat free cakes and biscuits*	Cakes,[†] biscuits,[†] buns, pastry for sweet and savoury foods, e.g. apple pie, quiche
Desserts	Jelly, meringue, sorbet, very low fat ice cream, skimmed milk puddings, e.g. rice, custard	Most desserts, e.g. whole milk puddings, trifle, cheesecakes, gateaux, mousse,[†] fruit pie or crumble
Fruit	Most varities – fresh, frozen, tinned, dried	Avocado pears, olives
Vegetables	All vegetables and salad Very low fat crisps*	Chips, crisps,[†] low fat crisps,[†] roast potato, potato or vegetable salad in mayonnaise or salad dressing, coleslaw[†]
Herbs and spices	Pickles, chutney Herbs, spices, salt, pepper	
Nuts and seeds		Nuts, peanut butter, seeds, e.g. sesame, sunflower
Sauces and gravies	Tomato ketchup, brown sauce, soy sauce, Marmite, Oxo, Bovril, very low fat gravy mixes Very low fat dressings and mayonnaise Minimal fat sauces (jars, tins, packets)	Gravy granules,[†] stock cubes[†] Salad cream, mayonnaise, oil and vinegar dressings Sauce mixes[†] (jars, tins, packets)
Soups	Some low calorie and 'healthy eating type' soups are very low fat	Most soups, cream soups
Confectionery	Boiled sweets, jelly sweets, fruit gums, pastilles, marshmallow, mints, ice-lollies fudge	Chocolate, chocolate covered sweets, toffee
Sugars and preserves	Sugar, golden syrup, jam, marmalade, honey, treacle	Lemon curd, chocolate spread
Baking products	Baking powder, bicarbonate of soda, yeast, arrowroot, essences, food colouring	
Drinks	Fruit juice, squash, fizzy drinks, milk shake flavourings, tea, coffee	Instant chocolate drinks,[†] cocoa, malted milk type drinks, e.g. Horlicks

* Intake of these foods may need to be restricted because of their fat content.
[†] These foods in the 'avoid list' often have very low fat equivalents which can be included in the diet.

from this alternative source of energy. MCT oil contains predominantly C8 and C10 fatty acids (96 g/100 g total fatty acids) and is suitable for children with long chain β-oxidation defects. MCT oil has a low smoke point compared with other cooking oils. Care must be taken to ensure it does not burn or become overheated as it develops a bitter taste and an unpleasant odour. The optimum cooking temperature for MCT is 160°C. MCT oil can be used for cooking and baking (e.g. cakes, biscuits and pastry). Recipes are available from SHS International Ltd.

EFA need to be provided in the diet and this can be provided from Monogen and/or walnut oil as described for infants. Supplements of fat-soluble vitamins (A, D and E) will also be needed unless the child remains on >600 mL/day Monogen. Intakes of iron, zinc and B_{12} should be regularly calculated as these can be low on minimal LCT diets. Forceval Junior capsules can provide an adequate intake of fat-soluble vitamins and minerals.

Lipolysis can be minimised by 3–4-hourly feeding during the day and continuous overnight tube feeds. The amount of glucose given overnight should at least equal basal glucose production rates for age (around 0.3–0.5 g CHO/kg/hour). It is not yet clear whether the night time feed should be changed to glucose polymer or whether it is helpful to continue some MCT at night (e.g. by using a mixture of glucose polymer and Liquigen; 52% MCT oil emulsion) [20]. In older children, it may be safe to stop the overnight feeds and substitute with one or more doses of UCCS. It is difficult to be sure, however, whether this treatment is as effective in preventing long term complications. UCCS is generally introduced at home to test its palatability and tolerance. Before changing management, it is the author's practice to assess the child's metabolic response by serial measurement of plasma free fatty acids, blood glucose and long chain 3-hydroxyacylcarnitines after a dose of UCCS. The results of these studies are used to plan how frequently a dose of UCCS needs to be given. Experience with a few older children (>8 years) has shown this to be around 6–9 hourly, the fasting tolerance increasing with age. Doses of cornflour used are 1–1.5 g/kg/dose in older children. It should be given raw because cooking or heating disrupts the starch granules and thus makes it much less effective. It is usually mixed with Monogen or skimmed milk.

The dose of UCCS is gradually increased, starting with 5 g and increasing in 5 g increments every few days or weeks to the full amount.

Feeding problems are common in children with long chain fatty acid oxidation disorders, particularly in early childhood and these can occur despite good metabolic and clinical condition [21]. Early recognition and management of feeding problems is important.

Exercise induced rhabdomyolysis occurs in many patients with long chain fatty acid oxidation defects, including adults with partial deficiencies of CPT II or VLCAD, who experience no other problems. As yet, no treatment has conclusively been shown to prevent rhabdomyolysis. Some patients appear to benefit from taking a high CHO drink before exercise; a low fat, high carbohydrate diet has also been reported to help these patients [22].

Minimal long chain fat, high CHO with frequent feeding diet – monitoring

Once an infant or child is established on dietary treatment, families need continued support and advice. Regular monitoring of this complex diet is essential to:

- Ensure an adequate intake of fat-soluble vitamins and EFA
- Ensure the overnight feeds provide adequate CHO
- Check the intake of long and medium chain fat
- Provide new ideas and information on low fat manufactured foods
- Check the emergency regimen for CHO concentration and volume and parents' understanding of its use

Clinical monitoring includes review of weight, growth, development, muscle and liver function. Cardiomyopathy usually resolves on institution of a minimal LCT diet supplemented with MCT. Thereafter cardiac function is usually monitored annually. Ophthalmological follow-up is important in LCHAD deficiency. Blood acylcarnitine concentrations may correlate with the outcome in these disorders. In LCHAD deficiency, for example, the long chain 3-hydroxyacylcarnitine concentrations appear to correlate with the progression of retinal disease [23]. Monitoring of acylcarnitines may therefore be useful in guiding dietary management. Fat-soluble vitamins, EFA and LCPUFA concentrations should probably be monitored but the optimal frequency is uncertain.

Diet during illness for long chain fatty acid oxidation disorders

If the child becomes unwell and has a reduced appetite the standard ER of very frequent feeds of glucose polymer, day and night, should be given (see p. 375). In patients with a gastrostomy or nasogastric tube, the drinks can be given via the tube if refused orally. The ER needs to be started promptly to inhibit the mobilisation of fatty acids as decompensation may be rapid. Long chain fat is strongly contraindicated and if the diet contains MCT it is best avoided initially. As the child improves, the normal diet can be resumed. While the normal diet is being reintroduced it is essential to maximise energy intake and continue with frequent feeding, usually 2 to 3-hourly by day and continuous tube feeds overnight.

Patients with cardiomyopathy should probably be admitted during any intercurrent illness because there is a risk of deteriorating cardiac function. Families should also be warned to look for dark urine, because illness can precipitate rhabdomyolysis with myoglobinuria and, occasionally, acute renal failure. As in MCAD deficiency, blood glucose monitoring by parents is not recommended because hypoglycaemia is a relatively late finding and treatment should be initiated long before this develops [7].

Multiple acyl-CoA dehydrogenase deficiency

Multiple acyl-CoA dehydrogenase deficiency (MADD, also known as glutaric aciduria type II) is caused by defects of ETF or ETF dehydrogenase. These molecules pass electrons from a number of dehydrogenase enzymes to the mitochondrial respiratory chain. The dehydrogenases include the acyl-CoA dehydrogenases of β-oxidation and also enzymes involved in choline metabolism and the breakdown of several amino acids (lysine, tryptophan and the branch chain amino acids). Impaired fatty acid oxidation seems to be responsible for most of the problems in patients with MADD.

MADD has a wide range of clinical severity. All forms of the disorder can cause hypoglycaemic encephalopathy. The most severely affected patients present with congenital malformations, such as renal cystic dysplasia leading to pulmonary hypoplasia (Potter's syndrome). Less severely affected patients may present with cardiomyopathy (usually as neonates) or with muscle weakness (at any age). Some mild cases show a clinical and biochemical response to riboflavin (100–200 mg/day). These patients usually present with progressive weakness as young adults, although there may be a long history of vague symptoms such as abdominal migraine [24].

Dietary management

In patients with severe congenital malformations, no treatment is effective or appropriate. At the other end of the spectrum, some patients respond completely to riboflavin and no dietary modification is necessary.

Most patients with MADD require a low fat diet. Severely affected patients may also profit from a modest protein restriction, because MADD affects the breakdown of some amino acids in addition to fatty acids. Designing an appropriate diet can be difficult and the degree of restriction needs to be tailored to the individual patient. Regular feeding with a high CHO intake is recommended to reduce lipolysis. Overnight fasting should be avoided in patients towards the severe end of the spectrum. A late night snack may be sufficient in some patients but others require a continuous overnight feed. UCCS could be substituted in older children to provide a 'slow release' source of glucose. It is essential to assess tolerance individually.

MCT should be avoided in MADD deficiency as it has appeared to have precipitated problems in some patients [25]. MCFA can enter the mitochondria independent of carnitine, bypassing CPT I, the step at which β-oxidation is normally regulated. High concentrations of toxic metabolites may therefore be generated.

Some patients with severe MADD have deteriorated despite the above dietary measures. Oral treatment with the ketone body, 3-hydroxybutyrate, has led to sustained clinical improvement in a few such patients [26].

Dietary guidelines are to provide:

- 65–70% energy from carbohydrate
- 8–10% energy from protein
- 20–25% energy from fat
- Frequent feeding to tolerance

During illness the standard emergency regimen of very frequent feeds, day and night, of glucose polymer should be given to minimise endogenous protein catabolism and lipolysis (see p. 375). These should be given via a tube if not managed orally. Fat should be avoided during the acute period. The usual diet can be introduced during the recovery period, but it is important to continue with frequent feeding and additional glucose polymer feeds until the normal diet is resumed.

3-Hydroxy-3-methylglutaryl-CoA synthase deficiency

Patients with 3-hydroxy-3-methylglutaryl-CoA (HMG-CoA) synthase deficiency present with hypoketotic hypoglycaemia during infancy or early childhood. They are generally thought to have a fatty acid oxidation defect until investigations exclude these conditions. Few patients have been reported as yet but outcomes appear to be good [27].

Dietary management

Patients do not require any dietary modification when they are well but prolonged fasting should be avoided. A standard ER (see p. 375) should be used during intercurrent illnesses, with frequent drinks containing glucose polymer, day and night. In the event of persistent vomiting, hospital admission is needed for an IV infusion containing glucose.

3-Hydroxy-3-methylglutaryl-CoA lyase deficiency

HMG-CoA lyase catalyses the final step in the synthesis of ketone bodies. HMG-CoA is formed predominantly using acetyl-CoA derived from fatty acid oxidation but it is also formed during the catabolism of leucine. Patients with HMG-CoA lyase deficiency normally present either in the early neonatal period or during an intercurrent illness later in infancy. Initial symptoms of vomiting and lethargy can progress to coma, with hypoketotic hypoglycaemia and lactic acidosis [28].

Dietary management

A standard emergency regimen (see p. 375) is used during intercurrent infections. This will prevent hypoglycaemia and reduce protein catabolism and lipolysis, limiting the production of potentially toxic metabolites. Patients can become anorexic at an early stage refusing all ER drinks. It is essential feeds are therefore given via a nasogastric tube at home or in hospital. If the child vomits or deteriorates despite taking feeds/drinks, an IV infusion containing glucose is necessary; sodium bicarbonate may also be required to correct acidosis. During the recovery phase the usual diet can be reintroduced over a period of a few days.

When well, patients can be on a normal diet but it is important to avoid prolonged fasting as this might lead to metabolic decompensation. It seems reasonable to continue a night time feed until the age of 1 year, as for MCAD deficiency. Older children tolerate overnight fasting without problems but they should be given a bedtime snack containing starch. Missed meals should be replaced with a high CHO drink. MCT should be avoided. Protein restriction has been recommended but this is probably not necessary as patients can do well without this (personal communication, J.V. Leonard). Carnitine supplements are often given but, again, their value is unproven.

Acknowledgement

I thank Dr Andrew Morris, Royal Manchester Children's Hospital, Manchester for his invaluable contribution to this chapter.

References

1   Roe C, Ding J Mitochondrial fatty acid oxidation disorders. In: Scriver C *et al.* (eds) *The Metabolic and*

Molecular Bases of Inherited Disease, 8th edn. New York: McGraw Hill, 2001, pp. 2297–326.

2 Seddon HR, Green A, Gray RGF *et al.* Regional variations in medium-chain acyl-CoA dehydrogenase deficiency (letter). *Lancet*, 1995, **345** 135–6.

3 Oerton J *et al* Newborn Screening for MCADD: preliminary findings from the UK Collaborative study. *Arch Dis Child*, 2006, **91** (Suppl 1) Abstract P2.

4 Iafolla AK, Thompson RJ, Roe CR Medium-chain acyl-CoA dehydrogenase deficiency: clinical course in 120 affected children. *J Pediatr*, 1994, **124** 409–15.

5 Touma EH, Charpentier C Medium-chain acyl-CoA dehydrogenase deficiency. *Arch Dis Child*, 1992, **67** 142–5.

6 Wilcken B, Hammond J, Silink M Mortality and morbidity in medium chain acyl-coenzyme A dehydrogenase deficiency. *Arch Dis Child*, 1994, **70** 410–12.

7 Morris AAM, Leonard JV Early recognition of metabolic decompensation. *Arch Dis Child*, 1997, **76** 555–6.

8 Heales SJR, Thompson GN, Massoud AF *et al.* Production and disposal of medium-chain fatty acids in children with medium-chain acyl-CoA dehydrogenase deficiency. *J Inherit Metab Dis*, 1994, **17** 74–80.

9 Wilcken B, Carpenter KH, Hammond J Neonatal symptoms in medium chain acyl-coenzyme A dehydrogenase deficiency. *Arch Dis Child*, 1993, **69** 292–4.

10 Preece MA, Chakrapani A, Reynolds F MCADD: The perils of alcohol! *BIMDG Bull*, 2004, Winter, 22.

11 Lee PJ, Harrison EL, Jones MG *et al.* L-carnitine and exercise tolerance in medium-chain acyl-coenzyme A dehydrogenase (MCAD) deficiency: a pilot study. *J Inherit Metab Dis*, 2005, **28** 141–52.

12 Huidekoper HH, Schneider J, Westphal T *et al.* Prolonged moderate-intensity exercise without and with L-carnitine supplementation in patients with MCAD deficiency. *J Inherit Metab Dis*, 2006, **29** 631–6.

13 Deschauer M, Weiser T, Zierz S Muscle carnitine palmitoyltransferase II deficiency clinical and molecular genetic features and diagnostic aspects. *Arch Neurol*, 2005, **62** 37–41.

14 Morris AAM, Turnbull DM Fatty acid oxidation defect in muscle. *Curr Opin Neurol*, 1998, **11** 485–90.

15 Jones PM, Butt Y, Bennett M Accumulation of 3-hydroxy-fatty-acids in the culture medium of long-chain-3-hydroxyacyl CoA dehydrogenase (LCHAD) and mitochondrial trifunctional protein-deficient skin fibroblasts: implications for medium chain triglyceride dietary treatment of LCHAD deficiency. *Pediatr Res*, 2003, **53** 783–7.

16 Gillingham MB, Connor WE, Matern D *et al.* Optimal dietary therapy of long-chain 3-hydroxyacyl-CoA dehydrogenase deficiency. *Mol Genet Metab*, 2003, **79** 114–23.

17 Roe CR, Sweetman L, Roe DS *et al.* Treatment of cardiomyopathy and rhabdomyolysis in long-chain fat oxidation disorders using an anaplerotic odd-chain triglyceride. *J Clin Invest*, 2002, **110** 259–69.

18 Department of Health Report on Health and Social Subjects No 41. *Dietary Reference Values for Food Energy and Nutrients for the United Kingdom.* London: The Stationery Office, 1991.

19 Lund AM, Dixon MA, Vreken P *et al.* Plasma and erythrocyte fatty acid concentrations in long-chain 3-hydroxyacyl CoA dehydrogenase deficiency. *J Inherit Metab Dis*, 2003, **26** 410–12.

20 Lund AM, Dixon MA, Vreken P *et al.* What is the role of medium chain triglycerides in the management of long-chain 3-hydroxyacyl-CoA dehydrogenase deficiency? *J Inherit Metab Dis*, 2003, **26** 353–60.

21 Lund AM, Leonard JV Feeding difficulties in long-chain 3-hydroxyacyl-CoA dehydrogenase deficiency. *Arch Dis Child*, 2001, **85** 487–8.

22 Orngreen MC, Ejstrup R, Vissing J Effect of diet on exercise tolerance in carnitine palmitoyl transferase II deficiency. *Neurology*, 2003, **61** 559–61.

23 Gillingham MB, Weleber RG, Neuringer M *et al.* Effect of optimal dietary therapy upon visual function in children with long-chain 3-hydroxyacyl CoA dehydrogenase and trifunctional protein deficiency. *Mol Genet Metab*, 2005, **86** 124–33.

24 Frerman FE, Goodman SI Defects of electron transfer flavoprotein and electron transfer flavoprotein ubiquinone oxidoreductase including glutaric acidaemia type II. In: Scriver C *et al.* (eds) *The Metabolic and Molecular Bases of Inherited Disease*, 8th edn. New York: McGraw Hill, 2001, pp. 2357–65.

25 Moore SJ, Hailes NE, Broom I *et al.* Acylcarnitine analysis in the investigation of myopathy. *J Inherit Metab Dis*, 1998, **21** 427–8.

26 Van Hove JL, Grunewald S, Jacken J *et al.* D,L-3-hydroxybutyrate treatment of multiple acyl-CoA dehydrogenase deficiency (MADD). *Lancet*, 2003, **361** 1433–5.

27 Thompson GN, Hsu BY, Pitt JJ *et al.* Fasting hypoketotic coma in a child with deficiency of mitochondrial 3-hydroxy-3-methylglutaryl-CoA synthase. *N Engl J Med*, 1997 **337** 1203–7.

28 Sweetman L, Williams JC Branched chain organic acidurias. In: Scriver C *et al.* (eds) *The Metabolic and Molecular Bases of Inherited Disease*, 8th edn. New York: McGraw Hill, 2001, pp. 2125–63.

20 Lipid Disorders

Patricia Rutherford

Introduction

There are three main types of lipid in the body: triglycerides, cholesterol and phospholipids. They are transported in the serum bound to specific proteins called apolipoproteins to form the four major lipoprotein families (Table 20.1). Each of these lipoproteins contain a different amount of cholesterol and triglyceride and have different functions:

- *Chylomicrons* carry dietary triglycerides from the intestine to peripheral tissues
- *Very low density lipoproteins (VLDL)* are synthesised by the liver and carry excess triglycerides produced by the liver to other tissues

- *Low density lipoproteins (LDL)* are formed from VLDL and transport cholesterol from the liver to the peripheral tissues
- *High density lipoproteins (HDL)* transport excess cholesterol from the cells to the liver for excretion in the bile

Disorders of lipid metabolism which are managed by dietary intervention can be classified into those in which serum lipoproteins are deficient or absent (hypolipoproteinaemia) or those in which they are increased (hyperlipoproteinaemia) (Tables 20.2 and 20.3). The nature of the lipid disorder

Table 20.1 Composition of lipoproteins.

Lipoprotein class	Principal lipids	Major apolipoproteins
Chylomicrons	Dietary triglycerides	A, B, C
VLDL	Endogenous triglycerides	B, C, E
LDL	Cholesterol ester and cholesterol	B
HDL	Cholesterol ester and phospholipid	A

HDL, high density lipoprotein; LDL, low density lipoprotein; VLDL, very low density lipoprotein.

Table 20.2 Classification and treatment of hypolipoproteinaemias.

Primary disorder	Lipoprotein class	Treatment
Abetalipoproteinaemia	Chylomicrons LDL	Very low fat diet Vitamin A, E, K supplements MCT not recommended
Hypobetalipoproteinaemia	LDL	None usually indicated Low fat diet if steatorrhoea is a problem

LDL, low density lipoprotein; MCT, medium chain triglyceride.

Table 20.3 Classification of hyperlipoproteinaemias.

Primary disorder	Lipoprotein class
Familial hyperchylomicronaemia (type I)	Chylomicrons
Familial hypercholesterolaemia (type IIa)	LDL
Familial combined hyperlipidaemia (type IIb)	LDL
	VLDL
Familial type III hyperlipidaemia (broad beta disease)	IDL
Familial hypertriglyceridaemia (type IV)	VLDL
Familial hyperlipoproteinaemia (type V)	Chylomicrons

IDL, intermediate density lipoprotein; LDL, low density lipoprotein; VLDL, very low density lipoprotein.

should be determined by measurement of serum lipoprotein fractions as well as total serum cholesterol and triglycerides.

Hyperlipidaemia, secondary to diabetes, nephrotic syndrome or glycogen storage disease, is treated by management of the underlying disease and specific dietary measures are not usually necessary. The dietary management of the primary disorders that are genetically inherited is reviewed. A brief description of the biochemical defect of each disorder is given; more detailed information on the biochemistry can be found in the references at the end of the chapter.

Hypolipoproteinaemias

All the primary hypolipoproteinaemias (Table 20.2) are rare and only abetalipoproteinaemia and occasionally hypobetalipoproteinaemia require dietary management.

Abetalipoproteinaemia

This is an autosomal recessive disorder characterised by the virtual absence of VLDL, LDL and chylomicrons from plasma. It is thought that abetalipoproteinaemia is caused by defects in the processing of β apolipoproteins or impairment of the assembly or secretion of triglyceride rich proteins [1]. The clinical features of abetalipopro-

teinaemia are diverse. The presenting clinical feature is usually severe fat malabsorption seen in the neonatal period as steatorrhoea and failure to gain weight. This is accompanied by low plasma levels of vitamins E, A and K. Other features are acanthocytosis of red blood cells, neurological lesions and ocular manifestations, predominantly retinitis pigmentosa.

The onset of neurological symptoms may be during the first year of life; ophthalmic symptom onset is variable but may begin during the first decade. The neurological and ophthalmic manifestations appear to be secondary to defects of transport of vitamin E; vitamin A deficiency may also contribute to retinopathy [1,2]. Despite the inability to secrete chylomicrons there does appear to be some absorption of long chain fatty acids [3]. These are probably transferred to the liver as free fatty acids. Levels of essential fatty acids are low in plasma and tissue although clinical deficiency is not reported. Treatment results in catch-up growth and further growth and development is normal.

Dietary management

The gastrointestinal symptoms respond to a low fat diet. The degree of fat restriction is determined by individual tolerance which increases with age and intake and can vary from 5 g/day in infants to 20 g/day in the older child. Although clinical deficiency of essential fatty acids (EFAs) has not been reported, a proportion of dietary fat should be provided as EFAs. Recommendations are that for infants, children and adults, linoleic acid should provide at least 1% of the total energy, and α-linolenic acid at least 0.2% of the total energy [4]. It should be borne in mind that these are minimum requirements for EFAs and their absorption will be impaired. At present there is no specific guidance for EFA supplementation in abetalipoproteinaemia and individual tolerance of total fat limits the amount of supplement that can be given. Individual monitoring of EFA status is recommended in order to optimise EFA supplementation.

Medium chain triglyceride
Fatty acids derived from medium chain triglyceride (MCT) do not require chylomicrons for absorption as they are transported via the hepatic portal system. Reports of hepatic fibrosis have, however,

Table 20.4   Minimal fat feed for infants for use in abetalipoproteinaemia.

Per 100 mL	Energy		Protein (g)	CHO (g)	Fat (g)	Sodium (mmol)	Potassium (mmol)
	(kJ)	(kcal)					
2 g Vitapro	30	7	1.5	0.2	0.12	<0.3	<0.4
15 g Glucose polymer	225	60	0	14	0	Trace	Trace
Water to 100 mL							
Total	255	67	1.5	14.2	0.12	<0.3	<0.4

CHO, carbohydrate.
1 Fat can be added to tolerance using a long chain fat (LCT) emulsion (e.g. Calogen), and the glucose polymer can be decreased accordingly.
2 Vitamins, minerals, trace elements and electrolytes must be supplemented to ensure individual requirements are met.
3 A source of essential fatty acids is required to be added to the feed.

been associated with the use of MCT in abetal-ipoproteinaemia and its use is not recommended [5]. A case has been described where a patient developed cirrhosis independent of the use of MCT oil [6]. This patient subsequently required liver transplantation after which fat malabsorption and steatorrhoea persisted because the primary defect, a mutant microsomal triglyceride transfer protein, remained expressed in the intestine.

Infancy
In infancy a low fat modular feed can be formulated (Table 20.4) using a protein source (e.g. Vitapro or skimmed milk powder) glucose polymer and an essential fatty acid source (e.g. walnut oil or soya oil; see p. 427). A long chain fat (LCT) emulsion (Calogen) can then be added to tolerance. This feed will require vitamin, mineral and trace element supplementation, which should be tailored to meet individual requirements.

Weaning
Weaning foods should be introduced at the usual age of around 6 months. Very low fat foods are suitable (e.g. baby rice, fruit, vegetables and pulses) (see p. 427). The infant should continue to take enough feed to ensure nutritional requirements are met.

Childhood and adolescence
It is necessary to continue with the use of glucose polymers to ensure sufficient energy is taken and normal growth and development are achieved. With increasing age children may maintain energy

intakes by regular consumption of carbohydrate foods (e.g. sugar, sweets, jam, fizzy drinks, bread, pasta, potatoes and rice).

Many low fat products (e.g. biscuits, cakes and savoury foods) can be made by adapting standard recipes. Regular dietary assessment should be undertaken throughout life to ensure the diet remains nutritionally adequate.

Non-compliance with treatment may arise in the teenage years and particular attention should be paid to rates of growth and plasma levels of fat-soluble vitamins during this period.

Vitamins A, E and K
The following therapeutic doses were recommended in 1983 by Professor Lloyd's group [7]. To date these recommendations are still used.

- *Vitamin A:* 7000 µg/day to maintain normal plasma concentrations.
- *Vitamin E:* 100 mg/kg/day. Concentrated preparations now permit the convenient administration of these doses.
- *Vitamin K:* 5–10 mg/day.

It is not necessary to supplement vitamin D.

Hyperlipoproteinaemias

The main types of primary hyperlipoproteinaemia are summarised in Table 20.3 and the typing system advocated by the World Health Organization is used. The two most commonly encountered in childhood are familial hyperchylomicronaemia (type I) and familial hypercholesterolaemia (type IIa). These two are discussed in detail. The other disorders, familial combined hyperlipidaemia (type IIb), familial type III hyperlipidaemia, familial hypertriglyceridaemia (type IV) and familial hyper-lipoproteinaemia (type V) are rarely expressed in childhood and treatment is therefore not described.

Familial hyperchylomicronaemia (type I)

The manifestation of the clinical features of this rare disorder varies greatly and often the child is asymptomatic. The asymptomatic child may be diagnosed by a chance finding of turbid plasma when a blood sample is taken for some other reason, or the finding of hepatomegaly or lipaemia retinalis in an older child. Alternatively, the child may present with attacks of acute abdominal pain resulting from pancreatitis and/or eruptive xanthomata and hepatosplenomegaly. The classic disorder is caused by a molecular defect in the activity of the enzyme lipoprotein lipase. There is a group of patients who have a distinct molecular abnormality in the apolipoprotein CII activator of the lipoprotein lipase enzyme complex. These patients tend to present later than those with classic lipoprotein lipase deficiency [8]. It is inherited as an autosomal recessive trait. There is a failure to clear chylomicrons at the normal rate which leads to an accumulation in the serum and there is a gross elevation of triglycerides (35–115 mmol/L, normal fasting level 0.5–2.2 mmol/L) and moderate elevation of cholesterol. There is no current evidence that the high triglyceride levels are associated with an increased risk of atherosclerosis in later life. Growth and development are normal and clinical deficiency of linoleic acid has not been reported.

Dietary management

The aim of the dietary treatment is to relieve the symptoms. Restriction of fat to 5 g/day will result in optically clear fasting serum and lowering of serum triglycerides. However, it is difficult to maintain this restriction long term, and fat intake is determined by tolerance. Triglycerides will remain high but as the condition is not associated with premature atherosclerosis there is no need for severe dietary restriction.

Acute episodes

During attacks of acute abdominal pain, a fat-free diet should be given: <5 g/day LCT (see Table 13.12). This will produce a rapid decrease in serum triglyceride levels within 5–7 days. A suitable feed for an infant is shown in Table 20.4. Older children should have frequent high carbohydrate drinks and very low fat foods as tolerated.

Long term management

Fat
Fat intake can be gradually increased to tolerance, which is usually around 20–30 g/day, although there is individual variation. Tolerance does not seem to increase with age. The fat should be equally distributed between meals. The serum triglyceride level will increase, but the restriction should be sufficient to avoid attacks of acute pancreatitis or the development of xanthomata. In infants an LCT emulsion (Calogen) can then be added to the low fat feed (Table 20.4) to tolerance.

Medium chain triglycerides
MCT emulsion (Liquigen) can also be used to provide additional energy. A number of MCT based formulas are available (see Table 7.20). The amount of LCT in some of these feeds may be too high for the acute phase. Feeds containing MCT should always be introduced slowly and care should be taken to ensure that the feed provides sufficient EFAs [9].

In older children MCT oils and emulsions can also be used to provide extra energy and to improve the palatability of the diet. They should always be introduced slowly. MCT oils and emulsions can be used in cooking and baking.

Energy
Energy requirements can be met by the use of MCT, refined carbohydrates, and glucose polymers if necessary.

Vitamins and minerals
For infants on modular feeds, supplementation is essential. MCT based complete infant formula feeds should provide adequate intakes provided sufficient volume is taken. Older children should have a supplement of fat-soluble vitamins.

Familial hypercholesterolaemia (type IIa)

Familial hypercholesterolaemia (FH) is the most common primary lipoprotein disorder of childhood and is inherited as an autosomal dominant trait. It is characterised by an elevated plasma LDL concentration and deposition of LDL cholesterol in tendons, skin (xanthomata) and arteries (atheromas). The primary defect is a mutation in the gene for the LDL receptor in the hepatic and extrahepatic cells. This results in a reduction in the rate of removal of plasma LDL which is then deposited in the cells producing xanthomata and atheromas. The incidence of homozygous FH is 1 in 1 000 000. It is characterised by severe hypercholesterolaemia (plasma cholesterol levels approximately 16–26 mmol/L) and coronary heart disease which begins in childhood; death from myocardial infarction frequently occurs before the age of 20 years. Cholesterol levels in children are generally considered to be normal up to a level of 5 mmol/L. However, reference ranges will differ between laboratories, and plasma cholesterol levels will change throughout childhood because of the influences of growth and puberty. Homozygotes for FH are generally resistant to dietary treatment, and radical therapy such as plasma LDL apheresis or liver transplantation may be considered. The incidence of heterozygous FH is approximately 1 in 500 and is one of the most common inborn errors of metabolism. Plasma cholesterol levels are typically 9–14 mmol/L from birth. Tendon xanthomata and coronary atherosclerosis usually develop after 20–30 years [10]. For the purpose of this chapter diet therapy will refer to the treatment of heterozygous FH.

Screening

Routine screening for FH is not currently undertaken. The recommendations of the British Hyperlipidaemia Association are as follows [11]:

- The use of selective screening based on a family history of FH or of premature coronary artery disease (premature defined as <50 years for men and <55 years for women).
- Measurement of non-fasting total cholesterol as a suitable screening test. If >5.5 mmol/L, then measure fasting total cholesterol, HDL cholesterol and triglyceride.

- In a child under 16, total cholesterol >6.7 mmol/L and LDL cholesterol >4.0 mmol/L on two occasions more than 1 month apart should be considered abnormal.
- Screening should not be carried out before 2 years of age but hypercholesterolaemia should be diagnosed before 10 years of age.
- Affected children should be referred for specialist care.

Dietary management

The aim of dietary management is to lower total serum and LDL cholesterol in an attempt to decrease the risk of cardiovascular disease in later life.

Energy intake
This should be based on age, weight and activity levels [4]. Obesity itself is a risk factor for coronary heart disease and if present then weight reduction must be the primary goal of diet therapy.

Total fat intake
The principal aim of the diet traditionally used in the treatment of FH has been to reduce the total dietary fat to 30–35% of total energy intake. This is achieved by avoidance of fried foods and those known to be high in fat. In addition, low fat dairy products (e.g. skimmed or semi-skimmed milk, low fat cheese and low fat yoghurt) are advocated. Lean meat is usually advised to be taken only once per day, using beans, pulses, poultry and fish as protein sources in preference. Eggs may be included as part of the total fat allowance.

Compliance with this dietary treatment is often poor because of its potentially bulky nature and low satiety value. In addition, energy from carbohydrate sources is substituted for fat which results in a reduction in both HDL and LDL cholesterol [12]. Although this reduces total plasma cholesterol levels it leaves the LDL : HDL ratio unaffected and may not reduce the risk of coronary heart disease [13].

Saturated fatty acids
Saturated fatty acids (SFAs) are limited to provide <10% of the total energy intake. There is some clinical and experimental evidence that shows that a diet high in SFAs is associated with increased plasma cholesterol concentrations.

Dietary cholesterol

Uncertainty remains as to whether dietary cholesterol requires restriction. In support of a restriction it is suggested that saturated fat down-regulates the LDL receptor especially when cholesterol is concurrently present. Conversely, there is the view that there is a negative feedback mechanism on the synthesis of cholesterol by the intake of dietary cholesterol. Where dietary cholesterol restriction is practised, foods low in saturated fat but high in dietary cholesterol (e.g. prawns and liver) are also excluded from the diet.

Polyunsaturated fatty acids

Polyunsaturated fatty acids (PUFAs) lower LDL cholesterol but there are concerns regarding their safety if used excessively. It is generally recommended that their intake should not exceed 10% of the total energy intake [4].

Monounsaturated fatty acids

Monounsaturated fatty acids (MUFAs) have been shown to have a hypocholesterolaemic effect when substituted for SFAs in the diet. Replacing energy with MUFAs rather than carbohydrate does not result in a reduction in plasma HDL [14]. Significant reductions in coronary heart disease have been shown using increased consumption of MUFAs from rapeseed margarine in a group of people after myocardial infarction [15]. There are many other reports of the beneficial effects of the Mediterranean diet which is high in MUFAs. Replacing energy lost from SFAs by MUFAs is currently used in some treatment centres. Anecdotally, compliance with diet is reported to be better than with that of a low total fat diet. The long term consequences of this type of diet therapy for children with FH are unknown and this practice should perhaps be treated with caution until more information regarding its use has been gathered.

Garlic, oats and soy protein

A systematic review of trials in the general population suggested that garlic may exert a cholesterol lowering effect; however, the evidence is not reliable because of flaws in these trials. Systematic reviews of studies in the general population evaluating oat and soy protein consumption showed a cholesterol lowering effect [16].

Fat-soluble vitamins

If a low fat diet is to be used then fat-soluble vitamin supplementation may be required.

Evidence for effectiveness of diet in the treatment of FH

In order to examine the evidence for diet therapy in children with FH, a systematic review was carried out and published on the Cochrane Library in 2001 [17]. The objectives for this review were to examine the evidence that in children and adults with FH a cholesterol lowering diet is more effective at lowering total serum cholesterol and LDL cholesterol and reducing the incidence of ischaemic heart disease than: (i) no intervention; (ii) other dietary interventions. The cholesterol lowering diet in this review was defined as one that used the following principles: a reduction in total fat intake; a reduction in the intake of saturated fatty acids; a reduction in dietary cholesterol intake; an increase in carbohydrate intake to replace the energy deficit of the low fat diet. The criteria for trial inclusion were: types of trial – randomised controlled trials (RCTs) both published and unpublished; types of participants – children and adults with FH; types of intervention – cholesterol lowering diet or any other dietary intervention intended to lower serum total and LDL cholesterol. A period of at least 6 months' dietary intervention was initially set; however, there were no trials identified that were longer than 6 months in duration. After consultation with review referees it was decided to include short term trials as information on change in serum lipid levels, nutritional status and nutritional intake from such trials could be considered useful.

Description of trials

Only seven of 355 trials met the inclusion criteria for the review. All of these were randomised controlled cross-over trials. All were short term trials with each arm lasting 1–3 months. One of these trials [18] studied a defined group of participants with FH alongside participants with other forms of hypercholesterolaemia. This assessed the efficacy of plant sterols and included 62 participants; however, the data were combined for both groups. The remaining six trials included a total of 100 participants. The interventions of the six trials were:

- Cholesterol lowering diet compared with no intervention [19]
- Manipulating dietary fat intake by increasing fish oil consumption [20]
- Effect of soy products [21]
- Effect of plant stanols [22]
- Effect of a high protein diet [23]
- Effect of dietary sterols [24]

Results of review

The results showed no significant differences between the comparisons assessed. All the trials were short term and did not assess long term outcomes. It was disappointing to see only one trial that assessed the effect of a cholesterol lowering diet compared with no dietary intervention as this is the current recommended dietary treatment for FH. No conclusions can be made about the short or long term effectiveness of the cholesterol lowering diet or any other dietary interventions suggested for FH because of the lack of adequate trial data. The Cochrane Review recommended current dietary treatment for FH should be continued, carefully observed and monitored until further evidence is available. Large parallel RCTs are needed to investigate the effectiveness of dietary interventions for FH.

Compliance

Compliance with diet is often poor as children with FH feel well and they find it difficult to motivate themselves to keep to a diet to avert symptoms that may not present clinically for 20 years or more. Inevitably, compliance is always greater in families where there has been a parental death from coronary heart disease.

Drug therapy

Dietary intervention is routinely used as the first line of treatment in children. The introduction of drug therapy is influenced by plasma cholesterol concentration and family history. In the majority of cases long term management will be by a combination of drugs and diet. Drugs currently licensed for children are fenofibrate and ion exchange resins (colestyramine and colestipol). Resins are available in powder form and can be mixed as a drink or with food. They are poorly tolerated. If they are used

then fat-soluble vitamins and folate must be prescribed [25].

Since the late 1980s a new class of cholesterol lowering drugs – the statins (3-hydroxy-3-methyl-glutaryl-CoA [HMG-CoA] reductase inhibitors) – have become available which can dramatically reduce plasma LDL cholesterol concentrations. Atorvastatin has recently been licensed for children aged 10 and over.

Follow-up

Children with FH should ideally be seen in a combined adult/paediatric clinic to ensure dietary advice is uniform and to encourage the incorporation of advice into the family meal plan.

Emphasis should also be placed on the reduction of other risks for coronary heart disease (i.e. avoidance of smoking, increasing exercise, watching weight and managing stress).

References

1   Kane JP, Havel RJ Disorders of the biogenesis and secretion of lipoproteins. In: Scriver CR *et al.* (eds) *The Metabolic and Molecular Basis of Inherited Disease*, 7th edn. New York: McGraw-Hill, 1995.
2   Desjeux JF Congenital transport defects. In: Walker *et al.* (eds) *Paediatric Gastrointestinal Disease*, 2nd edn. St Louis: Mosby, 1996.
3   Hoghwinkel GJM, Brwyn GW Congenital lack of betalipoproteins. A study of blood phospholipids in a patient and his family. *J Neurol Sci*, 1996, **3** 374.
4   Department of Health Report on Health and Social Subjects No. 41. *Dietary Reference Values for Food, Energy and Nutrients for the United Kingdom*. London: The Stationery Office, 1991.
5   Illingworth DR, Connor WE, Miller RG Abetalipoproteinaemia: report of two cases and review of therapy. *Arch Neurol*, 1980, **37** 659.
6   Braegger CP, Belli DC, Mentha G, Steinmann B Persistence of the intestinal defect in abetalipoproteinaemia after liver transplantation. *Eur J Paediatr*, 1998, **157** 576–8.
7   Muller DPR, Lloyd JK, Wolf OH Vitamin E and neurological function. *Lancet*, 1983, **1** 225–8.
8   Nyham WL, Ozand PT *Atlas of Metabolic Diseases*. London: Chapman and Hall, 1998.
9   FAO/WHO *Dietary Fats and Oils in Human Nutrition*. Rome: FAO of the United Nations, 1980, pp. 21–37.
10 Goldstein JL, Hobbs H, Brown M Familial hypercholesterolaemia. In: Scriver CR *et al.* (eds) *The*

Metabolic and Molecular Basis of Inherited Disease, 7th edn. New York: McGraw-Hill, 1995.

11   Wray R, Neil H, Rees J Screening for hyperlipidaemia in childhood. Recommendations of the British Hyperlipidaemia Association. *J R Coll Physicians, London*, 1996, Mar–Apr **30** 115–18.

12   Durrington PN Dietary fat and coronary heart disease. In: Poulter N, Sever P, Thom S (eds) *Cardiovascular Disease. Risk Factors and Intervention*. Oxford: Radcliffe Medical Press, 1993.

13   Clarke R, Frost C, Collins R *et al.* Dietary lipids and blood cholesterol: quantitative meta-analysis of metabolic ward studies. *Br Med J*, 1997, **314** 112–17.

14   Colquhoun DM, Moores D, Somerset SS *et al.* Comparison of the effects on lipoproteins of a diet high in monounsaturated fatty acids enriched with avocado and a high carbohydrate diet. *Am J Clin Nutr*, 1992, **56** 671–7.

15   De Longeril M, Renaud S, Mamelle N *et al.* Mediterranean alpha linolenic acid rich diet in secondary prevention of coronary heart disease. *Lancet*, 1993, **343** 1454–9.

16   NHS Centre for Reviews and Dissemination. University of York. *Effective Health Care, Cholesterol and Coronary Heart Disease: Screening and Treatment*. Latimer Trend & Co. Ltd., 1998, **4** 1.

17   Poustie VJ, Rutherford PJ Dietary treatment for familial hypercholesterolaemia. *Cochrane Database Syst Rev* 2001, **2** CD001918.DOI.

18   Neil HA, Meijer GW, Roe LS Randomised controlled trial of use by hypercholesterolaemic patients of a vegetable oil sterol-enriched fat spread. *Atherosclerosis*, 2001, **156** 329–37.

19   Chisholm A, Mann J, Sutherland W, Williams S, Ball M Dietary management of patients with familial hypercholesterolaemia treated with simvastatin. *Quart J Med*, 1992, **85** 307–8, 825–31.

20   Balestrieri GP, Maffi V, Sleiman I *et al.* Fish oil supplementation in patients with heterozygous familial hypercholesterolaemia. *Recenti Prog Med*, 1996, **87** 102–5.

21   Laurin D, Jaques H, Moorjani S *et al.* Effects of a soy protein beverage on plasma lipoproteins in children with famililal hypercholesterolaemia. *Am J Clin Nutr*, 1991, **54** 98–103.

22   Gylling H, Siimes MA, Miettinen TA Sitostanol ester margarine in dietary treatment of children with familial hypercholesterolaemia. *J Lipid Res*, 1995, **36** 1807–12.

23   Wolfe BM, Giovannetti PM High protein diet complements resin therapy of familial hypercholesterolaemia. *Clin Invest Med*, 1992, **15** 349–59.

24   Amundsen AL, Ose L, Nenseter MS, Ntanios FY Plant sterol ester-enriched spread lowers plasma total and LDL cholesterol in children with familial hypercholesterolaemia. *Am J Clin Nutr*, 2002, **76** 338–44.

25   Tonstad S, Kudtzan J, Sivertsom M *et al.* Efficacy and safety of cholestyramine treatment in peripubertal and prepubertal children with familial hypercholesterolaemia. *J Paediatr*, 1996, **129** 4–7.

Useful address

Heart UK
www.heartuk.org.uk

21 Peroxisomal Disorders

Refsum's Disease

Eleanor Baldwin

Peroxisomal disorders

Peroxisomal disorders can be divided into two groups:

- Peroxisomal biogenesis disorders (PBDs) including infantile Refsum's disease (IRD), neonatal adrenoleukodystrophy (nALD) and Zellweger syndrome (ZS), which affect the peroxisomal targeting signal 1 (PTS-1) imported proteins; and rhizomelic chondrodysplasia (RCDP) which affects the peroxisomal targeting signal 2 (PTS-2) proteins
- Single enzyme disorders of the peroxisome, which include adult Refsum's disease (ARD) and X-linked adrenoleukodystrophy (X-ALD)

The main difference between these groups is that the peroxisomal biogenesis disorders have several defective metabolic functions and tend to present in infancy with severe clinical symptoms (including mental and physical retardation), while in the single enzyme peroxisomal disorders presentation is often later and the peroxisomal structure is intact. In both groups of disorders there may be high levels of phytanic acid in the plasma and fat containing tissues. Plasma phytanic acid levels are in the range 100–6000 μmol/L at diagnosis of ARD. In RCDP, levels are variable but elevated in the range 100–1000 μmol/L. Levels are usually lower in the IRD-ZS continuum at 100–200 μmol/L.

Levels are normal in single enzyme peroxisomal deficiencies that do not affect alphaoxidation of fatty acids. Pristanic acid levels are elevated in PBDs, but are low or normal in ARD.

Reference values for plasma phytanic acid

Normal: 0–20 μmol/L (usually <10)
Heterozygote for ARD: 5–30 μmol/L
Peroxisomal disease: 0–320 μmol/L
ARD after 1 year of treatment: 20–1000 μmol/L
ARD untreated: 100–6000 μmol/L
ARD stable on diet: 0–400 μmol/L

Adult Refsum's disease

ARD is a rare inborn error of lipid metabolism inherited as an autosomal recessive trait [1]. The chief characteristics are retinitis pigmentosa, anosmia, peripheral neuropathy, deafness and ataxia. Other manifestations, usually associated only with extremely high levels of phytanic acid, include ichthyosis and cardiomyopathy. Skeletal abnormalities if present seem to be congenital.

Patients accumulate phytanic acid (3,7,11,15-tetramethyl-hexadecanoic acid) in plasma and all fat containing tissues [1–3]. This unusual isoprenoid 20 carbon branched chain fatty acid is normally rapidly degraded in the human body (Fig. 21.1).

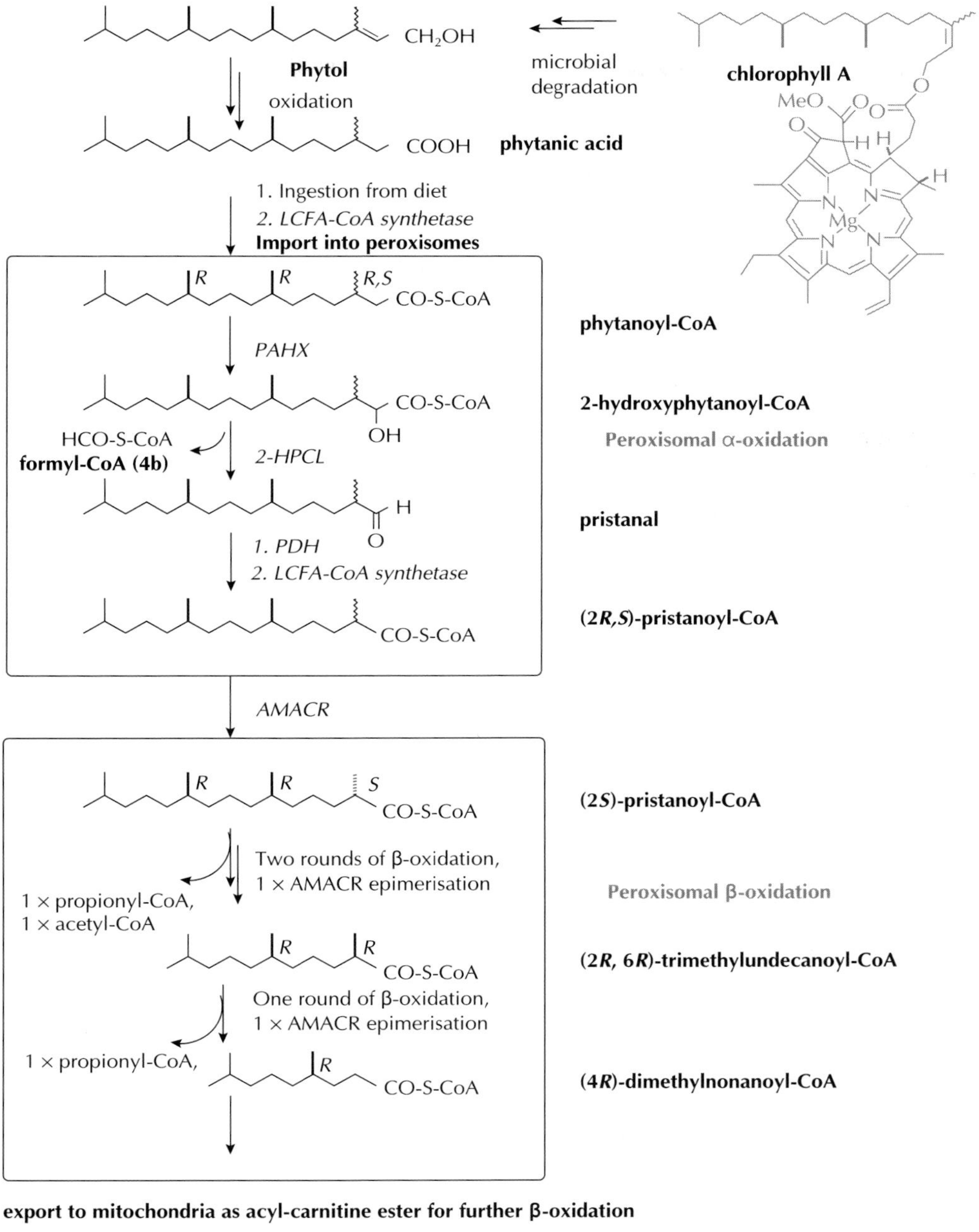

Figure 21.1   Metabolism of chlorophyll, phytol and metabolism of phytanic acid by α-oxidation.

Normal metabolism of phytanic acid involves peroxisomal α-oxidation, but an additional low capacity pathway through omega-oxidation and subsequent cycles of β-oxidation exist [4,5]. ARD

is mostly caused by a mutation of phytanoyl-coenzyme A hydroxylase (PhyH), which normally catalyses the second step in the breakdown of phytanic acid to pristanic acid using the CoA derivative as a substrate (the first step in α-oxidation is the conversion of phytanic acid to phytanoyl CoA by phytanoyl CoA ligase). The onset of symptoms is usually slow and diagnosis is often not made until the second to fifth decade of life, although some patients have been diagnosed in early childhood [1,6,7]. There is usually no developmental or mental retardation, but this has been reported in one child where symptoms presented at 7 months. It is possible this child was exposed to high phytanic acid levels *in utero* [7].

Phytanic acid is exogenous in origin being derived from the side-chain of chlorophyll and treatment is aimed at reducing plasma and tissue levels by means of a diet low in phytanic acid, which must be followed for life. Reduction of plasma phytanic acid levels significantly improves peripheral nerve function, ichthyosis and cardiac arrhythmias; it cannot, however, reverse the damage done to the sensory nerves, although further deterioration can be arrested. It is thought that in the case of young children, early diagnosis and treatment could delay or prevent the development of these irreversible lesions.

The clinical, biochemical and genetic features of ARD have been reviewed by Wierzbicki *et al.* and by Wanders *et al.* [1,2].

Peroxisomal biogenesis disorders

Patients with global peroxisomal biogenesis defects can also show raised plasma levels of phytanic acid [8]. These conditions (e.g. the IRD-nALD-ZS spectrum) must be distinguished from 'true' ARD. While patients with ARD appear to have an isolated enzyme defect, IRD is associated with many more defective metabolic functions including that of very long chain fatty acids (VLCFAs), especially hexacosanoic acid C26 : 0. These metabolic defects result in severe clinical symptoms, including mental and physical retardation, which present in infancy [8]. Some 5–10% of cases of ARD are caused by a mild phenotypic variant of RCDP caused by defective function of the peroxin-7 PTS-2 transporter, but clinically they are indistinguishable from ARD caused by mutations in PhyH [9,10].

A low phytanic acid diet may be requested for children with the IRD-nALD-ZS spectrum of

peroxisomal biogenesis defects and some improvement in behaviour has been claimed with this treatment. Restriction of C26 : 0 is generally advocated [11–13]. Supplementation with purified docasahexaenoic acid, mixed polyunsaturated fatty acids and erucic or oleic acids may be useful, but evidence is equivocal [14–19].

Because children with IRD also have abnormal metabolism of VLCFAs especially C26 : 0, as found in X-ALD, they might benefit from the dietary treatment applied in nALD. Similarly, although the severity of disease is greater in ZS there may be some benefit to diet strategies for reducing phytanic acid and C26 : 0 intake. There are few studies of the efficacy of low phytanic acid diets in RCDP but they are generally prescribed as PhyH function is impaired as part of this disorder. As some patients with classic ARD have a mild variant of RCDP and have benefited in terms of symptom alleviation and cessation of progression of disease, a low phytanic acid should be recommended for all patients with RCDP [10].

Dietary treatment of adult Refsum's disease

Although diagnosis is often not made until the second to fifth decade of life, some patients have been diagnosed in early childhood. The aims of dietary treatment are to:

- Avoid dietary sources of phytanic acid and free phytol. In patients compliant with diet plasma phytanic levels will halve approximately every 56 days until they stabilise [4]. However, fat-deposited phytanic acid is far more slowly released and may take years to be eliminated [20,21].
- Encourage appropriate weight gain and guard against weight loss (fasting and weight loss result in dramatic increases in the plasma phytanic acid levels as a result of the release of phytanic acid from the liver and from lipolysis in adipose tissue with a plasma phytanic acid doubling time of 29 hours) [4].
- Be aware that adrenergic stimulants (e.g. caffeine, theobromine, nicotine and cocaine) will result in increased hepatic and adipose tissue lipolysis with a consequent increase in plasma

phytanic acid levels [22]. Patients should be encouraged not to smoke and to maintain sensible consumption of caffeinated drinks.

- Ensure an adequate intake of all nutrients.

Dietary sources of phytanic acid

Phytanic acid derives from phytol, which is a part of the chlorophyll molecule. It is found in the fats of ruminant animals (cows, sheep and goats) and also of pelagic fish. The average western diet will provide 50–100 mg/day [20,23–25].

Free phytol in food is absorbed and metabolised to phytanic acid by humans and, therefore, potentially presents an additional source in the diet. Most phytol in food, however, is bound to chlorophyll which is poorly absorbed by humans [26,27]. The free phytol content of a typical western diet has been found to be <10% of the preformed phytanic acid [28]. The phytanic acid and free phytol content of some foods have been reported from various sources [25,29–33]. Varying values have been obtained for similar foods. This reflects the difficulty of the estimation and variation is expected when taking into account changes in the diet of animals, food processing methods (especially oils) and the composition of commercial food ingredients.

Little information is available on the phytol content of individual foods [33,34]. Again, published values show variation, reflecting perhaps the changes in food processing or the presence of other branched chain fatty acids. Initially, many fruits and vegetables were excluded from the diet as a potential source of phytol with the consequence that the diet was extremely restricted and unpalatable and vitamin supplements were necessary. In 1998 it was shown that fruit and vegetables could be introduced into the diet without any deterioration in clinical condition [33,34] and these are now permitted although some plant sources (e.g. peanuts) are rich in phytanic acid [34].

Patients with ARD have a residual capacity to metabolise phytanic acid by an alternative pathway involving omega-oxidation and subsequent cycles of beta-oxidation, resulting in the production of a variety of 3-methyl organic acids, including 3-methyl-hexadecanoic acid (Fig. 21.2). The capacity for omega-oxidation has been studied in adults with ARD. These small studies suggest a pathway with variable activity (6.9–30 mg phytanic acid may be metabolised daily by this route). The activity of this pathway seems to be increased when the plasma phytanic acid levels are high [4,5]. Accordingly, diets were devised to provide <10 mg/day phytanic acid based on published food analyses [25]. As recent analysis of foods has demonstrated the variability of these values foods are now simply placed in one of three groups. Actual values are in the literature [33].

Table 21.1 lists foods as presenting low, moderate or high risk for phytanic acid content based on recent analysis. Patients are advised to:

- Habitually choose low risk foods
- Avoid high risk foods altogether
- Limit their intake of moderate risk foods to one single choice (small portion, at the discretion and frequency suggested by the physician and dietitian)

Treatment on diagnosis

A child presenting with classic ARD may be anorexic and vomiting, making it very difficult to establish feeding. If plasma phytanic acid levels are very high, plasma exchange may be performed. It is vitally important to feed the child because any weight loss mobilises body fat stores, releasing further phytanic acid into the blood and exacerbating symptoms. If the child is not able to take adequate nutrition orally, then total or supplementary nasogastric feeding should be instituted as a matter of urgency.

Most commercial enteral feeding products are free from ruminant fats, but some contain fish oil, which is a rich source of phytanic acid. Suitable products are listed in Table 21.2 together with the origin of the vegetable oils used. The choice of feed should be made commensurate with the age and requirements of the child. If the child is able to eat, the diet should be devised to provide enough energy for growth appropriate for age and chosen from the low risk foods (Table 21.1). Weight gain is usually desirable at diagnosis and is, in itself, a useful means of reducing the plasma phytanic acid levels (by storing some phytanic acid in adipose tissue).

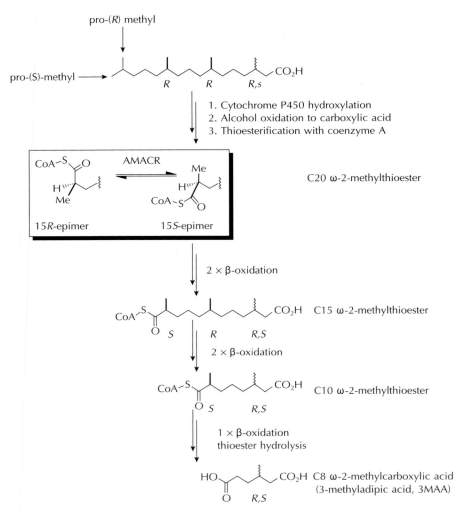

Figure 21.2   Alternative pathway of ω-oxidation of phytanic acid.

Supplements

Suitable nutritional supplements will almost certainly need to be prescribed to promote weight gain at the beginning of treatment. Their use can be discontinued at the discretion of the dietitian when the child is eating adequately and is clinically stable. It is useful for parents and carers to keep a store of these supplements for use during periods of intercurrent illness to prevent an acute exacerbation of ARD.

Supplements with a vegetable lipid source are suitable for a low phytanic acid diet; those containing fats from ruminants or fish oil should be excluded as they will contain phytanic acid. It has been suggested that oils that are high in linoleic acid are preferable because this has a faster metabolic turnover and would thus prevent further release of body stores of phytanic acid [24,25]. Sunflower and safflower oils have been favoured. The recent concern with ω6 : ω3 ratio of essential fatty acids (EFAs) perhaps points to the use of rapeseed and soya oils. Table 21.2 lists suitable supplements and the vegetable oil used where this is known.

Fresubin has been used successfully for adults and is suitable for children over 6 years of age. It is

Table 21.1   Sources of phytanic acid in food.

Low risk (no phytanic acid, allowed freely)	Moderate risk (up to 10 mg per serving)	High risk (more than 10 mg per serving)
Cereals and cereal products Wheat, rice, maize, oats, sago, tapioca Crispbreads, bran cereals Biscuits containing only vegetable and hydrogenated vegetable oils, e.g. Sainsbury Rich Tea		Biscuits with animal fat, e.g. shortbread
Dairy products Very low fat cottage cheese <1% fat Fat free fromage frais	Half fat cottage cheese	All cheeses including goat, sheep, cheese spreads, processed cheese
Skimmed milk and powder Very low fat yoghurt <1% fat Soya milks Soya based yoghurts, e.g. Alpro Non-dairy ice cream containing only vegetable fats Eggs	Semi-skimmed milk Low fat yoghurt	Full fat milk. Sheep, goat milks, evaporated milk Sheep and goat milk yoghurts, cream, Elmlea Infant formulas containing fish oil Dairy ice cream
Fats and oils Margarines and spreads containing only vegetable oils e.g. Pure Oils: corn, sunflower, safflower, soya, olive, rapeseed, arachis Lard		Margarines and spreads containing animal fats Butter Beef suet
Fish	Coley, cod (no skin), plaice, smoked haddock, tuna, crab, prawns	All fatty fish, e.g. herring, mackerel, sardines, salmon fresh and canned Fish oils, e.g. Maxepa, cod-liver oil Fish in sauces (boil in bag)
Meat Pork, pig liver, pig kidney Ham, bacon Chicken, chicken liver, turkey, duck Pork sausages	Rabbit	Beef and its offal Lamb and its offal Goat (not analysed) Beefburgers, other sausages (not analysed) All meat products (not analysed)
Vegetarian meat substitutes Soya based TVP products, e.g. Protoveg, soya chunks Sosmix Tofu Plain Quorn mycoprotein		
Vegetables Root vegetables, potatoes, crisps cooked in all vegetable oil Dried beans and pulses Green vegetables		Beef, cheese, prawn flavour crisps (not analysed)

continued on p. 448

Table 21.1   (Cont'd)

Low risk (no phytanic acid, allowed freely)	Moderate risk (up to 10 mg per serving)	High risk (more than 10 mg per serving)
Fruit All fresh and canned fruit	Dried fruit (possible phytol content)	
Nuts Almonds, coconut, Brazil, Tahini (sesame)	Walnuts Skins of nuts (possible phytol)	Peanuts
Miscellaneous Beverages – coffee, cocoa, drinking chocolate Supplements Chicken Oxo, Bisto, Marmite Clear vegetable soups	Tea in large amounts (phytol content)	Beef Oxo Cream soups
Confectionery Sugar based sweets containing no fat, e.g. boiled sweets, fruit gums, jellies, Turkish delight, marshmallows Plain chocolate with no butter fat, e.g. Waitrose continental plain chocolate Carob, e.g. Plamil raw sugar confection		Milk chocolate, e.g. Mars Bars, Cadbury's Dairymilk Plain chocolate with butter

Table 21.2   Tube and sip feed products free from animal fats.

Product	Fat source
Fresubin 1000 Complete	Soya, linseed, sunflower, MCT
Fresubin Original Drink	Sunflower, soya, linseed
Fresubin Energy Drink	Sunflower, soya, MCT, linseed
Frebini Energy Drink	Soya, MCT, linseed, sunflower
Resource Protein Extra	Soybean oil
Resource 2.0 Fibre	Rapeseed oil
Isosource Standard	Rapeseed, sunflower, MCT
Isosource Energy	Rapeseed, sunflower, MCT
Isosource Junior	Rapeseed, sunflower, MCT
Nutrison	Canola, sunflower
Nutrison Energy	Canola, sunflower
Nutrini	Canola, sunflower
Nutrini Energy	Canola, sunflower
Fortisip	Canola, sunflower
Clinutren Iso	Corn, rapeseed, soya
Ensure	High oleic safflower, canola, corn
Ensure Plus	Canola, corn, high oleic safflower
Jevity	High oleic safflower, canola, MCT, soy lecithin
Jevity 1.5 kcal	High oleic safflower, canola, MCT, soy lecithin
Osmolite	High oleic safflower, canola, MCT, soy lecithin

MCT, medium chain triglycerides.

available on prescription for patients with ARD. However, the composition of Fresenius enteral feeds has been altered and most Fresenius feeds now contain fish oil. The only Fresenius enteral feed suitable for Refsum's disease now is Fresubin 1000 Complete. The Fresenuis sip feeds do not contain fish oil and are therefore suitable. At the time of writing, the Refsum disease clinic group at the Chelsea & Westminster Hospital, London, are repeating and modernising the analyses of supplements, enteral feeds and common foods for their phytanic acid and free phytol content. Until these results are available, the choice of supplement, enteral and parenteral feed should be made according to the nutritional requirements of the patient and the known fat source of the feed. The *British National Formulary* has been notified of the feeds available on prescription that are suitable for patients with ARD.

Maintenance diet and long term management

Dietary treatment (sometimes together with plasma exchange) will usually lower plasma phytanic acid within a matter of weeks. The child will then be put on a diet low in phytanic acid and phytol which must be followed for life. Initially, the child is restricted to low risk foods only (Table 21.1). As the condition improves, one food from the moderate risk group may be allowed occasionally at the discretion of the physician. High risk foods must be avoided altogether. Attention to satisfactory growth (or weight maintenance in older children) is essential, because any weight loss mobilises stored phytanic acid from adipose tissue. With rigorous adherence to diet these adipose tissue stores can be gradually eliminated.

Special care is needed during infection or other intercurrent illness to maintain nutritional status and liquid supplements may need to be used at these times.

In general, the diet, if chosen from a variety of permitted foods, should be adequate in all nutrients. The exclusion of many saturated fats from animal sources shifts the diet of these patients towards a much higher polyunsaturated : saturated fat ratio than that of the general population. This means that the dietitian should check that there is an adequate intake of antioxidant nutrients, especially vitamin E. As beef and lamb must be excluded, iron intake may also be compromised.

The inclusion of convenience and manufactured foods in the diet of patients with adult Refsum's disease requires extreme vigilance in reading the ingredients list on food labels. Many commercial fats used in desserts and baked goods contain fish oils which are a rich source of phytanic acid. Patients are advised to look for and *avoid* the following: butter, cream, animal fats, full cream milk, cheese, butter, oil, ghee, beef, lamb, suet, milk fat, fish, fish products and fish oils.

Foods labelled as suitable for vegans are quickly and easily identified as safe (although labels must be checked and products containing walnuts or peanuts excluded). Most large retail food shops now issue lists of vegan foods on request. These are updated at regular intervals. The Vegan Society produces an Animal Free Shopper biannually, which lists foods by group (biscuits, etc.) and retailer.

Dietary treatment of infantile Refsum's disease

IRD is a global peroxisomal disease, which, unlike classic Refsum's, presents in infancy with more widespread biochemical deficiencies including raised plasma phytanic acid and abnormal levels of VLCFAs. There are also physical and mental abnormalities [8]. Despite the more complex nature of this condition, some paediatricians will prescribe a low phytanic acid diet. Some improvement has been claimed in lowering plasma phytanic acid but not for other parameters. Restriction of C26 : 0 is generally accepted [11–13] and supplementation with purified docasahexaenoic acid, mixed polyunsaturated fatty acids and erucic or oleic acids (p. 453) may be useful [14–19].

Infant feeding

If the mother is breast feeding this should be encouraged because human breast milk does not contain phytanic acid unless the mother is affected. Infant formulas should contain no ruminant fats (milk, beef, etc.) because the amount of phytanic acid in these is variable and could be significant. Soya based formulas have an acceptable fat content, but may not be the first choice of feed for young infants (see p. 95).

Suitable infant feeds are given in Table 21.3. The formulation of infant feeds is constantly being changed in line with new research. Concern about essential fatty acids has led to the introduction of milk fats and fish oils into some formulas. The ingredients should always be checked before use.

Table 21.3 Infant formulas free from ruminant fats and fish oil.

Manufacturer	Product
Cow & Gate	Plus
	Step-up
	Next Steps
	Comfort (1st infant milk and follow-on milk)
	Pepti-Junior
Farley's	Soy formula
Mead Johnson	Nutramigen 1 & 2
	Enfamil AR
SMA Nutrition	SMA Gold
	SMA White
	SMA Staydown

Nuts and seed oils (especially peanuts/arachis oil) have been shown to contain hexacosanoic acid (C26 : 0). VLCFAs (>20 carbon atoms) are synthesised and degraded in the peroxisome. Exogenous VLCFAs are considered toxic and should be restricted based on the experience in neonatal adrenoleukodystrophy [12,13]. The use of feeds containing medium chain triglyceride (MCT) oils, and which are also free of phytanic acid, might be of some benefit to patients with IRD as a source of energy for fat metabolism, but data on 2-hydroxy-sebacic acid excretion showing that the 2-R isomer is excreted in both premature and neonates with ZS after feeding with MCT [35] implies that peroxisomes have a role in MCT metabolism. Therefore MCT should be used with caution.

Solid food

The choice of weaning foods should be based on those shown in Table 21.1. Only low risk foods should be used. Proprietary baby foods should be checked for the presence of milk solids, milk fat, butter, cream, cheese, beef and beef fat, lamb and fish. These ingredients must be avoided. Products labelled as suitable for vegans are allowed.

Other peroxisomal biogenesis disorders

Although the severity of disease is greater in ZS than in IRD there may be some benefit to diet strategies for modifying phytanic acid and C26 : 0 metabolism in this condition. There are few studies of the efficacy of low phytanic acid diets in RCDP but they are generally prescribed as PhyH function is impaired as part of this disorder. As some patients with classic ARD have a mild variant of RCDP and have benefited in terms of symptom alleviation and cessation of progression of disease, a low phytanic acid should be recommended for all patients with RCDP [10]. As patients with RCDP have abnormal plasmalogens, supplementation with purified docasahexaenoic acid, mixed polyunsaturated fatty acids and erucic or oleic acids may be useful but evidence is equivocal [14–19].

X-linked Adrenoleukodystrophy

Anita MacDonald

X-linked adrenoleukodystrophy (X-ALD) is a rare, serious, progressive, peroxisomal β-oxidation disorder. The first clinical description of a child with this neurodegenerative disorder was as early as 1910 [36]. In X-ALD there is an accumulation of very long chain saturated fatty acids (VLCFAs), especially hexacosanoic acid (C26 : 0) in membrane and tissues [37] and they are particularly high in central nervous system myelin and the adrenal cortex. There is evidence that this accumulation contributes to the adrenoleukodystrophy (ALD) pathogenesis [38]. It is associated with central nervous system demyelination, peripheral nerve abnormalities, primary adrenal cortical insufficiency (Addison's disease) and, commonly, primary hypogonadism. In X-ALD there is an impaired capacity to β-oxidise these fatty acids [39] because of a deficiency of the peroxisomal enzyme lignoceroyl-CoA ligase [40]. It is caused by mutations in the ABCD1 gene that encodes a peroxisomal ATP-binding cassette protein [41].

X-ALD affects only males, although a small number of female carriers may develop a milder form of the disease. The disorder has been reported in all ethnic groups and geographical locations. The incidence of X-ALD is estimated to be 1 in 17 000 [42]. More than 500 distinct mutations in the defective gene have been identified and there is no evident correlation between genotype and the different neurological phenotypes [43]. It is not possible to predict outcome of young asymptomatic boys on the basis of mutation analysis. Even members of the same family present with different phenotypes [38].

Clinical features

There are several forms of X-ALD with at least

Table 21.4   Clinical phenotypes of X-linked adrenoleukodystrophy.

Clinical phenotype	Age of presentation (years)	Relative frequency (%)	Features	Progression
Childhood cerebral ALD	4–10	31–57	Behavioural disturbances, e.g. abnormal withdrawal or aggression, poor school performance, visual loss, deafness, poor co-ordination, melanoderma, dysarthria, dysphagia, seizures, spastic tetraplegia, progressive dermentia, Addison's disease	Rapid, rarely slowly
Adolescent ALD	11–21		Similar to childhood cerebral ALD	Rapid, rarely slowly
Adult cerebral ALD	>21	1–3	Similar to childhood cerebral ALD Symptoms resemble schizophrenia with dementia 50–70% have Addison's disease	Rapid, sometimes slowly
AMN	>18	25–40	Clumsiness, progressive spastic paraparesis (stiffness, weakness and or/paralysis) of the lower extremities, ataxia, testicular insufficiency, voiding dysfunction, scanty scalp hair	Slowly, sometimes rapidly
Addison's disease only	>2	8–14	Fatigue, hypotension, diffuse or focal bronzing of skin	–
Pre- or symptomatic ALD	–	4–10	Risk of developing neurological symptoms high, but some patients remain asymptomatic for many years	–

Source: adapted from van Geel *et al.* [44].
AMN, adrenomyeloneuropathy.

six known clinical phenotypes. They vary greatly in respect to phenotypic expression, age of onset, rate of progression and therapy (Table 21.4). X-ALD is a relatively common cause of Addison's disease [42].

Without treatment approximately 40% of boys with X-ALD will develop childhood cerebral disease, usually between 4 and 12 years [45]. This is the most severe phenotype, resulting in rapid neurological deterioration. Behavioural changes (withdrawn or hyperactive behaviour) and visual impairment are early symptoms. Unfortunately, in many cases diagnosis is made only after significant deterioration. Death may occur within 5 years of the onset of neurological symptoms [46] but some patients remain severely neurologically impaired, bedridden, blind and unable to eat or speak for several years [41].

Cerebral X-ALD can present in teenagers and adults but is rarer. The clinical features and progression resemble childhood cerebral ALD.

Adult cerebral X-ALD may be mistaken for a psychiatric disorder such as schizophrenia with dementia [42].

Forty to fifty per cent of patients with X-ALD (adrenomyeloneuropathy: AMN) present during their third or fourth decade with symptoms and signs of spinal cord involvement. Neurological disability is slowly progressive over several decades. Approximately half of the patients have normal magnetic resonance imaging (MRI) results although patients are at risk for developing the cerebral form of X-ALD. About 70% of men with AMN have impaired adrenocortical function at the time neurological symptoms are first noted [40].

Occasionally, symptoms occur in female carriers and include spastic paraparesis of the lower limbs, ataxia, hypertonia, mild peripheral neuropathy and urinary problems. Cerebral involvement is rare and adrenal insufficiency occurs in <1%. No specific therapy is available and diet is not advocated [45].

Diagnosis

X-ALD is probably underdiagnosed [41] and may be misdiagnosed as attention deficit or hyperactivity disorder in boys and as multiple sclerosis in men and women. Although laboratory evaluation of VLCFA concentrations is not the sole marker, it is a good indicator of X-ALD [47]. Almost all males (99.9% of hemizygous males) and 85% of heterozygous female carriers will have increased levels of VLCFAs in plasma [48]. Diagnosis may be confirmed by DNA analysis and fibroblast studies.

Genetic counselling of family members is essential in X-ALD and molecular genetic testing has been used primarily to determine carrier status in at-risk female relatives and for prenatal diagnosis when the nature of the familial mutation is known.

Treatment

Although the general prognosis for patients with childhood cerebral X-ALD is poor, there are some treatments available that may relieve clinical symptoms and prolong life. For boys with childhood cerebral X-ALD, treatment options include:

- Adrenal steroids for adrenal dysfunction
- Lorenzo's oil
- Hematopoietic stem cell transplantation in patients with early cerebral involvement

Dietary treatment

VLCFAs are derived from both dietary sources and by endogenous synthesis. Because of this, diet therapy has been developed to limit the intake of C26 : 0 fatty acids and to decrease their synthesis [49]. The diet is based on Lorenzo's oil and a moderate fat restriction. The aim is to achieve normal plasma C26 : 0 concentrations [38].

The diet is summarised in Table 21.5 and consists of:

- Lorenzo's oil
- Glycerol trioleate oil for cooking
- Moderately low fat diet
- Vitamin and mineral supplementation
- Essential fatty acids
- Energy supplementation

Table 21.5   Summary of diet therapy used in adrenoleukodystrophy.

Lorenzo's oil
Description
4 parts glycerol trioleate oil (GTO)
1 part glycerol trierucate (GTE)

Dose
20% of energy intake: some boys need less than this to normalise C26 : 0 levels

Administration
Give 2–3 times daily
Give neat as a medicine, or mixed with skimmed milk and flavouring or fruit juice
Can also be mixed with very low fat yoghurt
Not ACBS prescribable

Glycerol trioleate oil
Description
Rich in oleic acid; free of C26 : 0

Dose
No set dose

Administration
Use for frying potatoes, fish and meats, salad dressings
Not ACBS prescribable

Low fat diet
Description
Give 15% of dietary energy as fat (try not to exceed 35% energy from fat)
NB. No other dietary restrictions are necessary

Vitamin and mineral supplementation
Description
Diet low in fat-soluble vitamins and commonly trace elements

Type of supplements
Give comprehensive vitamin and mineral supplement, e.g. Forceval Junior capsules or Paediatric Seravit

Monitoring
Vitamin and mineral status must be monitored annually

Essential fatty acids
Description
Diet is low in essential fatty acids
Lorenzo's oil leads to reduced levels of omega 6 and omega 3 fatty acids

Type of supplements
Give 1–2% of total energy from essential fatty acid supplement
It should provide a source of linoleic acid and alpha-linolenic acid in the ratio 5 : 1, e.g. walnut oil (p. 427)

Energy supplements
Description
Energy intake may be low

Type of supplements
Useful ACBS energy supplements include glucose polymers, glucose drinks (liquid Polycal, liquid Maxijul) and fortified fat free fruit juice drinks (Fortijuce, Provide Xtra, Enlive Plus)

ACBS, Advisory Committee on Borderline Substances.

Historical perspective

The first diet, tried in 1981, limited C26 : 0 intake to <3 g/day but it was unsuccessful as it neither reduced plasma VLCFA levels nor inhibited disease progression [50]. As diet was not the only source of the accumulating VLCFA, attempts were made to reduce endogenous synthesis of VLCFA. Rizzo *et al.* [51] first identified that the addition of oleic acid, a monounsaturated fatty acid, decreased VLCFA in cultured fibroblasts by competing with the saturated fatty acids for the synthetase enzyme. Treatment was then based on glycerol trioleate oil (91% oleic acid) in combination with a low fat diet and was found to reduce plasma C26 : 0 levels by 50% in patients [52]. It was later shown that glyceryl trierucate produced a more striking reduction in VLCFA levels and a 4 : 1 ratio of glyceryl trioleate and trierucate normalised VLCFA blood concentration in 1 month [53]. The combination of these two fats in this ratio is known as Lorenzo's oil, named after the first boy with cerebral X-ALD to use it.

Lorenzo's oil

Fatty acid synthesis and elongation are complex highly regulated processes. Endogenous VLCFAs are synthesised in microsomes by a series of elongation steps that begin with palmitic acid (C16 : 0) and the successive addition of 2-carbon units [46]. Lorenzo's oil contains a high proportion of long-chain monounsaturated fatty acids and probably works by competitive inhibition of the microsomal elongation system for saturated long chain fatty acids [53]. In patients with ALD the rate of synthesis of C26 : 0 is increased and the ability to degrade saturated VLCFAs is impaired [54].

Lorenzo's oil (Table 21.6) is a blend of four parts glyceryl trioleate oil (GTO) and one part glyceryl trierucate (GTE). The GTE component is a solid fat at room temperature. It is about 93% erucic acid which is purified from rapeseed oil. When GTO and GTE are combined together, a clear yellow liquid is produced, although the GTE can solidify and form white sediment at ambient temperatures. Lorenzo's oil is 90% fat providing 8 kcal/mL (34 kJ/mL). It is recommended that 20% of the total energy intake is given from Lorenzo's oil and examples of calculated daily dosage are given in Table 21.7. Although this dosage normalises

Table 21.6   Composition of Lorenzo's oil.

Nutritional information	Composition (per 100 mL)
Energy kcal	807
kJ	3320
Protein (g)	Nil added
Carbohydrate (g)	Nil added
Fat (g)	89.7
Typical fatty acid profile	g/100 g fatty acids
C16 : 0	0.8
C17 : 0	0.16
C17 : 1	0.16
C18 : 0	2.4
C18 : 1	73
C18 : 2	3.25
C18 : 3	0.16
C20 : 1	0.48
C22 : 0	0.02
C22 : 1	19.1
C24 : 1	0.36
Other	0.14

Table 21.7   Suggested daily dosage of Lorenzo's oil.

Age (years)	Estimated average requirement for energy kcal/day (kJ/day) [55]	Daily requirement Lorenzo's oil (mL) (20% of energy intake)
1–3	1230 (5150)	30
4–6	1715 (7160)	45
8–10	1970 (8240)	50
11–14	2220 (9270)	55

plasma C26 : 0 levels, the figure of 20% is arbitrary. Because of an apparent dose–response effect of Lorenzo's oil on lowering C26 : 0 concentrations, it has no benefit unless substantial and sustained lowering of C26 : 0 concentrations are achieved [38,56].

The daily amount of Lorenzo's oil should be divided into two or three doses throughout the day. There is no evidence to suggest that its efficacy is affected if taken at different times to meals or in a single dose, although children may develop diarrhoea if the oil is taken in one dose. It is difficult to disguise the oily taste or consistency of Lorenzo's oil. Many children take their measured dose of Lorenzo's oil as a medicine, direct from a spoon or syringe without any additional flavouring. Some prefer to take it mixed with skimmed milk and milk shake flavouring or fruit juice. Unfortunately, the oil does not mix well with either. It may be easier to take the mixture in a covered cup or beaker to help mask the smell and the poorly dispersed fat. Others mix the oil with yoghurt or other low fat desserts. It is not recommended that Lorenzo's oil is used in cooking. It is not available on Advisory Committee Borderline Substances (ACBS) prescription.

Lorenzo's oil is not recommended before 18 months of age because it may lower the levels of docosahexaenoic acid (DHA) which has an important role in early retinal and brain development [56]. It is unclear at what age Lorenzo's oil therapy should be continued in patients who remain neurologically normal and there are no recommendations about stopping diet. Some patients are discontinuing in late teenage years; others are more cautious and remain on diet into the early adulthood.

Use and storage of Lorenzo's oil

The bottle of oil should be left at room temperature for 1 hour before use but otherwise should be stored in a refrigerator.

The bottle should be shaken very well until the white sediment of GTE is evenly distributed throughout the oil so that a homogenous dose of oil can be given.

Glycerol trioleate oil

GTO is often used in addition to Lorenzo's oil specifically as cooking oil. It is a pale yellow oil free of C26 : 0 and rich in oleic acid (Table 21.8). Like Lorenzo's oil it is 90% fat providing 8 kcal/mL (34 kJ/mL). It is useful in the preparation of salad dressings, GTO cakes and biscuits and for frying potatoes, crisps, fish and meats. It should be stored at 4°C under dry conditions. It is not currently available on ACBS prescription and is quite expensive to buy.

Moderately low fat diet

Intake of other dietary fats should be reduced to 15–20% of total energy [38]. Guidelines for daily fat intake are given in Table 21.9. Moser has suggested that a total fat intake in excess of 30–35% of total energy (from Lorenzo's oil and dietary fat) may counteract or nullify the C26 : 0 reducing

Table 21.8   Composition of glycerol trioleate oil.

Nutritional information	Composition (per 100 mL)
Energy kcal	819
kJ	3367
Protein (g)	Nil added
Carbohydrate (g)	Nil added
Fat (g)	91
Typical fatty acid profile	g/100 g fatty acids
C16 : 0	1
C17 : 0	0.2
C17 : 1	0.2
C18 : 0	3
C18 : 1	91
C18 : 2	4
C18 : 3	0.2
C20 : 1	0.4

Table 21.9   Guidelines on daily dietary fat intake.

Age (years)	Estimated average requirement for energy kcal (kJ)/day [55]	Approximate fat intake from food (g/day) (15% of energy intake)
1–3	1230 (5150)	20
4–6	1715 (7160)	30
8–10	1970 (8240)	35
11–14	2220 (9270)	40

effect of Lorenzo's oil. Table 21.10 gives examples of permitted foods on a moderately low fat diet. Children soon become bored with such a limited diet and imaginative use should be made of all freely allowed foods to try to prevent anorexia or cheating.

Energy supplementation

Although one-fifth of the total energy intake is from Lorenzo's oil and GTO can be incorporated into many dishes, appetite and energy intake is sometimes poor and growth may be affected. It is essential that both nutritional intake and status of patients are assessed at regular intervals and energy supplements given if needed. Energy supplements include glucose polymers; glucose drinks such as Polycal; milk shakes made from skimmed milk, glucose polymer and low fat milk shake flavourings. Fortunately, with increasing public

Table 21.10   Moderately low fat diet.

	Foods allowed	Foods not allowed
Meat and poultry	Extra lean beef, lamb, turkey, chicken, pork; lean ham, bacon	Fatty meat, sausages, salami, black pudding, corned beef
Fish	White fish, e.g. haddock, sole, plaice, whiting, prawns, shrimps, tuna, fish fingers	Oily fish, e.g. sardines, mackerel, kipper, fish canned in oil
Milk	Skimmed milk, low fat yoghurt, Quark, 'diet' low fat cheeses less than 3% fat	Whole milk, semi-skimmed milk, cream, full fat yoghurt
Eggs	Egg in moderation	
Pulses, nuts, seeds	Peas, beans, lentils, dhal	Nuts, seeds
Fruit	All fruits (except those on not allowed list)	Avocado, olives
Vegetables	All vegetables (except those on not allowed list) Low fat crisps (<5 g fat per bag): 1 bag per day	Chips, roast potato, regular crisps
Fats	Scraping of very low fat margarines Use GTO for cooking	All other fats, oils, butters and margarines
Bread, pasta, rice, cereals and breakfast cereals	All bread, chapatti, pasta, rice, tinned pasta, flours, most breakfast cereals	Breakfast cereals with nuts
Cakes and biscuits	Low fat cakes/biscuits/low fat cereal bars (but providing ⊁3 g fat/day in total)	Any other cakes, biscuits, pastries
Puddings and desserts	Jelly, sorbet, meringues, skimmed milk puddings, skimmed milk custard	Ice cream, milk puddings and desserts not made with skimmed milk
Sugar, preserves and spreads	All kinds of sugar Jam, marmalade, honey, syrup	Chocolate spread, peanut butter
Confectionery	Boiled sweets/lollies, gummy sweets, pastilles, jelly beans, marshmallows	Chocolate, toffee, fudge, carob
Soups	Low calorie and 'healthy eating' soups	Cream soups
Beverages	Fruit juice, squashes, tea, coffee, milk shake flavouring, low fat drinking chocolate	Malted milk drinks, cocoa, regular drinking chocolate

awareness of healthy eating, the number of suitable commercially available low fat products has greatly increased and can be incorporated into the diet.

Vitamin and mineral intake

Specific nutrients that may be low in the diet include the fat-soluble vitamins A, D and E, and vitamin C and folic acid. If appetite is poor a comprehensive vitamin and trace mineral supplement such as Paediatric Seravit or Forceval Junior capsules is advocated. If a child is eating well a source of fat-soluble vitamins may be all that is needed. The dosage and type of vitamin and mineral sup-

plement should be determined for the individual child.

Essential fatty acid supplementation

An essential fatty acid supplement is recommended for all X-ALD patients providing linoleic acid (C18 : 2ω6) and α-linolenic acid (C18 : 3ω3) in a ratio of between 4 : 1 and 10 : 1. Although GTO contains some linoleic and α-linolenic acid, and Lorenzo's oil contains some linoleic acid, the overall quantity of essential fatty acids obtained from a low fat diet and Lorenzo's oil is estimated to be approximately only 2% of total energy intake. It is

Table 21.11 Indications for treatment with Lorenzo's oil and moderately low fat diet in X-linked adrenoleukodystrophy.

Offer to male patients with ALD who are neurologically asymptomatic, have normal brain MRI results and are at risk of developing cerebral ALD

No benefit in X-ALD boys with neurological symptoms

No benefit in patients with AMN

No benefit in female carriers

ALD, adrenoleukodystrophy; AMN, adrenomyeloneuropathy; MRI, magnetic resonance imaging.

recommended to give a further 1–2% of essential fatty acids from supplements such as walnut oil; Moser recommends 5% [41]. It has been demonstrated that Lorenzo's oil therapy causes reduced levels of omega 6 and other omega-3 fatty acids in red blood cells [57,58].

Effectiveness of Lorenzo's oil

A summary of the indications for treatment with Lorenzo's oil is given in Table 21.11. It can reduce plasma C26 : 0 to normal levels in up to 86% of patients [59] within 1 month of diet therapy. It reduces C26 : 0 concentrations in the plasma, adipose tissue and liver [60], but the effect on C26 : 0 levels in the brain is variable [38]. It has been suggested that little erucic acid crosses the blood–brain barrier although in rodents C-labelled erucic acid does enter the brain [61].

A series of studies has shown that Lorenzo's oil does not halt the neurological progression in the cerebral form of childhood X-ALD [52,53,62,63] and AMN [62,64] so Lorenzo's oil has no real value in patients with established symptoms. In contrast, there is now evidence supporting the use of dietary therapy in asymptomatic boys to delay or prevent the onset of neurological disease. Two studies were conducted concurrently but independently from the USA (69 patients) and Europe (34 patients) on boys <6 years of age, with normal neurological examination and brain MRI at the time of enrolment. They were given 20% of energy intake as Lorenzo's oil and 10–15% of energy intake from dietary fat and were followed up for 2.6 and 4.3 years, respectively. Subjects (from both studies) were divided into two groups according to

lowering of plasma VLCFA: group 1 lowered mean annual plasma C26 : 0 concentrations within 2 SD of normal; and group 2 subjects, who were less compliant with diet, failed to do so. A positive association between the degree of lowering of C26 : 0 concentrations and clinical outcome in asymptomatic boys 2–10 years of age was demonstrated. The effect was only partial as 24% of group 1 patients developed neurological or MRI abnormalities. Delay in initiating the therapy increased the possibility of neurological involvement [64,65].

Moser *et al*. [38] continued to follow-up 89 children with asymptomatic X-ALD, treated with Lorenzo's oil and moderate fat restriction, for almost 7 years and examined disease progression. The mean age at baseline was 4.7 years. At the time of follow-up, 74% of the patients had normal neurological examination results and normal brain MRI results. Twenty four per cent of patients developed MRI abnormalities and only 11% had abnormal neurological and MRI results. In addition, all patients aged 7 years or older at the initiation of therapy remained neurologically and radiographically normal during the course of the study. Moser *et al*. compared clinical outcomes with C26 : 0 concentrations. There were significant associations between the development of MRI abnormalities and plasma C26 : 0 increases. A 0.6 µg/mL reduction in plasma C26 : 0 concentrations was associated with an approximately twofold reduction in the risk of developing MRI abnormalities. None of the patients with neurological involvement normalised their plasma C26 : 0 concentrations. Therefore, Moser *et al*. recommended Lorenzo's oil for all neurologically asymptomatic (with normal brain MRI results) male patients with biochemical evidence of X-ALD who are at risk of developing the childhood cerebral form of the disorder.

Complications associated with Lorenzo's oil

A number of side effects have been noted with Lorenzo's oil including mild increases in liver enzymes [59], thrombocytopenia [66–69], gastrointestinal complaints [59], gingivitis [59], decreased membrane anisotrophy [41] and a reduction of plasma essential fatty acids [57,58]. Platelet reduction has been noted in about 30–40% of patients [38,41]. Generally, the platelet reduction is not severe enough to warrant discontinuation of diet therapy in the majority of patients, but careful monitoring is recommended. It is Moser's policy to discontinue Lorenzo's oil when platelet count falls unacceptably low and the patients are then maintained on GTO as an alternative. This usually results in restoration of platelet count to pre-treatment levels when Lorenzo's oil is then resumed but at a lower dose [38].

Non-diet treatments

Eighty per cent of asymptomatic patients with ALD develop evidence of adrenal insufficiency [70] and it is essential that corticosteroid replacement treatment is provided. This does not change the neurological progression of the disorder [45].

Bone marrow transplant: haematopoietic stem cell transplantation is the treatment of choice in boys with very early symptoms and/or deteriorating MRI [71]. It is not recommended for patients with advanced disease. As it is impossible to predict the disease course in asymptomatic cases, transplants are only performed after the onset of symptoms. In patients with early neuropsychological deterioration, it has been shown to reverse or stabilise abnormalities on cerebral MRI [72,73] and may result in stability of mental ability.

Newer approaches to treatment that are being evaluated in the treatment of X-ALD include lovastatin [74], 4-phenylbutyrate [75], arginine butyrate [45], co-enzyme Q [45] and gene therapy [76].

Lovastatin: a lipid lowering drug that inhibits 3-hydroxy-3 methyl-glutaryl-coenzyme A reductase and normalises the VLCFA concentrations in fibroblasts and plasma from patients with X-ALD. However, when given to X-ALD protein deficient mice, it does not correct the accumulation of VLCFA in the plasma or tissues, including the brain and spinal cord [77].

Phenylbutyrate: this reduces the levels of VLCFA in the brain and adrenal gland in the X-ALD mouse model [75].

Monitoring

Regular monitoring of the following is important:

- Neurological function: for detecting early deterioration so boys who are potential candidates for haematopoietic stem cell transplantation are identified. Asymptomatic boys should be monitored serially for the earliest evidence of demyelination. Monitoring should include brain MRI, neurological examination, neuropsychological evaluation and evoked potentials.
- VLCFAs to monitor the effect and compliance with Lorenzo's oil. Ideally, these should be checked every 3 months. Most laboratories measure the absolute concentration of C26 : 0 as well as the C24 : 0 : C22 : 0 and C26 : 0 : C23 : 0 ratios [48].
- Platelet counts and liver function.
- Essential fatty acids.
- Adrenal function.

Other issues

In boys, once clinical neurological deterioration is evident, deterioration is usually rapid and it may be only a matter of months before the child is unable to eat or drink adequate amounts to sustain nutrition. Nasogastric or gastrostomy feeding is usually required with a standard enteral feed only; their nutritional management should be similar to other children with severe neurological impairment.

Acknowledgements

Eleanor Baldwin would like to acknowledge the collaboration of her colleagues in writing this chapter: the late F. Brian Gibberd, FRCP, Consultant Neurologist, who was a major contributor to research into Refsum's disease at the Chelsea & Westminster Hospital, London, and who strove to provide excellent care for the patients attending the Refsum Disease Clinic, and Anthony S. Wierzbicki, DM DPhil FRCPath, Consultant Chemical Pathologist, Refsum Disease Clinic, Chelsea & Westminster Hospital, London SW10 9NH, UK and Department of Chemical Pathology, St. Thomas' Hospital, London SE1 7EH, UK.

References

1 Wierzbicki AS, Lloyd MD, Schofield CJ *et al.* Refsum's disease: a peroxisomal disorder affecting

phytanic acid alpha-oxidation. *J Neurochem*, 2002, **80** 727–35.

2   Wanders RJA, Barth PG, Heymans HS Single perox-isomal enzyme deficiencies. In: Scriver CR, Beaudet AL, Sly WS, Valle D, Childs B, Kinzler KW *et al.* (eds) *The Metabolic and Molecular Bases of Inherited Disease*, 8th edn. New York, USA: McGraw-Hill, 2001. pp. 3219–56.

3   Mukherji M, Schofield CJ, Wierzbicki AS *et al.* The chemical biology of branched-chain lipid metabolism. *Prog Lipid Res*, 2003, **42** 359–76.

4   Wierzbicki AS, Mayne PD, Lloyd MD *et al.* Metabolism of phytanic acid and 3-methyl-adipic acid excretion in patients with adult Refsum disease. *J Lipid Res*, 2003, **44** 1481–8.

5   Komen JC, Duran M, Wanders RJ Characterization of phytanic acid omega-hydroxylation in human liver microsomes. *Mol Genet Metab*, 2005, **85** 190–5.

6   Dickson N, Mortimer JG, Faed JM *et al.* A child with Refsum's disease: successful treatment with diet and plasma exchange. *Dev Med Child Neurol*, 1989, **31** 92–7.

7   Herbert MA, Clayton PT Phytanic acid alpha-oxidase deficiency (Refsum disease) presenting in infancy. *J Inherit Metab Dis*, 1994, **17** 211–14.

8   Gould SJ, Raymond GV, Valle D The peroxisome biogenesis disorders. In: Scriver CR, Beaudet AL, Sly WS, Valle D, Childs B, Kinzler KW *et al.* (eds) *The Metabolic and Molecular Bases of Inherited Disease*, 8th edn. New York, USA: McGraw-Hill, 2001. pp. 3181–217.

9   Purdue PE, Skoneczny M, Yang X *et al.* Rhizomelic chondrodysplasia punctata, a peroxisomal biogenesis disorder caused by defects in Pex7p, a peroxisomal protein import receptor: a minireview. *Neurochem Res*, 1999, **24** 581–6.

10 Van Den Brink DM, Brites P, Haasjes J *et al.* Identification of PEX7 as the second gene involved in Refsum disease. *Am J Hum Genet*, 2003, **72** 471–7.

11 Van Duyn MA, Moser AE, Brown FR III *et al.* The design of a diet restricted in saturated very long-chain fatty acids: therapeutic application in adrenoleukodystrophy. *Am J Clin Nutr*, 1984, **40** 277–84.

12 Moser HW, Borel J Dietary management of X-linked adrenoleukodystrophy. *Ann Rev Nutr*, 1995, **15** 379–97.

13 Moser AB, Borel J, Odone A *et al.* A new dietary therapy for adrenoleukodystrophy: biochemical and preliminary clinical results in 36 patients. *Ann Neurol*, 1987, **21** 240–9.

14 Robertson EF, Poulos A, Sharp P *et al.* Treatment of infantile phytanic acid storage disease: clinical, biochemical and ultrastructural findings in two children treated for 2 years. *Eur J Pediatr*, 1988, **147** 133–42.

15 Martinez M Docosahexaenoic acid therapy in docosahexaenoic acid-deficient patients with disorders of peroxisomal biogenesis. *Lipids*, 1996, **31** (Suppl) S145–52.

16 Martinez M Restoring the DHA levels in the brains of Zellweger patients. *J Mol Neurosci*, 2001, **16** 309–16.

17 Schutgens RB, Wanders RJ, Heymans HS *et al.* Zellweger syndrome: biochemical procedures in diagnosis, prevention and treatment. *J Inherit Metab Dis*, 1987, **10** (Suppl 1) 33–45.

18 Moser HW, Raymond GV, Koehler W *et al.* Evaluation of the preventive effect of glyceryl trioleate-trierucate ('Lorenzo's oil') therapy in X-linked adrenoleukodystrophy: results of two concurrent trials. *Adv Exp Med Biol*, 2003, **544** 369–87.

19 Moser HW, Raymond GV, Lu SE *et al.* Follow-up of 89 asymptomatic patients with adrenoleukodystrophy treated with Lorenzo's oil. *Arch Neurol*, 2005, **62** 1073–80.

20 Steinberg D, Mize CE, Herndon JH Jr *et al.* Phytanic acid in patients with Refsum's syndrome and response to dietary treatment. *Arch Intern Med*, 1970, **125** 75–87.

21 Yao JK, Dyck PJ Tissue distribution of phytanic acid and its analogues in a kinship with Refsum's disease. *Lipids*, 1987, **22** 69–75.

22 Gibberd FB, Billimoria JD, Goldman JM *et al.* Heredopathia atactica polyneuritiformis: Refsum's disease. *Acta Neurol Scand*, 1985, **72** 1–17.

23 Steinberg D, Avigan J, Mize C *et al.* Conversion of U-C14-phytol to phytanic acid and its oxidation in heredopathia atactica polyneuritiformis. *Biochem Biophys Res Commun*, 1965, **19** 783–9.

24 Masters-Thomas A, Bailes J, Billimoria JD *et al.* Heredopathia atactica polyneuritiformis (Refsum's disease): 1. Clinical features and dietary management. *J Hum Nutr*, 1980, **34** 245–50.

25 Masters-Thomas A, Bailes J, Billimoria JD *et al.* Heredopathia atactica polyneuritiformis (Refsum's disease): 2. Estimation of phytanic acid in foods. *J Hum Nutr*, 1980, **34** 251–4.

26 Baxter JH. Absorption of chlorophyll phytol in normal man and in patients with Refsum's disease. *J Lipid Res*, 1968, **9** 636–41.

27 Mukherji M, Schofield CJ, Wierzbicki AS *et al.* The chemical biology of branched-chain lipid metabolism. *Prog Lipid Res*, 2003, **42** 359–76.

28 Steinberg D, Avigan J, Mize CE *et al.* Effects of dietary phytol and phytanic acid in animals. *J Lipid Res*, 1966, **7** 684–91.

29 Ackman RG, Harrington M *Fishery products as components of diets restricted in phytanic acid for patients with Refsum's syndrome*, 36th edn. 1975. pp. 50–3.

30 Ackman RG, Hooper SN *Isoprenoid fatty acids in the human diet: distinct geographical features in butterfat and*

importance in margarines based on marine oils, 6th edn. 1973. pp. 159–65.

31 Ratnayake WM, Olsson B, Ackman RG Novel branched-chain fatty acids in certain fish oils. *Lipids*, 1989, **24** 630–7.

32 Lough AK The phytanic acid content of the lipids of bovine tissues and milk. *Lipids*, 1977, **12** 115–19.

33 Brown PJ, Mei G, Gibberd FB *et al*. Diet and Refsum's disease. The determination of phytanic acid and phytol in certain foods and application of this knowledge to the choice of suitable convenience foods for patients with Refsum's disease. *J Hum Nutr Diet*, 1993, **6** 295–305.

34 Coppack SW, Evans R, Gibberd FB *et al*. Can patients with Refsum's disease safely eat green vegetables? *Br Med J (Clin Res Ed)* 1988, **296** 828.

35 Muth A, Mosandl A, Wanders RJ *et al*. Stereoselective analysis of 2-hydroxysebacic acid in urine of patients with Zellweger syndrome and of premature infants fed with medium-chain triglycerides. *J Inherit Metab Dis*, 2003, **26** 583–92.

36 Haberfield W, Spieler F Zur diffusen Hirn-Ruekenmarksclerose im Kindesalter. *Dtsch Z Nerventh*, 1910, **40** 436.

37 Ho JK, Moser H, Kishimota Y, Hamilton JA Interactions of a very long chain fatty acid with model membranes and serum albumin. Implications for the pathogenesis of adrenoleukodystrophy. *J Clin Invest*, 1995, **96** 1455–66.

38 Moser HW, Raymond GV, Lu SE *et al*. Follow-up of 89 asymptomatic patients with adrenoleukodystrophy treated with Lorenzo's oil. *Arch Neurol*, 2005, **62** 1073–80.

39 Korenke GC, Roth C, Krasemann E *et al*. Variability of endocrinological dysfunction in 55 patients with X-linked adrenoleucodystrophy: clinical, laboratory and genetic findings. *Eur J Endocrinol*, 1997, **137** 40–7.

40 Moser HW Clinical and therapeutic aspects of adrenoleukodystrophy and adrenomyeloneuropathy. *J Neuropathol Exp Neurol*, 1995, **54** 740–5.

41 Moser HW, Smith KD, Watkins PA *et al*. X-linked adrenoleukodystrophy. In: Scriver CR *et al*. (eds) *The Metabolic and Molecular Bases of Inherited Disease*, 8th edn. New York: McGraw-Hill, 2001, pp. 3257–302.

42 Moser HW, Raymond GV, Dubey P (2005) Adrenoleukodystrophy: new approaches to a neurodegenerative disease. *J Am Med Assoc*, 2005, **294** 3131–4.

43 Moser H, Dubey P, Fatemi A Progress in X-linked adrenoleukodystrophy. *Curr Opin Neurol*, 2004, **17** 263–9.

44 van Geel BM, Assies J, Wanders RJ, Barth PG X-linked adrenoleukodystrophy: clinical presentation, diagnosis, and therapy. *J Neurol Neurosurg Psychiatry*, 1997, **63** 4–14.

45 Mandel H Peroxosomal disorders. In: Blau N, Hoffmann GF, Leonard J, Clarke JTR (eds) *Physician's Guide to the Treatment and Follow-up of Metabolic Diseases*. Berlin: Springer-Verlag, 2006, pp. 267–77.

46 Ferri R, Chance PF Lorenzo's oil: advances in the treatment of neurometabolic disorders. *Arch Neurol*, 2005, **62** 1045–46.

47 Wanders JA, Barth PG, Poll-The BT Peroxisomal disorders. In Blau N, Duran M, Blaskovics ME, Gibson MK (eds) *Physicians Guide to the Laboratory Diagnosis of Metabolic Diseases*. Berlin: Springer-Verlag, 2003, pp. 481–508.

48 Kim JH, Kim HJ Childhood X-linked adrenoleukodystrophy: clinical-pathologic overview and MR imaging manifestations at initial evaluation and follow-up. *Radiographics*, 2005, **25** 619–31.

49 Singh I, Moser AE, Moser HW, Kishimoto Y Adrenoleukodystrophy: impaired oxidation of very long chain fatty acids in white blood cells, cultured skin fibroblasts, and amniocytes. *Pediatr Res*, 1984, **18** 286–90.

50 Moser AB *et al*. A new diet therapy for adrenoleukodystrophy: biochemical and preliminary clinical results in 36 patients. *Ann Neurol*, 1986, **21** 240–9.

51 Rizzo WB, Avigan J, Chemke J, Schulman JD Adrenoleukodystrophy: very long-chain fatty acid metabolism in fibroblasts. *Neurology*, 1984, **34** 163–9.

52 Moser AB, Borel J, Odone A *et al*. A new dietary therapy for adrenoleukodystrophy: biochemical and preliminary clinical results in 36 patients. *Ann Neurol*, 1987, **21** 240–9.

53 Rizzo WB, Leshner RT, Odone A *et al*. Dietary erucic acid therapy for X-linked adrenoleukodystrophy. *Neurology*, 1989, **39** 1415–22.

54 Tsuji S, Ohno T, Miyatake T *et al*. Fatty acid elongation activity in fibroblasts from patients with adrenoleukodystrophy (ALD). *J Biochem (Tokyo)*, 1984, **96** 1241–7.

55 Department of Health Report on Health and Social Subjects No. 41. Dietary Reference Values for Food, Energy and Nutrients for the United Kingdom. London: HMSO, 1991.

56 Moser HW, Raymond GV, Koehler W *et al*. Evaluation of the preventive effect of glyceryl trioleate-trierucate ('Lorenzo's oil') therapy in X-linked adrenoleukodystrophy: results of two concurrent trials. *Adv Exp Med Biol*, 2003, **544** 369–87.

57 Moser AB, Jones DS, Raymond GV, Moser HW Plasma and red blood cell fatty acids in peroxisomal disorders. *Neurochem Res*, 1999, **24** 187–97.

58 Ruiz M, Pampols T, Giros M Glycerol trioleate/glycerol trierucate therapy in X-linked adrenoleukodystrophy: saturated and unsaturated fatty acids in blood cells. Implications for the follow-up. *J Inherit Metab Dis*, 1996, **19** 188–92.

59 van Geel BM, Assies J, Haverkort EB *et al*. Progression of abnormalities in adrenomyeloneuropathy and neurologically asymptomatic X-linked adrenoleukodystrophy despite treatment with Lorenzo's oil. *J Neurol Neurosurg Psychiatry*, 1999, **67** 290–9.

60 Rasemussen M, Moser AB, Borel J, Moser HW Brain, liver, and adipose tissue erucic and very long chain fatty acid levels in adrenoleukodystrophy patients treated with glyceryl trierucate and trioleate oils (Lorenzo's oil). *Neurochem Res*, 1994, **19** 1073–82.

61 Murphy EJ Lorenzo's oil, adrenoleukodystrophy, and the blood brain barrier (abstract) *J Neurochem*, 2002, **81** (Suppl 1) 100.

62 Uziel G, Bertini E, Bardelli P *et al*. Experience on therapy of adrenoleukodystrophy and adrenomyeloneuropathy. *Dev Neurosci*, 1991, **13** 274–9.

63 Asano J, Suzuki Y, Yajima S *et al*. Effects of erucic acid therapy on Japanese patients with X-linked adrenoleukodystrophy. *Brain Dev*, 1994, **16** 454–8.

64 Aubourg P, Adamsbaum C, Lavallard-Rousseau MC *et al*. A two-year trial of oleic and erucic acids ('Lorenzo's oil') as treatment for adrenomyeloneuropathy. *N Engl J Med*, 1993, **329** 745–52.

65 Moser HW, Fatemi A, Zackowski K *et al*. Evaluation of therapy of X-linked adrenoleukodystrophy. *Neurochem Res*, 2004, **29** 1003–6.

66 Zierz S, Schroder R, Unkrig CJ Thrombocytopenia induced by erucic acid therapy in patients with X-linked adrenoleukodystrophy. *Clin Invest*, 1993, **71** 802–5.

67 Zinkham WH, Kickler T, Borel J, Moser HW Lorenzo's oil and thrombocytopenia in patients with adrenoleukodystrophy. *N Engl J Med*, 1993, **328** 1126–27.

68 Crowther MA, Barr RD, Kelton J *et al*. Profound thrombocytopenia complicating dietary erucic acid therapy for adrenoleukodystrophy. *Am J Hematol*, 1995, **48** 132–3.

69 Kickler TS, Zinkham WH, Moser A *et al*. Effect of erucic acid on platelets in patients with adrenoleukodystrophy. *Biochem Mol Med*, 1996, **57** 125–33.

70 Dubey P, Raymond GV, Moser AB *et al*. Adrenal insufficiency in asymptomatic adrenoleukodystrophy patients identified by very long-chain fatty acid screening. *J Pediatr*, 2005, **146** 528–32.

71 Mahmood A, Dubey P, Moser HW, Moser A X-linked adrenoleukodystrophy: therapeutic approaches to distinct phenotypes. *Pediatr Transplant*, 2005, **9** (Suppl 7) 55–62.

72 Shapiro E, Krivit W, Lockman L *et al*. Long-term effect of bone-marrow transplantation for childhood-onset cerebral X-linked adrenoleukodystrophy. *Lancet*, 2000, **356** 713–18.

73 Peters C, Charnas LR, Tan Y *et al*. Cerebral X-linked adrenoleukodystrophy: the international hematopoietic cell transplantation experience from 1982 to 1999. *Blood*, 2004, **104** 881–8.

74 Singh I, Pahan K, Khan M Lovastatin and sodium phenylacetate normalize the levels of very long chain fatty acids in skin fibroblasts of X- adrenoleukodystrophy. *FEBS Lett*, 1998, **426** 342–6.

75 Kemp S, Wei HM, Lu JF *et al*. Gene redundancy and pharmacological gene therapy: implications for X-linked adrenoleukodystrophy. *Nat Med*, 1998, **4** 1261–8.

76 Doerflinger N, Miclea JM, Lopez J *et al*. Retroviral transfer and long-term expression of the adrenoleukodystrophy gene in human CD34+ cells. *Hum Gene Ther*, 1998, **9** 1025–36.

77 Yamada T, Shinnoh N, Taniwaki T *et al*. Lovastatin does not correct the accumulation of very long-chain fatty acids in tissues of adrenoleukodystrophy protein-deficient mice. *J Inherit Metab Dis*, 2000, **23** 607–14.

22 Childhood Cancers

Evelyn Ward

Introduction

Childhood cancers differ from those seen in adults in both type and outcome [1]. In comparison with therapies used to treat adults, multimodal therapy and combination chemotherapy have been effective in vastly improving the outlook for children with cancer. Children have tumours that are chemotherapy responsive and they tolerate chemotherapy better than do adults [2]. Children differ metabolically as well and continued growth and development is desired throughout therapy which often spans several years. As more children are being treated for what is much of the time a chronic disease, there are increasing numbers of children who are subject to the nutritional problems caused by their disease and treatment.

Malnutrition and cancer cachexia are frequent consequences of paediatric cancer and therapy. A clear understanding of the metabolic alterations in the presence of malignancy which leads to cachexia and the value of maintaining nutritional equilibrium are a valuable part of managing these children. Nutritional support may enhance therapy, decrease complications, improve immunologic status and hopefully improve survival [3].

Types of cancers seen in childhood

The types of cancers seen in children can be divided into three main groups:

- Leukaemias
- Lymphomas
- Solid tumours

Leukaemias

Leukaemia is the most common neoplastic disease of infancy and childhood, accounting for 30–45% of all childhood cancers [4,5]. Acute lymphoblastic leukaemia (ALL) is the most common form of the disease in childhood, followed by acute myeloid leukaemia (AML) and then chronic myeloid leukaemia (CML). The cure rate (i.e. 5-year survival without relapse) is 85% with ALL and 65% with AML [5].

The leukaemias are fatal unless treated. At presentation pallor, fever, fatigue and aches and pains are the most common features. Haemorrhage, apart from easy bruising, is not common unless infection is present. Enlargement of the spleen and lymph nodes may be present [4].

Lymphomas

Lymphomas account for 9–15% of all childhood cancers [4,5]. In children the types of lymphomas seen are virtually limited to three types [6]:

- *Hodgkin's disease*, which affects the lymph glands causing them to enlarge.
- *Non-Hodgkin's lymphoma (NHL)*, which is a monoclonal neoplastic proliferation of lymphoid cells, usually B or T cells. It is more malignant than Hodgkin's.
- *Burkitt's lymphoma*, which is a malignant lymphoma of poorly differentiated lymphoblastic-type masses of immature lymphoid cells.

Solid tumours

Solid tumours account for 40% of childhood cancers. The most common solid tumours seen in children are [4,7]:

- *Brain tumours*, of which medulloblastoma is the most common. This is a tumour arising in the posterior fossa.
- *Wilm's tumour*, also known as nephroblastoma, which is a congenital highly malignant kidney tumour and can be bilateral.
- *Neuroblastoma*, which is another highly malignant tumour arising from the adrenal medulla from tissue of sympathetic origin. It can also arise from some parts of the abdominal, thoracic, pelvic or cervical chains of sympathetic ganglia.
- *Rhabdomyosarcoma*, which is a malignant tumour of striated muscle most commonly found in the orbital region, nose, mouth or pharynx and pelvic area.
- *Osteosarcoma*, which is a malignant tumour arising from bone. Any bone can be affected, but it usually occurs in the legs.
- *Ewing's sarcoma*, which is a very malignant tumour that can develop anywhere in the body, but usually starts in the bones, most commonly the pelvis, upper arm or thigh. It can develop in the soft tissue near bones.
- *Primitive neuroectodermal tumour* (PNET), which is a highly malignant tumour of neuroepithelial origin and can be thought of as being similar to a Ewing's sarcoma.

Incidence rates and survival rates for these tumours are given in Table 22.1 and Fig. 22.1.

Aetiology of malnutrition in children with cancer

The incidence of malnutrition in paediatric oncology patients ranges from 6 to 50% depending on the type, stage and location of the tumour [8,9]. Malnutrition is more severe with aggressive tumours in the later stages of malignancy, occuring in up to 37.5% of newly diagnosed patients with metastatic disease [10]. The greater the tumour burden and more intense the treatment, the higher the risk of nutritional morbidity. The initial nutritional problems resulting from the tumour may soon be compounded by iatrogenic nutritional abnormalities, the consequence of the treatment and its complications. Metabolic and psychological factors also have a role [11].

Malnutrition at diagnosis may be more common than previously thought because of nutritional assessment being based on measurement of height and weight, which may not be appropriate for assessing children with cancer. Many children with cancer have large tumour masses which inevitably add to their body weight, therefore weight : height ratios are distorted and, consequently, are unlikely to be a sensitive indicator of malnutrition [12]. The use of arm anthropometry (see p. 6) gives a more reliable indication of the presence of malnutrition at diagnosis and indicates that malnutrition is more common at diagnosis than previously realised [13].

Metabolic factors

Cancer cachexia is complex and multifactorial. It includes weight loss, anorexia, organ dysfunction and tissue wasting associated with significant alterations in protein, carbohydrate and lipid metabolism. The role of the cytokines remains unclear although tumour necrosis factor (TNF), interleukin-1 (IL-1), IL-6 and γ-interferon (IFN-γ) may have a role in cancer cachexia [14]. These cytokines are secreted by macrophages and lymphocytes and are thought to represent a host defence reaction to tumour cell invasion.

The normal response to starvation is to conserve

Table 22.1 UKCCSG registrations for children aged under 15 years by diagnostic group, 1982–2003.

Diagnosis	82	83	84	85	86	87	88	89	90	91	92	93	94	95	96	97	98	99	00	01	02	03	Total
ALL	287	288	291	297	293	308	327	329	370	361	368	395	377	383	384	376	431	388	374	368	455	255	8775
ANLL	54	41	60	61	64	65	62	71	63	66	55	75	81	67	81	77	65	85	68	72	80	60	1688
Hodgkin's disease	51	42	42	50	59	33	40	32	42	43	62	46	49	65	57	59	57	66	70	82	99	40	1361
NHL	57	51	67	67	66	69	84	75	81	76	87	79	74	95	73	93	104	92	95	78	102	56	1674
PNET	29	50	29	38	33	49	42	48	54	59	75	59	71	66	66	66	71	74	60	67	78	40	1364
Neuroblastoma	80	72	78	73	76	100	111	96	116	102	93	89	87	92	100	98	102	109	79	105	104	87	2307
Retinoblastoma	9	21	21	30	36	45	29	42	33	43	49	63	45	40	36	43	31	34	42	34	53	26	828
Wilm's tumour	64	69	64	63	70	83	76	69	94	72	75	81	91	67	85	91	81	67	82	88	97	59	1906
Osteosarcoma	20	20	13	16	22	19	23	14	21	21	19	37	30	46	37	29	28	33	32	33	44	23	650
Ewing's sarcoma	19	25	24	22	21	24	21	24	14	25	20	21	19	27	24	20	21	27	26	38	30	29	619
Rhabdomyosarcoma	51	50	60	67	50	68	55	52	67	70	61	78	55	63	65	55	51	56	54	42	52	50	1450

United Kingdom Children's Cancer Study Group Scientific Report, 2003. ALL, acute lymphoblastic leukaemia; ANLL, acute non-lymphoblastic leukaemia; NHL, non-Hodgkin's lymphoma; PNET, primitive neuroectodermal tumour.

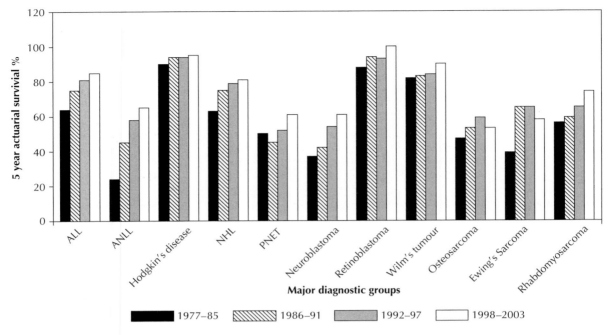

Figure 22.1   Survival rates in childhood cancer. ALL, acute lymphoblastic leukaemia; ANLL, acute non-lymphoblastic anaemia; NHL, non-Hodgkin's lymphoma; PNET, primitive neuroectodermal tumour.

energy (decreased energy expenditure) and protein reserves (decreased proteolysis and gluconeogenesis) at the expense of endogenous carbohydrate and fat stores (increased glycogenolysis and lipolysis). However, in children with cancers the result is a cascade of metabolic events which are typically characteristic of the acute metabolic stress response. Changes in the metabolism of fat, carbohydrate and protein have been demonstrated [15,16]. In addition to glycogenolysis and lipolysis, this response includes a marked increase in energy expenditure (hypermetabolism), proteolysis and gluconeogenesis (protein catabolism). This response results in an accelerated depletion of endogenous energy and substrate stores in the face of decreased exogenous fuel substrate provision [3].

Cachexia is more common in patients with solid tumours at diagnosis (33%) and during treatment (57%) compared with children with leukaemia (12% and 28%, respectively) [17]. Solid tumour patients developing cachexia during treatment were found to have a significantly raised sleeping energy expenditure at diagnosis whereas children

with leukaemia at risk of developing cachexia had no changes in energy expenditure at diagnosis [17]. Severe weight loss in children with leukaemia appears to be associated with more intensive treatment regimens such as those for AML [17] and more recently children treated on UKALL 2003 regimen C.

Malignant cachexia appears to result mainly from the increased metabolic demands imposed by the tumour burden itself, coupled with the acute stress response that malignancy evokes in the host.

With the ever increasing intensity of treatment regimens and treatment of relapsed patients there is a greater number of children at risk of the metabolic demands of their disease and treatment.

Complications of disease and treatment

Most of the malnutrition seen is a direct consequence of the disease progression and treatment. Table 22.2 shows the side effects that result in an increased risk of malnutrition.

Table 22.2   Side effects relating to treatment seen in paediatric oncology patients.

Side effect		Causative chemotherapeutic agent
Infection	Both chemotherapy and radiotherapy are known immune depressants; malnutrition also has an effect on immunity. The malnourished child with cancer and an uncontrolled infection can further deteriorate nutritionally from the side effects of cancer and infection leading to a vicious cycle	
Diarrhoea	This is the most common side effect and can be caused by mucositis and consequent malabsorption; tumour infiltration of the bowel; infection and prolonged use of antibiotics. Children are especially sensitive to the effects of drugs and radiotherapy to the intestinal tract	Actinomycin, Adriamycin, Methotrexate (high dose) Cytosine
Nausea and vomiting	This is another common side effect and some of the chemotherapy drugs are powerful inducers of vomiting	Actinomycin, Adriamycin, Carboplatin, Cisplatinum, Cyclophosphamide, Ifosfamide, Cytosine, Etoposide, Procarbazine
Stomatitis mucositis	Stomatitis or mucosal damage is a common side effect of chemotherapy and can be severe enough to prevent an adequate oral intake	Actinomycin, Adriamycin, Daunorubicin, Epirubicin, Bleomycin, Melphalan, Methotrexate
Renal damage and nutrient loss	A large number of chemotherapy drugs cause renal damage and hence significant protein and mineral losses	Cisplatin, Cyclophosphamide, Ifosfamide
Dysgeusia	This is often seen in advanced cancers, but is more often seen in adults	
Xerostomia	Xerostomia and poor oral hygiene can both be serious deterrents to an adequate oral intake	
Constipation	This can be a common problem in children with cancer	Vincristine

Psychological factors

Learned food aversion associated with treatment has been demonstrated in children with cancer and part of this behaviour is the phenomenon of anticipatory vomiting [18,19]. Parents can often become preoccupied with getting their children to eat. However, this preoccupation may reduce the child's appetite further, causing them to rebel against the parent and purposely not eat.

Identification of nutritional risk

Criteria for identifying children with cancer who are malnourished differ; however, determination of the nutritional risk of the child with cancer can be associated with the diagnosis of certain tumours and stages of the disease (Table 22.3) [20,21]. The following criteria can be used to identify children with cancer who are likely to require supplementary nutritional support [3]:

- Total weight loss of >5% relative to pre-illness body weight
- Weight for height <90%
- Serum albumin <32 mmol/L (in absence of recent acute metabolic stress within the last 14 days)
- A decrease in current percentile for weight (or height) of two major centiles
- Adipose energy reserves as determined by triceps skinfold thickness <5th percentile for age and sex

Table 22.3 Types of childhood cancers associated with high or low nutritional risk.

High nutritional risk	Low nutritional risk
Advanced diseases during initial intense treatment	Good prognosis acute lymphoblastic leukaemia
Stages III and IV Wilm's tumour and unfavourable histology Wilm's tumour	Non-metastatic solid tumours
Stages III and IV neuroblastoma	Advanced diseases in remission during maintenance treatment
Ewing's sarcoma	
Pelvic rhabdomyosarcoma	
Some non-Hodgkin's lymphoma	
Multiple relapse leukaemia	
Acute non-lymphoblastic leukaemia	
Some poor prognosis acute lymphoblastic leukaemia	
Medulloblastoma	

- Voluntary food intake <70% of estimated requirements for 5 days for well-nourished patients
- Anticipated gut dysfunction resulting from treatment for >5 days for well-nourished patients
- High nutritional risk patients based on tumour type and oncology treatment regimens
- Bone marrow transplant as a treatment for any tumour

The consequences of malnutrition are multiple and include a poorer outcome compared with children who are well nourished at diagnosis [8]. Malnutrition contributes to a reduced tolerance to therapy. Dose adjustments in chemotherapy have been seen most frequently in patients during a time of malnutrition [9]. Compromised nutritional status before initiation of therapy is associated significantly with relapse in solid tumour patients [22]. There also appear to be differences in the metabolism of chemotherapy agents between adequately nourished and inadequately nourished patients [23]. Malnutrition is associated with a higher risk of infectious complications and higher infection rates have been documented in malnour-

ished children [10]. The risk of opportunistic infection also appears to be increased in malnourished children with cancer.

Nutritional support

The main aims of nutritional support are to reverse the malnutrition seen at diagnosis, to prevent the malnutrition associated with treatment and to promote weight gain and growth rather than weight maintenance [24]. Nutritional support will improve immune competence, tolerance to treatment and quality of life [25]. A multidisciplinary approach, of which the dietitian is a key member, is the best way of providing safe, appropriate and effective nutritional support for this group of patients.

One of the questions that is often addressed in feeding cancer patients is the possibility that the nutrients given to replete the host may stimulate further growth of tumour mass [16]. Clinical studies of children with malignancy receiving nutritional support have failed to demonstrate increase in tumour growth or decreased survival despite improved host nutritional status [8]. Therefore, nutritional support should be considered a major part of therapy in order to prevent or reverse the effects of protein energy malnutrition and to increase the wellbeing of the child. If this is achieved then the aim of nutritional support has been reached even if the overall prognosis remains the same.

Oral feeding

In patients with a low nutritional risk, unless complicated by factors such as relapse, sepsis or major abdominal procedures, oral feeding is the best method if they are able to consume sufficient nutrients. However, the majority will need high energy supplements and specific advice on eating problems related to the side effects of their treatment (Table 22.4). Ideally, there should be flexibility with regard to menu choice, meal times and parental involvement. Some treatment centres are now moving towards meals being prepared at ward level. Studies have shown that a more flexible mealtime service can lead to a significant increase in the children's protein and energy intakes [28,29].

Table 22.4   Advice on nutritional problems associated with cancer and its treatment [26,27].

Problem	Suggested dietary advice
Loss of appetite	Offer small frequent meals/snacks 5–6/day Avoid rich fatty foods A soft diet may be better tolerated Avoid drinking just before and during mealtimes
Nausea	Offer small amounts of food at a time Cold food may be better tolerated Avoid fatty or greasy foods Offer dry foods, e.g. crackers, plain biscuits or toast Avoid very sweet foods Avoid hot and spicy foods Serve meals attractively Avoid favourite foods as the child may then develop a permanent dislike for them Sips of a cool, fizzy drink may help, e.g. soda water or ginger ale
Vomiting	Give mouth washes to help to remove the taste Avoid fluids or food until vomiting is controlled and then introduce clear fluids Avoid favourite foods Dry foods may be better tolerated
Sore mouth/throat	Offer soft, moist foods, e.g. mashed potato, scrambled egg, custard, yoghurt, ice cream If symptoms are severe blended/puréed foods may be more appropriate Use straws for drinking Keep foods moist by using butter, sauces, cream or yoghurt Avoid citrus fruits and fruit juices, spicy or salty foods Avoid rough or very dry foods
Dry mouth	Offer frequent drinks Crushed ice or cubes to suck may be useful Sucking fruit drops or boiled mints may stimulate saliva production Keep foods moist by using butter, sauces, cream, yoghurt, gravy
Taste changes and loss of taste	If the child complains of a 'metallic' taste when eating meat, then try poultry, fish, eggs or cheese instead Experiment using herbs and spices to flavour food Try cold sharp foods Offer foods familiar to and liked by the child Flavour gravy with Bovril, Marmite, soy and sweet and sour sauces Vary the colour and texture of the foods Emphasise the aroma of food
Diarrhoea	Avoid foods high in fibre Ensure the child continues to drink plenty, but avoid chilled drinks straight from the fridge Avoid any specific foods known to aggravate the diarrhoea
Intermittent constipation	Encourage foods high in fibre and plenty of fluids
Malabsorption	A low fat, low residue or lactose free diet as appropriate for the type of malabsorptive problem In some cases the enteral route will need to be avoided and the child will require total parenteral nutrition
Food aversion	Avoid favourite foods prior to chemotherapy Give carbohydrate based meals prior to chemotherapy rather then protein based meals Avoid making a big issue of the child's nutritional intake

Advice with regard to the use of high energy foods and small frequent meals should be given routinely to parents. Advice on the use of supplements (Table 11.3) should be given and how to modify them in order to improve their palatability; in this group of patients their liking for tastes changes very frequently.

Enteral nutrition

Whenever nutritional intervention is indicated it is preferable to use the enteral route. Enteral nutrition has numerous practical and psychological advantages over parenteral nutrition, including a low risk of infection and other catheter related complications, more normal play activities, and involves both parent and child. In addition, enteral feeding maintains gut integrity, reduces the risk of bacterial translocation and is more economical [8].

Studies report that nasogastric feeding during intensive treatment results in improved nutritional status with minimal complications [30–32]. It has been shown to improve energy intake and well-being and to result in a significant improvement in nutritional status as measured by mid upper arm circumference [33]. Even in children undergoing bone marrow transplant (BMT) where the nutritional insult is complex (as is its management), enteral nutrition when tolerated is effective in limiting the nutritional insult, leading to a better response and fewer complications [34,35].

While nasogastric feeding is effective, when there is a need for long term nutritional support the child may find it unacceptable psychologically so its usefulness may be limited. In some cases oral feeding is hindered by the presence of the tube. Other problems such as vomiting, thrombocytopenia and mucositis also result in a reduced acceptance of nasogastric feeding.

Whereas gastrostomy feeding has become the main method of providing long term nutritional support in other areas of paediatrics, until recently it has not been commonly used in children with cancer because of the perceived risk of infectious complications in immunosuppressed patients and tube related complications. However, the few published studies have shown it to be a safe and effective method of nutritional support in terms of cost and nutritional status. It appears to be associated with only minor complications such as site infection and over-granulation [36–39].

Nasojejunal or jejunostomy feeding should be considered in children with severe prolonged vomiting or gastric dysmotility following treatment.

Generally, a whole protein feed will be tolerated. However, following chemotherapy a protein hydrolysate or elemental feed may be more appropriate if malabsorption occurs and should be considered in children at risk of mucositis [40]. A child previously on total parenteral nutrition may not tolerate a whole protein feed initially when transferring to enteral feeding, so again a hydrolysate or elemental feed may be useful (see Tables 7.7, 7.9 and 7.12).

The majority of children receiving enteral feeding will require it throughout their intense treatment, but once they go on to maintenance treatment appetite usually improves and a conscious effort should be made to try and wean them off their feeds. Continuing support and monitoring is essential.

Parenteral nutrition

Parenteral nutrition (PN) should be reserved for those whose enteral feeding regimens cannot provide adequate nutrients, such as patients with abnormal gastrointestinal function related either to their tumour or following chemotherapy or radiotherapy treatments. Previously PN was often the feeding method of choice in children with cancer because they already had central venous access and it has been successful in preventing and correcting malnutrition [35]. It is now most commonly reserved for children with severe mucositis or neutropenic enterocolitis.

Children undergoing BMT or high dose therapy with peripheral blood stem cell rescue can have complex gastrointestinal damage and this may have profound nutritional consequences; PN is indicated in children with severe mucositis, in patients unable to tolerate adequate enteral nutrition because of diarrhoea and/or vomiting and in those with severe graft versus host disease involving the gut [41,42].

Although PN may be an appropriate method of renourishing children with cancer, some patients may not benefit from PN support because of overwhelming medical problems which may limit fluid intake, with medication and blood products taking precedence over nutrition.

Metabolic complications of PN are well documented [43] and are not significantly different between children with malignancies and other children requiring nutritional support. Monitoring of the patient's weight, fluid balance and biochemical parameters is essential. It is extremely important to check electrolyte levels daily, especially if the child has severe diarrhoeal losses or is receiving a course of chemotherapy containing drugs that impair renal function. Chemotherapy drugs such as cisplatin and ifosfamide can cause renal tubular damage. Cisplatin damage is common as the cumulative dose rises and is associated with excessive loss of magnesium, potassium and calcium. Cumulative doses of ifosfamide can cause Fanconi's renal syndrome leading to glycosuria and excessive bicarbonate, phosphate, potassium, magnesium and calcium losses through the kidney [44]. In this case, certain electrolytes will be required above normal maintenance level. Table 22.5 gives the side effects of low plasma electrolyte levels caused by chemotherapy agents.

Nutrition and the child with cancer undergoing bone marrow transplant

BMT is now widely used in children with malignancies and non-malignant illness. It is indicated for patients with high risk leukaemia or for patients with leukaemia who have disease recurrence. These patients undergo an allogenic transplant using donor (related or unrelated) marrow. Some children with solid tumours (e.g. stage IV neuroblastoma, stage IV rhabdomyosarcoma and Ewing's sarcoma) may undergo high dose therapy, usually melphalan or busulfan, supported with a peripheral blood stem cell transplant.

The priming chemotherapy used causes severe nausea, vomiting and oral ulceration and BMT in children is associated with diarrhoea, protein-losing enteropathy, hypoalbuminaemia and trace element deficiencies [34]. Transient intestinal failure following BMT is a common clinical problem as unlike other organ/tissue transplantation, BMT often requires the use of total body irradiation in addition to immunosuppression. Cells with a rapid turnover, such as haemopoietic cells and immature enterocytes, are well recognised as highly susceptible to the effects of radiation and chemotherapy [41].

Nutritional support is provided to minimise the nutritional morbidity of both the conditioning regimens, leading to mucositis of the gastrointestinal tract, and complications resulting from the procedure such as graft versus host disease or veno-occlussive disease of the liver.

PN continues to have a role in children who develop severe gastrointestinal toxicity or graft versus host disease. However, it has been demonstrated that adequate nutritional support can be provided enterally [34,35,45] and during periods of maximum gut toxicity an elemental feed or hydrolysed protein feed is recommended [40,45]. Children with severe graft versus host disease can become temporarily dissaccharide intolerant (mainly lactose) necessitating a lactose free diet and in some cases a low sucrose, low starch diet as well (see Tables 18.12 and 7.15).

The aetiology of nutritional compromise caused

Table 22.5 Effect of low plasma electrolyte levels caused by chemotherapy drugs.

Electrolyte affected	Side effect	Chemotherapy drug
Potassium	Muscular weakness Confusion Cardiac arrhythmias	Ifosfamide Cyclophosphamide Cisplatin Carboplatin
Phosphate	Anorexia, weakness, bone pain, joint stiffness	Ifosfamide Cyclophosphamide
	Further symptoms include muscle weakness, tremor, paraesthesia, confusion and coma	Cisplatinum Carboplatin
Calcium	Tetany Fitting Lethargy Osteomalacia	Ifosfamide
Magnesium	Muscle weakness Fasciculation Tetany Vertigo Depression	Cisplatin

by chemotherapy and total body irradiation is complex and nutritional support in this group of patients is challenging [46]. In addition to this the patient is severely neutropenic and needs to have a 'clean' diet in order to prevent gastrointestinal infection from foodborne pathogens [47]. The provision of a clean diet is described elsewhere (see p. 27).

Alternative diets

There is increasing awareness amongst parents of the role of alternative or complementary nutritional therapies, of which there are many, some of which claim to treat cancer. Examples include the Gerson treatment, the Kelley anticancer diet and the macrobiotic diet.

Most of these diets claim to rid the body of unnatural chemicals and to restore the efficiency of and strengthen the body's immune system by maximising the mineral, vitamin and enzyme systems. They are usually strictly vegetarian or vegan and, ideally, organic. The diets generally restrict animal products, salt and refined carbohydrate and allow only small quantities of fat. They often involve taking large amounts of vitamin and mineral supplements. They are bulky, low in energy, low in protein and totally inappropriate for the child with cancer who has a loss of appetite, nausea and vomiting who will find it extremely difficult to eat such a diet.

These diets are also very time consuming and costly to prepare and the high doses of vitamins and minerals may be harmful to children. It is essential that any parent contemplating putting a child on such a diet should be advised appropriately on the disadvantages of using such regimens in children. It is also worth noting that tumours in children have not been shown to be influenced by diet and if conventional curative treatment is displaced this will have a detrimental effect, because many childhood cancers are curable with conventional treatment [48].

Vitamins and minerals

Parents are also more aware of vitamin and mineral supplementation in the child being treated for cancer, in particular the role of the antioxidants. The rationale for antioxidant supplementation during chemotherapy is to compensate for treatment or tumour induced antioxidant depletion, and therefore an improvement in the effects of cytotoxic therapy and an alleviation of the side effects of treatment [49,50]. However, this may result in potential interactions with the efficacy of conventional treatment [48,49,51]. Some antioxidants may only be beneficial if taken as part of a normal diet and not as a supplement and high doses are potentially toxic.

Until further studies are published on the role and interactions of antioxidants it is prudent to advise the following: that supplementation of vitamins and minerals above the reference nutrient intake (RNI) (p. 10) is not recommended because of potential toxicity and interactions with the efficacy of conventional treatment. Children receiving enteral feeds or nutritionally complete oral sip feeds should not need additional vitamins or minerals. Children on less intensive treatment protocols who generally do not require nutritional support, but on occasion eat only a few foods and a limited intake of fruit and vegetables, may require a general multivitamin supplement.

Glutamine

Glutamine is a major fuel and important nitrogen source for enterocytes and has a key role in maintaining mucosal cell integrity and gut barrier function [52]. The use of many chemotherapy drugs, in particular anthrocyclines, actinomycin and high dose methotrexate, result in both structural and functional injuries to the gastrointestinal tract which results in mucositis severe enough to prevent an adequate oral intake. Therefore, glutamine may have a potential role in helping to reduce the incidence and severity of mucositis in at risk patients. Enteral feeds containing glutamine may help to protect the gut during chemotherapy and radiotherapy [40,53]. Some published studies have shown a significant decrease in the duration and severity of oral mucositis with oral doses of glutamine [54,55]. While the role of glutamine in the prevention of chemotherapy and radiotherapy toxicity continues to evolve, further studies are still required [56]. In a phase 1 pharmokinetic study an oral dose of 0.65 g/kg was shown to be an appropriate dose to use in paediatric oncology patients as determined by patient acceptability and by plasma glutamine and ammonia levels [57].

References

1   Van Eys J Nutritional therapy in children with cancer. *Cancer Res*, 1977, **87** 2457–61.
2   Van Eys J Malnutrition in pediatric oncology. In: Newell GR (ed.) *Nutrition and Cancer: Etiology and Treatment*. New York: Raven Press, 1981.
3   Andrassy RJ, Chwals WJ Nutritional support of the pediatric oncology patient. *Nutrition*, 1998, **14** 124–9.
4   Eden OB Paediatric oncology. *Hospital Update*, 1983, March, 779–88.
5   United Kingdom Children's Cancer Study Group *Scientific Report*. London: UKCCSG, 2003
6   Bury CL *Paediatric Pathology*, 2nd edn. Berlin: Springer-Verlag, 1989.
7   Mott MG, Burgess MF Paediatric malignancy: tumour types. *Medicine*, 1995, 460–63.
8   Donaldson SS, Wesley MN, DeWys WD *et al*. A study of nutritional status in paediatric cancer patients. *Am J Dis Child*, 1981, **135** 1107–12.
9   Van Eys J Malnutrition in children with cancer: incidence and consequences. *Cancer*, 1979, **43** 2030–5.
10 Smith DE, Stevenson MCG, Booth IW Malnutrition at diagnosis of malignancy in childhood; common but mostly missed. *Eur J Pediatr*, 1991, **150** 318–22.
11 Mauer AM, Burgess JB, Donaldson SS *et al*. Special nutritional needs of children with malignancies – a review. *J Parenter Enteral Nutr*, 1990, **14** 315–23.
12 Brennan B Sensitive measures of the nutritional status of children with cancer in hospital and in the field. *Int J Cancer* 1998, **Supp 11** 10–13.
13 Smith DE, Stevens MC, Booth IW Malnutrition in children with malignant solid tumours. *J Hum Nutr Diet*, 1990, **3** 303–9.
14 Tidsdale MJ Cancer cachexia; metabolic alterations and clinical manifestations. *Nutrition*, 1997, **13** 1–7.
15 Picton SV Aspects of altered metabolism in children with cancer. *Int J Cancer* 1998, **Suppl 11** 62–4.
16 Rossi-Fanelli F, Cascino A, Muscaritoli M Abnormal substrate metabolism and nutritional strategies in cancer management. *J Parenter Enteral Nutr*, 1991, **15** 680–3.
17 Picton SV, Eden OB, Rothwell NJ Metabolic rate, interleukin 6 and cachexia in children with malignancy. *Med Pediatr Oncol*, 1995, **5** 249 abstract 0–63.
18 Bernstein IL Learned taste aversions in children receiving chemotherapy. *Science*, 1978, **200** 1302–3.
19 Bernstein IL Physiological and psychological mecha-
nisms of cancer anorexia. *Cancer Res*, 1982, **42** 715S–20S.
20 Rickard KA, Coates TD, Grosfeld JL *et al*. The value of nutritional support in children with cancer. *Cancer*, 1986, **52** 587–90.
21 Rickard KA, Grosfeld JL, Coates TD *et al*. Advances in nutrition care of children with neoplastic disease – a review of treatment, research and application. *J Am Diet Assoc*, 1986, **86** 1666–75.
22 Rickard KA, Detamore CM, Coates TD *et al*. Effect of nutritional staging on treatment delays and outcome in stage IV neuroblastoma. *Cancer*, 1983, **52** 587–92.
23 Van Eys J Nutrition in the treatment of cancer in children. *J Am Coll Nutr*, 1984, **3** 159–68.
24 Rickard KA, Kirksey A, Baehner RL *et al*. Effectiveness of enteral and parenteral nutrition in the management of children with Wilm's tumours. *Am J Clin Nutr*, 1980, **33** 2622–9.
25 Van Eys J Benefits of nutritional intervention on nutritional status, quality of life and survival. *Inter J Cancer* 1998, **Suppl 11** 66–8.
26 *EAT* Paediatric Dietetic Department, St James's University Hospital, Leeds, UK, 1999.
27 Henry L Helping your child to eat. The Royal Marsden NHS Trust, London UK, 2004.
28 Williams R, Virtue K, Adkins A Room service improves patient food intake and satisfaction with hospital food. *J Pediatr Oncol Nurs*, 1998, **15** 183–9.
29 Kok K, Michaelsen KF, Vestergaard H *et al*. The effect of a new meal delivery system on the energy intake of children admitted with cancer. *Clin Nutr* 1992, **11** (Suppl 11) 92 abstract.
30 den Broeder E, Lippens RJJ, van't Hof MA *et al*. Effects of nasogastric feeding on nutritional status of children with cancer. *Eur J Clin Nutr*, 1998, **52** 494–500.
31 Pietsch P, Ford C, Whitlock JA Nasogastric feeding in children with high risk cancer: a pilot study. *J Pediatr Hematol Oncol*, 1999, **2** 111–14.
32 Deswarte-Wallace J, Firouzbakhsh S, Flinlestein JZ Using research to change practice: enteral feeding for pediatric oncology patients. *J Pediatr Oncol Nurs*, 2001, **5** 217–23.
33 Smith DE, Handy DJ, Holden CE *et al*. An investigation of supplementary naso-gastric feeding in malnourished children undergoing treatment for malignancy: results of a pilot study. *J Hum Nutr Diet*, 1992, **5** 85–91.
34 Papadopoulou A, MacDonald A, Williams MD *et al*. Enteral nutrition after bone marrow transplant. *Arch Dis Child*, 1997, **77** 131–6.
35 Papadopoulou A, Williams MD, Darbyshire PJ *et al*. Nutritional support in children undergoing bone marrow transplant. *Clin Nutr*, 1998, **17** 57–63.
36 Aquino V, Smyrl B, Hogg R *et al*. Enteral nutritional

support by gastrostomy tube in children with cancer. *J Pediatr*, 1995, **127** 58–62.

37   Mathew P, Bowman L, William R *et al.* Complications and effectiveness of gastrostomy feeding in pediatric cancer patients. *J Pediatr Hematol Oncol*, 1996, **18** 81–5.

38   Barron M, Duncan D, Green G *et al.* Efficacy and safety of radiologically placed gastrostomy tubes in pediatric haematology/oncology patients. *Med Paediatr Oncol*, 2000, **34** 177–82.

39   Bakish J, Hargrave D, Tariq N *et al.* Evaluation of dietetic intervention in children with medulloblastoma and supratentorial PNET. *Cancer*, 2003, **98** 1014–20.

40   Ward E. *Protocol for the management of mucositis in paediatric oncology: Nutritional care.* SHS International, Liverpool UK, 2003.

41   Papadopoulou A, Lloyd DR, Williams MD *et al.* Gastrointestinal and nutritional sequelae of bone marrow transplant. *Arch Dis Child*, 1996, **75** 208–13.

42   Papadopoulou A Nutritional considerations in children undergoing bone marrow transplant. *Eur J Clin Nutr*, 1998, **52** 863–71.

43   Shulman RJ, Philips J Parenteral nutrition in infants and children. *J Pediatr*, 2003, **36** 587–607.

44   Ladas EJ, Sacks N, Meacham L *et al.* A multidisciplinary review of nutrition considerations in the paediatric oncology population: A perspective from children's oncology group. *Nutr Clin Pract*, 2005, **20** 377–93.

45   Langdana A, Tully N, Molloy E *et al.* Intensive enteral nutrition in paediatric bone marrow transplant. *Bone Marrow Transplant* 2001, **27** 741–6.

46   Muscaritoli M, Grieco G, Capria S *et al.* Nutritional and metabolic support in patients undergoing bone marrow transplant. *Am J Clin Nutr*, 2002, **75** 183–90.

47   Henry L Immunocompromised patients and nutrition. *Prof Nurse*, 1997, **12** 655–9.

48   Weitzman S Alternative nutritional cancer therapies. *Int J Cancer* 1998, **Suppl 11** 69–72.

49   Ladas E, Jacobson S, Kennedy DD *et al.* Antioxidants and cancer therapy. *J Clin Oncol*, 2004, **22** 517–28.

50   Norman H, Bytrum RR, Feldman E *et al.* The role of dietary supplements during cancer therapy. *J Nutr*, 2003, **133** 3794S–9S.

51   Labriola D, Livingstone R Possible interactions between dietary antioxidants and chemotherapy. *Oncology*, 1999, **13** 1003–7.

52   Van Acker B, von Meyenfeldt MF, van der Hulst RRWJ *et al.* Glutamine: the pivot of our nitrogen economy. *J Parenter Enteral Nutr*, 1999, **23** S45–8.

53   Ward E, Kinsey S, Richards M Why do infants being treated for acute lymphoblastic leukaemia fail to thrive? *Arch Dis Child*, 2002, **87** 562.

54   Anderson P, Schroeder G, Anderson PM Oral glutamine reduces the duration and severity of stomatitis after cytotoxic cancer chemotherapy. *Cancer*, 1998, **83** 1433–9.

55   Skubitz K, Anderson P Oral glutamine to prevent chemotherapy induced stomatitis: a pilot study. *J Lab Clin Med*, 1996, **127** 223–5.

56   Savarese D, Savy G, Vahdat L *et al.* Prevention of chemotherapy and radiation toxicity with glutamine. *Cancer Treat Review*, 2003, **29** 501–13.

57   Ward E, Picton S, Reid U *et al.* Oral glutamine in paediatric oncology patients: a dose finding study *Eur J Clin Nutr*, 2003, **56** 1–6.

Useful addresses

Cancer BACUP
3 Bath Place, Rivington Streer, London, EC2A 3DR
www.cancerbacup.org.uk

Children's Cancer and Leukaemia Group (CCLG)
University of Leicester, Department of Epidemiology and Public Health, 22/28 Princess Road West, Leicester, LE1 6TP
www.cclg.org.uk

23 Eating Disorders

Dasha Nicholls

Introduction

Eating disorders are psychiatric disorders (generally considered to be emotional disorders) in which abnormalities of eating are the main behavioural symptoms. Hand-in-hand with abnormal eating behaviours go characteristic fears or beliefs, the so-called 'core psychopathology' of eating disorders. As with other psychiatric disorders, the diagnosis of an eating disorder depends on the presence of specific thoughts or ideas, *and* associated behavioural disturbance outside the range of what might be considered normal behaviour. These criteria distinguish the eating disorders from other abnormal eating behaviours, in which psychological disturbance may be present but is usually secondary, not primary. For example, low self-esteem and depression may be associated with obesity, but obesity is not a psychiatric disorder. Similarly, depression is often associated with loss of appetite, but the change in eating behaviour is secondary not primary.

The most widely recognised and well-described eating disorders are anorexia nervosa and bulimia nervosa. In both, the patient has an extreme preoccupation with (usually) her weight and/or shape and a specific 'morbid' fear of weight gain. In anorexia nervosa the associated behavioural disturbances are methods for achieving weight loss.

Most commonly, this is through dietary restriction, often coupled with excessive exercise; the so-called restrictive subtype of anorexia nervosa [1]. Alternatively, weight loss can be achieved by means of purging behaviours, such as self-induced vomiting, or laxative or diuretic abuse; the so-called binge–purge subtype.

In bulimia nervosa the same fears and beliefs about weight and shape exist, but the behavioural characteristics differ. The patient submits to intense cravings for large quantities of food – a binge – eaten over a short period of time. The binge is then often followed by extreme guilt about eating because of fear of weight gain. The patient will attempt to compensate for the additional calorie load through one or more 'compensatory behaviours'; either self-induced vomiting and purgative abuse (binge–purge subtype) or periods of fasting and exercising (restrictive subtype). An additional psychological feature of bulimia nervosa is the patient's sense of being unable to control her eating behaviour.

There is clearly much overlap between anorexia nervosa and bulimia nervosa, and indeed up to one-third of bulimia nervosa patients have had a previous episode of anorexia nervosa. Patients of bulimia nervosa are usually in the normal or slightly overweight range; if they were severely underweight they would be diagnosed as having anorexia nervosa – binge–purge subtype.

More recently, a third disorder has been described, binge-eating disorder (BED). In BED the patient has binge episodes, a sense of lack of control over food intake and a preoccupation with weight and shape, but does not utilise compensatory behaviours following a binge episode. BED can therefore be thought of as a distinct disorder in its own right or as a behaviour that reflects psychopathology among the obese [2].

There are a number of other disturbances of eating recognised as being severe enough to constitute disorder. These syndromes are of uncertain status, in terms of whether they are disorders in their own right or merely associated features of other disorders. In addition to the eating disorders described above, the International Classification of Diseases [3] includes: over-eating leading to obesity as a reaction to distressing events (*not* psychological disturbance as a consequence of obesity); vomiting associated with other psychological disturbances (e.g. dissociative disorders, hypochondriacal disorders or when emotional factors in pregnancy contribute); and other eating disorders such as pica and psychogenic loss of appetite in its eating disorders section.

In children there are a number of eating behaviours that are not currently classified at all, but which are nonetheless manifestations of, or cause, extreme psychological distress. There is no international consensus how to name these behaviours or how they should be classified [4]. The terms used in this chapter are therefore descriptive, but we have found them to be useful and meaningful in a clinical context working with children in the middle childhood and early adolescent age range. Most are clearly distinguishable from 'true' eating disorders [5].

Eating disorders in a developmental context

Eating is a key behaviour in developmental terms. Failure to make the transitions from milk through liquids to solids would raise suspicion of an organic or developmental disorder, or the possibility of severe abuse and neglect. Once established on solids, the developmental tasks are centred on increasing self-regulation on behalf of the child, with the gradual transition of control and responsibility for food intake from the parent to the child. Thus, by the age of 8 years or so, although a parent is the food provider, a child will usually feed themselves; usually select what of the provided food they will eat; and ask for more or stop eating when full (self-regulate quantity).

This process of transfer of responsibility is a careful balance of timing and encouragement – too much parental regulation and the child may rebel; too much autonomy for the child and he or she may not be able to cope. As such the transition from feeding to eating is highly susceptible to tension and conflict, particularly over issues of autonomy and control. It is also a point of communication between a child and his or her parent, and can therefore be a method for communicating distress or anxiety. In younger children, the importance of this partnership is recognised by the term 'feeding disorders' (conventionally requiring onset before the age of 6 years). In adolescents and adults, the term 'eating disorder' implies independence from carers, although one of the features of anorexia nervosa is that patients often revert to the need to be fed. The eating disturbances of middle childhood lie somewhere between the eating disorders and the feeding disorders of early childhood, and share some features of each.

When eating behaviour becomes the focus for distress or of significant harm (such as failure to thrive) help may be sought through a variety of means. Often a dietitian will be the first port of call, and it is important to be able to recognise the ways in which psychological distress can manifest through eating, and consider how to address these difficulties when encountered in clinical practice.

Anorexia nervosa

Both anorexia nervosa and bulimia nervosa are predominantly disorders of teenage girls and young women. However, anorexia nervosa can occur in boys and in children as young as 7 years. Both disorders are relatively common, with anorexia nervosa occurring in almost 1% of teenage girls. In the USA, anorexia nervosa is now the third most common chronic illness of adolescence [6]. While the figures in the UK are not quite so high, certain populations are more at risk (e.g. girls in high achieving academic environments and in high risk professions such as modelling and dancing). The prevalence of anorexia nervosa is probably not increasing [7], although the severity of the disorder may be [8]. Many of the complications of anorexia nervosa are related to the duration of illness and age of onset [9], and thus early diagnosis is important, particularly in growing children. The essential features of anorexia nervosa are as follow.

- *Weight loss (or failure of weight gain in growing children) sufficient for there to be physiological signs of underweight.* In post-menarcheal girls, this means weight loss sufficient for menses to have stopped for more than three cycles. In younger girls and in boys, signs of endocrine dysfunction are failure to onset or progress in puberty and slowing of linear growth. Both these signs can take months to become manifest. In practice, a child whose weight is not rising or is falling over a period of months can be assumed to be losing significant weight. The World Health Organization (WHO) definition of underweight and the diagnostic criteria for anorexia nervosa use a cut-off of 85% of weight for height to indicate low weight. This approximates to just above the second centile for body mass index (BMI) [10]. Rapid weight loss (>1 kg/week) is a poor prognostic sign and should be treated urgently.
- *Avoidance of food.* This may be evident simply as not eating (restraint) or by more surreptitious means such as hiding food, exercising to eliminate food, or purging (vomiting or laxative use). Patients may also indulge in rituals and compulsions to control their eating.
- *Morbid preoccupation with weight and/or shape.* The reason for avoiding food is a fear of weight gain and the changes in body shape that may accompany it. The individual may acknowledge this fear directly. Sometimes it may be inferred only by the specific avoidance of 'fattening' foods. Thus, the patient will often know more than their parents or even professionals about the calorific content of foods. In boys and young men the form of the preoccupation may differ slightly; females with anorexia nervosa see their stomach and thighs as particularly fat, whereas boys may be more concerned about their chest size and musculature.

Recognising anorexia nervosa

Eating disorders rarely present directly to specialists [11]. Atypical presentations and a particular lack of awareness that these conditions can arise in young children and boys may lead to delay in referral, diagnosis and treatment [12,13]. Recognition and diagnosis of eating disorders in children and adolescents needs to take into consideration the context of normal pubertal growth and adolescent development. While the problem may present as a result of concern from others, assessment of the young person alone is necessary to establish diagnosis, risk and attitude to help. Intervention should be considered not only in those who meet all the diagnostic criteria, but in young people with significantly abnormal eating attitudes and behaviours, such as those who vomit or take laxatives regularly but do not binge, or where rate of weight loss is of more concern than the degree of underweight.

The contrast between the patient's emaciated state and her irritable reluctance to acknowledge any difficulties is a good indicator of an eating problem. Protest that she is 'naturally thin' is not born out by a low pulse rate, low blood pressure and cold hands and feet. She is unlikely to present herself, but will be there at the behest of a family member, a friend, or because concerns have been expressed at school. While the patient may not want to be ill, she has an even greater desire not to be made to eat. She will therefore tend to avoid situations where her eating difficulties are most manifest (e.g. eating in public or social groups) and will avoid situations where she may be confronted about her weight. Adolescent patients typically present wearing many layers of clothes in all seasons, partly from a wish to hide their body and partly from feeling cold. Younger children, however, may not be self-conscious about their low weight and even seem to wish to display it at times.

After weighing and measuring height, the answers to a few key questions, asked in a non-judgmental manner, can be helpful in deciding whether further assessment is needed. Distress when asked about weight and food should heighten concern. If the degree of concern is equivocal, a return visit within a month is advisable. If in doubt, the simplest discriminator is food. When increased calorie intake is advised, the anorexia nervosa patient will need to increase food avoiding behaviours to counteract the effects on weight and shape, and/or will demonstrate greater distress/protest about eating. On a hospital ward this behaviour is quickly evident, particularly if there is a discrepancy between what the patient is thought to be eating and the weight changes that result.

Having recognised the problem, direct challenge or confrontation is unlikely to be helpful. Reasonable aims for a first meeting are to feedback findings from physical examination, including degree of underweight if relevant; establish weight monitoring, and a plan of action for if weight falls; discuss psychiatric risk as needed; and provide the family and young person with information about the nature, course and treatment of eating disorders [14]. There are a number of useful books available for parents and patients, although their use has not been evaluated as an adjunct to treatment. In the UK, the National Institute for Health and Clinical Excellence (NICE) has recently published guidelines on the treatment of eating disorders [15], which provide a useful overview of recognition and treatment for parents and professionals alike. Voluntary organisations such as the UK Eating Disorders Association also provide information for carers and patients.

For those under 16 years presenting alone, communication with parents and/or carers will need to be discussed. In general, the threshold for intervention in adolescents should be lower than in adults. Admission to a paediatric ward should be considered for patients with BMI or weight for height of 75% or below, or where there are signs of medical instability [16].

Overview of treatment

Whatever the eating disorder, the child's needs are essentially the same – to be able to eat enough to grow and develop normally, and to find a way of addressing her or his emotional needs through a medium other than food. Debate continues over which to tackle first: the eating behaviour or the emotional symptoms. A similar debate exists for the patient – 'the problem is not really about eating' alongside 'I can't bear to eat'. The main concern is that both are addressed.

In young people, eating behaviour is usually addressed first for a number of reasons. First, children dehydrate and physically decompensate very quickly. Secondly, the risk of complications such as growth failure, pubertal arrest and failure of bone accretion are related to age of onset and duration of illness. In a growing child, anorexia nervosa can have significant impact in as little as 6 months. In children and adolescents with eating disorders, growth and development should be closely monitored. Where development is delayed or growth is stunted despite adequate nutrition, paediatric advice should be sought [15]. Thirdly, responsibility for food intake will often lie with the parents and can therefore be established more quickly than when the patient needs to become self-motivated.

A multidisciplinary approach is essential because of the need to address the medical, nutritional and therapeutic needs of the young person and her family. Such an approach also minimises the risk of isolating the professional or their being drawn into colluding with the patient. Collusion is not uncommon, as the most difficult part of managing anorexia nervosa is agreeing mutually acceptable goals for treatment. Failure to agree goals, or failure to reach treatment goals are good indications for referral to a specialist eating disorders team. A number of specialist services exist nationwide, although availability of services for children and young adolescents is patchy. Anorexia nervosa is a disorder that can be treated under the Mental Health Act 1983 or under the Children Act 1989, if necessary. Specialist teams rarely, if ever, need to force-feed patients.

The mainstay of treatment for anorexia nervosa are various forms of psychotherapy, the type and intensity varying with the age of the patient and the chronicity of the problem. Behavioural techniques are not much use in isolation and, at worst, can be punitive. For patients under the age of 18 years with an illness of less than 3 years' duration, family therapy is the treatment of choice [15]. Family therapy aims to develop an alliance of parents and family members against the illness, and to support the young person in her attempts to communicate directly with her parents, explore areas of difference and negotiate issues around control and responsibility. The family is therefore seen as an important resource in the treatment [17]. There is no empirical evidence to suggest that families cause eating disorders, although there is no doubt that family functioning can become severely distorted as a result of the illness.

Role of the dietitian

Little has been said so far about specific nutritional aspects in the management of anorexia nervosa. In part this is because treatment for many eating disorders involves abandoning dietary rules rather than adopting them, and comes from a belief that it is more important to empower the parents or young person to determine their own food intake than for them to follow a prescribed regimen. In addition, wide cultural variations in eating habits as well as food content make it hard to contemplate a diet that would suit all. Nevertheless, nutritional counselling is an important component of the comprehensive care of young people with eating disorders. While the patient may know a great deal about the nutritional content of food, they will have a distorted view of their own dietary requirements and unrealistic weight goals. In order for parents and/or a young person to take responsibility for nutritional intake there is a need for factual information about daily nutritional requirements and some idea about energy balance, particularly if excessive exercising is one of the problem behaviours. In the nutritional management of children and adolescents with anorexia nervosa, carers should be included in any dietary education or meal planning [15].

Specific dietary expertise is needed when nasogastric or other feeding is necessary. This will usually be in an inpatient setting where monitoring for refeeding syndrome is possible. In most patients with anorexia nervosa, an average weekly weight gain of 0.5–1.0 kg in inpatient settings and 0.5 kg in outpatient settings should be an aim of treatment. This requires about 3500–7000 kcal (14.6–29.3 MJ) extra per week, but it is important to recognise the increased energy requirements of growth and development, such that growing adolescents' needs are often greater than those of adults. Regular physical monitoring, and in some cases treatment with a multivitamin/multimineral supplement in oral form, is recommended during treatment. Although iron, zinc and calcium deficiency have been reported in anorexia nervosa these all normalise with refeeding. Once a healthy weight is reached, children and adolescents need continued increased energy and nutrients in their diet to support further growth and development.

Osteoporosis is a recognised complication of prolonged anorexia nervosa. Traditional methods of oestrogen supplementation are of limited benefit, although they may be useful for damage limitation in persistent anorexia nervosa by preventing further bone loss [18]. Calcium supplements may help where intake is low, although evaluation suggests the impact is minimal. Vitamin D is usually unnecessary as patients are not usually deficient. Many patients with anorexia nervosa are, or have become, vegetarian. Treatment centres address this issue in different ways. However, it is possible that the risks of hypo-oestrogenism (and therefore low bone density) are increased in vegetarians compared with non-vegetarians who are not menstruating because of low weight (H. Jacobs, personal communication). Golden [19] provides a review of aspects of bone density in adolescent anorexia nervosa.

Bulimia nervosa

Bulimia nervosa is a disorder of over-eating rather than under-eating. It tends to onset slightly later in adolescence or early adulthood than anorexia nervosa and is less likely to come to medical attention until many months or years after onset. The prevalence is therefore probably underestimated, at around 2–3% of young women. Bulimia nervosa was first described in 1979 [20] as 'an ominous variant of anorexia nervosa'. Since 1979 there has been a rise in numbers of cases presenting for treatment [7]. The severity of purging behaviour can be extreme, with serious medical complications. In addition, the patient with bulimia nervosa is more likely to be overtly depressed than the anorexia nervosa patient. Overall, however, bulimia nervosa is generally considered a less severe illness than anorexia nervosa in terms of morbidity and mortality, and because of the availability of well-validated treatments that are effective in over 60% of patients [15].

Recognising and treating bulimia nervosa

Bulimia nervosa is less obvious than anorexia nervosa to recognise and may only come to light through suspicion of a family member or friend. Patients are normal weight and are usually ashamed of their eating difficulties, so may seek help for a different problem, with hints about food and dieting the only clues. Irregular periods, calouses on the knuckles of forefingers due to abrasions from self-induced vomiting (Russell's sign) or erosion of dental enamel from stomach acid may be picked up. Adolescents living at home may find it harder to hide bingeing and purging behaviour than adults living independently. There are no investigations that will confirm the diagnosis, only good interviewing skills. One or two simple screening questions can be helpful, such as 'Do you think you have an eating problem?' and 'Do you worry excessively about your weight?'

Once recognised and acknowledged, the patient may be able to use one of the well-validated self-help manuals: 'Overcoming binge eating' (Fairburn, 1995) or 'Getting Better Bit(e) by Bit(e): A survival kit for patients of bulimia nervosa and binge eating disorders' (Schmidt and Treasure, 1993). These are as effective as therapist led treatment in over half of cases and are a useful adjunct to treatment in the remainder. Antidepressant medication also has a role in bulimia nervosa, regardless of whether the patient is also clinically depressed. If these first steps are not sufficient, cognitive behaviour therapy for bulimia nervosa (CBT-BN) should be offered, involving the family for younger patients as appropriate. The course of treatment should be for 16–20 sessions over 4–5 months. Information about nutrition and control of appetite, and the establishment of regular mealtimes are important educational components. The key to treatment lies in the recognition of triggers for binges and the establishment of alternative responses to those triggers.

Other eating difficulties associated with weight loss

The term 'food avoidance emotional disorder' (FAED) was coined by Higgs and Goodyer [21] to describe those children who avoid food, sufficient to result in weight loss, for reasons other than fear of weight gain. Children with FAED can find it as difficult to eat as those with anorexia nervosa, although they often wish they could eat more. Depression may be present, but food avoidance can exist as an isolated symptom. Eating difficulties can

be part of other disorders such as depression, obsessive compulsive disorder and pervasive developmental disorders. In addition, physical illness may often be associated with manifest loss of appetite, to which psychological factors can significantly contribute [22]. We have come to use the term FAED when food avoidance is marked and merits treatment intervention in its own right. When co-morbid disorders exist, either physical or psychological, they need to be addressed in addition to the eating difficulty.

Unlike patients with anorexia nervosa, children with FAED know that they are underweight, would like to be heavier, and may not know why they find this difficult to achieve. They are more likely to have other medically unexplained symptoms and their parents may attribute weight loss to an undiagnosed physical disorder. Addressing these concerns with a comprehensive physical assessment and an open mind is essential for successful treatment. FAED patients are also more likely than anorexia nervosa patients to show anxiety in areas unrelated to food. It is likely that children with FAED are a heterogeneous group of children, a minority of whom will later develop anorexia nervosa. The term excludes children who are chronically low in weight (restrictive eating or failure to thrive) and those in whom the range of foods eaten is limited but weight is not generally compromised ('selective eating' – see below).

Phobias involving food occur in isolation (i.e. as simple phobias) or as part of a more generalised anxiety disorder and can result in rapid or slow weight loss. The nature of the specific fear will vary with, amongst other things, the child's developmental stage. Fears that are common are fear of vomiting (emetophobia), fear of contamination or poisoning, and fear of choking or swallowing (functional dysphagia). Functional dysphagia can be found clinically in patients with FAED, selective eating and sometimes anorexia nervosa, or it may be a new symptom following trauma. Common associated problems include depression, panic attacks, social anxiety, compulsions and difficulties with separation.

Food phobias are usually secondary events (i.e. follow a period of normal eating for developmental stage). Clear trigger events may be identified in some but not all cases (e.g. choking events) or in one case fear of cholesterol developed after the child saw his father die of a myocardial infarction [23]. Presenting features include rigid eating patterns and associated conflict, restricted range of foods and, in more extreme cases, restricted quantity of food leading to weight loss. Singer *et al.* [24] have described an approach to treatment of food phobias based on family involvement and anxiety management.

Failure to thrive should be considered when long term growth failure is seen in association with low weight, extending back to early childhood.

Recognising these more diffuse forms of food related anxiety can be harder than recognising anorexia nervosa and bulimia nervosa. Often the presentation will be 'unexplained' weight loss. The priority is to exclude organic disorder, but the risk is that the child loses further weight during the course of investigations, or is traumatised by them (as can occur, for example, with endoscopy for the investigation of functional dysphagia). Equally distressing can be the 'there's nothing wrong with you – go and see the psychiatrists' response. The most direct route to opening discussion about causes is to ask parents what they think is wrong with their child. If they have no opinion, it may be helpful to ask specifically whether they think it is a gut related problem, a cancer or other 'worst fear', or whether worry or an eating disorder may play some part. Psychological assessment can then be suggested as one of the possible investigations.

For all of these disorders, careful individualised assessment of the child and family is necessary in order to understand the origin and meaning of the symptom for the child in their particular context. A clear formulation of the problem is needed as a guide to treatment. Similarly, nutritional support may need to be carefully considered, taking into account the child's specific anxiety, and finding creative ways to encourage food intake while the child retains as much control as possible. In extreme cases nasogastric or other feeding can help take the pressure off while the child learns to overcome his or her fear of eating at his or her own pace.

Other eating difficulties associated with normal weight

'Faddy eating' occurs in over 20% of toddlers and can be considered normal at a particular developmental stage. In a small number, particularly boys, the behaviour persists into middle childhood and adolescence. This has been termed 'selective eating' [25], also known as 'picky eating' [26] or 'perseverative feeding disorder' [27]. In addition to the narrow range of foods, the consistent psychological characteristic is an extreme resistance or unwillingness to try new foods. Often selective eating exists as an isolated symptom. However, selective eating is found in a high number of children with neurodevelopmental difficulties such as autism. It is not unusual to find a mild degree of dyspraxia, language difficulty or social skills difficulty in a referred child with selective eating [28]. In addition, some show phobic anxiety about new things other than food and extreme sensory defensiveness is a common feature.

Because the energy content of the diet is usually adequate, the highly limited range of foods (generally 10 foods or less) seems to have no impact on growth and development, or on bone density. There have been no studies to date looking at the long term impact of the associated micronutrient deficiency. Reassurance that the child is not doing him or herself any damage may be all that is required. However, particularly with approaching adolescence, the young person may find himself socially disadvantaged by his or her eating, unable to go away on school trips or stay over at friends' houses. Alternatively, a parent may seek treatment anticipating social difficulties, while the child remains unconcerned.

For those children who are ready to change, a cognitive behavioural model of treatment, led by the child, can be rapidly effective. Over the years the child may have developed anticipatory nausea (with sight or smell triggers), fear of vomiting (textures) or a fear of choking at the sight of new foods. If the child is not committed to change trying new foods, treatment will re-evoke anxiety and may result in even greater food avoidance. Suggesting they return at a later date may be appropriate if the child is not yet ready for treatment.

Hyperphagic short stature (HSS) [29] is a distinctive disorder in which children will eat voraciously, often scavenging for food, gorging and vomiting. BMI is in the normal range. The characteristic associated feature is growth failure (height below third centile). Growth hormone secretion is suppressed, but returns to normal on removal from or reduction of stress [30]. HSS is not usually considered with the eating disorders, but there are continuities with failure to thrive during infancy as well as rumination disorders and pica.

Conclusions

Eating disorders are psychological disorders that manifest through disturbances in eating. Early recognition can prevent serious physical complications and also improves the outcome. Eating difficulties resulting in significant weight loss present the greatest risk. Nutritional counselling is one component of multidisciplinary team management and clear communication between members of the treating team can prevent professional isolation and collusion with the patient's anxiety. In early onset disorders, nutritional counselling and education may be more appropriately offered to the parents than to the young person themselves. The thrust of treatment for all eating disorders is to normalise eating as much as possible, while providing a context in which the underlying emotional issues can be addressed. Collaborative work involving parents and the child/adolescent as much as possible produces the best results.

References

1   American Psychiatric Association *Diagnostic and Statistical Manual of Mental Disorders – DSM IV*. Washington DC: American Psychiatric Association, 1994.
2   Devlin MJ, Goldfein JA, Dobrow I What is this thing called BED? Current status of binge eating disorder nosology. *Int J Eat Disord*, 2003, **34** (Suppl) S2–18.
3   WHO *ICD-10 Classification of Mental and Behavioural Disorders*. London: Churchill Livingstone, 1991.
4   Nicholls D, Bryant-Waugh R Children and young adolescents. In: Treasure J, Schmidt U, van Furth E (eds) *Handbook of Eating Disorders*. Chichester: John Wiley & Sons, 2003, pp. 415–33.
5   Cooper PJ, Watkins B, Bryant-Waugh R, Lask B The nosological status of early onset anorexia nervosa. *Psychol Med*, 2002, **32** 873–80.
6   Lucas AR, Beard CM, O'Fallon WM, Kurland LT Fifty year trends in the incidence of anorexia nervosa in Rochester, Minnesota: a population-based study. *Am J Psychiatry*, 1991, **148** 917–22.
7   Currin L, Schmidt U, Treasure J, Jick H Time trends in eating disorder incidence. *Br J Psychiatry*, 2005, **186** 132–5.
8   Moller-Madsen S, Nystrup J, Nielsen S Mortality of anorexia nervosa in Denmark during the period 1970–1987. *Acta Psychiatr Scand*, 1996, **94** 454–9.
9   Nicholls D, Stanhope R Medical complications of anorexia nervosa in children and young adolescents. *Eur Eating Disord Rev*, 2000, **8** 170–80.
10 Cole TJ, Freeman JV, Preece MA Body mass index reference curves for the UK, 1990. *Arch Dis Child*, 1995, **73** 25–9.
11 Fosson A, Knibbs J, Bryant-Waugh R, Lask B Early onset anorexia nervosa. *Arch Dis Child*, 1987, **62** 114–18.
12 Bryant-Waugh R, Lask B, Shafran R, Fosson A Do doctors recognise eating disorders in children? *Arch Dis Child*, 1992, **67** 103–5.
13 Jacobs BW, Isaacs S Pre-pubertal anorexia nervosa: a retrospective controlled study. *J Child Psychol Psychiatry*, 1986, **27** 237–50.
14 Nicholls D, Viner R Eating disorders and weight problems. *Br Med J*, 2005, **330** 950–3.
15 National Collaborating Centre for Mental Health *Core interventions in the treatment and management of anorexia nervosa, bulimia nervosa and related eating disorders*. 2004. The British Psychological Society and Gaskell.
16 Fisher M, Golden NH, Katzman DK, Kreipe RE *et al.* Eating disorders in adolescents: A background paper. *J Adolesc Health*, 1995, **16** 420–37.
17 Lock J, le Grange D, Agras S, Dare C *Treatment Manual for Anorexia Nervosa*. New York: Guilford Press, 2000.
18 Klibanski A, Biller BM, Schoenfeld DA *et al.* The effects of estrogen administration on trabecular bone loss in young women with anorexia nervosa. *J Clin Endocrinol Metab*, 1995, **80** 898–904.
19 Golden NH Osteopenia and osteoporosis in anorexia nervosa. *Adolesc Med*, 2003, **14** 97–108.
20 Russell GFM Bulimia nervosa: an ominous variant of anorexia nervosa. *Psychol Med*, 1979, **9** 429–48.
21 Higgs JF, Goodyer IM, Birch J Anorexia nervosa and food avoidance emotional disorder. *Arch Dis Child*, 1989, **64** 346–51.
22 Harris G, Blissett J, Johnson R Food refusal associated with illness. *Child Psychol Psychiatry Rev*, 2000, **5** 148–56.
23 Lifshitz F Nutritional dwarfing in adolescents. *Growth Genet Horm*, 1987, **3** 1–5.
24 Singer LT, Ambuel B, Wade S, Jaffe AC Cognitive-behavioral treatment of health-impairing food phobias in children. *J Am Acad Child Adolesc Psychiatry*, 1992, **31** 847–52.

25   Bryant-Waugh R Overview of the eating disorders. In: Lask B, Bryant-Waugh R (eds) *Anorexia Nervosa and Related Eating Disorders in Childhood and Adolescence.* Hove, East Sussex: Psychology Press, 2000, pp. 27–40.

26   Jacobi C, Agras WS, Bryson S, Hammer LD Behavioral validation, precursors, and concomitants of picky eating in childhood. *J Am Acad Child Adolesc Psychiatry*, 2003, **42** 76–84.

27   Harris G, Booth IW The nature and management of eating problems in pre-school children. In: Cooper PJ, Stein A (eds) *Feeding Problems and Eating Disorders in Children and Adolescents. Monographs in Clinical Pediatrics No. 5.* Harwood Academic Publishers, 1992, pp. 61–85.

28   Nicholls D, Christie D, Randall L, Lask B Selective eating: symptom, disorder or normal variant? *Clin Child Psychol Psychiatry*, 2001, **6** 257–70.

29   Skuse D, Albanese A, Stanhope R *et al.* A new stress-related syndrome of growth failure and hyperphagia in children, associated with reversibility of growth-hormone deficiency. *Lancet*, 1996, **348** 353–8.

30   Stanhope R, Adlard P, Hamill G *et al.* Physiological growth hormone (GH) secretion during the recovery from psychosocial dwarfism: a case report. *Clin Endocrinol (Oxf)*, 1988, **28** 335–9.

Further reading

Fairburn C *Overcoming Binge Eating.* New York: Guilford Press, 1995.

Schmidt U, Treasure J *Getting Better Bit(e) by Bit(e).* Hove, East Sussex: Psychology Press, 1993.

Useful address

Eating Disorders Association
Tel: (Helplines) 01603 621414
www.edauk.com

24

Epidermolysis Bullosa

Lesley Haynes

Introduction

Epidermolysis bullosa (EB) comprises a rare group of genetically determined, skin blistering disorders characterised by extreme fragility of the skin and mucous membranes. It is usually inherited either recessively or dominantly. EB is broadly classified into three main types:

- *Junctional (JEB):* Herlitz (formerly known as lethal) and non-Herlitz (formerly known as non-lethal)
- *Dystrophic (DEB):* dominant (DDEB) and recessive (RDEB, e.g. Hallopeau–Siemens)
- *Simplex (EBS):* Dowling–Meara, Koebner and Weber–Cockayne

Each type and subtype of EB result from structural defects in the skin which allow separation between different layers, causing blistering and ulceration [1] (Fig. 24.1). Individually, they vary greatly in their impact from death in infancy to relatively minor handicap (e.g. normal life expectancy, but with limited ability to walk because of painful foot blisters). Mild cases may remain undiagnosed, while the severely affected may die before a diagnosis is confirmed, hence it is difficult to assess prevalence. It is estimated from statistics in other countries that in the UK approximately 5–10 per million of the population have JEB, 5–20 per million DEB, 5–20 per million EBS Weber–Cockayne and 5–10 per million EBS Dowling–Meara [2].

EB affects the sexes equally and occurs in all ethnic groups; mental development is normal. Blisters or lesions may be present at birth or develop soon afterwards. Lesions generally occur as the result of mechanical trauma, particularly shearing forces. Delivery by caesarean section causes less damage to the neonate's skin than vaginal delivery and can give an initially misleading impression of disease severity. Throughout life, blisters are not self-limiting and continue to extend if they are not lanced as soon as they are detected. To minimise the area of the resultant raw lesion, carers are taught to pierce blisters, leaving the roof intact to protect the underlying wound. Non-adhesive dressings are applied both to damaged areas of skin and to protect areas vulnerable to injury. Lesions can remain permanently unhealed causing significant susceptibility to infection and greatly reduced

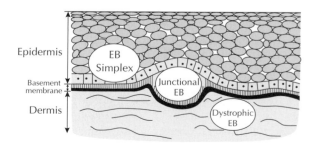

Figure 24.1 Cross-section of skin showing sites of main types of epidermolysis bullosa.

mobility because of both pain and contractures (fixed deformities resulting from pathological changes in a joint or muscle).

At present, there is no cure for any type of EB. A claim that one can be effected by an exclusion diet combined with topical and systemic treatments (the so-called Kozak regimen) was disproved in an open evaluation of the regimen [3]. Current management involves control of infection, wound management, pain relief, promotion of optimal nutritional status, surgical intervention and provision of best possible quality of life [1]. Nutrition support is a pivotal aspect of care in those with the more severe forms of EB. While improvements in nutritional status would be expected to lead to improved wound healing and lower infection rates, this is reported by only a minority. Disappointing though this is, it is important to remember that EB skin is intrinsically flawed and will never heal normally. This does not mean that nutrition has no role in the complex sequence of events surrounding wound healing and maintenance of optimal immune status. Assessment of wound healing in EB is highly subjective and fraught with confounding factors, most significantly infection and anaemia, and clinical trials need to be undertaken to monitor this more objectively. Much research is being undertaken to establish the molecular pathology of EB. Progress is slow, but researchers are cautiously optimistic that, within the lifetime of today's EB children, gene therapy will significantly improve the lives of many and perhaps provide a cure for others.

Some types of EB remain the most physically disabling and disfiguring of all diseases and although the dietitian may be shocked by the appearance (and sometimes the odour, caused by bacterial colonisation of the skin) of someone with EB, it is important not to show this. The dietitian cannot operate in isolation. Factors outside dietetic control, such as inadequate skin care, dental caries and periodontal disease, gastro-oesophageal reflux (GOR), chronic anaemia, faecal loading and overflow incontinence, psychological and psychosocial issues will sabotage the potential benefits of nutritional intervention if left unaddressed. The collective expertise of a multidisciplinary team is crucial to achieve a holistic approach to optimal management of EB [4]. Families need to feel confident that all their problems (which impinge both directly and indirectly on nutrition) are understood by those offering dietetic advice. Even despite rigorous attention to all the foregoing, the aetiology of EB is such that complications are inevitable to some extent. Parents experience huge pressures in caring for a child with severe EB [5] and goals must often be adjusted in accordance with families' priorities despite the clinical judgement of the dietitian.

Factors influencing nutritional status

Complications that compromise nutritional status occur mainly in RDEB, JEB and the Dowling–Meara subtype of EBS (Table 24.1). Inadequate dietary intakes with abnormal haematological and biochemical findings have been reported, not only in patients receiving no nutritional supplementation [6–8], but also in those receiving oral supplements and those receiving gastrostomy feeds [9]. The extent to which involvement of the internal mucosae is associated with nutritional deficiency is uncertain and it may be that the columnar epithelium of the gastrointestinal tract is affected [10]. Denudation of the intestinal epithelium has been said to lead to impaired absorption of amino acids and other nutrients [11]. Inflammatory bowel disease is suspected in a small number of patients with RDEB and JEB and it is associated with significant growth failure and suspected intolerance to whole protein feeds and to dietary components such as milk, egg, wheat and soya. However, many RDEB children thrive on whole protein feeds given via gastrostomy to complement oral intake (see p. 493). Strictures in the upper third of the oesophagus, where the diameter is narrowest, may result from the trauma of ingested food. Strictures in the distal oesophagus may reflect damage from reflux of gastric acid [12]. Although some adult RDEB patients report an improvement in dysphagia, many children and adults can tolerate only soft or puréed food and liquids. Several studies have demonstrated relief of dysphagia by oesophageal dilatation (see p. 494).

Two main factors potentially compromise nutritional status in EB:

- The hypercatabolic state in which open skin lesions with consequent losses of blood and serous fluid, increased protein turnover, heat loss and infection all contribute to increased requirements. As in the patient with thermal

Table 24.1 Main complications and nutritional interventions in different types of epidermolysis bullosa (EB).

EB type	Complications	Nutritional intervention
Dominant dystrophic EB	Usually mild lesions with minimal scarring. Anal erosions/fissures may cause painful and reluctant defaecation with/without constipation	Intervention is generally not indicated other than age-appropriate increase in fibre and fluid intakes
Recessive dystrophic EB	Recurrent moderate to severe lesions heal poorly with generalised scarring and contractures. Digits fuse. Internal contractures cause microstomia, dysphagia and oesophageal strictures. Anal erosions/fissures often cause painful and reluctant defaecation with/without constipation. Some patients develop IBD/colitis. Osteoporosis/osteopenia in immobile patients	Aim for up to 115–150% EAR for energy and up to 115–200% RNI for protein when catabolic. Supplementary iron, zinc, selenium, carnitine, calcium, vitamins (especially C & D) and fibre usually required. Gastrostomy feeding often indicated – apply DRV for age and sex in stable patients. Patients with IBD/colitis have been managed experimentally with specialised formula feeds and exclusion diets
Non-Herlitz junctional EB	Recurrent mild to severe lesions heal without scarring and contractures, but often very slowly. May be genitourinary involvement	As for recessive dystrophic EB. Gastrostomy placement may result in very poor healing around entry site and leakage of gastric contents necessitating removal/re-siting
Herlitz junctional EB	Recurrent moderate to severe lesions heal without scarring and contractures. Laryngeal involvement, hoarse cry. Pain relief often exacerbates constipation. Failure to thrive frequently follows initial good weight gain. Massive sepsis and respiratory complications are usual causes of early death. Survivors (unless form is mild) often profoundly anaemic and develop osteoporosis/osteopenia as a consequence of immobility/?malabsorption	Intervention is usually of limited benefit. Maintain hydration, feed to appetite, correct deficiencies. Experimentally, minimal fat diet with added MCT has been used. Gastrostomy placement is generally not undertaken for the reasons listed above
Dowling–Meara subtype of EB simplex	Mild to severe lesions heal without scarring and contractures. Feeding problems mainly resolve after infancy. Lesions tend later to become confined to hands and feet. Anal erosions/fissures lead to painful defaecation and constipation	Aim for up to 100–150% EAR for energy and up to 115–150% RNI for protein initially. Fibre, iron, zinc and vitamin supplementation may also be indicated. Beware of excess weight gain in later infancy/childhood
Weber–Cockayne subtype of EB simplex	Lesions usually confined to hands and feet, but may be severe, especially in hot weather	Supplementation is generally not indicated; but patients may require advice on weight reduction

DRV, dietary reference value; EAR, estimated average requirement; IBD, inflammatory bowel disease; MCT, medium chain triglycerides; RNI, reference nutrient intake.

burns, nutrient needs reflect the severity of lesions [13]; however, EB is a chronic condition and children can become overweight if fed overly enhanced energy intakes long term.

- The degree to which oral, oropharyngeal, oeso-phageal and gastrointestinal complications (ulceration with or without stricture) limit intake. Faecal loading, chronic constipation and painful defaecation (with or without consti-pation) are extremely common and frequently cause apathy and secondary anorexia [7].

The interactions between causes and effects of nutritional problems in severe RDEB are shown in Fig. 24.2.

General aims of nutrition support (modify for Herlitz JEB, see p. 487)

- To promote optimal quality of life
- To alleviate the stress associated with feeding difficulties

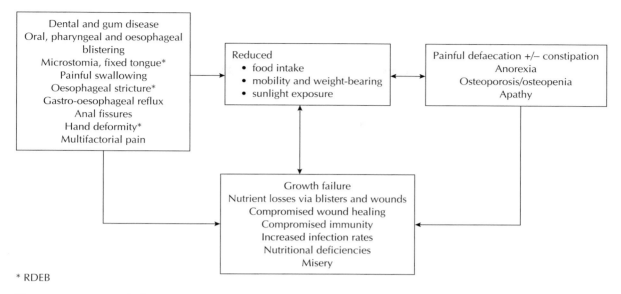

* RDEB

Figure 24.2   Causes and effects of nutritional problems in severe epidermolysis bullosa. RDEB, recessive dystrophic EB.

- To address macro- and micronutrient deficiencies (e.g. hypoproteinaemia, zinc and selenium deficiency)
- To alleviate painful defaecation and promote normal bowel function
- To promote optimal growth rates for age and sex
- To promote catch-up growth where required
- To promote optimal immune status
- To promote optimal wound healing

When widespread lesions are present, particularly in association with sepsis, nutritional requirements are likely to be raised [8], but the extent to which this occurs is unknown. Assessment of nutritional adequacy must currently depend on growth, haematological and biochemical indices (all of which should be age- and gender-appropriate) and assessment (albeit subjective) of wound healing. Regular monitoring and evaluation of interventions is crucial [4].

Energy requirements can be estimated using a calculation based on weight-for-height age and taking into account the degrees of blistering, sepsis and requirement for catch-up growth [14]. Although this method provides a working figure, the scoring of skin involvement is subjective and the formula is complex. Using a simpler method, based on Dietary Reference Values [15], increases in weight can be achieved by supplying 100–150% estimated average requirement (EAR) for energy and 115–200% reference nutrient intake (RNI) for protein, based on chronological age.

Growth

Measurements of weight and height velocity are generally the most practical means of assessing growth, and these should be plotted regularly. Children should be weighed and measured 3–6 monthly, preferably using the same equipment each time. The aim is for the child to grow according to his or her genetic (and ethnic) potential. However, pain and contractures around joints may lead to underestimated height measurements and a supine stadiometer or measuring mat may provide greater accuracy. Even this may not be possible in a severely contracted child and segmental measurements using specialised calipers or a metal tape may have to suffice. The traditional 'rule-of-thumb' that disparity between weight and height should not be greater than two major centiles is generally applicable. Optimal growth rates for children with severe EB can be difficult to gauge. Fox et al. [16] concluded that children with RDEB are of significantly lower birthweight than unaffected children, and that the compromise in growth seen throughout life in RDEB appears to begin *in utero*.

Nutrition support by gastrostomy feeding has definite advantages in EB, but tends to promote central fat deposition with poor linear growth. The reasons for this are likely to be multifactorial and inter-related, such as the disturbances in growth hormone production mediated by cytokines and increased cortisol production inherent in chronic inflammatory illness [17]. It is important to maintain a balance between promotion of mobility and optimal nutritional status. The EB child whose weight centile deviates upwardly by more than two centiles from his or her height centile may be less mobile and more likely to depend on a wheelchair. Significant wheelchair dependency is likely to compound abnormal bone mineralisation, leading to bone pain and fractures, and further reliance on wheelchair use. Further work is required to establish ideal growth rates when height is compromised. It may be beneficial to allow height to 'dictate' ideal weight provided that overall nutritional status is not adversely affected thereby impacting on immune status and attainment of puberty.

Importance of early nutrition support
(modify for Herlitz JEB, see p. 487)

The importance of providing optimal nutrition, starting as early as possible after birth, cannot be over-emphasised [4,7]. Unfortunately, this area of management may be neglected, with priority given to other critical issues such as skin care and control of infection. The assumption that either growth failure is an inevitable consequence of EB, or that catch-up can be achieved later, means that valuable time may be lost before a dietetic referral is made.

Energy requirements necessary to promote weight gain and wound healing seem to range from 130 to 180 kcal/kg (643–572 kJ/kg) actual body weight/24 hours (115–150% EAR), but can be as high as 225 kcal/kg (940 kJ/kg) if the skin is septic or growth failure is profound. Protein requirements tend to be 2.5–4 g/kg (115–200% RNI) and fluid 150–200 mL/kg. Babies with extensive blistering lose significant amounts of fluid from these open areas and may require correspondingly larger volumes of feeds.

Breast feeding an EB baby is possible, and if it permits normal weight gain should be encouraged for the many benefits it confers [18]. However, rooting may cause, or exacerbate, facial lesions and blistering of the fragile mucous membranes of the mouth, tongue and gums. Babies should be allowed to suckle on demand and applying white soft paraffin or Vaseline to the lips and to the nipple reduces friction. For all but mild cases of EB, breast milk alone often fails to satisfy increased requirements, demonstrated by failure to gain weight.

As soon as possible, measures should be taken to provide a more nutrient-dense feed. There are several ways in which this can be done (p. 15). Any feed modifications must be explained to parents and community medical and nursing personnel to avoid misunderstandings and conflicting advice. Alternatively, nutrient dense, ready-to-feed formulations such as SMA High Energy, Infatrini, Nutrini and Nutrini Extra can be used.

Weights should be recorded on alternate days while a feeding routine is established in hospital. Although nude weight is ideal, the skin damage incurred during handling usually precludes this. If such precision is required, the baby can be weighed before a dressing change and afterwards the weight of the soiled dressings subtracted from this first weight. Weighings can be reduced to once weekly and then less frequently once the baby is discharged from hospital. Values should be plotted on a growth chart so that any 'fall-off' can be detected early and appropriate measures taken to modify the feeds.

Feeding teats should be moistened with cooled, boiled water or Vaseline before feeding to avoid the teat sticking to the lips and causing damage when it is removed. A Habermann feeder (Athrodax Healthcare International) is extremely useful if the mouth is painful. The shape of this teat minimises trauma to the gum margin and the internal valve allows the carer to control the flow of feed, so that even a weak suck will deliver a satisfactory milk flow. Alternatively, the hole in a conventional teat can be enlarged using a sterile needle. Babies who cannot suck from a teat may need to be fed from a spoon or dropper or be fed by nasogastric (NG) tube (see p. 492). In babies with extensive lesions and significant blood losses, iron and zinc status should be assessed and supplemented as required (see p. 490).

Weaning (see also Recessive dystrophic EB)

Weaning foods should be offered at the same time as for unaffected babies. However, babies whose mouths are very fragile, or who have experienced GOR or aspiration of feed, are usually very reluctant to accept changes in texture or viscosity of foods. Carers should be reassured that this is not unusual, and advised that there is nothing to be gained, and everything to be lost, by force-feeding. Community personnel may be over-zealous in striving for 'normal' feeding milestones, and the practice of reducing the volume or the nutrient density of the feed to make the baby more hungry for solids is wholly inappropriate. Weaning foods of a suitable texture for unaffected babies are usually appropriate, although there is often aversion and fear of food composed of mixed textures (such as the soft lumps within a more liquid matrix found in many commercial baby foods); uniform textures are accepted more confidently. Hard or sharp foods such as baked rusks or crisp crusts are not suitable as these damage the fragile mucosa of the mouth and gums. If growth is poor, carers should be advised regarding ways to increase the protein and energy content of the diet without increasing its bulk (see *Nutrition for Babies with Epidermolysis Bullosa*, DebRA). Although there is no evidence to suggest that long term adherence to a liquid or puréed diet necessarily influences the course of dysphagia and oesophageal stricture, babies who demonstrate swallowing problems from early on may be best to remain indefinitely on very soft or puréed foods. The expertise of a speech and language therapist is often invaluable.

Herlitz junctional EB

The prognosis for Herlitz junctional EB (HJEB) is extremely poor, death usually occurring within the first year or two of life and often within weeks or months of birth. Paradoxically, skin lesions may initially be minimal, and weight gain deceptively good, on breast milk or normally reconstituted feeds. Almost invariably, however, this gives way

to growth failure as new areas of skin become denuded, infection sets in and laryngeal and respiratory problems increase [19]. The dietitian must be aware of the prognosis, to try to minimise the disappointment parents will feel when feed modifications have little or no impact on growth or healing. Nutritional intervention (as for RDEB, see below) should be offered as a means of enhancing the quality, rather than the quantity, of life. Protracted diarrhoea is often a hallmark of HJEB and it has been suggested that a deficiency of intestinal integrin is responsible [20]. It has been hypothesised that replacement of dietary long chain triglyceride (LCT) largely by medium chain triglyceride (MCT) using Monogen feeds may alleviate this.

Mothers who have established breast feeding a baby with HJEB and wish to continue should not be discouraged from doing so even if weight gain is poor, as this is one of the few positive things they can do for a terminally ill baby. Pain relief is an important aspect of terminal care, and regular weighing may be necessary to decide the best regimen. However, unless this is the case, parents and medical and nursing staff should be discouraged from routinely weighing the baby, as the disappointing result only adds to an already very distressing situation.

Non-Herlitz junctional EB

Some non-Herlitz junctional EB (NHJEB) patients are mildly affected and survive into adulthood with relatively little handicap. Others, however, experience extreme nutritional compromise because of extensive and chronic ulceration, both externally and internally. Associated pyloric atresia and genito-urinary disease have been reported [21]. Nutrition support is the same as that recommended for RDEB (below). A minimal LCT intake has been used experimentally, as for HJEB.

Recessive dystrophic EB

The complications of RDEB begin in infancy and, except in mild cases, progressively increase. In the more severe cases, prolonged and recurrent blisters with subsequent scarring gradually lead to tautness of the underlying joints known as contractures.

These progress to cause major walking difficulties and disability. Contractures in the mouth greatly limit opening and immobilise the tongue. Oesophageal scarring causes strictures and some patients experience periods when they are unable to swallow even their own saliva and require hospitalisation for rehydration. Anal scarring leads to fissures, extremely painful defecation and consequent faecal loading as defecation is postponed for lengthy periods [22,23]. Self-feeding is greatly limited when fingers become fused and contracted. Specialised surgery is available to separate the fingers although the benefits are temporary. In many cases, without oesophageal dilatation and/or gastrostomy placement, the resulting nutritional compromise leads to profound malnutrition and growth failure [14,24].

Patients with RDEB are at significantly increased risk of developing squamous cell (malignant) carcinoma, usually in early adulthood. Despite the surgical removal of affected areas, the tumours metastasise rapidly, and without early identification the prognosis is generally extremely poor. It has been proposed that chronic malnutrition indirectly contributes not only to the metastasis of cancer cells, but also to the development of primary skin malignacies [11]. Conversely, it has also been suggested that an inherent aspect of the cell leads to malignancy [25].

In the older child, a dietary assessment should be comprehensive and sensitively probing in order to elicit an authentic picture [4] and a demonstration of the child's maximum mouth opening capability and tongue mobility help to provide a complete picture. GOR and hiatus hernia are often neglected causes of dysphagia, the most serious complication of which is aspiration pneumonia [12,23]. A history suggestive of these must be fully explored and medically treated. Faecal loading (with or without constipation) is invariably present to a greater or lesser extent, often from infancy. This frequently exerts a disastrous effect on appetite and tolerance of feeds and supplements, especially iron. Parents regularly omit to report symptoms of these, probably because they do not appreciate their detrimental impact on nutritional intake.

The dietitian should not assume that the child's medical and surgical carers have investigated these issues. Other inexperienced professionals often fail to ask about such problems and parents do not mention them because they assume that they are inextricably linked to EB and therefore not treatable. What is frequently misinterpreted as noncompliant and manipulative behaviour or psychological disturbance is very often explained by complications such as GOR or faecal loading.

The form shown in Fig. 24.3 summarises the points to address when carrying out a dietary assessment. The RDEB child with significant oral and oesophageal complications seldom achieves even the EAR for most nutrients using normal foods. Liquidised foods tend to be low in all nutrients, unless large volumes are consumed. Advice, in the first instance, should aim to improve the nutritional value of the child's normal food intake (see *Nutrition in Epidermolysis Bullosa for Children over 1 year of age*, DebRA). As skin care and dressing changes can be extremely time-consuming, dietary modifications must be practical and realistic. The emphasis should be on increased protein and energy intakes, with improvements in vitamin and mineral intakes as indicated by dietary assessment and laboratory results. In practice, milk often figures prominently in the diets of EB children, so protein and calcium intakes are generally satisfactory. Conversely, the intakes of those who dislike milk and who have difficulties chewing and swallowing meat invariably fall below the RNI, and will require supplementation [7].

Realistically, few severely affected RDEB children can consume adequate quantities of normal foods and must rely heavily on multinutrient supplements to make up the deficit. Children who consume multinutrient supplements on a regular basis will generally receive extra vitamins from these. This should be taken into consideration before a further vitamin supplement is prescribed. Those with anything more than the mildest EB are likely to require extra vitamins [7,8] to achieve 150–200% of the RNI for age (see p. 490).

Children who can maintain adequate oral nutrition frequently do so only by the extreme efforts of their parents. These efforts invariably demand disproportionate amounts of time and are often detrimental to family life. While it is important to impress on parents the key part played by nutrition in overall management, it is also vital not to set unrealistic targets and so engender guilt when these are unattainable because of the complications of the condition rather than to lack of parental diligence. The effect of any intervention should be

NAME:		dob:		HOSPITAL NUMBER:			Date:	
WEIGHT:	kg		centile	**HEIGHT:**		cm	centile	

PREFERRED CONSISTENCY OF FOOD: Normal   Soft   Purée   Fluid

REASON(S)	Oral blistering	Microstomia	Fixed tongue
	Dental caries	Dysphagia	Oesophageal stricture
	Excess mucus production		Regurgitation G-O reflux

FREQUENCY OF DEFAECATION: x day   x week

	Pain	Bleeding p.r.	Stool consistency

LAXATIVE(S), PREBIOTIC(S), PROBIOTIC(S) etc   Preparation(s), dose, frequency

Senna	Movicol	Sodium picosulphate
Lactulose	Resource Benefiber	Other prebiotic Probiotic

TYPICAL	Breakfast:
	Snack:
MEAL	Lunch:
	Snack:
PATTERN	Evening:
	Bedtime

Time taken over an average meal: minutes   **Finishes amount offered**

GASTROSTOMY/other feeding tube *in situ*

NUTRIENT-DENSE/ENERGY-DENSE SUPPLEMENT(S)/GASTROSTOMY FEEDS:

Name of preparation(s), dose, frequency

OTHER SUPPLEMENT(S):   Name of preparation(s), dose, frequency

Iron	Zinc	Fluoride	Calcium +/– Vitamin D_3
Carnitine	Selenium	Other vitamins	Other

APPROX. DAILY INTAKE:	Protein	g (/kg)	Normal DRV* =	g (/kg)
	Energy	kcal (/kg)	Nomal DRV* =	kcal (/kg)

COMMENTS/ACTION

Figure 24.3   Suggested pro forma for recording factors affecting nutritional intake and other relevant information. DRV, dietary reference value.

monitored and an agreed time limit (e.g. 2–3 months) placed on assessing its efficacy. If significant improvement in nutritional intake is not achieved with oral supplementation, alternative intervention (e.g. oesophageal dilatation and gastrostomy placement) should be recommended. Percutaneous endoscopic gastrostomies (PEGs) are generally considered unsuitable because of the shearing damage to the oesophagus caused by their placement. Button devices inserted as a primary procedure are generally well tolerated, but should be placed via a laparotomy rather than endoscopically [26].

Dowling–Meara subtype of EB simplex

There is a wide range of severity in this type of EB. Death in the neonatal period is not uncommon, brought about by widespread blistering with associated hypoalbuminaemia and sepsis and feeding problems in which oropharyngeal blistering significantly compromises nutritional status. Nutritional support as outlined for RDEB should be provided at this time. Aspiration of feeds, believed to be caused by unco-ordinated swallowing, is common, and GOR may be significant [27]; fortunately, these complications and the tendency to blister generally lessen with time. Even infants whose survival was seriously jeopardised in the neonatal period usually proceed to thrive well. There may be some degree of lifelong disability because of persistent and extremely painful blistering of the hands and feet. This can lead to a very sedentary lifestyle and avoidance of weight-bearing exercise, often with significant reliance on a wheelchair. Excessive weight gain in later childhood is likely if measures are not taken to guard against this.

Vitamins

Infants who thrive on breast milk or normally reconstituted formula feeds tend to be those with minimal skin lesions, and their requirements for vitamins are unlikely to be greater than those of normal babies. However, if a satisfactory intake is in doubt, an age-appropriate multivitamin supplement should be given, provided that total intake (particularly of vitamin A) does not exceed recommended safe upper limits [15]. Although requirements have not been determined, it is suspected that more severely affected EB infants need increased amounts of all vitamins [8,14], especially vitamin C, whose role in enhancing iron absorption [28] and in collagen synthesis [29] is recognised. The provision of 150–200% of the RNI ensures that intakes are still within recommended safe limits.

Babies requiring feeds of increased concentration will automatically receive correspondingly increased amounts of all vitamins, possibly nearing 150% RNI if large volumes are consumed. Again, if a satisfactory intake is in doubt, and skin lesions are significant, a comprehensive preparation such as Ketovite liquid and tablets should be prescribed. Ketovite tablets can be crushed, mixed with a small amount of feed or water and given from a syringe or spoon. If this is not tolerated, a liquid preparation such as Abidec drops can be used, although this will not provide a complete range of vitamins. These preparations should be given at the normal recommended dose for age unless intake from other sources is substantial. When considering vitamin D intake, even fortified feeds may barely meet the normal RNI and it should be remembered that the skin of these babies may be largely covered with dressings and therefore receive minimal exposure to sunlight (see p. 491).

Older children who consume significant volumes of multinutrient supplements on a regular basis will receive correspondingly significant amounts of vitamins from these. In cases where vitamin intake falls below the RNI, a supplement should be prescribed. Although the protective role of antioxidant vitamins in the development of malignancy in EB is unproven, it seems prudent to recommend an enhanced intake of these, while keeping within the currently accepted safe upper limits [15]. The role of supplemental age-appropriate omega-6 and omega-3 fatty acids is currently unclear, but the benefits of their anti-inflammatory properties warrant consideration.

Biochemical and haematological estimations

Interpretation of blood tests in EB patients is never straightforward, mainly because of the inflammatory nature of the condition. Nevertheless, it is important to monitor certain parameters regularly. Table 24.2 lists the investigations that should be routinely carried out, with suggested sampling intervals. Frequency of sampling will vary depending on the disease severity of the individual case and the need to evaluate interventions such as selenium supplementation or gastrostomy placement with enhanced enteral nutrition. Care should be taken to ensure that results are compared with age-appropriate paediatric reference ranges.

Iron and anaemia

As with many other features of EB, the severity of anaemia depends on EB type. RDEB and JEB patients experience continual losses from skin lesions and from the upper gastrointestinal tract. In the Dowling–Meara subtype of EB simplex, lesions in infancy can be extensive and blood loss significant. The resulting anaemia is usually microcytic and hypochromic, and is believed to be related to the 'anaemia of chronic disease' [30]. This may not occur under 6 months of age in babies who were full term, presumably because of good iron stores at birth and an adequate iron intake from fortified baby milk and weaning foods. It is important that iron related parameters (Table 24.2) are checked

Table 24.2 Biochemical and haematological investigations in children with epidermolysis bullosa.

Investigation	Suggested frequency of sampling
Urea and electrolytes	6–12 monthly
Creatinine	6–12 monthly
Calcium, phosphate (+/– vitamin D$_3$)	6–12 monthly
Total protein, albumin	6–12 monthly
Alkaline phosphatase	6–12 monthly
Zinc, selenium	6–12 monthly
Vitamin B$_1$, carnitine	Yearly
Vitamin E	1–2 yearly
Serum iron, ferritin, full blood count	6–12 monthly
Hypochromic red blood cell	6–12 monthly
Transferrin receptors	6–12 monthly
Mean corpuscular volume (MCV)	6–12 monthly
Reticulocytes, red cell folate	6–12 monthly
Erythrocyte sedimentation rate (ESR)	6–12 monthly
Free erythrocyte protoporphyrin (FEP)	6–12 monthly
Vitamin B$_{12}$, folate	Yearly

The above is a guide. Sampling frequency depends on individual disease severity and the need to evaluate impact of intervention.

before this time, and iron should be supplemented if deficiency is indicated. Care is required in the interpretation of laboratory results because factors such as infection can produce spuriously raised ferritin. If extra iron is indicated, a liquid form is preferable (e.g. Sytron).

Opinion is divided as to the merits of daily [31] versus weekly iron administration [32]. The latter view relies on the hypothesis that a mucosal 'block' occurs in intestinal cells which then cannot absorb therapeutic daily doses of iron until they are renewed by cell turnover at roughly 3-day intervals. Because, in practice, medications given on a less than daily basis are more likely to be forgotten, it is probably safer to prescribe a daily dose so that administration is a part of the regular routine. Compliance is often poor because of the association between iron and constipation and gastric irritation. Dividing a daily dose into two may ease undesirable side effects. Constipation can be significantly reduced by an increase in fibre intake and appropriate prescription of laxatives and/or stool softeners [22]. To improve iron absorption, children whose oral mucosa is not irritated by a source of vitamin C should be advised to take this with the

iron supplement. The debate continues surrounding the joint administration of iron and zinc supplements [33]. These micronutrients have the potential to interact, leading to potentially reduced absorption of both. A recent review article concluded that, although some trials have shown that joint iron and zinc supplementation has less of an effect on biochemical or functional outcomes than does supplementation with either mineral alone, there is no strong evidence to discourage joint supplementation [34].

Zinc

Zinc has a vital role in growth, wound healing, immune function and membrane stability where its antioxidant properties are crucial [35,36]. These processes are especially important in EB, and zinc should be supplemented when skin lesions are severe, in regimens recommended in publications such as the *British National Formulary*. Biochemical estimation should be undertaken to provide a baseline and dosage adjustments made in the light of subsequent laboratory results and wound healing response. However, the interpretation of plasma zinc concentration is notoriously difficult. For example, a low albumin level will cause an associated low zinc result. In this situation, energy and protein intake should also be increased and a zinc supplement concurrently prescribed. It is illogical and probably futile to do the latter without the former. For ease of administration, a liquid supplement is preferable. To optimise absorption and minimise nausea, the daily dose should ideally be split into two. Some patients find that flavoured zinc lozenges, e.g. Holland & Barratt (23 mg zinc per lozenge) cause less nausea. These dissolve slowly in the mouth although the chalky 'mouth feel' may be unacceptable (see above for information regarding joint versus separate administration of zinc with iron).

Calcium and vitamin D, osteoporosis and osteopenia

Children with the more severe forms of EB have low bone mass and are at risk of abnormal bone mineralisation and fractures. This is believed to be due to factors such as poor nutrition, delayed puberty, reduced levels of mobility and weight-bearing exercise, and reduced exposure to sunlight [37]. Although EB children receiving enteral feeds via gastrostomy obtain their theoretical age-appropriate requirements for calcium, elevated cytokine concentrations secondary to chronic infection or inflammation may adversely affect bone turnover and gastrointestinal complications may interfere with absorption. Current management involves determination of bone mass by dual X-ray absorptiometry (DEXA scan), biochemical estimation of calcium and vitamin D status and administration of bisphosphonates with a combined calcium and vitamin D preparation such as Cacit D3.

Selenium and carnitine

A small number of severely affected RDEB children have developed a fatal dilated cardiomyopathy, thought to be associated with deficiencies of selenium and carnitine [38]. However, these children had been suffering from long-term generalised malnutrition, so the cause of their cardiomyopathy was likely to have been multifactorial. More recent work [39] supports the hypothesis that selenium and carnitine are implicated, although evidence remains inconclusive. Until more information is available, it is prudent to monitor selenium and carnitine status in all EB children whose nutrition is compromised and/or who rely on nutritional support (e.g. gastrostomy feeding) [9]. Biochemical evidence of selenium deficiency is rarely seen in those <2 years who have been receiving a proprietory formula containing it. Deficiency should be addressed by supplementation of pure selenium; currently this is available only as a 50-µg/day tablet, and cannot be prescribed by a GP or dispensed by a community pharmacist but must be prescribed and dispensed from hospital. It must be carefully crushed and mixed with water if it is to be given via gastrostomy, but this is time-consuming and any undissolved pieces can block the device. A liquid formulation of selenium is more practical (e.g. Selenase Oral Solution) and provides 500 µg/10 mL. This is prescribable on Form FP10, but contains no preservative and its very short shelf-life makes its use prohibitive. Selenium preparations in combination with vitamin A should not be

recommended if intake of vitamin A from other sources is significant and provides intakes above the accepted safe level. Biochemical evidence of carnitine deficiency should be addressed by giving 50–100 mg/kg/day Carnitor Paediatric Solution.

Gastro-oesophageal reflux

GOR is common in all types of EB and the corrosive action of gastric acid on the delicate oesophageal and oropharyngeal mucosae can cause severe, extensive and permanent scarring. Anecdotal evidence strongly suggests that unaddressed GOR is significantly responsible for much of the aversion to eating seen in the more severe forms of EB. Barium studies, milk scans and pH studies are difficult to perform in EB and, if GOR is suspected, anti-reflux medication should be prescribed even in the absence of positive results from such tests [27]. For infants, it may also be beneficial to provide thickened feeds in addition to medication (see Table 7.27).

Nasogastric feeding

Except as a short-term measure, NG feeding should not be undertaken routinely in EB because external as well as internal damage can occur in the securing and passing of the tube. It is inappropriate for children whose skin condition already attracts stares and questions to be subjected to further attention and scrutiny by the presence of an NG tube. If a long-term feeding problem seems likely, insertion of a gastrostomy should be considered (see p. 493). Temporary NG feeding is indicated for babies who do not take satisfactory volumes of oral feeds and those whose mouths become excessively traumatised by suckling. It is also useful as an interim measure in the older RDEB or non-lethal JEB child who it is believed would benefit from gastrostomy placement, but who needs, or whose carers need, evidence of the effects of improved nutrition before agreeing to surgery. A 6–8-week period of NG feeding should be sufficient to demonstrate benefit.

A further indication for temporary NG feeding is in RDEB, where dental procedures frequently cause significant peri- and postoperative oral and pharyngeal blistering. Because invasive dental procedures are undertaken under general anaesthetic, an NG tube can be passed in the operating theatre and the child fed by this route until an adequate oral intake is resumed. Whatever the age of the patient, the tube used should be as soft and of as narrow a gauge as possible, and it should not be re-sited at every feed, but left *in situ*. Tubes should never be fixed to the skin with adhesive tape, because skin will be removed with the tape. Tubes can be secured with a minimally adhesive dressing such as Mepiform or tape Mepitac or a non-adhesive dressing such as Tubifast, the tube being secured by winding a length of Tubifast around it where it enters the nostril. The edge of the nostril can be protected from trauma by applying Vaseline. The ends of the dressing are then tied together behind the head.

Gastrostomy feeding

For many severely affected EB children, oral feeding is stressful, tedious and often painful. In RDEB particularly, oral nutrition is compromised as much by oesophageal stricturing as by oral complications and, in some children, serial oesophageal dilatations can postpone or obviate gastrostomy placement. However, difficulties with chewing (especially meat), compliance with medications and maintenance of a satisfactory fibre intake are issues that are likely to continue.

The decision to proceed with gastrostomy placement should ideally be taken before the child's growth deteriorates. Although children with growth failure can achieve varying degrees of catch-up, they are often reluctant to persevere with oral nutrition, preferring to rely heavily on gastrostomy feeds. The most recent reviews of gastrostomy feeding in EB [4,26] were based on data collected almost a decade ago, and information gained more recently suggests that gastrostomy feeding can simply replace some problems with others. Interestingly, despite negative aspects such as leakage or infection around entry site and bedwetting, parents' views are such that they would still recommend gastrostomy placement to other EB families [author's unpublished work]. Gastrostomy placement is not a panacea and families' priorities should be established and detailed discussions regarding the pros and cons undertaken before surgery takes place.

Some parents initially view the recommendation of a gastrostomy as a sign of their failure to nourish the child adequately and request continued information regarding alternative oral supplements. In fact, delaying placement only adds to their stress and frustration, engendering increased feelings of failure. With early intervention, in association with oesophageal dilatation (OD), the child is more likely to continue with oral nutrition, albeit in small and varying quantities. This is important, not only for social reasons but also in anticipation of a time, after the pubertal growth spurt, when they may be able to take sufficient nutrition orally and the gastrostomy can be reversed. A nutrient-dense feed containing a mixed fibre source (e.g. Nutrini Multi Fibre, Nutrini Energy Multi Fibre or Jevity Plus) should be chosen. The choice of daytime bolus versus pumped overnight gastrostomy feeds will depend on the individual child and family dynamics; some prefer a combination. To optimise feed tolerance and promote continuing oral intake, it is advisable to begin with small volumes; this may mean as little as 200–250 mL of a 1.5 kcal/mL (6 kJ/mL) continuous feed for a child under 5 years, and 300–500 mL for an older child.

Painful defaecation with/without constipation

Several references deal with the subject of constipation in EB [4,10,22,23], yet chronic constipation (often more accurately termed faecal loading) with painful defaecation remains one of the most frequent, and underestimated, complications of all types of EB. Even a moderately bulky stool can tear the delicate anal skin causing fissuring and extreme pain with subsequent bowel movements. Fear of defaecation leads to infrequent and incomplete bowel emptying and the gradual accumulation of hard faeces. It should be treated without delay if the vicious cycle of pain, conscious ignoring of the gastrocolonic reflex and secondary anorexia (Fig. 24.2) is to be avoided. In babies, extra fluid should be offered in the form of water or, if this is refused, one teaspoon of fresh fruit juice diluted in 100 mL water or ready-to-feed baby juice diluted with an equal volume of water. Alternatively, one teaspoon of sugar (anecdotal evidence suggests that brown sugar is more effective than white) can be added to each feed. Lactulose should be prescribed, starting with 2.5 mL once daily to 2.5 mL twice daily. A pure fibre source (e.g. Resource Benefiber) or a fibre-containing feed such as Paediasure with Fibre or Nutrini Fibre can be introduced from 6–8 months. Whether the infant is constipated or not, it is prudent to introduce a fibre source at 9–12 months of age, because constipation is such a likely complication of all types of EB, plus a stool softener such as lactulose or Movicol Paediatric. If the child then progresses onto a diet sufficiently high in fibre to promote comfortable defaecation, the fibre source can be phased out.

Overflow incontinence is often mistaken for diarrhoea, and the prescribed laxative therapy is stopped, inadvertently exacerbating the situation. Oral lesions, dysphagia and requirement for a low bulk, nutrient-dense intake preclude the consumption of a conventional high fibre diet. An increase in fibre intake is important, however, and a fibre containing feed (preferably one based on a mixed fibre source) should be introduced, orally or by gastrostomy, but only after the extent of faecal loading has been investigated and addressed.

The incorporation into feeds or foods of a pure fibre source is extremely successful in normalising stool consistency and frequency of defaecation. In the absence of UK recommended intakes of fibre for children and adolescents, the US formula of age (years) plus 5–10 g/day [40] is a useful guideline. For example, a 3-year-old child will require 8–13 g/day fibre. It is important to note that, if such preparations are introduced while the child remains faecally loaded, problems such as abdominal pain, GOR and vomiting will invariably ensue and compliance will be jeopardised. Therefore, first, intestinal transit time should be assessed. This can be done by giving a carmine dye marker and noting the time taken for it to appear in the stools. Then, depending on the degree of faecal loading, this can be addressed by giving either a bowel-prep solution such as Klean-Prep as a hospital inpatient, or a strong laxative such as Picolax. Thereafter, some permutation of stool softener and/or laxative is generally necessary in the long term.

Dental aspects

Tooth enamel in JEB is more porous and pitted than normal, making it more susceptible to acid attack [41]. The oral mucosa of patients with JEB and RDEB is generally too fragile to allow the use of a normal brush and access is often difficult because of contractures causing microstomia. Plaque collects around the teeth, leading to chronic marginal gingivitis. Because the tongue is immobilised by scar tissue, it cannot perform the normal cleansing action along the tooth–gum margin and food débris accumulates there. The removal of badly decayed teeth from a mouth with limited opening may be extremely difficult even under general anaesthesia and often results in increased oral ulceration and scarring [42].

Unless a gastrostomy has been placed, a diet sufficiently high in energy to fulfil energy requirements generally means the consumption of considerable quantities of fermentable carbohydrate, especially sucrose, at regular intervals throughout the day. The frequency of such foods, especially coupled with the complications noted above, is highly conducive to the development of dental caries. This apparent conflict of interests between dietitian and dentist can lead to contradictory advice to the child and the carers. However, compromise is possible, and families should be taught from early on the importance of good oral hygiene. The advice of an experienced dentist should be followed regarding a fluoride supplement, fluoride toothpaste and a plaque-inhibiting mouthwash. Sweets and chocolate biscuits should ideally be restricted to the end of mealtimes and continuous sipping of sugary drinks outside mealtimes discouraged. However, in a severely affected child who relies on oral nutrition, this may be impossible as eating and drinking are extremely slow and one mealtime unavoidably merges into the next.

Oesophageal dilatation and colonic interposition

For many RDEB patients, dysphagia and oesophageal strictures are significant reasons for their failure to consume sufficient nutrition. OD of the narrowed segment can relieve much of the problem. However, the pharyngeal and oesophageal mucosae are extremely fragile and may rupture. Fatalities have occurred when these procedures were undertaken using an endoscope [43] when shearing forces are applied. Balloon dilatations (which apply mainly radial forces) undertaken while being viewed radiologically appear to be much safer [44]. Colonic interposition and oesophago-colonoplasty (where a section of colon is inserted into the oesophagus) have been undertaken with success in a small number of patients [45], but considering the technical complexity of the procedure and the significant mortality risk, this currently remains a last resort for those whose nutritional status cannot be maintained by any other means [45,46].

References

1 Pai S, Marinkovich MP Epidermolysis bullosa new and emerging trends. *Am J Clin Dermatol*, 2002, **3** 371–80.

2 Horn HM, Priestley GC, Tidman MJ Epidemiology of epidermolysis bullosa in Scotland. *Br J Dermatol*, 1995, **133** 1005.

3 Haber RM, Ramsay CA, Boxall LBH Epidermolysis bullosa. Assessment of a treatment regimen. *Int J Dermatol*, 1985, **24** 324–8.

4 Haynes L Nutritional support for children with epidermolysis bullosa. *J Hum Nutr Diet*, 1998, **11** 163–73.

5 Fine J-D, Johnson LB, Weiner M *et al.* Impact of inherited epidermolysis bullosa on parental interpersonal relationships, marital status and family size. *Psychodermatol*, 2004, **152** 1009–14.

6 Lechner-Gruskay D, Honig PJ, Pereira G *et al.* Nutritional and metabolic profile of children with epidermolysis bullosa. *Pediatr Dermatol*, 1988, **5** 22–7.

7 Allman SM, Haynes L, MacKinnon P *et al.* Nutrition in dystrophic epidermolysis bullosa. *Pediatr Dermatol*, 1992, **9** 231–8.

8 Fine J-D, Tamura T, Johnson L Blood vitamin and trace metal levels in epidermolysis bullosa. *Arch Dermatol*, 1989, **125** 374–9.

9 Ingen-Housz-Oro S, Blanchet-Bardon C, Vrillat M *et al.* Vitamin and trace metal levels in recessive dystrophic epidermolysis bullosa. *J Eur Acad Dermatol Venereol*, 2004, **18** 649–53.

10 Sehgal VN, Rege VL, Ghosh SK *et al.* Dystrophic epidermolysis bullosa. Interesting gastrointestinal manifestations. *Br J Dermatol*, 1977, **96** 389–91.

11 Fine J-D, McGuire J Altered nutrition and inherited epidermolysis bullosa. In: Fine J-D, Bauer EA, McGuire J, Moshell A (eds) *Epidermolysis Bullosa. Clinical, Epidemiologic and Laboratory Advances and the Findings of the National Epidermolysis Bullosa Registry*. Baltimore: Johns Hopkins University Press, 1999, pp. 225–35.

12 Ergun G, Schaefer RA Gastrointestinal aspects of epidermolysis bullosa. In: Lin AN, Carter DM (eds) *Epidermolysis Bullosa: Basic and Clinical Aspects*. New York: Springer-Verlag, 1992, pp. 169–84.

13 Gamelli RL Nutritional problems of the acute and chronic burn patient; relevance to epidermolysis bullosa. *Arch Dermatol*, 1988, **124** 756–9.

14 Birge K Nutrition management of patients with epidermolysis bullosa. *J Am Diet Assoc*, 1995, **95** 575–9.

15 Department of Health Report on Health and Social Subjects No 41. *Dietary Reference Values for Food Energy and Nutrients for the United Kingdom*. London: The Stationery Office, 1991.

16 Fox AT, Alderdice F, Atherton DJ Are children with recessive dystrophic epidermolysis bullosa of low birthweight ? *Pediatr Dermatol*, 2003, **20** 303–6.

17 Van den Berghe G Dynamic neuroendocrine responses to critical illness. *Front Neuroendocrinol*, 2002, **23** 370–91.

18 Department of Health and Social Security Report on Health and Social Subjects No. 32. *Present Day Practice in Infant Feeding*. London: The Stationery Office, 1988.

19 Lin AN, Carter DM Junctional epidermolysis bullosa: a clinical overview. In: Lin AN, Carter DM (eds) *Epidermolysis Bullosa: Basic and Clinical Aspects*. New York: Springer-Verlag, 1992, pp. 118–34.

20 Lachaux A, Bouvier R, Loras-Duclaux I *et al.* Isolated deficient $\alpha6\beta4$ integrin expression in the gut associated with intractable diarrhea. *J Pediatr Gastroenterol Nutr*, 1999, **29** 395–401.

21 Berger TG, Maj MC, Detlefs RL *et al.* Junctional epidermolysis bullosa, pyloric atresia and genitourinary disease. *Pediatr Dermatol*, 1986, **3** 130–4.

22 Haynes L, Atherton DJ, Clayden G Constipation in epidermolysis bullosa: successful treatment with a liquid fiber-containing formula. *Pediatr Dermatol*, 1997, **14** 393–6.

23 Clayden GS Dysphagia and constipation in epidermolysis bullosa. In: Priestley GC *et al.* (eds) *Epidermolysis Bullosa: A comprehensive review of classification, management and laboratory studies*. Berkshire: Dystrophic Epidermolysis Bullosa Research Association (DebRA), 1990, pp. 67–71.

24 Tesi D, Lin AN Nutritional management of the epidermolysis bullosa patient. In: Lin AN, Carter DM (eds) *Epidermolysis Bullosa: Basic and Clinical Aspects*. New York: Springer-Verlag, 1992, pp. 261–6.

25 Arbiser JL, Fine J-D, Murrell D *et al.* Basic fibroblast growth factor: a missing link between collagen VII, increased collagenase and squamous cell carcinoma in recessive dystrophic epidermolysis bullosa. *Mol Med*, 1998, **4** 191–5.

26 Haynes L, Atherton DJ, Ade-Ajaye N *et al.* Gastrostomy and growth in dystrophic epidermolysis bullosa. *Br J Dermatol*, 1996, **134** 872–9.

27   Atherton DJ, Denyer J *Epidermolysis Bullosa. An Outline for Professionals*. Berkshire: Dystrophic Epidermolysis Bullosa Research Association (DebRA), 2003.

28   Seshadri A, Shah A, Bhade S Haematological response of anaemic pre-school children to ascorbic acid supplementation. *Hum Nutr Appl Nutr*, 1985, **39A** 151–4.

29   Levene CI, Bates CJ Ascorbic acid and collagen synthesis in cultured fibroblasts. *Ann N Y Acad Sci*, 1975, **258** 288–305.

30   Giardina PJ, Lin AN Hematologic problems in epidermolysis bullosa. In: Lin AN, Carter DM (eds) *Epidermolysis Bullosa: Basic and Clinical Aspects*. New York: Springer-Verlag, 1992, pp. 191–7.

31   Hallberg L Combating iron deficiency: daily administration of iron is far superior to weekly administration. *Am J Clin Nutr*, 1998, **68** 213–17.

32   Beard JL Weekly iron intervention: the case for intermittent iron supplementation. *Am J Clin Nutr*, 1998, **68** 209–12.

33   Whittaker P Iron and zinc interactions in humans. *Am J Clin Nutr*, 1998, **68** (Suppl) 442S–6S.

34   Walker CF, Kordas K, Stoltzfus RJ *et al.* Interactive effects of iron and zinc on biochemical and functional outcomes in supplementation trials. *Am J Clin Nutr*, 2005, **82** 5–12.

35   Halstead JA Zinc deficiency in man, the Shiraz experiment. *Am J Med*, 1972, **53** 277–84.

36   Shankar AH, Prasad AS Zinc and immune function: the biological basis of altered resistance to infection. *Am J Clin Nutr*, 1998, **68** (Suppl) 447S–63S.

37   Reyes LM, Cattani A, Gajardo H *et al.* Bone metabolism in children with epidermolysis bullosa. *J Pediatr*, 2002, **140** 467–9.

38   Melville C, Atherton D, Burch M *et al.* Fatal cardiomyopathy in dystrophic epidermolysis bullosa. *Br J Dermatol*, 1996, **135** 603–6.

39   Sidwell RU, Yates R, Atherton DJ Dystrophic epidermolysis and dilated cardiomyopathy. *Arch Dis Child*, 2000, **83** 59–63.

40   Williams CL, Bollella M, Wynder EL A new recommendation for dietary fiber in childhood. *Pediatr*, 1995, **96** 985–8.

41   Kirkham J, Robinson C, Strafford SM *et al.* The chemical composition of tooth enamel in junctional epidermolysis bullosa. *Arch Oral Biol*, 2000, **45,** 377–86.

42   Harris JC, Bryan RAE, Lucas VS *et al.* Dental disease and caries related microflora in children with dystrophic epidermolysis bullosa. *Am Acad Pediatr Dent*, 2001, **23** 43–3.

43   Griffin R, Mayou B The anaesthetic management of patients with dystrophic epidermolysis bullosa. A review of 44 patients over a ten year period. *Anaesthesia*, 1993, **48** 810–15.

44   Inal M, Soyupak S, Akgul E *et al.* Fluoroscopically guided endoluminal balloon dilatation of esophageal stricture due to epidermolysis bulllosa dystrophica. *Dysphagia*, 2002, **17** 242–5.

45   Gryboski JD, Touloukian R, Campanella RA Gastrointestinal manifestations of epidermolysis bullosa in children. *Arch Dermatol*, 1988, **124** 746–52.

46   Fine J-D, Bauer EA, McGuire J The treatment of inherited epidermolysis bullosa. Nonmolecular approaches. In: Fine J-D, Bauer EA, McGuire J, Moshell A (eds) *Epidermolysis Bullosa. Clinical, Epidemiologic and Laboratory Advances and the Findings of the National Epidermolysis Bullosa Registry*. Baltimore: Johns Hopkins University Press, 1999, pp. 374–406.

Useful address

Dystrophic Epidermolysis Bullosa Research Association (DebRA)

DebRA House, 13 Wellington Business Park, Dukes Ride, Crowthorne, Berkshire, RG45 6LS. Tel. 01344 771961; Fax 01344 762661

e-mail: debra@debra.org.uk

DebRA is a charity that exists to help people with all types of EB. DebRA also funds research into all aspects of EB care as well as dedicated nursing and social support.

Nutrition information booklets published by DebRA:

Haynes L *Nutrition in Epidermolysis Bullosa, for children over 1 year of age* (2002).

Haynes L *Nutrition for babies with Epidermolysis Bullosa*, 2003. (This information may be suitable for babies with EBS Dowling–Meara and non-Herlitz JEB, but not Herlitz JEB.)

Useful fora, websites

www.internationalebforum.org (international multidisciplinary professionals' forum). This includes the International Network of Dietitians in Epidermolysis Bullosa (INDEB)

www.debra.org.uk (DebRA UK website)

www.debra.org (DebRA of America website)

www.ebanusa.org (US EB Action Network)

www.ebinfoworld.com (US website, compiled by the parent of an EB child)

www.ryanlewiscottrell.emuconnie.co.uk/index.htm (UK website, compiled by the parent of an EB child)

25 Burns

Helen McCarthy & Claire Gurry

Introduction

It is estimated that approximately 250 000 people suffer from a burns injury each year in the UK. Children under the age of 4 years account for 20% of this total and a further 10% are children aged 5–14 years. Approximately 500 children each year sustain a major burns injury requiring fluid resuscitation [1,2].

Assessment of injury

Burns are assessed from an accurate history of the incident. This should include the cause of the injury, the depth and surface area of the wound and whether there has been any smoke inhalation. The main causes and types of burns injury in children and adolescents are listed in Table 25.1. Approximately 70% of thermal injuries sustained by children under 4 years of age are scalds [3].

Burn depth is classified as:

- Partial thickness (superficial, superficial dermal, deep dermal)
- Full thickness

Burns are dynamic injuries that are rarely uniform in depth and therefore require continual reassessment [4]. The total body surface area (TBSA) is determined using Lund and Browder charts; in children, a major burn is defined as an injury covering an area >10% TBSA [5].

Metabolic response to burn injury

Recent evidence suggests that adults with major burns injuries develop a hypermetabolic state in the first 5 days post-injury. This hypermetabolism

Table 25.1 Causes and types of burn injury.

Type of burn	Cause of burn
Water	Kettle, teapot, cup, mug, bath, saucepan
Contact	Radiator, iron, oven, hot-water bottle
Flame	House fire, chip pan, electric/coal fire, barbecue
Fat	Chip pan, oven trays
Chemical	Cement, hair dye, cleansing agents, cytotoxic drugs
Electrical	Electrical appliances, overhead and underground cables
Other	Over-exposure to radiotherapy, frostbite, animal manure

is present throughout the acute period and has been observed to persist for up to 12 months post-injury [6–8]. Modern medical and nursing management including early excision and grafting; increased use of artificial skin and other novel wound coverings; regular analgesia; and control of ambient temperature have had beneficial effects on the metabolic response to the burns injury [9,10].

Aims of nutritional support

The aim of nutritional support is to provide appropriate intervention in order to promote optimal wound healing and to maintain normal growth. It is well documented that improved nutritional status in the critically ill patient reduces the likelihood of complications (e.g. infection, poor wound healing) and length of stay in hospital [11–14].

Assessment of nutritional requirements

Factors influencing the nutritional requirements of a child with a thermal injury are listed in Table 25.2. A full assessment of nutritional requirements should be made, taking these and any additional factors into consideration.

Energy requirements

Several researchers have investigated energy requirements in children with thermal injuries. Although the ideal way of calculating energy requirements would be to measure them on a daily basis, using indirect calorimetry and adjusting all

Table 25.2   Factors influencing nutritional requirements.

Age
Sex
Weight
Height/length
Pre-injury nutritional status
Current nutritional status
Percentage burn surface area
Thickness of burn
Grafted area
Extent of healing

Table 25.3   Hildreth formula for energy requirements.

Infants <1 year	2100 kcal (8.8 MJ)/m^2 (SA) + 1000 kcal (4.2 MJ)/m^2 (BSA)
Children <12 years	1800 kcal (7.5 MJ)/m^2 (SA) + 1300 kcal (5.4 MJ)/m^2 (BSA)
Children >12 years	1500 kcal (6.3 MJ)/m^2 (SA) + 1500 kcal (6.3 MJ)/m^2 (BSA)

BSA, burn surface area; SA, surface area.

nutritional support to meet these figures, this is impractical.

The Hildreth formula (Table 25.3), which takes account of age, weight, total body surface area and percentage burn surface area, can be calculated at the bedside [15,16]. Energy requirements in children with burns rarely rise above the estimated average requirement (EAR) in the first 24 hours post-burns injury [17,18]. An alternative may therefore be to aim for the EAR for energy in injuries of a small surface area. Any formula is only a guideline and provides a starting point for estimating requirements. Frequent reassessment and adjustment of requirements are needed for an uneventful course and successful outcome.

Protein requirements

Protein requirements for children with burns injuries remain unclear. Losses of lean muscle mass and negative nitrogen balance have both been recognised in studies investigating the nutritional needs of this patient group. Cunningham *et al.* [19] suggest that appropriate wound healing is achievable in children receiving 2–3 g protein/kg/day. It has also been suggested that higher protein intakes may have beneficial outcomes in thermally injured children [20,21]. However, a more recent review by Herndon and Tompkins [6] states that protein intakes of 3 g/kg/day may raise urea production without improvement in muscle protein synthesis.

Moderate hypoalbuminaemia is common in children with thermal injuries and the literature suggests that this can be well tolerated. Increases in protein provision may be required to correct this. If the serum albumin level falls too low despite the calculated protein requirement being met, then albumin infusions should be considered [22].

Vitamin and mineral requirements

This area is still very much under debate as there are few studies that specifically look at the requirements for vitamins and minerals in children with burns. It can be assumed, however, that requirements are increased for certain vitamins and minerals because of their role in the metabolic pathways of the body. When assessing the requirements in burns patients, the following should be considered:

- Vitamin A may have a role in the prevention of stress ulcers [23]
- Vitamin C is vital to collagen synthesis [23]
- B group vitamins are required proportional to energy intake
- Low levels of serum iron in most cases are not diet related and may have a protective effect against infection [24]
- Both zinc and copper have a role in the wound healing process; however, the methods and benefits of supplementation require further investigation [25]

Recently, the increased incidence of fractures reported in children post-burns injury has led to a raised awareness of vitamin D deficiency. It has been suggested that risk factors for vitamin D deficiency include lack of sunlight exposure, reduced intake and poor absorption [26,27]. Before a vitamin and mineral supplement is considered it is important to check the nutritional composition and bioavailability of enteral and/or parenteral nutrition intervention, in conjunction with the appropriate biochemical parameters. Excessive supplementation may result in a nutritional imbalance, which could potentially result in toxicity of certain nutrients or interfere with the utilisation of others.

Novel substrates

These include immune-enhancing nutrients such as antioxidants, omega-3 fatty acids, glutamine, arginine and nucleotides. The limited studies available have focused on their use in adults and recommendations have yet to be made regarding their use in children. Antioxidant therapy (vitamins A, C, E) has been shown to reduce burns and burns sepsis mortality in adult burns patients [28]. Omega-3 fatty acids may improve wound healing [29]. Glutamine deficiency is known to occur in children with burns injuries, but the significance of this is unknown [30]. Supplementation appears to have a protective effect on protein synthesis and tissue repair in adults. Glutamine is also the main fuel source for gut enterocytes preserving mucosal integrity and reducing bacterial translocation [31,32]. Arginine is known to have many potential beneficial effects in stressed patients; arginine deficiency has been documented in adults post-burns injury [33].

Meeting nutritional goals

Several factors need to be considered before deciding upon the most appropriate method of achieving nutritional requirements. These are listed in Table 25.4.

Minor burns (<10%)

Children with minor burns should be encouraged to start eating and drinking as early as possible. Nutritious fluids such as milk, milk shakes and proprietary dietary supplements should be offered in preference to juice or fizzy drinks. Every effort should be made to provide familiar foods in order to promote the child's appetite.

Daily food and fluid intake should be accurately recorded by nursing staff. If this highlights difficulties in meeting the dietary targets alternative nutritional intervention may be necessary.

Table 25.4   Factors influencing the achievement of nutritional requirements.

Percentage burn surface area
Site of injury
Pre-existing clinical conditions
Previous nutritional status
Special dietary needs
Gastrointestinal function
Pain management and sedation
Pyrexia
Periods of fasting
Psychological distress

Major burns (>10%)

In major burns, a nasogastric or nasojejunal feeding tube should be passed within the first few hours of treatment when other invasive procedures are taking place. Enteral feeds should then be commenced as early as possible and balanced against oral intake. It has been well documented that early enteral feeding of burns patients (within the first 6 hours) reduces the incidence of paralytic ileus and may moderate the hypermetabolic response. Other benefits of early enteral feeding include maintenance of gut integrity and a reduction in bacterial translocation, as well as improvements in immune status and wound healing [6,34–36].

Continuous enteral feeding should be commenced at a low rate and increased as tolerated, aiming to achieve full requirements within the first 24 hours post-injury [35]. Feeding regimens must take into account fasting periods related to surgical intervention, dressing changes, physiotherapy and medications. Nasogastric feeding is routinely used in many centres, but where this is poorly tolerated, transpyloric feeding should be considered. The use of gastrostomy feeding has been reported where long term enteral nutritional support has been required in burns patients [37].

Well-recognised complications of enteral feeding include increased gastric aspirates and diarrhoea. Gastric aspirates in excess of the hourly feed rate are closely correlated with infection and sepsis [38]. Diarrhoea occurs frequently in paediatric burns patients, but appears to be unrelated to the osmolality or volume of feed [39]. Because broad spectrum antibiotics are often used in this patient group, it has been suggested that the use of pre- and probiotics may have a beneficial effect on gut flora [40,41].

Parenteral nutrition (PN) should only be considered when there is prolonged paralytic ileus or where poor tolerance of enteral feeding prevents nutritional requirements from being met by this route alone. However, where possible, minimal enteral feeds should continue to be infused at a very low rate (as little as 2 mL/hour) to maintain the brush border integrity of the gastrointestinal tract [42,43]. The complications of PN are well recognised and as infection risks are already high in burns patients special care must be taken when

Table 25.5   Suitable feeds for paediatric patients.

0–1 year	Low birth weight formula; infant formula; follow-on milk; high energy infant formula; protein hydrolysate formula
Younger children 8 kg up to 30 or 45 kg (depending on feed)	Paediatric enteral feeds; high energy paediatric enteral feeds; paediatric fibre feeds; age appropriate sip feeds
Older children 30–45 kg upwards (depending on feed)	Paediatric enteral feeds as above; adult enteral feeds; high energy adult feeds; adult fibre feeds; critical care enteral feeds; oral sip feeds
Others	Glucose polymers; fat emulsions; protein supplements; novel substrates

considering PN. Other issues, such as electrolyte imbalances and hyperglycaemia, also require particularly close monitoring. Further guidance on enteral and parenteral nutrition support in children may be found in Chapters 3 and 4.

Choice of oral and enteral feeds

The choice of feed will vary depending on the age of the child, the calculated requirements, any underlying medical condition and the clinical course during admission. Some of the products available for use in the nutritional management of paediatric burns patients are outlined in Table 25.5. There is some evidence to suggest that the use of high carbohydrate feeds may improve protein synthesis and muscle mass accretion, although such feeds are not routinely used in the UK at the present time [6,33].

Monitoring

Burns injuries are dynamic and this patient group has constantly changing nutritional needs related to the healing of their wounds. As the percentage burn surface area changes so the nutritional requirements should be reassessed.

● Regular weights (without dressings) should be recorded and plotted on appropriate centile charts. These should be compared with pre-admission measurements where available. It is important to remember that oedema may mask true weight early in the clinical course.

- Routine biochemistry should be monitored. Frequency will vary depending on the child's clinical course. Vitamin, mineral and trace element status should also be monitored in extensive burns injuries. The recommendation for adult burns patients by the Burns Interest Group of the British Dietetic Association can be used as a guide at this time [23].
- Raised serum levels of C-reactive protein predict sepsis in children with burns injuries [44]. This would suggest that it is included in routine monitoring in major burns where there is an increased risk of infection.
- Bowel motions should be recorded accurately indicating frequency and consistency. Adjustments to feeding regimens may be beneficial in normalising bowel habit.

Monitoring of nutritional intake and overall nutritional status should continue post-discharge. Changes in the medical management of burns patients now results in an early discharge home, even for quite major injuries. These children are still at risk of inadequate nutritional intake and therefore growth failure once at home [45,46]. It should also be noted that even with adequate nutritional intake, poor growth often continues to be an issue. In these circumstances children exhibit increased body fat stores but no significant increase in lean body mass. This should be monitored closely in children with major burns injuries post-discharge.

Case study

An 18-month-old toddler has sustained a 15% partial thickness scald as a result of pulling a jug of freshly boiled water over himself. His weight and length on admission are on the 25th centile for age.

A dietary history indicates that he takes approximately 500–600 mL of a follow-on milk, recommended as the family follows a lacto-vegetarian diet. There is no history of iron deficiency anaemia. He eats three meals plus supper daily and has no noted dislikes or food intolerance.

Calculating requirements

Energy: 1800 kcal (7.5 MJ)/m^2 (SA) + 1300 kcal (5.4 MJ)/m^2 (burn SA)
= $(1800 \times 0.48) + (1300 \times 0.072)$
= 958 kcal

Protein: 2–3 g protein/kg
= 24–36 g protein

SA, surface area.

Achieving requirements

The following need to be considered:

- Site of injury – facial injury, therefore oral feeding may be compromised; a feeding tube should be passed on admission prior to facial swelling
- Percentage burn area – this is >10% and is therefore a major burn
- There is no previous medical history of note
- Previous nutritional status – good
- Special dietary needs – lacto-vegetarian
- No gastrointestinal problems
- Pain management – as a result of the injury the child is in a great deal of pain and has commenced opiate-based pain relief
- Pyrexia – none noted yet
- The child is scared and unsure of what is happening to him

Method of feeding

An enteral feeding tube should be passed during the resuscitation period. Enteral feeds should commence within 6 hours of admission via this route, until such a time as the child is able to feed orally. Enteral feeds should gradually be replaced by oral intake to meet full nutritional requirements. Good oral hygiene should be maintained throughout.

Choice of feed

- A normal follow-on milk supplemented with glucose polymer and fat emulsion. The advantage of this option is familiarity, which eases the transition from enteral to oral feeding. The disadvantages are incomplete nutritional composition of the feed and the increased infection risk resulting from feed modification.

- A standard 1 kcal/mL (4 kJ/mL) paediatric enteral feed. The advantage of this option is a nutritionally complete feed that will meet all nutritional requirements without modification. The disadvantages are the unfamiliarity of the product and palatability for oral feeding.

The final feeding regimen should be planned in conjunction with medical and nursing management.

Monitoring

- Dressings are changed twice weekly. The child should be weighed and the degree of healing assessed on each of these occasions. Nutritional support should be reassessed according to these criteria.
- Nutritional biochemical markers should be requested and monitored as necessary to 'fine tune' dietetic intervention and promote a positive outcome.
- A possible side effect of analgesia is constipation; bowel habits should be monitored closely and fibre enriched feeds considered.

Acknowledgements

We acknowledge the input of Dearbhla Hunt for her work on the previous version of this chapter and John Stanton for his comments on this version.

References

1   Hettiaratchy S, Dziewulski P ABC of Burns. Introduction. *Br Med J*, 2004, **328** 1366–8.
2   Wilkinson E The epidemiology of burns in secondary care, in a population of 2.6 million people. *Burns*, 1998, **24** 139–43.
3   Hettiaratchy S, Dziewulski P ABC of Burns. Pathophysiology and types of burns. *Br Med J*, 2004, **328** 1427–9.
4   Hettiaratchy S, Papini R ABC of Burns. Initial management of a major burn: II – assessment and resuscitation. *Br Med J*, 2004, **329** 101–3.
5   Lund CL, Browder ND The estimation of areas of burns. *Surg Gynecol Obstet*, 1944, **78** 352.
6   Herndon DN, Tompkins RG Support of the metabolic response to burn injury. *Lancet*, 2004, **363** 1895–902.
7   Dickerson RN *et al.* Accuracy of predictive methods to estimate resting energy expenditure of thermally-injured patients. *J Parenter Enteral Nutr*, 2002, **26** 17–29.
8   Hart DW *et al.* Persistence of muscle catabolism after severe burn. *Surgery*, 2000, **128** 312–19.
9   Papini R ABC of Burns. Management of burn injuries of various depths. *Br Med J*, 2004, **329** 158–60.
10 King P Artificial skin reduces nutritional requirements in a severely burned child. *Burns*, 2000, **26** 501–3.
11 Bagley SM Nutritional needs of the acutely ill with acute wounds. *Crit Care Nurs Clin North Am*, 1996, **22** 159–67.
12 Kiyama T *et al.* The route of nutrition support affects the early phase of wound healing. *J Parenter Enteral Nutr*, 1998, **22** 276–9.
13 Wallace E Feeding the wound: nutrition and wound care. *Br J Nurs*, 1994, **3** 662.
14 Kings Fund Centre *A Positive Approach to Nutrition as a Treatment*. London: Kings Fund, 1992.
15 Hildreth M *et al.* Calorie requirement of patients with burns under one year of age. *J Burn Care Rehabil*, 1993, **14** 108–12.
16 Hildreth M *et al.* Current treatment reduces calories required to maintain weight in paediatric patients with burns. *J Burn Care Rehabil*, 1990, **11** 405–9.
17 Childs C Studies in children provide a model to reexamine the metabolic response to burn injuries in patients treated by contemporary burn protocol. *Burns*, 1994, **20** 291–300.
18 Dept of Health Report on Health and Social Subjects No. 41. *Dietary Reference Values for Food Energy and Nutrients for the UK*. London: The Stationery Office: 1991.
19 Cunningham JJ *et al.* Calorie and protein provision for recovery from severe burns in infants and young children. *Am J Clin Nutr*, 1990, **51** 553–7.
20 Prelack K *et al.* Energy and protein provisions for thermally injured children revisited: an outcome-based approach for determining requirements. *J Burn Care Rehabil*, 1997, **18** 177–81.
21 Alexandra JW *et al.* Beneficial effects of aggressive protein feeding in severely burned children. *Ann Surg*, 1980, **192** 505–17.
22 Sheridan RL Physiologic hypoalbuminaemia is well tolerated by severely burned children. *J Trauma*, 1997, **43** 448–52.
23 Glencorse C *et al.* Thermal injury. In: *A Pocket Guide to Clinical Nutrition*, 3rd edn. Birmingham: British Dietetic Association, 2004.
24 Ward CG *et al.* Iron and infection: new developments and their implications. *J Trauma*, 1996, **41** 356–64.
25 Cunningham JJ *et al.* Low ceruloplasmin levels during recovery from major burn injury: influence of open wound size and copper supplementation. *Nutrition*, 1996, **12** 83–8.

26 Mayes T *et al*. Four-year review of burns as an etiologic factor in the development of long bone fractures in pediatric patients. *J Burn Care Rehabil*, 2003, **24** 279–84.

27 Gottschlich MM *et al*. Hypovitaminosis D in acutely injured pediatric burn patients. *J Am Diet Assoc*, 2004, **104** 931–41.

28 Horton JW Free radicals and lipid peroxidation mediated injury in burn trauma: the role of antioxidant therapy. *Toxicology*, 2003, **189** 75–88.

29 Abribat T *et al*. Decreased serum insulin-like growth factor-1 in burn patients: Relationship with serum insulin-like growth factor binding protein-3 proteolysis and the influence of lipid composition in nutritional support. *Crit Care Med*, 2000, **28** 2366–72.

30 Gore DC, Jahoor F Deficiency in peripheral glutamine production in pediatric patients with burns. *J Burn Care Rehabil*, 2000, **21** 172–7.

31 Saffle JR *et al*. Randomized trial of immune enhancing enteral nutrition in burns patients. *J Trauma*, 1997, **42** 793–800.

32 Houdijk AP *et al*. Randomised trial of glutamine enriched enteral nutrition on infectious morbidity in patients with multiple trauma. *Lancet*, 1998, **353** 772–6.

33 Andel H *et al*. Nutrition and anabolic agents in burned patients. *Burns*, 2003, **29** 592–5.

34 Chiarelli A *et al*. Very early nutritional supplementation in burned patients. *Am J Clin Nutr*, 1990, **51** 1035–9.

35 McDonald WS *et al*. Immediate enteral feeding in burn patients is safe and effective. *J Parenter Enteral Nutr*, 1991, **15** 578–9.

36 Hansbrough JF Enteral nutritional support in burn patients. *Gastrointest Endosc Clin N Am*, 1998, **42** 645–67.

37 Sefton EJ *et al*. Enteral feeding in patients with major burn injury: the use of nasojejunal feeding after the failure of nasogastric feeding. *Burns*, 2002, **28** 386–90.

38 Wolfe SE *et al*. Enteral feeding intolerance: an indicator of sepsis-associated mortality in burned children. *Arch Surg*, 1997, **132** 1310–14.

39 Thakkar K *et al*. Diarrhea in severely burned children. *J Parenter Enteral Nutr*, 2005, **29** 8–11.

40 Bleichner G *et al*. *Saccharomyces boulardii* prevents diarrhea in critically ill tube-fed patients. *Intensive Care Med*, 1997, **23** 517–23.

41 D'Souza AL *et al*. Probiotics in the prevention of antibiotic associated diarrhoea: meta-analysis. *Br Med J*, 2002, **324** 1361–4.

42 ASPEN Guidelines for the use of parenteral and enteral nutrition in adults and pediatric patients. *JPEN*, 2002, **26** 1SA–138SA.

43 Ziegler TR *et al*. Tropic and cytoprotective nutrition for intestinal adaptation, mucosal repair, and barrier function. *Ann Rev Nutr*, 2003, **23** 229–61.

44 Neely AN *et al*. Efficiency of a rise in C-reactive protein serum levels as an early indicator of sepsis in burned children. *J Burn Care Rehabil*, 1998, **19** 102–5.

45 Mittendorfer B *et al*. The 1995 clinical research award. Younger paediatric patients with burns are at risk for continuing post discharge weight loss. *J Burn Care Rehabil*, 1995, **16** 589–95.

46 Windle EM Audit of successful weight maintenance in adult and paediatric survivors of thermal injury at a UK regional burn centre. *J Hum Nutr Diet*, 2004, **17** 435–41.

26 Autistic Spectrum Disorders

Zoe Connor

Introduction

Autistic spectrum disorders (ASD), also known as autism spectrum disorders or pervasive developmental disorders (PDD), are a range of complex lifelong developmental disabilities that affect the way a person communicates and relates to people around them. At the core is a disorder in the capacity for social understanding. Some people with an autistic spectrum disorder have severe learning disabilities, some may never speak, whereas some have an average or above average IQ, and acquire spoken language at the same age as typically developing children.

ASD is a common disorder occurring in at least 60 in every 10 000 children under 8 years, with boys up to four times more affected than girls [1]. The term autism is often used interchangeably with ASD to mean the full spectrum of disorders.

This chapter aims to help dietitians work more effectively with this patient group by:

- Describing the aspects of ASD that make this a challenging group to work with
- Suggesting strategies for the management of dietetic issues commonly found in this group
- Summarising the evidence for and against therapeutic dietary interventions

Diagnosis and co-morbidities

ASD is an umbrella term for a spectrum of three more common diagnoses:

- Autism, also known as classic autism and Kanner's autism
- Pervasive development disorder not otherwise specified (PDDNOS), sometimes known as atypical autism
- Asperger's syndrome

and two rarer conditions:

- Rett's syndrome, which affects primarily girls and is characterised by severe mental and physical regression
- Childhood disintegrative disorder (CDD), which is characterised by 'normal' development of communication and social relationship skills until at least the age of 2 years, followed by regression to display severely autistic characteristics

These five conditions are sometimes known collectively as pervasive development disorders rather than autistic spectrum disorders, with only the first three diagnoses classified as ASD.

Individuals with ASD have three main areas of difficulty, known as the 'triad of impairments':

- *Social interaction:* difficulty with social relationships, e.g. appearing aloof and indifferent to other people and difficulty with understanding others' viewpoints and intentions
- *Social communication:* difficulty with verbal and non-verbal communication
- *Imagination:* difficulty with interpersonal play and imagination (e.g. having a limited range of imaginative activities, possibly copied and pursued rigidly and repetitively)

For a diagnosis of ASD, there must be impairments in each of these three areas. In addition to this triad, repetitive behaviour patterns and resistance to change in routine are often characteristic.

The differentiation between autism, PDDNOS and Asperger's depends on the number and distribution of impairments within the triad as specified by international descriptors [2,3]. As a crude generalisation, children with Asperger's have developed speech by the age of 3 years, autism is often seen as the more severe end of the spectrum with PDDNOS falling in between the two.

The diagnosis of ASD is made by recognising patterns of behaviour rather than by medical investigations and is a process of observation by a multidisciplinary team typically consisting of a paediatrician, speech and language therapist and psychologist. A diagnosis is often made between the age of 18 months and 3 years, although diagnoses are commonly sought and obtained throughout the school life and sometimes into adulthood. There are a number of 'scales' and 'tools' for diag-

nosis. Their use, and access to professionals adequately trained in carrying out assessments, varies around the UK [2].

Co-morbidities common to ASD include learning difficulties, attention deficit hyperactivity disorder (ADHD), motor co-ordination problems, anxiety and epilepsy. Very few people with ASD have the savant abilities that are often associated with ASD in the media.

Sensory issues

Impairment in perception of sensory stimuli is commonly reported in children and people with ASD. Under-sensitivity may result in actions such as spinning, rocking or hand-flapping which are forms of self-stimulation. Other children may demonstrate over-sensitivity by being aversive to touch, light and/or sound. Considerations of possible sensory issues can help to understand a child's behaviour. Table 26.1 demonstrates examples that could affect food intake and mealtimes.

Table 26.1 Examples of sensory issues that could affect food preferences and mealtime behaviour.

Sense	Hypersensitivity	Hyposensitivity
Taste	Strong preference for bland tasting foods Aversion to spicy foods	Preference for strong tasting spicy foods Licking objects
Smell	Distracted or disturbed by food smells Ability to detect smells that others may not, e.g. protein foods	
Visual	Distracted by lighting, movement or colours at mealtimes Preference for bland coloured foods Preference for different foods to be presented separately Disturbed by foods not presented in the usual way Aversion to certain coloured foods	
Auditory	Dislike of crunchy foods Distracted or disturbed by background sounds, some of which may not be obvious, e.g. fluorescent light tubes	Preference for foods that make sounds when you eat, e.g. crunchy ones
Touch	Dislike of mixed textures in mouth Dislike of hot or cold foods and drinks Dislike of some cutlery in mouth Dislike of tooth brushing	Preference for lumpy or crunchy foods Preference for very hot or very cold foods and drinks (possibility of burning self as hyposensitive to pain) Tendency to frequently put foods and other objects to the mouth
Proprioception	Alterations can contribute to clumsiness in eating or drinking, or being distracted by arm movements during eating	
Vestibular attention	Alterations can cause child to be distracted by moving or not moving self, or by body position during a meal	

Causes of ASD

The original theory that ASD could be attributed to parenting has been completely disproved by research. A small proportion of cases of ASD can be attributed to known medical causes which include herpes simplex encephalitis, rubella, intrauterine exposure to thalidomide or valproate, fragile-X syndrome, Angelman's syndrome, untreated PKU or tuberous sclerosis [4]. The majority of cases have no known cause. It is thought that there could be an inherited predisposition to increased sensitivity to an environmental trigger such as an infection or immunological reaction.

Treatment and management

ASD is a life-long developmental disability; children with the condition grow up into adults with the condition. However, with appropriate intervention early in life, specialised education and structured support, a child can be helped to maximise their skills and achieve their full potential as adults. Many individuals can get to the point where they will 'function normally' socially.

Medical treatment is usually focused on managing common co-morbidities such as ADHD, anxiety or epilepsy. Treatment for the traits of ASD is often focused on the early implementation of education and behaviour interventions, where these services are available. These interventions focus on teaching the individual (or helping parents to teach the individual) with ASD the appropriate responses to social situations they struggle with, and also focus on developing communication methods.

Strategies commonly advocated for use with individuals with ASD are:

- Creating a structured routine (which reduces the anxiety a person with ASD may feel at the unpredictable environment around them).
- Care with use of verbal communication. People with ASD are likely to take things very literally, and so may misunderstand idioms (e.g. 'I'll be back in a second', 'Eating that will put hairs on your chest'). It is recommended to use simple language and positive commands rather than negative (e.g. 'Sit down there' rather than 'Don't stand over there').

- Using visual tools to complement any verbal instructions (e.g. signing), the use of objects or (commonly) the use of picture symbols (p. 520).

EarlyBird is a programme developed by the National Autistic Society and is available on the National Health Service in some areas of the UK. It is a 3-month programme run by licensed professionals which combines group training sessions for parents or pre-school children and individual home visits. There are many different programmes of intervention available privately including: Applied Behavioural Analysis (ABA); Lovaas; the Hanen programme; the Son-Rise program; Options; Treatment and Education of Autistic and Related Communication Handicapped Children (TEACCH).

Gastrointestinal issues and ASD

A nested case–control study carried out from the UK General Practice Research Database found that at the time of diagnosis of autism children were no more likely to have had a history of defined gastrointestinal disorder (coeliac disease, chronic gastroenteritis, regional enteritis, malabsorption, ulcerative colitis, food intolerance or recurrent gastrointestinal symptoms on three occasions in 6 months) than children without autism [5].

Many parents of children with ASD, however, report gastrointestinal problems such as constipation, diarrhoea, excessive wind and abdominal pain. Hovarth et al. [6] stated that unrecognised gastrointestinal disorders may contribute to behavioural problems in non-verbal autistic patients; in a sample of 36 children with ASD with frequent gastrointestinal complaints 69% were found to have reflux oesophagitis, 42% chronic gastritis, 67% chronic duodenitis and 58% low intestinal carbohydrate digestive enzyme activity (but normal pancreatic function).

There is a range of published data exploring gastrointestinal problems as possible aetiologies for ASD summarised in Table 26.2 and detailed below.

Constipation

This has been reported to be a frequent, significant and under-recognised problem in children with

Table 26.2 Summary of reported gastrointestinal abnormalities in autistic spectrum disorders.

Frequent, significant constipation
Autistic enterocolitis
Increased gut permeability to lactulose
Altered upper and lower intestinal flora

Table 26.3 Summary of reported metabolic abnormalities in autistic spectrum disorders.

Lower sulphation capacity
Low zinc : copper ratios
Low serum ferritin levels
Low plasma magnesium levels
Abnormal levels of plasma phospholipid fatty acids
Dysregulated amino acid metabolism
Increased oxidative stress
High plasma vitamin B_6 levels

autism, with abdominal X-rays recommended in aiding the assessment of the degree of constipation because of the difficulty in obtaining an accurate history [7].

'Autistic enterocolitis'

Researchers have also reported a novel gastro-enterocolitis in children with ASD which has been named 'autistic enterocolitis', characterised by ileo-colonic lymphoid nodular hyperplasia and mucosal inflammation [8]. The significance of this finding to clinical practice or the possible contribution to the cause of some cases of ASD is not yet clear.

Gut permeability

D'Eufemia *et al.* [9] reported that 43% of a sample of 21 autistic children had an increased intestinal permeability for lactulose compared to none in 40 controls. They proposed that the elevated permeability reflected damage to the tight junctions linking the intestinal epithelial cells in the affected autistic patients. Further research needs to be carried out in this area.

Intestinal flora

Finegold *et al.* [10] and Parracho *et al.* [11] report significant alterations in the upper and lower intestinal flora of children with 'late-onset' autism, characterised by increased amount and number of clostridial species. These organisms produce toxins that may contribute towards gut dysfunction and other systemic effects [11]. Further research needs to be carried out in this area to verify these preliminary findings. There are two detailed reviews of gastrointestinal factors in ASD [12,13].

Nutritional or metabolic abnormalities in ASD

There is no evidence that children with ASD have increased requirements for macro- or micronutrients. However, there are some published data that suggest abnormalities in nutrient levels or metabolism in small groups of individuals with ASD or in closely related co-morbidities. This is summarised in Table 26.3 and detailed below.

Sulphation

Researchers in Italy have found that children with ASD (sample size 20) had a significantly lower sulphation capacity than that of a control group [13]. It is hypothesised that this would cause an inability to effectively metabolise compounds that could be toxic to the central nervous system, such as phenolic compounds that are derived from dietary sources. Different non-professional organisations recommend either taking the supplement methyl sulphonyl methane or magnesium sulphate orally, or bathing in magnesium sulphate (Epsom salts) as therapeutic measures.

Zinc

A study of 500 children with ASD reported low zinc : copper ratios [14]. Zinc has been shown in placebo controlled, blind studies to reduce ADHD symptoms [15,16].

Urinary peptides

The University of Sunderland, Autism Research Unit carry out urine peptide analysis by post for a non-profit fee. The urine peptide profiles often show peaks which are hypothetically linked in the returned report to abnormal casein and/or gluten derived peptides. There have been no published data to support this. Reports that the levels of another peptide seen in this analysis – indolyl-3-acryloylglycine – were higher in people with ASD than in the wider population have been discounted [16]. Many parents use this service before making the decision to trial therapeutic removal of gluten and casein from their child's diet. The centre also advocates the trial of many other dietary interventions: 'The Sunderland Protocol' [17].

Iron

In a study of 53 children with ADHD, 84% were found to have low serum ferritin levels compared to 18% of an age- and sex-matched control group of 27 [18]. One recently published case study demonstrates reduced ADHD symptoms after treating with iron supplements [19].

Magnesium

A study of 34 children with ASD found significantly lower plasma concentrations of magnesium compared to 14 control subjects [20].

Essential fatty acids

Researchers in France [21] found abnormal levels of plasma phospholipid fatty acids in individuals with autism compared to controls. Bell *et al.* [22] found abnormal levels of fatty acids in red blood cell membranes of patients with autism and Asperger's syndrome. They also reported a high level of clinical signs of fatty acid deficiency as reported by parents [22]. Similar abnormalities have been reported in other disorders: dyslexia [23], ADHD [24] and mood disorders [25]. The abnormal levels of highly unsaturated fatty acids in Bell's ASD sample was linked to abnormal levels of a phospholipid enzyme, which resolved with eicosapentaenoic acid (EPA) supplementation [24].

Plasma amino acids

Researchers in Birmingham have reported a dysregulated amino acid metabolism in individuals with ASD, and their family members, evidenced by abnormal plasma amino acid levels [26].

Increased oxidative stress

Researchers in the USA have found an increased vulnerability to oxidative stress and a decreased capacity for methylation in 20 children with autism compared to 33 control children. Supplementation with folinic acid, betaine and methylcobalamin normalised this metabolic imbalance [27].

Vitamin B_6

A recent study of 35 children with ASD found them to have 75% higher plasma levels of total vitamin B_6 than 11 'typical children' [28]. None of each group was on supplements. It is hypothesised that children with ASD have an impaired ability to convert vitamin B_6 to pyridoxal-5-phosphate, an active cofactor for amongst other things, the formation of key neurotransmitters.

Dietetic challenges in ASD

ASD-friendly consultations

The National Autism Plan [29] recommends that professionals working with children have training in ASD awareness and that additional training should be provided for all staff delivering specific ASD interventions. Additionally, a National Autistic Society information sheet for professionals makes the following suggestions [30]:

- Be aware that a child may find lights, noises and new surroundings overwhelming and may use walking around, flapping their hands, rocking, putting their hands over their ears or closing their eyes to calm themselves
- Try to give the first or last appointment of the day, to reduce the anxiety of waiting
- If necessary provide a quiet room for the family to wait in, rather than a busy waiting room or corridor, or allow the family to wait in their car until you call them in
- Use clear, simple language with short sentences
- Avoid idioms, irony, metaphors and words with double meaning
- Give direct requests

- Do not assume that a non-verbal patient cannot understand what you are saying
- Explain what you are going to do clearly before taking any measurements, and if possible show a picture or doll to explain what you are going to do
- Avoid using body language, gestures or facial expressions without verbal instruction
- A person with ASD may not make eye contact, and may invade your personal space or climb over you

Selective eating

Children with ASD have been shown to have significantly more feeding problems and eat a significantly narrower range of foods that children without autism [31]. DeMeyer [32] found 94% of parents with children with autism reported feeding difficulties compared with 59% of normally developing pre-school children. These feeding problems often present to general paediatric clinics as faddy eating, but are often chronic and extremely selective or perseverant eating. An audit of children seen in an interdisciplinary clinic in the USA found children with autism to have a high prevalence of selectivity by type of food: 62% of autistic clinic attenders ($n = 26$) compared to 21% of total clinic attenders ($n = 349$); and selectivity by texture (31% compared to 26%) [33]. An audit of 17 children with ASD in the UK found 59% to have a selective diet; 18% ate less than eight different foods in total, and 41% ate between 10 and 19 different foods [34]. Because of the nature of ASD the management of selective eating can be challenging and complex.

Commonly reported aspects of selective eating in ASD are:

- Texture preferences/difficulty with transition to textured foods
- Distress at trying new foods/food neophobia
- Strong preference for foods of a particular colour
- Acceptance only of foods with familiar packaging
- Distress in some mealtime environments (e.g. it may be too noisy; too quiet; too bright; distressed by smells or look of other people's food; distressed by being around other people)

- Demands that food is presented in a consistent way (e.g. same plate and cutlery, positioning of food on plate)
- Seeming not to recognise their own thirst or hunger

Some parents report that their child ate well until the age of 1–2 years, when they regressed to only eating baby food textures and self-restricting the range of foods they would accept. This often coincides with the time at which the parents feel their child's social skills deteriorated. Parents sometimes report this regression coincided with a vaccination or illness. Some texts suggest that this 'regressive' form of ASD, which makes up 15–40% of cases, may be classified as a subtype of ASD in the future [1].

Some of the characteristics of ASD can help to explain why selective eating is so common:

- Indifference to social cues (i.e. not copying parents' and peers' eating behaviour)
- Resistance to new experiences, such as trying new foods
- Preference for rigid routines, such as eating the same food from the same plate in same place
- Distraction by change (e.g. usual preference for the regular shaped and coloured crisps but reluctant to eat one with a brown 'bit', distracted by crumb on table or unable to eat foods that touch each other on a plate)
- Obsession with familiarity, such as one particular make and flavour of yoghurt

Dietetic assessment of a child with selective eating

As with any child with faddy eating, a standard dietetic assessment would include monitoring of growth, assessment of nutritional adequacy of diet through diet history, and recommendation of dietary changes to ensure adequacy, including supplements where needed. Further objectives of dietetic consultations can be:

- Helping to identify the underlying factors causing the selective eating
- Helping parents and other carers to understand these factors in light of the characteristic features of ASD in their child

- Advising on strategies to help change their child's diet
- Co-ordinating a multidisciplinary approach to changing the child's dietary intake

Continued refusal of family foods can cause great distress to families. Often one of the key things parents are seeking from a dietetic consultation is reassurance that their child is growing well and although eating an apparently unvaried diet is getting foods from the different food groups and is not deficient in any nutrients. A UK study of 3-day food recalls of 17 children with ASD reported to have eating problems found them to have surprisingly adequate nutritional intakes despite an apparently unvaried diet. Forty-seven per cent of them met the reference nutrient intake (RNI) for all nutrients and only 6% were under the lower RNI for iron, and 18% for dietary vitamin D [35]. It can also help reassure parents that their problem is not unique. A useful resource for parents and professionals is the book, *Can't eat, won't eat*, written by a mother of a child with selective eating and Asperger's syndrome, which includes the detailed results of a survey the author carried out of other parents of children with selective eating.

Tooth decay can be a problem for children who favour sugary foods and drinks, and resist tooth brushing. Tooth decay can lead to pain which further limits their intake. Some areas have specialist dental services with staff experienced in dealing with children with ASD and their help can be invaluable.

Strategies for dealing with selective eating

Typically, parents with children with ASD and chronic selective eating will report that they have tried the standard behavioural advice for toddlers with faddy eating, and not found this to be helpful. Parents often need individualised advice to deal with the ASD specific selectiveness of their children or indeed intensive interventions such as those offered by multidisciplinary feeding clinics, to see even small progressions in their child's diet.

The following are suggestions for strategies for parents to use.

Make mealtimes more predictable

- Establish a structured eating routine. As with

other children with faddy eating, this is key. Try to make mealtimes a predictable occurrence for the child in terms of time and place and situation.
- Use visual timetables. Again to make mealtimes more predictable and a less anxious occasion for a child, write a timetable detailing when and where they will eat and what will be eaten. The timetable can be supplemented with picture symbols or photographs.
- Use visual schedules. Written or picture symbol schedules detailing behaviour expected at meal time or foods to be tried at a meal time. Some children with ASD seem to follow written visual instructions well.

Deal with underlying issues that may be exacerbating eating problems

- As with any child, medical problems may reduce appetite (e.g. pain; dental problems; gastrointestinal problems; medications, such as methylphenidate).
- The expertise of other professionals may need to be sought for physical problems such as positioning at mealtimes and swallowing issues.
- Take into account sensory issues in creating a calm, comfortable eating environment (e.g. eating in quiet place versus eating with a video or music on; eating meals with others versus alone).
- Involve an occupational therapist, physiotherapist or speech and language therapist trained in sensory integration therapy to help to identify and address sensory perception problems that may be causing aversions to certain foods. Interventions may involve special seating, messy play and other activities to desensitise to different foods and activities such as massage and touching around the mouth and face.
- Devise a slow step-by-step programme for introducing new foods which minimises anxiety where a child is extremely food phobic.

Find ways to motivate

This can be extremely difficult with some children, as commonly advised motivators such as praise, affection and star charts may not have any effect. Parents and other caregivers can be helped to think of things that have motivated other changes (e.g. toilet training). Some things that have been found to help:

- 'Eat it up' books. Written list or picture symbol lists of foods liked, foods parents want the child to try and the foods the child is going to try next. Foods can be moved gradually up the lists.
- Use of 'social stories'. A specially written story in simple language explaining to a child/young person with learning difficulties or ASD how and why to do something (see p. 520).
- Using 'special interests' to motivate. Children with ASD often have 'obsessive' interests (e.g. watching the same part of a particular Thomas the Tank engine video).
- Using a specially devised board game where specific squares instruct to try a different food [36].

Involve other caregivers

Some class teachers or classroom support assistants may be willing to devise programmes to introduce new foods at school, and to find ways of improving the mealtime environment for a child who is not eating well. Some areas have specialised education staff experienced in working with children with ASD who can advise class teachers and parents and help to devise programmes appropriate to individual children.

Excessive weight gain

The prevalence of obesity in children with ASD has not been found to be higher than of that of the general population [35]. However, as effecting lifestyle change is very challenging in many children and young people with ASD, the management of overweight can be very difficult.

Some underlying issues that may be present in an overweight child with ASD:

- Selective eating and self-selecting calorific snacks, drinks, meals and puddings
- Free access to foods and helping themselves throughout the day
- Aggressively demanding their favoured foods
- Self-stimulating by continually eating (e.g.

enjoying the feel or taste or sound of food in the mouth)
- Being very sedentary as a result of medication, lack of ability to be active safely, or dislike of movement because of hypersensitivity to vestibular feedback
- Some behaviour management programmes use foods as motivators so that snack foods such as biscuits are being used a number of times a day to teach communication and other skills

Useful strategies for managing overeating include:

- Using a visual timetable to dictate set snack and meal times
- Helping parents to find strategies to say no to their child's demands
- Keeping tempting foods out of the house or locked away
- Getting other caregivers and school staff to give consistent messages

Biomedical interventions: therapeutic diets for ASD

Interest in the use of dietary manipulation in the treatment of ASD dates back nearly 50 years and a great number of different nutritional interventions are implemented by families affected by ASD. Surveys in the USA report that 17–43% of children with ASD are on a micronutrient supplement for treatment of ASD and 16–27% are on a modified diet [37,38].

The amount of information available to parents via the Internet, books, parent networks and other organisations can be overwhelming and often contradictory. 'Biomedical interventions' are recommended to parents as a therapeutic option to alleviate symptoms of ASD and some suggest that they are a near cure. Interventions include various exclusion diets, named or trade-marked special diets, supplementation with vitamins, minerals or fats, probiotics and enzymes. Some advocates of biomedical interventions recommend a number of different interventions to be followed in steps, which can lead to children being on heavily restricted diets and megadoses of different supplements. Biomedical interventions described in more detail in this text are summarised in Table 26.4.

Table 26.4   List of biomedical interventions: therapeutic diets for autistic spectrum disorders.

Some supporting literature (mixed quality) for use in ASD	Some supporting literature (mixed quality) for use in ASD-related conditions (e.g. ADHD)	No supporting literature for use in ASD
Gluten and casein free diet	Fish oil supplementation	Feingold diet
Ketogenic diet	Avoidance of aspartame	Rotation diet
High dose vitamin B$_6$ and magnesium	Avoidance of MSG	DMG supplementation
High dose vitamin C	Avoidance of artificial colours and benzoates	Intravenous secretin
Fish oil supplementation		Body ecology diet
Avoidance of phenolic compounds		Specific carbohydrate diet
Vitamin A supplementation		Probiotics
		Digestive enzymes
		Yeast free diet

ADHD, attention deficit hyperactivity disorder; DMG, dimethylglycine; MSG, monosodium glutamate.

Role of dietitians in therapeutic diets for ASD

Despite the lack of high quality evidence for any therapeutic diets for ASD, there are many anecdotal reports of dramatic improvements available to parents, and understandably they will often try out one or a number of these with or without the support of professionals.

Dietitians have a role in helping families to navigate safely through the considerable 'trial and error' of diet therapy in ASD. Scientific evidence may be weak, but there is too much of it and little conclusive evidence against these interventions for them to be discounted.

The multiagency guidance document, the National Autism Plan [31], found insufficient evidence to recommend the use of any 'alternative' therapies, but recommended that parents wishing to explore the use of these therapies for their child 'should do so with the support and knowledge of their named senior clinician from the base service and their key worker'.

As with any restricted diet, a dietitian has a key role in assessing the adequacy of a child's diet, monitoring growth and advising on products and supplements where necessary to maintain adequate nutritional intake. Some children will be very resistant to taking nutritional supplements, or including recommended foods in their diets.

Additionally, a dietitian's role can be to provide parents (and other professionals) with quality information to help them weigh up the benefits of trying different nutritional interventions with the difficulties they are likely to face, and any potential harm, and to support them in attempting any dietary manipulations in a safe and objective way.

Implementing and monitoring dietary interventions

Parents can be advised to undertake any intervention in clear steps:

- *Baseline period:* follow their regular diet for an agreed specified time period while keeping a diary of behavioural and bowel habits.
- *Preparation:* start introducing the intervention gradually to get the child used to the new foods or supplements. Some families may decide against the intervention at this stage as they find it unrealistic to implement. Decide how long they are planning on trialling the intervention (2 weeks may be adequate, although many organisations recommend 3–12 months to see behavioural improvements).
- *Exclusion period:* strict implementation of therapeutic dietary intervention for an agreed specified time period. Behavioural and bowel monitoring as in the baseline period should continue. Ideally, no other new interventions should be started at this time. This is often not practical for parents as they are often keen to

carry out interventions as early as possible after diagnosis to maximise their effects.

- *Reintroduction:* regular diet to be reintroduced (or dietary supplements to be stopped) in a systematic way with behavioural and bowel habit monitoring as before. This step is key to help determine whether the diet has been effective, but parents who have seen improvements in their child are often very reluctant to take this step, and parents who have seen no or only subtle changes are often keen to continue as different organisations report that it can take up to a year to see improvements.

Keeping a detailed diary before, during and after any dietary intervention can help a family to be objective about any perceived outcomes, and help them to convince any sceptical professionals of any improvements they have seen. Details they might like to record:

- Intervention – what is being avoided/introduced/challenged
- Factors that might affect the intervention (e.g. illness, any items taken contrary to diet, change in routine, medications taken)
- Objective observations:
  Bowel symptoms: any bloating or wind, number of times bowels opened and form of stool
  Sleeping: number of time woken during night and for how long
  Challenging behaviour: self-injury, aggressiveness to other people, handling of urine or faeces, masturbation
- Less objective observations:
  Social interaction: seeking aloneness, ignoring people, eye contact, effort to communicate verbally or non-verbally, use of facial expressions and gestures, use of repetitive sounds
  Other ASD characteristics: inappropriately relating to inanimate objects, ritual use of objects, resisting change, stereotypical movements, restlessness, signs of anxiety, moodiness, abnormal attention, bizarre responses to stimuli

Dietary manipulations

Exclusion of gluten and casein

The most popular and best known dietary intervention for ASD is the use of a gluten and casein free diet (GFCF). Some organisations advise to cut both out at once, others to try one at a time. Avoidance usually includes oats as well as the gluten containing grains, and some families will not use wheat derived gluten free foods as they feel the traces of gluten may cause a toxic reaction. All mammalian milk and products are avoided. ASD is not an indicated use of gluten free prescribable products and therefore the cost of this diet is completely borne by the family, although some GPs will prescribe products at their discretion.

One proposed mechanism of action of this therapeutic restriction is 'the opioid theory' – that poorly digested casein and gluten provide 'opioid like' peptides that are absorbed into the blood stream through an abnormally permeable or 'leaky' gut. These peptides then cross the blood–brain barrier, where they interfere with various neurological processes [39]. In theory, the 'leaky' gut is caused by yeast overgrowth, or enzyme deficiency in the gut leading to inadequate breakdown of casein and gluten into these abnormal peptides. This is seen as distinct from an allergic or intolerance reaction.

Studies have demonstrated improvements in communication and cognitive function, with regression on dietary challenge [38,40]. The only paper to meet the inclusion criteria of a Cochrane review is a randomised control study which found a significant reduction in 'autistic traits' in the diet group compared to controls [41]. The Cochrane review found insufficient evidence to recommend GFCF diets in the treatment of ASD, but acknowledged that it is an important area of future investigation.

The professional consensus statement of a national group of dietitians working with children and adults with ASD, Dietitians' Autistic Spectrum Interest Group (DASIG) [42], recommends that gluten and casein free diets should not be recommended as a general treatment for ASD, because of the current lack of well-constructed, adequately powered, randomly controlled research, in line with the professional code of conduct. However, it is recommended that a dietitian should provide support for those who wish to embark on a dietary trial, as part of a multidisciplinary team.

Exclusion of phenolic compounds and salicylates

Linked to the findings of a small sample of children with ASD having impaired sulphation capacity

[14], some organisations advocate the avoidance of foods high in compounds broken down by sulphur dependent enzymes, as their consumption may inhibit the body's usual sulphation detoxification pathways [43], and lead to raised levels of neurotransmitters such as serotonin.

Foods that are often excluded are cheese, chocolate, tomatoes, oranges, bananas, yeast extract, some food colourings and foods high in salicylates. Salicylates are found naturally in fruit and vegetables and levels vary according to varieties and growing conditions. Children following a low salicylate diet are often avoiding a wide variety of fruits and vegetables. Lists of those foods to avoid are often obtained from the organisations that advocate their use.

Exclusion of various food additives

There has been little good quality research on the affect of food additives on people with ASD, although the avoidance of particular substances is very common. A trial exclusion of any or all of aspartame, monosodium glutamate, artificial food colours and benzoate preservatives is a low risk, manageable form of diet therapy that can often be carried out before considering more complex special diets.

Aspartame
Published papers have linked the intake of the artificial sweetener aspartame with worsening of depression [44], altered brain activity in people with epilepsy [45] and migraine [46–48]. There is a significant amount of (scientifically unsubstantiated) information on the Internet claiming aspartame to be highly toxic.

Monosodium glutamate (MSG, E621)
One paper links the intake of the flavour enhancer monosodium glutamate (MSG) with migraine [49].

Artificial colours and benzoates
A double blind, placebo controlled trial of 400 healthy pre-school children found an increase in hyperactive behaviour when given a drink of sunset yellow (E110), tartrazine (E102), carmoisine (E122), ponceau 4R (E124) and sodium benzoate (E211) compared with placebo [50]. A meta-analysis of 15 double blind, placebo controlled, cross-over trials reported that removing artificial food colours is

30–50% as effective in improving ADHD symptoms as stimulant medication, without side effects [51].

Nitrates and nitrites (E249–E252)
There are no published papers linking these preservatives with ASD or its common co-morbidities.

Yeast free diet with antifungal treatment

It has been proposed that yeast proliferation in the gut following antibiotic use causes 'leaky gut syndrome', behavioural and allergic reactions and a greater susceptibility to food allergies [52]. Antifungal treatment in the form of metronidazole, vancomycin or grapefruit seed extract is recommended, followed by 'dietary control of yeast overgrowth', i.e. elimination of natural and refined sugars (including all fruit for a month), with the simultaneous use of antifungals and vitamin B$_6$ and magnesium supplementation. A 'die-off reaction' may occur in the first 3–7 days after antifungal treatment commences and it is suggested that this reaction is a result of the release of toxins from *Clostridia* and can include heart palpitations, fever and extreme tiredness.

In the same publication, a more restrictive regimen of anti-yeast therapy, nystatin plus a 2–4 stage dietary intervention, is recommended:

1 Elimination of barley malt, vinegar, chocolate, pickled foods, alcohol, aged cheese, soy sauce, Worcestershire sauce, cottonseed oil, nuts, apples, grapes, coffee, processed meats for 4–6 weeks
2 In addition, for 4–6 weeks elimination of goods baked with yeast, corn and rye, vanilla extract, dried fruit, fruit juice, MSG, aspartame, maple syrup, bananas, all meat and fish except veal, spices, mushrooms, soda drinks, various cooking oils, sugar, margarine, buttermilk
3 If deemed necessary, for 4–6 weeks additional elimination of gluten and casein
4 In severe cases, for 4–6 weeks additional elimination of most fruits, onions, all meat except veal, and canned goods

Other dietary manipulations

Ketogenic diet
A well-designed pilot study of 30 children with

ASD found improvements on the Childhood Autism Rating Scale in all 18 who tolerated the diet. For 10 children, the improvement was average to significant [53]. Ketogenic diets are described in Chapter 16.

Feingold diet
This involves the elimination of artificial colourings, flavourings and preservatives, aspartame and salicylates [54].

Rotation diets
This involves the avoidance of eating the same food again within a number of days (e.g. 3–5 days). There is no evidence for its use in ASD.

The body ecology diet
This advocates eating a diet of foods that are kept as close to their natural state as possible, with gluten excluded, and a number of special foods that are purported to re-establish the intestinal flora and heal the body, such as fermented coconut juice and raw butter [55].

The Specific Carbohydrate Diet™
This advocates the elimination of grains, sucrose and lactose with the theory that this will modify intestinal bacteria growth [56]. There is no published evidence for its use.

Therapeutic supplementation

Some organisations suggest that people with ASD need particularly high 'therapeutic' doses of individual vitamins and minerals because of metabolic and biochemical abnormalities. Sometimes the suggested doses exceed the safe upper limit for adults and little is known about long term high doses in children [57].

Vitamin B_6 and magnesium

Several investigators have reported significant improvement in behaviour following doses of 15–30 mg/kg/day pyridoxine (700–1000 mg/day), and 10–15 mg/kg/day magnesium (380–500 mg/day) [58,59]. A Cochrane review concluded that these studies were inadequately designed and too small to make any recommendations [60]. The usual doses used in these reports exceed the safe upper limit for vitamin B_6 (10 mg/day). Long term doses >200 mg/day have been associated with neuropathy, low serum folic acid, night restlessness and rashes, and >2000 mg/day can cause nerve damage. In most, but not all reported cases, the damage has been reversible [61]. Advocates of vitamin B_6 therapy purport that the side effects of neuropathy are rare and the concurrent use of magnesium could be protective against these. They hypothesise that the therapeutic effect of B_6 and magnesium is caused by an abnormal metabolism or a deficiency and advise that if no improvements are seen within 4 weeks, therapy is unlikely to help and should be stopped. It would be particularly ill advised to give high doses of vitamin B_6 to children who are unable to communicate feelings of neuropathy.

Vitamin C

Researchers in the USA reported improvement in sensory motor symptoms in a double blind, placebo controlled trial of 20 children with autism given high doses of ascorbic acid (8 g/70 kg body weight/day) [62]. The researchers proposed a dopaminergic mechanism of action.

Vitamin A

Two case studies report improvements of social skills after treatment with natural *cis* forms of vitamin A in cod liver oil [63]. The paper hypothesises that autism 'may be a disorder linked to the disruption of the G-alpha protein, affecting retinoid receptors in the brain'. At a cost this protocol can be obtained from the website for use by paediatricians [64].

Dimethylglycine

Dimethylglycine (DMG), a non-essential amino acid, is anecdotally reported to improve behaviour and communication in some children and adults with ASD in doses of 60–600 mg/day. A double blind, placebo controlled, cross-over pilot study of low dose DMG and placebo in eight autistic males did not find any significant differences [65]. DMG is sometimes known as pangamic acid, calcium pangamate or 'vitamin B_{15}'.

Multivitamin and mineral supplementation

'Moderate dose' of vitamins and minerals was associated with significant improvements in children with ASD compared to control subjects given placebo [66]. However, the study used a supplement with doses of B_6 and zinc that were well above the RNI.

Fish oil and other fat supplements

Fish oil supplements are widely used by families affected by ASD. Anecdotal accounts of positive impact are common, but there is only one published case study describing the positive impact of fish oil on a patient with ASD [67], and there are no randomised controlled trials. Some fairly well-designed studies suggest a positive effect in other neurodevelopmental disorders [68,69], mood disorders [70,71] and learning difficulties [69]. A recent trial showed that an EPA rich fish oil supplement (of approximately 550 mg EPA/day for 8-year-olds) produced highly significant improvements in behaviour, reading and spelling in a group of children with developmental co-ordination disorder (DCD) compared with placebo [72]. Few side effects were experienced at this dose. The Department of Health recommendation of two portions of fish a week equates to an intake of <200 mg/day EPA.

It is hypothesised that omega-3 rich fish oil supplements improve the composition and function of the phospholipid bilayer in cell membranes and have a subsequent effect on nerve transmission and brain function [73]. Because of this theory, families are advised to wait 3 months to see any improvements in behaviour or function as oils take time to build up in the fatty tissue. The cost of fish oil supplements can be high and they are not prescribable for ASD.

Some organisations advocate the use of hemp oil rubbed into the skin as a therapeutic option, but there is no evidence for this.

Probiotics

Probiotics are commonly taken as yogurt drinks or powders. There is no research to indicate they have any therapeutic effect in ASD.

Enzymes

Numerous digestive enzyme products aimed at ASD are available. There is no evidence that they have a useful role.

Intravenous secretin

Secretin is a peptide secreted by duodenal cells in response to lowered pH on stomach emptying. It stimulates secretion of water and bicarbonate from the pancreas and there have been reports of improved language and behaviour in children with ASD after intravenous secretin. A Cochrane review found insufficient evidence for this to be used as an intervention and advised against its use [74].

Summary of evidence for the use of therapeutic diets

Few dietary interventions used in ASD stand up to the scrutiny of reviews such as the Cochrane Reviews. ASD is a label for a collection of behaviours and may incorporate subgroups with shared biochemical and physiological problems. It seems reasonable that there might be particular subgroups that would be more likely to respond to a particular intervention (e.g. those with bowel problems or those with the 'regressive subtype'). Outlining clear outcomes of positive interventions for ASD is problematic as, although some improvements may be objective (such as bowel symptoms), behavioural changes are more subjective.

In conclusion, none of these dietary interventions are based on adequate evidence for a dietitian to recommend their use with confidence. However, it is clear that improvements are seen in some children undertaking some of these interventions, and so supervised trials may be advised in some cases (e.g. in those whose symptoms have been linked to particular dietary components). Providing professional support and advice as part of a multidisciplinary team may help to ensure that a family wishing to pursue dietary interventions will do this with a logical approach that ensures that the effect of any intervention is clear and that the child is not adversely affected nutritionally.

Table 26.5 qualitatively summarises the advantages and disadvantages of different interventions in ASD.

Table 26.5 Qualitative comparison of therapeutic diets in autistic spectrum disorders.

Intervention	Difficulty in following intervention	Supporting evidence	Negative impact on nutrition/health
Exclusion of gluten and casein	Moderate/high*	Some	Possible
Other exclusion diets	Moderate/high*	None	Possible
Other named diets	Moderate/high*	None	Possible
Individual vitamin and mineral supplementation	Low/high*	None/some for vitamin B_6	Possible side effects at high doses
Fish oil supplements	Low/high*	None/some for DCD	Unlikely
Probiotics	Low/high*	None	Unlikely
Enzymes	Low/high*	None	Unlikely

DCD, developmental co-ordination disorder.

* Ease of intervention is greatly decreased if child is resistant to changes in diet/resistant to taking supplements.

Acknowledgements

This chapter was written with the kind help of members of DASIG and numerous other colleagues experienced in working with children with ASD. A major contribution to the section on dietary interventions was drafted by David Rex.

References

1 Medical Research Council Review of Autism Research Epidemiology and Causes, 2001.

2 World Health Organization. *The ICD-10 Classification of Mental and Behavioural Disorders. Clinical Descriptors and Diagnostic Guidelines*, 10th edn, Geneva: WHO, 1992.

3 American Psychiatric Association. *Diagnostic and Statistical Manual of Mental Disorders*, 4th edn. Washington DC: American Psychiatric Association, 1994.

4 Rapin I Diagnosis and management of autism in: David TJ (ed.) *Recent advances in Paediatrics: No. 18*, London: Harcourt Publishers, 2000, pp. 121–34.

5 Black C, Kaye JA, Jick H Relation of childhood gastrointestinal disorders to autism: nested case–control study using data from the UK General Practice Research Database. *Br Med J*, 2002, **325** 419–21.

6 Horvath K, Papadimitriou JC, Rabsztyn A *et al.* Gastrointestinal abnormalities in children with autistic disorder. *J Pediatr*, 1999, **135** 559–63.

7 Afzal N, Murch S, Thirrupathy K, Berger L *et al.* Constipation with acquired megarectum in children with autism. *Pediatrics*, 2003, **112** 939–42.

8 Wakefield AJ, Ashwood P, Limb K *et al.* The significance of ileo-colonic lymphoid nodular hyperplasia in children with autistic spectrum disorder. *Eur J Gastroenterol Hepatol*, 2005, **17** 827–36.

9 D'Eufemia P, Celli M, Finocchiaro R *et al.* Abnormal intestinal permeability in children with autism. *Acta Paediatr*, 1996, **85** 1076–9.

10 Finegold SM, Molitoris D, Song Y *et al.* Gastrointestinal microflora studies in late-onset autism. *Clin Infect Dis*, 2002, **35** (Suppl 1) S6–S16.

11 Parracho HM, Bingham MO, Gibson GR *et al.* Differences between the gut microflora of children with autistic spectrum disorders and that of healthy children. *J Med Microbiol*, 2005, **54** 987–91.

12 White JF Intestinal pathophysiology in autism. *Exp Biol Med*, 2003, **228** 639–49.

13 Alberti A, Pirrone P, Elia M *et al.* Sulphation deficit in 'low functioning' autistic children: a pilot study. *Biol Psychol*, 1999, **46** 420–4.

14 Walsh W Metallothionein promotion therapy in autistic spectrum disorders. In: Rimland B (ed.) *DAN! (Defeat Autism Now!)* Spring conference practitioner training, San Diego, CA: Autism Research Institute, 2002.

15 Akhondzadeh S, Mohammadi-Reza M, Khademi M Zinc sulfate as an adjunct to methylphenidate for the treatment of attention deficit hyperactivity disorder in children: A double blind and randomized trial. *BMC Psychiatry*, 2004, **4** 9.

16 Wright B, Brzozowski AM, Calvert E *et al.* Is the presence of urinary indolyl-3-acryloylglycine associated with autism spectrum disorder? *Dev Med Child Neurol*, 2005, **47** 190–2.

17 Shattock P, Whiteley P The Sunderland Protocol: A logical sequencing of biomedical interventions for the treatment of autism and related disorders. http://osiris.sunderland.ac.uk/autism/durham2.htm Accessed February 2006.

18 Konofal E, Lecendreux M, Arnulf I, Mouren MC Iron deficiency in children with attention-deficit/hyperactivity disorder. *Arch Pediatr Adolesc Med*, 2004, **158** 1113–15.

19 Konofal E, Cortese S, Lecendreux M *et al*. Effectiveness of iron supplementation in a young child with attention-deficit/hyperactivity disorder. *Pediatrics*, 2005, **116** 732–4.

20 Strambi M, Longini M, Hayek J *et al*. Magnesium profile in autism. *Biol Trace Elem Res*, 2006, **109** 97–104.

21 Vancassel S, Durand G, Barthelemy C *et al*. Plasma fatty acid levels in autistic children. *Prostaglandins Leukot Essent Fatty Acids*, 2001, **65** 1–7.

22 Bell JG, MacKinlay EE, Dick JR *et al*. Essential fatty acids and phospholipase A2 in autistic spectrum disorders. *Prostoglandins Leukot Essent Fatty Acids*, 2004, **71** 201–4.

23 MacDonell LEF, Skinner FK, Ward PE *et al*. Increased levels of cytosolic phospholipase A2 in dyslexics. *Prostoglandins Leukot Essent Fatty Acids*, 2000, **63** 37–9.

24 Stevens LJ, Zentall SS, Deck JL *et al*. Essential fatty acid metabolism in boys with attention deficit hyperactivity disorder. *Am J Clin Nutr*, 1995, **62** 761–8.

25 Horrobin DF Fatty acid levels in the brains of schizophrenics and normal controls. *Biol Psychol*, 1991, **30** 795–805.

26 Aldred S, Moore KM, Fitzgerald M *et al*. Plasma amino acid levels in children with autism and their families. *J Autism Dev Disord* 2003, **33** 93–7.

27 James SJ, Cutler P, Melnyk S *et al*. Metabolic biomarkers of increased oxidative stress and impaired methylation capacity in children with autism. *Am J Clin Nutr*, 2004, **80** 1611–17.

28 Adams JB, George F, Audhya T Abnormally high plasma levels of vitamin b(6) in children with autism not taking supplements compared to controls not taking supplements. *J Altern Complement Med*, 2006, **12** 59–63.

29 Le Couteur A National Autism Plan for Children (2003). The National Autistic Society for NIASA in collaboration with The Royal College of Psychiatrists (RCPsych), The Royal College of Paediatrics and Child Health (RCPCH) and the All Party Parliamentary Group on Autism (APPGA). http://www.nas.org.uk/content/1/c4/34/54/NIASARep.pdf Accessed February 2006.

30 National Autistic Society. Patients with autistic spectrum disorders – information for health professionals http://www.nas.org.uk/nas/jsp/polopoly.jsp?d=306&a=8521 Accessed February 2006.

31 Schreck KA, Williams K, Smith A comparison of eating behaviors between children with and without autism. *J Autism Dev Disord*, 2004, **34** 433–8.

32 DeMeyer MK *Parents and Children With Autism*, New York: Wiley,

33 Field D, Garland M, Williams K Correlates of specific childhood feeding problems *J Paediatr Child Health*, 2003, **39** 299–304.

34 Cornish E A balanced approach towards healthy eating in autism. *J Hum Nutr Diet*, 1998, **11** 501–9.

35 Curtin C, Bandini LG, Perrin EC *et al*. Prevalence of overweight in children and adolescents with attention deficit hyperactivity disorder and autism spectrum disorders: a chart review. *BMC Pediatrics*, 2005, **5** 48.

36 Gillis L Use of an interactive game to increase food acceptance – a pilot study. *Child Care Health Dev*, 2003, **29** 373–5.

37 Witwer A, Lecavalier LJ Treatment incidence and patterns in children and adolescents with autism spectrum disorders. *Child Adolesc Psychopharmacol*, 2005, **15** 671–81.

38 Lucarelli S, Frediani T, Zingoni AM *et al*. Food allergy and infantile autism. *Panminerva Med*, 1995, **37** 137–41.

39 Reichelt KL, Knivsberg AM, Lind G *et al*. The probable etiology and possible treatment of childhood autism. *Brain Dysfunction*, 991, **4** 308–19.

40 Whiteley P, Rodgers J, Savery D *et al*. A gluten free diet as an intervention for autism and associated spectrum disorders: preliminary findings. *Autism*, 1999, **3** 45–65.

41 Knivsberg AM, Reichelt KL, Nodland M *et al*. A randomised, controlled study of dietary intervention in autistic syndromes. *Nutr Neurosci*, 2002, **5** 251–61.

42 Isherwood E, Thomas K Professional consensus statement on the dietary management of autism spectrum disorder. members area www.bda.uk.com Accessed September 2002.

43 Harris RM, Waring RH Dietary modulation of human platelet phenolsulphotransferase activity. *Xenobiotica*, 1996, **26** 1241–7.

44 Walton RG, Hudak R, Green-Waite RJ Adverse reactions to aspartame: double-blind challenge in patients from a vulnerable population. *Biol Psychol*, 1993, **34** 13–17.

45 Camfield PR, Camfield CS, Dooley JM *et al*. Aspartame exacerbates EEG spike-wave discharge in children with generalized absence epilepsy: A double blind controlled study. *Neurology*, 1992, **42** 1000–3.

46 Van den Eeden SK, Koepsell TD, Longstreth WT Jr *et al*. Aspartame ingestion and headaches: A randomized cross-over trial. *Neurology*, 1994, **44** 1787–93.

47 Lipton RB, Newman LC, Cohen JS *et al*. Aspartame as a dietary trigger of headache. *Headache*, 1989, **29** 90–2.

48 Koehler SM, Glaros A The effect of aspartame on migraine headache. *Headache*, 1998, **28** 10–14.

49 Yang WH, Drouin MA, Herbert M *et al*. The monosodium glutamate symptom complex: Assessment

in a double blind, placebo-controlled, randomized study. *J Allergy Clin Immunol*, 1997, **99** 757–62.

50 Bateman B, Warner JO, Hutchinson E *et al.* The effects of a double blind, placebo controlled, artificial food colourings and benzoate preservative challenge on hyperactivity in a general population sample of pre-school children. *Arch Dis Child*, 2004, **89** 506–11.

51 Schab DW, Trinh NH Do artificial food colors promote hyperactivity in children with hyperactive syndromes? A meta-analysis of double-blind placebo-controlled trials. *J Dev Behav Pediatr*, 2004, **25** 423–34.

52 Shaw W *Biological Treatments for Autism and PDD: What's Going On? What Can You Do about It?* USA, Great Plains Laboratory, 1998.

53 Evangeliou A, Vlachonikolis I, Mihailidou H *et al.* Application of a ketogenic diet in children with autistic behavior: pilot study. *J Child Neurol*, 2003, **18** 113–18.

54 www.feingold.org Accessed February 2003.

55 www.bodyecologydiet.com Accessed February 2003.

56 www.breakingtheviciouscycle.info Accessed February 2003.

57 Food Standards Agency *Expert Group on Vitamins and Minerals. Safe Upper Levels for Vitamins and Minerals.* London: Crown Copyright, 2003.

58 Rimland B, Callaway E, Dreyfus P The effect of high doses of vitamin B6 on autistic children: A double-blind crossover study. *Am J Psychiatry*, 1978, **135** 472–5.

59 Findling RL, Maxwell K, Scotese-Wojtila L *et al.* High-dose pyridoxine and magnesium administration in children with autistic disorder: An absence of salutary effects in a double-blind, placebo-controlled study. *J Autism Dev Disord*, 1997, **27** 467–78.

60 Nye C, Brice A Combined vitamin B6-magnesium treatment in autism spectrum disorder. *Cochrane Database Syst Rev* 2005, **19** 4.

61 Food Standards Agency Expert Group on Vitamins and Minerals 2003 Risk assessment vitamin B6 (pyridoxine). http://www.food.gov.uk/multimedia/pdfs/evm_b6.pdf Accessed February 2006.

62 Dolske MC, Spollen J, McKay S *et al.* A preliminary trial of ascorbic acid as supplemental therapy for autism. *Prog Neuropsychopharmacol Biol Psychiatry*, 1993, **17** 765–74.

63 Megson MN Is autism a G-alpha protein defect reversible with natural vitamin A? *Med Hypotheses*, 2000, **54** 979–83.

64 www.megson.com Accessed February 2003.

65 Bolman WM, Richmond JA A double-blind, placebo-controlled, crossover pilot trial of low dose dimethylglycine in patients with autistic disorder. *J Autism Dev Disord*, 1999, **29** 191–4.

66 Adams J, Holloway C Pilot Study of a moderate dose multivitamin/mineral supplement for children with autistic spectrum disorder. *J Altern Complement Med*, 2004, **10** 1033–9.

67 Hollander E, Johnson SM Evidence that eicosapentaenoic acid is effective in treating autism. *J Clin Psychol*, 2003, **64** 7.

68 Richardson AJ, Montgomery P The Oxford–Durham Study: a randomized controlled trial of dietary supplementation with fatty acids in children with developmental co-ordination disorder. *Paediatr*, 2005, **115** 1360–6.

69 Richardson AJ, Puri BK A Randomized double-blind, placebo-controlled study of the effects of supplementation with highly unsaturated fatty acids on ADHD-related symptoms in children with specific learning difficulties. *Prog Neuropsychopharmacol Biol Psychiatry*, 2002, **26** 233–9.

70 Su KP, Huang SY, Chiu CC, Shen WW Omega 3 fatty acids in major depressive disorder. A preliminary double blind, placebo controlled trial. *Eur J Neuropsychopharmacol*, 2003, **13** 267–71.

71 Peet M, Brind J, Ramchand CN, Shah S, Vankar GK Two double blind placebo controlled pilot studies of eicosapentaenoic acid in the treatment of schizophrenia. *Schizophrenia Res*, 2001, **49** 243–51.

72 Richardson AJ, Montgomery P The Oxford-Durham Study: a randomized controlled trial of dietary supplementation with fatty acids in children with developmental co-ordination disorder. *Pediatrics*, 2005, **115** 1360–6.

73 Richardson AJ, Ross MA Fatty acid metabolism in neurodevelopmental disorder: a new perspective on associations between attention-deficit/hyperactivity disorder, dyslexia, dyspraxia and the autistic spectrum. *Prostoglandins Leukot Essent Fatty Acids*, 2000, **63** 1–9.

74 Williams KW, Wray JJ, Wheeler DM Intravenous secretin for autism spectrum disorder. *Cochrane Database Syst Rev*, 2005, **20** 3.

Further reading

Campbell-McBride N *Gut and Psychology Syndrome: Natural Treatment for Autism, ADD/ADHD, Dyslexia, Dyspraxia, Depression, Schizophrenia.* Medinform Publishing, 2004.

Early Support Programme Leaflet *Information for parents: Autistic spectrum disorders (ASDs)* accessed from http://www.earlysupport.org.uk Feb 2006.

Ernsperger L, Stegen-Hansen T *Just Take A Bite: Easy, Effective Answers to Food Aversions and Eating Challenges!* Arlington, TX: Future Horizons, USA, 2004.

Gray C *The New Social Story 2000.* Arlington, TX: Future Horizons, USA, 2004.

Le Breton M *Diet Intervention and Autism: Implementing the Gluten Free and Casein Free Diet for Autistic Children and Adults: A Practical Guide for Parents*. London: Jessica Kingsley Publishers, 2001.

Legge B *Can't eat, won't eat: dietary difficulties and ASDs*. London: Jessica Kingsley Publishers, 2001.

Shaw W *Biological Treatments for Autism and PDD: What's Going On? What Can You Do about It?* Great Plains Laboratory, USA, 1998.

Useful addresses

Professional networking and resources

Dietitians' Autistic Spectrum Interest Group (DASIG)
(formerly ASIG) linked with BDA Paediatric Group and BDA Mental Health Group
e-mail: nicky.calow@lnds.nhs.uk or dasiglistserv-owner@yahoogroups.com

National Autistic Society
www.nas.org.uk

Picture symbols
www.dotolearn.com/

Social stories
www.thegraycenter.org/Social_Stories.htm

Sensory Processing Disorder
www.out-of-sync-child.com and www.sinetwork.org

Resources advocating dietary interventions

University of Sunderland Autism Research Unit
http://osiris.sunderland.ac.uk/autism

Autism Induced Allergy (AiA)
www.autismmedical.com

Autism Network for Dietary Intervention (ANDI)
www.autismndi.com

Autism Research Institute
www.autism.com/ari/

Autism Unravelled
www.autism-unravelled.org

Gluten Free Casein Free (GFCF) Diet Support Group
www.gfcfdiet.com

Part 4

Community Nutrition

27 Healthy Eating

Judy More

Introduction

Infants, toddlers and school children need to satisfy their energy and nutrient requirements for normal growth, development and activity through eating a varied and balanced diet. The UK Department of Health's Dietary Reference Values [1] can be used as a guideline for the healthy child (see Table 1.9). In addition, the Food Standards Agency (FSA) have set maximum guideline daily amounts of sodium and salt consumption for babies and children [2] in order to tackle the longer term problems of hypertension and cardiovascular disease found in the adult population (Table 27.1).

The Government's White Paper *Choosing Health* [3] states that 'Nutrition is a key component of a healthy start in life' and emphasises healthy eating through a number of initiatives:

- Promoting breast feeding
- Broadening the nutritional support given to low income families through the Sure Start and Healthy Start schemes
- Widening children's exposure to fruit and vegetables through the School Fruit and Vegetable Scheme
- Introducing healthy eating as a key component in the National Healthy Schools Programme
- Revising school meals standards and introducing standards to cover provision of food across the school day, including vending machines and tuck shops

Infants

Breast feeding

Breast feeding is the ideal way to feed infants and is considered nutritionally adequate up until 6 months for healthy term babies [4].

Colostrum is the breast milk produced by the mother in the first few days after birth and is particularly high in proteins, especially immunoglobulins which confer maternal immunity against infection. It is low in fat and energy and newborn babies generally take small volumes infrequently

Table 27.1 Guideline daily amounts of sodium and salt.

Age	Reference Nutrient Intake [1] Sodium (g/day)	Daily recommended maximum intake [2] Sodium (g/day)	Salt (g/day)
0–12 months	0.21–0.35	0.4	1
1–3 years	0.5	0.8	2
4–6 years	0.7	1.2	3
7–10 years	1.2	2.0	5
11+ years	1.6	2.4	6

[5]. The composition changes from about day 3 postpartum to transitional milk which usually coincides with the infant demanding feeds more frequently. Mature breast milk is produced about 3 weeks postpartum.

The energy composition of breast milk is estimated to be 69 kcal/100 mL (289 kJ/100 mL) [6] but this varies throughout the feed: fore milk is low in fat and higher in lactose and satisfies the baby's thirst; hind milk is produced towards the end of a feed and is higher in fat, is more energy dense and satisfies the baby's hunger. Provided there is no restriction on how much a baby can breast feed (i.e. demand feeding is practised), no extra water is needed in addition to breast milk, even in very hot weather, as the baby will simply feed more frequently to obtain more fluid when thirsty.

Mothers should be encouraged to let their baby drink as much as desired from the first breast before offering the second breast; this way the baby gets its full quota of energy from both fore and hind milk. Less milk (or none at all) may be taken from the second breast offered. At each feed the first breast offered should be alternated so that both breasts receive equal stimulation and drainage. Babies may need to be woken by cuddling them upright and changing their nappy after finishing at the first breast before being offered the second breast.

Breast feeding offers several advantages over infant formula feeding:

- Less infections particularly those of the gastrointestinal tract, respiratory system and urinary tract [7–12]
- Improved cardiovascular health in the long term [8,13]
- Improved cognitive development [13,14]
- Lower risk of atopy in those with a family history [13]
- Potential protection against insulin dependent diabetes [15]
- Potentially improved bone development [16]
- Potentially reduced risk of obesity later in life [13,17]

Formula feeding

Up until 12 months of age the only nutritionally adequate alternatives to breast milk are infant

Table 27.2 Energy densities of breast milk.

per 100 g	Hosoi *et al.* 2005 [19]	McCance and Widdowson 1991 [22]
Colostrum	57 kcal (238 kJ)	56 kcal (236 kJ)
Transitional milk	63 kcal (263 kJ)	67 kcal (281 kJ)
Mature breast milk	64 kcal (268 kJ)	69 kcal (289 kJ)

formulas which comply with government regulations based on European Union (EU) Directives. These Directives are based on expert advice from the EC Scientific Committee for Food and the European Society of Paediatric Gastroenterology, Hepatology and Nutrition (ESPGHAN), and implement the 1981 World Health Organization International Code of Marketing of Breast Milk Substitutes as appropriate to the EU. Current regulations are available from the Infant and Dietetic Food Association (IDFA) website [18].

Recent research suggests that infant formulas may contain too high an energy level for normal growth. The energy content of breast milk may be lower than current accepted estimations and the higher energy density of infant formulas may account for the different growth patterns in breast fed compared with formula fed infants (Table 27.2) [6,19–22].

The infant formulas available in the UK are listed in Table 1.11. Those with a high whey : casein ratio (60 : 40) are the most similar in nutrient compostion to breast milk. Those with a higher casein content and lower whey : casein ratio (20 : 80) are marketed as more suitable for hungry babies; this is probably because the curd formed by the higher casein level slows gastric emptying. Formula fed babies should be demand fed just as breast fed babies are and offered adequate feed to satisfy their hunger and growth needs. The hungry whey dominant formula fed baby should be offered a larger volume of feed rather than changing them to a casein dominant formula.

Making up infant formula from powder

Tap water or bottled waters which comply with the EU standards for tap water [23] may be used for making up infant formula. Up to 200 mg/L sodium is allowed in tap water which will add 0.9 mmol sodium/100 mL feed. This extra sodium will not matter for most infants and powdered feeds on sale in the UK will still comply with the EU Directive's acceptable sodium content if made up with water containing this level of sodium. Bottled mineral waters may contain excess amounts of sodium or other electrolytes and should not be used for making up infant formula. Just as tap water must be boiled before being used for reconstituting formula feeds so must any bottled water. Carbonated fizzy water is not suitable for making up formula feeds.

Infant formula powder is not sterile and may contain microorganisms such as salmonella and *Enterobacter sakazakii* [24]. Neonates, particularly those who are preterm, of low birthweight or immunocompromised, are most at risk. To minimise the risk of gastroenteritis from these bacteria:

- Feeds should be made up using boiled water >70°C (that has been left to cool in the kettle for no more than half an hour).
- This water is measured into a sterile bottle and the appropriate number of scoops of powder are then added (1 level unpacked scoop of powder per 30 mL/1 fluid ounce water). The bottle should then be sealed with a sterilised cap and shaken to mix the powder; the feed must then be cooled (by holding the sealed bottle under cold running water) and the temperature tested before giving to the baby.
- Bottles should be made up fresh for each feed.
- Any left over milk at the end of the feed should be thrown away.
- Parents who require a feed for later are advised to use liquid ready-to-feed formula which is sterile. Alternatively they could keep water they have just boiled in a sealed flask and make up fresh formula milk when needed [24].

If parents choose to ignore this advice and make up feeds for up to 24 hours in advance, the bottles of formula should be cooled quickly and stored in a refrigerator at <5°C. These feeds can be warmed just before use by standing the bottle in a container of hot water. Microwave ovens must not be used as the milk is not uniformly heated and hot spots in the milk could burn the baby's mouth [25].

Feeds should be made up using boiled water and sterile bottles or cups until 1 year of age because of the potential risk of bacterial growth. This risk is enhanced if bottles, teats and cups are not cleaned properly.

In the case where a baby is prescribed a multi-ingredient feed the dietitian may deem it safer, from the point of view of accuracy of feed reconstitution, for the parent to make up 24 hours' worth of feeds at one time. It is incumbent on the dietitian to give advice about scrupulous hygiene, rapid cooling and safe storage at <5°C if feeds are to be made up in advance. Any remaining milk not completed after 1 hour of feeding should be discarded.

Follow-on milks

The infant formula companies in the UK and Republic of Ireland, as IDFA members, have voluntarily agreed that follow-on formulas should only be marketed as suitable for infants over the age of 6 months. This policy is more restrictive than the law requires as European legislation permits follow-on formulas to be marketed as suitable from 4 months and this occurs in other European countries. These milks (see Table 1.12) have higher levels of protein, minerals and some vitamins than the infant formulas designed for feeding from birth. Some mothers choose to use them but it is not generally necessary. They can be used to give additional nutrients to children who do not eat solids very well and they have been shown to reduce iron deficiency anaemia in inner city deprived populations [26–30].

Weaning

An infant feeding survey in the UK in 2000 showed that babies are weaned anytime from before 6 weeks up to 9 months of age [31] despite recommendations of starting between 4 and 6 months [25].

In 2001, the World Health Organization recommended exclusive breast feeding until 6 months (26 weeks) of age as it offers protection against gastroenteritis, and breast milk is considered nutritionally adequate for most babies until 6 months [32]. The Department of Health has recommended since 2003 that exclusive breast feeding (or formula feeding) is ideal until 6 months but should parents choose to introduce solids earlier than this then weaning should not commence before 17 weeks (4 calendar months) [24].

Table 27.3 Developmental stages of weaning.

Stage	Age guide	Skills to learn	New food textures to introduce
1	6 months, but not before 4 months (17 weeks) if parents choose to begin earlier	Taking food from a spoon Moving food from the front of the mouth to the back for swallowing Managing thicker purées and mashed food	Smooth purées Mashed foods
2	6–9 months	Moving lumps around the mouth Chewing lumps Self-feeding using hands and fingers Sipping from a cup	Mashed food with soft lumps Soft finger foods Liquids in a lidded beaker or cup
3	9–12 months	Chewing minced and chopped food Self-feeding attempts with a spoon	Hard finger foods Minced and chopped family foods

It is generally accepted that a better indication as to when babies are ready to be weaned is when they reach certain developmental stages:

- Able to sit up and support their head, which reduces the risk of choking
- Taking an interest in other people eating
- Mouthing toys [33]

During the weaning period infants learn new skills and will progress through the developmental stages of weaning as they are given the opportunities to learn. Some progress faster than others. Table 27.3 gives a rough guide.

Weaning usually begins with 1–2 teaspoons of a smooth purée or mashed food being offered at just one meal a day. The addition of solids to bottles of milk is not advised in the UK [33]; however, this is accepted practice in other European countries.

As the baby learns to manage solid food and begins to take a larger quantity, a second meal and then a third meal can be introduced. Once three meals are established a variety of foods from the four main food groups should be included [25]. Table 27.4 shows the food groups and recommended servings. Meals should be nutrient dense and contain iron rich foods. Foods high in fat and sugar do not have a place in the early weaning diet. It is recommended that [33]:

- Salt and sugar should not be added to baby foods
- If weaning begins before 6 months foods containing gluten, eggs, fish and shellfish should be avoided until after 6 months because of the potential for allergic reactions to these foods

- Liver should be avoided before 6 months because of its high vitamin A content
- Honey should not be given before 12 months as there is a small risk of infant botulism
- Peanuts should not be given to infants (or any child under 3 years) with a family history of atopy

Cow's milk is the most common potential food allergen in infancy. While fresh cow's milk should not be used in weaning solids before 6 months of age, milk may be an ingredient of commercial weaning foods used before 6 months of age (and is, of course, the source of protein in normal infant formulas); the heat treatment during the manufacturing processes reduces the allergic potential of the cow's milk protein.

Early weaning meals should finish with the usual milk feed. Milk based desserts can be given to replace the feed at one and then two meals as the baby takes more food and two courses are offered. The amount of breast milk or infant formula consumed by the infant will gradually reduce to about 500–600 mL/day towards the end of the first year.

The majority of infants will try a wide variety of tastes and textures and they learn to like the foods they are offered [34]. The frequency with which they are offered a food, rather than the amount they eat, determines how quickly they will learn to like it. By the end of their first year infants should be eating family foods and the more variety they have been offered by around 12 months the wider the range of foods they will be familiar with and accept before food neophobia begins in their second year (see below).

Table 27.4 Food groups and recommended servings. Based on recommendations of the Paediatric Group of the British Dietetic Association.

Food Group	Foods included	Main nutrients supplied	Recommendations		
			Infants 6–12 months [25]	Toddlers and preschoolers 1–4 years	School children 5–18 years
1. Bread, other cereals and potatoes	Bread, chapatti, breakfast cereals, rice, couscous, pasta, millet, potatoes, yam, and foods made with flour such as pizza bases, buns, pancakes	Carbohydrate B vitamins Fibre Some iron, zinc and calcium	3–4 servings a day	Serve at each meal and some snacks	Serve at each meal and some snacks
2. Fruit and vegetables	Fresh, frozen, tinned and dried fruits and vegetables. Also pure fruit juices	Vitamin C Phytochemicals Fibre Carotenes	3–4 servings a day	Offer at each meal and aim for about 5 small servings a day	Aim for 5 servings a day
3. Milk, cheese and yoghurt	Breast milk, infant formulas, follow-on milks, cow's milk, yoghurts, cheese, calcium enriched soya milks, tofu	Calcium Protein Iodine Riboflavin	Demand feeds of breast milk or infant formula as main drink (about 500–600 mL/day). Some yoghurt and cheese	3 servings a day 1 serving is • 120 mL milk in a beaker or cup • 1 pot yoghurt or fromage frais • a serving of cheese in an sandwich or on a pizza • a milk based pudding • a serving of tofu	3 servings a day 1 serving is • 1 glass milk 150–250 mL • 1 pot yoghurt or fromage frais • a serving of cheese in an sandwich or on a pizza • a milk based pudding • a serving of tofu
4. Meat, fish and alternatives	Meat, fish, eggs, pulses, dhal, nuts, seeds	Iron Protein Zinc Magnesium B vitamins Vitamin A Omega 3 long chain fatty acids: EPA and DHA from oily fish	1–2 servings a day 2–3 for vegetarians	2 servings a day 3 for vegetarians Fish should be offered twice per week and oily fish at least once per week*	2 servings a day 3 for vegetarians Fish should be offered twice per week and oily fish at least once per week*
5. Foods high in fat and/or sugar	Cream, butter, margarines, cooking and salad oils, mayonnaise, chocolate, confectionery, jam, syrup, crisps and other high fat savoury snacks	Some foods provide: Vitamins D & E, omega 3 fatty acids (α-linolenic acid)		In addition to but not instead of the other food groups	In addition to but not instead of the other food groups
Fluid	Drinks	Water Fluoride in areas with fluoridated tap water	Water or well diluted fruit juice with meals, and milk feeds	6–8 drinks per day and more in hot weather or after extra physical activity	6–8 drinks per day and more in hot weather or after extra physical activity
Vitamin supplements			Vitamins A & D for breast fed infants, and formula fed infants drinking less than 500 mL formula milk/day	Vitamins A & D up to 5 years	Folic acid for adolescent girls who could become pregnant. Vitamin D for pregnant teenagers

Serving sizes of food and drinks will increase as children grow. Examples of average portion sizes for different ages are shown in Table 2.1.
* see p. 535.

Parents should allow their baby to decide on the quantity of food they eat and should not coerce them to eat more when they have indicated they have had enough. Force feeding is counterproductive to developing a positive attitude to food.

Commercial weaning foods

The energy density and composition of homemade weaning foods varies widely [35]. By contrast, commercial weaning foods must conform to EU Directives which govern their composition. There are British Regulations based on these guidelines [36]. The regulations governing pesticide residues in all commercial weaning foods are very strict. However, many parents choose to use commercial organic baby foods, which allow no pesticides to be used in their culture and preparation, and these have become popular in recent years. Organic regulations prohibit iron fortification and consequently organic savoury baby foods are much lower in iron content than non-organic savoury baby foods, which are usually fortified with iron sulphate:

- Iron fortified non-organic savoury jar 1.4 mg iron/100 g
- Organic savoury jar 0.6 mg iron/100 g [37]

Fluids

Milk

Breast milk or infant formula should be given as the main milk drink up until 12 months of age. Infants changed onto cow's milk before 12 months are at higher risk of iron deficiency and anaemia [38].

Water

Before weaning, cooled boiled water can be offered to formula fed babies in very hot weather if they seem to be thirsty. Breast fed infants do not need this as they will demand more frequent feeds and satisfy their thirst with the extra fluid in the fore milk.

Once weaning is established water should be offered from a cup or beaker with meals. This water does not have to be boiled for babies over 6 months old but can be freshly drawn tap water or bottled water given from a clean cup.

Juices

Infants do not need fruit juices or baby fruit juices as:

- Both breast milk and infant formula are nutritionally complete until 6 months and contain adequate vitamin C
- A balanced weaning diet for infants over 6 months will include fruit and vegetables

Many parents give baby fruit juices which are sold in a concentrated form or prediluted and ready to feed. All fruit juices (including baby juices), even when diluted, are acidic and contain non-milk extrinsic sugars. They can cause dental erosion so if offered:

- Should be given at a suggested dilution of 1 in 10 with water [33]
- Should be served only at meal times in a cup or beaker, never a bottle
- Drinking times should be kept short
- They should not be given at or after bedtime
- Infants should never be left alone with juices as they may choke

Other fluids

Tea and coffee should not be given as the tannins and polyphenols in them inhibit iron absorption. Sugary drinks should not be given as they cause dental caries especially when taken frequently from a bottle.

Vitamin supplementation

The Department of Health recommends a supplement of vitamins A and D for:

- Breast fed infants from 6 months (or from 1 month if there is any doubt about the mother's nutritional status during pregnancy)
- Formula fed infants over 6 months when they are taking <500 mL/day formula

This recommendation is particularly important for infants at risk of low vitamin D status and includes those living in northern areas of the UK and those of Asian, African and Middle Eastern origin [25]. Vitamin drops containing vitamins A, C and D are available free for infants in some low income families under the Healthy Start scheme [39] (p. 531).

Vitamin drops should always be given from a spoon, not added to bottles, to ensure the full dose is taken.

Toddlers and young children under 5 years of age

Toddlers' diets should be based on a combination of foods from the first four food groups in Table 27.4 and can include some foods that are high in fats and sugars. There are differences to both the diet offered to infants and that for older children and adults:

- Less milk than the infant diet
- More fat and less fibre than the healthy eating recommended for older children over 5 years and adults
- A meal pattern of three meals and 2–3 snacks per day as toddlers may only take small quantities of food at a time

How easily this is managed depends to some extent on parental knowledge and parenting skills. At the same time developmental changes in toddlers affect how they respond to food and meals.

The most recent National Diet and Nutrition Survey (NDNS) of $1^1/_2$ to $4^1/_2$-year-olds [40] indicated that the nutrients most at risk in toddlers' diets are vitamins A, C, D, iron and zinc (Table 27.5).

Neophobia

During their second year toddlers develop a neophobic response to food which means they become wary of trying new foods. The origin of this is may

be a survival mechanism to prevent the mobile toddler from poisoning themselves. This neophobic response usually peaks around 18 months and is more evident in some toddlers than others. If toddlers are being offered a wide variety of foods by around 12 months then they will enter their second year with a wider range of foods they recognise, like and readily accept [41].

Disgust and contamination fears

Between 3 and 5 years young children may develop disgust fears and stop eating foods they may have previously enjoyed [42]. They will refuse a food on sight if it resembles something they find disgusting (e.g. they may find spaghetti suddenly looks like worms). Contamination fears occur around the same time; if a disliked food is put on a plate next to a liked food the toddler may refuse both foods.

Learning to like new foods

The neophobic response dissipates slowly throughout the rest of childhood and adolescence [43,44]. Toddlers and young children can be helped to pass through this stage by eating in social groups, as they learn by copying adults and other children. It is therefore important that families eat together as often as possible and that toddlers are praised when they eat well. Toddlers may also learn to eat new foods when eating with other children at nursery or with friends. Some toddlers need to be offered a new food more than 10 times before they accept it as a liked food [41,45].

Some toddlers have more problems than others [46] and there are two main reasons for this in healthy individuals:

- Some become very rigid about the foods they will eat. They tend to be more emotional and more stubborn about what they will or will not do. They do not copy other children and so will not copy other people's eating behaviour.
- Others may be more sensory sensitive and have extreme reactions to touch, taste and smell. They may have problems with different textures of food and may have taken longer to progress from purée to lumpy food and on to more difficult textures. They may worry about

Table 27.5 Nutrients most at risk in toddlers' diets

Nutrient	Toddlers below RNI (%)	Toddlers below LRNI (%)
Vitamin A	50	7
Vitamin C	35	1
Vitamin D	95	
Iron	84	16
Zinc	72	14

LRNI, lower reference nutrient intake; RNI, reference nutrient intake [1].

getting their hands and face dirty and find it difficult to handle food and feed themselves.

Toddlers who experience faltering growth as a result of this will need to be referred to specialists who can assess and advise.

Exacerbating food refusal

Parental anxiety when toddlers only eat a limited variety of foods can exacerbate the problem, especially if parents try to coerce or force feed the child with food they are wary of or dislike. Up until 4–5 years young children's appetites are determined mainly by their energy and growth needs. They will eat well at some times and less so at other times and should always be allowed to decide the quantity they eat themselves. Some parents expect their toddlers to eat more than they need and coerce their toddler when they are actually signalling that they have had enough food. As mealtimes develop into a battle ground between toddler and parent, the toddler can lose their appetite just by becoming anxious as the mealtime approaches.

Around 5 years of age children learn to modify their eating according to social rules and will learn to finish what is on their plate, eat when others are eating even if they are not hungry, and they will also begin to comfort eat.

Balanced meals and snacks

A balanced and varied diet should be offered with meals and snacks based mainly on the first four food groups in Table 27.4. Two courses at each meal, a savoury course followed by a sweet course, ensures a wider variety of foods and nutrients will be offered. Parents should be encouraged to think of the sweet course as a second opportunity to offer energy and nutrients and should not offer it only as a reward for finishing the savoury course.

The food groups

Starchy carbohydrates

A mixture of some white and some wholegrain varieties should be offered as the fibre load from only wholegrain cereals would be too high for toddlers. Excess fibre can fill up the stomach and reduce their food intake thereby restricting energy and nutrient intake.

Fruit and vegetables

Fruit and vegetables should be offered at each meal and some snacks. Toddlers may be averse to the bitter taste in some vegetables and may eat a limited variety in this food group. This should not be a cause for concern as this age should be seen as a time for learning to like fruit and vegetables and parents should encourage their toddlers to eat these foods by setting an example and eating and enjoying these foods themselves.

Milk and milk products

Milk intake should reduce to 350–500 mL during the second year. During the pre-school years three servings of milk, yoghurt and cheese per day will ensure calcium requirements are met. An excess of milk in the diet usually means less iron rich foods are eaten and iron deficiency and anaemia are associated with toddler diets with an excess of milk [47,48].

Toddlers up to 2 years of age should have whole (full fat) milk for the extra energy and fat-soluble vitamins it contains. After 2 years toddlers can change to semi-skimmed milk if they are eating well and growing normally.

Follow-on and toddler milks marketed for this age group are enriched with more iron, zinc and vitamin D than that found in cow's milk and can provide a nutritional safety net for toddlers who are not eating well. They are lower in certain nutrients than cow's milk: calcium, phosphorus, iodine and riboflavin.

Meat, fish and alternatives

Many toddlers do not like the texture of chewy meat and prefer soft tender cuts or meat products made from minced meat such as sausages, burgers and meatballs. As long as these foods are made from good quality ingredients with a high lean meat and low salt content they will make a valuable contribution to a healthy diet. Chicken, which often has a softer texture than red meat, is popular with this age group.

Fish should be offered twice a week and one portion should be oily (see Food Safety below for maximum limits). Most toddlers enjoy fish when served as fish cakes or fish and potato pie.

Dhal is commonly used by some Asian cultures and a variety of other pulses can be used in soups and stews. Hummus and nut butters can be used as spreads.

Foods high in fat and/or sugar

These high energy foods give toddlers extra energy to satisfy their high requirements and help to reduce the bulk in the diet. Small amounts of them can be given in addition to the other food groups, not instead of them. An excess of these foods will increase the likelihood of obesity which is now increasing in this age group.

Drinks

Bottles for milk or other drinks should have been discontinued by around 12 months as sucking on a bottle can become a comfort habit that is hard to break. Children who drink sweet drinks from bottles have a higher risk of dental caries [49]. Water and some milk are preferred drinks and should be given in a cup, beaker or glass. Six to eight drinks of about 100–120 mL can be offered throughout the day, with meals and snacks (see Table 1.13). More may be needed in very hot weather or after a lot of physical activity. Drinks containing artificial sweeteners should be kept to a minimum and be well diluted.

Dental care

In 2003, 40% of 5-year-olds had experience of dental decay and 53% had signs of tooth erosion [50]. The incidence of dental disease is lower in children who brush their teeth twice a day with a pea-sized amount of fluoride toothpaste. A smear of toothpaste is enough for babies whose teeth should also be brushed twice a day by their parents from the time teeth appear. Reducing the amount of time and the number of times per day that teeth are exposed to sugary foods and sugary and acidic drinks will decrease the risk of dental caries and tooth erosion.

Vitamin supplements

A supplement of vitamins A and D is recommended for children up to the age of 5 years [25]. As for infants this recommendation is particularly important for children at risk of low vitamin D status and includes picky fussy eaters, those living in northern areas of the UK and those of Asian, African and Middle Eastern origin [25].

Social support for toddlers in low income families

Healthy Start

Healthy Start replaced the Welfare Food Scheme in England, Wales, Northern Ireland and Scotland in 2006. Families who qualify for this scheme are those in receipt of Income Support, Income-based Jobseeker's Allowance or Child Tax Credit (but not Working Tax Credit) with an income below £14 155 a year (in 2006–07). They are entitled to vouchers that can be exchanged for cow's milk, fresh fruit and vegetables and infant formula (Table 27.6). Children up to 4 years in these families are also entitled to free vitamin drops containing vitamins A, C and D (see p. 18). Details of entitlement and how to access the scheme can be found on the Healthy Start website [39].

Nursery Milk

Children under 5 years are entitled to 1/3 pint (200 mL) milk per day if they attend a nursery or are with a registered childminder for more than 2 hours per day.

Table 27.6 Voucher entitlement for infants and children through *Healthy Start*.

	No. of vouchers valued at £2.80/week*
Term infants up to 12 months	2
Preterm infants up to 12 months after EDD	2
Children 1–3 years	1

EDD, estimated date of delivery.
* Voucher value as defined in 2006.

Sure Start

This is a government initiative in areas of deprivation and low income that is intended to support families with young children. One aim is to help overcome the barriers to feeding young children a healthy diet and dietitians have been involved in:

- Training Sure Start workers, community food assistants and play workers on weaning and healthy eating messages
- Developing food policies with parents and staff.
- Developing resources with parents
- Education sessions for parents on cooking, shopping, weaning. Cook and eat sessions are popular and developing literacy skills has become part of some shopping and cooking sessions
- Holiday play schemes
- Clinical input and home visits

Current schemes and activities can be accessed on the Sure Start website [51].

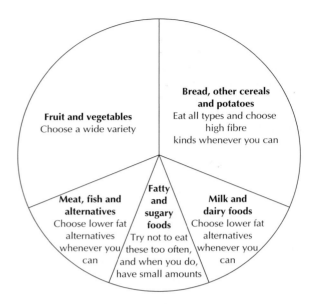

Figure 27.1   The Balance of Good Health (© The Food Standards Agency).

Primary and secondary school children

From around the age of 5 years the principles of healthy eating which are recommended for the adult population should be introduced:

- At least 50% of energy from total carbohydrates
- A maximum of 11% of energy from non-milk extrinsic sugars
- A maximum of 35% of energy from fat
- A maximum of 11% of energy from saturated fat
- About 15% energy from protein [1]

Combining the five food groups in the proportions represented in the Balance of Good Health underlies the basis of healthy eating (Fig. 27.1). In order to satisfy the nutrient requirements of children the recommendations need to be more specific than those given by the FSA for the adult population: see recommendations from the Paediatric Group of the British Dietetic Association on which Table 27.4 is based.

During childhood many children remain neophobic, preferring to eat foods they are familiar with. They must be motivated to taste new foods. Work in this field continues to show that the number of times children are exposed to food increases

the likelihood they will try the food and then learn to like it [52].

The most recent National Diet and Nutrition Survey showed that the 'at risk' nutrients for primary age school children (4–10 years of age) are zinc and vitamin A (Table 27.7) [53].

During adolescence teenagers develop their own autonomy, rejecting their parents' values and developing their own. Values around food and

Table 27.7   Population groups with nutrient intakes more than 10% below the lower reference nutrient intake (LRNI) [1].

	Girls	Boys
4–6 years	Zinc	Zinc
7–10 years	Vitamin A, zinc	
11–14 years	Vitamin A, riboflavin, iron, calcium, magnesium, zinc, potassium, iodine	Vitamin A, calcium, magnesium, zinc, potassium
15–18 years	Vitamin A, riboflavin, iron, calcium, magnesium, zinc, potassium	Vitamin A, potassium, magnesium

meals are no exception to this and many teenagers change their eating habits so that they are different to the rest of their family. Some become vegetarian, others increasingly eat more food outside the home [43]. Their choices include a lot of high fat, high sugar foods and the NDNS survey showed many, particularly girls, have diets deficient in several nutrients (Table 27.7).

Vegetarian diets

A vegetarian diet is based around the same food groups shown in Table 27.4. Within the milk, cheese and yoghurt group, calcium enriched soya milk and yoghurts and tofu can be substituted for cow's milk. Within the meat, fish and alternatives group eggs, nuts, pulses and seeds will be eaten. At least three servings are needed each day to provide an adequate iron intake as the bioavailability of iron from eggs and plant sources is much lower than that of haem iron found in meat and fish.

Nutritional initiatives in schools

Food and drinks taken at school can make a large contribution to a child's nutrient intake. Poor nutrient intakes in school children, particularly those at secondary school [53], have resulted in a number of nutritional initiatives in schools including:

- The national fruit and veg scheme. All 4–6-year-old children in Local Education Authority maintained infant, primary and special schools are entitled to a free piece of fruit or vegetable each school day [54].
- Subsidised school milk is available for primary school children. In England schools choose whether they wish to offer it, but in Wales children up to 7 years of age are entitled to $1/3$ pint (200 mL) milk free per day [55].
- School Nutrition Action Groups are a central component to ensure the whole school approach to healthier eating and drinking in schools. This may be via the development of a School Food policy. Groups usually include senior teaching staff, pupils, parents, caterers and school nurses. A community dietitian may be involved.
- Wired for Health is a series of websites developed by the Department of Health and the Department for Education and Skills. Health information, including healthy eating, is provided for a range of audiences which relates to the National Curriculum and the National Healthy Schools Programme [56].
- Healthy eating became one of the four themes of the National Healthy Schools Programme. The other themes are physical activity; personal, social and health education, including sex and relationship education and drug education; emotional health and wellbeing (including bullying). The programme aims to guide schools towards being a health promoting environment with the Government target that all schools will be Healthy Schools by 2009.
- The Food in Schools Toolkit [57] is funded by the Department for Education and Skills and offers guidelines on improving food and drinks offered on school sites. Recommended items for improved vending in machines and tuck shops are:
  Fresh fruit, prepared fruit salads and dried fruits
  Filled rolls, sandwiches and baguettes
  Fruit or cheese scones
  Salads
  Pasta mixes
  Breakfast cereals, with semi-skimmed milk
  Yoghurts, fromage frais
  Pizza slices (with thick bases and less cheese)
  Semi-skimmed milk (plain or flavoured)
  Water, fruit juices and drinking yoghurts
  Baked corn snacks or unsalted popcorn
- The School Food Trust is an independent body set up by government in 2005 and aims to transform school food and food skills to improve health and education in England.

School meals

Current recommendations in England, Wales and Northern Ireland [58,59] are based on the food groups in Table 27.4 and specify that at least one item or a choice of two items from each food group is available throughout the meal service. Recent research has shown that these standards have failed to have a positive effect on healthy food choices and nutrient intakes in primary and secondary schools [60,61]. Scotland has introduced nutrient based standards specifying the amounts of certain nutrients that must be provided on average over a week [62]. Currently, the other three home countries are considering whether similar nutrient based standards should be adopted. They are likely to be based on the Caroline Walker Trust recommendations [63].

Breakfasts are offered in many schools and have the potential to improve nutrient intakes and improve concentration and school performance depending on the foods offered [63–65]. This can make a difference to the large numbers of school children who leave home without breakfast.

Foods eaten on the way to and from school are also a significant part of school children's nutrient intake. A survey produced every 2 years by a large international school caterer reported that in 2005:

- £519 million was spent by school children on their way to and from school
- Main purchases were sweets, crisps and savoury snacks, chocolate, canned fizzy drinks, chewing gum, other soft drinks, cigarettes, bottled water, chips and ice cream [66]

Adolescent growth spurt

The adolescent growth spurt lasts approximately 2 years and takes place, on average, around 12 years of age for girls and 14 for boys, but can be 2 years earlier or later. The peak height velocity can be up to 13 cm/year for boys and 10 cm/year for girls [67]. Growth rate then declines until full height is reached. During this time adolescents' energy requirements will be noticeably higher and appetite may be larger. Extra snacks often make up this difference but the NDNS showed those snacks are often from food group 5, the high fat, high sugar foods, rather than food groups 1–4 [53].

Implications of the teenage diet on future risk of osteoporosis

Even after the growth spurt calcification of bones

continues as peak bone mass is not reached until the early twenties. Three large servings of milk, cheese or yoghurt will ensure that calcium and phosphorus requirements are being met to ensure bone deposition [68]. This applies for Caucasian teenagers but not necessarily for other minority ethnic groups [69]. Adequate calcium intakes at this age may protect against osteoporosis in later life [70].

Sports nutrition

Meeting the higher energy needs for adolescents undertaking sports training is essential and may require specialist input from an Accredited Sports Dietitian. Energy requirements should be calculated to support the training programme using Basal Metabolic Rate and Physical Activity Level and adding in 60–100 kcal/day (250–420 kJ/day) to allow for extra growth [1]. Monthly height measurement can be used to assess when the growth spurt is taking place. Adolescents in sports training should eat a high carbohydrate snack or meal, containing some protein, within an hour of finishing training to ensure good glycogen stores within muscles (as should any other athlete).

Teenage girls of child bearing age

All women of child bearing age should have a nutritious diet with an adequate intake of folic acid. The Department of Health recommends a supplement of 400 μg folic acid for any woman or teenager who could become pregnant. Because most teenage pregnancies are unplanned, a diet rich in folic acid should be recommended to all teenage girls.

Pregnancy

Pregnancy during the teenage years places extra nutritional requirements on girls who may not have finished growing themselves and who will not have attained their peak bone mass. Nutrient requirements have not been specified for these young mothers but a healthy balanced diet with folic acid and vitamin D supplementation would be a minimum requirement. For those eating poorly a multivitamin and mineral supplement (not containing vitamin A) could be recommended. Under the Healthy Start scheme all pregnant girls under 18 are entitled to benefits regardless of their financial circumstances [39].

Food safety

Good food hygiene and storage is extremely important for young children particularly infants and children under 5 years. To offset any risks of poisoning from *Salmonella*, the FSA recommends that eggs are cooked until both the yolk and white are hard for this age group [71].

Dioxins levels in oily fish

Varying levels of dioxins accumulate in the fatty tissues of oily fish and to limit their intake the FSA recommends that boys have a maximum of four portions of oily fish per week. A maximum limit of two portions is set for girls to reduce the amounts they will have accumulated in their tissues as they enter their child bearing years [71].

Mercury levels in large fish

Large fish – shark, swordfish and marlin – live for many years and can accumulate high levels of mercury in their flesh. The FSA recommends that pregnant women, babies and young children under 5 years do not eat these fish [71].

High vitamin A levels in liver

Although liver is a very good source of several nutrients, particularly some 'at risk' nutrients discussed above (e.g. iron and zinc), it contains very high levels of vitamin A. The Scientific Advisory Committee on Nutrition has recommended that no-one should increase their consumption of liver beyond one portion per week [72]. Although no recommendations were made for young children and babies it would be prudent to avoid giving liver to babies who are weaned early, before 6 months, and to limit it to once per week in older infants and young children.

Organic foods

Many parents are now choosing to buy organic food for their babies and children despite the extra expense; the majority of commercially prepared baby foods sold are now organic. Parents do this to avoid the possible detrimental effects that pesticide residues found in foods from non-organic sources may have on the developing organs and systems of babies and children. This remains a controversial issue as food safety bodies in the UK and Europe only allow pesticides at levels that are judged to be non-harmful in conventional baby foods. However, advocates of organic food point out that there may be toxic effects of ingesting combinations of several different chemicals which may have been harmless when tested individually. Many of these chemicals are new, having only been synthesised in the last few decades, so their potential cumulative effects are unknown.

Studies linking pesticide or synthetic chemical exposure in children with an increased incidence of cancer [73], hormone disruption [74] and impaired cognitive function [75] have been published. *In utero* exposure of the fetus to these chemicals may be the most damaging [76].

Controversial issues around nutrients and foods

Omega-3 fatty acids and learning skills

Optimum brain functioning and sight are dependent on an adequate intake of the omega-3 long chain polyunsaturated fatty acids (LCPs), eicosapentaenoic acid (EPA) and docosahexaenoic acid (DHA) during fetal growth and early infancy [77,78]. They are present in breast milk and are added to all whey dominant and most casein dominant infant formulas (see Table 1.11). Whether their presence in food or supplements for older infants and children influences brain function, behaviour or the risk of atopy remains controversial. A weekly serve of oily fish will ensure an adequate intake of omega-3 LCPs. Walnuts and linseeds as well as rapeseed, walnut, linseed and soya oils are good sources of the omega-3 essential fatty acid, α-linolenic acid. Current research has not shown that children with adequate dietary intake of omega-3 fats will benefit from extra supplements. However, omega-3 supplements and foods that have been enriched with omega-3 fats are now subject to high level marketing following anecdotal evidence of children's learning skills improving with omega-3 LCP supplementation [79].

Food advertising

Much controversy surrounds the issue of advertising poor nutrient quality foods to children. The food industry argues that advertising does not affect food choices and nutritional intakes, but there are studies that cast doubt on this and point towards its contribution to rising levels of childhood obesity [80–82]. The Government is working with Ofcom and the Committee on Advertising Practice to introduce tighter restrictions on the advertising to children of foods high in fat, salt and sugar. The Government will monitor closely the impact of Ofcom and other measures – across all media – in order to see whether or not there is a change in the nature and balance of food promotion to children. An interim review will be conducted in 2007, and working with Ofcom, a more detailed review in 2008. On that basis, the Government will decide whether or not future action through new or existing legislation is required.

Genetic modification

The long term effects of genetic modification (GM) of foods are as yet unknown and remain controversial. The nutritional content of GM and non-GM foods sold in the UK are comparable and therefore do not affect a baby or child's nutritional intake. Many parents choose not to give GM food to their children, but they may not always be aware of the extent to which GM ingredients are used in processed foods.

References

1 Department of Health Report on Health and Social Subjects No. 41. *Dietary Reference Values for Food Energy and Nutrients for the United Kingdom.* London: The Stationery Office, 1991.

2 www.salt.gov.uk Accessed April 2006.

3 Department of Health *Choosing Health: Making healthier choices easier.* London: The Stationery Office, 2004.

4 Scientific Advisory Committee on Nutrition (SACN). SCMN/03/08. *Introduction of Solid Foods,* 2003. http://www.sacn.gov.uk/meetings/subgroups/maternal/2003_09_29.html 2003 Accessed April 2006.

5 Dollberg S, Lahav S, Mimouni FB A comparison of intakes of breast-fed and bottle-fed infants during the first two days of life. *J Am Coll Nutr,* 2001, **20** 209–11.

6 Food Standards Agency *McCance and Widdowson's The Composition of Foods,* 6th summary edition. Cambridge: Royal Society of Chemistry, 2002.

7 Howie PW, Forsyth JS, Ogston SA *et al.* Protective effect of breast-feeding against infection. *Br Med J,* 1990, **300** 11–16.

8 Wilson AC, Forsyth JS, Greene SA *et al.* Relation of the infant diet to childhood health: seven year follow up of cohort of children in Dundee infant feeding study. *Br Med J,* 1998, **316** 21–5.

9 Cesar JA, Cesar GV, Barros FC *et al.* Impact of breast feeding on admission for pneumonia during post-neonatal period in Brazil: nested case–control study. *Br Med J,* 1999, **318** 1316–20.

10 Aniansson G, Alm B, Andersson B *et al.* A prospective cohort study on breast-feeding and otitis media in Swedish infants. *Pediatr Infect Dis J,* 1994, **13** 183–8.

11 Marild S, Hansson S, Jodal U *et al.* Protective effect of breastfeeding against urinary tract infection. *Acta Paediatr,* 2004, **93** 164–8.

12 Kramer MS, Chalmers B, Hodnett ED *et al.* PROBIT Study Group (Promotion of Breastfeeding Intervention Trial). Promotion of Breastfeeding Intervention Trial (PROBIT): a randomized trial in the Republic of Belarus. *J Am Med Assoc,* 2001, **285** 413–20.

13 Fewtrell MS The long-term benefits of having been breastfed. *Curr Paediatr,* 2004, **14** 97–103.

14 Angelsen NK, Vic T, Jacobsen G, Bakketeig LS Breastfeeding and cognitive development at ages 1 and 5 years. *Arch Dis Child,* 2001, **85** 183–8.

15 Sadauskaite-KuehneV, Ludvigsson J, Pagaiga Z *et al.* Longer breastfeeding as an independent protective factor against development of type 1 diabetes mellitus in childhood. *Diabetes Metab Res Rev,* 2004, **20** 150–7.

16 Jones G, Riley M, Dwyer T Breastfeeding in early life and bone mass in prepubertal children: a longitudinal study. *Osteoporosis Int,* 2000, **11** 146–52.

17 Arnez S, Ruckeri R, Koletzko B, von Kries R Breastfeeding and childhood obesity: a systematic review. *Int J Obes,* 2004, **28** 1247–56.

18 www.idfa.org.uk Accessed April 2006.

19 Hosoi S, Honma K, Daimatsu T *et al.* Lower energy content of human milk than calculated using conversion factors. *Pediatr Int,* 2005, **47** 7–9.

20 Butte NF Energy requirements of infants. *Public Health Nutr,* 2005, **8** (7A) 953–67.

21 Butte NF, Wong WW, Hopkinson JM *et al.* Infant feeding mode affects early growth and body composition. *Pediatrics*, 2000, **106** 1355–66.

22 Ministry of Agriculture, Fisheries and Food and the Royal Society of Chemistry *McCance and Widdowson's The Composition of Foods, 5th edition*. Cambridge: Royal Society of Chemistry, 1991.

23 www.dwi.gov.uk Accessed April 2006.

24 http://www.dh.gov.uk/PolicyAndGuidance/ HealthAndSocialCareTopics/ MaternalAndInfantNutrition/fs/en Accessed April 2006.

25 Department of Health Report on Health and Social Subjects No. 45. *Weaning and the Weaning Diet*, London: The Stationery Office, 1994.

26 Wall CR, Grant CC, Taua N *et al.* Milk versus medicine for the treatment of iron deficiency anaemia in hospitalised infants. *Arch Dis Child*, 2005, **90** 1033–8.

27 Morley R, Abbott R, Fairweather-Tait S *et al.* Iron fortified follow on formula from 9 to 18 months improves iron status but not development or growth: a randomised trial. *Arch Dis Child*, 1999, **81** 247–52.

28 Gill DG, Vincent S, Segal DS Follow-on formula in the prevention of iron deficiency: a multicentre study. *Acta Paediatr*, 1997, **86** 683–9.

29 Daly A, MacDonald A, Aukett A *et al.* Prevention of anaemia in inner city toddlers by an iron supplemented cows' milk formula. *Arch Dis Child*, 1996, **75** 9–16.

30 Williams J, Wolff A, Daly A *et al.* Iron supplemented formula milk related to reduction in psychomotor decline in infants from inner city areas: randomised study. *Br Med J*, 1999, **318** 693–8.

31 Hamlyn B, Brooker S, Oleinkova K, Wands S. *Infant feeding 2000*. Office for National Statistics. London: The Stationery Office, 2002.

32 World Health Organization Document A54/INF. DOC./4 (1 May 2001) Fifty-Fourth World Health Assembly Available at www.who.int/gb/ebwha/ pdf_files/WHA54/ea54id4.pdf

33 Department of Health *Birth to Five. Your complete guide to parenthood and the first five years of your child's life*. London: Central Office of Information, 2006.

34 Pliner P The effects of mere exposure on liking for edible substances. *Appetite*, 1982, **3** 283–90.

35 Stordy BJ, Redfern AM, Morgan JB Healthy eating for infants – mothers' actions. *Acta Paediatr*, 1995, **84** 733–41.

36 www.food.gov.uk/multimedia/pdfs/ babyfoodcerealsidraft2004.pdf Accessed May 2006.

37 More J Organic Babyfood. *J Fam Health Care*, 2003, **13** 6–8.

38 Male C, Persson LA, Freeman V *et al.* Euro-Growth Iron Study Group. Prevalence of iron deficiency in 12-mo-old infants from 11 European areas and influence of dietary factors on iron status (Euro-Growth study). *Acta Paediatr*, 2001, **90** 492–8.

39 www.healthystart.nhs.uk Accessed April 2006.

40 Gregory JR, Collins DL, Davies PSW *et al. National Diet and Nutrition Survey: children aged $1^1/_2$ to $4^1/_2$ years. Volume 1: Report of the diet and nutrition survey*. London: The Stationery Office, 1995.

41 Addessi E, Galloway AT, Visalberghi E, Birch LL Specific social influences on the acceptance of novel foods in 2–5-year-old children. *Appetite*, 2000, **45** 264–71.

42 Koivisto U-K, Sjödén P-O Reasons for rejection of food items in Swedish families with children aged 2–17. *Appetite*, 1996, **26** 83–103.

43 Hill AJ Developmental issues in attitudes to food and diet. *Proc Nutr Soc*, 2002, **61** 259–66.

44 Pliner P, Loewen ER Temperament and food neophobia in children and their mothers. *Appetite*, 1997, **28** 239–54.

45 Birch L, Marlin DW I don't like it, I never tried it: Effects of exposure to food on two-year-old children's food preferences. *Appetite*, 1982, **3** 353–60.

46 Harris G, Blissett J, Johnson R Food refusal associated with illness. *Child Psychol Psychiatry Rev*, 2000, **5** 148–56.

47 Cowin I, Emond A, Emmett P ALSPAC Study Group. Association between composition of the diet and haemoglobin and ferritin levels in 18-month-old children. *Eur J Clin Nutr*, 2001, **55** 278–86.

48 Thane CW, Walmsley CM, Bates CJ *et al.* Risk factors for poor iron status in British toddlers: further analysis of data from the National Diet and Nutrition Survey of children aged 1.5–4.5 years. *Public Health Nutr*, 2000, **3** 433–40.

49 Hinds K, Gregory JR *National Diet and Nutrition Survey: children aged $1^1/_2$ to $4^1/_2$ years. Volume 2. Report of the Dental Survey*. London: The Stationery Office, 1995.

50 Department of Health *Children's Dental Health in the United Kingdom 2003*. London: The Stationery Office, 2005.

51 www.surestart.gov.uk Accessed April 2006.

52 Cooke L The development and modification of children's eating habits. *Br Nutr Found Nutr Bull*, 2004, **29** 31–5.

53 Gregory J, Lowe S, Bates CJ *et al. National Diet and Nutrition Survey: young people aged 4 to 18 years. Volume 1: Report of the diet and nutrition survey*. London: The Stationery Office, 2000.

54 www.5aday.nhs.uk/sfvs/default.aspx Accessed May 2006.

55 www.milkforschools.org.uk Accessed May 2006.

56 www.wiredforhealth.gov.uk Accessed May 2006.

57 www.foodinschools.org/fis_toolkit.php Accessed May 2006.

58   www.dfes.gov.uk/schoollunches Accessed May 2006.
59   www.deni.gov.uk/schools/index.htm Accessed May 2006.
60   Nelson M, Nicholas J, Suleiman S *et al. School Meals in Primary Schools in England.* London: Department for Education and Skills Research Report RR753, 2006.
61   Nelson M, Bradbury J, Poulter J *et al. School Meals in Secondary Schools in England.* London: Department for Education and Skills Research Report RR557, 2004.
62   www.scotland.gov.uk/Publications/2003/05/17090/21740 Accessed May 2006.
63   Crawley H *Eating Well at School Nutritional and Practical Guidelines.* London: The Caroline Walker Trust & National Heart Forum, 2005.
64   Belderson P, Harvey I, Kimbell R *et al.* Does breakfast-club attendance affect schoolchildren's nutrient intake? A study of dietary intake at three schools. *Br J Nutr*, 2003, **90** 1003–6.
65   Grantham-McGregor S Can the provision of breakfast benefit school performance? *Food Nutr Bull*, 2005, **26** (Suppl 2) S144–58.
66   Sodexho Ltd. The Sodexho School Meals and Lifestyle Survey. London: Sodexho Ltd, 2005.
67   Kelnar CJH, Butler G Endocrine gland disorders and disorders of growth and puberty. In: McIntosh N, Helms PJ, Smyth RL (eds) *Forfar and Arneil's Textbook of Paediatrics*, 6th edn. London: Churchill Livingstone, 2003.
68   Teegarden D, Lyle RM, Proulx WR *et al.* Previous milk consumption is associated with greater bone density in young women. *Am J Clin Nutr*, 1999, **69** 1014–17.
69   Opotowsky AR, Bilezikian JP Racial differences in the effect of early milk consumption on peak and postmenopausal bone mineral density. *J Bone Miner Res*, 2003, **18** 1978–88.
70   Kalkwarf HJ, Khoury JC, Lanphear BP Milk intake during childhood and adolescence, adult bone density, and osteoporotic fractures in US women. *Am J Clin Nutr*, 2003, **77** 257–65.
71   www.eatwell.gov.uk Accessed April 2006.
72   Scientific Advisory Committee on Nutrition on behalf of the Food Standards Agency and the Department of Health. *Review of Dietary Advice on Vitamin A.* London: The Stationery Office, 2005.
73   Meinert R, Schuz J, Kaletsch U *et al.* Leukemia and non-Hodgkin's lymphoma in childhood and exposure to pesticides: results of a register-based case–control study in Germany. *Am J Epidemiol*, 2000, **151** 639–46.
74   Colon I, Caro D, Bourdony CJ, Rosario O Identification of phthalate esters in the serum of young Puerto Rican girls with premature breast development. *Environ Health Perspect*, 2000, **108** 895–900.
75   Guillette EA, Meza MM, Aguilar MG *et al.* An anthropological approach to the evaluation of preschool children exposed to pesticides in Mexico. *Environ Health Perspect*, 1998, **106** 347–53.
76   Garry VF, Schreinmachers D, Harkers ME, Griffith J Pesticide applicators, biocides and birth defects in rural Minnesota. *Environ Health Perspect*, 1996, **104** 394–9.
77   Koletzko B, Agostoni C, Carlson SE *et al.* Long chain polyunsaturated fatty acids (LC-PUFA) and perinatal development. *Acta Paediatr*, 2001, **90** 460–4.
78   Gil A, Ramirez M, Gil M Role of long-chain polyunsaturated fatty acids in infant nutrition. *Eur J Clin Nutr*, 2003, **57** (Suppl 1) S31–4.
79   www.durhamtrial.org Accessed May 2006.
80   Lobstein T, Dibb S Evidence of a possible link between obesogenic food advertising and child overweight. *Obes Rev*, 2005, **3** 203–8.
81   Carter OB The weighty issue of Australian television food advertising and childhood obesity. *Health Promot J Austr*, 2006, **1** 5–11.
82   Halford JC, Gillespie J, Brown V *et al.* Effect of television advertisements for foods on food consumption in children. *Appetite*, 2004, **42** 221–5.

Further reading and information

Infants and preschool children

Unicef Babyfriendly Initiative
www.babyfriendly.org.uk

National Childbirth Trust
www.nctpregnancyandbabycare.com

Association of Breast Feeding Mothers
www.abm.me.uk

La Leche League
www.lalecheleague.org

Breast Feeding Network
www.breastfeeding.co.uk

National Service Framework for Children
www.dh.gov.uk/childrensnsf

Crawley H *Eating Well for Under-5s in Childcare.* London: Caroline Walker Trust, 2006.

Crawley H *Eating Well for Under-5s in Childcare: Training materials.* London: Caroline Walker Trust, 2006.

Dyson L, Renfrew M, McFadden A *et al. Effective Action briefing on the intitiation and duration of breastfeeding* 2006 www.nice.org.uk

Hall DMB, Elliman D *Health for all children*, 4th edn, Oxford: Oxford University Press, 2003.

Infant and Toddler Forum. Toddler Fact Sheets. Available at: www.infantandtoddlerforum.org

Morgan J, Dickerson JWT *Nutrition in Early life*. Chichester: John Wiley, 2003.

Nutritional guidance for early years: food choices for children aged 1–5 years in early education and child-care settings. Scottish Executive, 2006. Available at: www.scotland.gov.uk/publications/2006/01/18153659/0

Nutrition matters for the early years: Healthy Eating for the Under Fives in Childcare. Health Promotion Agency for Northern Ireland, 2006. Available at: www.healthpromotionagency.org.uk; Resources/nutrition/pdfs/nutmatters2006.pdf

Studies from the Avon Longitudinal Study of Pregnancy and Childhood www.alspac.bris.ac.uk

School children

School Food Trust
www.schoolfoodtrust.org.uk

Health Education Trust
www.healthedtrust.com

Couch kids: the continuing epidemic. British Heart Foundation, 2004. Available at: www.bhf.org.uk

Kids and schools catalogue. British Heart Foundation, 2006. Available at: www.bhf.org.uk/publications

Nutrition and Schoolchildren. British Nutrition Foundation, London, 2003.

Young People in Wales: Findings from the Health Behaviour in School-aged Children (HBSC) Study 1986–2000. Technical Report 1. Cardiff: Welsh Assembly Government, 2002.

Adolescents

BMA Board of Science and Education. *Adolescent Health*. London: BMA Publications, 2003.

Report from Maternity Alliance and Food Commission *Good Enough to Eat? The Diet of Pregnant Teenagers*, 2003. Available at: www.foodcomm.org.uk

Sproston K, Primatesta P *Health Survey for England 2002. The Health of Children and Young People*. London: The Stationery Office, 2003.

28 Children from Ethnic Groups and those following Cultural Diets

Sue Wolfe

Introduction

The UK is the home to a multicultural and multi-ethnic society. Immigration occurred mainly during the late 1950s and early 1960s in response to labour shortages. Therefore the main ethnic communities are situated near large industrialised cities. These ethnic groups have introduced a wide variety of cultures, including dietary beliefs and practice which have had to fit into their new lifestyles. Achieving nutritionally adequate diets became a challenge with people finding themselves in an environment very different from their homeland.

Infants and children of any age have special dietary requirements. It is therefore essential that religious and cultural attitudes towards diet are understood by health care professionals when they are initiating any dietary intervention, in order to achieve optimal growth and development in these children. Assessment of intake must be accurate and any advice given must be relevant to dietary custom so that it is both realistic and achievable.

Children are subject to many outside influences and often start to develop westernised dietary ideas. With time these ideas are taken home and adopted by other members of the family. The extent of adoption of dietary practices differing from traditional customs is variable, therefore all diets must be individually assessed.

Vegetarian and vegan diets

Vegetarianism and veganism are common dietary practices among many religious and ethnic groups. In addition, increasing numbers of the indigenous population are restricting their intake of meat and animal products for either humanitarian, ethical or health reasons. Table 28.1 gives a classification of vegetarian and vegan diets. Providing careful attention is given to ensuring nutritional adequacy, these diets will support normal growth and development [1–3]. In general, the greater the degree of dietary restriction the greater the risk of nutritional deficiency [4].

Infant feeding

Breast feeding is commonly practised amongst the indigenous vegetarian and vegan population. Providing the maternal diet is adequate, breast milk will be nutritionally complete for the first 6 months of life for most infants. Specific attention must be paid to the mother's vitamin D, calcium and iron intakes. Vegan mothers may require supplementation with additional vitamin B_{12} [5]. Vitamin B_{12} deficiency resulting in neurological damage [6], irritability, faltering growth, apathy, anorexia and developmental regression has been reported in breast fed infants of vegan mothers [7].

Table 28.1   Classification of vegetarianism and veganism.

	Foods excluded	Protein source		Nutrient at risk of deficiency
Partial vegetarian	Red meat Offal Milk Cheese Yoghurt	Poultry Fish Eggs	Beans Lentils Nuts	Iron
Lacto-ovo vegetarian	Red meat Offal Fish Poultry	Milk Cheese Yoghurt Eggs	Beans Lentils Nuts	Iron
Lacto vegetarian	Red meat Offal Poultry Fish Eggs	Milk Cheese Yoghurt	Beans Lentils Nuts	Iron Vitamin D
Vegan	Red meat Offal Fish Poultry Eggs Milk Cheese Yoghurt Honey	Beans Lentils Nuts		Protein Energy Iron Fat-soluble vitamins Vitamin B_2 Vitamin B_{12} Calcium Zinc

Table 28.2   Infant formulas suitable for vegetarian and vegan children.

Milk based	Soya based
Cow & Gate Premium	InfaSoy*
Cow & Gate Plus	Wysoy*
Cow & Gate Organic first milk	ProSobee*
Cow & Gate Organic second milk	Farley's soya formula*
SMA Gold	Isomil*
SMA White	
Farley's First Milk	
Farley's Second Milk	
Aptamil First	
Aptamil Extra	
Enfamil Lacto free	
Enfamil AR	

Protein hydrolysates (for therapeutic use only)
Pepti
Pepti-Junior
Pregestimil
Nutramigen 1 and 2
Nan HA (partial hydrolysate)
Comfort (partial hydrolysate)
Neocate* (amino acid based feed)

* Suitable for vegans.

If the infant is not breast fed a suitable infant formula must be given (Table 28.2). The Chief Medical Officer for the UK has recently commented on the phytoestrogen content of infant soya formulas and has advised that soya infant formulas 'may be given to infants of vegan parents who are not breast-feeding' (see p. 95). Infants should not be given nutritionally deficient homemade or unmodified soya milks [5].

Some vegetarian families choose to give their babies goat's milk or ewe's milk in the belief that these confer health benefits and are preferable to cow's milk. These milks are contraindicated because of their nutritional inadequacy, high renal solute load and doubtful microbiological safety [5,7]. Nanny Infant Formula approaches the nutritional profile of infant formulas that are based on cow's milk, but has no health benefits over normal infant formulas. Infant formulas based on goat's milk are not available in the UK.

Weaning

Breast milk or infant formula will provide sufficient nutrition until the infant is 6 months of age (p. 525). After this period, solids should be gradually introduced, increasing flavours and textures with time (Table 28.3). Fruit, vegetables and pulses should be cooked with the skin on to preserve nutrients. This should then be removed to avoid an excessive fibre intake, which adds too much bulk to the diet and may bind certain trace minerals, inhibiting their absorption [8]. Pulses must be thoroughly cooked to destroy toxins such as trypsin inhibitors and haemaglutinins which may cause diarrhoea and vomiting [5]. Breast feeding or infant formula should be continued until 1 year of age. As the child gets older he or she should be encouraged to take at least 500 mL/day full fat cow's or approved fortified soya milk (see p. 99), or the equivalent in cheese or yoghurt in order to provide enough calcium [5].

Table 28.3 Suitable vegetarian and vegan weaning foods [5,14].

Around 6 months	Baby rice*
	Fruit and vegetable purées (cooked)
6–7 months	Rusk*
	Weetabix
	Pulse and lentil purées (well cooked)
	Pulse and vegetable purées
	Pulse and cereal purées
	Fruit purées
	Milk puddings or custards
	(cow's† or soya milk based)
7–9 months	Introduce lumps to the above foods
	Wholegrains
	Bread (white and wholemeal)
	Pasta and rice
	Finely ground nuts
	Dried fruits
	Cheese, e.g. cheese sauces†
	Eggs, e.g. savoury egg custards†
	Tofu and Quorn†

* Milk-free varieties for vegans.
† Suitable for vegetarians only.

Table 28.4 Sample vegetarian or vegan menu plan.

Breakfast	Cereal milk or milk substitute
	Wholemeal or white bread, margarine, peanut butter or yeast extract
	Egg*
	Diluted fresh orange juice
Dinner	Bean or nut based dish or cheese* based dish
	Vegetables or salad
	Bread, potato, pasta or rice
	Fruit or fruit crumble/pie/sponge*, custard (cow's* or soya milk) or milk pudding (cow's milk* or soya based)
Tea	Lentil or bean burgers or bean soup or baked beans or egg*
	Bread, margarine
	Fruit or yoghurt or fromage frais (cow's milk* or soya based)
Snacks	Nuts, toast, biscuits, crisps, fruit, cake

* Suitable for vegetarians only.

Children

Vegan diets are typically high in fibre and low in fat, so care must be taken to ensure an adequate energy intake to support growth. There have been many conflicting studies examining the dietary intake and growth of vegan children [9,10].

To provide optimal nutrition a vegetarian or vegan diet should be well balanced, containing two or three protein foods and cereals, vegetables, fruits and fats daily (Table 28.4). Vegetable and pulse proteins have a lower concentration and range of essential amino acids than protein from animal or fish sources. Therefore, careful planning of menus with pulse and cereal combinations is necessary to provide sufficient protein of high biological value [5]. The protein and energy content of the diet can be increased by the use of nuts, beans and oils [5].

The main micronutrients at risk of deficiency in the vegan diet are shown in Table 28.5. A daily vitamin supplement such as Abidec or Dalivit is beneficial for both vegetarian and vegan children and

should be given from the age of 6 months to 5 years [7]. In addition, vegan children may require a daily supplement of 1–2 µg vitamin B_{12} [5].

The increased intake of phytate containing legumes and wholegrains may lead to poor bioavailability of zinc [11] and iron [12], therefore a higher intake than is usually advised may be required. It is also important to ensure that a food rich in vitamin C is given alongside the iron containing food to increase its bioavailability.

When considering the COMA [13] recommendations for dietary fat, a vegan diet is often regarded as 'healthy'. However, the vegan diet may, as well as being low in total fat, also contain a very poor quality of fat. The essential fatty acid, docosahexaenoic acid (22 : 6n-3), has been found to be absent from vegan diets [1]. Docosahexaenoic acid has an important role in growth, the health of the retina, central nervous system and skin. Vegans should therefore use oils with a low linoleic : α-linolenic acid ratio such as rapeseed, flax and linseed oils [9].

Zen macrobiotic diets

The Zen macrobiotic principle originates from Japan and is based on the correct balance between Yin (positive) and Yang (negative) foods. This

Table 28.5   Sources of nutrients at risk of deficiency in a vegan diet [10,14,24].

Nutrient	Vegan sources	
Riboflavin	Wheat germ Almonds[†] Green leafy vegetables Mushrooms	Avocados Soya beans Fortified soya milk Yeast extracts* e.g. Marmite, Tastex
Vitamin B$_{12}$	Fortified cereals Fortified soya milk Soya meat analogues	Yeast extracts* Tofu
Vitamin D	Fortified margarine Fortified soya milk	Fortified cereals Sunlight
Calcium	Fortified soya milk Green leafy vegetables Legumes White bread Cashew nuts[†]	Hard water Sunflower seeds[†] Sesame seeds Almonds[†]
Iron	Fortified cereals Wholegrain cereals Wholegrain bread Green leafy vegetables Pulses Legumes Tofu	Nuts[†] Dried fruit Molasses Cocoa Curry powder
Iodine	Wholegrains Vegetables	Seaweed
Essential	Oils	Nuts[†]
Fatty acids	Wholegrains	Seeds

* Should be used with care in children under the age of 2 years because of high salt content.
[†] Should not be given to children under the age of 2 years unless finely ground.

balance is believed to keep spiritual, mental and physical wellbeing. There are 10 levels of dietary elimination. Animal products, fruits and vegetables are gradually removed from the diet until the ultimate goal is achieved of consuming only brown rice. Fluids are also severely restricted [14].

This type of diet is nutritionally inadequate for a child of any age. Marked growth retardation, associated with muscle wasting and a delay in gross motor and language development, have been documented in infants fed macrobiotic weaning diets [15,16]. Growth failure [17] and reduced bone mass [18] have also been documented in older children. Deficiencies of vitamins B$_{12}$, D and thiamin, and of

calcium and iron have also been observed [19–22]. Improved growth has been reported following the addition of fatty fish and dairy products to the macrobiotic diet [23].

Fruitarian diets

Fruitarian diets are based on fruit and uncooked fermented cereals and seeds. These diets are nutritionally inadequate for children of any age and can lead to severe protein energy malnutrition, anaemia and multiple vitamin and mineral deficiencies.

Asian diets

The Asian community represents the largest ethnic group in the UK. The communities consist of people who migrated directly from India, Pakistan and Bangladesh and those who came via East Africa [25]. Traditional dietary customs are largely based on the religious and cultural beliefs of the three main religious groups: Hindus, Muslims and Sikhs. Dietary variance is observed within these groups, as income and geographical area [25,26] have an influence on the diet.

Hindus

Approximately 30% of the Asian population in the UK are Hindu. The majority originally came from the Gujarat region of India, although some are from the Indian Punjab and East Africa [25,26]. Hindus believe that the soul is eternal and therefore believe in reincarnation.

Dietary customs

The caste system dictates who can prepare and serve food [25] and dietary restrictions are laid down in the Bhagavad Gita. A restriction on eating beef was introduced in 800 BC because Hindus regard the cow as sacred. It is also unusual for pork to be eaten as the pig is thought to be unclean (Table 28.6). Devout Hindus believe in the doctrine of Ahisma (not killing) and are vegetarian. Some will eat dairy products and eggs, while others refuse

Table 28.6 Asian religious groups [25,26].

Group	Religion	Language	Staple	Dietary customs
Hindus	Hinduism	Hindi Gujarati	Millet Wheat Rice	No beef Often no pork No alcohol Often vegetarian or vegan
Muslims	Islam	Urdu Bengali Gujarati Punjabi	Rice Millet Wheat	No pork Halal meat No alcohol No fish without scales
Sikhs	Sikhism	Punjabi Hindi	Wheat	No beef Often no pork No Halal meat

eggs on the grounds that they are potential sources of life. A minority of Hindus practice veganism.

Wheat is the staple food eaten by Hindus in the UK. It is used to make chapattis, puris and parathas. Oil and ghee (clarified butter), which is believed to sanctify food, are used extensively in cooking [25]. Alcohol is forbidden.

Most Hindus fast on 3 days a year to celebrate the birthdays of the Lords Shiva (March), Rama (April) and Krishna (August). Orthodox Hindus may also fast once or twice every week (often on Tuesdays and Fridays). Fasting lasts from dawn to dusk and varies from avoiding all foods except those considered pure (e.g. rice, fruit and yoghurt) to total food exclusion [25,27].

Muslims

Approximately 30% of the Asian population in the UK are Muslim, the majority originating from Pakistan and Bangladesh [25]. Muslims practice the Islamic religion; Allah is their god and the prophet Mohammed his final messenger.

Dietary customs

The Koran provides Muslims with their food laws. The consumption of Haram foods: pork, carnivorous animals, fish without scales, some birds and alcohol is strictly prohibited [25]. All meat and poultry must be ritually slaughtered (bled to death and then blessed) to render it Halal making it legitimate

to eat [25]. Wheat, usually in the form of chapattis, is the staple cereal eaten by Muslims from Pakistan, whereas those from Bangladesh eat more rice [25,26]. Cooking oil is used in preference to ghee.

During the lunar month of Ramadan, Muslims fast between sunrise and sunset. Children under the age of 12 years and the elderly are exempt from fasting. People who are ill, pregnant, menstruating or on a long journey are also excused, but are expected to fast at a later date. Unfortunately, many pregnant women fast with the rest of the family during Ramadan as they find it more convenient [25,27]. The Koran also dictates that children should be breast fed up to the age of 2 years [25].

Sikhs

The remaining 40% of the Asian population in the UK are Sikh. Sikhism is a relatively new religion, originating as a reformist movement of Hinduism, in the Indian Punjab in the sixteenth century. Sikhs believe in reincarnation and in one personal god who is eternal, the creator of the universe and the source of all being [25,27]. Devout Sikhs undergo Amarit, a special kind of confirmation where certain practices must be followed. Prayers must be said every day and Sikhs must not drink alcohol, smoke or eat Halal meat. They must also adhere to a strict ethical code and wear the five signs of Sikhism: Kesh (uncut hair), Kara (steel or silver bangle), Kanga (comb), Kirpa (small symbolic dagger) and Kaccha (special undergarments).

Dietary customs

Most Sikhs will not eat pork or beef but some will eat lamb, poultry, fish, eggs and dairy produce. Vegetarianism is common, with eggs and dairy produce usually being eaten [25,27].

Wheat and, to a lesser extent, rice are the main staples eaten and ghee and oil are used in cooking [25]. Devout Sikhs fast once to twice weekly and most will fast on the first day of the Punjabi month or when there is a full moon. This again varies from total food exclusion to eating only pure foods [27].

Common Asian dietary customs

Many of the Asian people in the UK share dietary

Table 28.7   Foods commonly eaten by the Asian population in the UK [24,28,29].

Food	Nutrients	Method of cooking	
Cereals			
Wheat	Energy	Chapatti	Samosa
	B vitamins	Paratha	Pakora
		Poppodom	Poori
		Bhagi	Fried
Rice		Boiled	
Semolina		Porridges	
Ground rice		Sweetmeats	
Tubers			
Arvi/colocasia root	Energy	Boiled	
Cassava		Fried	
Taro tuber		Curries	
Yam			
Vegetables			
Ackee Okra	Vitamin A	Boiled	
Bringal Pepper	Riboflavin	Fried	
Cho cho/chayote	Folic acid	Curries	
Fenugreek leaves	Vitamin C	Chutneys	
Bitter gourd/darela	Iron	Pickles	
Kantola	Calcium		
Patra leaves	Fibre		
Spinach			
Peas, beans and nuts			
Balor/valor beans	Energy	Curries	Dhals
Blackgram/urad gram	Protein		
Chickpeas/bengal gram	B vitamins		
Cluster beans/guar	Iron		
Coconut	Calcium		
Red lentils/masur dhal	Fibre		
Mung/moong beans			
Papri beans			
Pigeon peas/red gram			
Lima beans			
Fruits			
Guava, lychee, mango	Vitamin A	Raw	
Paw paw/papaya	Vitamin C	Curries	
Indian gooseberries	Fibre	Chutneys	
Dried fruits			
Meat and fish			
Many types	Protein	Curries	
(see Table 28.6)	Fat-soluble	Roast	
	vitamins		
	Iron		
Dairy products			
Milk	Energy	Drinks	
Yoghurt	Protein	Raw	
Cheese/paneer	Vitamin A	Boiled	

Table 28.7   (*Cont'd*)

Food	Nutrients	Method of cooking
Eggs	Riboflavin	Fried
	Nicotinic	
	acid	
	Vitamin D	
	Iron	
	Calcium	
Fats and oils		
Ghee/clarified butter	Energy	Frying
Vegetable oil	Essential	Spreading
Margarine	fatty acids	

customs, despite their varying religious and geographical background (Table 28.7). Older members of the Asian community, especially those originating from Pakistan and Bangladesh, tend to retain traditional dietary customs. However, there is an increasing consumption of westernised foods, especially convenience foods. The extent of adoption of these foods is variable, tending to be greater in the younger generations who were born in the UK and in those who have lived in the UK for some time [25].

At breakfast time chapattis, parathas, bread and occasionally hard boiled or fried eggs are traditionally eaten. The two main meals are based around the staple, usually served with a vegetable, pulse or nut based curry [26,27]. Most foods, including spices, are usually fried before adding to the curry, which is then served with homemade chutneys, side salads of tomatoes and onions and yoghurt [27]. Very little hard cheese is eaten; paneer, an Indian soft curd cheese, is preferred [27]. Meals are usually served with tea, which is made with hot milk and sugar, although English tea is becoming popular [27]. Traditionally, Asians rarely eat snacks, although western snack foods are increasing in popularity. Traditional Asian savoury snacks (usually reserved for celebrations only) are high in fat and the sweets are often very high in refined sugar.

Many Asians believe that foods have heating and cooling effects on the body. These hot and cold foods should be eaten in the correct balance to achieve a healthy state. Certain hot foods cause symptoms such as constipation, sweating and body fatigue, while certain cold foods lead to strength and happiness. Foods may also be used to treat a condition, for example hot foods should be avoided during pregnancy and cold ones avoided when breast feeding [27].

Infant feeding

Early studies reported lower breast feeding rates among Asians in the UK compared with the Caucasian population [30,31] and Asians in the Indian subcontinent [32]. However, high incidences of breast feeding among Bangladeshi, Indian and Pakistani mothers compared with white mothers have more recently been reported in 1997 [33]. In this large survey, which sampled 95% of the Asian population in the UK, Bangladeshi and Pakistani mothers were less likely to continue breast feeding their babies beyond 8 weeks of life. Interestingly, of mothers who were born outside the UK, 30–40% who bottle fed initially or who stopped breast feeding to bottle fed reported that they would have fed their babies differently had the babies not been born in the UK. Unfortunately, for some bottle feeding is perceived as the western ideal and therefore better for the baby. There is also often a lack of education promoting breast feeding in the Asian community [25,31]. This problem is compounded by communication difficulties and overcrowded housing [5], making it difficult for a mother to breast feed in privacy.

Weaning

Social disadvantage, the varying quality, expense and availability of familiar Asian weaning foods and the pressures of westernisation may compromise good weaning practice [34]. Late weaning and prolonged breast feeding are common in infants who are born on the Indian subcontinent and those who have only been in the UK for a short time [30–32,35]. In the UK late weaning may be partly because of the poor availability of suitable foods and the lack of adequate and appropriate advice [33]. Some Asian infants born in the UK are weaned earlier [31,32], but are commonly given sweet commercial weaning foods that are low in protein and iron [30,31,34,35]. This mainly occurs because many mothers do not know the composition of

Table 28.8 Suitable Asian weaning foods.

Around 6 months	
Puréed	Cauliflower and potato*
	Cauliflower and pea*
	Pea and potato*
	Aubergine and potato*
	Green vegetable and potato*
	Vegetable and cheese*
	Lentil and rice*
	Chickpea and marrow*
	Porridge
	Fruit

7–12 months
Introduce small lumps to the above foods
Mild spices, e.g. cumin and coriander may be used
Introduce finger foods, e.g. small pieces of chapatti

* A small amount of meat, poultry or fish may be added if eaten.

savoury weaning products and will not use them unless they are vegetarian [25]. Because of these problems, mothers should be encouraged to cook savoury weaning foods at home. Suitable homemade Asian weaning foods are given in Table 28.8. The practice of sweetening milk and adding foods such as rusk, honey, Weetabix and baby rice to bottles is also common [25,31,33] and should be discouraged.

Many Asian infants are given cow's milk from the age of 5 months [25,33]. This results in a higher saturated fat and salt intake and a reduced vitamin D and iron intake than if breast milk or infant formula were continued [8]. Feeding development is often delayed because of late conversion from bottle to cup and very late progression onto family foods [25,31,33,35]. It is not unusual for a 2-year-old to derive the majority of their nutrition from bottles of cow's milk and sweetened fruit drinks.

Very few differences have been reported between the diets of first and second generation Asians [36]. It has been suggested that this may be because of the cohesive nature of the community and because all young children are subject to similar dietary and cultural expectations and pressures. Therefore, infant feeding practices among the Asian population can still be improved:

- The teaching curriculum of all catering and health-related training should include ethnic cultures, food and diet, so that effective education on all aspects of infant feeding can be given [35]. This training should be updated regularly [31].

- Practical demonstrations, the use of bilingual interpreters and written advice in the Asian languages should be available [25,31,35].
- Education promoting breast feeding should reach the parents before pregnancy, and support should be given while breast feeding [31].
- Breast or formula milk should be given up to 1 year of age [31].
- Sugary drinks should be avoided [31].
- Infants should be weaned around 6 months of age.
- Weaning advice should include the use of appropriate family foods in addition to commercial baby foods [25,31].
- Salt, sugar, honey or hot spices should not be added to bottles or weaning foods.
- Advice should be given on foods rich in vitamin C, vitamin D and iron, as these nutrients may be at risk of deficiency [31].
- The cup should be introduced between 6 months and 1 year of age [31].
- Vitamin drops should be given from the age of 6 months up to 2 years and preferably up to 5 years [8].

Nutritional problems commonly found in Asian children

Faltering growth

Dietary intake, family income, housing standards, maternal education, psychological distress and morbidity all influence growth [25,30]. Low birth weight has been reported in the Asian population, both in this country and in the homeland [32,37]. Birth weight has, however, increased over the last 15 years. Longer birth intervals, fewer teenage pregnancies and improved nutrition are thought to be contributing factors [25].

Despite lower birth weights, some studies show that Asian babies and children grow as well as the indigenous population [25,32,33,37–39]. In contrast, others suggest that growth failure is still common [40]. These conflicting observations highlight the importance of individually assessing the need for nutritional supplementation.

Iron deficiency anaemia

Iron deficiency anaemia has been described in Asian infants [41,42]. Contributing factors include maternal iron deficiency during pregnancy, premature delivery and low birthweight. Inadequate dietary intake of iron is commonly related to the early introduction and excessive use of unfortified cow's milk [25]. Prolonged use of a baby bottle and the mother being born outside the UK have also been shown to have a negative influence on the iron status of Asian children [42]. Advice should include information on the use of foods rich in iron and vitamin C, as the diets of Asian children are unlikely to regularly contain fresh vegetables [33].

Megaloblastic anaemia

Megaloblastic anaemia resulting from vitamin B_{12} deficiency has been observed in some strict vegetarian and vegan Asians [43]. Education regarding vitamin B_{12} sources in the vegetarian diet is required and supplementation may be needed in the vegan diet.

Rickets

The steady decline in rickets in the UK was halted in the late 1960s and early 1970s when a number of cases appeared in immigrant families, mainly of Asian origin [35,44,45]. There is now evidence that the incidence is in decline again following large scale vitamin D supplementation [25]. However, low plasma vitamin D levels are still observed in some members of the Asian population, especially those of Pakistani origin and those who do not take routine vitamin supplements [46–48].

In addition to the dietary intake of vitamin D, other factors such as low sunlight exposure, skin pigmentation, late weaning, high fibre and high phytate intakes may also contribute to the development of rickets in Asian children [25]. The weaning diets of infants should include foods rich in vitamin D such as milk, milk products, eggs, oily fish, liver, fortified cereals and margarine [5,49,50]. Vitamin D supplementation is advisable for infants, young children and deficient pregnant women to prevent neonatal hypocalcaemia and rickets [5,25,49]. In addition, children should be encouraged to play outside [50].

Dental caries

Traditionally, sugary foods are reserved for celebrations and therefore do not have a major role in Asian diets. However, with increasing westernisation, over-consumption of refined sugar leading to a high incidence of dental caries has been observed in Asian pre-school children [51]. Asian mothers often add sugar to babies' bottles and give sweetened drinks via the bottle for prolonged periods. These drinks, as well as having a high sugar content, are acidic which can lead to tooth decay [31]. Education regarding infant feeding with the restriction of quantity and frequency of sugar intake, the use of fluoride-containing drops and toothpaste and frequent dental visits will help to reduce the incidence of dental caries.

Obesity and diabetes

With the increasing consumption of high sugar and high fat foods the prevalence of obesity is increasing. The incidence of obesity and diabetes is now higher in Asian children than in Caucasian children (see pp. 176, 588). In addition to restricting these foods, advice on acceptable Asian food alternatives and appropriate cooking techniques must be given. The dietary fat intake can be reduced by avoiding deep fried foods, reducing the amount of oil or ghee used in cooking and restricting or not adding fat to chapattis. Avoiding the popular sweet sugary tea and Asian sweetmeats will reduce dietary sugar.

Afro-Caribbean diets

The Afro-Caribbean community is the second largest ethnic minority group in the UK [25,52].

Dietary patterns

The two main meals are taken at breakfast time and in the evening [53,54]. Traditional breakfasts include fried plantain, cornmeal dumplings and fried dumplings. However, many dietary practices have now been adopted from British culture, with toast and cereals largely replacing these foods. The evening meal is more likely to contain traditional foods, especially with the younger generation who seem keen to retain their identification and culture. Cereals and tubers such as rice, green banana, yam and sweet potato form the main part of the diet [52]. These starchy foods are served with small amounts of meat or fish [53]. The tropical climate in the homeland makes it difficult to keep foods fresh and therefore preserved meat, fish and milk are eaten [52]. Peas, beans, nuts and green leafy vegetables are widely used, often being made into homemade soups and stews which are well seasoned with herbs and spices (Table 28.9) [25].

Rastafarians

A minority of the Afro-Caribbean population within the UK are Rastafarians. Dietary beliefs are based on laws laid down by Moses in Genesis which state that certain types of meat should be avoided. However, many Rastafarians avoid meat completely to obey the commandment 'thou shalt not kill'. Vinegar, raisins, grapes and wine are also avoided by some Rastafarians as the Nazarite law states that fruits of the vine should not be eaten. Dietary restrictions are followed with varying degrees of strictness. The most orthodox follow a vegan diet and will only eat 'Ital' (natural) foods; chemicals and additives are thought to pollute the body and soul [52]. In addition, salt is also prohibited. All food must be fresh rather than processed and fruit and vegetables must be organic. Many Rastafarians are socially deprived and find it difficult to provide adequate nutrition for their children within the dietary code [25]. Less orthodox Rastafarians, although accepting the central tenets of 'Ital', will eat dairy products, small amounts of fish with scales, sea salt and other seasonings. The nutritional adequacy of these diets is much easier to achieve.

Infant feeding

Infant feeding is mainly influenced by the place of birth, knowledge of traditional practices and advice from relatives. In the homeland over 90% of women breast feed their babies initially. However, even in Africa, this is often short-lived and exclusive breast feeding is rare [52]. The large scale marketing of infant formulas and the early return of women

Table 28.9   Foods commonly eaten by the Afro-Caribbean population in the UK [52,55].

Food	Nutrients	Method of cooking
Cereals		
Wheat	Energy	Boiled
Oats	B vitamins	Dumplings
Maize		Porridges
Rice		Bread
Tubers		
Green banana	Energy	Mashed
Sweet potato	B vitamins	Fried
Bread fruit	Vitamin C	Roasted
Yams		Stewed
Cassava		
Plantain		
Peas, beans and nuts		
Red peas	Protein	Stews
Pigeon peas	B vitamins	Boiled
Coconut	Calcium	
Almonds	Iron	
Sesame seeds	Fibre	
Black eyed peas		
Broad beans		
Channa		
Cashews		
Pumpkin seeds		
Dark green leafy vegetables		
Cabbage	Vitamin A	Stews
Carrot	Vitamin C	Stir fry
Egg plant	Calcium	
Okra	Iron	
Callaloo		
Dasheen leaves		
Karela		
Pumpkin		
Fruit		
Avocado	Vitamin C	Fresh
Cashewfruit		Stewed
Guava		
Oranges		
Paw-paw		
Sapodilla		
Mango		
Cane sugar		
Grapefruit		
Oteheite apple		
Passion fruit		
Pineapple		
Soursop		
Coolie		
Meat and fish		
Mainly chicken	Protein	Fry
Many types of fish	Fat-soluble	Steam

Table 28.9   (*Cont'd*)

Food	Nutrients	Method of cooking
	vitamins	Roast
	Iron	Boil
		Stewed
		Bake
Eggs		
	Protein	Scrambled
	Vitamin A	Cake
	Vitamin D	Fritters
	Iron	Puddings
Fats and oils		
Coconut oil	Essential	Frying
Olive oil	fatty acids	Spreading
Margarine		Baking
Lard		
Vegetable oil		
Butter		
Suet		

to work are implicated. Many Afro-Caribbean mothers avoid giving their infants colostrum and in its place give water, which is thought to cleanse the body before the breast milk is given. This practice may reduce breast milk production and therefore also contribute to the low exclusive breast feeding rate both in this country and in Africa.

Weaning

Infants are traditionally weaned as early as 1 month of age and 45% are reported to be receiving food by 3 months [52–54]. In contrast, late weaning is commonly observed within the orthodox Rastafarian population [5]. Common weaning solids include high starch foods with a low nutrient density such as cornmeal, oats or rice porridge. This practice may lead to energy, protein, vitamin and mineral deficiencies if continued for a long time [5,27,56,57]. More suitable weaning foods are shown in Table 28.10. The common practice of adding thin porridge to bottles should be discouraged as it can lead to a delay in the weaning process. It is also common for infants to be given bush teas (infusions of herbs and leaves) as a cure for minor ailments [53]. Care should be taken to ensure that these are not given instead of milk.

Table 28.10   Suitable Afro-Caribbean weaning foods.

Around 6 months
Rice or oat porridge
Puréed fruit
Puréed vegetables, e.g. yam, peas, okra
Puréed vegetables and meat or fish
Puréed rice and vegetable
Egg custard

7–12 months
Introduce:
   Small lumps to the above foods
   Mashed family foods avoiding highly seasoned foods
   Finger foods, e.g. toast, biscuits, fruit

By the age of 9 months most infants are eating family foods with the diet having both traditional and western influences [53].

Nutritional problems found in Afro-Caribbean children

Obesity and diabetes

With the adoption of British dietary customs there has been an increase in the consumption of high sugar and high fat convenience foods and drinks. This has led to an increased prevalence of obesity and diabetes in Afro-Caribbean children compared to Caucasian children (see pp. 176, 588).

Iron deficiency anaemia

Iron deficiency anaemia has been observed in Afro-Caribbean children living in the UK. The main causes are thought to be prolonged bottle feeding, late weaning onto foods with a low iron content and the early introduction and excessive use of cow's milk [25].

Megaloblastic anaemia

There have been reports of megaloblastic anaemia in Rastafarian children living in Jamaica [58,59]. Vegan children may require vitamin B_{12} supplementation.

Rickets

Rickets has been seen in Afro-Caribbean children

[25,57]. Advice on dietary sources of vitamin D and calcium and vitamin D supplementation is beneficial.

Lactose intolerance

There is a high incidence of lactose intolerance because of hypolactasia among the Afro-Caribbean population. A reduction in, and occasionally the avoidance of, the consumption of milk and other foods containing lactose will usually reduce symptoms (see p. 404).

Chinese diets

Chinese people represent the third largest ethnic group in the UK [60]. Over 25% are British born; the rest originate from the Caribbean, Hong Kong, Taiwan, China, Malaysia and Singapore [60]. Dietary habits vary according to the country and region of origin.

Dietary patterns

Very few foods are avoided, with the exception of pork, which is not eaten by the Chinese Muslim population. Eggs are highly valued as they are regarded as food for the brain. Northern China has a cool climate favouring the growth of wheat, maize, sorghum and millet. These staples are often made into steamed bread, dumplings, pancakes or noodles [27,60]. Meals are often based on root vegetables such as sweet potato and turnip, with very little meat being eaten. In contrast, because of its high rainfall, rice is the staple in southern China. Fresh vegetables and fruit are also found in abundance [60]. In the east, because of the long coastline, fish and shellfish are plentiful. In the west, livestock are reared and therefore the consumption of meat, milk and cheese is much higher [60].

Traditional breakfasts include rice porridge (congee), served either plain or with liver, meat, salted fish, salted eggs or Chinese cheese and a soup made from rice and meat [27,60]. These traditional foods are, however, slowly being replaced by western alternatives. The midday and evening meals consist of boiled rice or noodles and a variety of highly seasoned dishes such as fried or steamed meat and fish and stir-fried vegetables. Raw food is rarely eaten, as fertiliser in China commonly contains human manure. Meals are usually served with either China tea or a thin soup and then followed with fruit. Sweet foods are usually reserved for special occasions [27,60].

The main health concern is the high salt intake associated with many of the preserved foods, seasonings and soya sauce. A high fat and refined sugar intake associated with the increasing consumption of western foods, especially by the younger generation is also of concern [60]. A high incidence of lactose intolerance, because of hypolactasia, is also becoming apparent with the increasing consumption of milk and other dairy products [60].

Yin and Yang foods

To Chinese people health is perceived as the maintenance of a sound body and mental state, rather than absence of disease. Traditional Chinese medicine states that good health relies on the body's balance of two opposite elements, Yin (cold), which represents female energy, and Yang (hot), which represents male energy [27,60]. In illness the balance becomes disturbed and the body becomes either too hot or too cold. Tolerance of Yin and Yang increases with age; thus an adult can eat a much wider variety of foods than can a child. The classification of foods varies: in general meat, duck, goose, oily fish, potatoes, coffee, chocolate, sugar, nuts, herbs, spices, alcohol and fats are regarded as hot foods; chicken, milk, rice and some vegetables are neutral foods; fish, shellfish, soya beans, certain fruits and vegetables and barley water are cold foods. Stewing, deep fat frying, grilling and roasting makes foods hotter, steaming neutralises and boiling and stir-frying have a cooling effect [27,60]. The Chinese believe that a healthy diet should be three parts Yang and two parts Yin. The balance should be changed for certain illnesses (e.g. for hyperactivity more Yin foods should be eaten than Yang foods).

During pregnancy and after childbirth the woman's body is thought to become cool and therefore cold foods are avoided. Alcohol, ice cream, mutton, beef and fizzy drinks are also avoided. In addition, if the woman is breast feeding, green vegetables and fruit are avoided because of concern that they may give the baby diarrhoea. As a consequence

breast feeding mothers often have a high protein intake [60].

Infant feeding

In the UK, Chinese women often return to work soon after childbirth, which has led to a decrease in the rate and duration of breast feeding. Low breast feeding rates in the Chinese population living in other countries have also been observed [61,62]. Soya bean oil, which is a poor source of essential fatty acids, is a major source of fat in the Chinese diet. Because of this, breast milk has been found to have a low concentration of docosahexaenoic acid (DHA) and arachidonic acid (AA) [63]. It has, therefore, been suggested that mothers who are breast feeding their infants should supplement their diet with a good source of DHA and AA such as fish oil.

Because infant formula is regarded as hot, bottle fed babies are often given frequent cooling drinks such as water and barley water. Most infants are weaned at 3 months of age. Traditionally, rice based porridges are introduced but more recently commercial baby foods are being used [60]. A study examining westernisation of the nutritional pattern of Chinese children living in France reported that at 1 year of age Chinese children mainly consumed a traditional diet. The intake of dairy products and fresh fruit was very low and that of soft drinks high, resulting in suboptimal calcium and vitamin C intakes [61]. In general, infants are thought to have a hot equilibrium and therefore neutralising or cooling foods are considered best for them. It is common practice for children to be given afternoon tea consisting of cooling foods such as bread, biscuits, cake, barley water and herb teas to counteract the heating effect of school meals [60].

Vietnamese diets

Some 75% of Vietnamese settlers in the UK are ethnic Chinese and, therefore, share many of the Chinese traditions [60].

Food habits

The Vietnamese diet is typically high in

carbohydrate and low in fat [64]. Vietnam borders the ocean and has an extensive river system and therefore fish and shellfish are staple parts of the traditional diet. There are no forbidden foods; however, certain unfamiliar foods such as lamb, ox liver, tinned or cooked fruit and some root vegetables may be avoided [27]. Rice is the main staple food and is served either boiled or fried with small amounts of meat or fish. Like Chinese food, main dishes are often heavily seasoned and vegetables are lightly steamed or stir-fried in oil or lard. The resultant high sodium intake is the main health issue. Very little fresh milk, butter, margarine and cheese are used, because of their lack of availability in Vietnam and the high incidence of lactose intolerance. Snacks of roasted nuts, sweet potatoes, rice or noodle soup, spring rolls and fresh fruit are frequently eaten. Common beverages include tea, coffee and fruit juice and alcohol is taken on special occasions [27]. With increasing westernisation, the intake of high sugar and high fat snack foods is increasing, especially in the younger generation. This has led to an increase in dental caries and obesity in the Vietnamese population, both in the UK [65] and other countries [66]. Unfortunately, obesity is traditionally seen as a sign of prosperity.

The Vietnamese people observe hot and cold food principles, similar to the Chinese. In contrast to the Chinese, however, pregnancy is regarded as a hot condition and therefore women eat less red meat and fish. A traditional stew called Keung Chow, made from pigs' trotters, boiled eggs, vinegar and ginger, is given to women after childbirth to help recovery and to celebrate the birth of the child. After childbirth, women are encouraged to eat hot foods to regain their strength [27].

Infant feeding

Since their arrival in westernised countries, including the UK, Vietnamese mothers have abandoned traditional infant feeding practices in favour of more modern bottle feeding methods [66–69]. In addition, many Vietnamese women believe that breast feeding will cause their breasts to sag. Hence the incidence of breast feeding is low and there is a need for culturally sensitive health education programmes to support breast feeding in this group. Infants are typically given a rice based porridge at

around 6 months, minced meat and vegetables are given at 9 months and more solid food at 1 year.

Nutrients at risk of deficiency

Iron

There is an increased risk of iron deficiency in young Vietnamese children [70]. This is particularly associated with a high milk intake and poor body weight.

Calcium

Children are at risk of calcium deficiency, especially if minimal milk and associated products are eaten [27]. The rice traditionally grown in Vietnam is a good source of calcium, but is unavailable in Britain. Traditional Vietnamese fruit and vegetables also contain more calcium than British varieties [27].

Vitamin D

Deficiency of vitamin D has been noted in Vietnamese children. For this reason children may need vitamin D supplementation [27].

Somalian diets

The Somalis first settled in the UK in 1914 when they were recruited to fight in the First World War. They are now thought to be the oldest African community in London. Later arrivals included Somalian asylum seekers who fled the civil unrest in their country and settled around the main cities in the UK. Today there are second, third and fourth generation Somalis living in the UK.

Dietary patterns

Somalis are of Arab-African ethnicity and their faith is Islam. They therefore share many of the Islamic (Muslim) dietary customs. Somalia was formed in 1960 from a British Protectorate and an Italian Colony. As a result many Southern Somalis eat Italian food and spaghetti is a national dish. The Somalian diet tends to be relatively high in protein.

Breakfast usually consists of 2–3 pieces of injera (a fermented pancake-like Somali bread made from corn and wheat) with ghee or butter and tea. Lunch is the main meal and usually consists of spaghetti or rice with a meat sauce (beef or goat) and mixed vegetables. Food is often flavoured with aromatic spices (cumin powder, cinnamon, cloves, cardamon, garlic, cilantro, parsley). Pork is avoided and chicken, fish and eggs are not usually eaten. The evening meal consists of injera or bread with butter and jam, or a traditional meal of rice, beans, butter and sugar. Desserts and snacks are not considered as part of the daily diet. Sweets are usually given to children but are not usually eaten by adults. Children usually drink cow's or goat's milk three times or more each day. From the age of 3 years, sweetened tea is usually added to the milk.

During pregnancy Somali women tend to decrease their meals to ensure an easier delivery. They believe that too much food will make the baby grow too big and it will be hard to deliver normally. The diet usually improves during the third trimester although most women do not take prenatal vitamins.

Infant feeding

Almost all women breast feed, often for 2–3 years. Breast milk is not offered in the first 24 hours when infants may be given sugar water or fresh cow's or goat's milk. Colostrum is thought to have a poor nutritional value or to be unhealthy, and it often expressed and discarded. A mixture of rice and cow's milk is introduced at 6 months of age and drinks from a cup are offered at 6–8 months [71].

Nutrients at risk of deficiency in the Somalian diet

Calcium and vitamin D

The traditional Somalian diet is low in vitamin D and calcium and could give rise to poor bone mineralisation and the development of osteoporosis [72]. Vitamin D deficiency has been reported in 82% of Somalis living in Liverpool [72]. Dietary advice should therefore focus on improving the intake of these nutrients from dietary sources and considera-

tion should be given to additional supplementation with vitamin D where appropriate.

References

1   Mesina V, Mangels AR Considerations in planning vegan diets: children. *J Am Diet Assoc*, 2001, **101** 661–9.
2   Hebbelinck M, Clarys P, De Malsche A Growth, development, and physical fitness of Flemish vegetarian children, adolescents, and young adolescents. *Am J Clin Nutr*, 1999, **70** 579S–85S.
3   Sanders TA Vegetarian diets and children. *Pediatr Clin North Am*, 1995, **42** 955–65.
4   Hackett A, Nathan I, Burgess L Is a vegetarian diet adequate for children? *Nutr Health*, 1998, **12** 189–95.
5   Wardley BL, Puntis JWL, Taitz LS Cultural and ethnic diets. In: *Handbook of Child Nutrition*, 2nd edn. Oxford: Oxford University Press, 1997, pp. 113–29.
6   Weiss R, Fogelman Y, Bennett M Severe vitamin B_{12} deficiency in an infant associated with a maternal deficiency and strict vegetarian diet. *J Pediatr Hematol Oncol*, 2004, **26** 270–1.
7   Roschitz B *et al*. Nutritional infantile vitamin B_{12} deficiency: pathobiochemical considerations in seven patients. *Arch Dis Child Fetal Neonatal Ed* 2005, **90** F281–2.
8   Committee on Medical Aspects of Food Policy *Present day practice in infant feeding*. Report of a Working Party of the Panel on Child Nutrition. London: The Stationery Office, 1988.
9   Sanders TAB, Manning J The growth and development of vegan children. *J Hum Nutr Diet*, 1992, **5** 11–21.
10 Sanders TA Growth and development of British vegan children. *Am J Clin Nutr*, 1988, **48** 822–5.
11 Gibson RS Content and bioavailability of trace elements in vegetarian diets. *Am J Clin Nutr*, 1994, **59** 1223–32.
12 Hunt JR Bioavailability of iron, zinc and other trace minerals from vegetarian diets. *Am J Clin Nutr*, 2003, **78** 633S–9S.
13 Committee on Medical Aspects of Food Policy *Diet and Cardiovascular Disease*. DHSS Report on Health and Social Subjects. London: The Stationery Office, 1984.
14 Thomas B (ed.) Vegetarianism and veganism. In: *Manual of Dietetic Practice*, 3rd edn. Oxford: Blackwell Science, 2001, pp. 304–14.
15 Dagnelie PC *et al*. Nutritional status of infants aged 4–18 months on macrobiotic diets and matched omnivorous control infants: a population based mixed longitudinal study. II: Growth and psychomotor development. *Eur J Clin Nutr*, 1989, **43** 325–38.

16   Dagnelie PC *et al.* Do children on macrobiotic diets show catch up growth? A population based cross sectional study in children aged 0–8 years. *Eur J Clin Nutr*, 1988, **42** 1007–16.

17   Van Dusseldorp *et al.* Catch-up growth in children fed a macrobiotic diet in early childhood. *J Nutr*, 1996, **126** 2977–83.

18   Parsons TJ *et al.* Reduced bone mass in Dutch adolescents fed a macrobiotic diet in early life. *J Bone Miner Res*, 1997, **12** 1486–94.

19   Herens MC *et al.* Nutrition and mental development of 4–5 year old children on macrobiotic diets. *J Hum Nutr Diet*, 1992, **5** 1–9.

20   Dagnelie PC *et al.* Nutritional status of infants aged 4–18 months on macrobiotic diets and matched omnivorous control infants: a population based mixed longitudinal study. I: Weaning patterns, energy and nutrient intake. *Eur J Clin Nutr*, 1989, **43** 311–23.

21   Dagnelie PC *et al.* Increased risk of vitamin B_{12} and iron deficiency in infants on macrobiotic diets. *Am J Clin Nutr*, 1989, **50** 818–24.

22   Dagnelie PC *et al.* High prevalence of rickets in infants on macrobiotic diets. *Am J Clin Nutr*, 1990, **51** 202–8.

23   Dagnelie PC *et al.* Effects of macrobiotic diets on linear growth in infants and children until 10 years of age. *Eur J Clin Nutr*, 1994, **48** S103–11.

24   Food Standards Agency *McCance and Widdowson's The Composition of Foods*, 6th summary edn. Cambridge: Royal Society of Chemistry, 2002.

25   Health Education Authority *Nutrition in Minority Ethnic Groups: Asians and Afro-Caribbeans in the United Kingdom*. London: HEA, 1991.

26   Price SR Observations on dietary practices in India. *Hum Nutr Appl Nutr*, 1984, **38A** 383–9.

27   Thomas B (ed.) People from ethnic minority groups. In: *Manual of Dietetic Practice*. Oxford: Blackwell Science, 2001, pp. 283–303.

28   Tan SP, Wenlock RW, Buss DH *Immigrant Foods*. The Second Supplement to *McCance and Widdowson's The Composition of Foods*. London: The Stationery Office, 1985.

29   Jaffrey M *Indian Cookery*. London: BBC Books, 1988.

30   Warrington S, Storey DM Comparative studies on Asian and Caucasian children. 2: Nutrition, feeding practices and health. *Eur J Clin Nutr*, 1988, **42** 69–80.

31   Sahota P *Feeding Baby: Inner City Practice*. Bradford: Horton Publishing, 1991.

32   McNeill G Birth weight, feeding practice and weight/age of Punjabi children in the UK and in the rural Punjab. *Hum Nutr Clin Nutr*, 1985, **39C** 69–72.

33   Thomas M, Avery V *Infant Feeding in Asian Families*. Office for National Statistics. London: The Stationery Office, 1997.

34   Sarwar T Infant feeding practices of Pakistani mothers in England and Pakistan. *J Hum Nutr Diet*, 2002, **15** 419–28.

35   Jones VM Current weaning practices within the Bangladeshi community in the London Borough of Tower Hamlets. *Hum Nutr Appl Nutr*, 1987, **41A** 349–52.

36   Parsons S *et al.* Are there intergenerational differences in the diets of young children born to first- and second-generation Pakistani Muslims in Bradford, West Yorkshire? *J Hum Nutr Diet*, 1999, **12** 113–22.

37   Warrington S, Storey DM Comparative studies on Asian and Caucasian children. 1: Growth. *Eur J Clin Nutr*, 1988, **42** 61–7.

38   Duggan MB, Harbottle L The growth and nutritional status of healthy Asian children aged 4–40 months living in Sheffield. *Br J Nutr*, 1996, **76** 183–97.

39   Gatrad AR, Birch N, Hughes M Preschool weights and heights of Europeans and five subgroups of Asians in Britain. *Arch Dis Child*, 1994, **71** 207–10.

40   Rona R, Chinn S National study of health and growth: social and biological factors associated with height of children from ethnic groups living in England. *Ann Hum Biol*, 1986, **13** 453–71.

41   Ehrhardt P Iron deficiency anaemia in young Bradford children from different ethnic groups. *Br Med J*, 1986, **292** 90–3.

42   Lawson MS, Thomas M, Hardiman A Iron status of Asian children aged 2 years living in England. *Arch Dis Child*, 1998, **78** 420–6.

43   Chanarin I *et al.* Megaloblastic anaemia in a vegetarian Hindu community. *Lancet*, 1985, **2** 1168–72.

44   Goel KM *et al.* Reduced prevalence of rickets in Asian children in Glasgow. *Lancet*, 1985, **ii** 405–7.

45   Dunnigan MG *et al.* Prevention of rickets in Asian children: assessment of the Glasgow campaign. *Br Med J*, 1985, **291** 239–42.

46   Lawson MS, Thomas M, Hardiman A Dietary and lifestyle factors affecting plasma vitamin D levels in Asian children living in England. *Eur J Clin Nutr*, 1999, **53** 268–72.

47   Lawson M, Thomas M Vitamin D concentrations in Asian children aged 2 years living in England: population survey. *Br Med J*, 1999, **318** 28.

48   Iqbal SJ *et al.* Continuing clinically severe vitamin D deficiency in Asians in the UK (Leicester). *Postgrad Med J*, 1994, **70** 708–14.

49   Department of Health. *Nutrition and Bone Health: With particular reference to calcium and vitamin D.* Report on Health and Social Subjects 49. London: The Stationery Office, 1998.

50   Wharton BA Low plasma vitamin D in Asian toddlers in Britain. *Br Med J*, 1999, **318** 2–3.

51   Holt RD *et al.* Caries in pre-school children in Camden 1993/94. *Br Dent J*, 1996, **181** 405–10.

52 Douglas J *Caribbean Food and Diet*. Cambridge: National Extension College for Training in Health and Race, 1987.

53 Kemm J, Douglas J, Sylvester V Afro-Caribbean diet survey interim report to the Birmingham inner city partnership programme. *Proc Nutr Soc*, 1986, **45** 87A.

54 Kemm J, Douglas J, Sylvester V A survey of infant feeding practice by Afro-Caribbean mothers in Birmingham. *Proc Nutr Soc*, 1986, **45** 87A.

55 Holland B, Unwin ID, Buss DH *Vegetables, herbs and spices*. Fifth supplement to *McCance & Widdowson's The Composition of Foods*, 4th edn. London: Royal Society of Chemistry/MAFF, 1991.

56 Springer L, Thomas J Rastafarians in Britain: a preliminary study of their food habits and beliefs. *Hum Nutr Appl Nutr*, 1983, **37A** 120–7.

57 James JA, Clark C, Ward PS Screening Rastafarian children for nutritional rickets. *Br Med J*, 1985, **290** 899–900.

58 Campbell M, Lofters WS, Gibbs WN Rastafarianism and the vegan syndrome. *Br Med J*, 1982, **285** 1617–18.

59 Close GC Rastafarians and the vegan syndrome. *Br Med J*, 1983, **286** 473.

60 Goodburn PC, Falshaw M, Hughes H *Chinese Food and Diet*. Cambridge: National Extension College for Training in Health and Race, 1987.

61 Roville-Sausse FN Westernization of the nutritional pattern of Chinese children living in France. *Public Health*, 2005, **119** 726–33.

62 Leung S, Davies DP Infant feeding and growth of Chinese infants: birth to 2 years. *Paediatr Perinat Epidemiol*, 1994, **8** 301–13.

63 Xiang M, Lei S, Li T, Zetterstrom R Composition of long chain polyunsaturated fatty acids in human milk and growth of young infants in rural areas of northern China. *Acta Paediatr*, 1999, **88** 126–31.

64 Carlson E, Kipps M, Thomson J An evaluation of a traditional Vietnamese diet in the UK. *Hum Nutr: Appl Nutr*, 1982, **36** 107–15.

65 Todd R, Gelbier S Dental caries prevalence in Vietnamese children and teenagers in three London Boroughs. *Br Dent J*, 1990, **168** 24–6.

66 Harrison R *et al*. Feeding practices and dental caries in an urban Canadian population of Vietnamese preschool children. *ASDC J Dent Child*, 1997, **64** 112–17.

67 Rossiter JC Promoting breast feeding: the perceptions of Vietnamese mothers in Sydney, Australia. *J Adv Nurs*, 1998, **28** 598–605.

68 Sharma A, Lynch MA, Irvine ML The availability of advice regarding infant feeding to immigrants of Vietnamese origin: a survey of families and health visitors. *Child Care Health Dev*, 1994, **20** 349–54.

69 Nguyen ND *et al*. Growth and feeding practices of Vietnamese infants in Australia. *Eur J Clin Nutr*, 2004, **58** 352–62.

70 Nguyen ND *et al*. Iron status of young Vietnamese children in Australia. *J Pediatr Child Health*, 2004, **40** 424–9.

71 www.ethnomed.org Accessed 10 March 2006.

72 Maxwell SM, Salah SM, Bunn JEG Dietary habits of the Somali population in Liverpool, with respect to foods containing calcium and vitamin D: a cause for concern? *J Hum Nutr Diet*, 2006, **19** 125–7.

29 Faltering Growth

Zofia Smith

Introduction

The term 'failure to thrive' (FTT) was used to describe infants and young children who fail to achieve expected growth as assessed by measurements of weight and height. In the early 1920s, the poor growth and miserable state of many deprived infants and young children was observed in institutions. During the 1940s, Spitz termed this disorder 'hospitalism' [1], suggesting that understimulation, emotional deprivation and poor nutrition were all contributing factors to 'retarded growth'.

Traditionally, FTT had been subdivided into the two categories of 'organic' and 'non-organic' failure to thrive. This division is no longer thought to be appropriate as the two categories are not mutually exclusive, and undernutrition is now accepted as the primary cause of poor growth in infancy [2].

Medical conditions such as gastrointestinal disease, neurological disorders or congenital heart disease may be a contributing factor in failure to thrive. However, only 5% of children who are failing to thrive have an underlying medical condition [3]. In the absence of physical disease, a combination of factors can contribute to poor growth in young infants at a time when energy needs are extremely high.

In more recent years, the term failure to thrive has itself been criticised for being pejorative. Parents perceive themselves to be failures, rather than the child's growth, and feel blamed for a child's inadequate intake. Although 'failure to thrive' is still used by health professionals, other terms such as slow weight gain, undernutrition and faltering growth have been suggested as alternatives, with the latter being accepted and used more widely today [4].

When does faltering growth become a cause for concern?

Normal growth is usually defined in relative terms. Centile charts allow a child's growth to be viewed in relation to the growth of a normal population (see Chapter 1). Corrections for prematurity should be made up to the age of 2 years. The child's maximum weight centile achieved between 4 and 8 weeks may be a better predictor of the centile at 12 months than the birth centile [5].

It is now recognised that infants show considerable weight variability in the early weeks with very large and small babies showing regression to the mean. The infant on the second centile is likely to show catch-up growth, whereas the 98th centile infants tend on average to catch-down [6]. Therefore, babies who gain weight slowly or whose weight chart gradually crosses centile lines in the first year of life may simply be adopting a growth trajectory that is normal for them.

Patterns of weight gain differ between breast fed and bottle fed infants. Breast fed babies tend to gain more weight than formula fed infants in the first 2 months of life, but then progressively fall behind them. Charts have been developed which show the weight gain centile for breast fed babies (see p. 7), but further work is required to determine their applicability to the general population of breast fed infants [7].

Abnormal growth patterns and faltering growth

Traditionally, concern has been shown for children below the third centile, but a fall across centiles, plateauing or fluctuating weight are more worrying and require further assessment. Batchelor and Kerslake [8] have described several patterns of faltering growth:

- *Falling centiles* A downward deviation in weight across two or more major centile lines.
- *Poor parallel centiles* When growth falters, a child's centile position initially falls, and growth for both height and weight follows a lower parallel centile line as the child has adapted to poor nutrition.
- *Height and weight centiles markedly discrepant* Where there is a marked discrepancy between height and weight centiles and between the individual child and other family members, growth faltering should be suspected.
- *Discrepant family patterns* Children whose growth falters frequently show marked discrepancies from the parents' attained height centiles. Parental height is influenced by a number of factors including whether the parents failed to thrive as children.
- *Retrospective rise* Improvement in the child's centile position may occur if nutrition is improved, demonstrating catch-up growth.
- *Saw-tooth pattern* This is also referred to as 'dipping', whereby a child's weight fluctuates, crossing and recrossing centile positions. Dips in weight may be related to episodes of intercurrent illness but may reflect other problems such as family stress around life events.

Recognition of faltering growth

Identification of faltering growth and an assessment

of the severity of the nutritional state are important to recognise in children at risk, and to provide appropriate intervention. Faltering growth is usually identified from weight and this is still the most reasonable marker for diagnosis [9]. Early work in poor growth looked predominantly at weight below a low centile. A study from Batchelor and Kerslake [8] showed that 1 in 3 children whose weight had fallen below the third centile were not recognised by health professionals as children who had faltering growth. The reasons for non-recognition included:

- A general lack of awareness of the problem
- Social class – a child from an owner-occupying two parent family was more likely to be considered naturally small
- No signs of physical neglect and a well-cared for child
- No reported feeding difficulties
- Underuse of growth charts
- Lack of treatment facilities

Weight measurement is now routinely recorded at birth, at the 6–8 week check, at other reviews and at the times of immunisations. This should be sufficient to identify most cases of faltering weight gain [7]. Length/height is not measured routinely in clinics but advised at 6–8 weeks for low birthweight infants or where there are concerns about health or growth.

It is good clinical practice to measure, and plot onto the growth chart, the weight, length/height and head circumference of any child where there are concerns about growth.

Height centile should be compared to the parental height as weight gain has been shown to correlate with parental height, suggesting that smaller parents have infants with poor weight gain [10]. Mid upper-arm circumference (MUAC), which indirectly assesses nutritional status by estimating body fat and muscle bulk, is also a useful measurement (Table 29.1).

Table 29.1 Mid upper-arm circumference of 1–5-year-olds [11].

<14.0 cm	Very likely to be a significantly malnourished child
14.0–15.0 cm	May be malnourished (likelihood greater if age nearer to 5 than 1 year)
>15.0 cm	Nutrition likely to be reasonable

Conventional growth charts identify infants who are light and whose weight is below the bottom centile but does not detect those with a slow weight velocity. Although not universally used, charts have been developed based on the 3-in-1 weight monitoring system, a combination of distance, velocity and conditional charts derived by Cole [12], which addresses this problem. It has the usual nine centiles plus extra curves called thrive lines that mark poor weight gain (see p. 8). The slope, not the position of the thrive line, identifies either adequacy of weight gain or cause for concern. A growth chart for children aged 0–5 years which includes projected growth patterns for weights with a standard deviation (z) score of –5.0 are also available [13].

The routine use and correct interpretation of growth charts, proactive health care and acknowledgement of abnormal growth patterns will allow early intervention before poor patterns of nutrition and growth become firmly entrenched.

Consequences of faltering growth

Nutrition in the early years of life is a major determinant of growth and development, and it influences future adult health [14]. When growth falters, deficits may also be seen in the child's emotional and later intellectual development [15]. A child's growth, including brain growth, is rapid in the first 2 years of life. Evidence from studies indicates that faltering growth in infancy is associated with adverse intellectual outcomes sufficiently large to be of importance at a population level [16].

Prevalence of faltering growth

The prevalence of faltering growth in the population depends very much on how faltering growth is defined. It is suggested that it affects 5% of infants in deprived inner city areas but also occurs across a wide social range [17].

Contributing factors

Faltering growth is caused by inadequate energy intake, which can arise when food is not available

Table 29.2   Organic factors in faltering growth.

Inability to digest or absorb nutrients
  – coeliac disease
  – cystic fibrosis
Excessive loss of nutrients
  – vomiting
  – chronic diarrhoea
  – protein-losing enteropathy
Increased nutrient requirements due to underlying disease
  – chronic cardiac or respiratory failure
  – chronic infection
Inability to fully utilise nutrients
  – metabolic disease
Inability to achieve adequate intake
  – functional problems
  – suck/swallow inco-ordination
  – oral hypersensitivity

or is taken in insufficient amounts. The aetiology of faltering growth is complex and many factors may inter-relate and contribute to the problem. In some children, medical conditions are clearly the principal reason for undernutrition (Table 29.2).

Despite an often seemingly adequate intake, gastrointestinal disorders may lead to faltering growth because of malabsorption (e.g. in coeliac disease). Children with congenital cardiac or respiratory defects may show poor growth resulting from decreased nutritional intake because of anorexia, breathing problems or increased energy requirements brought about by their disease. Children with metabolic disorders can present with faltering growth as a result of poor feeding or inability to utilise energy correctly. Children with neurological dysfunction may have problems with oral motor development which can affect the ability to suck and swallow. They may also suffer from oral hypersensitivity and therefore refuse to feed. Faltering growth is common in infants born preterm. Their special nutritional needs and oral motor problems are reviewed separately.

For the children with poor weight gain and no organic problem, an inadequate intake of energy is still the underlying cause. When growth falters in an infant, the causes that limit or affect intake are often complex, with many factors contributing to the problem (Table 29.3).

Table 29.3 Factors contributing to faltering growth.

Parental factors	Child factors
Parental attitude and cultural beliefs	Progression through weaning
Child management/coercive behaviour	Appetite
Maternal influence/family difficulties	Feeding difficulties
Poverty	Excess fluid
Neglect and abuse	Dental caries

Weaning

The earliest months of life require high energy intakes with a significant proportion needed for growth. Growth in a child can falter at any age, but for many the problem starts around the time of weaning when a young infant's oral motor skills develop, allowing the acceptance of new tastes and textures. If this opportunity is missed, the progression through weaning and the acceptance of more solid textures can be difficult, leading to overdependence on milk. Intake is then restricted, inappropriate for age and with insufficient energy for normal growth. Excessive consumption of fluids whether milk or juice can also exacerbate the problem [18,19].

Feeding problems

Difficulty with feeding is the most commonly cited reason for faltering growth. One study examined whether inefficient sucking was related to faltering growth, and concluded that early sucking difficulties could just be a transitory problem, whereas ongoing feeding difficulties are more suggestive of faltering growth [20]. In a population based study, children with faltering growth had significantly more feeding problems, with infants being introduced to solids later than controls as well as showing undemanding behaviour, low appetite and poor feeding skills [21]. Many parents with children whose growth has faltered report feeding difficulties in their children such as holding food in the mouth, spitting food out or vomiting [22]. The child may show no signs of being hungry, nor any

apparent eagerness to feed when food is offered [23]. There are many reasons for food refusal including dental caries, excessive temperatures of food, inappropriately sized pieces, insensitive feeding or reluctance of parents to allow the child to feed itself and make the inevitable 'mess'.

Maternal influence

A number of studies over the years have suggested that mothers of children with faltering growth may have some of the following characteristics: depression, anxiety, social isolation, low intelligence level, eating disorders and a family cycle in which the mother received inadequate nurturing during her own childhood. However, it must be noted that the presence of these factors are not necessarily identifiable as risk factors of poor growth.

Maternal attitudes towards food and feeding also have an influence on the eating habits of children. McCann *et al.* [24] reported that mothers of children whose growth faltered showed greater dietary restraint both concerning what they ate themselves and what they were prepared to offer their children.

Family problems

Many studies have focused on psychosocial characteristics of the family and the environment of the child who has faltering growth. Parents' inability to provide emotional nurturing may well contribute to the problem. Family conflict before the age of 7 has been shown to have a strong and significant association with slow growth [25]. Faltering growth may occur amidst a range of parenting problems such as difficulties with feeding, poor routine, disorganised, disrupted or chaotic lifestyles and, in the extreme, cases of alcohol or substance abuse.

Poverty

There is little direct evidence to suggest that deprivation and poverty are important social factors for faltering growth [26]. A recent study of a 1 year birth cohort in Newcastle-upon-Tyne, UK, found that the relative risk for faltering growth was about twice as high in deprived as in the intermediate areas, but it was also substantially higher in affluent areas [6]. It has been shown that children from severely deprived backgrounds, devoid of almost all stimulation, recovered weight rapidly when energy intake was 50% greater than normal requirements [27]. Poverty is not a factor in isolation and there is little to suggest an increased risk of faltering growth in the poorest, but there is a strong suggestion that larger families constitute a risk [10].

Neglect and abuse

Two population studies found that 5–10% of children who had faltering growth had been considered at risk of abuse or neglect [21,28]. It is thought that children in abusing or neglecting families are probably at an increased risk of poor growth but these families are only a small proportion of all faltering growth cases.

Behavioural feeding difficulties

Behavioural feeding problems, including food refusal, can occur in early life with many contributing factors [29].

Poor parent–child interaction

One of the earliest forms of infant communication occurs during feeding. In the interaction between the carer and infant, each mutually responds and reacts to the other by adapting their behaviour. The child needs to control his own behaviour (e.g. to signal satiety). If the parent does not respond to these satiety signals, the child may then increase behaviours such as screaming, turning away, spitting or throwing food. Once a child is showing signs of satiety and refusing any more food, further attempts to get the child to eat more are unlikely to succeed.

Developmental stage

A young infant, particularly as weaning progresses, will show increasing independence, wanting to self-feed and refusing both to be fed and to accept new foods.

Learned food aversion

The child may have had an experience of vomiting, which is then associated with ingestion of a particular food, which can contribute to food aversion even though the vomiting may not have been caused by the food. Other difficulties such as insensitive feeding or force-feeding by overly anxious parents can contribute to the problem.

Behavioural feeding problems often frustrate parents who will differ in their ways of coping with it. The nature of the interaction between the child and parent can affect the child's behaviour at mealtimes and consequently the child's intake. In addition, the parental anxiety about insufficient weight gain and the frequently associated feeding problems can cause great distress and disruption to family life. These may well contribute to the onset and persistence of faltering growth.

Management of faltering growth

Faltering growth is a common problem of early childhood, needing practical yet effective intervention. Health visitors, with appropriate support and training, are ideally placed to work with families and young children. An assessment (preferably undertaken at home) may reveal obvious dietary issues which if acted upon can result in an improvement in intake and consequently growth. Further input from the community paediatric dietitian to clarify and ensure nutritional adequacy may be necessary.

For the child where poor growth continues, there is much to recommend a multidisciplinary team approach to its management, where the medical and psychosocial aspects are combined into a clear focus on food and feeding [30,31]. This will allow for assessment of medical and nutritional status, feeding history, dietary intake, oral function and psychosocial and developmental aspects. Potential members of a multidisciplinary feeding team are given in Table 29.4. Joint working enables discussion of individual cases, and close co-operation between professionals.

Parents need to be listened to and their concerns should be taken into account. Medical investigations are undertaken to exclude organic disease rather than to diagnose the cause of faltering growth. A full paediatric assessment should be

Table 29.4 Multidisciplinary feeding team.

Paediatrician
General practitioner
Community paediatric dietitian
Clinical psychologist
Speech and language therapist
Nurse
Social worker
Health visitor
Others, e.g. nursery key worker, family aide worker

Table 29.5 Mealtime observation.

Observation of child	Observation of parents
Interest in own and others' food	Awareness of child's needs
Desire to feed or drink by themselves	Ability to tolerate mess
Quantity, texture and type of food eaten	Quantity, texture and type of food offered
Ability to concentrate and persevere	Management style, e.g. force, encouragement
Ability to communicate needs	Emotional state, e.g. frustration, anxiety
Reaction to parent's behaviour	Control over child's behaviour

undertaken if there are any suggestions of organic symptoms.

Dietary assessment

There is little research on dietary intake of children with faltering growth. One study raised the difficulties in collecting dietary information and suggested that only a minority of children with faltering growth will have dietary histories that are obviously inadequate but that wider ranging nutritional assessment will be more revealing [32].

It is important to construct a complete picture of all aspects of, and influences on, the child's feeding. Dietary assessment will include early feeding history, dietary recall of present intake and the completion of a food diary.

Early feeding from birth, including the start and progression of solids, will help to identify if there were problems within the first year of life. Dietary recall, information on the variety and the frequency of foods offered and eaten, mealtime routines and drinks taken through the day will all help to look at the child's current intake. Information on the purchasing of food and its preparation within the home may also be revealing.

Food diaries are a very useful tool in nutritional assessments, revealing invaluable quantitative information as well as helping to establish the nature of dietary inadequacies [33] (see p. 3). Health conscious parents may report a high fibre, low fat diet which is unsuitable for young children [34]. Some parents report what they would like their children to eat and record excessively large quantities at any one meal. These are seen as 'food lies' and can be recorded for many reasons which need to be investigated. The information shared from the diaries is not used to judge or criticise, but to explore issues sensitively.

Feeding assessment

In many cases of faltering growth, the lack of adequate nutritional intake is compounded by the child's behavioural feeding problems. Observation of the child being fed by the parent or carer in the normal feeding environment will provide crucial information about how the child feeds, parent–child interaction and the emotions surrounding feeding (Table 29.5).

A clinical psychologist can provide valuable input into assessments of interactions between parent and child during playing and feeding as well as working with families to address behavioural difficulties.

Assessment of oral motor function

For a small number of children who have neurodevelopmental problems or continue to exhibit food refusal and faltering growth, it is important for a speech and language therapist to assess oral motor function. Such assessments, often in conjunction with video-fluoroscopy, will identify children who are unable to co-ordinate the suck–swallow reflex. These children are likely to aspirate feeds and may require nasogastric or gastrostomy feeding.

The assessment will also detect oral hypersensitivity and be able to help with desensitisation programmes.

Nutritional management

Assessment of requirements

Following feeding assessment, a strategy for catch-up growth should be planned. The main objectives are:

- To improve energy intake
- To promote weight gain enabling catch-up and allowing optimum growth
- To correct nutritional deficiencies and achieve an adequate nutritional intake
- To empower and support parents through dietary changes

Diets that only meet age-specific requirements for energy and protein [35] will not provide for catch-up growth. Diets based on normal requirements will usually allow for maintenance of growth along the centile to which the child has fallen. Additional protein and energy will be required for catch-up growth.

Healthy infants require 7–12% of their energy to come from protein. To support catch-up growth the percentage of energy supplied from protein should be about 9% (see p. 16) although care must be taken when advising high protein intakes if there is any risk of renal insufficiency. Providing a lower percentage of energy from protein has been associated with higher rates of fat deposition [36].

A formula for predicting energy requirements for catch-up growth in infants and young children has been suggested [37]:

$$\text{kcal (kJ)} / \text{kg} = \frac{120 \times \text{ideal weight for height (kg)}}{\text{actual weight (kg)}}$$

This may mean an intake of 1.5–2 times the normal recommended energy requirements for age.

Anaemia is common in children who are failing to thrive and in one study in Leeds, one-third of the sample had iron deficiency anaemia [38]. Vitamins, minerals and trace element requirements are increased during periods of rapid growth and a suitable supplement should be included if the child's intake is thought to be inadequate. No guidelines exist, but intakes should be at least appropriate for the proposed energy intake.

Achieving nutritional requirements

Working in partnership with parents and engaging them in any decisions on intervention is crucial. If a child is underweight for height and failing to gain weight at the expected rate, whatever they are consuming is insufficient for their needs.

In a young breast fed infant where growth is faltering, the maternal diet needs to be assessed and its quantity and quality improved. Supplementation of breast feeds may be necessary but this should be carried out under dietary supervision and with caution as it may suppress production of breast milk. For formula fed infants, options include increasing the volume of feed, supplementing infant feeds, concentrating the infant formula or the use of a high energy formula (see Table 1.14). A study in Birmingham showed the benefits of using a ready-to-feed high energy formula rather than adding energy supplements to standard infant formula [39].

In general, young children have a high energy requirement relative to their size. In cases of poor growth, when catch-up growth is the aim, requirements are even higher. This is difficult to achieve as many children have small appetites, consuming small food portions at any one time. The following ways of increasing energy intake must be considered:

- Regular meals
- Frequent snacks
- Use of energy dense foods
- Fortification of foods
- Supplements

Regular feeding

Children need a good routine of regular meals, which include energy dense foods. It is advisable to start with small quantities and offer realistic portions of every day family foods, with the opportunity for the child to be given more if they can manage. Emphasis needs to taken off mealtimes and the importance of total intake emphasised.

Frequent snacks

Meals alone will usually not enable catch-up growth. One study showed that when children with faltering growth were offered a high energy snack, they took more at the next meal than the control group where there were no concerns about growth [40]. In clinical practice, regular snacks as well as meals are advised to increase interest in food, improve appetite and therefore energy intake. Excess juice consumption encountered in many young children should be discouraged and solids should be offered first.

Energy dense foods

Children still need to consume as wide a variety of foods as possible from the five food groups: bread, other cereals and potatoes; meat, fish and alternatives; full fat milk and dairy foods; fruit and vegetables; fatty and sugary foods (see Table 27.4), with a greater emphasis on the energy dense foods. Foods high in fibre are bulky and may contain high phytate levels compromising both energy intake and the bioavailability of micronutrients.

Fortification of foods

Energy dense products, such as butter, margarine and cheese, can be added to popular foods. Dried full fat milk powder can be used to fortify puddings, soups and milk. If necessary the iron status of young children can be improved initially by giving iron supplements and, in the longer term, encouraging children to consume iron containing foods.

Supplements

The use of dietary supplements is not recommended for children with non-organic poor growth. The use of these products can medicalise the problem and give the impression to parents or carers that they do not have a role in helping their child to improve nutritional intake.

For children who are unable to take an adequate oral intake, dietary supplements may be necessary and can be prescribed. Supplements of carbohydrate, fat or protein can be used to enrich foods or prepacked nutrient and energy dense drinks (sip feeds) may be more suitable (see Tables 1.15, 1.17

and 11.3). The principle of frequent feeding, regular meals and snacks, use of energy dense foods and fortification of solids with extra energy still applies.

For all children with poor growth, advice tailored to individual needs is extremely important, starting with the foods that the child is happy to eat. Initially, weight gain may be rapid, followed by a gradual deceleration until the child's normal centile is reached.

Use of enteral feeding

If the child has severe growth faltering and it is not possible to achieve a reasonable intake orally, enteral feeding (nasogastric or gastrostomy) may be initially required. The use of overnight feeds is preferred as this allows oral feeding to be established during the daytime.

Behavioural management

Faltering growth in a number of children can be compounded by behavioural problems. Any attempts to improve nutritional intake and to achieve catch-up growth should be backed up by behavioural management techniques. Parents should be helped in a sensitive way, offering support and constructive advice, with no blame attached and no criticism of their parenting. Behavioural management includes:

- No force feeding
- Relaxed mealtimes
- Positive reinforcement of good feeding behaviour; aberrant behaviour should be ignored, e.g. by turning the face away from the child
- A time limit for mealtimes
- Closely spaced mealtimes are a possibility, to maximise the opportunity for feeding practice and to reduce the pressure to eat at any one meal

Social services

In some families, where there has been no improvement in weight, a referral to social services requesting input from a social worker under the category of a 'child in need' is necessary. This will enable a better assessment of the family and allows input and support from a wider range of services. Social work referral is very important whenever there are concerns about a child's care, safety or wellbeing [41].

Faltering growth can affect physical, intellectual, emotional and social growth. To thrive, children need adequate nutrition and appropriate nurturing.

Many factors contribute to a child's poor growth and intervention benefits from a multidisciplinary team approach encompassing diagnosis of underlying organic causes, assessment of nutritional intake, feeding patterns, oral motor function and behavioural difficulties. Early intervention is crucial, with a clear focus on improving the child's nutrition to enable catch-up growth. It is important to acknowledge parental concerns, avoid blame, build on strengths and wherever possible work in partnership with families.

References

1 Spitz RA Hospitalism. *Psychoanal Study Child*, 1945, **1** 55–74.
2 Skuse D Failure to thrive: current perspectives. *Curr Paediatr*, 1992, **2** 105–10.
3 Wright C, Callum J, Birks E *et al.* Effect of community based management in failure to thrive: randomized control trial. *Br Med J*, 1998, **317** 571–4.
4 Underdown A, Birks E *Faltering growth: taking the failure out of failure to thrive*. Professional briefing paper. London: CPHVA & The Children's Society, 1999.
5 Edwards AGK, Halse PC, Parkin JM *et al.* Recognising failure to thrive in early childhood. *Arch Dis Child*, 1990, **65** 1263–5.
6 Wright CM, Waterston A, Matthews JNS *et al.* What is the normal weight gain in infancy? *Acta Paediatr*, 1994, **83** 351–6.
7 Hall DMB, Elliman D *Health for All Children*, 4th edn. Oxford: Oxford University Press, 2003.
8 Batchelor J, Kerslake A *Failure to Find Failure to Thrive*. London: Whiting & Birch, 1990.
9 Raynor P, Rudolf M Anthropometric indices of failure to thrive. *Arch Dis Child*, 2000, **82** 364–5.
10 Blair PS, Drewett RF, Emmett PM *et al.* Family, socioeconomic and prenatal factors associated with failure to thrive in the Avon Longitudinal Study of Parents and Children (ALSPAC). *Int J Epidemiol*, 2004, **33** 839–47.
11 Hobbs CJ, Hanks HGI, Wynne JM *Child Abuse and Neglect: A Clinician's Handbook*. Edinburgh: Churchill Livingstone, 1999.
12 Cole TJ 3-in-1 weight monitoring chart, *Lancet*, 1997, **349** 102–3.
13 Wright C, Avery A, Epstein M *et al.* New chart to evaluate weight faltering. *Arch Dis Child*, 1998, **78** 40–3.
14 Barker DJP The fetal and infant origins of adult disease. *Br Med J*, 1990, **301** 1111.
15 Dowdney L, Skuse D, Hepinstall E *et al.* Growth retardation and developmental delay amongst inner city children. *J Child Psychol Psychiatry*, 1987, **28** 529–40.
16 Corbett SS, Drewett RF To what extent is failure to thrive in infancy associated with poorer cognitive skills? A review and meta-analysis. *J Child Psychol Psychiatry*, 2004, **45** 641–54.
17 Wright CM, Waterston A, Aynsley-Green A Effect of deprivation on weight gain in infancy. *Acta Pediatr*, 1994, **83** 357–9.
18 Smith MM, Lifshitz F Excess fruit consumption as a contributing factor in non-organic failure to thrive. *Pediatrics*, 1994, **93** 438–43.
19 Hourihane JO'B, Rolles CJ Morbidity from excess intake of high energy fluids: the 'squash drinking syndrome'. *Arch Dis Child*, 1995, **72** 141–3.
20 Ramsey M, Gisel E, McCusker J *et al.* Infant sucking inability, non-organic failure to thrive, maternal characteristics, and feeding practices: a prospective cohort study. *Dev Med Child Neurol*, 2002, **44** 405–15.
21 Wright C, Birks E Risk factors for failure to thrive: a population-based survey. *Child Care Health Dev*, 2000, **26** 5–16.
22 Iwaniec D, Herbert M, McNeish AS Social work with failure to thrive children and their families. Part 1: Psychological factors. *Br J Social Work*, 1985, **15** 243–59.
23 Skuse D, Reilly S, Wolke D Psychological adversity and growth during infancy. *Eur J Clin Nutr*, 1994, **48** (Suppl 1) S113–30.
24 McCann JB, Stein A, Fairburn CG *et al.* Eating habits and attitudes of mothers of children with non-organic failure to thrive. *Arch Dis Child*, 1994, **70** 234–6.
25 Montgomery SM, Bartley M, Wilkinson R Family conflict and slow growth. *Arch Dis Child*, 1997, **77** 326–30.
26 Skuse D Epidemiological and definitional issues in failure to thrive. *Child Adolesc Psychiatr Clin N Am*, 1993, **2** 37–59.
27 Whitten CF, Pettit MG, Fischhoff J Evidence that growth failure from maternal deprivation is secondary to undereating. *J Am Med Assoc*, 1969, **209** 1675–82.
28 Skuse D, Gill D, Reilly S *et al.* Failure to thrive and the risk of child abuse: a prospective population study. *J Med Screen*, 1995, **2** 145–9.

29   Harris G, Booth IW The nature and management of eating disorders in pre-school children. In: Cooper P, Stein A (eds) *Monographs in Clinical Paediatrics; Feeding Problems and Eating Disorders*. Switzerland: Harwood Academic Publishers, 1991.

30   Hobbs C, Hanks HGI A multidisciplinary approach for the treatment of children with failure to thrive. *Child Care Health Dev*, 1996, **22** 273–84.

31   Blithoney WG, McJunkin J, Michalek J *et al*. The effect of a multidisciplinary team approach on weight gain in non-organic failure to thrive children. *Dev Behav Pediatr*, 1991, **12** 254–8.

32   Wright CM, Loughridge J, Moore J Failure to thrive in a population context: two contrasting studies of feeding and nutritional status. *Proc Nutr Soc*, 2000, **59** 37–45.

33   Moores J Non-organic failure to thrive – dietetic practice in a community setting. *Child Care Health Dev*, 1996, **22** 251–9.

34   Department of Health Report on Health and Social Subjects No. 45. *Weaning and the Weaning Diet*. London: The Stationery Office, 1994.

35   Department of Health Report on Health and Social Subjects No. 41. *Dietary Reference Values for Food Energy and Nutrients for the United Kingdom*. London: The Stationery Office, 1991.

36   Dewey KG, Beaton G, Fjeld C *et al*. Protein requirements of infants and young children. *Eur J Clin Nutr*, 1996, **50** (Suppl 1): S119–50.

37   Maclean WC *et al*. Nutritional management of chronic diarrhoea and malnutrition: primary reliance on oral feeding. *J Pediatr*, 1990, **97** 316–23.

38   Raynor P, Rudolf MCJ What do we know about children who fail to thrive? *Child Care Health Dev*, 1996, **22** 241–50.

39   Clarke SE *et al*. Impaired growth and nitrogen deficiency in infants receiving an energy supplemented standard infant formula. Proceedings of the Royal College of Paediatrics and Child Health Annual Meeting, 1998, Abstract G132.

40   Kasese-Hara M, Wright C, Drewett R Energy compensation in young children who fail to thrive. *J Child Psychol Psychiatry*, 2002, **43** 449–56.

41   Wright C, Talbot E Screening for failure to thrive: what are we looking for? *Child Care Health Dev*, 1996, **22** 223–34.

Further reading

Iwaniec D *Children who fail to thrive – A practice guide*. Chichester: Wiley, 2004.

30 Feeding Children with Neurodisabilities

Sarah Almond, Liz Allott & Kate Hall

Introduction

Neurodisability, according to the Royal College of Paediatrics and Child Health [1], is an umbrella term used to describe conditions affecting the brain and central nervous system (CNS) and includes muscular, developmental, motor, sensory, learning and neuropsychiatric disorders. CNS damage can be brought about by disease, genetics, oxygen deprivation or acquired brain injury amongst other causes, and can occur antenatally, neonatally or at any stage in a child's life. The majority of research is on children with motor disorders or cerebral palsy (CP) as their primary diagnosis, which is also the most common cause of neurodisability [2]. However, these children often have neurological involvement of other body systems as part of their condition [3].

Examples of neurodisabilities include CP, Down's syndrome, muscular dystrophy and degenerative disorders. Irrespective of diagnosis, if the child has difficulties with eating and drinking, they are likely to have nutritional concerns which will need to be addressed [4]. Those with motor, physical or sensory impairments are more likely to struggle [2]. It is known that the more severe the disability, the more likely the child is to be at nutritional risk [5]. Feeding dysfunction is common in CP and can affect 60–90% of children [2,6–9].

The ability of infants, children and adolescents to achieve their potential for growth and development will depend on the intervention provided in critical time periods. In the past, multidisciplinary teams did not focus on nutrition, which resulted in recognition of children with malnutrition only when it was very evident. This was often later rather than earlier in life; for example, when the child had difficulty maintaining their centile curves during growth spurts, or did not enter puberty at the expected time [2]. A recent study highlighted that 64% of children with neurodevelopmental delay had never had their feeding and nutrition assessed. Furthermore, the same authors concluded that, 'Many children with neurological impairment would benefit from individual nutritional assessment and management as part of their overall care' [10].

Previously it was accepted that children with neurodisability were small as part of their condition. With the evolution of enteral feeding it became evident that children had the potential to grow if adequate nutrition was provided. However, at present dietetic resources are limited so children often are only identified as needing dietetic input when malnutrition becomes marked [11].

National Service Framework for Children and the social context

Specific standards for the health and social care of disabled children is laid out in the National Service

Framework for Children, Young People and Maternity Services (NSF) [12]. In addition 'Every Child Matters' [13] states that such children should be able to achieve the five key outcomes outlined for the nation's children.

A child's need for the services that attendance at a special school can provide is usually determined by the severity of the disability and the therapy input required. Many children are integrated into mainstream education, either on a full time basis or part time combined with days at a special school. Some special schools offer residential accommodation and the child may board either full time or during the school week only, going home at weekends. A multidisciplinary team from health, social care and extended family often supports these children. Liaison with all involved is essential when planning care. The social context affects the lives of children and should be taken into account when planning nutritional interventions.

Medical conditions

Cerebral palsy

CP is non-progressive brain damage in the cerebral cortex. CP lesions cause neuromuscular problems producing abnormal muscle tone resulting in disorders of movement and posture. CP includes a variety of conditions. There are four main types, which correspond to injuries to different parts of the brain [14]:

1 Children with spastic CP find that some muscles become very stiff and weak, especially under effort. They also have high muscle tone. This can affect their control of movement.
2 Children with hypotonic CP have low muscle tone with little or no resistance to movement. These children frequently have feeding difficulties.
3 Children with athetoid CP have some loss of control of their posture and they tend to make unwanted movements. They have a mixture of high and low muscle tone and often have a high requirement for energy.
4 Children with ataxic CP usually have problems with balance. They may also have shaky hand movements and irregular speech. Their muscle tone tends to be low but can fluctuate.

A child with CP may have one distinct type or more commonly a mixture of these. The distribution of CP can be limited to one limb (monoplegia), diplegia with two limb involvement or quadriplegia where all four limbs affected.

Those children more severely affected are likely to have multiple co-morbidities including sensory impairments (vision, hearing, touch), perceptual difficulties resulting in impaired sensory interpretation, learning disabilities, limited communication and medical conditions such as respiratory difficulties, seizure disorders and gastro-oesophageal reflux (GOR). The incidence of cerebral palsy is 2–3 in every 1000 live births and the likelihood of feeding problems is very high [15].

A large multicentre study of 230 children and young people with moderate to severe CP living in the community showed that the level of feeding dysfunction was directly related to degree of undernutrition, and even those who had mild feeding dysfunction had poor growth and limited fat stores. Therefore, a child requiring any modified consistency of food and fluids can be at risk of nutritional compromise [5]. It has also been documented that 89% of children with CP need help with feeding and 55% regularly choke at mealtimes [2].

Almost one-third of children with CP were found to have a height-for-age below the 25th centile in a study by Vik *et al.* [16] while 7% were classified as being obese (weight above the 97.5th centile).

Down's syndrome

For every 1000 babies born, one will have Down's syndrome and approximately 600 babies with Down's syndrome are born in the UK each year. It is estimated that there are around 60 000 people with Down's syndrome living in the UK [17].

Down's syndrome is the most common autosomal trisomy and genetic cause of learning disabilities [18]. Many children with Down's syndrome are born with congenital abnormalities such as heart defects (40%); they also have gastrointestinal problems (15%), recurrent respiratory infections, joint problems, endocrine dysfunction, vitamin malabsorption, constipation, GOR and feeding difficulties [19].

A number of studies have been carried out to ascertain the frequency of feeding problems in children with Down's syndrome [20,21]. American based studies suggest that eating problems are common but are usually minor in nature. Subsequently, Spender *et al.* [22] have found significant impairments in oral motor function among children with Down's syndrome. Surveys of parents suggest that 60% are totally independent in feeding by early childhood [20] and the most common problems are slight oral hypotonia, tongue thrust, difficulties in chewing, poor lip seal, and choking and gagging on food. However, it is noted that this feeding success may be partly as a direct result of feeding programmes and not simply a natural developmental step, thus reinforcing the need for assessment and management programmes. Hopman *et al.* [23] noted that solids were introduced at a later stage compared with controls, possibly because of low parental expectations of developmental ability. Foods requiring less chewing were given, further inhibiting oral motor development. Frazier and Friedman [24] found that children with Down's syndrome have increased oral sensitivity, interfering with the acceptance of new foods and a high incidence of aspiration, which is possibly related to the high incidence of respiratory disease.

Severe feeding difficulties secondary to hypotonia, placidity, weak suckling and rooting reflex may occur at birth as a result of multiple cranial skeletal differences. The palate is often short and narrow, and this underdevelopment of the maxilla may alter the position of the muscles used for chewing. The tongue may be large or appear large because of a small oral cavity secondary to midfacial hypoplasia. Many children with Down's syndrome are mouth breathers, because of a small oral cavity, enlargement of the tonsils and/or decreased nasal passages. This will have an effect on the development of efficient oral skills. Generalised facial/oral hypotonia also contributes to poor lip closure, poor suck, poor tongue control and difficulties with jaw stability.

In addition, infants with Down's syndrome and congenital heart defects may have the combined problems experienced by infants with heart abnormalities and poor oral skills stated above. Other medical problems that may be present and have a direct effect on nutrition assessment are compromised immune systems and hypothyroidism. Down's syndrome has also been associated with immune-related disorders such as a high incidence of coeliac disease [25,26].

Anthropometric assessment of children with Down's syndrome is complicated because the disorder is associated with a number of abnormalities related to growth such as short stature, decreased head circumference and altered growth patterns. Cronk [27,28] suggests that while height in people with Down's syndrome is significantly lower than the norm, the period in which most significant growth failure occurs is during the first 5 years of life. Growth rate is reduced by one-fifth between the ages 3 and 36 months in both sexes. Longitudinal studies [29] corroborate this but show that growth velocity of children aged 7–18 years was not significantly different to the norm. Growth charts for children with Down's syndrome based on these studies are available from the Child Growth Foundation (see p. 20).

Despite an energy intake below the normal requirement, there is a high prevalence of obesity in children and adults with Down's syndrome [15,30,31]. A 10–15% lower resting metabolic rate, but equivalent expenditure above resting, has been found in pre-pubescent children with Down's syndrome [30]. Crino *et al.* [32] report 66% of pubertal children with Down's syndrome were obese.

Lower energy and micronutrient intakes compared with a control group have been described [30]; 20% were considered to be at risk of vitamin A and C deficiency and 50% for vitamin E deficiency.

Low levels of calcium have been reported [33] which may be related to poor vitamin D absorption. A study using analysis of trace metal levels in hair reported lower levels of calcium, copper and manganese [34]. There is no consistent evidence of vitamin deficiencies but the reported deficiencies of certain vitamins and minerals in some of the literature has been proposed to be caused by malabsorption of nutrients rather than dietary insufficiency. There is little clinical evidence to suggest that megadoses of vitamin supplementation have significant beneficial effects on health outcome or intellectual functioning [35,36].

Neuromuscular disorders

There are approximately 60 different types of muscular dystrophy and related neuromuscular conditions. Congenital neuromuscular disorders in children include spinal muscular atrophy and muscle disorders such as Duchenne muscular dystrophy and congenital muscular dystrophies.

These conditions are characterised by the loss of muscle strength, as progressive muscle wasting or nerve deterioration occurs. They are mainly inherited, can cause shortened life expectancy and there are currently no cures. It is estimated that there are about 30 000 people in the UK with neuromuscular conditions [37].

Neuromuscular disorders are caused by disorders of the lower motor pathway [18]. Feeding difficulties are common in young children with neuromuscular disorders, in particular swallowing problems and associated choking and vomiting, which can lead to undernutrition [38,39]. As the condition progresses, overnutrition becomes a more prevalent concern. Feeding difficulties, including oral motor and gastrointestinal changes, become evident in the last years of life and focus once again shifts to undernutrition.

Duchenne muscular dystrophy is the most frequently occurring of the childhood muscular dystrophies, affecting predominantly males whom can be mildly to moderately delayed [19]. The prevalence of obesity is 54% by 13 years of age and can be related to lower resting energy expenditure and reduced physical activity [40]. In addition, these children, as they get older, can also be at risk of malnutrition which has been reported in 54% of boys by the time they are 18 years old [41]. Where weight has been appropriately managed, improved mobility and less pressure on already weakened muscles has been demonstrated [42].

Progressive degenerative disorders

These are extremely rare conditions in which neurological deterioration progresses with time. There are a large number of different diagnoses (e.g. Batten's disease, Cockayne's syndrome, tuberous sclerosis and Rett's syndrome). Some conditions progress at a steady rate while others degenerate in phases. Because of the very nature of these conditions, the nutritional status of the child is also likely to change with every progressive step. The key here is to ensure frequent monitoring and regular dietetic follow-up. All of these rare progressive degenerative disorders require the dietitian to conduct a literature search at the time of dietetic review for the most up-to-date information.

Nutritional concerns

The main nutritional concerns seen in children with neurodisabilities are:

- Faltering growth
- Gastro-oesophageal reflux disease
- Constipation
- Micronutrient deficiency
- Dental problems

Faltering growth

Faltering growth, or low weight for height, has been well documented for children with neurodisabilities [43–46]. Studies have been published showing the positive impact of nutrition intervention for children with CP [47–50]. Sanders et al.'s [47] prospective study demonstrated the importance of early intervention during the first year of CNS damage in order to prevent or reverse growth deficits. Some studies have proposed that growth failure in children with CP is independent of nutrition [51,52]. In addition, beliefs that it is 'normal' for children with severe disabilities, particularly children with CP, to have poor stature and low weights has often been ascribed to their underlying cerebral deficit or physical inactivity rather than to chronic malnutrition [47,51,52].

Growth data for children with CP must be interpreted with care, as no large studies to date have been completed to establish normal growth profiles for these children. Normal parameters for identifying faltering growth may not be appropriate. Stallings [53], in her summary of nutritional assessment, states:

'Nutrition and growth status in children and adults with CP and other severe types of developmental disabilities is an essential component of care. While data are not available to provide precise definitions of the levels of severity of malnutrition and growth failure and their effect on long-term outcome, it is clear that many patients with moderate and severe CP and other disabilities have malnutrition and growth failure as the result of inadequate caloric intake.'

There is evidence that the severity of feeding problems in children with CP is directly related to the degree of faltering growth in children who are not enterally fed [5]. Resulting malnutrition is linked to poorer health status and reduced ability to participate in normal daily activities [54]. Vik et al. [16] found almost one-third of children with CP to have a height-for-age below the 25th centile.

Gastro-oesophageal reflux disease

GOR is the passage of stomach contents into the oesophagus and mouth. Gastro-oesophageal reflux disease (GORD) is GOR with secondary complications such as faltering growth, oesophagitis and feeding difficulties. GORD is commonly documented in children with severe neurological impairment [55]. Its mechanism is attributed to the motility disorder present in the upper gastrointestinal tract including the oesophagus and oesophageal sphincter, which leads to regurgitation of stomach contents. It is often associated with foregut dysmotility secondary to vagal nerve dysfunction or an anatomical abnormality [56]. GORD differs from vomiting, the emetic reflex following ingested toxins that acts as a protective mechanism. Diagnosis is made by pH study where a pH probe is inserted into the oesophagus and recordings are taken over a 24-hour period. This is effective in diagnosing acid reflux; however, non-acid reflux will be missed. Barium studies are also sometimes used although they are now normally considered to be more useful at ruling out any anatomical abnormality as the cause of GORD [57].

Treatment of GORD is initially managed by drug therapy and success can be attained using a combination of prokinetic agents (domperidone), H_2 receptor antagonists (ranitidine) and proton pump inhibitors (omeprazole, lanzoprazole). Where drug therapy fails the child may be offered anti-reflux surgery, a fundoplication (see p. 129). Often a gastrostomy tube is placed at the same time as, post-fundoplication, the gastric anatomy will be altered making future gastrostomy placement a difficult procedure. Success rates in children with neurodisability are variable and may result in additional complications [58–61] such as gastric dysmotility causing diarrhoea, excessive gas bloating, disabling retching and dumping syndrome [62]. Moreover, the underlying oesophageal dysmotility still remains and if retching or attempted vomiting are not controlled by continuing drug therapy, slippage or unwrapping of the fundoplication can occur [63]. Because of these symptoms, establishing enteral feeding post-fundoplication can be troublesome.

Constipation

Constipation is a common problem for children with neurodevelopmental disabilities [2,64]. It may be as a result of inadequate fluid intake, excessive fluid loss via spillage, poor lip closure, poor head control or dribbling. Immobility, incorrect positioning, abnormal gut motility, side effects of medication and lack of the urge to defaecate also impact on bowel function but occasionally a lack of dietary fibre may be the reason [19,65]. As a consequence, constipation will have a negative effect on appetite, behaviour and general wellbeing; anecdotally it has been reported to trigger seizures. Dietetic assessment and treatment is necessary in order to avoid further nutritional compromise [66] and supplementation with dietary fibre from food, enteral feeds or commercial preparations may help to normalise bowel function. However, often simply increasing the child's fluid intake can have the most success [67–72].

Micronutrient deficiency

Studies on vitamin and mineral intakes and deficiencies in children with feeding problems are not well documented. However, nutritional assessment often highlights inadequate intakes because of poor variety, small quantities of food eaten and potential vitamin losses through liquidising foods or long cooking methods. Sodium and potassium intakes tend to be low; however, current opinion is that a level between the reference nutrient intake (RNI) and lower RNI (LRNI) for height age, is acceptable provided urine and blood biochemical parameters are within normal ranges. It is also important to ensure an adequate calcium intake because of the high incidence of fractures seen in non-weight bearing disabled children.

Dental problems

Dental caries can be caused by a number of factors:

- Poor dental hygiene because of hypersensitivity to teeth cleaning
- Medications
- Inability to clear the mouth of food after eating
- Reduced saliva production
- GORD
- Frequent consumption of cariogenic foods

Small, energy dense meals and drinks are often encouraged throughout the day in order to improve nutritional intake, although this is often contrary to dental advice given to prevent caries. A discussion with the community dental service may facilitate compromise at the same time as preventing contradictory messages. Often, alternative preventative dental treatment can be suggested in its place. Boyd *et al.* [73] conclude that, 'Developmentally delayed children have the greatest diversity in nutritional and oral health needs' and that 'the special needs child will require early anticipatory guidance and intensive preventive dental therapy with frequent prophylaxis'. Dental treatment can be dangerous, time-consuming and very frightening for some children and therefore prevention should always be considered. Oral sensitivity can cause the child to be intolerant of having things in or near their mouth [73]. In addition, the child with dental caries who cannot communicate pain will more than likely exhibit negative behaviours around food and drink thus increasing his or her feeding difficulties.

Feeding difficulties

Importance of eating and drinking

The development of eating and drinking skills is important for several reasons, only one of which is nutrition [74]:

- It is essential that the child eats efficiently in order to consume adequate nutrition orally

- The movements of the jaw, lips and tongue, in synchronisation with breathing while eating and drinking, will influence the level of mature speech and saliva control
- Development and fine tuning of posture, head control and eye–hand co-ordination is practised at mealtimes
- Mealtimes provide an opportunity for creating an environment for learning and practising communication skills
- Mealtimes are ideal settings in which rules for social interaction are learned and rehearsed
- Giving choice and control at mealtimes allows the child to develop self-esteem and independence

Oral dysfunction

Oral dysfunction may result from either structural abnormalities such as high roof of the mouth, enlarged tongue, abnormal dentition or motor difficulties such as those seen in CP. There are five stages of eating and drinking, all of which need to be functioning correctly for the safe and efficient passage of fluid or solids to the stomach.

Anticipatory stage

This includes all the activities taking place before feeding occurs and is extremely important as the entire swallowing process can be disrupted if the child is not prepared to receive the food or drink. The child with neurodisability needs as much information as possible about the mealtime in order to organise the movements of the jaw, lips, tongue and breathing. Before the meal, the child should be involved by being offered a reasonable choice. They also need to know who their helper will be and this person should be consistent throughout. If the child can feed assisted, this should be encouraged as the hand to mouth action will help with anticipation. In terms of the food, verbalising the sight, smell, taste, texture and temperature of the food is necessary and is especially important for those who have sensory impairments.

Oral preparatory stage

This begins once the food has reached the lips and

is prepared in the mouth before swallowing. The process consists of head and jaw movements including voluntary opening of the mouth, lip closure around the utensil or biting food, transferring the food around the mouth including chewing, sorting and mixing to form a bolus and holding on to this bolus ready for swallowing. Problems with altered muscle tone, which affect this stage, include an inability to open the mouth voluntarily; inadequate lip closure and so loss of foods and fluids; tongue thrust because of low tone; and possible aspiration. Oral hypersensitivity indicated by food refusal or hyposensitivity indicated by poor trigger of swallow is also seen.

Oral stage

This relates to the initiation of the swallow and involves elevation of the front of the tongue to seal the mouth, propulsion of the bolus by the tongue to the back of the mouth and raising the soft palate to provide a nasopharyngeal seal. Difficulties seen at this stage include lack of co-ordination of tongue movement, incomplete nasopharyngeal seal and risk of aspiration.

Pharyngeal stage

This is an involuntary stage triggered by the closure of the pharynx. The bolus of food is transported through the pharynx and into the oesophagus by peristalsis. Closure of the vocal fold prevents aspiration. Indications of problems at this stage include coughing, choking, gagging and aspiration and can be caused by ineffective function of peristalsis or any part of the pharyngeal anatomy.

Oesophageal stage

This depends on the peristaltic action of oesophageal muscles to propel the bolus of food into the stomach and the contraction of the criopharyngeus muscle to prevent reflux. Difficulties arising at this stage include oesophageal obstruction and GOR.

Abnormal movement and reflexes

From infancy to childhood, as the CNS matures, certain reflexes usually disappear. Children with physical disabilities may keep some of these and when coupled with abnormal movement patterns, can make it difficult to co-ordinate the passage of food and fluids to the mouth. Table 30.1 summarises the effect of abnormal movement on eating.

Sensory and perceptual difficulties

Sensory impairments, such as visual abnormalities and perceptual difficulties resulting in an altered interpretation of the senses, impact on eating and drinking skills. The use of prompts can be extremely useful in these cases as it will clarify the child's expectation of the mealtime experience. Verbal prompts such as a running commentary of the meal can be particularly useful for the visually impaired child.

Posture

The child's position at mealtimes is fundamental to the quality of their eating and drinking skills. There are a variety of positions that can be used at mealtimes depending on the age, size and abilities of the child. An occupational therapist, physiotherapist and speech and language therapist should all be involved in assessing the optimum posture for mealtimes.

Communication

A child or young person with a severe neurodisability may not be able to verbalise or signal their wish for food. This inability to make their request leads to an increased risk of insufficient nutrition, as they are unable to make the same demands that their non-disabled counterparts can do.

As a child grows older or their condition progresses, oral motor abilities may also change which can result in difficulties with managing food and drinks. Children with unrecognised feeding difficulties may be incorrectly interpreted at mealtimes. Often, rejection of certain textures or consistencies can be mistaken for the child being fussy, disliking the food, being lazy or badly behaved. They may

Table 30.1   Abnormal movements and reflexes affecting eating and drinking.

Name	Description	Effect on mealtimes
Asymmetrical tonic neck reflex	Caused by turning the head and triggers extension of the limbs on the side which the head is rotated and an increase flexion of the opposite side	Posture: the child can be difficult to position Feeding: the child may be unable to look at their hand and bring their hand to mouth Swallow: head turned severely to one side may prevent an effective swallow
Extensor thrust	Voluntary or involuntary strong push back of head and trunk	Posture: the child can be difficult to position Swallow: chin thrust inhibits effective swallow, may cause choking Oral: jaw thrust prevents mouth closure and can obstruct suckling and chewing
Startle reflex	Sudden extension of arms and opening of hands, stimulated by sudden noise or unexpected movements	Posture: the child can be difficult to position for self or assisted feeding Feeding: the sudden loss of posture may rouse feelings of insecurity Swallow: associated with a fast intake of breath which may cause choking
Rooting reflex	When cheek is touched, the head turns to that side	Oral: when head is out of midline, the configuration of the mouth changes including the jaw and lip positioning
Bite reflex	When mouth touched there is a sudden jaw closure	Oral: can not co-ordinate jaw movement in order to introduce or withdraw utensil
Tongue thrust	Tongue moves in direction when touched	Oral: difficult to introduce food, retain food and deal with it in the mouth

even display self-injurious behaviour or pica as a sign of distress. Furthermore, an inability to vocalise means that carers may not recognise when eating and drinking causes discomfort. The child's way of displaying this may initially be food refusal or passive behaviour at mealtimes or if in extreme discomfort or pain can result in confused nonverbal signals, excessive movements and spasm. When a child is reported to be fussy or badly behaved at mealtimes, thorough investigation of exactly what is happening is needed, as the possibilities of misinterpreting intentions are very great.

Medication

Some children may be on medication with side effects that directly or indirectly have a negative effect on their nutrition. Some anticonvulsant therapy can cause taste changes, affect appetite, cause drowsiness, induce nausea and gastrointestinal irritation. In addition, changes in medication may negatively or positively impact on oral skills (e.g. the introduction of a muscle relaxant may improve the position of the child during feeding). Oral medications, especially in liquid forms, often have unpleasant flavours and cause reluctance in accepting food in which the child suspects it is hidden.

Social issues

The social issues affecting a disabled child in terms of eating and drinking are the same as for any other child and disability intensifies the effect. Financial difficulties are known to be greater in a family where there is a disabled child. Social eating such as eating out, picnics and barbecues are limited unless careful arrangements are made prior to the event. Thus, the opportunity to learn normal mealtime behaviour is reduced.

Government guidance encourages children with disabilities and their families to live as 'ordinary' a life as possible [12]:

NSF Standard 8 Disabled children and young people and those with complex health needs: '[should] receive co-ordinated, high quality child and family-centred services which are based on assessed needs, which promote social inclusion and, where possible, enable them and their families to live ordinary lives'.

The pressure on the carer of the child is enormous. Expectations to provide a nutritionally balanced, correct consistency diet while helping the child develop oral motor skills can understandably be stressful. Time is a major consideration, as it takes longer to feed a child with feeding difficulties. Gisel and Patrick's [75] study of children with CP and oral motor dysfunction showed some required up to 18 times longer per mouthful of food.

Nutrition screening

At present there is no nutrition screening tool designed specifically for children with neurodisability. While the need is recognised and data collection to produce a nutrition screening tool is underway [76], there are a number of practices that can be followed to highlight those children most likely to need assessment by a dietitian. There is a direct relationship between severity of oral motor dysfunction and increased likelihood of malnutrition. It is important for a speech and language therapist (SLT) to be involved in assessing eating and drinking. School nurses should measure the child's weight and height regularly and alert the dietitian when deviation from a centile arises.

Funding for dietetic input to neurodisability is limited and intervention often only occurs when the child is referred in a malnourished state. It is inevitable that dietetic workloads will increase as screening becomes established and education of other health care professionals to initiate first line nutritional advice is essential.

Multidisciplinary assessment

Current literature highlights the importance of the multidisciplinary approach to nutritional assessment of children with neurodisabilities [5,77–81]. In the absence of a validated nutrition screening tool, nutrition and feeding problems are identified by measuring children, observing mealtimes and questioning parents, carers and nursing staff. A multidisciplinary feeding assessment draws together the skills and expertise from parent, carer and a range of health care professionals.

Speech and language therapist

A feeding assessment by an SLT should always be incorporated into the nutritional assessment of a child with neurodisability [82]. Assessment of feeding competence provides vital information for identifying children at risk from poor nutritional status. Feeding dysfunction is related to nutritional risk and it has been shown that even those who have mild dysfunction are still lighter and shorter than their peers [5,83]. The assessment will also highlight any problems with drooling or excess salivation, which will need to be factored into calculation of fluid requirements.

Occupational therapist

The occupational therapist takes a particular interest in the child's position for eating and drinking, their level of independence and any special equipment that may aid the child. A child will need to have a secure base and symmetrical position to obtain optimum trunk, limb, head and oral control. The position may be either on the carer's lap for infants and small children or in adapted seating. The assessment should also involve the carer's needs so they adopt a position that is comfortable, safe for their back and facilitates the techniques necessary to help the child. Sometimes this will require the parent or carer to experiment with different positions until they have the best arrangement for them both.

The child's position during mealtimes can affect their ability to swallow safely. Young babies are usually fed in a reclined position. Children should generally eat and drink in an upright position to ensure a safe swallow. If a degree of tilt is required on their seating system a reassessment of their ability to swallow safely should be carried out.

There is a wide range of specialised equipment available on the market to assist with eating and drinking for children with special needs. A joint assessment between the child's occupational therapist and SLT is required to ensure the correct equipment is selected.

Clinical psychologist

The input of a clinical psychologist is necessary for the maximum benefit to be derived from a feeding assessment. A child's early feeding experiences may impact on how they currently feed, particularly those children who have experienced distress because of early feeding practices. This can sometimes result in a learned aversive behaviour often mistaken for a dislike of food or a poor appetite, which can only be resolved with adequate psychological support. The psychologist will consider factors influencing feeding including:

- The environment where the child usually eats
- Parents' eating history and attitude to food
- Early attachment difficulties, especially with an ill child
- Marital/family stress, life events, social support, family networks
- General parenting skills
- Parent–child relationship and interaction
- Past and present parental mental health
- Parental level of anxiety and obsessions

Parents and carers

Health care professionals use the information from parents and carers as a basis for their assessments, providing invaluable details about the child. However, the dietitian should always check the reliability of the information supplied as dietary reports are known to be inaccurate [5,83,84].

Nutritional assessment

A systematic review of the literature revealed that there were no randomised controlled trials on dietetic assessment to ascertain nutritional status in children with neurodisability. Thus, the following information has been developed as a consensus guideline of what is felt to be best practice based on the most current literature [85]. Most research is concerned with children with CP, therefore, caution must be taken when extrapolating these recommendations to children with other neurodisabilities.

Weight

Weight should be measured routinely on the most appropriate weighing equipment for the individual child or situation. These include wheelchair scales and sitting scales for the child, as well as the carer holding the child on the scales and then their weight being subtracted. There is no evidence comparing the accuracy of the various weighing methods, thus all should be accepted as of equal value. The chosen method should be recorded and used in subsequent weighings. Weight measures should be plotted on growth charts. The frequency of measurements will be dependent on local practice and the child's individual circumstances, but should be a minimum of every 6 months for older children and young people, but more frequently for children under the age of 2 years.

Height

Accurate height measures are often difficult to obtain in disabled children and young people because of scoliosis or kyphosis caused by a twisted posture or contractures of the spine. Where this is not a problem, a standing height is preferable, but a supine length is an acceptable second choice. It is important to note, however, that a supine length will measure longer than a standing height and serial measures should not be confused.

Where a length or height is not possible there are three suggested alternatives: upper arm length, lower leg length and knee height, all of which have been found to correlate with actual height [85].

Upper arm length

Upper arm length (UAL) is measured from the acromion to the head of the radius (Fig. 30.1). It should be measured on the right or the least affected side. Two measurements are taken and then averaged. Research suggests it can only be taken accurately using an anthropometer. The measurement can be converted into a height measure

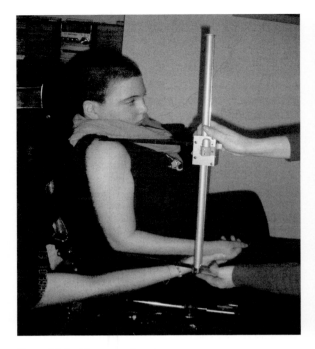

Figure 30.1   Upper arm length.

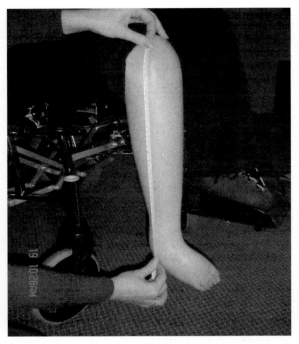

Figure 30.2   Lower leg length.

and plotted on a normal growth chart, using the following formula:

Stature $= (4.35 \times \text{UAL}) + 21.8$

The technical error is ± 1.7 cm

Lower leg length

The lower leg length, also know as the tibial length (TL), is measured from the lower border of the medial malleolus to the medial tip of the tibia. It requires the child to be sitting and is taken on the right side or the least affected side. This measurement can be taken accurately with an anthropometer or steel tape measure (Fig. 30.2). Two measurements should be taken and averaged. The measurement can be converted into a height measure and plotted on a normal growth chart, using the following formula:

Stature $= (3.26 \times \text{TL}) + 30.8$

The technical error is ± 1.4 cm

Knee height

Knee height (KH) is measured with the child sitting down and the knee and ankle bent to 90°. Using a sliding caliper the distance between the heel to the superior surface of the knee over the femoral condyle is measured on the left side or least affected side (Fig. 30.3). Two measurements should be taken and averaged. The measurement can be converted into a height measure and plotted on a normal growth chart, using the following formula:

Stature $= (2.69 \times \text{KH}) + 24.2$

The technical error is ± 1.1 cm

When an alternative length measurement is taken, note of which limb the measurement was taken from should be made, and this should be consistently used for all subsequent measures. There are centiles specifically for each of the alternative measurements based on American data by Snyder *et al.* [86] but these tables are presently not widely available within the UK; thus, conversion to a

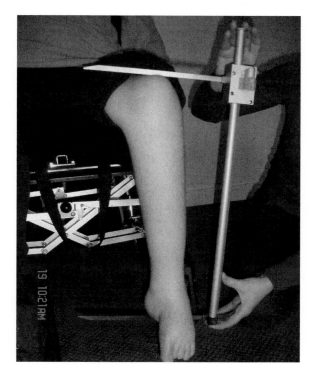

Figure 30.3   Knee height.

height measure and plotting on a standard growth chart is recommended.

Body mass index

There is no evidence to support the use of body mass index (BMI) in children with neurodisability, and one study found BMI to be a poor indicator of low body fat in children with CP [87].

Body composition

There is good evidence that body composition of disabled children can be ascertained by measuring skinfold thickness. Triceps and subscapular skinfold thickness in particular correlates highly with true fat and fat free mass. However, in routine practice, it can be difficult to take accurate skinfold thickness measurements. For example, a subscapular skinfold thickness measurement may be

impractical because of the need to remove clothing or spinal jackets. In practical terms, annual serial measurements of mid arm circumference and triceps skinfold thickness can be a useful monitoring tool [85] when plotted on Tanner–Whitehouse skinfold charts.

Growth charts

The standard UK 1990 charts (available from the Child Growth Foundation) should be used for monitoring weight and height centiles for the majority of disabled children [85], the exception being conditions where disease specific charts have been published (e.g. Down's syndrome). Charts for children with CP have been suggested for use by Krick *et al.* [52]; however, these charts have not been reproduced for clinical use and were based on a small study sample size and poor method of data collection so should not be used in routine practice.

Dietary assessment

Current evidence to support the methods of assessing food intake is poor. There are three common methods of assessment: food diaries, dietary recall and food frequency questionnaires. All available evidence emphasises that no method gives accurate information on food intake and over-reporting is the main problem. This can be as high as 54% more than the child's actual intake so calculating food intake is likely to be inaccurate and is not routinely recommended [85].

However, dietary assessments are useful for assessing meal patterns and the types of food offered and eaten, in relation to the food groups. Observation of a child at a mealtime may be more useful and can highlight other factors that affect dietary intake such as the child's posture and the mealtime environment [85].

Nutritional requirements

Energy

Disabled children have lower resting energy expenditure because of reduced mobility so their total requirement for energy is often lower. Prediction equations and Dietary Reference Values therefore overestimate needs [88–90]. This has been seen in projects carried out by the Oxford Feeding Study research team, where disabled children tended to lay down stores of fat rather than muscle when gastrostomy fed beyond their requirement [91,92].

Previously, a prediction equation by Krick *et al.* [93] was advocated as a method of calculating nutritional requirements. This was a complicated equation using muscle tone, activity and growth in its formula. A modified simpler version was published in the second edition of this textbook, but this is no longer recommended. A recent review paper by Hogan [88] suggests a number of formulas for calculating energy requirements of children with CP, but on critical appraisal none are appropriate for application to this client group.

What is known is that children with neurodisability are smaller than their non-disabled counterparts. Until further research becomes available, dietetic consensus opinion is to use height age as a basis to estimate energy needs. Height age is a crude estimation of bone age and bone age is used as the basis for calculating nutritional requirements. This should be adjusted depending on whether weight loss or weight gain is needed. A child entering their pubertal growth spurt will require more energy than one who is not. In practice, the energy requirement is often no more than 75% of the estimated average requirement (EAR) for height age and is often considerably less.

The exceptions to this are those children with mixed CP that includes an athetoid component. Excessive involuntary movements will mean that their energy requirements may actually be higher and closer to the EAR for height age.

For children with Down's syndrome it is suggested that energy requirements are calculated on kcal/cm height. Culley *et al.* [94] have advocated 16.1 kcal/cm/day (67 kJ/cm/day) for boys and 14.3 kcal/cm/day (60 kJ/cm/day) for girls. Patterson and Walberg Ekvall [95] endorse this figure in their nutrition assessment of children with Down's syndrome.

Protein and micronutrients

There are no studies advising what the requirement for these nutrients should be. However, as it is known that disabled children tend to be smaller than their non-disabled peers, dietary reference values for actual age are likely to be too high. Height age should be used as a basis for estimations and it is advisable to meet at least the LRNI.

Fluid

Actual body weight is used to calculate fluid requirement and should be based on those recommended by Great Ormond Street Hospital for Children [96] (see p. 14). However, it is interesting to note that many children appear well hydrated on a fluid intake lower than that calculated. This applies to children over the age of 2 years.

Fibre

Currently there are no UK recommendations for fibre intake in children. In the absence of these, some dietitians may refer to the American recommendations which suggest the calculation of fibre intake in grams: age (years) + 5–10 g [97].

Nutritional management

Oral nutrition

Mealtimes need to be enjoyable for the child, otherwise they are unlikely to be able to eat and drink to their best ability. When the child is alert and healthy they will manage a more challenging consistency of food than if they are tired or unwell and the carer needs to be sensitive to the child's needs on each eating or drinking occasion.

Texture

An SLT should assess the food texture required by the child. The National Descriptors for Texture Classification (produced jointly by the British Dietetic Association and Royal College of Speech and Language Therapists) give clear definitions of texture [98]. The required texture should be described to the carer, giving plenty of examples of ways of achieving the desired texture. The dietitian will also need to discuss the effect that cooling or warming the food may have on texture, the effect of stirring the food repeatedly and how saliva from the spoon will thin the consistency during a prolonged meal.

Presentation

The way food is presented to the child is important for success. Food should be given slowly and rhythmically allowing time to finish each mouthful and anticipate the next one. Small mouthfuls are more likely to be successful; for some children the food needs to be heaped towards the tip of the spoon to provide sensory cues for the lips. The spoon should normally be presented horizontally from the front. Depending on the techniques being practised at the time to encourage chewing, the food may be placed centrally or towards the side of the mouth. Scraping food off the spoon with the top teeth should be avoided. The SLT or occupational therapist can advise appropriate methods for the child to remove food from the spoon and achieve lip closure.

Prompts

The use of prompts at mealtimes prepares a child for eating or drinking. It helps understanding of what is expected and therefore is more likely to be successful. Prompts can be given visually (e.g. an environment with other people eating, mirrors, and seeing, smelling and hearing the food being prepared or arriving at the table). Physical prompts such as the smell of food; stroking the lower lip with the spoon; giving very small amounts so allowing time for the child to experience the taste, texture and temperature of the food can all be used. Verbal prompts promote the awareness of the concepts of eating; asking the child how they would like to be fed, telling the child what is going to happen next, explaining what is being done as it occurs. Repetitive phrases throughout the meal help the child know what they are doing (e.g. 'bite', 'chew' and 'swallow'). Object recognition, such as a spoon being placed in the child's hand prior to each meal helps the child to understand and anticipate that a food is on its way. Assessment will suggest which combination the child will prefer; however, consistency by all helpers is important.

Eating with other people

Eating with other people is important for children with feeding difficulties. However, limitations may prevent this from happening; for instance, the special chair may not fit under the family table. Such problems should be identified in a multidisciplinary mealtime assessment. In some cases the carer may find it easier to give the child their meal before everyone else. Practical ways in which the child can join in with family mealtimes need to be identified. Eating out may be a problem and familiarisation with popular commercial menus will provide ideas for the carer. For example, many venues serve thick shakes which, if transferred to the appropriate cup, can provide a perfect consistency for some children requiring thickened drinks.

Helpers

All people who could possibly be involved with feeding the child should be identified. Total reliance on one main carer should be discouraged as this can make the child dependent on one person's feeding technique. Other members of the family, grandparents, friends, respite care, social service family support, students and volunteers can all give support at mealtimes. The carer should be encouraged to let another person help with at least one meal a week. Training and support should be offered to the helpers and they should be involved in the assessment and review process. Clear details of the programme such as a 'mealtime guidance sheet' must be accessible to all involved with feeding.

Small goals

Skills should be broken down into small, short term goals as these are more likely to enable the child to succeed. Regular review of the child's progress will provide the baseline for building on these skills. Ideally, more small goals will be added according to the child's needs, speed of learning and opportunity to practise. When a child has been unable to achieve a goal it needs to be assessed whether the goal was realistic, whether he or she has been given long enough to practise, whether the task has been impractical for the carer to carry out and why and whether the carer has understood the purpose of carrying out the task. The same goals need to be followed by all involved.

Demonstrating technique

A model of how the task is best carried out provides the carer with a clear picture of what is expected. Also, this can increase the empathy of the demonstrator by briefly experiencing the difficulties experienced by the feeder at every meal.

Support literature

Pre-printed diet sheets rarely accommodate the needs of children with feeding difficulties. Individualised lists of foods of the correct consistency, including suggestions and/or recipes for meals and snacks, are the most useful to a carer. This is particularly important if a child cannot eat commonly used foods such as bread. Foods that can quickly be added to instant mashed potato (e.g. grated cheese, cream cheese, mashed tinned fish, corned beef, paté, avocado pear, frozen chopped spinach) all provide variety without too much preparation time. Some convenience foods can be included when compiling food and drinks lists in order to help reduce the time involved with the preparation of foods and to help reduce the guilt that some carers may feel when relying heavily on convenience foods. Carers should be helped to select value-for-money convenience foods that can be easily modified to the correct texture for the child. There could also be discussion about foods that can be prepared in bulk and frozen in single meal portions.

Food fortification

This should be based on the same dietetic principles as for other children whose growth is faltering. The energy content of food should be increased by using high energy foods and the effect monitored. Energy dense foods need to be of the correct consistency for the child's oral motor skills. Carers familiar with current healthy eating messages are often concerned about the use of high fat foods and re-education is important.

Fluids

Inadequate consumption or excessive fluid loss is a feature common to many children with feeding difficulties. Advice should be based on assessment of why the child is not able to consume adequate fluids. Children with poor lip seal and those who lose fluid from the mouth will need to be offered drinks more frequently. The occupational therapist and SLT can identify the best drinking method, allowing the child to drink enough fluid safely.

For some children thickened fluids can enable more successful drinking. Proprietary pre-thickened drinks are available (Table 30.2). Other fluids can be thickened using food products such as thick yoghurts, ice cream, instant powdered desserts, instant sauce granules and smooth puréed fruit. A range of proprietary thickening agents are also available on prescription (Table 30.2). Many carers have fears about offering thick drinks as they

Table 30.2 Prescribable thickeners and pre-thickened drinks.

	Manufacturer	Product	Suitable for
Thickeners	Cow & Gate	Carobel Instant	Infants and small children
	Nestlé	Nestargel	Infants and small children
	Novartis	Resource ThickenUp	Over 1 year old
	Fresenius Kabi	Thick and Easy	Over 1 year old
	Sutherland	Thixo-D original	Over 1 year old
	Vitaflo	Vitaquick	Over 1 year old
	Nestlé	Clinutren Thickener	Over 3 years old
	Nutricia	Nutilis	Over 3 years old
Thickened drink	Nestlé	Clinutren Thickened Drinks	Over 3 years old
	Novartis	Resource Thickened Drink	Over 1 year old
	Novartis	Resource Thickened Squash	Over 1 year old
	Fresenius Kabi	Thick and Easy Thickened Juices	Over 1 year old
	Fresenius Kabi	Thick and Easy Dairy	Over 2 years old

perceive this as not as thirst quenching, and their use should be fully discussed.

For children who manage food better than fluids, a method of increasing their fluid intake is to offer foods with a high water content between meals (e.g. puréed fruit, thick yoghurts, fromage frais, ice cream and ice lollies). Jelly can be useful, but it dissolves immediately on entering the mouth resulting in the same problems as thin fluids.

Monitoring an increase in fluid intake includes asking whether there have been more wet nappies, less urinary tract infections, and softer or more regular bowel movements. Despite all efforts some children still find it extremely difficult to achieve an acceptable fluid intake.

Increasing fibre

Increasing the child's intake of fruit and vegetables is the most effective way of increasing fibre intake. Puréed fruit can be added to breakfast cereal, yoghurt, custard or given as a fruit smoothie, and extra vegetables can be incorporated in gravy, mashed potato, casseroles and thick soups.

The use of cereal fibre to help with constipation should only be considered if the child is consuming adequate fluids. Breakfast cereals (e.g. Weetabix, Shreddies, Readybrek) softened with hot milk or incorporated into desserts, or soft wholemeal breadcrumbs added to main courses can be eaten by some children. The use of natural bran or high bran foods should be avoided. Prescribable sources of fibre can also be considered.

Supplementation

Prescribed supplements (sip feeds) may be appropriate for some children (Table 11.3). The child's current nutritional intake should be assessed first to ensure that the supplement with the desired composition is selected. The use of supplements should be reviewed regularly. Supplements can be thickened if this has been recommended by the SLT.

Enteral nutrition

Disabled children form the largest group of children requiring long term home enteral tube feeding (HETF) in the UK [99]. Recent data from the British Artificial Nutrition Survey (BANS) shows that this group make up 41% of all children receiving HETF with a large proportion requiring feeding for longer than 1 year.

Short or long term feeding should be considered for children who are faltering in growth with severe feeding difficulties. This must be weighed against the evidence that tube feeding has a severe impact upon the child. The Norah Fry Research Centre study [100] documents the problems encountered by disabled children, their families and those providing health, social care and education services, suggesting 'serious and unintended social deprivations resulting from the need to be tube fed'. This national survey showed a lack of both co-ordination of services and health/social policy resulting in the provision of ineffective support to the child and families. The recommendations from this study to improve the services to children who are tube fed should be encompassed by all statutory agencies nationally.

The choice of nasogastric versus gastrostomy feeding has to be carefully assessed for the child with feeding difficulties. The first is highly likely to interfere with the child's already compromised oral motor skills and respiratory patterns, such as increasing sensitivity and gagging. A gastrostomy can increase the opportunities to improve oral and enteral intake but has surgical risks. Given the right information and support, children with feeding difficulties and their families can find that tube feeding enhances health and quality of life [101].

When the child must receive all of their nutrition by tube feeding, as a result of medical confirmation of aspiration of food/fluids, it must be remembered that this will not prevent aspiration of oral secretions or gastric contents. In some children the placement of a tube will result in a reduction in the lower oesophageal sphincter pressure and subsequent development or increase of GOR. Thorough assessment of the presence or potential development of GOR prior to tube feeding should be carried out.

The decision to initiate enteral feeding is an emotive one which has many ethical considerations. The decision must be in the best interests of the child from a medical point of view and in terms of quality of life and ensuring dignity is maintained. Parents are often reluctant to consent to placement of a gastrostomy tube for feeding, as it can be perceived as having failed to nurture their child by providing food, one of the basic fundamentals of life. Parents should be given all the information they need to reach an informed decision and the process should not be rushed [102,103].

In children with neurodisabilities it has been shown that enteral feeding as well as being well tolerated can improve energy and protein intake, improve weight gain and nutritional status in addition to improving the parental/carers' perceptions of their child's health and quality of life [104–108].

Feeds

An enteral feed should be chosen that supplies the best match with the child's estimated nutritional requirements. This is not an easy task and often it is necessary to look beyond those marketed for specific age and weight ranges (see Table 3.3). It is important not to assume that an age-matched feed will supply adequate levels of nutrients; children with neurodisabilities are a unique group and it is necessary to calculate feeds to ensure all macro- and micronutrients are provided in a reduced energy intake. A lower energy feed specifically designed for children may be the most appropriate. In some situations a feed designed for the older paediatric age range, with more concentrated nutrients, may be more appropriate for the younger child who has low energy requirements and a smaller volume of this type of feed will provide their micronutrient requirements while restricting energy intake. Some children with very low energy requirements may benefit from a small volume of a high protein adult feed and this can be used in children as young as 1 year of age if it is the best nutritional fit. Those adult feeds that are nutritionally complete in a reduced volume (Nutrison 1200 Complete Multi Fibre, Nutrison 1000 Complete Multi Fibre, Fresubin 1000 Complete, Jevity Promote) are worth considering in smaller volumes for children. As constipation is also often an issue a feed containing fibre is always worthwhile using.

Sometimes, if energy requirements are very low, it may not be possible to meet micronutrient requirements in a small volume of any feed. In this instance supplements need to be considered such as Paediatric Seravit for vitamins and minerals, Dioralyte for sodium and potassium, and the various protein powders (e.g. Vitapro, Protifar).

Feeding regimens

Feeding regimens should be decided on discussion with the child, their family and carers. Common choices are:

- Continuous
- Bolus
- Slow bolus via pump

The choice of regimen will also be affected by whether the child is still allowed to eat and drink. The feed may be used merely as a top up after meals or it may replace all oral intake. Commonly, children who are at risk of aspiration are still allowed to take small tastes of food for pleasure but this should be directed by the SLT. If the enteral feed is to be the sole or major source of nutrition, it is common to feed a small volume via a pump at each mealtime to replace the psychological and physiological effects of a meal. Overnight feeding can accompany this type of regimen if a larger volume is required, but this should be discouraged if the child has a nasogastric tube because of the risk of displacement and aspiration, particularly as disabled children often have irregular postures when lying down. Overnight gastrostomy feeding can only be offered if the child can maintain a safe sleeping position, propped up at least 30°. The use of a sleep system can help with safe positioning. The choice of feeding regimen may depend on the child's tolerance, particularly if GORD is present.

Overweight

Sometimes children become very overweight when enteral feeds have not been carefully monitored, or higher volumes (and hence higher energy) have been given to ensure a supply of minimum levels of protein and micronutrients. This can be a very difficult problem to rectify and has led to the precaution of underestimating energy requirements rather than overestimating these when feeds are initially started. The low energy paediatric feed, Nutrini Low Energy Multi Fibre, or a reduced volume of an older paediatric or adult feed can be useful in terms of providing a weight reducing diet via an enteral feed.

Nutritional monitoring

Nutritional   monitoring   of   children   with

neurodisability is actually the reassessment of their nutritional needs. Since their last dietetic review, the child may or may not have grown, because of the difficulty in predicting nutritional requirements in this group.

Monitoring children is as lengthy a process as the initial assessment, but there is often insufficient dietetic provision for this monitoring to happen regularly, if at all. Many of these children may be lost to follow-up once they have had their initial dietetic intervention, as was supported by the results of a recent survey highlighting the potential shortfall in dietetic care for these children [11]. Ideally, adequate time should be allocated for monitoring and this concept should be highlighted in dietetic business case planning.

Weight gain is a crude guide to assessing whether the right amount of nutrition has been prescribed. Often the subjective opinion of the parent or carer on how well nourished their child appears is also sought as a guide. However, these children tend to put on weight as fat rather than muscle and often do not grow taller no matter how much additional nutrition is provided [92]. Measuring body composition by taking skin fold thickness measurements can help clarify this quandary.

The rate of growth and weight gain can be tracked using the child's growth chart. It is normal for many of these children to be tracking below the 0.4th centile for both height and weight and this is acceptable providing they are following the shape of the curve.

The frequency of monitoring has been discussed by Stewart et al. [85] in their consensus guideline for dietetic assessment of children with special needs. They found no evidence to suggest what the optimum frequency should be but have recommended the following:

- *Weight* The frequency of measurements will be dependent on local practice and individual circumstances; weight should be taken a minimum of every 6 months and plotted on the growth chart. Children under 2 years of age should be measured more frequently.
- *Height, length or alternative measure* The frequency of measurements will be dependent on local practice and individual circumstances; height should be taken a minimum of every 6 months and plotted on the growth chart.

- *Triceps skin fold thickness and mid-arm circumference* Measurements should be taken as a minimum every 12 months. Where possible other anthropometric measurements such as subscapular skin fold thickness should be taken.

References

1 Education and Training Subgroup of the Royal College of Paediatrics and Child Health Standing Committee on Disability Training Pack for specialist registrars aiming to be consultants with special responsibility for Paediatric Neurodisability. www.bacdis.org.uk/new/download/training_pack.pdf October 2003.

2 Sullivan PB, Lambert B, Ford-Adams M *et al.* Prevalence and severity of feeding and nutritional problems in children with neurological impairment: Oxford feeding study. *Dev Med Child Neurol*, 2000, **42** 674–80.

3 Almond S Challenges in feeding children with neurodisabilities. *Complete Nutr*, 2005, **5** 37–9.

4 Straus DJ, Shavelle RM, Anderson TW Life expectancy of children with cerebral palsy. *Pediatr Neurol*, 1998, **18** 143–9.

5 Fung E, Samson-Fang L, Stallings V *et al.* Feeding dysfunction is associated with poor growth and health status in children with cerebral palsy. *J Am Diet Assoc*, 2002, **102** 361–73.

6 Reilly S, Skuse D, Poblete X Prevalence of feeding problems and oral motor dysfunction in children with cerebral palsy: a community survey. *J Pediatr*, 1996, **129** 877–82.

7 Dahl M, Thommesen M, Rasmussen M *et al.* Feeding and nutritional characteristics in children with moderate or severe cerebral palsy. *Acta Paediatr*, 1996, **85** 697–701.

8 Del Giudice E, Staiano A, Capano G *et al.* Gastrointestinal manifestations in children with cerebral palsy. *Brain Dev*, 1999, **21** 307–11.

9 Gonzalez L, Nazario CM, Gonzalez MJ Nutrition-related problems of pediatric patients with neuromuscular disorders. *Puerto Rico Health Sci J*, 2000, **19** 35–8.

10 Sullivan P, Juszczak E, Lambert B *et al.* Impact of feeding problems on nutritional intake and growth: Oxford feeding study II. *Dev Med Child Neurol*, 2002, **44** 461–7.

11 Hartley H, Thomas JE Current practice in the management of children with cerebral palsy: a national survey of paediatric dietitians. *J Hum Nutr Diet*, 2003, **16** 219–24.

12 Department of Health *National Service Framework*

for Children, Young People and Maternity Services. Crown copyright, 2004.

13 HM Government. *Every Child Matters: Change for Children.* www.everychildmatters.gov.uk/aims/ 2003.

14 Scope www.scope.org.uk/helpline/cp.shtml Accessed August 2006.

15 Cronk C, Fung E, Stallings V Body composition in children with special health needs. In: Preedy VR, Grimble G, Watson R (eds) *Nutrition in the Infant. Problems and Practical Procedures.* London: GMM, 2001, pp. 31–8.

16 Vik T, Skrove MS, Dollner H *et al.* Feeding problems and growth disorders among children with cerebral palsy in south and north Trondelag. *Tidsskr Nor Laegeforen*, 2001, **121** 1570–4.

17 Down's Syndrome Association www. downssyndrome.org.uk/DSA_Faqs.aspx#faq45 Accessed August 2006.

18 Lissauer T, Clayden G Neurological disorders. In: *Illustrated Textbook of Paediatrics.* London: Mosby, 1997, pp. 291–312.

19 Parkman Williams C (ed) *Pediatric Manual of Clinical Dietetics.* Developed by the Pediatric Nutrition Practice Group. American Dietetic Association, 1998.

20 Van Dyke D *et al.* Problems in feeding. In: Van Dyke DC *et al.* (eds) *Clinical Perspectives in the Management of Down Syndrome.* New York: Springer-Verlag, 1990.

21 Lucas BL In: With Feucht SA, Grieger LE (eds) *Children with Special Health Care Needs.* Chicago, IL: American Dietetic Association, 2004.

22 Spender Q, Stein A, Dennis J *et al.* An exploration of feeding difficulties in children with Down syndrome. *Dev Med Child Neurol*, 1996, **38** 681–94.

23 Hopman E, Csizmadia CG, Bastiani WF *et al.* Eating habits of young children with Down syndrome in the Netherlands: adequate nutrient intakes but delayed introduction of solid food. *J Am Diet Assoc*, 1998, **98** 790–4.

24 Frazier JB, Friedman B Swallow function in children with Down syndrome: a retrospective study. *Dev Med Child Neurol*, **38** 695–703.

25 Jansson U, Johanson C Down's syndrome and coeliac disease. *J Paediatr Gastroenterol Nutr*, 1995, **21** 443–5.

26 Gale L, Wilmalaratra H, Brotodiharjo A *et al.* Down's syndrome is strongly associated with coeliac disease. *Gut*, 1997, **40** 492–6.

27 Cronk C, Crocker AC, Pueschel SM *et al.* Growth charts for children with Down syndrome 1 month to 18 years of age. *Pediatrics*, 1988, **81** 102.

28 Cronk CE Growth of children with Down syndrome: birth to age 3 years. *Pediatrics*, 1978, **61** 564.

29 Rarick GL, Seefeldt V Observations from longitudinal data on growth in stature and sitting height of children with Down's syndrome. *J Mental Defic Res*, 1974, **18** 63.

30 Luke A, Sutton M, Schoeller DA *et al.* Nutrient intake and obesity in prepubescent children with Down syndrome. *J Am Diet Assoc*, 1996, **96** 1262–7.

31 Rubin SS, Rimmer JH, Chicoine B *et al.* Overweight prevalence in persons with Down syndrome. *Ment Retard*, 1998, **36** 175–81.

32 Crino A, Diagilio MC, Ciampalini P *et al.* Growth pattern and pubertal development in Down syndrome: a longitudinal and cross sectional study. *Dev Brain Dysfunction*, 1996, **9** 72–9.

33 Cabana MD, Capone G, Fritz A *et al.* Nutritional rickets in a child with Down syndrome. *Clin Pediatr*, 1997, **36** 235–7.

34 Barlow PJ, Sylvester PE, Dickerson JW Hair trace metal levels in Down's syndrome patients. *J Ment Defic Res*, 1981, **25** 161.

35 Smith GF, Spiker D, Peterson CP *et al.* Use of megadoses of vitamins in Down syndrome. *J Pediatr*, 1984, **105** 228–34.

36 Weathers V Effects of nutritional supplementation on IQ and certain other variables associated with Down syndrome. *Am J Ment Defic*, 1983, **88** 214–17.

37 Muscular Dystrophy Campaign www.musculardystrophy.org/ Accessed August 2006.

38 Willig TN, Paulus J, Lacau Saint Guily J *et al.* Swallowing problems in neuromuscular disorders. *Arch Phys Med Rehabil*, 1994, **75** 1175–81.

39 Jaffe KM, McDonald CM, Ingman E *et al.* Symptoms of upper gastrointestinal dysfunction in Duchenne muscular dystrophy: case–control study. *Arch Phys Med Rehabil*, 1990, **71** 742–4.

40 Hankard R, Gottrand F, Turck D *et al.* Resting energy expenditure and energy substrate utilization in children with Duchenne muscular dystrophy. *Pediatr Res*, 1996, **40** 29–33.

41 Willig TN, Carlier L, Legrand M *et al.* Nutritional assessment in Duchenne muscular dystrophy. *Dev Med Child Neurol*, 1993, **35** 1074–82.

42 Griffiths RD, Edwards RH A new chart for weight control in Duchenne muscular dystrophy. *Arch Dis Child*, 1988, **63** 1256–8.

43 Karle IP, Bleiler RE, Ohlson MA Nutritional status of cerebral palsied children. *J Am Diet Assoc*, 1961, **38** 22–6.

44 Krick J, Van Duyne M The relationship between oral-motor involvement and growth: a pilot study in paediatric population with cerebral palsy. *J Am Diet Assoc*, 1984, **84** 555–9.

45 Tobis J, Saturen P, Larios G *et al.* A study of growth patterns in cerebral palsy. *Arch Phys Med*, 1961, **42** 475–81.

46 Thommessen M, Heiberg A, Kase BF *et al*. Feeding problems, height and weight in different groups of disabled children. *Acta Paediatr Scand*, 1991, **80** 527–33.

47 Sanders KD, Cox K, Cannon R *et al*. Growth response to enteral feeding by children with cerebral palsy. *J Parenter Enteral Nutr*, 1990, **14** 23–6.

48 Thommessen M, Kase BF, Riis G *et al*. The impact of feeding problems on growth and energy intake in children with cerebral palsy. *Eur J Clin Nutr*, 1991, **45** 470–87.

49 Corwin DS, Isaccs JS, Georgeson KE *et al*. Weight and length increase in children after gastrostomy placement. *J Am Diet Assoc*, 1996, **96** 874–9.

50 Samson-Fang, Stevenson R Linear growth velocity in children with cerebral palsy. *Dev Med Child Neurol*, 1998, **40** 874–9.

51 Stevenson RD, Hayes RP, Virgil Cater L *et al*. Clinical correlates of linear growth in children with cerebral palsy. *Dev Med Child Neurol*, 1994, **36** 135–42.

52 Krick J, Murphey-Miller P, Zeger S *et al*. Pattern of growth in children with cerebral palsy. *J Am Diet Assoc*, 1996, **96** 680–5.

53 Stallings V Nutritional assessment of the disabled child. In: *Feeding the Disabled Child*. Clinics in Developmental Medicine no 140. Sullivan P, Rosenbloom L. London: Mackeith Press, 1996 pp. 62–76.

54 Samson-Fang L, Fung E, Stallings VA *et al*. Relationship of nutritional status to health and societal participation in children with cerebral palsy. *J Pediatr*, 2002, **141** 637–43.

55 Sondheimer JM, Morris BA Gastroesophageal reflux among retarded children. *J Paeditr*, 1979, **94** 710–14.

56 Kawahara H, Dent J, Davidson G Mechanisms responsible for gastroesophageal reflux in children. *Gastroenterol*, 1997, **113** 339–408.

57 Rudolph CD, Mazur LJ, Liptak SJ Guidelines for evaluation and treatment of gastroesophageal reflux in infants and children: Recommendations of the North American Society for Pediatric Gastroenterology and Nutrition. *J Pediatr Gastroenterol Nutr*, 2001, **32** S1–31.

58 Spitz L, Roth K, Kiely EM *et al*. Operation for gastro-oesophageal reflux associated with severe mental retardation. *Arch Dis Child*, 1993, **68** 347–51.

59 Stringel G, Delgado M, Guertin L *et al*. Gastrostomy and Nissen fundoplication in neurologically impaired children. *J Pediatr Surg*, 1989, **24** 1044–8.

60 Kimber C, Keily EM, Spitz L The failure rate of surgery for gastro-oesophageal reflux. *J Pediatr Surg*, 1998; **33** 64–6.

61 Sullivan P Annotation: Gastrostomy feeding in the disabled child: when is an antireflux procedure required? *Arch Dis Child*, 1999, **81** 463–4.

62 Hussain S Z, Di-Lorenzo C Motility disorders. Diagnosis and treatment for the paediatric patient. *Paediatr Clin North Am*, 2002, **49** 27–51.

63 Hassall E Outcomes of fundoplication: causes for concern, newer options. *Arch Dis Child*, 2005, **90** 1047–52.

64 Bohmer CJM, Taminiau JAJM, Klinkenberg-Knol EC *et al*. The prevalence of constipation in institutionalised people with intellectual disability. *J Intellect Disab Res*, 2001, **45** 212–18.

65 Chong SKF Gastrointestinal problems in the handicapped child. *Curr Opin Pediatr*, 2001, **13** 441–6.

66 Clayden G Constipation in disabled children. In: *Feeding the Disabled Child*. Clinics in Developmental Medicine no 140. Sullivan P, Rosenbloom L. London: Mackeith Press, 1966, pp. 106–16.

67 Liebl BH, Fischer MH, Van Calcar SC *et al*. Dietary fiber and long-term large bowel response in enterally nourished nonambulatory profoundly retarded youth. *J Parenter Enteral Nutr*, 1990, **14** 371–5.

68 Tolia V, Ventimiglia J, Kuhns L Gastrointestinal tolerance of a pediatric fiber formula in developmentally disabled children. *J Am Coll Nutr*, 1997, **16** 224–8.

69 Staiano A, Simeone D, Del Giudice E *et al*. Effect of the dietary fiber glucomannan on chronic constipation in neurologically impaired children. *J Pediatr*, 2000, **136** 41–5.

70 Trier E, Wells JCK, Thomas AG Effects of a multifibre supplemented paediatric enteral feed on gastrointestinal function. *J Pediatr Gastroenterol Nutr*, 1999, **28** 595.

71 Tse PWT, Leung SSF, Chan T *et al*. Dietary fibre intake and constipation in children with severe developmental disabilities. *J Paediatr Child Health*, 2000, **36** 236–9.

72 Daly A, Johnson T, MacDonald A Is fibre supplementation in paediatric sip feeds beneficial? *J Hum Nutr Diet*, 2004, **17** 365–70.

73 Boyd LD, Palmer C, Dwyer JT Managing oral health related nutrition issues of high risk infants and children. *J Clin Pediatr Dent*, 1998, **23** 31–6.

74 Chailey Heritage. *Eating and Drinking Skills for Children with Motor Disorders*. 1998. Chailey Heritage Clinical Services, Beggars Wood Road, North Chailey, Lewes, East Sussex, BN8 4JN.

75 Gisel E, Patrick J Identification of children unable to maintain a normal nutritional state. *Lancet*, 1998, **1** 283–6.

76 Almond S Design and validation of a nutrition screening tool for children aged 3–19 years with neurodisability. Thesis, University of Brighton.

77 Miles A, Reed G Feeding challenges in children with neurologic impairment. *Support Line*, 2004, **25** 16–23.

78   Chong, Sonny KF Gastrointestinal problems in the handicapped child. *Curr Opin Pediatr*, 2001, **13** 441–6.

79   Schwarz S Feeding disorders in children with developmental disabilities. *Infants and Young Children*, 2003, **16** 317–30.

80   Samson-Fang L, Fung E, Stallings V *et al*. Relationship of nutritional status to health and societal participation in children with cerebral palsy. *J Pediatr*, 2002, **141** 637–43.

81   Manikam R, Perman JA Paediatric feeding disorders. *J Clin Gastroenterol*, 2000, **30** 34–6.

82   Troughton K, Hill AE Relation between objectively measured feeding competence and nutrition in children with cerebral palsy. *Dev Med Child Neurol*, 2001, **43** 187–90.

83   Reilly JJ, Hassan TM, Braekken A *et al*. Growth retardation and undernutrition in children with spastic cerebral palsy. *J Hum Nutr Diet*, 1996, **9** 429–35.

84   Stallings VA, Zemel BS, Davies JC *et al*. Energy expenditure of children and adolescents with severe disabilities: a cerebral palsy model. *Am J Clin Nutr*, 1996, **64** 627–34.

85   Stewart L, Mckaig N, Dunlop C *et al*. Guidelines on dietetic assessment and monitoring of children with special needs with faltering growth. British Dietetic Association, Birmingham, 2006.

86   Synder RG, Golomb DH, Schork MA Anthropometry of infants, children and youths to age 18 for product Safety Design. UM-HSRI-77-17. 1977. Bethesda MD, Consumer Product Safety Commission.

87   Samson-Fang L, Stevenson RD Identification of malnutrition in children with cerebral palsy: poor performance of weight-for-height centiles. *Dev Med Child Neurol*, 2000, **42** 162–8.

88   Hogan, SE Energy requirements of children with cerebral palsy. *Can J Diet Pract Res*, 2004, **65** 124–30.

89   Bandini LG, Schoeller DA, Fukagawa NK *et al*. Body composition and energy expenditure in adolescents with cerebral palsy or myelodysplasia. *Pediatr Res*, 1991, **29** 70–7.

90   Azcue MP Zello GA, Levy LD *et al*. Energy expenditure and body composition in children with spastic quadriplegic cerebral palsy. *J Pediatr*, 1996, **129** 870–6.

91   Vernon-Roberts A Bachlet A, Warner J *et al*. Energy balance and body composition in children with cerebral palsy. *J Pediatr Gastroenterol Nutr*, 2002, **34** 478.

92   Bachlet A, Vernon-Roberts A, Stirling L *et al*. Body composition in severely disabled children fed either orally or via gastrostomy. *J Pediatr Gastroenterol Nutr*, 2003, **36** 525.

93   Krick J, Murphy PE, Markham JFB *et al*. Proposed formula for calculating energy needs of children with cerebral palsy. *Dev Med Child Neurol*, 1996, **43** 481–7.

94   Culley W, Goyal K, Jolly DH *et al*. Caloric intake of children with Down's syndrome (mongolism). *J Pediatr*, 1965, **66** 722.

95   Patterson B, Walberg Ekvall S. Down syndrome. In: *Pediatric Nutrition in Chronic Diseases and Developmental Disorders: Prevention, Assessment and Treatment*. New York: Oxford University Press, 1993.

96   Great Ormond Street Hospital for Children NHS Trust. *Nutritional Requirements for Children in Health and Disease*, 3rd edn. 2000.

97   Williams CL, Bollella M, Wynder EL A new recommendation for dietary fibre in children. *Pediatrics*, 1995, **96** 985–8.

98   www.bda.uk.com/members/professionalguidancedocuments/dysphagia Accessed August 2006.

99   Jones B, Stratton R, Holden C *et al*. Trends in home artificial nutrition support in the UK during 2000–2003. A Report by the British Artificial Nutrition Survey (BANS), a committee of the British Association for Parenteral and Enteral Nutrition. Redditch, Worcs. 2005.

100   Townsley R, Robinson C *Food for Thought? Effective support for families caring for a child who is tube fed*. Bristol: Norah Fry Research Centre, 2000.

101   McCurtin A *The Manual of Paediatric Feeding Practice*. Bicester, Oxon: Winslow Press, 1997.

102   Isaacs JS, Georgeson KE, Cloud HH *et al*. Weight gain and triceps skinfolds fat mass after gastrostomy placement in children with developmental disabilities. *J Am Diet Assoc*, 1994, **94** 849–54.

103   Wilkinson D Response to 'Nutrition in children with cerebral palsy'. *J Paediatr Child Health*, 2004, **40** 308–10.

104   Brant CQ, Stanich P, Ferrari AP Jr Improvement of children's nutritional status after enteral feeding by PEG: an interim report. *Gastrointest Endosc*, 1999, **50** 183–8.

105   Brant CQ, Smith SW, Camfield C *et al*. Living with cerebral palsy and tube feeding: A population-based follow-up study. *J Pediatr*, 1999, **135** 307–10.

106   Rogers B, Wood K, Almeida J *et al*. Feeding method and growth of children with cerebral palsy. *Dev Med Child Neurol*, 2000, **42** (Suppl 83) abstract E1.

107   Sullivan PB, Thomas AG, Eltumi M *et al*. Gastrostomy-tube feeding improves quality of life in caregivers of disabled children. *J Pediatr Gastroenterol Nutr*, 2002, **34** 485(A34).

108   Samson-Fang L, Butler C, O'Donnell M Effects on gastrostomy feeding in children with cerebral palsy: an AACPDM evidence report. *Dev Med Child Neurol*, 2003, **45** 415–26.

Useful addresses

Cerebra
13 Guildhall Square, Camarthen, SA31 1PR
www.cerebra.org.uk

Scope for People with Cerebral Palsy
6 Market Road, London, N7 9PW
Tel. 020 7619 7100
www.scope.org.uk

The Bobath Centre for Children with Cerebral Palsy
Bradbury House, 250 East End Road, London, N2 8AU
Tel. 020 8444 3355

Crisp
NICOD, Malcolm Sinclair House, 31 Ulsterville Avenue, Belfast, BT9 7AS
Tel. 01232 666188

National Institute of Conductive Education
Cannon Hill House, Russell Road, Moseley, Birmingham, B13 8RD
Tel. 0121 449 1569
www.conductive-education.org.uk

Advisor Service Capability Scotland (ASCS)
111 Ellersly Road, Edinburgh, EH12 6HY
Tel. 0131 346 7864

The Scottish Centre for Children with Motor Impairments
Craighalbert Centre, 1 Craighalbert Way, Cumbernauld, G68 0LS
Tel. 01236 456 100

Norah Fry Research Centre
3 Priory Road, Bristol, BS8 ITX
Tel. 0117 923 8137
www.bris.ac.uk/Depts/NorahFry/

Rett Syndrome Association UK
113 Friern Barnet Road, London, N11 3EU
Tel. 020 8361 5161
www.rettsyndrome.org.uk

31 Obesity

Laura Stewart

Introduction

Obesity is the most common childhood nutritional disorder worldwide and is widely acknowledged as having become a global epidemic [1,2]. The prevalence of childhood obesity has followed the trend of the disease in adults and in the UK has dramatically increased over a short number of years during the 1990s [3,4]. In the UK the importance of finding effective strategies for the prevention and treatment of childhood obesity has gained national significance with the publication of various expert reports and evidence based guidelines [5–7] as well as government reviews and reports [8–10].

Aetiology

The aetiology of obesity is complex and multifactorial: it has become generally well recognised that the causes of childhood obesity are an interaction between our obesogenic environment and individual lifestyle choices. Increases in the amount of energy dense foods eaten (particularly fast foods), more time spent watching television and playing computer games with a simultaneous decrease in the amount of physical activity undertaken by children have all been mooted as causes of the current epidemic [8,10,11]. Because excess weight gain occurs in a state of positive energy balance, the aetiology of obesity is most likely a combination of these factors.

There is an increasing understanding of genetics in the aetiology of obesity although further research is required. There is evidence that some genes may predispose certain people to obesity although this predisposition cannot explain the rapid increase in prevalence over such a short time. Work on monogenetic obesity also continues but the numbers of people affected by this is extremely small.

Organic causes of obesity such as Cushing's syndrome and hypothyroidism are rare. Prader–Willi syndrome is often associated with obesity and this condition is dealt with separately at the end of this chapter.

Within the UK prevalence studies have shown that there are certain groups that appear to be more 'at risk' of childhood obesity: lower social economic groups (V and IV) [12,13]; certain ethnic groups (as detailed in the UK Health of the Nation Survey of ethnic minority groups) [13], in particular Asians [14] and Africans or Afro-Caribbeans; and children and adolescents with special needs [15]. There also appears to be a higher prevalence in Scotland and Wales than in England [14].

Definition

Body mass index (BMI) is generally recognised as

the most appropriate measure for defining and diagnosing childhood obesity and overweight [2,5,16]. Because normal BMI in childhood changes with age and differs between the sexes, it is only meaningful when plotted correctly on age and sex specific centile charts. UK BMI centile charts have been available since the early 1990s and all health professionals working with obese children should use these charts for diagnosis and monitoring of treatment [17]. They are available from the Child Growth Foundation (CGF; see pp. 20, 596).

As in adulthood any definition of childhood overweight and obesity needs to define not only body fatness but also the clinical relevance of this body fat: at what level of BMI is there a significant increase in the consequences of childhood obesity? Currently there is much debate, both nationally and internationally, over the most appropriate centile cut-off points for defining childhood overweight and obesity. There are essentially two schools of thought: those who favour the use of the 95th centile on the UK BMI 1990 charts for epidemiological studies (and importantly the 98th centile for clinical use) to define obesity [5], and the 85th centile (91st centile for clinical use) to define overweight; and those who advocate the use of an 'international cut-off point' which on the UK 1990 charts is close to the 99th centile for obesity for both boys and girls and around the 90th centile for overweight [18].

This debate is likely to continue for some time. However, studies are continuing to appear that support the 95th centile cut-off as more specific and sensitive for diagnosis as well as more clinically significant than the international cut-off point [19,20].

Consequences

There are a number of consequences of childhood obesity that are seen in childhood, adolescence and later in life. Clustering of cardiovascular risk factors have been reported in children and adolescents: high blood pressure, dyslipidaemia, abnormalities in left ventricular mass and/or function, abnormalities in endothelial function and hyperinsulinaemia and/or insulin resistance. There is a body of evidence that these cardiovascular risk factors are seen in adults who were obese children or

adolescents [19,21]. There is also a growing number of reports of type 2 diabetes being seen in adolescents [22,23], a previous unknown condition in this age group. Psychological problems, particularly in girls, have been reported in relation to low self-esteem and behavioural problems. There are also long term consequences of social and economic effects particularly in women achieving a lower income [19,21].

There is good evidence to suggest that childhood and adolescent obesity does persist (or track) into adulthood. This risk of persistence into adulthood is affected by a number of factors, the most significant being:

- Parental obesity; high risk if one parent is obese, higher if both are obese
- Level of obesity; increasing risk with increasing level of obesity
- Obesity in adolescence [19,21]

Assessment

At the first clinic visit, baseline measurements should be obtained for weight and height and plotted on centile charts (UK 1990 charts, CGF). BMI should be calculated [weight (kg) ÷ height $(m)^2$] and plotted at the correct age on the appropriate centile chart for sex (UK 1990 chart, CGF). Although used regularly in research in clinical practice, arm anthropometry such as triceps skinfold measurement and mid arm circumference are rarely used. The use of waist measurements in children has gained support in recent years and UK waist circumference centile charts [24] are now available from the CGF. Dietitians should be aware, however, that there is no agreed cut-off point for defining those at health risk [2]. Taking the waist measurement can be difficult in obese children but is felt by some to be a useful tool in monitoring progress in weight management.

At this first visit it is most important to get a detailed dietary history from both the child and the parent or carer. It is advisable to ask specifically about takeaway meals, snack foods and drinks consumed between meals and outside of the house because these are often overlooked. Other details such as age of onset of obesity, eating patterns and family dynamics are most helpful.

It is essential to ascertain the levels of physical activity that are normally undertaken as well as time spent watching television and playing computer or video games.

Management

In recent years there have been a number of systematic reviews and guidelines on childhood obesity [5–8,25,26]. Surprisingly, there is a lack of good quality evidence on successful treatment of childhood obesity. There is, however, consensus on the following points:

- Treatment should only be commenced when the parents are ready and willing to make lifestyle changes
- Treatment should be family based with at least one of the parents involved
- Lifestyle changes in diet, physical activity and sedentary behaviours should be targeted
- Weight maintenance is an acceptable goal of treatment, with height increasing and the BMI decreasing over time
- For children over 7 years slow weight loss of 0.5 kg/month may be advised [5,6,27]

The role of the dietitian (whether in the community or hospital setting, individually or as part of a multidisciplinary team), is to educate the child and family on the necessary lifestyle changes and to help facilitate behavioural modifications. It is important that this is done in a positive, enthusiastic, non-judgmental and sensitive manner. The

dietitian should encourage healthy eating and healthy lifestyle messages are conveyed to both parents, other family members, teachers and other carers. The whole family should be encouraged to make any necessary lifestyle changes.

Some dietitians may work with individual children and their families or hold group sessions. Where group sessions are used it is not uncommon for there to be some separate sessions for the children and parents. Indeed, some parents appreciate the opportunity to discuss problems they have encountered with fellow parents and the dietitian without the child being present.

Diet

Children and their families should be encouraged to reduce the amount of foods high in sugar and fat in their diet (Table 31.1) and replace them with foods lower in energy such as fruit and vegetables (Table 31.2). Calorie counting is not normally used with children. The dietitian should consider the number of takeaway meals the child and family have, the amount and types of snacks the child eats and the amount of pocket money the child has to freely spend. Many parents find food labelling confusing and appreciate advice and help with understanding what to look for and interpret and how to read labels on packets.

It is important to ensure that normal growth occurs when dietary intake is restricted. Adequate quantities of protein, vitamins and minerals should be taken; some children who dislike certain foods

---

Table 31.1 General guidelines for reducing energy intake.

Avoid fried foods (including chips and crisps) and added fat during cooking
Remove visible fat from meat and choose low fat product (e.g. low fat mince, sausages)
Use butter and margarine sparingly on bread and crispbread; a low fat spread is preferable
Do not add butter or alternatives to foods (e.g. cooked vegetables)
Avoid adding sugar to foods and drinks. An energy free artificial sweetener (e.g. aspartame) may be used if required
Exclude as far as practical chocolate, sweets, cakes and biscuits
Give vegetables or salad at each meal
Use fruit (fresh, frozen, tinned in natural juice), low calorie yogurt and sugar free jelly in place of desserts
Use low energy drinks and squash
Use semi-skimmed or skimmed milk (with care in children under 5 years); do not exceed 600 mL/day
Use low fat cheese in place of full fat; use low fat fromage frais in place of cream
Avoid using diabetic foods except fruit squash

Table 31.2 Low energy foods allowed freely.

All vegetables
All fruit

Miscellaneous
Artificial sweeteners (e.g. saccharin, aspartame)
Sugar free drinks
Coffee
Tea
Herbs
Spices
Seasonings
Vinegar
Sugar free jelly and chewing gum
Mineral and soda water
Stock cubes

Table 31.3 Healthy intake for weight management.

Milk – aim to give 300 mL/day, with a maximum of 600 mL.
Semi-skimmed or skimmed can be used. Low fat yogurts, low
fat hard cheese will all provide calcium if milk is disliked
as a drink

Meat, fish, poultry, egg, cheese, beans and lentils – two
portions should be given from this group daily. Low fat meats
should be used, and meat should be grilled or baked, not fried

Cereal foods – breakfast cereal, wholemeal bread, brown rice,
wholegrain pasta and crackers – at least one portion should be
included at each meal. Avoid adding extra fat and sugar

Vegetables and fruit – aim for five portions daily, raw or
cooked

Sample menu

Breakfast	Wholegrain unsweetened cereal, porridge or muesli with semi-skimmed milk (no sugar) Bread or toast with small amount of spread Semi-skimmed milk or unsweetened fruit juice
Snack	Plain cracker or piece of fruit Water or low calorie squash
Lunch	Roll or bread, filled with tuna, meat, egg, low fat cheese or peanut butter/baked beans on toast Chopped salad or cooked vegetables Low calorie yogurt or fruit
Snack	Fruit, raisins or small sandwich Water or low calorie squash
Evening meal	Meat, fish, cheese or pulse dish Vegetables or salad Potatoes, rice or pasta Fruit or low energy dessert
Bedtime	Semi-skimmed milky drink (unsweetened)

and do not consume a nutritionally adequate diet
may need a supplement of vitamins or minerals
(particularly iron and calcium). Written information including a list of unrestricted foods and a list
of foods allowed should be given to the parents and
child (Tables 31.2 and 31.3).

The question of school dinners should be
addressed as many overweight children regularly
consume foods high in fat and sugar for lunch at
school. Government initiatives to improve school
meals and encourage healthy eating such as
'Hungry for Success' in Scotland [28] should help
improve this situation (see p. 533). Fruit and low
calorie yogurt are a good replacement for dessert
and the child should be advised to avoid second
helpings. It is easier to provide suitable food in the
form of a packed lunch, although a certain amount
of swapping of items often takes place.

The suggestion that money previously spent on
foods such as sweets, chocolate, crisps can be used
for other items of the child's choice (e.g. games,
books, clothing) is sometimes useful, particularly
for indulgent grandparents. However, the use of a
food 'treat' on a weekly or daily basis, if necessary,
can help the child psychologically and provide
motivation.

Physical activity

Children should be encouraged to increase their
overall activity levels, aiming for a minimum of
30 minutes increasing to 60 minutes of moderate–
vigorous activity per day [5]. Many overweight and
obese children dislike team sports and physical
education at school so it is important for the dietitian to help the child and family find local activities
that they enjoy and are not embarrassed to take part
in. Research has shown that increasing 'lifestyle
activities' such as walking, taking the stairs rather
than lifts can be particularly effective in controlling
weight on a long term basis [29].

Sedentary behaviours

Recommendations are that the amount of time
children spend watching TV or playing video/
computer games should be decreased to under
2 hours/day or an average of 14 hours/week

[5,30,31]. Some children and parents may find this difficult and the dietitian needs to discuss how this reduction can be attained over time.

Behavioural modification

Many clinics have a high drop out rate [32] and dietitians need to think very carefully about their manner and approach with the child and family. The use of behavioural change techniques such as goal setting, recording and rewards might be considered [7,29,33–36]. Successful treatment of obesity demands a sustained commitment and effort from the whole family and the dietitian must endeavour to maintain a positive attitude and help motivate the child and family towards weight control.

The management outlined above is relevant for all age groups; however, there are two groups that require particular consideration.

Infants and pre-school children

It is difficult to overfeed a breast fed infant, but bottle fed infants can be persuaded to consume a greater volume than they require; in addition feeds can be made more concentrated than recommended or items such as cereal can be added to the bottle [37]. An infant naturally has more body fat than at other times in the lifespan; body fat content begins to decline after the first year of life. There is usually no need to restrict an infant's diet but advice may be needed if feeding practices are inappropriate or a slowing of weight gain is thought to be necessary.

The following advice may be helpful:

- Make sure that parents react appropriately to the infant's crying; often crying is perceived as indicating hunger, when in fact the baby may be bored, tired or uncomfortable.
- Avoid any additions to the infant's bottle (e.g. sugar or cereal).
- Make certain that the feed dilution is correct and that volume is appropriate for age.
- Solids should not be introduced before the age of 6 months.
- Weaning solids should have a low energy density (e.g. vegetables and unsweetened fruit).

- Reduced fat products can be used in the weaning diet (e.g. low fat yogurts, reduced fat cheese).
- When a greater variety of foods are being consumed (e.g. lean meat, white fish and wholegrain cereals), the quantity of milk (breast or formula) should be decreased.
- Infants should be introduced to a cup or teacher beaker from about 7–8 months and bottles omitted by 1 year of age. More formula is generally consumed when feeding from a bottle.
- Whole cow's milk can be used as the main milk drink from 1 year of age. Generally, skimmed and semi-skimmed milk should not be used before the ages of 5 and 2 years, respectively. However, these lower fat milks are a useful way of decreasing energy intake in the overweight toddler. It is important that a supplement of vitamins A and D are given with these milks.
- Drinks of water should be offered with and in between meals. If the child is reluctant to drink water, pure unsweetened fruit juice, well diluted, can be given once or twice daily, with meals, although if the vitamin C content of the diet is adequate there is no nutritional need for this.

Physical activity should be increased among the less active families/children; on occasions parents may be seen who still use a pushchair for an overweight child of 3–4 years because he or she walks too slowly!

Adolescents

Adolescents present dietitians with their greatest challenge. Normal adolescent behaviours and peer pressure for consumption of snack foods dense in fat and sugar is high and can lead to resistance towards lifestyle changes. The lifestyle advice as outlined above should be given but the dietitian needs to carefully consider their approach and ensure that the adolescent feels ownership of goal setting and all stages towards behavioural change.

'Slimming' foods and drinks as a replacement for a meal are not appropriate, as they generally contain insufficient protein, minerals and micronutrients to meet the high requirements for this age group.

Drug therapy

'New generation' drugs for the treatment of obesity (orlistat, sibutramine) are being used in adults but at present these have not been licensed for use in children or adolescents in the UK.

Prevention

Promotion of a healthy lifestyle must start in childhood if we are to reverse the present trend and current government initiatives around healthy eating and increasing physical activities at schools may be helpful in the future. Prevention strategies need to focus on the complex issues around childhood obesity involving diet, physical activity, sedentary behaviour, family lifestyle and environment. These interventions must therefore engage complex behavioural changes such as in the school based 'Planet Health' project [38]. The most recent Cochrane review on interventions for preventing childhood obesity found a limited number of well-conducted studies and the review recommends that future interventions consider sustainability and environmental changes along with individual and family lifestyle [39].

Prader–Willi syndrome

Prader–Willi syndrome (PWS) is a rare genetic disorder; the main characteristics are hypotonia, short stature, hypogonadism, varying degrees of mental retardation, short stature and poor emotional and social development. Children with PWS have an insatiable appetite (hyperphagia) leading to gross obesity if not controlled. The prevalence has been estimated at 1 in 25 000 births [40] making PWS the most common genetic cause of obesity.

There are two distinct phases that are characteristic of this syndrome – at birth infants present with hypotonia and feeding difficulties and subsequently fail to thrive (Fig. 31.1). Tube feeding may be required during this period, which is typically from birth to approximately 2 years of age. It is from around 2–3 years onwards that weight is likely to escalate [41].

The combination of behavioural and nutrition problems requires a multidisciplinary team approach

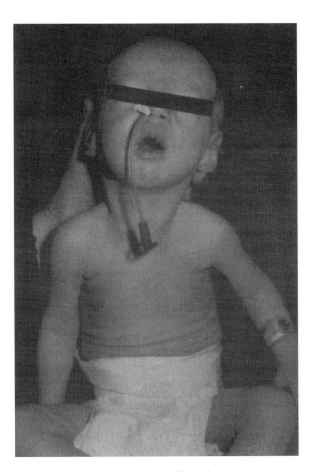

Figure 31.1   Infant with Prader–Willi syndrome.

to the management of PWS [42]. It is important that dietary intervention and advice is given before the onset of weight gain in order that excessive weight gain is curtailed. Consistent dietary advice from all professionals must be given to parents and carers and the need to adhere to this explained. This can prove very difficult because of the hyperphagia. Gross obesity often occurs during adolescence (Fig. 31.2) and behavioural problems encountered during this period can add to the difficulties of treatment [43–45]. Weight can be controlled with comprehensive management. In addition, growth hormone treatment has been shown to be beneficial in reducing BMI significantly in PWS children [46]. Interestingly, Crnic et al. [47] believe that maintenance of a lower body weight will improve intellectual performance.

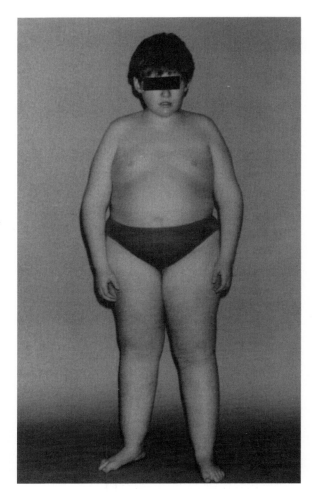

Figure 31.2   Adolescent with Prader–Willi syndrome (same boy as Fig. 31.1). With kind permission of Dr J.K. Brown.

Dietary treatment

As a result of low muscle tone and abnormal body composition the child with PWS requires a considerably lower energy intake than his or her normal peers (this can be as little as 50% of requirements for age). The precise calorie intake required by a PWS child will be dependent on their BMI and level of physical activity.

Much encouragement is required, but weight loss can be achieved with great vigilance. Weight should be monitored at constant and regular intervals. The diet presents great difficulty for the child,

family, carers and school; because of the insatiable appetite, food is uppermost in the thoughts of most people with PWS. Attempts should be made to check any potential sources of food (e.g. from neighbours or friends). Foraging for food is common and parents should be advised to lock the kitchen, cupboards and refrigerator. Many children get up during the night to eat, and inappropriate foods such as bread for the birds or dog and cat food are commonly eaten. Interestingly, however unsuitable the foods are that may be eaten, stomach upsets are rare.

Increasing physical activity levels can increase energy expenditure and overall feeling of well-being. Some activities are physically difficult for the PWS child because of poor muscle strength, but walking and swimming can be accomplished by most and should be encouraged to increase energy expenditure. Contrary to some views it has been shown that during exercise, individuals with PWS require as much energy as other obese individuals for the same level of work [48].

Dietitians must be aware that medical and other health workers may not have encountered PWS previously and may lack the understanding necessary to give proper support to the family. Communication with other health professionals is essential to avoid misunderstanding.

There is a parents' self-help group which parents may find helpful and supportive.

References

1   World Health Organization Diet, Nutrition and the Prevention of Chronic Diseases. WHO TRS 916. 2003. Geneva, WHO/FAO.

2   Lobstein T, Baur L, Uauy R for the IASO International Obesity Task Force. Obesity in children and young people: a crisis in public health. *Obes Rev*, 2004, **5** (Suppl 1) 4–85.

3   Reilly JJ, Dorosty AR Epidemic of obesity in UK children. *Lancet*, 1999, **354** 1874–5.

4   Chinn S, Rona RJ Prevalence and trends in overweight and obesity in three cross sectional studies of British children, 1974–94. *Br Med J*, 2001, **322** 24–6.

5   Scottish Intercollegiate Guideline Network (SIGN) *Management of Obesity in Children and Young People.* Edinburgh: SIGN 69, 2003.

6   Gibson P, Edmonds L, Haslam DW *et al.* An approach to weight management in children and adolescents (2–18 years) in primary care (RCPCH). *J Fam Health Care*, 2002, **12** 108–9.

7   NICE Guideline Obesity: the prevention, identification, assessment and management of overweight and obesity in adults and children. National Institute for Health and Clinical Excellence, London, 2007.

8   Mulvihill C, Quigley, R The management of obesity and overweight: an analysis of reviews of diet, physical activity and behavioural approaches. Evidence briefing. London: NHS Health Development Agency, 2003.

9   Postnote. Childhood obesity 2003. Parliament Office of Science and Technology. www.parliament.uk/post/pn205.pdf

10 House of Commons Health Committee *Obesity Third Report of Session 2003–04*, Vol. 1. London: The Stationery Office, 2004.

11 Prentice AM, Jebb SA Obesity in Britain: gluttony or sloth? *Br Med J*, 1995, **311** 437–9.

12 Kinra S, Nelder RP, Lewendon GJ Deprivation and childhood obesity: a cross sectional study of 20 973 children in Plymouth, United Kingdom. *J Epidemiol Community Health*, 2000, **54** 456–60.

13 Health Survey for England 2004. Health of Ethnic Minorities. www.ic.nhs.uk.pubs/hlthsvyeng2004ethnic

14 Jebb SA, Rennie KL, Cole TJ Prevalence and demographic determinants of overweight and obesity among young people in Great Britain. *Int J Obes*, 2003, **27** 59.

15 Stewart L, Nwafor N, Jackson P *et al.* Children and teenagers with special needs: highest population risk group for paediatric obesity in the UK. *Arch Dis Child*, 2005, **90** A15 G24.

16 Reilly JJ, Wilson ML, Summerbell CD *et al.* Obesity: diagnosis, prevention, and treatment; evidence based answers to common questions. *Arch Dis Child*, 2002, **86** 392–5.

17 Cole TJ, Freeman JV, Preece MA Body mass index reference curves for the UK, 1990. *Arch Dis Child*, 1995, **73** 25–9.

18 Cole TJ, Bellizzi MC, Flegal KM *et al.* Establishing a standard definition for child overweight and obesity worldwide: international survey. *Br Med J*, 2000, **320** 1–6.

19 Reilly JJ Descriptive epidemiology and health consequences of childhood obesity. *Best Pract Res Clin Endocrinol Metab*, 2005, **19** 327–41.

20 Neovius MG, Linne YM, Barkeling BS *et al.* Sensitivity and specifity of classification systems for fatness in adolescents. *Am J Clin Nutr*, 2004, **80** 597–603.

21 Reilly JJ, Methven E, McDowell ZC *et al.* Health consequences of obesity. *Arch Dis Child*, 2003, **88** 748–52.

22 Drake AJ, Smith A, Betts PR *et al.* Type 2 diabetes in obese white children. *Arch Dis Child*, 2002, **86** 207–8.

23 Sinha R, Fisch G, Teague B *et al.* Prevalence of impaired glucose tolerance among children and adolescents with marked obesity. *N Engl J Med*, 2002, **346** 802–10.

24 McCarthy HD The development of waist circumference percentiles in British children aged 5–16.9 years. *Eur J Clinl Nutr*, 2005, **55** 902–7.

25 Summerbell CD, Ashton V, Campbell KJ *et al.* Interventions for treating obesity in children. *Cochrane Database Syst Rev*, 2003, **3** CD01872.

26 National Health and Medical Research Council. Clinical practice guidelines for the management of overweight and obesity in children and adolescents. 2003. Commonwealth of Australia. www.health.gov.au/internet/wcms/publishing.nsf/Content/obesityguidelines-guidelines-children.htm

27 Barlow SE, Dietz WH Obesity evaluation and treatment: expert committee recommendations. *Pediatrics*, 1998, **102** 1–11.

28 Hungry for Success: A whole school approach to school meals in Scotland. Scottish executive Publications. www.scotland.gov.uk/Publications/2003/02/16273/17566

29 Epstein LH, Wing RR, Valoski AM Childhood obesity. *Pediatr Clinics North Am* 1985, **32** 363–79.

30 Epstein LH, Paluch RA, Gordy CC *et al.* Decreasing sedentary behaviors in treating pediatric obesity. *Arch Pediatr Adolesc Med*, 2000, **154** 220–6.

31 Gortmaker SL, Must A, Sobol AM *et al.* Television viewing as a cause of increasing obesity among children in the United States, 1986–1990. *Arch Pediatr Adolesc Med*, 1996, **150** 356–62.

32 Stewart L, Deane M, Wilson DC Failure of routine management of obese children: an audit of dietetic intervention. *Arch Dis Child*, 2004, **89** A13–16.

33 Epstein LH, Valoski AM, Wing RR *et al.* Ten-year outcomes of behavior family-based treatment for childhood obesity. *Health Psychol*, 1994, **13** 373–83.

34 Robinson TN. Behavioural treatment of childhood and adolescent obesity. *Inl J Obesity* 1999, **23** S52–7.

35 Lask B Motivating children and adolescents to improve adherence. *J Pediatr*, 2003, **Oct** 430–3.

36 Stewart L, Houghton J, Hughes AR *et al.* Dietetic management of pediatric overweight: development of a practical and evidence-based behavioral approach. *J Am Diet Assoc*, 2005, **105** 1810–15.

37 Taitz LS *The Obese Child*. Oxford: Blackwell Science, 1983.

38 Gortmaker SL, Peterson K, Wiecha J *et al.* Reducing obesity via a school based interdisciplinary intervention among youth: Planet Health. *Arch Pediatr Adolesc Med*, 1999, **151** 409–18.

39 Summerbell CD, Waters E, Edmonds L *et al.* Interventions for preventing obesity in children. *Cochrane Databse Syst Rev*, 2005.

40 Bray GA The Prader–Willi syndrome: a study of 40

patients and a review of the literature. *Medicine*, 1983, **62** 69–80.

41   Wollmann HA, Shultz U, Grauer ML *et al.* Reference values for height and weight in Prader–Willi syndrome based on 315 patients. *Eur J Pediatr*, 1998, **157** 634–42.

42   Wodarski LA, Bundschuh E, Forbus WR Interdisciplinary case management: a model for intervention. *J Am Diet Assoc*, 1988, **88** 332–5.

43   Whitman B, Accardo P Emotional symptoms in Prader–Willi syndrome adolescents. *Am J Med Genet*, 1987, **28** 897–905.

44   State MW, Dykens EM, Rosner B *et al.* Obsessive-compulsive symptoms in 'Prader–Willi and Prader–Willi-like' patients. *J Am Acad Child Adolesc Psychiatry*, 1999, **38** 329–34.

45   Dykens EM, Kasari C Maladaptive behavior in children with Prader–Willi syndrome, Down's syndrome, and non-specific mental retardation. *Am J Ment Retard*, 1997, **102** 228–37.

46   Lindgren AC, Hagenas L, Muller J *et al.* Growth hormone treatment of children with Prader–Willi syndrome affects linear growth and body composition favorably. *Acta Paediatr*, 1998, **87** 28–31.

47   Crnic KA, Sulzbacher S, Snow J *et al.* Preventing mental retardation associated with gross obesity in Prader–Willi syndrome. *Pediatrics*, 1980, **66** 787–9.

48   Holm VA, Pipes PL Food and children with Prader–Willi syndrome. *Am J Dis Child*, 1976, **130** 1063–7.

Useful resources and addresses

RU Ready 2 Change?
Leaflet produced by Paediatric Group of the BDA available from:
Cambertown Ltd (Paediatric Gp), Cambertown House, Commercial Road, Goldthorpe Industrial Estate, Goldthorpe, Rotherham, S63 9BL
www.cambertown.com

The Right Choice
Series of leaflets produced by the Scottish Nutrition and Dietetic Resource initiative (SNDRi) available from:
John McCormick & Co Ltd, 46 Darnley St, Glasgow, G41 2TY
www.jmccormick.co.uk

Child Growth Foundation
Growth and BMI centile charts available from:
Harlow Printing Ltd, Maxwell St, South Shields, Tyne & Wear, NE33 4PU
www.harlowprinting.co.uk

Prader–Willi Syndrome Association (PWSA) (UK)
125a London Rd, Derby, DE1 2QQ
www.pwsa.co.uk

32 Prevention of Food Allergy

Kate Grimshaw & Carina Venter

Introduction

Allergic diseases, such as asthma, rhinitis, eczema and food allergies, are increasing worldwide [1,2]. It is reported that infants born to families with a history of atopy are more at risk of developing allergic diseases than those born to non-atopic families [3], with genetic influences most definitely playing a part [4]. In the UK, allergic disease currently accounts for 6% of general practice consultations and 10% of the prescribing budget [5]. Add to this the impact allergic disease has on quality of life of both patients and carers and that there is currently no cure, then it is natural that attention is turning to possible prevention strategies. Prevention of the first stage of the allergic march seems the obvious course of action when trying to reduce the prevalence of allergic diseases. This is called primary prevention and its main aim is to prevent allergic sensitisation (i.e. the production of IgE antibodies). Such strategies focus on pregnancy and the first year of life.

Strategies during pregnancy

Despite a number of research studies looking at the maternal avoidance of allergenic foods through pregnancy [6–8], restricting the maternal diet during pregnancy is not advised as no benefit has been shown and dietary restrictions may have nutritional consequences for the mother and child [9]. Table 32.1 summarises results of studies of allergy prevention during pregnancy.

However, in 1998 the Committee on Toxicity of Chemicals in Food, Consumer Products and the Environment (COT) issued guidelines to women suggesting they may 'wish to' avoid nuts and peanuts during pregnancy and lactation if they or their partner suffered from any allergic disease [11]. This recommendation is partly based on a study carried out by Hourihane *et al.* [12]. The COT report is currently under review by the Food Standards Agency.

Other studies have also looked at whether maternal diet can affect the allergic status of the child. One of the nutrients of interest is omega-3 polyunsaturated fatty acids (n-3 PUFAs). A study looking at the relationship between fish oil supplementation and allergic sensitisation showed there may be a reduction in infant allergy after maternal supplementation with n-3 PUFAs [13]. These diets are rich in linolenic acid, a precursor of arachidonic acid which promotes prostaglandin E_2 (PGE_2) production. This in turn promotes interleukin-4 (IL-4), the main cytokine involved in immunoglobulin E (IgE) [14]. This is thought to be due to the fact that

Table 32.1 Intervention studies during pregnancy.

Intervention	Timing	Outcome
Avoid milk, egg	From 28 weeks' gestation until term	At 5 years: persistent food allergy to egg was significantly more common in children of the mothers who avoided milk and egg [6]
Four diets ranging from a diet free from egg and cow's milk to a diet containing intake of one egg and 1 L/day milk	Last trimester of pregnancy	No significant difference in terms of maternal or cord blood IgE to ovalbumin, ovomucoid and beta-lactoglobulin [7]
Avoid egg	From 16–20 weeks' gestation until term	At 6 months: the infants of those mothers with low and high egg intake were less likely to be atopic than those with moderate egg intake [10]

prostaglandins and interleukins produced from n-3 PUFAs have weaker inflammatory properties than those produced from n-6 PUFAs. By increasing the amount of n-3 PUFAs in the diet, less potent prostaglandins and leukotrienes predominate in the immunological milieu. This work needs to be replicated but encouraging mothers to at least meet their requirements for n-3 fatty acids while pregnant (currently 2–3% of total energy intake) [15] appears to be a sensible recommendation.

In terms of the prevention of allergy, there has been some evidence that a high intake of vegetable oil and fat during pregnancy [16] may be related to the development of allergy in the infant. Another maternal dietary factor thought to be related to the later development of allergic diseases is a poor intake of fruit and vegetables [17,18] and although there is little evidence to support this theory, there can be little harm in advocating that pregnant women try and meet the recommended five portions a day of fruit and/or vegetables a day.

Two studies suggested that vitamins E and C taken as food rather than supplements may have a role in reducing prevalence of allergic disease [19,20], whereas two further studies have suggested that supplementation of vitamin D could lead to an increased prevalence of allergy [21,22].

Some research has been carried out into supplementing pregnant mothers' diets with probiotics. Kalliomäki *et al.* [23] supplemented a group of mothers from allergic families with a Gram-positive probiotic, *Lactobacillus rhamnosus* (*Lactobacillus GG*) during the last 4 weeks of pregnancy and the infants' first 6 months of life. The prevalence of eczema was reduced by 50% in the intervention group when compared with a control group.

However, these findings need to be repeated in similar studies using more readily available products before mothers are advised to take probiotics during pregnancy.

Infant feeding strategies

In 2001 at the 54th World Health Assembly, the World Health Organization (WHO) recommended exclusive breast feeding for the first 6 months of an infant's life and the nutrient adequacy of exclusive breast feeding for the term infant during this period is documented [24]. The UK's Scientific Advisory Committee on Nutrition [25] has supported this and stated that there is sufficient evidence to suggest that exclusive breast feeding for 6 months is nutritionally adequate.

The recommendations of WHO for exclusive breast feeding are based on nutrient adequacy in terms of functional outcomes (e.g. growth, immune response, neurodevelopment). Breast milk strengthens the immune system of the infant because of the hormones, growth factors, colony-stimulating factors and nutrients present in it [26]. In addition to this, breast milk promotes gastro-intestinal mucosal maturation, decreases the incidence of infection and has immunomodulatory and anti-inflammatory functions [27]. Although the human gut is anatomically and functionally mature at birth in the full term infant, immaturities in digestion, absorption and protective function still exist. This may predispose the infant during the first 6 months of life to age-related gastrointestinal disease. Exclusive breast feeding provides both passive and active support of the infant's gut function during the first 6 months of life and should therefore be recommended for general health [28]. It is unclear at present whether this is applicable for allergy prevention *per se*.

Breast milk composition

Breast milk not only provides nutrients but also provides biologically active compounds that affect the developing immune system. These compounds include immunoglobulins and other cells involved in the immune system, prebiotics (i.e. oligosaccharides), nucleotides and long chain fatty acids [29]. However, the levels of nutritive and bioactive factors in milk varies according to the nutritional and atopic status of the mother [30,31]. Atopic mothers have a lower level of omega-3 fatty acid levels and CD14 cells in their breast milk [30,32].

Infant feeding and allergy prevention

There are three points regarding infant feeding and allergy prevention that need to be considered:

- The effect of breast feeding on allergy prevention
- Maternal diet during breast feeding and allergy prevention

- Which formula to choose when mother cannot or wishes not to breast feed

Breast feeding and the development of allergic disease

Some studies show breast feeding to have a beneficial effect on the allergic outcome of the infant [33,34], whereas others show breast feeding to be associated with an increased risk of atopy [35]. This may be because of differences in study design or breast milk composition of the mother. Reverse causality means that when considering the aetiology of breast feeding and allergy, breast feeding groups may contain more infants at high risk compared to groups who choose not to breast feed. It is also well reported that up to one-third of infants will develop cow's milk allergy during exclusive breast feeding, probably brought about by the cow's milk protein in breast milk [36]. However, breast feeding is still the recommended feeding method for all infants because of its nutritional, immunological and psychological benefits.

Maternal diet and breast feeding

A number of randomised controlled trials in high-risk infants have investigated the effect of different dietary allergy prevention programmes during breast feeding and pregnancy and these are summarisd in Tables 32.2 and 32.3. A recent review

Table 32.2   Intervention studies during pregnancy and lactation.

Intervention	Timing	Outcome
Avoid milk, egg, peanut ($n = 108$, 103 intervention) [8]	Last trimester of pregnancy and lactation	12 months: less atopic dermatitis and urticaria 24 months: less food sensitisation Reduced the cumulative incidence of food allergy from 1–4 years, but point prevalence at age 3 and 4 years was the same for the two groups
Avoid milk and egg [37]	Group 1: Intervention – last trimester of pregnancy and lactation ($n = 30$) Group 2: Intervention – only during lactation ($n = 33$) Group 3: Control group ($n = 41$) Group 4: Using hydrolysed formula ($n = 34$)	No difference in atopic dermatitis and skin prick tests to egg and milk at 6 and 12 months between the different groups
Avoid milk and egg [6]	From 28 weeks' gestation and reduced intake of these foods during lactation	No difference in skin prick tests, IgE levels and blinded examination

Table 32.3 Intervention studies during lactation only.

Intervention	Timing	Outcome
Avoid milk (*n* = 24, 12 intervention) [38]	Late pregnancy and lactation Group 1: Atopic – intervention Group 2: Atopic – control Group 3: Non-atopic	Lower incidence of allergy at 18 months
Avoid milk, eggs, fish, peanuts and soybeans [39]	Lactation	Less atopic dermatitis (less common and milder) at 18
Avoid milk, egg, fish and nuts plus house dust mite [40]	Lactation	Less allergic disorders at 12 months, less wheeze and nocturnal cough at 8 years
Group 1: Mothers and infants on whey hydrolysate Group 2: Exclusively breast fed Group 3: Cow's milk formula [41]	Lactation	Less atopic dermatitis and cow's milk allergy

paper by the European Academy of Allergy and Clinical Immunology (EAACI) concludes that there is no evidence for maternal dietary intervention during pregnancy or lactation in the prevention of allergic disease [42].

Infant formula and allergy prevention

If a mother is unable to breast feed, choosing the right formula could be difficult. It is known that early exposure to cow's milk can increase prevalence of cow's milk allergy [43,44] and that gut maturation and development of the gut mucosal barrier is delayed with early cow's milk feeding [45]. EAACI therefore recommends that if a mother is not breast feeding she should use an infant formula with reduced allergenicity, defined as a formula that significantly reduces the prevalence of allergic disease when compared with other formulas [42]. This recommendation applies only to infants born into high risk families (i.e. either mother, father or sibling suffers from documented allergic disease) [42].

Both extensively hydrolysed formulas (Nutramigen, casein based; Pepti-Junior, whey based) and partially hydrolysed formulas (Nan HA) have shown an allergy preventative effect. A recent study showed that both an extensively hydrolysed (casein based) and partially hydrolysed formula led to less allergic disease in the offspring compared to the infants receiving a standard infant formula [46]. Further analysis of the results, however, showed that only the extensively hydrolysed formula (casein based) led to less allergic disease when the mother herself had atopic dermatitis.

It is advised that soya formula should not be given as an alternative to cow's milk formula for the prevention of allergy in infants under 6 months of age as it has been considered by some that soy protein is as allergenic as cow's milk protein in infant formulas [47]. The UK's Chief Medical Officer has advised against the use of soya formula in infants unless there is a specific medical indication (see p. 95) [48], so the debate about the use of soya formula in allergy prevention has become academic.

Weaning strategies

This is an area of great confusion. What is widely agreed is that infants should receive no solid food until they are at least 4 months (17 weeks) of age. The Department of Health has stated that 26 weeks is the recommended age for the introduction of solids for healthy term infants [49] in order to support the promotion of exclusive breast feeding for the first 6 months of life. If it is necessary to introduce solids into an infant's diet before this age then that food should be of low allergenicity [50]. After 6 months there is no reason to delay the introduction of the most potentially allergenic foods because delayed introduction of solids into the diet to prevent the development of allergic disease has not been shown to be beneficial. Despite this, delayed or staged introduction of foods is commonly advised by both specialist texts for professionals working in the field and books designed for the general public [51,52].

Observational studies looking at the role of weaning in allergy prevention can be divided into three groups:

- Introduction of solids before 3–4 months increases the risk of allergic disease in both high risk [53] and unselected [54,55] cohorts of children
- Delaying introduction of solids beyond 3.5–6.0 months increases the risk of allergic disease in both high risk [56] and unselected [57] cohorts of children
- Early feeding practices has no effect on allergic symptoms [58]

In summary, from these observational studies we can learn that weaning both before the age of 3 months and beyond the age of 6 months may increase the risk of allergic disease. Whether weaning at 3–4 months as opposed to 6 months poses a higher risk for developing allergic disease was unanswered until very recently. Zutavern et al. [59] have looked at this much discussed topic in a prospective study in 2,612 infants. They found that introduction of solid foods after 4 months decreased the odds ratio for atopic dermatitis. Delaying solid food introduction beyond 6 months did not provide any additional benefits.

Where there is allergy in the family it is prudent to introduce allergenic foods one at a time into the diet and, in the case of egg, to give it initially in a well cooked form such as an ingredient in a biscuit [60]. The COT report advises that peanuts and tree nuts should not be introduced into the diet of a child with allergy in the family until they are 3 years of age [11].

Studying the age of introduction of a particular food and the subsequent development of food allergy seems to suggest that the earlier introduction of peanut (before 12 months) [61], milk (in the first few days of life) [43,62] and egg (before 6 months) [63] may cause sensitisation or clinical allergy. However, only a few studies, some with small numbers or possible recall bias, have been published in this area.

Environmental strategies

An association between passive smoking has not only been shown between tobacco smoke exposure and asthma [64], but also to other allergic diseases [65]. An important allergy prevention measure is to avoid smoking during pregnancy and to ensure the baby is not exposed to tobacco smoke.

Exposure to high levels of house dust mite should also be avoided. Following anti-dust mite procedures such as covering the mattress, ventilation of the infant's room, regular vacuuming and cleaning with a damp cloth have been shown to reduce sensitisation to house dust mites at 1 year of age [66]. It remains to be proved that these measures will lead to a reduced incidence of allergic disease, but follow-up research is planned in order to investigate this.

Recommendations

Although more research needs to be carried out in order to offer definitive allergy prevention advice, a number of recommendations can be made from the evidence base at this time. These are as follow:

- No avoidance of allergens during pregnancy or lactation (except the COT advice that those with a history of allergy in the mother's or father's family may wish to avoid peanuts and tree nuts).
- A healthy balanced maternal diet with sufficient portions of fruits, vegetables and n-3 fatty acids.
- Exclusive breastfeeding for at least 4 months (preferably 6).
- If breast feeding is not possible, the infant with a family history of allergy should have a hydrolysed formula (of proven reduced allergenicity) until the age of 6 months.
- Delay of the introduction of all solid foods until at least 17 weeks (4 months) and preferably 6 months, with high allergenic foods such as wheat, egg and milk not being introduced until over 6 months of age.
- In families with a history of atopy introduction of allergenic foods one at a time.
- Initially, introduction of eggs in a well cooked form (e.g. as an ingredient in biscuits).
- Avoidance of exposure to cigarette smoke during pregnancy as well as to the infant after birth.

- Avoidance of exposure to high levels of house dust mite by using special dust mite protection mattress covers, using a high efficiency vacuum cleaner, cleaning with a damp cloth, and keeping rooms well ventilated with low humidity levels. Also consideration of removing carpets and using blinds instead of curtains in the infant's bedroom.

References

1 Austin JB, Kaur B, Anderson HR *et al.* Hay fever, eczema, and wheeze: a nationwide UK study (ISAAC, international study of asthma and allergies in childhood). *Arch Dis Child*, 1999, **81** 225–30.

2 Dennis R, Caraballo L, Garcia E *et al.* Asthma and other allergic conditions in Colombia: a study in 6 cities. *Ann Allergy Asthma Immunol*, 2004, **93** 568–74.

3 Kurukulaaratchy R, Fenn M, Matthews S *et al.* The prevalence, characteristics of and early life risk factors for eczema in 10-year-old children. *Pediatr Allergy Immunol*, 2003, **14** 178–83.

4 Van Eerdewegh P, Little RD, Dupuis J *et al.* Association of the ADAM33 gene with asthma and bronchial hyperresponsiveness. *Nature*, 2002, **418** 426–30.

5 A report of the Royal College of Physicians Working Party on the provision of allergy services in the UK. *Allergy: the unmet need. A blueprint for better patient care.* Royal College of Physicians, London, 2003.

6 Falth-Magnusson K, Kjellman NI Allergy prevention by maternal elimination diet during late pregnancy: a 5-year follow-up of a randomized study. *J Allergy Clin Immunol*, 1992, **89** 709–13.

7 Lilja G, Dannaeus A, Falth-Magnusson K *et al.* Immune response of the atopic woman and foetus: effects of high- and low-dose food allergen intake during late pregnancy. *Clin Allergy*, 1988, **18** 131–42.

8 Zeiger RS, Heller S, Mellon MH *et al.* Effect of combined maternal and infant food-allergen avoidance on development of atopy in early infancy: a randomized study. *J Allergy Clin Immunol*, 1989, **84** 72–89.

9 Host A, Halken S Primary prevention of food allergy in infants who are at risk. *Curr Opin Allergy Clin Immunol*, 2005, **5** 255–9.

10 Vance GH, Grimshaw KE, Briggs R *et al.* Serum ovalbumin-specific immunoglobulin G responses during pregnancy reflect maternal intake of dietary egg and relate to the development of allergy in early infancy. *Clin Exp Allergy*, 2004, **34** 1855–61.

11 Committee on Toxicity of Chemicals in Food, Consumer Products and the Environment. *Peanut allergy.* Department of Health, 1998. Crown Copyright.

12 Hourihane JO, Dean TP, Warner JO Peanut allergy in relation to heredity, maternal diet, and other atopic diseases: results of a questionnaire survey, skin prick testing, and food challenges. *Br Med J*, 1996, **313** 518–21.

13 Dunstan JA, Mori TA, Barden A *et al.* Fish oil supplementation in pregnancy modifies neonatal allergen-specific immune responses and clinical outcomes in infants at high risk of atopy: a randomized, controlled trial. *J Allergy Clin Immunol*, 2003, **12** 1178–84.

14 Naito Y, Endo H, Arai K *et al.* Signal transduction in Th clones: target of differential modulation by PGE2 may reside downstream of the PKC-dependent pathway. *Cytokine*, 1996, **8** 346–56.

15 Makrides M, Neumann MA, Gibson RA Is dietary docosahexaenoic acid essential for term infants? *Lipids*, 1996, **31** 115–19.

16 Ushiyama Y, Matsumoto K, Shinohara M *et al.* Nutrition during pregnancy may be associated with allergic diseases in infants. *J Nutr Sci Vitaminol*, 2002, **48** 345–51.

17 Heinrich J, Holscher B, Bolte G *et al.* Allergic sensitization and diet: ecological analysis in selected European cities. *Eur Respir J*, 2001, **17** 395–402.

18 Stazi MA, Sampogna F, Montagano G *et al.* Early life factors related to clinical manifestations of atopic disease but not to skin-prick test positivity in young children. *Pediatr Allergy Immunol*, 2002, **13** 105–12.

19 Fogarty A, Lewis S, Weiss S *et al.* Dietary vitamin E, IgE concentrations, and atopy. *Lancet*, 2000, **356** 1573–4.

20 Martindale S, McNeill G, Devereux G *et al.* Antioxidant intake in pregnancy in relation to wheeze and eczema in the first two years of life. *Am J Respir Crit Care Med*, 2005, **171** 121–8.

21 Matheu V, Back O, Mondoc E *et al.* Dual effects of vitamin D-induced alteration of Th1/Th2 cytokine expression: enhancing IgE production and decreasing airway eosinophilia in murine allergic airway disease. *J Allergy Clin Immunol*, 2003, **112** 585–92.

22 Hypponen E, Sovio U, Wjst M *et al.* Infant vitamin D supplementation and allergic conditions in adulthood: northern Finland birth cohort 1966. *Ann N Y Acad Sci*, 2004, **1037** 84–95.

23 Kalliomaki M, Salminen S, Arvilommi H *et al.* Probiotics in primary prevention of atopic disease: a randomised placebo-controlled trial. *Lancet*, 2001, **357** 1076–9.

24 Butte NF, Lopez-Alarcon MG, Garza, C *Nutrient adequacy of exclusive breastfeeding for the term infant during the first six months of life.* World Health Organization, Geneva, 2002.

25 Scientific Advisory Committee on Nutrition. *Optimal Duration of Exclusive Breastfeeding and Introduction of Weaning.* www.sacn.gov.uk SACN 01/07. 2004.

26 Oddy WH The impact of breastmilk on infant and child health. *Breastfeed Rev*, 2002, **10** 5–18.

27 Field CJ The immunological components of human

milk and their effect on immune development in infants. *J Nutr*, 2005, **135** 1–4.

28 Goldman AS, McNeilly AS, Naylor AJ *et al. Wellstart. Reviews of the Relevant Literature Concerning Infant Gastrointestinal, Immunologic, Oral Motor and Maternal Reproductive and Lactational Development.* Naylor AJ, Morrow A (eds) 2001, pp. 1–4.

29 Das UN Essential fatty acids as possible enhancers of the beneficial actions of probiotics. *Nutrition*, 2002, **18** 786.

30 Yu G, Duchen K, Bjorksten B Fatty acid composition in colostrum and mature milk from non-atopic and atopic mothers during the first 6 months of lactation. *Acta Paediatr*, 1998, **87** 729–36.

31 Hoppu U, Kalliomaki M, Laiho K *et al.* Breast milk: immunomodulatory signals against allergic diseases. *Allergy*, 2001, **56** (Suppl 67) 23–6.

32 Jones CA, Holloway JA, Popplewell EJ *et al.* Reduced soluble CD14 levels in amniotic fluid and breast milk are associated with the subsequent development of atopy, eczema, or both. *J Allergy Clin Immunol*, 2002, **109** 858–66.

33 Saarinen UM, Kajosaari M Breastfeeding as prophylaxis against atopic disease: prospective follow-up study until 17 years old. *Lancet*, 1995, **346** 1065–9.

34 Bergmann RL, Diepgen TL, Kuss O *et al.* Breastfeeding duration is a risk factor for atopic eczema. *Clin Exp Allergy*, 2002, **32** 205–9.

35 Sears MR, Greene JM, Willan AR *et al.* Long-term relation between breastfeeding and development of atopy and asthma in children and young adults: a longitudinal study. *Lancet*, 2002, **360** 901–7.

36 Jarvinen KM, Suomalainen H Development of cow's milk allergy in breast-fed infants. *Clin Exp Allergy*, 2001, **31** 978–87.

37 Herrmann ME, Dannemann A, Gruters A *et al.* Prospective study of the atopy preventive effect of maternal avoidance of milk and eggs during pregnancy and lactation. *Eur J Pediatr*, 1996, **155** 770–4.

38 Lovegrove JA, Hampton SM, Morgan JB The immunological and long-term atopic outcome of infants born to women following a milk-free diet during late pregnancy and lactation: a pilot study. *Br J Nutr*, 1994, **71** 223–38.

39 Hattevig G, Sigurs N, Kjellman B Effects of maternal dietary avoidance during lactation on allergy in children at 10 years of age. *Acta Paediatr*, 1999, **88** 7–12.

40 Arshad SH, Matthews S, Gant C *et al.* Effect of allergen avoidance on development of allergic disorders in infancy. *Lancet*, 1992, **339** 1493–7.

41 Fukushima Y, Iwamoto K, Takeuchi-Nakashima A *et al.* Preventive effect of whey hydrolysate formulas for mothers and infants against allergy development in infants for the first 2 years. *J Nutr Sci Vitaminol*, 1997, **43** 397–411.

42 Muraro A, Dreborg S, Halken S *et al.* Dietary prevention of allergic diseases in infants and small children. Part III: Critical review of published peer-reviewed observational and interventional studies and final recommendations. *Pediatr Allergy Immunol*, 2004, **15** 291–307.

43 Saarinen KM, Juntunen-Backman K, Jarvenpaa AL *et al.* Supplementary feeding in maternity hospitals and the risk of cow's milk allergy: A prospective study of 6209 infants. *J Allergy Clin Immunol*, 1999, **104** 457–61.

44 Host A Importance of the first meal on the development of cow's milk allergy and intolerance. *Allergy Proc*, 1991, **12** 227–32.

45 Arvola T, Rantala I, Marttinen A *et al.* Early dietary antigens delay the development of gut mucosal barrier in preweaning rats. *Pediatr Res*, 1992, **32** 301–5.

46 von Berg A, Koletzko S, Grubl A *et al.* The effect of hydrolyzed cow's milk formula for allergy prevention in the first year of life: The German Infant Nutritional Intervention Study, a randomized double-blind trial. *J Allergy Clin Immunol*, 2003, **111** 533–4.

47 Host A, Koletzko B, Dreborg S *et al.* Dietary products used in infants for treatment and prevention of food allergy. Joint Statement of the European Society for Paediatric Allergology and Clinical Immunology (ESPACI) Committee on Hypoallergenic Formulas and the European Society for Paediatric Gastroenterology, Hepatology and Nutrition (ESPGHAN) Committee on Nutrition. *Arch Dis Child*, 1999, **81** 80–4.

48 Department of Health *Chief Medical Officer Update 37.* 2004.

49 Department of Health *Infant Feeding Recommendation.* 2004.

50 Paediatric Group Position Statement on breastfeeding and weaning onto solid foods. Birmingham: British Dietetic Association, 2004.

51 Sampson HA Food Allergy. Part 2: Diagnosis and Management. *J Allergy Clin Immunol*, 1999, **103** 981–9.

52 Scott-Moncrieff C *Overcoming Allergies.* London: Collins and Brown, 2002.

53 Kajosaari M, Saarinen UM Prophylaxis of atopic disease by six months' total solid food elimination. Evaluation of 135 exclusively breast-fed infants of atopic families. *Acta Paediatr Scand*, 1983, **72** 411–14.

54 Fergusson DM, Horwood LJ, Shannon FT Early solid feeding and recurrent childhood eczema: a 10-year longitudinal study. *Pediatrics*, 1990, **86** 541–6.

55 Morgan J, Williams P, Norris F *et al.* Eczema and early solid feeding in preterm infants. *Arch Dis Child*, 2004, **89** 309–14.

56 Zutavern A, von Mutius E, Harris J *et al.* The introduction of solids in relation to asthma and eczema. *Arch Dis Child*, 2004, **89** 303–8.

57   Saarinen KM, Savilahti E Infant feeding patterns affect the subsequent immunological features in cow's milk allergy. *Clin Exp Allergy*, 2000, **30** 400–6.

58   Gustafsson D, Sjoberg O, Foucard T Development of allergies and asthma in infants and young children with atopic dermatitis: a prospective follow-up to 7 years of age. *Allergy*, 2000, **55** 240–5.

59   Zutavern A, Brockow I, Schaaf B *et al.* Timing of solid food introduction in relation to atopic dermatitis and atopic sensitization: results from a prospective birth cohort study. *Pediatrics*, 2006, **117** 401–11.

60   Food Allergy and Intolerance Group *Practical dietary prevention strategies for infants at risk of developing allergic diseases*. Birmingham: British Dietetic Association, 2005.

61   Frank L, Marian A, Visser M *et al.* Exposure to peanuts in utero and in infancy and the development of sensitization to peanut allergens in young children. *Pediatr Allergy Immunol*, 1999, **10** 27–32.

62   Host A, Husby S, Osterballe O A prospective study of cow's milk allergy in exclusively breast-fed infants. Incidence, pathogenetic role of early inadvertent exposure to cow's milk formula, and characterization of bovine milk protein in human milk. *Acta Paediatr Scand*, 1988, **77** 663–70.

63   Kocijancic LB Relationship between early exposure of hen's egg yolk and atopic dermatitis in 18 month old Slovene children. XXIII EAAACI Conference, Amsterdam, Netherlands, 2004.

64   DiFranza JR, Aligne CA, Weitzman M Prenatal and postnatal environmental tobacco smoke exposure and children's health. *Pediatrics*, 2004, **113** (4 Suppl) 1007–15.

65   Kramer U, Lemmen CH, Behrendt H *et al.* The effect of environmental tobacco smoke on eczema and allergic sensitization in children. *Br J Dermatol*, 2004, **150** 111–18.

66   Halmerbauer G, Gartner C, Schierl M *et al.* Study on the Prevention of Allergy in Children in Europe (SPACE): allergic sensitization at 1 year of age in a controlled trial of allergen avoidance from birth. *Pediatr Allergy Immunol*, 2003, **14** 10–17.

Appendix I

Manufacturers of Dietetic Products

A full list of drugs and their manufacturers appears in the *British National Formulary* (BNF), a joint publication of the British Medical Association and the Royal Pharmaceutical Society of Great Britain.

Abbott Laboratories Ltd
Abbott House, Norden Road, Maidenhead, Berkshire SL6 4XE

Alliance Pharmaceuticals Ltd
Avonbridge House, 2 Bath Road, Chippenham, Wiltshire SN15 2BB

Aventis
(*see* Sanofi-Aventis)

Axcan Pharma
22 Inverness Center Parkway, Birmingham, AL 35242, USA

Baxter Healthcare Ltd
Caxton Way, Thetford, Norfolk IP24 3SE

Bio Diagnostics Ltd
Upton Industrial Estate, Rectory Road, Upton-under-Severn, Worcestershire WR8 0XL

B Braun (Medical) Ltd
Brookdale Road, Thorncliffe Park Estate, Sheffield S35 2PW

Chefaro UK Ltd
Unit 1, Tower Close, St Peter's Industrial Park, Huntingdon, Cambridgeshire PE29 7DH

Cow & Gate Nutricia Ltd
White Horse Business Park, Trowbridge, Wiltshire BA14 0XQ

Farley
(*see* Heinz)

Fate Special Foods
Unit E2, Brook Street Business Centre, Brook Street, Tipton, West Midlands DY4 9DD

Firstplay Dietary Foods Ltd
338, Turncroft Lane, Offerton, Stockport, Cheshire SK1 4BP

Fresenius Kabi Ltd
Parenteral Nutrition Division, Davy Avenue, Knowlhill, Milton Keynes MK5 8PH

General Dietary Ltd
PO Box 28, Kingston upon Thames, Surrey KT2 7YP

Gluten Free Foods Ltd
Unit 10 Honeypot Business Park, Parr Road, Stanmore, Middlesex HA7 1NL

Heinz H J Co Ltd
Hayes Park, Hayes, Middlesex UB4 8AL

Janssen-Cilag Ltd
PO Box 79, Saunderton, High Wycombe, Buckinghamshire HP14 4HJ

KoRa Healthcare Ltd
Frans Maas House, Swords Business Park, Swords, Co. Dublin, Ireland

Mead Johnson Nutritionals
Division of Bristol-Myers Squibb Pharmaceuticals Ltd, 141–149 Staines Road, Hounslow, Middlesex TW3 3JA

Merck Pharmaceuticals
Harrier House, High Street, West Drayton, Middlesex UB7 7QG

Milupa Ltd
White Horse Business Park, Trowbridge, Wiltshire BA14 0XQ

Nestlé Clinical Nutrition
St George's House, Croydon, Surrey CR9 1NR

Novartis Consumer Health
Wimblehurst Road, Horsham, West Sussex RH12 5AB

Nutricia Clinical Care
Nutricia Ltd, White Horse Business Park, Trowbridge, Wiltshire BA14 0XQ

Orphan Europe (UK) Ltd
Isis House, 43 Station Road, Henley-on-Thames, Oxfordshire RG9 1AT

Paines & Byrne Ltd
Yamanouchi House, Pyrford Road, West Byfleet, Surrey KT14 6RA

Sanofi-Aventis Ltd
1 Onslow Street, Guildford, Surrey GU1 4YS

SHS International Ltd
100 Wavertree Boulevard, Wavertree Technology Park, Liverpool L7 9PT

SMA Nutrition
Huntercombe Lane South, Taplow, Maidenhead, Berkshire SL6 0PH

Solvay Healthcare Ltd
Mansbridge Road, West End, Southampton SO18 3JD

Sutherland Health Ltd
Unit 1 Rivermead, Pipers Way, Thatcham, Berkshire RG19 4EP

UCB Pharma Ltd
Star House, 69 Clarendon Road, Watford, Hertfordshire WD1 1DJ

Ultrapharm Ltd
PO Box 18, Henley-on-Thames, Oxfordshire RG9 2AW

Vitaflo Ltd
11 Century Building, Brunswick Business Park, Liverpool L3 4BL

Vitaline Pharmaceuticals UK Ltd
8 Ridge Way, Drakes Drive, Crendon Business Park, Long Crendon, Buckinghamshire HP18 9BF

Appendix II

Dietetic Products

Abidec	Chefaro UK
Adamin G	SHS
Additrace	Fresenius Kabi
ADEK	Axcan Pharma
Aminex	Gluten Free Foods Ltd
Aminogran Food Supplement	UCB Pharma
Aminogran PKU tablets	UCB Pharma
Aproten	Ultrapharm
Bi-Aglut	Novartis
Calogen	SHS
Caloreen	Nestlé
Calshake	Fresenius Kabi
Caprilon	SHS
ClinOleic	Baxter
Clinutren 1.5	Nestlé
Clinutren Dessert	Nestlé
Clinutren Fruit	Nestlé
Clinutren ISO	Nestlé
Clinutren Thickened Drinks	Nestlé
Clinutren Thickener	Nestlé
Comfort	Cow & Gate
Complete Amino Acid Mix (Code 124)	SHS
Cow & Gate Nutriprem 1	Cow & Gate
Cow & Gate Nutriprem 2	Cow & Gate
Cow & Gate Nutriprem breast milk fortifier	Cow & Gate
Cow & Gate Plus	Cow & Gate
Cow & Gate Premium	Cow & Gate
Cow & Gate Step-Up	Cow & Gate
Creon 10000	Solvay
Creon 25000	Solvay
Creon Micro	Solvay
Dalivit	LPC
Dialamine	SHS
Dialyvit Paediatric	Vitaline
Dioralyte	Aventis
Dioralyte Relief	Aventis
Duobar	SHS
Duocal	SHS
Easiphen	SHS
Electrolade	Baxter
Elemental 028	SHS
Elemental 028 Extra	SHS
Emsogen	SHS
Ener-G	General Dietary Ltd
Energivit	SHS
Enfamil	Mead Johnson
Enfamil AR	Mead Johnson
Enfamil Lactofree	Mead Johnson
Enlive Plus	Abbott
Enrich	Abbott
Ensure Plus	Abbott
Essential Amino Acid Mix	SHS
Farley's First Milk	Farley/Heinz
Farley's Follow-on Milk	Farley/Heinz
Farley's Second Milk	Farley/Heinz

Farley's Soya Formula	Farley/Heinz	Lipofundin MCT/LCT	B Braun
Fate Low Protein	Fate Special Foods	Liquigen	SHS
Forceval	Alliance Pharmaceuticals	Locasol	SHS
		Lophlex	SHS
Formance	Abbott	Lophlex LQ	SHS
Fortijuce	Nutricia	Loprofin	SHS
Fortimel	Nutricia	Loprofin PKU Drink	SHS
Fortini	Nutricia	Lorenzo's Oil	SHS
Fortini Multi Fibre	Nutricia	lp-drink	Milupa
Fortisip	Nutricia	Mapleflex	SHS
Fortisip Multifibre	Nutricia	Maxijul	SHS
Frebini Energy	Fresenius Kabi	Maxijul Liquid	SHS
Frebini Energy Fibre	Fresenius Kabi	MCT Duocal	SHS
Frebini Original	Fresenius Kabi	MCT Oil	Mead Johnson
Frebini Original Fibre	Fresenius Kabi	MCT Pepdite	SHS
Fresubin Energy	Fresenius Kabi	MCT Pepdite 1+	SHS
Fresubin Energy Fibre	Fresenius Kabi	MCT Step 1	Vitaflo
Fresubin 1000 Complete	Fresenius Kabi	Metabolic Mineral Mixture	SHS
Galactomin 17	SHS		
Galactomin 19	SHS	Milupa Aptamil Extra	Milupa
Generaid	SHS	Milupa Aptamil First	Milupa
Generaid Plus	SHS	Milupa Aptamil Forward	Milupa
Glucogel	SHS	Milupa Pre-Aptamil	Milupa
Glycerol Trioleate Oil	SHS	Minaphlex	SHS
HCU Express	SHS	MMA/PA Express	SHS
HCU Gel	SHS	MMA/PA Gel	SHS
Hcu lv	SHS	Modulen IBD	Nestlé
Heparon Junior	SHS	Monogen	SHS
Hepatamine	SHS	MSUD Aid III	SHS
Hepatical	SHS	MSUD Analog	SHS
Hydrolysed whey protein/ maltodextrin mixture	SHS	MSUD Express Cooler	Vitaflo
		MSUD Gel	Vitaflo
InfaSoy	Cow & Gate	MSUD Maxamaid	SHS
Infatrini	Nutricia	MSUD Maxamum	SHS
Instant Carobel	Cow & Gate	Nan HA	Nestlé
Intralipid	Fresenius Kabi	Neocate	SHS
Isomil	Abbott	Neocate Active	SHS
Isosource Energy	Novartis	Neocate Advance	SHS
Isosource Energy Fibre	Novartis	Nepro	Abbott
Isosource Fibre	Novartis	Nestargel	Nestlé
Isosource Junior	Novartis	Novasource Forte	Novartis
Isosource Standard	Novartis	Novasource GI Control	Novartis
Jevity	Abbott	Nutilis	Nutricia
Jevity 1.5	Abbott	Nutramigen 1	Mead Johnson
Jevity Plus	Abbott	Nutramigen 2	Mead Johnson
Jevity Promote	Abbott	Nutriflex	B. Braun
Juvela	SHS	Nutrini	Nutricia
Ketocal	SHS	Nutrini Energy	Nutricia
Ketovite	Paines & Byrne	Nutrini Energy Multi Fibre	Nutricia
Kindergen	SHS		

Nutrini Low Energy Multi Fibre	Nutricia	Polycose	Abbott
Nutrini Multi Fibre	Nutricia	Pregestimil	Mead Johnson
Nutrison 1000 Complete Multi Fibre	Nutricia	Prejomin	Milupa
		Pre Nan	Nestlé
Nutrison 1200 Complete Multi Fibre	Nutricia	PremCare	Farley/Heinz
		Primene	Baxter
Nutrison Energy	Nutricia	Promin	Firstplay Dietary Foods Ltd
Nutrison Energy Multi Fibre	Nutricia	ProMod	Abbott
		ProSobee	Mead Johnson
Nutrison MCT	Nutricia	Protifar	Nutricia
Nutrison Multi Fibre	Nutricia	Provide Xtra	Fresenius
Nutrison Pepti	Nutricia	Pulmocare	Abbott
Nutrison Soya	Nutricia	Rapolyte	Provalis
Nutrison Standard	Nutricia	Renamil	KoRa
Nutrizym 22	Merck	Renilon	Nutricia
Nutrizym GR	Merck	Renapro	KoRa
OliClinomel	Baxter	Resource Benefiber	Novartis
Osmolite	Abbott	Resource Energy Dessert	Novartis
Osmolite Plus	Abbott	Resource Fruit Flavour Drink	Novartis
Osterprem	Farley/Heinz	Resource Junior	Novartis
Pancrease	Janssen-Cilag	Resource Protein Extra	Novartis
Pectigel	Vitaflo	Resource Shake	Novartis
Paediasure	Abbott	Resource Thickened Drink	Novartis
Paediasure with Fibre	Abbott		
Paediasure Plus	Abbott	Resource Thickened Squash	Novartis
Paediasure Plus with Fibre	Abbott	Resource ThickenUp	Novartis
Paediatric Seravit	SHS	Rite-Diet	SHS
Peditrace	Fresenius Kabi	Scandishake	SHS
Pepdite	SHS	Seravit	SHS
Pepdite 1+	SHS	SMA breast milk fortifier	SMA Nutrition
Peptamen	Nestlé	SMA Gold	SMA Nutrition
Peptamen Junior	Nestlé	SMA Gold Prem	SMA Nutrition
Peptide Module (Code 767)	SHS	SMA High Energy	SMA Nutrition
Pepti	Cow & Gate	SMA Lactofree	SMA Nutrition
Pepti-Junior	Cow & Gate	SMA Progress	SMA Nutrition
Phlexy 10 Exchange System	SHS	SMA Staydown	SMA Nutrition
		SMA White	SMA Nutrition
Phlexy-vits	SHS	Sno-Pro	SHS
PK Aid 4	SHS	Solvito	Fresenius Kabi
PK Foods	Gluten Free Foods Ltd	Sucraid	Orphan Europe
PKU 2	Milupa	Suplena	Abbott
PKU 3	Milupa	Tentrini	Nutricia
PKU Express	Vitaflo	Tentrini Energy	Nutricia
PKU Cooler 15	Vitaflo	Tentrini Energy Multi Fibre	Nutricia
PKU Gel	Vitaflo		
Polycal	Nutricia	Tentrini Multi Fibre	Nutricia
Polycal Liquid	Nutricia	Thick and Easy	Fresenius Kabi

Thick and Easy Dairy	Fresenius Kabi	XMet Maxamaid	SHS
Thick and Easy		XMet Maxamum	SHS
Thickened Juices	Fresenius Kabi	XMTVI Analog	SHS
Thixo-D	Sutherland	XMTVI Asadon	SHS
Tyr Express	Vitaflo	XMTVI Maxamaid	SHS
Tyroflex	SHS	XMTVI Maxamum	SHS
Tyr Gel	Vitaflo	XP Analog	SHS
Ultra	Ultrapharm	XP Analog LCP	SHS
Valpiform	Gluten Free Foods Ltd	XP Maxamaid	SHS
Vamin 9 Glucose	Fresenius Kabi	XP Maxamaid Bar	SHS
Vaminolact	Fresenius Kabi	XP Maxamum	SHS
Vita-Bite	Vitaflo	XPhen, Tyr Analog	SHS
Vitajoule	Vitaflo	XPhen, Tyr, Met Analog	SHS
Vitapro	Vitaflo	XPhen, Tyr Maxamaid	SHS
Vitaquick	Vitaflo	XPhen, Tyr Maxamum	SHS
Vitlipid Infant	Fresenius Kabi	XPhen, Tyr,	
Wysoy	SMA Nutrition	Met Maxamaid	SHS
XLYS, Low Try Analog	SHS	XPhen, Tyr,	
XLYS, Low Try		Met Maxamum	SHS
Maxamaid	SHS	XPT Tyrosidon	SHS
XMet Analog	SHS	XPTM Tyrosidon	SHS
XMet Homidon	SHS	X Tyr Maxamum	SHS

Index